Complimentary Access

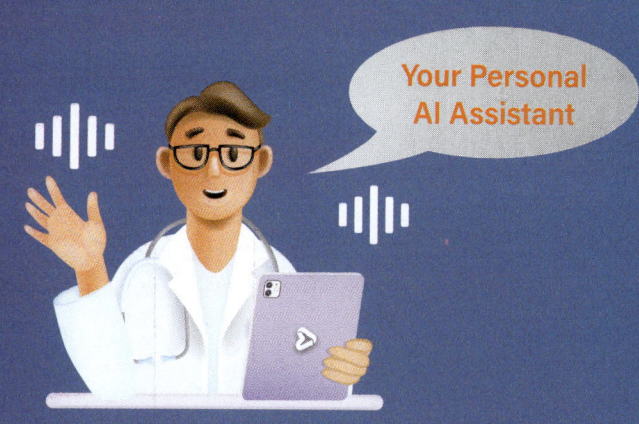
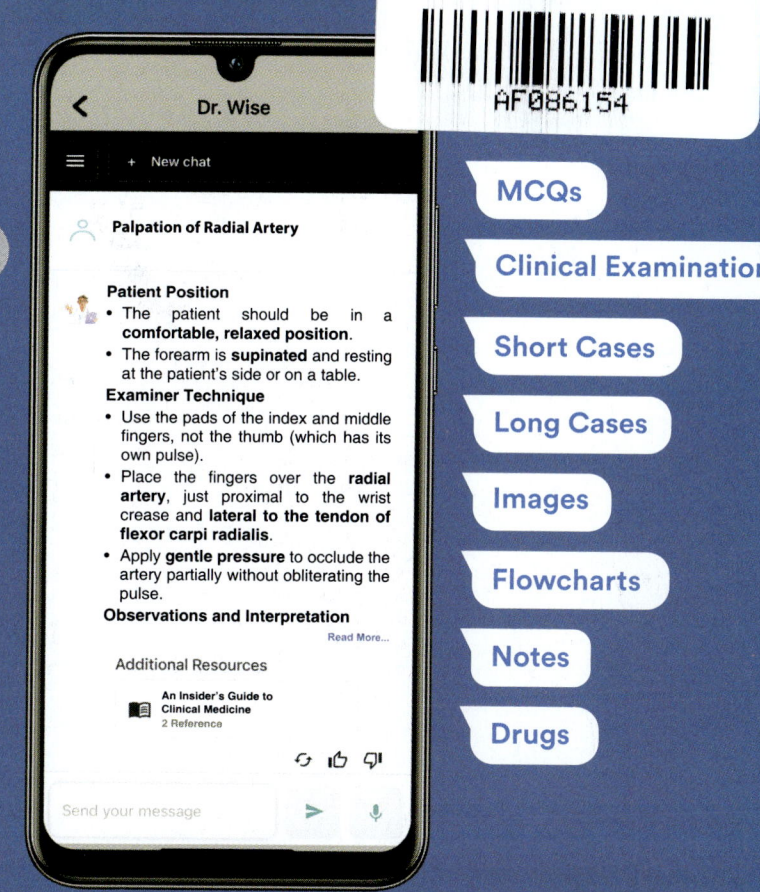

Your Personal AI Assistant

Dr. Wise
Be Wise, Ask Dr. Wise!
You can search Anything, Anywhere, Anytime

- MCQs
- Clinical Examination
- Short Cases
- Long Cases
- Images
- Flowcharts
- Notes
- Drugs

Precisely Crafted Answers with References!
Concepts with Detailed Explanation

Easy Steps to Access Dr. Wise Features

New User:
1. Scan the QR code to Install App
2. Click redeem and enter the redemption code
3. Create account to access Dr. Wise
4. If you are an existing user of learn.Ejaypee, login with same email & password and follow point 2 below

Existing User/Add New Book in Dr. Wise App:
1. Login with Dr. Wise email & password
2. In more options, redeem code to add new book

DOWNLOAD APP

Download on the App Store

GET IT ON Google Play

An Insider's Guide to Clinical Medicine

Part-1

As per the Revised Competency-based Medical Education Curriculum (NMC)

Third Edition

Archith Boloor
MBBS MD (Internal Medicine)
Additional Professor and HOU
Department of Medicine
Kasturba Medical College, Mangaluru
Manipal Academy of Higher Education
Karnataka, India
archithb@gmail.com

Anudeep Padakanti
MBBS MD (Internal Medicine) DM (Medical Oncology)
Department of Medical Oncology
MNJ Institute of Oncology and Regional Cancer Centre
(Osmania Medical College)
Hyderabad, Telangana, India
anudeeppadakanti.aigcm@gmail.com

Foreword
RN Sharma

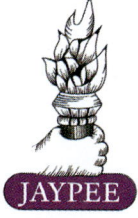

JAYPEE BROTHERS MEDICAL PUBLISHERS
The Health Sciences Publisher
New Delhi | London

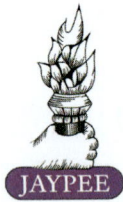

Jaypee Brothers Medical Publishers (P) Ltd

Headquarters
EMCA House
23/23-B, Ansari Road, Daryaganj
New Delhi 110 002, India
Landline: +91-11-23272143, +91-11-23272703
+91-11-23282021, +91-11-23245672
E-mail: jaypee@jaypeebrothers.com

Overseas Office
J.P. Medical Ltd
83 Victoria Street, London
SW1H 0HW (UK)
Phone: +44 20 3170 8910
E-mail: info@jpmedpub.com

Corporate Office
4838/24, Ansari Road, Daryaganj
New Delhi 110 002, India
Phone: +91-11-43574357
Fax: +91-11-43574314
E-mail: jaypee@jaypeebrothers.com

EU GPSR Authorised Representative
Logos Europe, 9 rue Nicolas Poussin
17000, La Rochelle, France
Phone: +33 (0) 6 67 93 73 78
E-mail: contact@logoseurope.eu

Website: www.jaypeebrothers.com
Website: www.jaypeedigital.com

© 2026, Jaypee Brothers Medical Publishers

The views and opinions expressed in this book are solely those of the original contributor(s)/author(s) and do not necessarily represent those of editor(s) and publisher of the book.

All rights reserved. No part of this publication may be reproduced, stored or transmitted in any form or by any means, electronic, mechanical, photocopying, recording or otherwise, without the prior permission in writing of the publishers.

All brand names and product names used in this book are trade names, service marks, trademarks or registered trademarks of their respective owners. The publisher is not associated with any product or vendor mentioned in this book.

Medical knowledge and practice change constantly. This book is designed to provide accurate, authoritative information about the subject matter in question. However, readers are advised to check the most current information available on procedures included and check information from the manufacturer of each product to be administered, to verify the recommended dose, formula, method and duration of administration, adverse effects and contraindications. It is the responsibility of the practitioner to take all appropriate safety precautions. Neither the publisher nor the author(s)/editor(s) assume any liability for any injury and/or damage to persons or property arising from or related to use of material in this book.

This book is sold on the understanding that the publisher is not engaged in providing professional medical services. If such advice or services are required, the services of a competent medical professional should be sought.

Every effort has been made where necessary to contact holders of copyright to obtain permission to reproduce copyright material. If any have been inadvertently overlooked, the publisher will be pleased to make the necessary arrangements at the first opportunity.

Inquiries for bulk sales may be solicited at: jaypee@jaypeebrothers.com

An Insider's Guide to Clinical Medicine

First Edition: 2020

Second Edition: 2022

Third Edition: **2026**

ISBN: 978-93-6616-760-2

Printed in India

Dedicated to

All the young budding doctors who shall be the future caretakers of our society

Contributors

Nikhil Kenny Thomas MD DM DrNB
Department of Gastroenterology and Hepatology
St. Luke Hospital, Pathanamthitta
Dr KM Cherian Institute of Medical Sciences
Chenganur, Kerala, India

Mohamed Faizan Thouseef MD DNB
Department of Internal Medicine
Kasturba Medical College, Mangaluru
Manipal Academy of Higher Education
Karnataka, India

PS Gayathri Thampi MD
Department of Internal Medicine
Kasturba Medical College, Mangaluru
Manipal Academy of Higher Education
Karnataka, India

Raghavendra P Desai MD
Department of Medical Gastroenterology
Institute of Gastroenterology Sciences and
Organ Transplant
Victoria Hospital Campus
Bengaluru, Karnataka, India

Varun M Nair MD
Department of Internal Medicine
Kasturba Medical College, Mangaluru
Manipal Academy of Higher Education
Karnataka, India

Ashwini MV MD DM
Department of Cardiology
Kasturba Medical College, Manipal
Manipal Academy of Higher Education
Karnataka, India

Sriraksha R Nayak DPM MD
Department of Psychiatry
PES University Institute of Medical Sciences and Research
Electronic City
Bengaluru, Karnataka, India

Prajwal Pai MD
Department of Medical Gastroenterology
Kasturba Medical College, Manipal
Manipal Academy of Higher Education
Karnataka, India

Deepti Agarwal MD DM
Consultant Rheumatologist
JJM Medical College
Davangere, Karnataka, India

Mohammed Shaheen
Department of Emergency Medicine
Hamad Medical Corporation
Doha, Qatar

Sheetal Raj M MD
Department of Internal Medicine and Program
Director—Geriatric Medicine Fellowship
Kasturba Medical College, Mangaluru
Manipal Academy of Higher Education
Karnataka, India

Manoj Kumar Devera MD
Department of Internal Medicine
Sri Venkateswara Institute of Medical Sciences
Tirupati, Andhra Pradesh, India

Vivek Hari MD
Department of Nephrology
Vardhman Mahavir Medical College and
Safdarjung Hospital
New Delhi, India

Sagi Pranathi MD
Department of Neurology
Andhra Medical College
Visakhapatnam, Andhra Pradesh, India

Saladi Sri Vijay Sasikanth
Department of Internal Medicine
Kasturba Medical College, Mangaluru
Manipal Academy of Higher Education
Karnataka, India

Vidarshan Mathavan
Department of Internal Medicine
Kasturba Medical College, Mangaluru
Manipal Academy of Higher Education
Karnataka, India

Madhav H Hande MD DrNB
Department of Nephrology
Manipal Hospital, Whitefield
Bangaluru, Karnataka, India

Vivek K Koushik MD DrNB
Department of Nephrology
Prashanth Hospitals, Kolathur
Chennai, Tamil Nadu, India

Abu Thajudeen MD
Department of Neurology
Father Muller Medical College
Mangaluru, Karnataka, India

Foreword

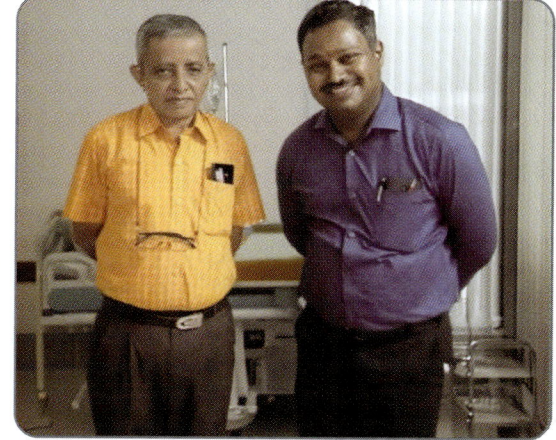

I am very much delighted to write a forward for the book *An Insider's Guide to Clinical Medicine*. It is written by Dr Archith Boloor, a reputed teacher who has bagged many awards and coauthored by Dr Anudeep Padakanti.

The book is a must possess for medicine students. Clinical examination has been dealt with extensively in all systems. It is written in an easy-to-understand format, so that both undergraduates and postgraduates can grasp the ideas and concepts very clearly. There are innumerable charts and tables, which make the book more attractive. Large number of splendid photographs depicting methods of clinical examination and abnormal findings are the unique captivating factor of the book.

Great effort has been invested by both authors to make the book student friendly. Large volume of clinical information has been incorporated into the book in an orderly manner. Apart from above-mentioned features, authors have taken utmost care to impart information regarding case sheets submitted in the practical examination. Hence, it is a valuable tool of learning both for undergraduates and postgraduates, especially from examination point of view.

I regularly use this book as a reference book for taking postgraduate class in medicine. It is an invaluable asset particularly for the postgraduate students. It should find a place in every departmental library of medicine. Every faculty in department of medicine will find it useful as a reference book.

My hearty congratulations to the authors for bringing out such a book in clinical medicine, which is the need of the hour.

Best wishes

RN Sharma MD
Emeritus Professor, Department of Medicine, Pushpagiri Institute of Medical Sciences, Thiruvalla, Kerala, India
Former Head, Department of Medicine (Government Medical College, Kottayam, AIMS, Kochi and Pushpagiri Institute of Medical Sciences)
Former Dean, Faculty of Medicine, MG University, Kottayam, Kerala, India
Former Chair Person, Postgraduate Studies, Faculty of Medicine, MG University Kottayam
rnsharmasaimsdept@gmail.com

Preface to the Third Edition

The beauty of life is in its infinite tendency to give you time. To learn, to heal, and to get better: In whatever capacity that may be. As students of medicine, we are very often pressured to get things right on the first try. To be perfect and to not leave any stone unturned; yes, we agree that the stakes are a lot different for us than it is for a chef or an actor. But understand that as 20-somethings learning medicine in an environment that is very service-centric, you are not helping anyone by adding an extra layer of troubles to your existing mountain of troubles. Give yourself some breathing space, take it easy and relish that second chance.

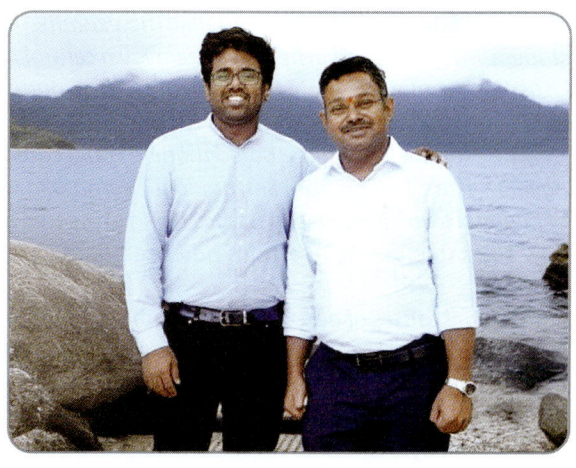

The more mistakes you make, the more chances you get to correct them. Every senior doctor that you have met will have innumerable stories of how they have made fools of themselves in medical school. We too have several anecdotes of our own, with which we could regale our students to several hours of mirth. But let's digress. What we really want to shine light on is the importance of chances and taking them when they are thrown at you. With the pandemic having pushed admissions and examinations and opportunities by several years, it is important for you students to reflect on the progress you have made in your journey as a doctor and it is imperative that you accept second chances, with open arms. It is even more important to accept with open, lab-coat laden arms, these second chances.

We have received another chance with this book. The crux of this book largely remains the same, along with some finer adjustments. Font sizes, color, and page breaks have been adjusted to make reading easier. We have added a more detailed section on history-taking with some much-needed adjustments, especially with respect to patients that are different from the masses. The highlights from the previous book, the positive points which most of you gave very good feedback about have been left as it is—complete case sheets on all organ systems, with added emphasis on the common examination cases. A plethora of pictures make the visual experience of this book what it is, it also gave many of my interns a very interesting past time activity to run around the wards with a camera and a consent form. While we worked on the different case sheets, both short and spot cases, we have included model cases and classical presentations to help you to arrive at a diagnosis earlier than most. X-rays, Spotters, Common Drugs, and Instruments take up their own spot in this book, deservedly so.

As students of medicine, you may very often find yourself, lost in a maze of facts and clinical experiences. This book is designed to help you to best navigate the maze, that is the world of medicine, while keeping an astute eye on the requirements for passing your clinical examination. We hope you enjoy reading and comprehending the finer concepts and learn to love this book as much as we enjoyed bringing to you this second edition. We welcome your suggestions, criticisms, and feedback, wholeheartedly and look forward to enriching your learning in the times to come.

Archith Boloor
Anudeep Padakanti

Preface to the First Edition

The clock had struck a solid 1:30 PM. The examiner was hungry, the last student was jittery and in between them lay a central nervous system (CNS) case that was going to determine whether a four-and-half-year ripe child of medicine would be prefixed with a "Dr" or not.

The examiner was more bored than he could care to admit. Lakshman, aged 32 years, hailing from Shivamogga, Karnataka with chief complaints of bilateral lower limb weakness was being presented for the 14th time that day. The same boring questions had been asked in the same uninspired fashion.

"List the causes of neck pain", the examiner asked.

A little taken aback, but the student realized that the question was within the realm of a CNS case. After gathering his thoughts for a moment, he began listing out, "Meningitis causing neck muscle spasm, cervical spondylosis, cervical spondylolisthesis..." his voice trailing off in response to the examiner's unimpressed face.

"Go ahead, what else?"

Not to lose face in front of the examiner, the student once again reset his thoughts, and a few umms and ahhs later continues: "Sir, other cervical causes like cervical intraepithelial neoplasia and cervical cancer can also cause neck pain".

Jokes apart, getting psyched for an examination is an absolutely normal and foreseeable predicament. We often notice the most brilliant students fumbling to show off years' worth of hard work simply, because the psyche overpowers their preparation. As the saying goes "For most diagnoses, all that is needed is an ounce of knowledge, an ounce of intelligence, and a pound of thoroughness." With that very thought in mind, it is our pleasure to present to you a simple, comprehensive, and exam-oriented clinical manual—a compass to guide you through the art of clinical medicine.

The practical examinations pose a real challenge to the medical student—he has to finish writing an entire case sheet, elicit the expected clinical findings and finally arrive at a proper diagnosis. All this to be done before the examiner has even made eye contact with the student. The catch here being the limited availability of what we all take for granted—time. One asks the wrong questions, examines the wrong systems, latches on to the wrong points, and before we realize, we are knee-deep in heaps of unorganized information that has no head or tail. Having been in the same shoes at some point in the past, this book was made to solve those problems: Complete case sheets on all organ systems, with added emphasis on the common examination cases have been incorporated. We hope it will teach the reader to anticipate questions that are asked in different contexts. The book is as visually charged as we could possibly make it, because we believe that seeing is learning. We have dealt with spot and short cases, which are meant to test a student's take on the bigger picture of diseases. The diagnostic clues given in this book will help the student to arrive at a definitive decision sooner. X-rays, spotters, and instruments are dealt with extensively and in exquisite detail.

We have read several clinical books in an attempt to make this one different. In doing so, we have found that this is one single guide which can be safely relied upon to deal with the practicals of Final MBBS Part II. We hope that the fruit of our labor becomes as close to your bookshelf as it is to our hearts. Any suggestions and/or constructive criticism is always welcome, and we hope you enjoy reading *An Insider's Guide to Clinical Medicine*.

Archith Boloor
Anudeep Padakanti

Remembering the Father of Modern Medicine

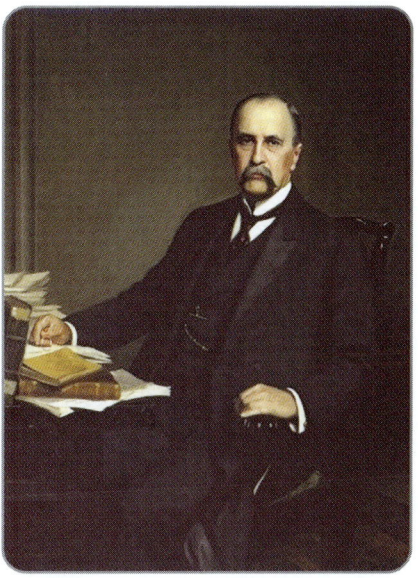

"Medicine is a science of uncertainty and an art of probability."

"The best preparation for tomorrow is to do today's work superbly well."

"Every patient you see is a lesson in much more than the malady from which he suffers. Listen to your patient. He is telling you the diagnosis."

"He who studies medicine without books sails an uncharted sea, but he who studies medicine without patients does not go to sea at all."

"The good physician treats the disease; the great physician treats the patient who has the disease."

"We are here to add what we can to life. Not to get what we can from life."

"Too many men slip early out of the habit of studious reading and yet that is essential."

"Look wise, say nothing, and grunt. Speech was given to conceal thought."

"One of the duties of the physician is to educate the masses not to take medicine."

"The practice of medicine is an art. Not a trade; a calling. Not a business: A calling in which your heart will be exercised equally with your head."

"Happiness lies in the absorption in some vocation which satisfies the soul. To have striven. To have made the effort. To have been true to certain ideals this alone is worth the struggle."

"Acquire the art of detachment, the virtue of method and the quality of thoroughness but above all the grace of humility."

"Think not of the amount to be accomplished, the difficulties to be overcome, or the end to be attained, but set earnestly, at the little task at your elbow, letting that be sufficient for the day."

"In science, the credit goes to the man who convinces the world, not to the man to whom the idea first occurs."

"The very first step towards success in any occupation is to become interested in it."

"To do today's work well and not to bother about tomorrow is the secret of accomplishment."

Sir William Osler
(July 12, 1849 – December 29, 1919)

Acknowledgments

With immense gratitude we place on record our heartfelt thanks for the appreciation our book *An Insider's Guide to Clinical Medicine* has received from students and teachers all over India. With inputs and feedback from all we set to compile the second edition. The task was not easy. Working as frontline healthcare workers, along with our peers we managed to find time to compile this edition, the experience of which has been infinitely memorable.

Firstly, we would like to thank our families—the unwavering pillars of strength that have supported us throughout every challenge in our life. Our friends, colleagues, and well-wishers who have always supported our work were not an exception this time too. Lastly, we want to thank all our students, each and every one, because without their unrelenting urge to learn, we would not have the drive to compile our teachings in the form of a book.

We thank the faculty of medicine in colleges around India for recommending my book to your students.

We remain profoundly grateful to Professor RN Sharma for his gracious foreword. To have his thoughtful words precede this work is both a privilege and an enduring honor. His endorsement lends this endeavor a depth of meaning that far exceeds the written page.

We are thankful to all our friends whose contributions and knowledge flowed seamlessly at a very short notice. We thank Dr Nikhil Kenny Thomas, Dr Mohamed Faizan Thouseef, Dr Mohammed Shaheen, Dr Madhav H Hande, Dr Vivek K Koushik, Dr Abu Thajudeen, Dr Sheetal Raj M, Dr Prajwal Pai, Dr Raghavendra P Desai, Dr Deepti Agarwal, Dr Sriraksha R Nayak, Dr Saladi Sri Vijay Sasikanth, Dr Manoj Kumar Devera, Dr Vidarshan Mathavan, Dr PS Gayathri Thampi, Dr Varun M Nair, Dr Ashwini M V, Dr Vivek Hari, and Dr Sagi Pranathi for their contribution.

We are thankful to our editor and the whole team of M/s Jaypee Brothers Medical Publishers (P) Ltd, New Delhi, India, who helped and guided us. We are also thankful to Shri Jitendar P Vij (Group Chairman), Mr Ankit Vij (Managing Director), Mr MS Mani (Group President), Dr Madhu Choudhary (Director–Educational Publishing), Ms Pooja Bhandari [Director–Production (Books and Journals)], Mr Ajay Kumar Sharma [Deputy General Manager (Books and Journals)], Dr Aditya Tayal (Senior Editorial Manager–Content Strategy), Mr Vijay Kumar Bhatia (Manager–Production), Mr Bishan Singh (Production Manager–Press), Ms Seema Dogra (Cover Visualizer), Ms Neha Verma (Graphic Designer–Cover), Mr Laxmidhar Padhiary (Team Lead–Production), Mr Akshay Thakur (DTP Operator), Mr Sumit Kumar (Team Lead–Graphic Designer), and their team members, for their dedication, expertise, and tireless efforts to bring this project to life. Their constructive feedback and keen insights were crucial in refining our manuscript into the book it is today.

To our readers and students thank you for picking up this book and embarking on this journey with us. To all who trust this book as part of their preparation, thank you. It is your determination and commitment to excellence that inspired us to compile this work. We hope this book becomes a reliable companion on your journey to success.

A very special gratitude goes out to all our teachers, who are solely responsible for what we are today and for having ignited the passion of teaching and writing in us.

Lastly, we thank God Almighty, for what was, what is, and what will be.

Archith Boloor
Anudeep Padakanti

Contents

1. **Introduction** 1
   - The Importance of History Taking *1*
   - Prerequisites for Practical Examination *5*
   - Checklist for Practical Examination *5*
   - Format of Clinical Examination *6*
   - Common Examination Cases *6*

2. **General Examination** 7
   - **A. Case Sheet Format** *7*
     - Body Mass Index *7*
     - Vitals Examination *7*
     - Physical Examination *7*
     - Others *7*
   - **B. Vitals Examination** *8*
     - Pulse *8*
     - Respiration *16*
     - Blood Pressure *18*
     - Ankle-Brachial Index *21*
     - Jugular Venous System *22*
     - Body Temperature *26*
     - Pain: The Fifth Vital Sign *29*
   - **C. Physical Examination** *31*
     - Pallor *31*
     - Icterus *32*
     - Cyanosis *34*
     - Clubbing (Hippocrates Fingers) *35*
     - Edema *38*
     - Lymphadenopathy *40*
     - Nutritional Assessment *46*
     - Nail Changes *48*
   - **D. Anthropometry** *49*
     - Height *49*
     - Arm Span *50*
     - Upper Segment and Lower Segment *50*
     - Skinfold Thickness *51*
     - Body Mass Index *52*
     - Waist-Hip Ratio *52*
     - Mid-Arm Circumference *52*
     - Neck Circumference *52*
     - Neck Height Ratio *53*
     - Miscellaneous Topics *53*
     - Marfan's Syndrome: Diagnostic Criteria and Features *54*

3. **Respiratory System Examination** 55
   - **A. Case Sheet Format** *55*
     - History Taking *55*
     - General Examination *56*
     - Systemic Examination *56*
   - **B. Diagnosis Format** *60*
     - Anatomical Diagnosis *60*
     - Pathological Diagnosis *60*
     - Etiological Diagnosis *60*
     - Complications *60*
     - Examples *60*
   - **C. Discussion on Cardinal Symptoms** *61*
     - Cough *61*
     - Expectoration/Sputum *62*
     - Hemoptysis *63*
     - Dyspnea *64*
     - Timing of Dyspnea *67*
     - Chest Pain *68*
     - Other Symptoms *68*
   - **D. Discussion on Examination** *70*
     - General Examination *70*
     - Examination of Respiratory System *72*
     - The Most Important Examination Finding is to Check for Hemithorax Expansion and Hemithorax Measurement *81*
   - **E. Respiratory System: Summary of Findings in Common Respiratory Diseases** *91*

4. **Cardiovascular System Examination** 93
   - **A. Case Sheet Format** *93*
     - History Taking *93*
     - General Examination *94*
     - Systemic Examination *95*
     - Other System Examination *96*
   - **B. Diagnosis Format** *97*
     - Acquired/Congenital Heart Disease *97*
   - **C. Discussion on Cardiac Cycle** *98*
     - Systole and Diastole *98*
     - Events of Cardiac Cycle *98*
     - Cardiac Murmurs—Timing with Other Cardiac Events *99*
     - ECG Waveform—Timing with Other Cardiac Events *100*
     - Standard Representation of All Cardiac Events in Cardiac Cycle *100*
   - **D. Discussion on Cardinal Symptoms** *102*
     - Chest Pain *102*
     - Palpitations *104*
     - Dyspnea *105*
     - Syncope *105*
     - Pedal Edema *106*
   - **E. Discussion on Examination** *109*
     - General Examination *109*
     - Physical Examination *109*

- Systemic Examination *111*
- Cardiac Cycle and Heart Sounds *119*
- Third Heart Sound (S3) *122*
- Pericardial Knock *122*
- Fourth Heart Sound (S4) *122*
- Clicks and Snaps *123*
- Pericardial Rub *123*
- Summary of Auscultation of Heart Sounds *124*
- Murmurs *124*
- Summary of Heart Murmurs *131*
- Other System Examination *132*
- Pulsatile Liver *132*

F. **Summary of Findings in Common Cardiovascular Diseases 135**

5. **Gastrointestinal System 137**
   A. **Case Sheet Format 137**
   - History Taking *137*
   - General Examination *138*
   - Systemic Examination *138*

   B. **Diagnosis Format 141**
   - Cirrhosis/Liver Disease *141*
   - Example *141*

   C. **Discussion on Cardinal Symptoms 142**
   - Abdominal Swelling *142*
   - Jaundice *142*
   - Gastrointestinal Bleeding *142*
   - Nausea and Vomiting *143*
   - Diarrhea *144*
   - Constipation *145*
   - Dyspepsia *145*
   - Dysphagia *146*
   - Odynophagia *146*
   - Pain in Abdomen *146*

   D. **Discussion on Examination 151**
   - General Examination *151*
   - Oral Cavity Examination *156*
   - Systemic Examination *157*
   - Auscultation *160*
   - Palpation and Percussion of the Abdomen *161*
   - Examination of Individual Organs *161*
   - Inspection *161*
   - Renal Angle *170*
   - Murphy's Kidney Punch (Costovertebral Angle Tenderness) *170*
   - Complications of Cirrhosis *177*
   - Sites of Portosystemic Anastomosis *179*
   - Classification of Portal Hypertension *179*

6. **Nervous System 181**
   A. **Case Sheet Format 181**
   - History Taking *181*
   - Higher Mental Function *181*
   - Cranial Nerve Dysfunction *181*
   - Motor Dysfunction *181*
   - Sensory Dysfunction *182*
   - Cerebellar History *182*
   - History Suggesting Meningitis/Raised Intracranial Pressure *182*
   - History Suggesting Autonomic Dysfunction *182*
   - Review of Common Neurological Symptoms *182*
   - General Examination *183*
   - Nervous System Examination *184*
   - Higher Mental Functions *184*
   - Motor System *185*
   - Reflexes *186*
   - Sensory System *186*
   - Cerebellar Signs *186*
   - Gait *187*
   - Soft Neurological Signs *187*
   - Other Systems *187*

   B. **Diagnosis Format 188**
   - General Format *188*
   - For Cerebrovascular Accident *188*
   - For Neuropathy *188*
   - For Spinal Cord Disease *188*
   - For Extrapyramidal (Parkinson's Disease) *188*
   - For Ataxia *188*

   C. **Central Nervous System: Discussion on Cardinal Symptoms 189**
   - Discussion on Cardinal Symptoms *189*
   - Higher Mental Function *189*
   - Cranial Nerve Dysfunction *189*
   - Motor Dysfunction *189*
   - Sensory Dysfunction *191*
   - Cerebellar Examination *191*
   - Autonomic Dysfunction *192*
   - Meningeal Signs *192*
   - Others *192*
   - Neck Pain *192*
   - Backache *193*
   - Red Flags for Acute Low Back Pain *193*

   D(i). **General Examination in Neurology 195**
   - General Physical Examination in Nervous System *195*
   - Neurocutaneous Syndromes/Phakomatoses *195*
   - Nerve Thickening *197*

   D(ii). **Higher Mental Functions 200**
   - Nervous System Examination *200*
   - Consciousness *200*
   - Orientation *201*
   - Appearance/Behavior *201*
   - Memory *201*
   - Attention *202*
   - Intelligence/Calculation *202*
   - Cognition Assessment Tool *202*
   - Speech *202*
   - Aphasias *204*
   - Dysarthrias *205*
   - Apraxia *206*
   - Agnosia *206*
   - Delusions *206*
   - Hallucinations *206*

D(iii). Cranial Nerves 209
- Cranial Nerve I—Olfactory Nerve 209
- Cranial Nerve II—Optic Nerve 210
- Stages of Diabetic Retinopathy 214
- Stages of Hypertensive Retinopathy 214
- Causes of Optic Atrophy 214
- Cranial Nerves III, IV and VI—Oculomotor, Trochlear and Abducens 215
- Ocular Movement Testing 218
- Diplopia 218
- Strabismus/Squint 221
- Pupillary Abnormalities 222
- Ophthalmoplegia 226
- Nystagmus 228
- Cranial Nerve V—Trigeminal Nerve 228
- Facial Nerve 233
- Facial Nerve Palsy 236
- Cranial Nerve VIII—Vestibulocochlear Nerve 239
- Cranial Nerve IX and X: Glossopharyngeal and Vagus 243
- Glossopharyngeal Nerve IX 243
- Cranial Nerve X—Vagus 244
- Cranial Nerve XI—Spinal Accessory 245
- Cranial Nerve XII—Hypoglossal Nerve 246
- Multiple Cranial Nerve Palsies 248

D(iv). Motor System Examination 250
- Attitude 250
- Muscle Bulk/Nutrition 250
- Muscle Tone 252
- Motor Power 254
- Examination for Subtle Hemiparesis 263

D(v). Reflexes 265
- Definition 265
- Mechanism of Reflex Generation 265
- Types of Reflexes 265
- Grading of Reflexes (for DTRs) NINDS Scale 265
- Reinforcement Mechanism and Methods 265
- Deep Tendon Reflexes 266
- Superficial Reflexes 272
- Plantar Reflex and Variations 272
- Latent Reflexes of Upper Limb 275
- Primitive Reflexes 275
- Inverted and Perverted Reflexes 277
- Signs to Identify Hysterical Weakness 277

D(vi). Sensory System Examination 278
- Primary Modalities 278
- Secondary Modalities 281
- Homunculus, Sensory Pathway, Dermatomes and Clinical Patterns of Sensory Loss 283
- Sensory Dermatomes 284
- Nonorganic Sensory Loss 285

D(vii). Cerebellum and Coordination 287
- Signs of Cerebellar Disorders 287
- Heel Knee Test 288
- Toe Finger Test 289
- Nose-Finger-Nose Test 290
- Dysdiadochokinesia 291
- Foot Tapping/Foot Pat Test 292
- Straight Line Walking 292
- Tandem Walking 292
- Approach to Ataxia 293
- Cerebellar Ataxia 293
- Causes of Cerebellar Ataxia 293
- Localization of Cerebellar Lesions 294

D(viii). Gait 295
- Normal Gait Cycle 295
- Abnormalities of Gait 295
- Gait Abnormalities Analysis 298
- Bedside Tests to Diagnose Pes Cavus and Pes Planus 299

D(ix). Approach to Involuntary Movements 300
- Movement Disorders 300
- Tremor 301
- Chorea 301
- Athetosis 301
- Hemiballismus 301
- Myoclonus 302
- Tic 302
- Dystonia 302
- Myokymia 302
- Akathisia 302
- Restless Legs Syndrome/ "Ekbom's Syndrome" 302
- Synkinesis/Mirror Movements 302
- Fasciculations 303

D(x). Meningeal Signs, Skull, and Spine 304
- Signs of Meningeal Irritation 304
- Meningism 305
- Examination of Skull 306
- Examination of Spine 306
- Autonomic Nervous System Testing 306
- Diseases Associated with Autonomic Dysfunction 308

7. Rheumatology 309
A. Case Sheet Format 309
- History Taking 309
- Examination 310

B. Diagnosis Format 312
- Examples 312

C. Discussion on Symptomatology and Examination 313
- Discussed in the Following Headings 313
- Symptomatology 313
- Examination of Skin, Hands, and Eyes 314
- Examination Pattern of Musculoskeletal System 317
- Examination of Upper Limbs 319
- Examination of Lower Limb 323
- Examination of Spine 325
- Examination of Other Joints 327
- Examination of Other Systems in Rheumatological Disorders 327

- Discussion on Common Rheumatological Diseases *328*
- Scoring Systems for Severity of Disease *332*

8. **Comprehensive Geriatric Assessment** 335
   Case Sheet Format *335*
   - History Taking *335*

   Diagnosis Format *337*

   Discussion *338*
   - Frailty Syndrome *339*
   - Dementia *339*
   - Incontinence *340*
   - Falls in the Elderly *341*

9. **Approach to Psychiatric Illness** 342
   Case Sheet Format *342*
   - History *342*
   - Examination *342*

   Diagnosis Format *344*

   Discussion on History and Examination *345*
   - Salient Points in History *345*
   - Salient Points in General Physical and Systemic Examination *346*
   - Mental Status Examination *346*
   - Delusion *347*
   - Obsessions *348*
   - Mood and Affect *348*
   - Illusions *348*
   - Hallucination *348*
   - Pseudohallucination *348*

   Discussion on Diagnosis of Psychiatric Disorders *350*
   - Approach to Diagnosis in Psychiatry *350*
   - Clinical Institute Withdrawal Assessment for Alcohol (CIWA-A) Scale *353*
   - General Outline of Plan of Management of Psychiatric Disorders *354*

10. **Semilong Cases** 355
    - Semilong/Therapeutic Cases *355*

11. **Simplified Approach to ECG (Reading and Diagnosis)**............................ 362
    - Conduction System of the Heart *362*
    - ECG Waveforms and Intervals *362*
    - Reading 12-Lead ECGS *364*
    - Types of LVH *373*
    - ECG Changes in Myocardial Infarction *374*
    - Electrolytes and ECG *376*
    - Examples *377*

12. **A Systematic Approach to Chest X-rays**.. 414
    - Approach to Chest X-rays *414*
    - Discussion on Common X-rays *427*
    - Computed Tomography *436*
    - Magnetic Resonance Imaging *437*
    - Contrast Agents *438*

13. **Basic Instruments and Procedures in Viva**...................................... 439
    - Gastric Lavage Tube *439*
    - Laryngoscope *440*
    - Metal Tracheostomy Tube *440*
    - Endotracheal Tube *441*
    - Oropharyngeal Airway *441*
    - Ambu Bag *442*
    - Ryles Tube—Nasogastric Tube *442*
    - Suction Catheter *443*
    - Foleys Catheter *443*
    - Sahli's Hemoglobinometer *444*
    - Neubauer Chamber/Hemocytometer *444*
    - Insulin Syringe *444*
    - Tuberculin Syringe *444*
    - Vim Silverman Liver Biopsy Needle *445*
    - Trucut Biopsy Gun *445*
    - Bone Marrow Aspiration Needle *446*
    - Bone Marrow Biopsy Needle (Jamshidi Needle) *446*
    - Lumbar Puncture Needle *446*
    - Intravenous Drip Set *447*
    - Intravenous Cannula *448*
    - Oxygen Mask *449*
    - Nasal Cannula *449*
    - Venturi Mask *449*
    - Non-rebreather Mask *449*
    - Inhaler Devices *450*
    - Nebulizers *451*
    - Urinometer *451*
    - Westergren Tube *452*
    - Peak Flow Meter *452*

14. **Spotters**... 454

15. **Discussion on Drugs and Medical Emergencies** 464
    - Antimalarials *464*
    - Antitubercular *465*
    - Antiepileptics *466*
    - Antihistaminics *466*
    - Antiarrhythmics *467*
    - Antianginal and Antiplatelets *468*
    - Antiparkinson *470*
    - Antipsychotics and Antidepressants *471*
    - Analgesics *472*
    - Diuretics *473*
    - Drugs for Asthma *474*
    - Antihypertensives *476*
    - Drugs Acting on Autonomic System *479*
    - Endocrine *480*
    - Antibiotics *484*
    - Antiviral Oseltamivir *488*
    - Antiretroviral *488*
    - Anticoagulation *490*
    - Fibrinolytic *491*
    - Disease-Modifying Antirheumatic Drugs *491*
    - For Inflammatory Bowel Disease *492*

- Antiencephalopathy *493*
- COVID-19 Drugs *493*
- Antifungal *494*
- For *H. pylori* *494*
- For Diarrhea *495*
- Toxicology *495*
- Intravenous Fluids *496*
- Common Drugs Used in Emergencies *497*

16. Annexures 499

A. Miscellaneous Topics *499*
- Pedigree Analysis *499*
- Alcohol Use *501*
- Smoking *503*

B. Definitions *504*
- Pulse *504*
- Blood Pressure *504*
- Hypertension *504*
- Resistant Hypertension *505*
- Refractory Hypertension *505*
- Pseudoresistant Hypertension *505*
- Pseudohypertension *505*
- Secondary Hypertension *505*
- Masked Hypertension *505*
- White Coat Hypertension *505*
- Hypertensive Crisis *505*
- Hypertensive Emergency *505*
- Malignant Hypertension *505*
- Hypertensive Urgency *505*
- Jugular Venous Pressure *505*
- Anemia *505*
- Erythrocytosis and Polycythemia *505*
- Jaundice *506*
- Cyanosis *506*
- Clubbing *506*
- Fever *506*
- Fever of Unknown Origin *506*
- Revised Definition of Fever of Unknown Origin *506*
- Hyperpyrexia *506*
- Hyperthermia *506*
- Heatstroke *507*
- Dyspnea *507*
- Orthopnea *507*
- Paroxysmal Nocturnal Dyspnea *507*
- Platypnea *507*
- Orthodeoxia *507*
- Trepopnea *507*
- Bendopnea *507*
- Palpitations *507*
- Tachycardia *507*
- Bradycardia *507*
- Apex Beat *507*
- Acute Coronary Syndrome *507*
- Pulmonary Hypertension *508*
- Heart Failure *508*
- Dilated Cardiomyopathy *508*
- Cough *508*
- Massive Hemoptysis *508*
- Lung Sounds *508*
- Chronic Obstructive Pulmonary Disease *508*
- Chronic Bronchitis *509*
- Emphysema *509*
- Chronic Cor Pulmonale *509*
- Asthma *509*
- Bronchiectasis *509*
- Unintentional Weight Loss *509*
- Dysphagia *509*
- Dyspepsia *509*
- Nausea *509*
- Retching *509*
- Vomiting *509*
- Regurgitation *509*
- Diarrhea *509*
- Constipation *510*
- Fecal Incontinence *510*
- Hematemesis *510*
- Malena *510*
- Hematochezia *510*
- Severe Gastrointestinal Bleeding *510*
- Occult Gastrointestinal Bleeding *510*
- Obscure Gastrointestinal Bleeding *510*
- Acute Liver Failure *510*
- Cirrhosis of Liver *511*
- Portal Hypertension *511*
- Hepatic Encephalopathy *511*
- Polyuria *511*
- Nocturia *511*
- Oliguria *511*
- Anuria *511*
- Hematuria *511*
- Moderately Increased Albuminuria *511*
- Severely Increased Albuminuria *511*
- Acute Kidney Injury *511*
- Chronic Kidney Disease *511*
- Nephrotic Syndrome *512*
- Uncomplicated UTI and Complicated UTI *512*
- Asymptomatic Bacteriuria *512*
- Neutropenia and Agranulocytosis *512*
- Febrile Neutropenia *512*
- Lymphadenopathy *512*
- Generalized Lymphadenopathy *512*
- Massive Splenomegaly *512*
- Hypersplenism *512*
- Stupor *512*
- Coma *513*
- Confusion *513*
- Dementia *513*
- Delirium *513*
- Akinetic Mutism *513*
- Locked in Syndrome *513*
- Abulia *513*
- Attention and Concentration *513*
- Memory *513*
- Amnesia *513*
- Agnosia *513*

- Insomnia 513
- Aphasia 514
- Dysarthria 514
- Aphonia and Dysphonia 514
- Agraphia/Dysgraphia 514
- Alexia 514
- Echolalia 514
- Palilalia 514
- Perseveration 514
- Neologisms 514
- Idioglossia 514
- Dyslogia 514
- Confabulation 514
- Tone 514
- Rigidity 514
- Cogwheel Rigidity 515
- Akathisia 515
- Asterixis 515
- Athetosis 515
- Chorea 515
- Dystonia 515
- Hemiballismus 515
- Myoclonus 515
- Myokymia 515
- Restless Leg Syndrome 515
- Tics 515
- Tremor 515
- Agraphesthesia 516
- Allodynia 516
- Alloesthesia 516
- Analgesia 516
- Asterognosis 516
- Anesthesia 516
- Dysesthesias 516
- Extinction 516
- Hypalgesia 516
- Hyperalgesia 516
- Hyperpathia 516
- Kinesthesia 516
- Pallesthesia 516
- Paresthesias 516
- Neglect 517
- Anosognosia 517
- Constructional Apraxia 517
- Ataxia 517
- Paralysis and Paresis 517
- Apraxia 517
- Stroke 517
- Transient Ischemic Attack 517
- Lacunar Stroke 517
- Epileptic Seizure 517
- Epilepsy 517
- Syncope 518
- Metabolic Syndrome 518
- Sepsis 518
- Systemic Inflammatory Response Syndrome 518
- Acute Respiratory Distress Syndrome 518
- Macule 518
- Patch 518
- Papule 518
- Nodule 519
- Tumor 519
- Plaque 519
- Vesicle 519
- Pustule 519
- Bulla 519
- Wheal 519
- Telangiectasia 519
- Lichenification 519
- Scale 519
- Crust 519
- Erosion 519
- Ulcer 519
- Excoriation 519
- Atrophy 519
- Scar 519
- Purpuric Lesions 519
- Gynecomastia 520

C. Grading Systems 521
- 1952 MRC Breathlessness Scale 521
- Modified MRC Dyspnea Scale 521
- MRC Muscle Scale 521
- NYHA Breathlessness 521
- Canadian Cardiovascular Society—Grading of Angina Pectoris 522
- NINDS Myotactic Reflex Scale 522
- Freeman and Levine Grading of Systolic Murmur 522
- ABCD and ABCD2 Scores 523
- BODE Index 523
- COPD Assessment Test 524
- CHADS2 524
- CHADS-VASC 524
- HAS-Bled 524
- EHRA Score 525
- Child-Turcotte-Pugh Score 525
- Framingham Heart Failure Criteria 525
- GCS 525
- West Haven Grading of Hepatic Encephalopathy 526
- CKD Stages 526
- 2015 Revised Jones Criteria 527
- Modified Duke's Criteria 527
- Cage Questionnaire 528
- Light's Criteria 528
- qSOFA 528
- SOFA 529
- CURB 65 529
- Forrest Grading of Gastrointestinal Ulcers 529
- Severity Index for Ulcerative Colitis 529

D. Laboratory Values of Clinical Importance 530
- Hematology and Coagulation 530

E. Short List of Routinely Used Formulas in Medicine 535

Index 537

List of QR Codes

List of QR Codes for Clinical Signs Videos, Examination Videos and Auscultation Audios

Video display name	Chapter number	Page number
Clubbing	Chapter 2	36
Aorta Palpation	Chapter 2	15
Apex Pulse Deficit	Chapter 2	9
Axillary LN Examination	Chapter 2	43
Blood Pressure Measurement	Chapter 2	19
Carotid Pulse	Chapter 2	15
Cervical Lymph Node Examination	Chapter 2	41
Collapsing Pulse	Chapter 2	13
Cyanosis	Chapter 2	35
Dorsalis Pedalis Artery	Chapter 2	16
Femoral Pulse	Chapter 2	15
Icterus	Chapter 2	33
JVP and Carotid Pulse	Chapter 2	23
JVP Measurement	Chapter 2	23
Pallor	Chapter 2	31
Pedal Edema	Chapter 2	38
Popliteal Artery	Chapter 2	16
Posterior Tibial Artery	Chapter 2	16
Radial Pulse Examination	Chapter 2	8
AP and Transverse Measurements	Chapter 3	81
Auscultation of Respiratory System	Chapter 3	86
Chest Expansion	Chapter 3	80
Fissures of Lungs	Chapter 3	72
Forced Expiratory Time	Chapter 3	90
Hemithorax Measurements	Chapter 3	81
Respiratory Movements	Chapter 3	78
Respiratory Percussion	Chapter 3	83
Respiratory System General Examination 1	Chapter 3	72
Respiratory System General Examination 2	Chapter 3	72
Shifting Dullness Chest	Chapter 3	85
Spinoacromial Distance	Chapter 3	82
Spinoscapular Distance	Chapter 3	82
Tidal Percussion	Chapter 3	85
Tracheal Examination	Chapter 3	77
Tracheal Tug (Oliver's Sign)	Chapter 3	78
Vocal Fremitus	Chapter 3	82
Normal Breath Sound	Chapter 3	87
Crackles Sound	Chapter 3	89
Pleural Rub Sound	Chapter 3	89
Wheeze Sound	Chapter 3	88
Early Diastolic Murmur Auscultation	Chapter 4	126
Epigastric Pulsations	Chapter 4	115
Mid Diastolic Murmur Auscultation	Chapter 4	126
Parasternal Heave	Chapter 4	114
Percussion of Heart Borders	Chapter 4	117
Pulsatile Liver	Chapter 4	132
Aortic Regurgitation Sound	Chapter 4	136
Apex Beat	Chapter 4	112
Aortic Stenosis Early Sound	Chapter 4	136
Aortic Stenosis Severe Sound	Chapter 4	124
Atrial Septal Defect Sound	Chapter 4	136
Dynamic Auscultation	Chapter 4	95
Heart Sound 3	Chapter 4	122
Heart Sound 4	Chapter 4	122
Heart Sound Split 2	Chapter 4	121
Mitral Regurgitation Sound	Chapter 4	136
Mitral Stenosis Sound	Chapter 4	136
Normal Heart Sound	Chapter 4	120
Patent Ductus Arteriosus Sound	Chapter 4	136
Pericardial Rub Sound	Chapter 4	123
Ventricular Septal Defect Sound	Chapter 4	136
Valsalva Maneuver	Chapter 4	132

List of QR Codes

Video display name	Chapter number	Page number
Abdominal Bruits	Chapter 5	160
Abdominal Quadrants and Regions	Chapter 5	158
Ascites Tap	Chapter 5	175
Ascites	Chapter 5	171
Asterixis	Chapter 5	155
Dilated Veins	Chapter 5	176
Face in Liver Disease	Chapter 5	156
Fluid Thrill	Chapter 5	174
Hands in Liver Diseases	Chapter 5	151
Kidney Palpation and Renal Angle	Chapter 5	169
Liver Palpation	Chapter 5	161
Liver Percussion and Liver Span	Chapter 5	162
Overview of Abdomen	Chapter 5	157
Shifting Dullness	Chapter 5	171
Spider Nevi	Chapter 5	152
Spleen Palpation	Chapter 5	165
Spleen Percussion	Chapter 5	166
Beevor's Sign	Chapter 6A	186
Bell's Phenomenon	Chapter 6D (iii)	238
CN IX and X—Deviation of Uvula	Chapter 6D (iii)	243
Corneal Reflex	Chapter 6D (iii)	232
Facial Nerve Examination	Chapter 6D (iii)	236
Hypoglossal Nerve	Chapter 6D (iii)	246
Nystagmus	Chapter 6D (iii)	228
Tongue Fasciculations	Chapter 6D (iii)	246
UMN Facial Palsy	Chapter 6D (iii)	238
Abdominal Muscles	Chapter 6D (iv)	261
Abductor Digiti Minimi	Chapter 6D (iv)	261
Abductor Pollicis Brevis	Chapter 6D (iv)	259
Adductor Pollicis Brevis	Chapter 6D (iv)	255
Biceps Muscles	Chapter 6D (iv)	257
Brachioradialis Muscle	Chapter 6D (iv)	257
Cog Wheel Rigidity	Chapter 6D (iv)	253
Dorsal Interossei Muscles	Chapter 6D (iv)	260
Extensor Carpi Radialis Longus	Chapter 6D (iv)	257
Extensor Carpi Ulnaris	Chapter 6D (iv)	258
Extensor Hallucis Longus	Chapter 6D (iv)	263
Extensor Pollicis Brevis	Chapter 6D (iv)	255
Extensor Pollicis Longus	Chapter 6D (iv)	255
Flexor Carpi Radialis	Chapter 6D (iv)	258
Flexor Carpi Ulnaris	Chapter 6D (iv)	258
Flexor Digiti Minimi	Chapter 6D (iv)	261
Flexor Digitorum Profundus	Chapter 6D (iv)	260
Lead Pipe Rigidity	Chapter 6D (iv)	253
Lumbricals	Chapter 6D (iv)	260
Neck Extension	Chapter 6D (iv)	256
Neck Flexion	Chapter 6D (iv)	255
Neck-Back Extensors	Chapter 6D (iv)	261
Palmar Interossei	Chapter 6D (iv)	260
Pectoral Muscles	Chapter 6D (iv)	257
Serratus Anterior Muscle	Chapter 6D (iv)	256
Shoulder Muscles 1	Chapter 6D (iv)	256
Shoulder Muscles 2	Chapter 6D (iv)	256
Triceps Muscles	Chapter 6D (iv)	257
Abdominal Reflex	Chapter 6D (v)	272
Ankle Clonus	Chapter 6D (v)	271
Ankle Reflex	Chapter 6D (v)	269
Biceps Reflex	Chapter 6D (v)	267
Finger Flexion Reflex	Chapter 6D (v)	270
Glabella Tap	Chapter 6D (v)	276
Grading of Reflexes	Chapter 6D (v)	265
Knee Reflex	Chapter 6D (v)	269
Plantar Reflexes	Chapter 6D (v)	273
Primitive Reflexes	Chapter 6D (v)	275
Supinator Reflex	Chapter 6D (v)	268
Triceps Reflex	Chapter 6D (v)	268
Ataxia	Chapter 6D (vii)	293
Circumduction Gait	Chapter 6D (vii)	295
Classical Ataxic Gait	Chapter 6D (vii)	296
Classical Scissoring Gait	Chapter 6D (vii)	297
Dysdiadochokinesia	Chapter 6D (vii)	291
Finger-Nose-Finger Test	Chapter 6D (vii)	290
Heel Shin Test	Chapter 6D (vii)	288
High Stepping Gait	Chapter 6D (vii)	296
Parkinson's Gait	Chapter 6D (vii)	297
Parkinson's Shuffling Gait	Chapter 6D (vii)	297
Pendular Knee Jerk	Chapter 6D (vii)	287
Scanning/Staccato Speech	Chapter 6D (vii)	287
Wide-based Gait	Chapter 6D (vii)	287
Titubation	Chapter 6D (vii)	288

Abbreviations

°C	:	Degree Celsius		
°F	:	Degree Fahrenheit		
ABPA	:	Allergic bronchopulmonary aspergillosis		
ACA	:	Anterior cerebral artery		
ACD	:	Anemia of chronic disease		
ACE	:	Addenbrooke's cognitive examination		
ACEI	:	Angiotensin converting enzyme inhibitor		
ACPA	:	Anticitrullinated protein antibody		
ACR	:	American College of Rheumatology		
ACS	:	Acute coronary syndrome		
ACTH	:	Adrenocorticotropic hormone		
ADC	:	Apparent diffusion coefficient		
ADHD	:	Attention deficit hyperactivity disorder		
ADHF	:	Acute decompensated heart failure		
ADL	:	Activities of daily living		
ADR	:	Adverse drug reaction		
AEM	:	Ambulatory electrocardiogram monitoring		
AF	:	Atrial fibrillation		
AGN	:	Acute glomerulonephritis		
AI	:	Aortic insufficiency		
AICA	:	Anterior inferior cerebellar artery		
AICD	:	Automated implantable cardioverter defibrillator		
AIDP	:	Acute inflammatory demyelinating polyneuropathy		
AION	:	Anterior ischemic optic neuritis		
AKI	:	Acute kidney injury		
ALL	:	Acute lymphoblastic leukemia		
ALL	:	Acute lymphoblastic leukemia		
ALS	:	Amyotrophic lateral sclerosis		
AML	:	Acute myeloid leukemia		
ANS	:	Autonomic nervous system		
AP	:	Anteroposterior		
APB	:	Atrial premature beat		
APLA	:	Antiphospholipid antibody syndrome		
ARB	:	Angiotensin receptor blocker		
ARDS	:	Acute respiratory distress syndrome		
ARF	:	Acute renal failure		
ARVD	:	Arrhythmogenic right ventricular dysplasia		
ASCVD	:	Atherosclerotic cardiovascular disease		
ASD	:	Atrial septal defect		
AVF	:	Arteriovenous fistula		
AVM	:	Arteriovenous malformation		
AVNRT	:	AV nodal re-entrant tachycardia		
AVR	:	Aortic valve replacement		
AVRT	:	Atrioventricular re-entrant tachycardia		
B/L	:	Bilateral		
BADL	:	Basic activities of daily living		
BAL	:	Bronchoalveolar concentration		
B-ALL	:	B-cell acute lymphoblastic leukemia		
BAV	:	Bicuspid aortic valve		
BBB	:	Bundle branch block		
BC	:	Bone conduction/blood culture		
BCAT	:	Brief cognitive assessment tool		
BER	:	Benign early repolarization		
BIH	:	Benign intracranial hypertension		
BLS	:	Basic life support		
BM	:	Bone marrow		
BMI	:	Body mass index		
BMV	:	Bag and mask ventilation/balloon mitral valvotomy		
BP	:	Blood pressure		
BSA	:	Body surface area		
BT	:	Bleeding time		
BUN	:	Blood urea nitrogen		
BVP	:	Biventricular pacing		
Bx	:	Biopsy		
C/L	:	Contralateral		
C/O	:	Complaints of		
CABG	:	Coronary artery bypass graft		
CAD	:	Coronary artery disease		
CAMCOG	:	Cambridge cognitive examination		
CAUTI	:	Catheter-associated UTI		
CBC	:	Complete blood count		
CBD	:	Common bile duct		
CBE	:	Clinical breast examination		
CCA	:	Common carotid artery		
CCCU	:	Critical coronary care unit		
CCF	:	Congestive cardiac failure		
CCS	:	Canadian Cardiovascular Society		
CDAI	:	Clinical disease activity index		
CDC	:	Centers for disease control and prevention		
CGA	:	Comprehensive geriatric assessment		
CHB	:	Complete heart block		
CHF	:	Congestive heart failure		
CIDP	:	Chronic inflammatory demyelinating polyneuropathy		
CKD	:	Chronic kidney disease		
CLD	:	Chronic liver disease		
CLL	:	Chronic lymphoid leukemia		
CML	:	Chronic myeloid leukemia		
CMT	:	Charcot–Marie–Tooth disease		
CMV	:	Cytomegalovirus		
CN	:	Cranial nerve		
CNS	:	Central nervous system		

COPD	: Chronic obstructive pulmonary disease	GERD	: Gastroesophageal reflux disease
COST	: Cognitive state test	GH	: Growth hormone
CP angle	: Cerebellopontine angle	GI	: Gastrointestinal
CPB	: Cardiopulmonary bypass	HAI	: Hospital-acquired infection
CPR	: Cardiopulmonary resuscitation	Hb	: Hemoglobin
CRF	: Chronic renal failure	HBV	: Hepatitis B virus
CRP	: C-reactive protein	HCC	: Hepatocellular carcinoma
CSF	: Cerebrospinal fluid	HD	: Huntington's disease
CT	: Computed tomography	HDL	: C-High density lipoprotein cholesterol
CVA	: Cerebrovascular accident	HDS	: Hemodynamically stable
CVP	: Central venous pressure	HE	: Hepatic encephalopathy
CVS	: Cardiovascular system	HIT	: Heparin-induced thrombocytopenia
CXR	: Chest X-ray	HIV/AIDS	: Human immunodeficiency virus/acquired immunodeficiency syndrome
DAS	: Disease activity score		
DDx or D/D	: Differential diagnosis	HL	: Hodgkin lymphoma
DIC	: Disseminated intravascular coagulation	HMF	: Higher mental functions
DIP joint	: Distal interphalangeal joint	HOCM	: Hypertrophic obstructive cardiomyopathy
DKA	: Diabetic ketoacidosis	HTN	: Hypertension
DLCO	: Diffusion lung capacity for carbon monoxide	HUS	: Hemolytic uremic syndrome
DLE	: Disseminated lupus erythematosus	IADL	: Instrumental activities of daily living
DM	: Diabetes mellitus	IBD	: Inflammatory bowel disease
DNR	: Do not resuscitate	IBS	: Irritable bowel syndrome
DPI	: Dry powder inhaler	ICA	: Internal carotid artery
DR	: Diabetic retinopathy	ICD	: Intercostal drain
DSM	: Diagnostic and statistical manual of mental disorders	ICH	: Intracerebral hemorrhage
		ICP	: Intracranial pressure
DTA	: Descending thoracic aorta	ICS	: Intercostal space/inhaled corticosteroid
DTR	: Deep tendon reflex	ICSOL	: Intracranial space-occupying lesion
DVT	: Deep venous thrombosis	IDDM	: Insulin-dependent diabetes mellitus—Type 1 diabetes
DWI	: Diffusion weighted imaging		
EAT	: Ectopic atrial tachycardia	IGF	: Insulin-like growth factor-1
ECA	: External carotid artery	IHD	: Ischemic heart disease
ECD	: Endocardial cushion defects	IJV	: Internal jugular vein
ECF	: Extracellular fluid	ILD	: Interstitial lung disease
ECG	: Electrocardiogram	IMN	: Infectious mononucleosis
ECHO	: Echocardiogram	INH	: Isoniazid
ECMO	: Extracorporeal membrane oxygenation	INO	: Internuclear ophthalmoplegia
EDH	: Extradural hematoma	INR	: International Normalized Ratio
EDM	: Early diastolic murmur	IP joint	: Interphalangeal joint
EF	: Ejection fraction	IPPV	: Intermittent positive pressure ventilation
EM	: Erythema multiforme	ITP	: Immune thrombocytopenic purpura
EOM	: Extraocular muscles/movement	IV	: Intravenous
EPO	: Erythropoietin	IVC	: Inferior vena cava
EPS	: Extrapyramidal system	IVH	: Intraventricular hemorrhage
ESM	: Ejection systolic murmur	JME	: Juvenile myoclonic epilepsy
ESRD	: End-stage renal disease	JRA	: Juvenile rheumatoid arthritis
ESV	: End-systolic volume	JVP	: Jugular venous pressure
ET	: Endotracheal tube	KDIGO	: Kidney disease improving global outcomes
EULAR	: European League Against Rheumatism	KF Ring	: Kayser–Fleischer ring
FBS	: Fasting blood sugar	KUB	: Kidney, ureters, and bladder
FEV1	: Forced expiratory volume in first second	L/A	: Local anesthetic
FMS	: Fibromyalgia syndrome	LDL	: C-Low density lipoprotein cholesterol
FTT	: Failure to thrive	LGIB	: Upper gastrointestinal bleed
FVC	: Forced vital capacity	LMN	: Lower motor neuron
GBS	: Guillain–Barré syndrome	LOC	: Loss of consciousness
GCS	: Glasgow Coma Scale	LP	: Lumbar puncture

LQTS	: Long QT syndrome	PDA	: Patent ductus arteriosus
LSM	: Late systolic murmur	PE	: Pulmonary embolism
LV	: Left ventricle	PEEP	: Positive end expiratory pressure
LVE	: Left ventricular enlargement	PEFR	: Peak expiratory flow rate
LVF	: Left ventricular failure	PICA	: Posterior inferior cerebellar artery
LVH	: Left ventricular hypertrophy	PIP Joint	: Proximal interphalangeal joint
MAP	: Mean arterial pressure	PLS	: Progressive lateral sclerosis
MAT	: Multifocal atrial tachycardia	PMI	: Point of maximal impulse
MCA	: Middle cerebral artery	PND	: Paroxysmal nocturnal dyspnea
MCP joint	: Metacarpophalangeal joint	pO_2/paO_2	: Partial pressure of oxygen
MCTD	: Mixed connective tissue disease	PPBS	: Post-prandial blood sugars
MCTD	: Mixed connective tissue disease	PUO/FUO	: Pyrexia (fever) of unknown origin
MDI	: Metered dose inhaler	PVC	: Premature ventricular contractions
MDM	: Mid-diastolic murmur	QSART	: Quantitative sudomotor axon reflex test
MDS	: Myelodysplastic syndrome	qSOFA	: Quick sequential organ failure assessment
MI	: Myocardial infarction	RA	: Rheumatoid arthritis
MLF	: Medial longitudinal fasciculus	RAI scan	: Radioactive iodine scan
mMRC	: Modified Medical Research Council	RAPD	: Relative apparent pupillary defect
MMSE	: Mini-mental state examination	RAS	: Reticular activating system
MND	: Motor neuron disease	RCC	: Renal cell carcinoma
MoCA	: Montreal cognitive assessment	RCM	: Restrictive cardiomyopathy
MODS	: Multiorgan dysfunction syndrome	RDW	: Red cell distribution width
MRC	: Medical Research Council	REM	: Rapid eye movement
MRI	: Magnetic resonance imaging	REMS	: Regional examination of musculoskeletal system
MS	: Mitral stenosis/multiple sclerosis		
MSA-C	: Multisystem atrophy—cerebellar	RF	: Rheumatoid factor
MSA-P	: Multisystem atrophy—Parkinson's	RHD	: Rheumatic heart disease
MVP	: Mitral valve prolapse	RLN	: Recurrent laryngeal nerve
MVR	: Mitral valve replacement	RR	: Respiratory rate
NASH	: Non-alcoholic steatohepatitis	RS	: Respiratory system
NCV	: Nerve conduction velocity	RSOV	: Ruptured sinus of Valsalva
NG Tube	: Nasogastric tube	RS3PE	: Remitting seronegative symmetrical synovitis with pitting edema
NHL	: Non-Hodgkin lymphoma		
NMJ	: Neuromuscular junction	RV	: Right ventricle
NPH	: Normal pressure hydrocephalus	RVF	: Right ventricular failure
NPPV	: Noninvasive positive pressure ventilation	RVH	: Right ventricular hypertrophy
NREM	: Non-rapid eye movement	SAAG	: Serum–ascites albumin gradient
NSAIDs	: Nonsteroidal anti-inflammatory drugs	SACD	: Subacute combined degeneration of cord
NST	: Non-stress test	SAH	: Subarachnoid hemorrhage
NSTEMI	: Non-ST-elevation myocardial infarction	SANRT	: Sinoatrial node re-entrant tachycardia
NTS	: Nucleus tractus solitarius	SCM	: Sternocleidomastoid
NYHA	: New York Heart Association	SDAI	: Simplified disease activity index
O/E	: On examination	SDH	: Subdural hematoma
OA	: Osteoarthritis	SIRS	: Systemic inflammatory response syndrome
OP	: Organophosphorus	SLE	: Systemic lupus erythematosus
OSA	: Obstructive sleep apnea	SLICC	: Systemic Lupus International Collaborating Clinics
PA	: Posteroanterior		
paCO2	: Partial pressure of carbon dioxide	SLRT	: Straight leg raise test
PAH	: Pulmonary artery hypertension	SMA	: Spinal muscular atrophy
PAH	: Pulmonary artery hypertension	SOFA	: Sequential organ failure assessment
PAN	: Polyarteritis nodosa	SSPE	: Subacute sclerosing pan-encephalitis
PCA	: Posterior cerebral artery	SSR	: Sympathetic skin response
PCI	: Percutaneous coronary intervention	STEMI	: ST-elevation myocardial infarction
PCV	: Packed cell volume	STMS	: Short test of mental status
PCWP	: Pulmonary capillary wedge pressure	SV	: Stroke volume
PD	: Parkinson's disease	SVC	: Superior vena cava

SVT	: Supraventricular tachycardia	UMN	: Upper motor neuron
TAPVC	: Total anomalous pulmonary venous connection	URTI	: Upper respiratory tract infection
TB	: Tuberculosis	US/USG	: Ultrasonogram
TBI	: Traumatic brain injury	UTI	: Urinary tract infection
TG	: Triglycerides	V/Q	: Ventilation/perfusion
TIA	: Transient ischemic attack	VAP	: Ventilator-acquired pneumonia
TIN	: Tubulointerstitial nephritis	VC	: Vital capacity
TMJ	: Temporomandibular joint	VDRL	: Venereal Disease Research Laboratory
TSH	: Thyroid stimulating hormone	VPC	: Ventricular premature contractions
TST	: Thermoregulatory sweat test	VSD	: Ventricular septal defect
U/L	: Unilateral	VT	: Ventricular tachycardia
UA	: Unstable angina	VUR	: Vesicouretreric reflux
UGI	: Upper gastrointestinal	WHO	: World Health Organization
UGIB	: Upper gastrointestinal bleed	WPW	: Wolff–Parkinson–White syndrome
UIP	: Usual interstitial pneumonitis	ZES	: Zollinger–Ellison syndrome

Competency Table

Number	COMPETENCY The student should be able to	Core (Y/N)	Suggested teaching learning method	Chapter number	Page number
GM1.8	Elicit document and present an appropriate history that will establish the diagnosis, cause and severity of heart failure including: presenting complaints, precipitating and exacerbating factors, risk factors exercise tolerance, changes in sleep patterns, features suggestive of infective endocarditis	Y	Bedside clinic	4	93
GM1.9	Perform and demonstrate a systematic examination based on the history that will help establish the diagnosis and estimate its severity including: measurement of pulse, blood pressure and respiratory rate, jugular venous pulses, peripheral pulses, conjunctiva and fundus, lung, cardiac examination including palpation and auscultation with identification of heart sounds and murmurs, abdominal distension and splenic palpation	Y	Bedside clinic, DOAP	2, 4	8, 102
GM1.10	Demonstrate peripheral pulse, volume, character, quality and variation in various causes of heart failure	Y	Bedside clinic, DOAP	2	8
GM1.11	Measure the blood pressure accurately, recognize and discuss alterations in blood pressure in valvular heart disease and other causes of heart failure and cardiac tamponade	Y	Bedside clinic, DOAP	2	18
GM1.12	Demonstrate and measure jugular venous distension	Y	Bedside clinic, DOAP	2	44
GM1.13	Identify and describe the timing, pitch quality conduction and significance of precordial murmurs, their variations, use of dynamic auscultation	Y	Bedside clinic, DOAP	4	125
GM1.15	Order and interpret diagnostic testing based on the clinical diagnosis including 12 lead ECG, chest radiograph, blood cultures	Y	Bedside clinic, DOAP	11	362
GM1.16	Perform and interpret a 12-lead ECG	Y	Bedside clinic DOAP	11	362
GM1.26	Elicit document and present an appropriate history, demonstrate correctly general examination, relevant clinical findings and formulate document and present a management plan for an adult patient presenting with a common form of congenital heart disease		SGT, bedside clinic	4	110, 135
GM2.6	Elicit document and present an appropriate history that includes onset evolution, presentation risk factors, family history, comorbid conditions, complications, medication, history of atherosclerosis, IHD and coronary syndromes	Y	Bedside clinic/DOAP	4	102
GM2.7	Perform, demonstrate and document a physical examination including a vascular and cardiac examination that is appropriate for the clinical presentation	Y	Bedside clinic/DOAP	4	109
GM2.8	Generate document and present a differential diagnosis based on the clinical presentation and prioritize based on "cannot miss", most likely diagnosis and severity	Y	SGT/bedside clinic	4	109
GM2.9	Distinguish and differentiate between stable and unstable angina and AMI based on the clinical presentation	Y	Bedside clinic/DOAP	4	103
GM2.10	Order, perform and interpret an ECG	Y	Bedside clinic/DOAP	11	362
GM2.11	Order and interpret a chest X-ray and markers of acute myocardial infarction		Bedside clinic/DOAP	12	414
GM3.4	Elicit document and present an appropriate history including the evolution, risk factors including Immune status and occupational risk	Y	Bedside clinic, DOAP	3	55
GM3.5	Perform, document and demonstrate a physical examination including general examination and appropriate examination of the lungs that establishes the diagnosis, complications and severity of disease	Y	Bedside clinic, DOAP	3	70
GM3.6	Generate document and present a differential diagnosis based on the clinical features, and prioritize the diagnosis based on the presentation	Y	Bedside clinic, DOAP	3	91

Competency Table

Number	COMPETENCY The student should be able to	Core (Y/N)	Suggested teaching learning method	Chapter number	Page number
GM3.15	Select, describe and prescribe based on the most likely etiology, an appropriate empirical antimicrobial based on the pharmacology and ant microbial spectrum	Y	Bedside clinic, tutorial	15	464
GM3.16	Select, describe and prescribe based on culture and sensitivity appropriate empirical antimicrobial based on the pharmacology and antimicrobial spectrum	Y	Bedside clinic, SGT	15	464
GM4.10	Elicit document and present a medical history that helps delineate the etiology of fever that includes the evolution and pattern of fever, associated symptoms, immune status, comorbidities, risk factors, exposure through occupation, travel and environment and medication use	Y	Bedside clinic, DOAP	2	27
GM4.11	Perform a systematic examination that establishes the diagnosis and severity of presentation that includes: general skin mucosal and lymph node examination, chest and abdominal examination (including examination of the liver and spleen)	Y	Bedside clinic, DOAP	2	31
GM4.12	Generate a differential diagnosis and prioritize based on clinical features that help distinguish between infective, inflammatory, malignant and rheumatologic causes	Y	Bedside clinic, SGT	2	27
GM5.8	Elicit document and present a medical history that helps delineate the etiology of the current presentation and includes clinical presentation, risk factors, drug use, sexual history, vaccination history and family history in patients with liver disease	Y	Bedside clinic, DOAP session	5	137
GM5.9	Perform a systematic examination that establishes the diagnosis and severity that includes nutritional status, mental status, jaundice, abdominal distension ascites, features of portosystemic hypertension and hepatic encephalopathy	Y	Bedside clinic, DOAP session	5	151
GM5.10	Generate a differential diagnosis and prioritize based on clinical features that suggest a specific etiology for the presenting symptom in patient with liver disease	Y	Bedside clinic, SGT	5	151
GM5.13	Outline a diagnostic approach to liver disease based on hyperbilirubinemia, liver function changes and hepatitis serology	Y	LGT/bedside clinic/SGT, tutorial	5	151
GM7.8	Elicit document and present a medical history that will differentiate the etiologies of disease	Y	Bedside clinic, DOAP	7	309
GM7.9	Perform a systematic examination of all joints, muscle and skin that will establish the diagnosis and severity of disease	Y	Bedside clinic, DOAP	7	309
GM7.10	Generate a differential diagnosis and prioritize based on clinical features that suggest a specific etiology	Y	Bedside clinic, SGT	7	309
GM7.16	Select, prescribe and communicate appropriate medications for relief of joint pain and preventive therapy for crystalline arthropathies	Y	DOAP	7	309
GM8.8	Elicit document and present a medical history that includes: duration and levels, symptoms, comorbidities, lifestyle, risk factors, family history, psychosocial and environmental factors, dietary assessment, previous and concomitant therapy	Y	Bedside clinic, DOAP	4	93
GM8.10	Generate a differential diagnosis and prioritize based on clinical features that suggest a specific etiology	Y	Bedside clinic, DOAP	4	93
GM8.16	Perform and interpret a 12-lead ECG	Y	DOAP	11	362
GM9.3	Elicit document and present a medical history that includes symptoms, risk factors including GI bleeding, prior history, medications, menstrual history, and family history	Y	Bedside clinic, DOAP	5	142
GM9.4	Perform a systematic examination that includes: general examination for pallor, oral examination, DOAP of hyperdynamic circulation, lymph node and splenic examination	Y	Bedside clinic	5	151
GM9.5	Generate a differential diagnosis and prioritize based on clinical features that suggest a specific etiology	Y	Bedside clinic, DOAP	5	151
GM10.9	Elicit document and present a medical history that will differentiate the etiologies of disease, distinguish acute and chronic disease, identify predisposing conditions, nephrotoxic drugs and systemic causes	Y	Bedside clinic, DOAP	10	357

Competency Table

Number	COMPETENCY The student should be able to	Core (Y/N)	Suggested teaching learning method	Chapter number	Page number
GM10.10	Perform a systematic examination that establishes the diagnosis and severity including determination of volume status, presence of edema and heart failure, features of uremia and associated systemic disease	Y	Bedside clinic, DOAP	10	357
GM10.11	Generate a differential diagnosis and prioritize based on clinical features that suggest a specific etiology	Y	DOAP, SGT	10	357
GM10.14	Identify the ECG findings in hyperkalemia	Y	DOAP, SGT	11	362
GM11.7	Elicit document and present a medical history that will differentiate the etiologies of diabetes including risk factors, precipitating factors, lifestyle, nutritional history, family history, medication history, comorbidities and target organ disease	Y	LGT, SGT	10	355
GM11.8	Perform a systematic examination that establishes the diagnosis and severity that includes skin, peripheral pulses, blood pressure measurement, fundus examination, detailed examination of the foot (pulses, nervous and deformities and injuries)	Y	LGT, SGT	10	355
GM12.4	Elicit document and present an appropriate history that will establish the diagnosis cause of thyroid dysfunction and its severity	Y	Bedside clinic, skill lab	10	358
GM12.5	Perform and demonstrate a systematic examination based on the history that will help establish the diagnosis and severity including systemic signs of thyrotoxicosis and hypothyroidism, palpation of the rhythm abnormalities neck palpation of the thyroid and lymph nodes and cardiovascular findings	Y	Bedside clinic, skill lab	10	358
GM12.7	Generate a differential diagnosis based on the clinical presentation and prioritize it based on the most likely diagnosis	Y	Bedside clinic, SGT	10	358
GM12.9	Identify atrial fibrillation, pericardial effusion and bradycardia on ECG	Y	Bedside clinic, DOAP	11	362
GM12.14	Describe and discuss the indications of thionamide therapy, radioiodine therapy and surgery in the management of thyrotoxicosis	Y	Bedside clinic	15	480
GM15.4	Elicit and document and present an appropriate history that identifies the route of bleeding, quantity, grade, volume loss, duration, etiology, comorbid illnesses and risk factors	Y	Bedside clinic/tutorial	5	142
GM15.5	Perform, demonstrate and document a physical examination based on the history that includes general examination, volume assessment and appropriate abdominal examination	Y	Bedside clinic/tutorial	5	142
GM16.4	Elicit and document and present an appropriate history that includes the natural history, dietary history, travel, sexual history and other concomitant illnesses in a patient with diarrhea	Y	Bedside clinic, SGT	5	144
GM16.5	Perform, document and demonstrate a physical examination based on the history that includes general examination, including an appropriate abdominal examination	Y	Bedside clinic, DOAP session	5	151
GM16.6	Distinguish between diarrhea and dysentery based on clinical features	Y	Bedside clinic, SGT	5	144
GM16.7	Generate a differential diagnosis based on the presenting symptoms and clinical features and prioritize based on the most likely diagnosis	Y	Bedside clinic, SGT	5	151
GM17.2	Elicit and document and present an appropriate history including aura, precipitating aggravating and relieving factors, associated symptoms that help identify the cause of headaches	Y	Bedside clinic, SGT	6	182
GM17.4	Demonstrate a detailed neurologic examination in a patient of headache and raised intracranial tension including signs of meningitis	Y	Bedside clinic, SGT	6	182
GM17.5	Generate, document and present a differential diagnosis based on clinical features in a patient with headache	Y	Bedside clinic, SGT	5	182
GM18.3	Elicit and document and present an appropriate history in a cerebrovascular patient including onset, progression, precipitating and aggravating relieving factors, associated symptoms that help identify the cause of the cerebrovascular accidents	Y	Bedside clinic, SGT	6	188
GM18.4	Perform, demonstrate and document physical examination that includes general and a detailed neurologic examination as appropriate, based on the history in a stroke patient	Y	Bedside clinic, DOAP	6	188
GM18.5	Distinguish the lesion based on upper verses lower motor neuron, side, site and most probable nature of the lesion in a given patient with neurological symptoms/signs	Y	LGT, bedside clinic, DOAP	6	233

Number	COMPETENCY The student should be able to	Core (Y/N)	Suggested teaching learning method	Chapter number	Page number
GM18.6	Elicit, document and present clinical examination of a stroke patient with speech disorder. Enumerate and describe the points for distinguishing the various disorders of speech based on site of lesion	Y	Bedside clinic, DOAP	6	188
GM18.7	Describe and distinguish, based on the clinical presentation, the types of bladder dysfunction seen in neurological diseases	Y	LGT, bedside clinic, SGT	6	192
GM19.3	Elicit and document and present an appropriate history including onset, progression precipitating, aggravating and relieving factors, associated symptoms that help identify the cause of the movement disorder	Y	Bedside clinic, SGT	7	309
GM19.4	Perform, demonstrate and document a physical examination that includes a general examination and a detailed neurologic examination using standard movement rating scales	Y	Bedside clinic, SGT	7	309
GM19.5	Generate, document and present a differential diagnosis based on the history and physical examination in a patient with movement disorder	Y	Bedside clinic, SGT	7	309
GM19.6	Document and describe clinical diagnosis regarding the anatomical location, nature and cause of the lesion based on the clinical presentation and physical examination in a patient with movement disorder	Y	Bedside clinic, SGT	7	309
GM25.2	Describe the multidimensional geriatric assessments that includes medical, psychosocial and functional components	Y	Bedside clinic, DOAP	8	335
GM26.3	Elicit document and present a medical history that helps delineate the etiology of infectious diseases that includes the evolution and pattern of symptoms, risk factors, exposure through occupation and travel	Y	Bedside clinic, DOAP	3	55
GM26.4	Perform a systematic examination that establishes the diagnosis and severity of presentation that includes: general skin, mucosal and lymph node examination, chest and abdominal examination (including examination of the liver and spleen)	Y	Bedside clinic, DOAP	3	55
GM27.5	Elicit, document and present an appropriate medical history that includes risk factor, contacts, symptoms including cough, fever, anorexia, weight loss, hemoptysis and symptoms of extra-pulmonary manifestations	Y	Bedside clinic, DOAP session	3	55
GM27.6	Demonstrate and perform a systematic examination that establishes the diagnosis based on the clinical presentation that includes: (a) general examination, (b) examination of the chest and lung including loss of volume, mediastinal shift, percussion and auscultation of lung sounds and added sounds, (c) examination of the lymphatic system and (d) relevant CNS examination	Y	Bedside clinic, DOAP session	3	55
GM27.8	Generate a differential diagnosis based on the clinical history and evolution of the disease that prioritizes the most likely diagnosis in patient with history/examination findings suggestive of tuberculosis	Y	Bedside clinic, small group discussion	3	55
GM27.13	Describe and discuss the pharmacology of various anti-tuberculous agents, their indications, contraindications, interactions and adverse reactions	Y	LGT, SGT discussion	15	465
GM28.8	Elicit document and present a medical history that will differentiate the etiologies of obstructive airway disease, severity and precipitants	Y	Bedside clinic, DOAP	3	70
GM28.9	Perform a systematic examination that establishes the diagnosis and severity that includes measurement of respiratory rate, level of respiratory distress, effort tolerance, breath sounds, added sounds, identification of signs of consolidation, pleural effusion and pneumothorax	Y	Bedside clinic, DOAP	3	70
GM28.10	Generate a differential diagnosis and prioritize based on clinical features that suggest a specific etiology	Y	Bedside clinic, DOAP session	3	70
GM28.17	Develop a therapeutic plan including use of bronchodilators and inhaled corticosteroids	Y	Bedside clinic, SGT, DOAP session	15	474
GM28.18	Develop a management plan for acute exacerbations including bronchodilators, systemic steroids, antimicrobial therapy	Y	Bedside clinic, SGT, DOAP session	15	474

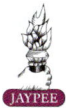
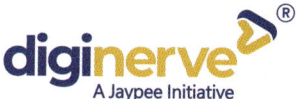

DigiNEET

Simplify your undergraduate studies and NEET PG preparation with this comprehensive program covering all 19 subjects. Crafted by India's top faculty, it includes video lectures, printed notes, OSCEs, a QBank, test series, and the innovative Dr. Wise AI Chatbot.

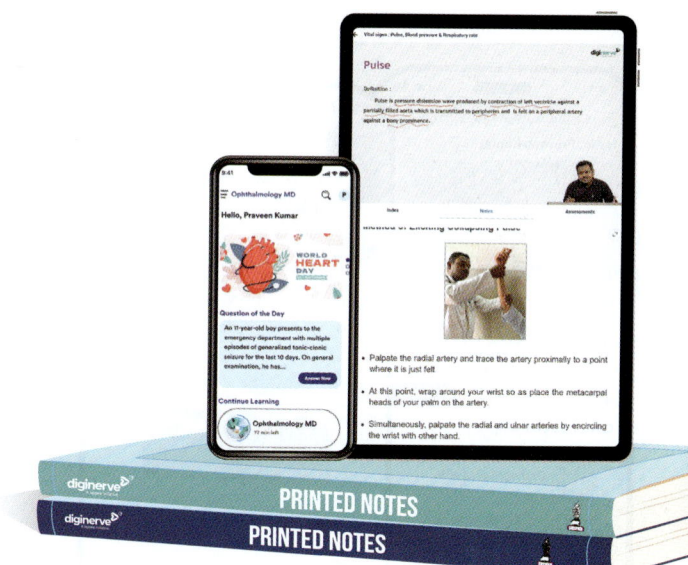

Course Features

 1400+ hrs Video Lectures

 1500+ Topics in Notes

 15000+ Questions in QBank

 1800+ GEMS

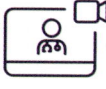 450+ OSCEs

 Test Series

 Dr. Wise AI Chatbot

 Drug Chart

Regular Webinars by Esteemed Faculty

Access Anytime, Anywhere

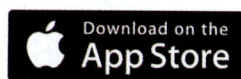
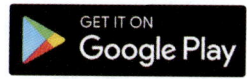

Scan to Download

+91-8800-418-418   marketing@diginerve.com

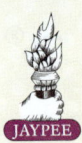
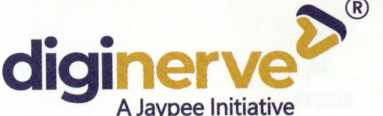

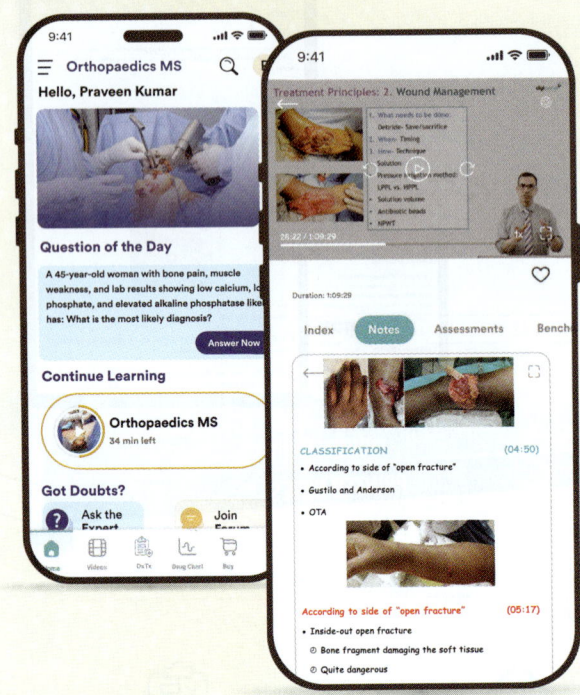

Premium Medical Content, Anytime, Anywhere

Trusted by 150K+ Users

20+ Courses | **3600+** Hrs of Video Content | **790+** Mentors

---

A host of features for **UnderGrads, PostGrads** and **Professionals**

Available on

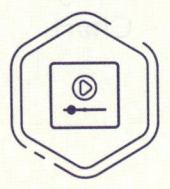 **Video Lectures**

 **Notes**

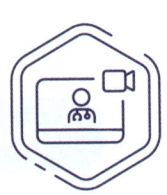 **OSCEs**

 **Drug Chart**

 **Question Bank**

 **Dr. Wise AI Chatbot**

📞 +91-8800-418-418   ✉ marketing@diginerve.com

CHAPTER 1

Introduction

THE IMPORTANCE OF HISTORY TAKING

"Listen to your patient, he is telling you the diagnosis."
— Sir William Osler, *Father of Modern Medicine*

A good history and detailed examination form the foundation of medical practice. Whether you are a physician, a surgeon, an emergency medical technician or a first responder; an extensive, precise and accurate initial assessment sets the pace for further care, evaluation and testing. From a clinical standpoint, the decision making of the patient's treatment depends solely on the information gathered during your history and examination. These are also the skills that a medical professional carries with them till the end of their practice. As one garners more experience, you will become faster, more concise and will be able to derive more information out of less questions.

With more and more emphasis being placed on the integration of health care across specialties; the basics of medical knowledge have become irreplaceable. Each of your patients are going to be different, unique individuals–spanning various ages, gender identities, sexualities, socio-economic backgrounds and ethnicities. The essentials of health care: empathy, listening, clinical reasoning and deduction—are skills that will help you to understand the psyche and the state of every patient. History taking and examination is a vital first step in developing a meaningful therapeutic relationship with your patient.

- Primary tool for diagnosis—Provides 70–80% of diagnoses.
- Guides examination and investigations—Makes them focused and efficient.
- Builds doctor–patient trust—Essential for effective communication.
- Saves time and resources—Reduces unnecessary tests and treatments.
- Legal protection—Well-documented history acts as a defense in medicolegal cases.
- Holistic care—Considers social, psychological, and family factors.
- Enhances clinical reasoning—Strengthens diagnostic and logical thinking.

Detailed Assessments vs Problem-focused Assessments

While encountering a patient for the first time, one should make the decision of doing a detailed assessment or a problem-focused assessment. It is also always prudent to make adjustments into your history as you go along; if a patient presents with a fresh wound, you may start with a problem-based approach. But as you take history, you may find out that the patient is diabetic, in which case you may need to go into further detail.

As students of medicine, it is encouraged to do a detailed history. This helps you develop pace and flow, two very important qualities when interviewing a patient. However, the ground reality is very different. As you become interns and residents, you may have to allocate time and resources to your patient based on the urgency of their problem. This equity of health care is what we refer to as triaging: The patient that needs attention the most gets it first. In such situations, a short, focused history is preferred.

Detailed	*Problem-focused*
Essential for forming the initial framework of a patient's symptoms	Essential for returning patients, emergent patients or follow-up cases
Provides a baseline for future reference	Saves time in dire situations for quick intervention
Holistic approach to the patient as an individual	Assessment of only a particular system with respect to the chief symptom

Writing a Case Sheet

In the era of evidence-based medicine, documentation has become a skill that doctors need to master. A good, crisp case sheet can make the difference in pattern of care; especially in larger hospitals where a patient is treated upon by a team of healthcare professionals. Even in smaller clinics, it is impractical to expect a doctor or a nurse to remember every detail about every patient. Hence, good documentation paves the way for good clinical outcomes.

Unfortunately for the students, like most things in medicine, a universally accepted format for case sheets does not exist. Keep in mind that it is more important to include everything than to nitpick about the order of the information presented. Students are always encouraged to find a format that is comfortable for them and stick to that while taking history, so that they do not miss out on any vital information. The final case sheet can then be tailored to the hospital, clinic or institution's requirement.

Around the world, different countries practice different ways of case sheet writing. However, the one thing that is always common is the S-O-A-P approach.

The subjective: The first part of the case sheet always consists of the subjective history provided by the patient. These include all the information that is given by the patient verbally and more often than not, cannot be verified by the clinician. A patient might tell you that he feels like a rat gnawing away in his stomach. This is his subjective way of expressing his discomfort to you. As a clinician, you have no way of confirming this. The subjective part includes the Chief Complaints, History of Presenting Illness, Past, Personal and Family Histories.

The objective: The objective part of the case sheet includes all the information that is elicited by the doctor which he can verify. This usually means the examination findings and their interpretations. A patient may tell you that his legs have been feeling weak for a month, this is subjective. However, once you test the power in his lower limbs and verify that he cannot move his leg against resistance, it is an objective finding. The objective part usually includes the General Physical Examination and the Systemic Examination.

The assessment: The assessment is the part of the case sheet which consists of the summarization of the subjective and the objective findings. A concise summary with all the positive findings, a preliminary diagnosis and any recent investigations or reports may be included in the assessment portion.

The plan: The plan is the part of the case sheet which outlines the diagnostic and therapeutic interventions that the patient must receive under your care. This includes all the investigations, interventions, procedures and the drug charting that need to be done. If the patient is admitted in your facility, then it is of utmost importance to include a daily follow-up note. The follow-up note consists of the patient's general condition, relevant examination findings and any changes to their initial plan that may be recommended as per the patient's prognosis.

Though it is rare that doctors will encounter this terminology in India, in several countries, the case sheet itself is known as the SOAP note. As members of a quickly growing global health network, this was added here in an attempt to sensitize the Indian healthcare community towards this format. It is also good to notice that it is not very different from what we follow in India.

Etiquette During History Taking

More often than not, medical professionals are accused of taking their position of respect for granted. This is definitely not an appreciable quality. As doctors, we must hold ourselves to an extremely high standard, especially when we deal with patients and their families. It is imperative that we follow all the general rules of social etiquette: dress well, talk empathetically and use respectful language. It is always recommended to introduce yourself to the patient before the interview, state the purpose of the interview and approximately how long it will take. This is also a good time to ask if the patient has any pressing concern which needs immediate attention. Reassure the patient that all the information provided during this interview is completely confidential.

Components of History Taking

Initial Information

The initial information during history taking entails the date and time of evaluation. In situations where several clinicians are handling multiple cases, it may also be prudent to add the name of the evaluating physician. This is exceptionally important in emergency situations where the physician performing the initial assessment needs to be readily available for assistance.

Personal Details

This includes all the details that help us in identifying the patient. A good rule of thumb to follow is name, age, gender identity, occupation and marital status. In a multicultural society like India, the patient's native village or town is also a good point of identification. If the patient is referred from a different center, that can also be entered here.

Source of History and Reliability

The source of history or reliability is usually a must-have in pediatric cases. Though not always necessary, it is a good practice to mention this in adult history taking as well. This is exceptionally useful when the patient himself is poorly oriented or unable to give clear history. It reflects the accuracy of the information in the case sheet.

Chief Complaints

The chief complaint is the immediate, emergent complaint which brings the patient to you. Try to use the patient's own words when writing the chief complaint. Arranging the chief complaints chronologically can also help to streamline your thought process while interpreting your case sheet at a later time.

A point to keep in mind is that more often than not; it is the history-taker's duty to arrange and make sense out of the information. Do not be afraid to ask leading questions to clarify the time and intensity of each symptom. For example, a patient may present with a fluid-filled abdomen as his chief complaint for one month. It may strike as odd to you that the patient noticed his abdomen enlarging for an entire month and decided to come to the hospital on this particular day. However, upon further probing it will be clear that the patient's family brought him to the hospital because he was somnolent since 2 days.

History of Presenting Illnesses

This column provides the descriptive aspect of the chief complaints. It is a comprehensive, clear and chronological account of the patient's problems. This includes all the details that come with the famous mnemonic OLD-CHART:
- **Onset:** Sudden, insidious, immediate or emergent.
- **Location:** Site of the symptom.
- **Duration:** How long has the symptom been bothering the patient?
- **Character:** Any descriptive words that the patient may use to help narrow down the cause of his symptom. A common example is seen in pain, where patients can describe it as stabbing, crushing, burning, dull-aching, etc.
- **Aggravating factors:** Are there any actions that increase the symptom?
- **Relieving factors:** Are there any actions that reduce the symptom?
- **Temporal pattern:** Does the intensity of the symptom change throughout the day? This can also be extrapolated to seasonal variations also.

As illnesses affect different parts of the body, and many illnesses may be multi-system, it is important to ask about connected symptoms. You need to cover the following areas:
- **Respiratory system:** Dyspnea, wheeze, cough, sputum, hemoptysis, chest pain
- **Cardiovascular system:** Chest pain, orthopnea, paroxysmal nocturnal dyspnea, ankle swelling, palpitations and intermittent claudication
- **Gastrointestinal system:** Abdominal pain, nausea, vomiting, hematemesis, bowel habit, blood P/R, melena
- **Urogenital system:** Frequency, nocturia, polydipsia, loin pain, hematuria
- Menarche, menopause, cycle, intermenstrual bleeding, postcoital bleeding
- **Central nervous system:** Headaches, visual disturbances, sleep, hearing, tinnitus, light headedness, blackouts, fits, unsteady gait, weakness and paresthesia's
- **Musculoskeletal:** Myalgia, arthralgia, back pain, joint swelling
- **Psychiatric:** The mental state examination will be taught more formally in your psychiatric attachment. Remember, depression is common and may often co-exist with physical ill health.

The best way to round out a good history of presenting illness note is to include relevant positive history and relevant negative history. There are several commonly encountered cases which are diagnoses of exclusions. Noting down these "points of exclusion" (often called negative history in clinical practice) is the mark of a good clinician.

Past (Medical or Surgical) History

Broadly, the past medical or surgical history can be divided into three categories: childhood illnesses, adult illnesses and screening tests. Childhood illnesses are usually not mentioned in the past history, unless there is a significant residual morbidity or chronicity of the condition.

In order to give a complete picture of the patient's health status, adult past history can be divided into medical, surgical, obstetric/gynecological and psychiatric. In each of these categories, always focus on the past illnesses which might give a clue to the patient's current ailment. A great rule of thumb to follow is disease-duration-drug, i.e., name of the ailment, followed by duration, and then the therapeutic intervention that was used.

In elderly patients, screening tests are done to rule out certain predictable age-dependent conditions. The results of these screening tests can be mentioned in the past history. This saves both time and resources for the treating clinician as these tests need not be repeated again.

Personal History

In personal history, we comment on the person's temperament. An additional note on the patient's appetite, sleep, bowel and bladder habits is encouraged, especially if there is any variation from his normal patterns. If the patient is sexually active, the clinician should elicit history about his sexual practices and evaluate whether the patient engages in high-risk sexual behavior.

Lastly, it is always prudent to ask the patient about his addictions and allergies. Tobacco usage, drug addictions, alcohol consumption are all commonly encountered addictions which can alter or change the course of both the patient's condition and your treatment. When eliciting such history, it is always important to be open-minded and to make the patient feel safe enough to share that information with you.

A common situation that can be encountered is family members and patient bystanders asking prying questions about the patient's addictions, sexuality or gender identity. Similarly, an employer or manager may contact you in order to gain information about the patient's condition. Handling these situations tactfully is of paramount importance. Trust is the foundation of a good doctor-patient relationship. It is therefore extremely necessary to keep the information furnished in the personal history between the treating doctor and his patient. Learning to intersperse questions about personal details within regular history taking is very helpful to establish the rapport with the patient.

Family History

Under family history, outline the present or past health conditions of any immediate family member. These include but are not limited to hypertension, cardiovascular disease, diabetes, cancer, autoimmune conditions and untimely deaths. If the patient has a known genetically transmitted disease, a pedigree chart may also be added.

Review of Systems

Review of systems is an additional column that can be added when a clinician is evaluating a patient for a routine health checkup. It is very similar to the "head-to-toe" examination part except that questions are asked pertaining to the patient's general health status. Go from the head to the toe of the patient, asking questions that may be significant to his quality of life such as "How is your vision?" and "How is your hearing?" and "Do you have any skin rashes?"

Do keep in mind that when a patient presents with a chief complaint, the history and your line of questions will be streamlined to include all the details that contribute to his current ailment. As such, a review of systems is not necessary in those situations since all those points would have been covered previously.

Examination of the Patient

Setting up the Examination

Before you examine the patient, take your time and prepare yourself for the sequence in which you wish to go about. Approach the patient with calmness and be as professional as one can be. Introduce yourself as a student, ask if they have any urgent discomfort which needs attending and then request the patient to let you examine them.

Once the patient has agreed to the examination, it is both your responsibility and your best interest to make the patient feel as comfortable as possible. It is very common for patients to feel vulnerable and uneasy during examination. This may be in anticipation of pain or the uncertainty of what the doctor may find. But an uncomfortable patient begets an uncomfortable doctor. Adjust the height of the bed, the lighting and your stance based on the patient's requirement. Take extra steps to protect the patient's modesty. The extra work done in preparation tells a patient that you are genuinely concerned about their health and the patients will show their appreciation in the form of cooperation.

"A doctor is one of the only jobs where you can ask someone to take off their clothes and they will do it without question". This trust is a unique aspect of the doctor-patient relationship which is your responsibility to safeguard. Close the doors, place blinds or partitions, ask the patient if they want anyone in the room to leave and comply with their requests. Wash and warm your hands before you touch the patient.

During the Examination

A seasoned clinician completes the physical examination in a quick, thorough and gentle manner. He notices the body language and the mannerisms of the patient, empathizes with his condition and provides reassurance in the best way possible. It is very normal to forget a particular part of the examination during the process. Go back to the patient and request his permission to do the parts that you missed out.

During examination, it might take time for you, as a student, to appreciate certain findings. No clinician expects a second- or third-year student to properly diagnose a heart murmur. As such, if you find yourself spending some extra time trying to learn the nature of a finding, it is always a good practice to inform the patient that you are doing so because of your desire to learn and not because there is something wrong with them.

Another common happening in the wards is the patient or their bystanders asking you to interpret your findings to them. In the eyes of the patient, you are another doctor and they can use your knowledge as a "secondary opinion". As an inexperienced doctor who is not the patient's primary clinician, you may find yourself in a situation trying to give information that you yourself are unsure of. Be respectful and mindful of the patient bystanders concerns but also be gracious enough to accept what you know and do not know. As a student, it is more fruitful to share findings with your peers and your professors. Discuss the diagnosis and plan with them so that you can be an active part of the treating team.

After the Examination

Write down your findings in a streamlined and systemic manner. Go through your pre-examination list and fill in any gaps in your case sheet. It is also good practice to thank the patient for his cooperation and to offer them some positive reassurance.

Protecting yourself: Hygiene for the healthcare worker.

In a hospital, your chances of being cured of a disease and your chances of contracting a disease are both extremely high. Healthcare workers are constantly at the risk of life-threatening illnesses because of the close proximity with which they work with sick patients. Even after countless years of research, effort and studies, hospital infections are an occupational hazard that we may never be able to completely eliminate due to the nature of our jobs. Hence, it is always important for a doctor to adopt certain practices to put their health and safety first.

> **CDC recommendations for hand hygiene**
> - Key situations where hand hygiene should be performed include:
>   - Before touching a patient, even if gloves are worn;
>   - Before exiting the patient's care area after touching the patient or the patient's immediate environment;
>   - After contact with blood, body fluids, or excretions, or wound dressings;
>   - Prior to performing an aseptic task (e.g., placing an intravenous drip, preparing an injection);
>   - If hands are moving from a contaminated-body site to a clean-body site during patient care; and
>   - After glove removal.
> - Use soap and water when hands are visibly soiled (e.g., blood, body fluids), or after caring for patients with known or suspected infectious diarrhea (e.g., *Clostridium difficile*, norovirus). Otherwise, the preferred method of hand decontamination is with an alcohol-based hand rub.

Universal precautions are a set of guidelines by the CDC that have been recommended in an effort to reduce the risk of parenteral, mucous membrane and noncontact exposure of healthcare workers to harmful blood-borne pathogens. The following body fluids are considered potentially harmful: blood, blood products, semen, vaginal secretions, synovial fluid, pleural fluid, peritoneal fluid, pericardial fluid and amniotic fluid. All healthcare workers must be cautious to prevent injury through needle-stick and exposure to these hazards. Further, with the rise of Sars-Cov-2 or the coronavirus, it is now more important than ever to maintain a strict level of hand and hospital hygiene.

Patient-Doctor Privilege

As a doctor, it is a very natural and expected part of your profession to ask extremely embarrassing, secretive and personal information. Your clinical reasoning relies entirely upon your ability to convince a patient that they can trust you with the most intimate parts of their lives; information which they have perhaps not shared with anyone else. It is very important for you, as a doctor, to be receptive to such information and to accept it with an open mind. These may include sensitive information pertaining to their daily habits, drug addictions, sexual activity, sexuality, gender identity, criminal activity or prior illnesses. The conversation between a doctor and a patient is not the place for prejudice or judgment, especially if it is against your cultural and religious beliefs. If you feel like you cannot get past your inhibition when dealing with a patient, be respectful and ask a peer or colleague to take over.

Furthermore, if a patient provides you with such information, it is your duty to keep that information a secret. This is exceptionally important when a patient bystander, distant relative or employer asks you for details pertaining to the patient's condition. In the western countries, it is illegal for you to provide confidential details even to the next of kin without the patient's consent. However, in the Indian scenarios, due to the close-knit nature of families and communities, privacy is often taken for granted. As a doctor, it is your responsibility to uphold the patient's dignity.

Always ask for the patient's consent before sharing sensitive information to their family, friends or employers. When the patients are teenagers or under-aged, ask the patient if they need some time to speak alone away from their parents. It is always good practice to ask the patient bystanders to leave during the examination process. This is the ideal time to elicit sensitive history from the patient.

PREREQUISITES FOR PRACTICAL EXAMINATION

Clinical skills, such as the physical examination remain an important instrument in the physician's armamentarium and assessment of these skills form the basis of the final clinical examination. Every student appearing for the examination will be under a lot of stress, which even though justifiable becomes detrimental for the performance of the student. Here are some suggestions:

- The first and foremost is preparation. Try to have a timetable and cover all important cases well in advance. You have a set of cases that are usually kept for the examination and most of the questions asked are also predictable. Do not keep any important things pending to read on the day prior to examination.
- Sleep is of utmost importance on the day prior to the examination. You need to sleep for a **minimum 4–5 hours on the day prior to the examination**. The curriculum being vast, compromising a few hours of sleep would do more harm than good.
- Have a **light breakfast**. Hypoglycemia hampers your thought process, delays your reaction time and severely impairs the performance. Agreed that the feel of examination may be like undergoing a surgery, but nil per oral (NPO) status is not needed.
- Attire is important. Be neatly groomed and dressed. Wear a clean apron with a number badge.
- Carry all your instruments.
- Write a detailed case sheet. Examine each case thoroughly. Never rely on expert's diagnosis. Make your own diagnosis. Always justify it with your own views.
- Stick to the set time limits. Do not waste time.
- Be gentle to the patient when you examine. The more cooperative the patient is, the better will be your performance. Always take the permission of the patient and explain before examining and do not forget to thank them at the end.
- Never forget to wish the examiner good morning/evening. If you do not know an answer, say sorry! (Most of the examiners will change the question or give you a clue). Always finish with a thank you!
- Confidence is of paramount importance. Practice presenting cases without referring to the case sheet.
- Be clear in the order of presentation, both history and examination. Stress on relevant important findings. To be expressive is important, but not over expressive. Eye contact is essential. Answer clearly and to the point. Do not speak about rare causes. When demonstrating signs, do it clearly.
- Most importantly, have faith in yourself and your preparation. You shall succeed.

CHECKLIST FOR PRACTICAL EXAMINATION

1. Clean apron with roll number tag
2. Hall ticket
3. Stationery
4. Stethoscope with a bell
5. Knee hammer
6. Key (to test plantar reflex, stereognosis)
7. Wristwatch with seconds needle
8. Measuring tape
9. Two scales
10. Pins
11. Glass slides
12. Two small boxes for testing smell (soap and coffee)
13. Four boxes for testing taste (sugar, salt, bitter and sour)
14. Four cards with the words "sweet", "sour", "bitter" and "salt" written on them.
15. Snellen's chart
16. Ishihara's chart
17. Cotton
18. Tuning forks (128 Hz and 512 Hz)
19. Divider
20. Ophthalmoscope with full batteries
21. Torch with full batteries
22. Thermometer
23. Tongue depressor
24. Cotton wick/throat swab stick—gag reflex
25. Two test tubes preferably aluminum for temperature testing (glass test tubes may be used if aluminum test tubes are not available)
26. Pulse oximeter (not mandatory)
27. Gloves
28. Mask
29. Hand rub

FORMAT OF CLINICAL EXAMINATION

The general format of cases in the examination is as follows:

Type of case	Time given for examination of patient	Time for clinical viva	Marks
Long	45–60 min detailed case sheet needed	15–20 min	50/40 marks
Short	15 min	7–10 min	20 marks
Semi-long	15 min	7–10 min	20 marks
Spotters	1 min	2–3 min	5 marks each
Charts (laboratory data, clinical)	1 min	2–3 min	5 marks each
OSCE (any clinical sign)	5 min	5 min—observed	5–10 marks each
Viva voce	• 4 table vivas, each carrying 5 marks, each timed for 5 minutes • Topic—X-rays, ECG, instruments, drugs, charts, general viva		

COMMON EXAMINATION CASES

Respiratory system

Long case	Short case
• Bronchial asthma • Emphysema • Chronic bronchitis • Bronchiectasis • Pleural effusion/empyema • Lung abscess • Bronchial carcinoma • Consolidation • Pneumothorax • Hydropneumothorax • Collapse of the lung • Diffuse parenchymal lung disease/interstitial lung disease • Fibrosis/fibrocavity • Fibrothorax	• Bronchial asthma • Emphysema • Chronic bronchitis • Bronchiectasis • Pleural effusion/empyema • Lung abscess • Bronchial carcinoma • Consolidation • Pneumothorax • Hydropneumothorax • Collapse of the lung • Diffuse parenchymal lung disease/interstitial lung disease • Fibrosis/fibrocavity • Fibrothorax

Cardiovascular system

Long case	Short case
• Mitral stenosis • Mitral regurgitation • Mixed mitral stenosis with mitral regurgitation • Aortic stenosis • Aortic regurgitation • Mixed aortic stenosis and regurgitation • Multivalvular heart diseases • Subacute bacterial endocarditis • Eisenmenger's syndrome • Tetralogy of Fallot • Ventricular septal defect • Atrial septal defect • Patent ductus arteriosus • Hypertrophic cardiomyopathy • Dilated cardiomyopathy • Congestive cardiac failure	• Mitral stenosis • Mitral regurgitation • Mixed mitral stenosis with mitral regurgitation • Aortic stenosis • Aortic regurgitation • Mixed aortic stenosis and regurgitation • Hypertension • Subacute bacterial endocarditis • Rheumatic fever • Eisenmenger's syndrome • Tetralogy of Fallot • Ventricular septal defect • Atrial septal defect • Patent ductus arteriosus • Coarctation of aorta • Hypertrophic cardiomyopathy • Dilated cardiomyopathy • Congestive cardiac failure

Gastrointestinal system

Long case	Short case
• Jaundice • Acute/chronic hepatitis • Chronic liver disease (cirrhosis of liver) • Liver abscess • Ascites • Hepatomegaly • Splenomegaly • Hepatosplenomegaly • Polycystic kidney disease	• Jaundice • Acute/chronic hepatitis • Chronic liver disease (cirrhosis of liver) • Liver abscess • Ascites • Hepatomegaly • Splenomegaly • Hepatosplenomegaly • Polycystic kidney disease

Nervous system

Long case	Short case
• Cerebrovascular disease • Ataxia • Peripheral neuropathy • Guillain–Barré syndrome • Chronic inflammatory demyelinating polyneuropathy • Myasthenia gravis • Spastic paraplegia (cord compression) • Transverse myelitis • Myopathy • Parkinsonism • Motor neuron disease • Multiple sclerosis	• Motor system examination • Facial nerve palsy • Foot drop • Claw hand • Examination of cranial nerves • Cerebellar signs • Involuntary movements • Sensory system examination

Semi-long cases/therapeutic cases

Renal	• Nephrotic syndrome • Glomerulonephritis • Chronic kidney disease
Rheumatology	• Systemic lupus erythematosus • Rheumatoid arthritis • Ankylosing spondylitis • Systemic sclerosis
Endocrine	• Diabetes mellitus • Hypothyroidism • Graves' disease (with thyrotoxicosis) • Cushing's syndrome • Addison's disease • Hypopituitarism • Acromegaly • Obesity • Short stature
Hematology	• Anemia • Bleeding disorders • Hepatosplenomegaly • Lymphadenopathy
General	• Pyrexia of unknown origin • Hypertension • Edema • Heart failure • Dyspnea • Comprehensive geriatric assessment

CHAPTER 2

General Examination

A. CASE SHEET FORMAT

Patient is
- Conscious
- Oriented
- Cooperative
- Obeying commands.

BODY MASS INDEX (BMI)
- Weight (kg)/height (m^2)
- Grading according to World Health Organization (WHO) for Southeast Asian countries.

VITALS EXAMINATION
- Pulse
  - Rate
  - Rhythm
  - Volume
  - Character
  - Vessel wall thickening
  - Radio-radial delay and radio-femoral delay
  - Peripheral pulses
- Blood pressure
  - Right arm
  - Left arm
  - Both legs
- Respiration
  - Rate
  - Abdominothoracic (male) or Thoracoabdominal (female)
  - Use of accessory muscles
- Jugular venous pulse
  - Waveform
- Jugular venous pressure
  - _____ cm of blood/water above sternal angle (+ 5 cm water from right atrium)
- Temperature _____ °C or °F measured at _____ site
- Pulse oximetry saturation
- Pain

PHYSICAL EXAMINATION
- Pallor
- Icterus
- Cyanosis
- Clubbing
- Lymphadenopathy
- Edema

OTHERS

Note: General physical examination findings relevant to each system shall be discussed in the respective chapters.

B. VITALS EXAMINATION

PULSE

Definition

Pulse is defined as a pressure distension wave produced by the contraction of the left ventricle against a partially filled aorta which is transmitted to peripheries and is felt on a peripheral artery against a bony prominence.

Assessment of arterial pulse	
Characteristics	Best assessed by palpating
Rate	Radial artery
Rhythm	
Volume	Carotid artery
Character or quality	Carotid artery **Exceptions:** ■ Collapsing pulse, pulsus alternans and pulsus paradoxus are appreciated at the radial artery ■ Pulsus bisferiens best appreciated in brachial artery
Radio-radial and radio-femoral delay	
Whether all peripheral pulses are felt	
Condition of vessel wall	

Example: 72 beats per minute, regular rhythm, normal volume and character, all peripheral pulses are well felt, no radio-radial or radio-femoral delay, no vessel wall thickening.

Method of Palpation of Radial Artery (Fig. 2B.1)

The radial pulse is felt using three fingers. The pads of the fingers are placed along the radius bone. The distal finger is to prevent the backflow (to obliterate retrograde pulsations from palmar arch), proximal finger is to stabilize artery on the bone and middle finger is used to feel and count the pulse (three-finger method). Another accepted method of palpating the pulse is by using two fingers.

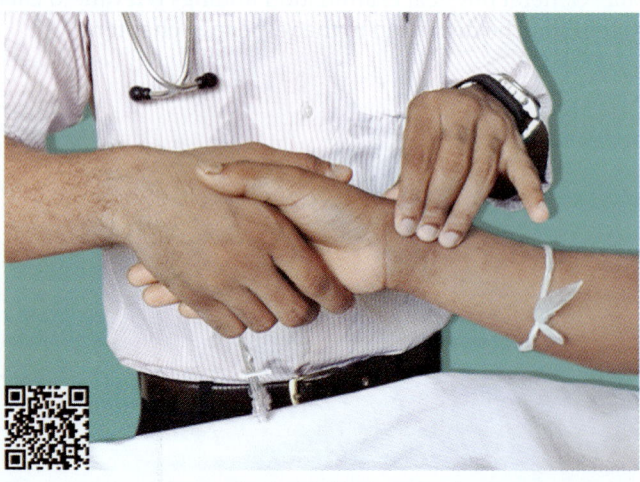

Fig. 2B.1: Method of palpation of radial artery.

Pulse Rate

Calculate the rate by counting the radial pulse for **one full minute**. Normal heart rate is 60–100 beats per minute.

<60 (bradycardia)	>100 (tachycardia)
Physiological: Athletes, sleep **Pathological:** ■ Severe hypoxia ■ Hypothyroidism/myxedema ■ Obstructive jaundice ■ Hypothermia ■ Sick sinus syndrome ■ Drugs—β-blockers, verapamil, and digoxin ■ Heart block ■ Raised intracranial tension (Cushing's reflex)	**Physiological:** Infants, children, emotion, exertion, anxiety and pregnancy **Pathological:** ■ Tachyarrhythmias ■ High output states: Severe anemia, thyrotoxicosis, beriberi, Paget's disease of the bone, cirrhosis of liver, AV fistula ■ Cardiac failure ■ Cardiogenic shock ■ Drugs (e.g., atropine, nifedipine, salbutamol, terbutaline, nicotine, and caffeine)

Relationship between pulse and temperature	
For every °C rise in temperature, the pulse rate increases by 10—**Liebermister rule**	
Relative tachycardia	Relative bradycardia

■ Acute rheumatic carditis
■ Diphtheric myocarditis
■ Tuberculosis
	■ Yellow fever (**Faget's sign**)
	■ Dengue fever
	■ First week of enteric fever
	■ Pyogenic meningitis/intracerebral abscess
	■ Brucellosis
	■ Legionella
	■ Psittacosis
	■ Typhus
	■ Q fever
	■ Leptospirosis
	■ Noninfectious:
	  • Patients on β-blockers
	  • Lymphomas
	  • Factitious fever
	  • Drug fever

Rhythm

Rhythm is assessed by palpating the radial pulse. The normal rhythm is regular.

Causes of irregular rhythm
Regularly irregular ■ Atrial tachyarrhythmias with fixed AV blocks, sinus arrhythmia, partial/second degree atrioventricular (AV) blocks ■ Ventricular bigeminy and trigeminy **Irregularly irregular** ■ Ventricular ectopics/ventricular premature complexes (VPCs) ■ Atrial fibrillation (AF) ■ Atrial tachyarrhythmia with varying AV blocks **Regular with occasional irregularity** ■ Extrasystoles

Arrhythmias with regular rhythm
1. Atrial flutter 2. Ventricular tachycardia 3. First degree heart block 4. Second degree heart block

General Examination

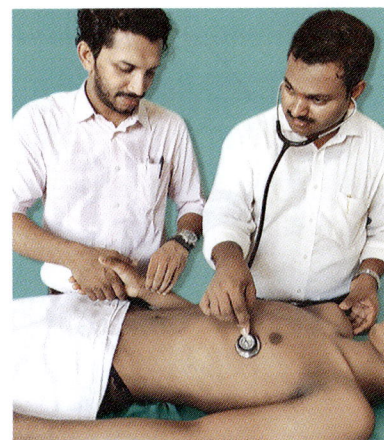

Fig. 2B.2: Demonstration of apex pulse deficit.

Pulse deficit (apex-pulse deficit) (Fig. 2B.2) is the difference between the heart rate (counted by auscultation) and pulse rate when counted simultaneously for one full minute by two individuals.

When two people are not available, only one person can simultaneously feel the radial pulse and auscultate for the apex—only the missed beats are counted.

Causes

Pulse deficit of more than 10/minute occurs in atrial fibrillation (AF) and less than 10/minute may be found with ventricular premature beats or slow/controlled AF. In AF, each ventricular contraction may not be sufficiently strong to transmit an arterial pulse wave through the peripheral artery, so we get apex pulse deficit.

Differences Between Atrial Fibrillation and Ventricular Premature Complexes (VPCs)

	Atrial fibrillation	VPCs
Apex pulse deficit	Usually, >10	Usually, <10
JVP 'a' wave	Absent	Normal
S_1	Variable intensity	Normal
Effect of exercise/ hand grip	Irregularity persists	Pulse becomes regular

Volume of the Pulse

Volume of the pulse is a measure of the pulse pressure. The pulse pressure is the difference between systolic and diastolic blood pressure (SBP-DBP)

Normal pulse pressure is 30–60 mm Hg	
<30 mm Hg (low volume) hypokinetic pulse	>60 mm Hg (high volume) hyperkinetic pulse
<ul><li>Congestive cardiac failure</li><li>Hypovolemia</li><li>Shock</li><li>Mitral stenosis</li><li>Aortic stenosis **(pulsus minimus)**</li><li>Constrictive pericarditis</li></ul>	**Physiological:** Fever, pregnancy, alcoholism, and exercise **Pathological:**<ul><li>**High output states:** Anemia, beriberi, hypercarbia</li><li>Cirrhosis liver (hypoproteinemia) thyrotoxicosis,</li><li>Arteriovenous (AV) fistula</li><li>Paget's disease of the bone</li></ul>

Contd...

Contd...
- **Cardiac causes (pulsus magnus):**
  - Aortic regurgitation
  - Severe mitral regurgitation
  - Complete heart block
  - Patent ductus arteriosus (PDA)
  - Rupture of sinus of valsalva and aortopulmonary window

Varying volume: Seen in atrial fibrillation
Anisosphygmia: Varying volume of pulses in bilateral brachial/radial vessels. Seen in Takayasu's arteritis
Coanda effect: In supravalvular aortic stenosis, pulse volume is better in the right upper limb compared to left due to the selective jet of the blood directed to the right subclavian vessel.
Note: Pulsus alternans, pulsus bigeminus, and pulsus paradoxus are also abnormalities in volume (described under the section of character of pulse).

Grading of Pulse

The examination of the arterial pulses is tabulated using a scale as follows:

Grade	Description
0	Complete absence of pulsation
1	Small or feeble/reduced pulsation
2	Palpable but diminished as compared to other side
3	Normal pulsation
4	Large or high volume/bounding pulsation

Character of Pulse

Best assessed in the carotids.

Exceptions:
- Collapsing pulse which is appreciated better at radial artery
- Pulsus bisferiens best appreciated in brachial artery.

Trisection Method

Varying degrees of pressure are applied with the finger pads of the thumb or first two fingers to assess upstroke, systolic peak and diastolic slope of the **pulse**.

Components of pulse wave **(Figs. 2B.3A and B):**

Individual components of pulse waveform	
Wave	Description
Percussion wave	It is due to arrival of the impulse generated by LV ejection
Tidal wave	It is due to the reflected waves from the upper part of the body
Dicrotic wave	It is due to the reflected waves from the lower part of the body
Dicrotic notch or incisura	This corresponds to S_2 (closure of aortic and pulmonary valves)

Normal contour of pulse (normal arterial pulse): The normal carotid pulse has a smooth, rapid upstroke or ascending limb to a smooth, dome-shaped summit. Then a downstroke occurs that is somewhat less rapid than the

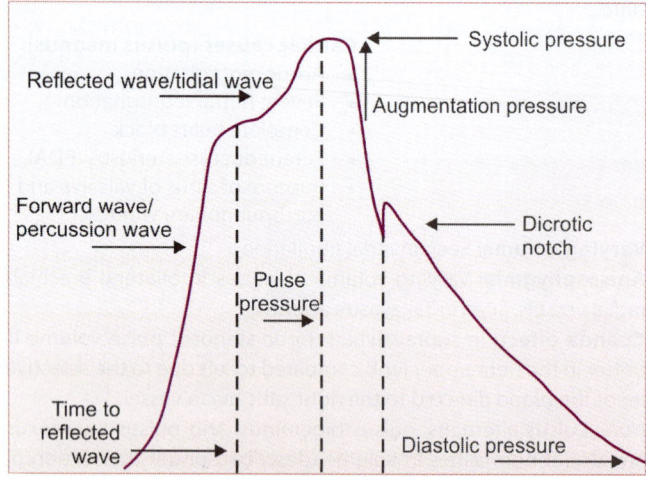

Fig. 2B.3A: Arterial pulse tracing.

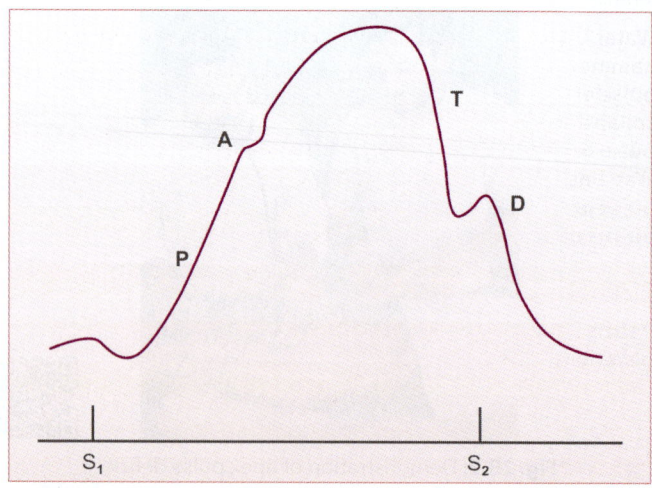

Fig. 2B.3B: Waveform showing different components of pulse wave.

upstroke. The dicrotic notch and secondary diastolic wave are usually not felt but can be palpable in some normal individuals, particularly during fever, exercise, or excitement. The dicrotic notch usually occurs approximately 300 milliseconds after the onset of the pulse wave when corrected for heart rate.

Graphic recordings of the arterial pulses frequently show two positive deflections during systole, the first shoulder being referred to as the percussion wave and the second as the tidal wave. In the normal proximal aortic pulse, the percussion wave is caused by arrival of the impulse generated by LV ejection, the tidal wave can represent its echo from the upper part of the body, and the dicrotic or diastolic wave is a reflection from the lower part of the body **(Fig. 2B.3A)**.

Speed of Pulse Wave and Time Taken to Reach the Peripheral Arteries

Speed of pulse wave	5 m/sec
Speed of blood flow	0.5 m/sec

Contd...

Time taken for transmission of pulse to	
Carotid	30 ms
Brachial	60 ms
Femoral	75 ms
Radial	80 ms

Normally radial pulse is felt 5–10 m/sec later than femoral pulse.

Characters of pulse (Fig. 2B.4)		
Character	Description	Condition seen
Catacrotic pulse	It is the normal character of the pulse	
Pulsus parvus et tardus	A low amplitude pulse (parvus) with a slow rising and late peak (tardus)	Severe aortic stenosis (AS)
Pulsus anacroticus	Single peak low volume	Severe aortic stenosis
Spike and Dome pulse	Seen in HOCM	

Contd...

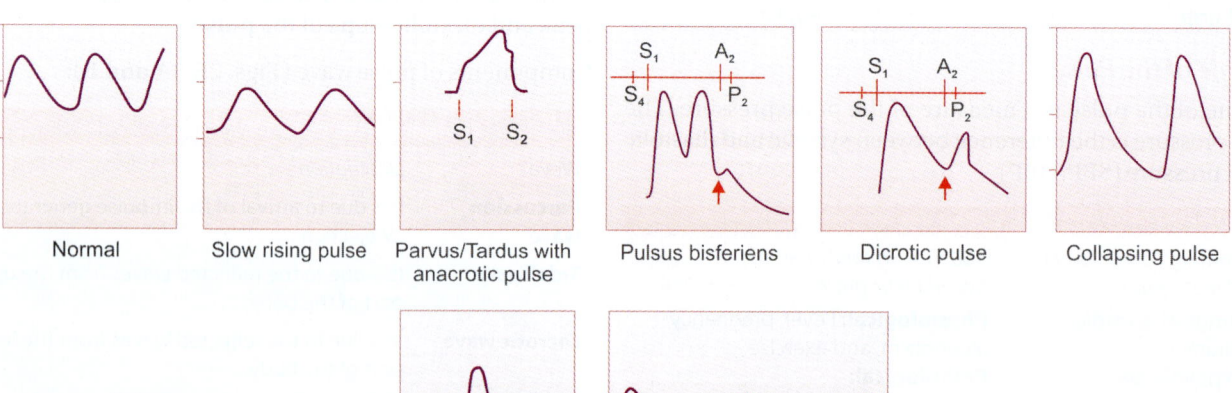

Fig. 2B.4: Image showing different pulse waveforms.

General Examination

Contd...		
Water hammer pulse or collapsing pulse or Watsons pulse or pulsus celer	▪ High (large) volume pulse ▪ Sharp rise (systolic pressure is high) ▪ Ill-sustained, sharp fall (diastolic pressure is low) ▪ Pulse pressure is at least 60 mm Hg	Aortic regurgitation, patent ductus arteriosus (PDA), aortopulmonary window, rupture of sinus of Valsalva, arteriovenous fistula, severe mitral regurgitation
Twin beating pulse		
Pulsus bisferiens	Two peaks in systole	▪ Severe aortic regurgitation (AR) ▪ Moderate AR + AS ▪ Hypertrophic obstructive cardiomyopathy (HOCM)
Pulsus dicroticus	One peak in systole, another peak in diastole. Seen when pulse rate and diastolic pressure is low	▪ Typhoid fever ▪ Severe left ventricular failure (LVF) ▪ Pulse is intra-aortic balloon counter pulsation ▪ Dehydration ▪ Dilated cardiomyopathy endotoxic shock
Alternating volume pulses		
Pulsus alternans	▪ Alternating high volume and low volume pulse ▪ Regular rhythm ▪ Korotkoff sounds double on lowering cuff pressures	Left ventricular failure
Pulsus bigeminus	Pulse wave with normal beat followed by a premature beat and a compensatory pause, occurring in rapid succession, resulting in alteration of the strength of pulse	Digoxin toxicity
Pulsus paradoxus		
Pulsus paradoxus	Systolic blood pressure falls more than 10 mm Hg during inspiration (exaggeration of normal phenomenon)	**Physiological:** ▪ Obesity ▪ Pregnancy **Respiratory system:** ▪ Bronchial asthma ▪ Emphysema ▪ Chronic obstructive pulmonary disease (COPD) ▪ Large bilateral pleural effusion **Cardiovascular system:** ▪ Cardiac tamponade ▪ Constrictive pericarditis (one-third)

Contd...

	▪ Hypovolemic shock ▪ Pulmonary embolism ▪ RV Infarct ▪ Cardiomyopathy ▪ SVC obstruction ▪ Post-thoracotomy

Reverse pulsus paradoxus (inspiratory rise in pulse volume and pressure): Seen in intermittent positive-pressure ventilation in the presence of left ventricular failure, hypertrophic obstructive cardiomyopathy (HOCM) and isorhythmic AV dissociation—atrial activity precedes QRS during inspiration and marches into QRS during expiration. The atrial activity during inspiration increases the stroke volume and its lack during expiration decreases the stroke volume and systolic pressure.

Absent pulsus paradoxus in constrictive pericarditis: If associated with large atrial septal defect/ventricular septal defect/aortic regurgitation/(ASD/VSD/AR)/pericardial adhesions

Method of Eliciting Pulsus Paradoxus (Fig. 2B.5)

Paradox about the pulse is absence of pulse during inspiration but presence of heart sounds and was coined by Adolph Kussmaul in 1873.

Suspected if the pulse varies with inspiration in all accessible arteries.

- **Misnomer**—the term paradoxus is that normally there is a fall in BP during inspiration (4–6 mm Hg) which in PP is exaggerated (>10 mm Hg).
- Patient is placed in a semi recumbent position; respirations should be normal. *Do not instruct them to change their breathing pattern as the depth of respiration influences the magnitude of pulsus paradoxus and will be amplified in patients with pulmonary disease.*
- The blood pressure cuff is inflated to at least 20 mm Hg above the systolic pressure and slowly deflated until the first Korotkoff sounds are heard.
- Initially sounds will be heard only during expiration. Note the level.
- As the cuff is further deflated, the first Korotkoff sound will be heard during both inspiration and expiration. Note this level.
- If difference between the two is more than 10 mm Hg, then it is pulsus paradoxus.
- This is not a true paradox as it is an exaggeration of normal phenomenon of fall of BP during inspiration.

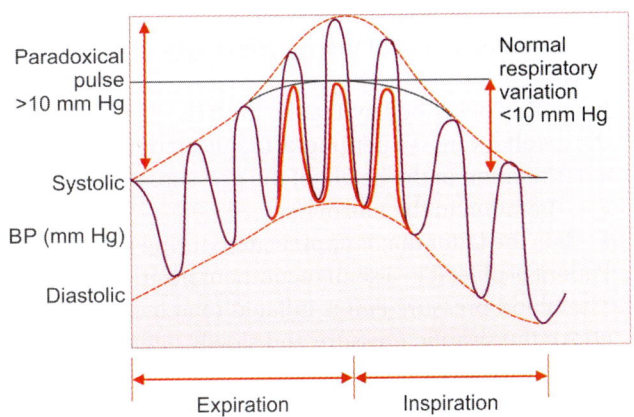

Fig. 2B.5: Pulsus paradoxus.

Then, What is the Paradox?

The paradox is that, in patients with constrictive pericarditis, during inspiration the blood pressure might drop significantly enough that the peripheral pulses will be absent; however, the heart sounds will still be heard.

Mechanism of Pulsus Paradoxus
- LV filling is reduced during inspiration because exaggerated RV filling causes
  - Leftward shift of IVS reducing LV volume and diastolic compliance
  - Elevated intrapericardial pressure which is transmitted to the LA but not the extraparenchymal pulmonary veins and hence a decreased pulmonary vein—LA pressure gradient
- Inspiratory pooling of blood in the pulmonary bed produces decline in LA and LV filling.

[Under filled LV may be operating in the steep ascending limb of starling curve so that any inspiratory reduction of LV filling results in marked depression of the LV stroke volume and the systolic pressure].

> **Other Paradoxes in Medicine**
> - **French paradox:** The observation that the French suffer a relatively low incidence of coronary heart disease, despite having a diet relatively rich in saturated fats.
> - **"Thrombotic paradox" of hypertension (or) "Birmingham paradox":** Hypertension is a prothrombotic state, hence paradoxically thrombotic strokes are more common than hemorrhagic.
> - **Venous paradox**—Kussmaul sign is a paradoxical rise in jugular venous pressure (JVP) on inspiration, or a failure in the appropriate fall of the JVP with inspiration.
> - **Ulnar paradox:** Higher the lesion minimal is the deficit.
> - **Paradoxical respiration:** It causes the chest to contract while inhaling and to expand during exhaling, the opposite of how it should move. The causes of paradoxical breathing include chest trauma and diaphragmatic paralysis. Neurological problems that can paralyze the diaphragm.
> - **Kinesia paradoxa:** Seen in parkinsonism, patients who generally cannot move but under certain circumstances exhibit a sudden, brief period of mobility (walking or even running).

Method of Elicitation of Pulsus Alternans (Fig. 2B.6)
- Beats occur at regular intervals but in which there is a regular attenuation of the systolic height of the pressure pulse.
- It was first described by Traube in 1872.
- Pulsus alternans is a peripheral manifestation of LV failure
  - Alteration in the height of the pressure pulse
  - Alteration in the rate of rise
  - It is the latter that is appreciated during palpation.
- Patient is placed in a semi recumbent position.
- The blood pressure cuff is inflated to at least 20 mm Hg above the systolic pressure and slowly deflated until the first Korotkoff sounds are heard.
- Initially, the Korotkoff's sounds due to the high-volume pulses will be heard.

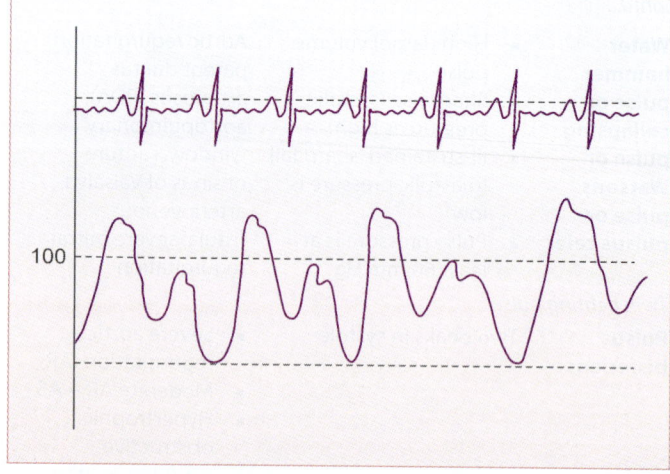

Fig. 2B.6: Pulsus alternans.

- On lowering the blood pressure, Korotkoff sounds will be heard due to both high volume and low volume pulses.
- This will produce doubling of Korotkoff's sounds.
- Can be brought out or exaggerated by decreasing venous return by
  - Sitting
  - Standing
  - Head up tilting
- It is usually associated with S_3.

Mechanism
- It is due to alteration of the contractile state of at least part of the myocardium, caused by failure of electromechanical coupling in some cells during weaker contraction.
- Alternate more and a smaller number of contractile elements participate in each contraction.
- Correlates with alteration in intensity of Korotkoff sounds.

Causes
- LV failure of any cause
- Myocarditis, dilated cardiomyopathy (DCM)
- Acute pulmonary embolism
- Severe AS with failure
- Severe PS with failure
- Severe aortic regurgitation with failure, especially after aortic valve replacement.
- Briefly during or after supra ventricular tachycardia
- Severe systemic hypertension
- Transient right ventricular outflow occlusion during balloon dilatation of pulmonary stenosis.

Types of Pulsus Alternans
- **Total:** When the weak beat is not perceived at all or when involving both sides of the heart.
- **Partial:** When involving only RV (as in PE) or LV (as in AS).
- **Concordant alternans:** Simultaneous alternans of right and left ventricles.
- **Discordant alternans:** Alternating alternans of right and left ventricles.

Differentiating Pulsus Alternans from Bigeminy
- Pulsus alternans is associated with LV S_3
- In PA the interval between the weak and strong beats are equal

General Examination

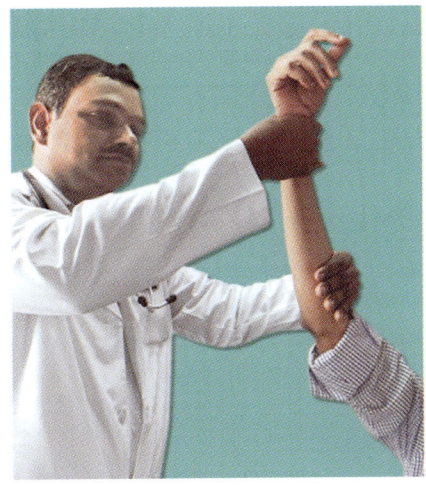

Fig. 2B.7: Demonstration of collapsing pulse.

Causes of Collapsing Pulse

With aortic run off: Aortic regurgitation, patent ductus arteriosus, aortopulmonary window, rupture sinus of Valsalva into right side and AV fistula.

Cyanotic congenital heart disease:
- Truncus arteriosus with truncal run off into PA or truncal insufficiency
- Pulmonary atresia with AP collaterals
- TOF with AP collaterals/associated PDA/associated AR/after BT shunt

Hyperkinetic states
Pregnancy, anemia, thyrotoxicosis, beriberi, fever, Paget's disease of bone

Normal volume collapsing pulse
- Mitral regurgitation
- Ventricular septal defect

- In pulsus bigeminy the weaker beats arise prematurely, and the stronger beats occur after a pause resulting in ventricular cycles that are alternatively short and long.

Method of Eliciting Collapsing Pulse (Fig. 2B.7)

- Thomas Watson (1844) coined the term after Victorian toy
- Palpate the radial artery and trace the artery proximally to a point where it is just felt
- At this point, wrap your wrist around the patient's forearm, so as to place the heads of the metacarpals over the artery.
- Simultaneously, palpate the radial and ulnar arteries by encircling the patient's wrist with your other hand.
- Now, abruptly raise the patient's hand above the shoulder (artery becomes in line with the central aorta, allowing direct systolic ejection and diastolic backflow).
- In collapsing pulse, both radial and ulnar arteries are felt distinctly and, there is an abrupt thrust/knock and collapse under the metacarpal heads on elevation.
- Thrust produced is similar to the one produced by tilting of water hammer toy.
- It is due to diastolic run-off in aortic regurgitation.

> **Collapsing pulse** is characterized by rapid upstroke (percussion wave) followed by rapid descent (collapse) of the pulse wave without dicrotic notch, which reflects low systemic vascular resistance.
> - Rapid upstroke is due to the rapid ejection of greatly increased stroke volume.
> - The rapid descent or collapsing character is due to:
>   - Diastolic "run-off" (backflow) into the left ventricle
>   - Reflex vasodilation mediated by carotid baroreceptors secondary to large stroke volume
>   - The rapid run-off to the periphery due to decreased systemic vascular resistance.
>
> **Corrigan's pulse/sign** is largely used to describe the abrupt distension and quick collapse of carotid pulse in aortic regurgitation, whereas the term **Watson's water hammer pulse** is used for the characteristic pulse seen in peripheral arteries like the radial artery.

Note: Make sure the patient does not have shoulder pain before doing this.

Method of Eliciting Pulsus Bisferiens

- The bisferiens (from the Latin twice beating) pulse has a waveform characterized by two positive waves during systole.
- Normally percussion wave is felt but not the tidal wave. In all the conditions where percussion wave is prominent, tidal wave also becomes prominent.
- The pulse wave upstroke rises rapidly and forcefully, producing the first systolic peak (percussion wave). A brief decline in pressure is followed by a smaller and somewhat slower-rising positive pulse wave (tidal wave). Abnormalities of LV ejection and reflected waves from peripheral arteries contribute to the prominence of the second systolic wave in the bisferiens pulse. The bisferiens pulse is sometimes more easily palpable in a brachial or radial artery. The bisferiens pulse can be elicited by maneuvers that decrease the LV size or increase its contractility.
- Felt by applying **graded pressure**
- With fingers press and occlude the brachial artery
- On slowly releasing the pressure, the double peaking of the pulse is appreciated.

Mechanism

- In combined AS and AR, the stenotic component permits a jet, and lateral to the jet there is a fall in pressure (Bernoulli phenomenon), this results in a dip or inward movement in the pulse with secondary outward movement in a pulse or tidal wave **(Fig. 2B.8A)**.
- In HOCM, the initial part of left ventricular ejection is rapid, resulting in rapid upstroke. As obstruction to the outflow starts later in the systole, due to SAM, a sudden interruption to left ventricular ejection occurs resulting in a dip in the pressure pulse followed by the slow rising pulse wave, which is characteristic of HOCM (spike and dome pattern). The percussion wave is more prominent than tidal wave in HOCM **(Fig. 2B.8B)**.

Condition of Vessel Wall

Vessel wall thickening is assessed by using Osler's sign (described under the pseudohypertension in chapter blood pressure).

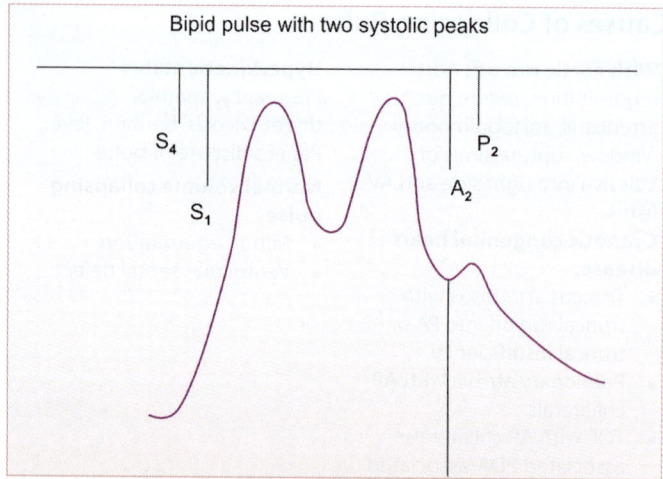

Fig. 2B.8A: Pulsus bisferiens in severe AR.

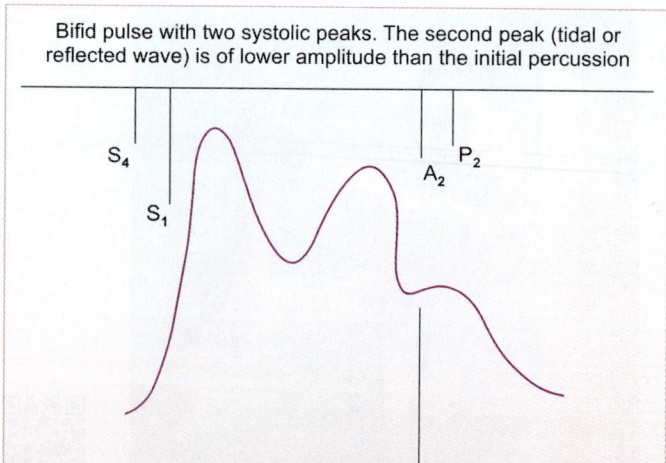

Fig. 2B.8B: Pulsus bisferiens in HOCM.

Absent Pulses

- Absence of a pulse could suggest occlusion by thrombus, embolus, or dissection.
- Unilateral absence of a pulse can aid in the diagnosis of a dissected aortic aneurysm.
- History and physical examination findings can help assess the level of arterial obstruction in lower extremity claudication.
- Auscultation for aortic and femoral artery bruits should be routinely done. Carotid and vertebral bruit are important in cases of stroke.
- A cervical bruit is a poor indicator of the degree of carotid artery narrowing, and the absence of a bruit does not exclude significant luminal compromise. Extension of a bruit into diastole or a thrill generally indicates severe stenosis.
- Abnormal pulse oximetry, defined by a more than 2% difference between finger and toe oxygen saturation, can also indicate lower extremity peripheral arterial disease (PAD) and is comparable to the ankle brachial index (ABI) (likelihood ratio [LR]: 30; 95% confidence interval [CI]: 7.6–121.0 vs. LR: 24.8; 95% CI: 6.2–99.8).

Branham sign/Nicoladoni-Israel-Branham sign
Compression of the arterial supply to an arteriovenous fistula causes a decrease in pulse and increase in blood pressure if there is a significant circulation through the fistula. This test can be used to clinically test the patency of AV fistula.

Peripheral Pulses

Refer **Figure 2B.9**.

Palpation of Carotid Pulse (Figs. 2B.10A and B)

- Ask the patient to relax the neck.
- Palpate the right carotid artery by placing your left thumb near the upper neck between the sternomastoid and trachea roughly at the level of cricoid cartilage.
- Note the character of the pulse.
- Now, repeat the procedure on other side by placing your right thumb over the patients left carotid.
  Note: Make sure not to compress the carotid sinus.

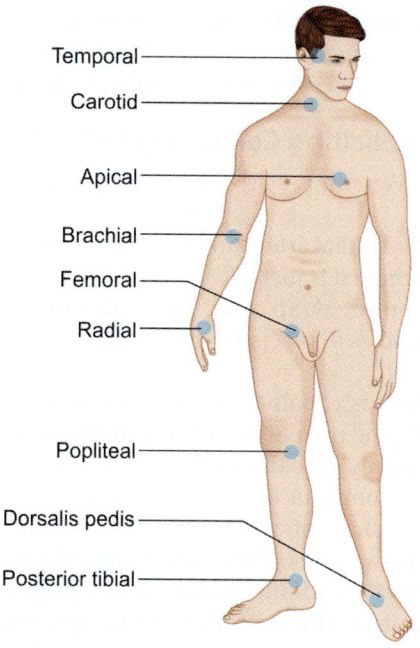

Fig. 2B.9: Image showing site of different peripheral pulses.

- It is advisable to auscultate for carotid bruit prior to palpation, to prevent possible dislodgement of the atherosclerotic plaque (if present).

Palpation of Brachial Pulse (Fig. 2B.11)

- To examine the *brachial artery* in the right arm, the examiner supports the patient's forearm in his left hand.
- Patient's upper arm abducted, the elbow slightly flexed, and the forearm externally rotated.
- The examiner's right hand is then curled over the anterior aspect of the elbow to palpate along the course of the artery just medial to the biceps tendon and lateral to the medial epicondyle of the humerus.
- The position of the hands should be switched when examining the opposite limb.

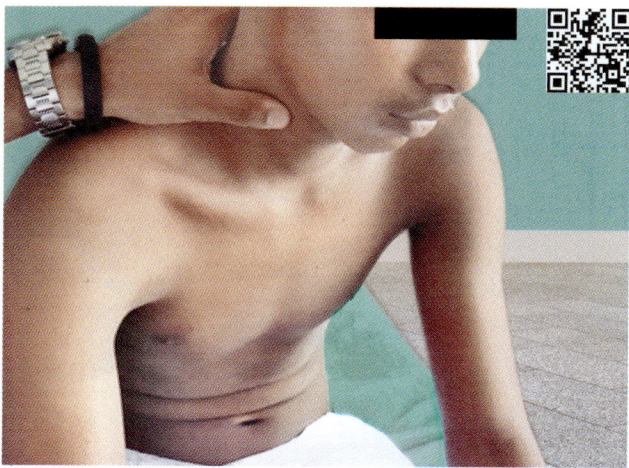

Fig. 2B.10A: Demonstration of palpation of right carotid pulse.

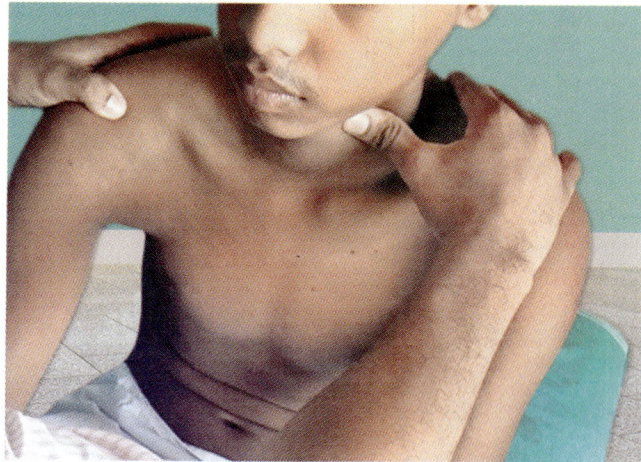

Fig. 2B.10B: Demonstration of palpation of left carotid pulse.

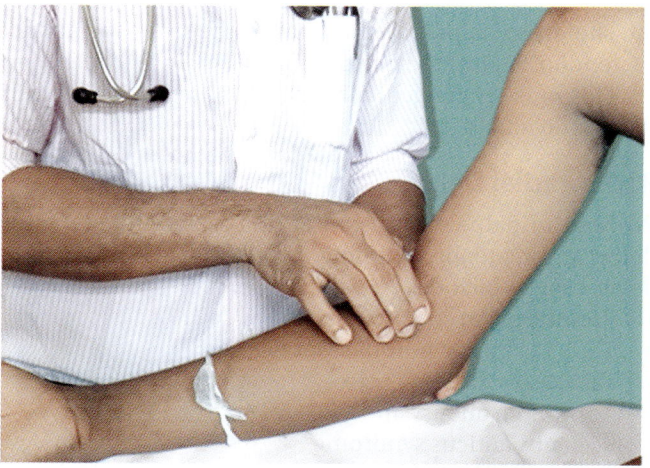

Fig. 2B.11: Demonstration of palpation of brachial pulse.

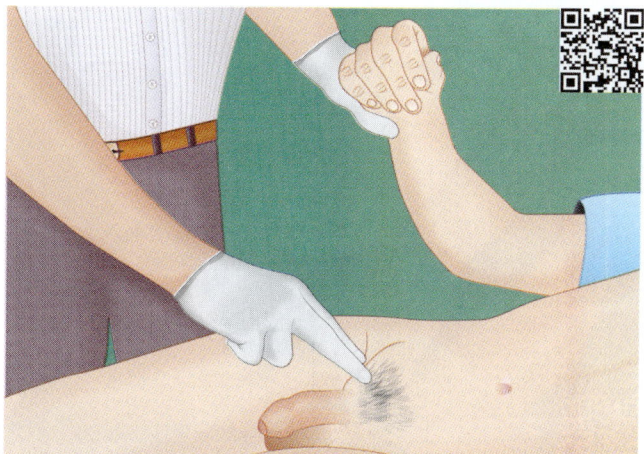

Fig. 2B.12: Site of examination of femoral pulse.

Palpation of Abdominal Aorta

- The *abdominal aorta* is best palpated by applying firm pressure with the flattened fingers of both hands to indent the epigastrium toward the vertebral column.
- For this examination, it is essential that the subject's abdominal muscles be completely relaxed; such relaxation can be encouraged by having the subject flex the hips and by providing a pillow to support the head.
- In extremely obese individuals or in those with massive abdominal musculature, it may be impossible to detect aortic pulsation.

Palpation of Common Femoral Artery (Fig. 2B.12)

- The *common femoral artery* emerges into the upper thigh from beneath the inguinal ligament one-third of the distance from the pubis to the anterior superior iliac spine.
- It is best palpated with the examiner standing on the ipsilateral side of the patient and the fingertips of the examining hand pressed firmly into the groin.

Palpation of Popliteal Artery (Fig. 2B.13)

- The *popliteal artery* passes vertically through the deep portion of the popliteal space just lateral to the mid plane.
- Generally, this pulse is felt most conveniently with the patient in the supine position and the examiner's hands encircling and supporting the knee from each side.
- The pulse is detected by pressing deeply into the popliteal space with the supporting fingertips.
- Since complete relaxation of the muscles is essential to this examination, the patient should be instructed to let the leg "go limp" and to allow the examiner to provide all the support needed.

Palpation of Posterior Tibial Artery (Fig. 2B.14)

- The *posterior tibial artery* lies just posterior to the medial malleolus.
- It can be felt most readily by curling the fingers of the examining hand anteriorly around the ankle, indenting the soft tissues in the space between the medial malleolus and the Achilles tendon, above the calcaneus.
- The thumb is applied to the opposite side of the ankle in a grasping fashion to provide stability.

Palpation of Dorsalis Pedis Artery (Fig. 2B.15)

- The *dorsalis pedis artery* is examined with the patient in the recumbent position and the ankle relaxed.

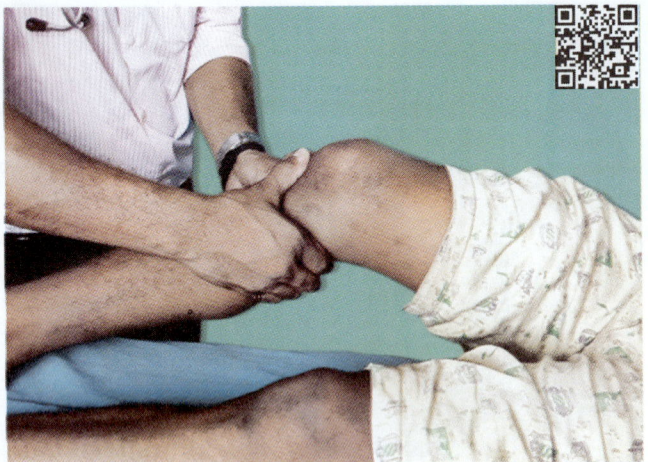

Fig. 2B.13: Demonstration of palpation of popliteal artery.

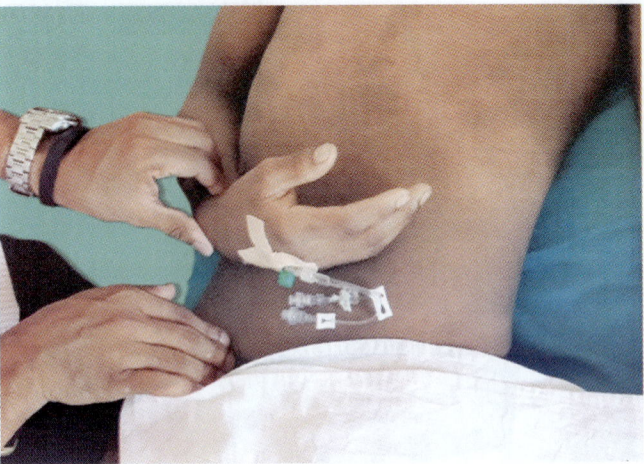

Fig. 2B.16: Demonstration of radio-femoral delay.

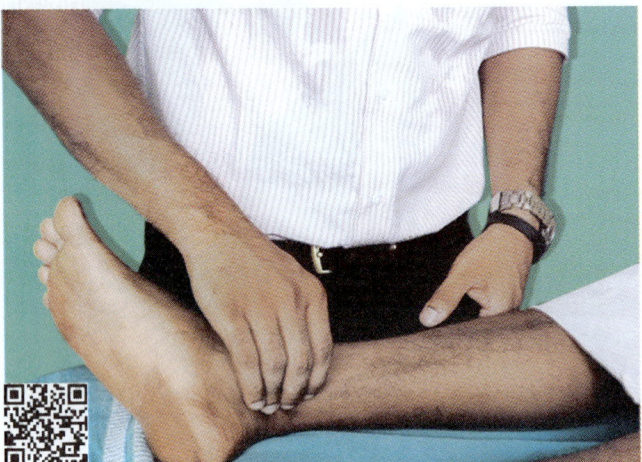

Fig. 2B.14: Demonstration of palpation of posterior tibial pulse.

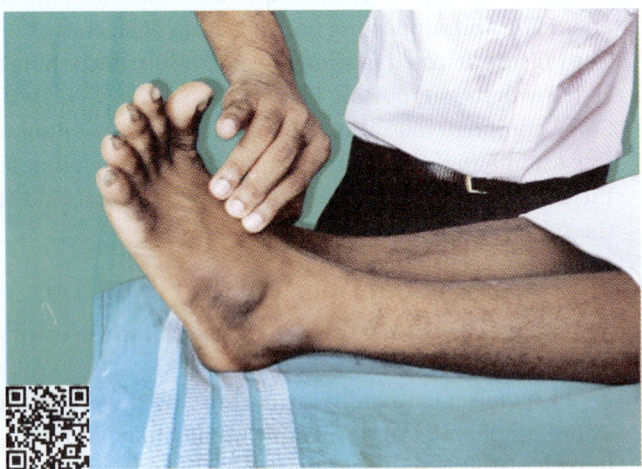

Fig. 2B.15: Demonstration of palpation of dorsalis pedis artery.

- The examiner stands at the foot of the examining table and places the fingertips across the dorsum of the forefoot near the ankle.
- The artery is palpated lateral to the extensor hallucis tendon, against the navicular bone.
- This pulse is congenitally absent in approximately 10% of individuals.

Radio-radial Delay

Proceed to palpate both radial pulses simultaneously to detect any inequality in timing. This is known as radio-radial delay. Causes include:
- Presubclavian coarctation
- Thoracic inlet syndrome: Cervical rib
- Takayasu's disease
- Aortic arch aneurysm
- Scalenus anticus syndrome
- Anomalous right subclavian artery
- Aberrant course of radial artery.

Radio-femoral Delay (Fig. 2B.16)

Normally the time taken for the pulse wave to reach the radial artery after the cardiac systole is 80 milliseconds and for the femoral artery it is 75 milliseconds. If the femoral pulse is delayed compared to radial pulse it is called radio-femoral delay.

This is a sign of coarctation of aorta. It is not the delayed arrival of the femoral pulse wave but instead a slow rate of rise to a delayed peak.

This can rarely be seen with occlusive disease of the bifurcation of the aorta, common iliac or external iliac arteries like aortoarteritis.

Right radio-femoral delay can be seen in supravalvular aortic stenosis.

RESPIRATION

Respiratory Rate

Counted by placing the examiner's palm over the patient's abdomen, noting the rise and fall of the abdomen. Simultaneously divert the patient's attention by measuring the patient's pulse with your other hand (**Fig. 2B.17**).

General Examination

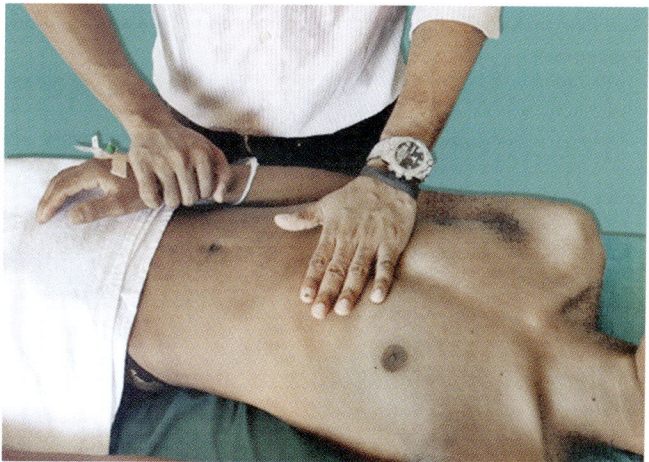

Fig. 2B.17: Method of calculating respiratory rate.

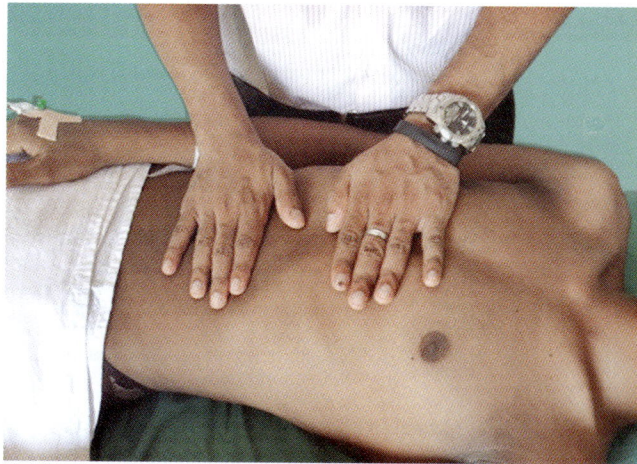

Fig. 2B.18: Method of assessing type of respiration.

Normal pulse rate: respiratory rate = 4:1

Normal (16–20)	
Tachypnea >20	*Bradypnea <10*
Physiological: - Anxiety - Exertion **Pathological:** - Emphysema - Pneumothorax - Acute respiratory distress from infections - Pleurisy - Pulmonary embolism - Metabolic acidosis - Cardiac insufficiency - Anemia - Hyperthyroidism - Weakness of respiratory muscles - Obesity - Restrictive chest wall disease	- CNS-depressant drugs (e.g., opiates, benzodiazepines, barbiturates, alcohol) - Uremia - Increased intracranial pressure - Hypothermia - Hypothyroidism

Muscles of Respiration

Inspiration	*Expiration*
Main: - External intercostal muscle - Diaphragm	Predominantly passive process
Accessory muscles: - Serratus anterior - Sternocleidomastoid (SCM) - Scalenus anterior - Pectoralis - Trapezius	**Accessory muscles (used in forceful expiration):** - Internal intercostals - Abdominal muscles - Quadratus lumborum - Latissimus dorsi

Type of Respiration

Keep two hands flat, one on the chest and other on the abdomen and watch for movements of hand **(Fig. 2B.18)**.
- **In abdominothoracic**—movements of hand over the abdomen are more prominent.
- **In thoracoabdominal**—movements of hand over the thorax are more prominent.

Contd...

Contd...

Abdominothoracic	*Thoracoabdominal*
Due to well-developed abdominal muscles	Well-formed internal intercostal muscles
Seen in males	Seen in females

Variants

Purely thoracic	*Purely abdominal*
Abdominal movement during respirations is absent - Peritonitis - Pregnancy - Ascites/ovarian cyst	**Thoracic movement during respiration is absent** - Pleuritic chest pain - Defective chest wall - Respiratory muscle paralysis [neurogenic, neuromuscular junction (NMJ), and muscular]

Abnormal Patterns of Breathing (Fig. 2B.19)

Regular	*Irregular*
Cheyne–Stokes (periods of apnea alternating with hyperpnea) - Cardiac failure (LVF)—most common cause - Raised intracranial pressure (ICP) - Brainstem lesions	**Biot breathing** (an uncommon variant of Cheyne-Stokes respiration. Periods of apnea alternate irregularly with a series of breaths of equal depth that terminates abruptly) - Meningitis
Kussmaul's (rapid deep breathing) - Metabolic acidosis [diabetic ketoacidosis (DKA) and renal failure]	**Ataxic** - Brainstem disorders **Apneustic** - Pontine lesions

Pursed Lip Breathing

- Seen with chronic obstructive pulmonary disease (COPD)
- Mechanism of auto-positive end-expiratory pressure (PEEP)
- The purpose of this breathing is to slow down the air flow during the exhalation to build up back pressure in the airway to avoid a sudden drop in intrapulmonary pressure resulting in alveolar and airway collapse.

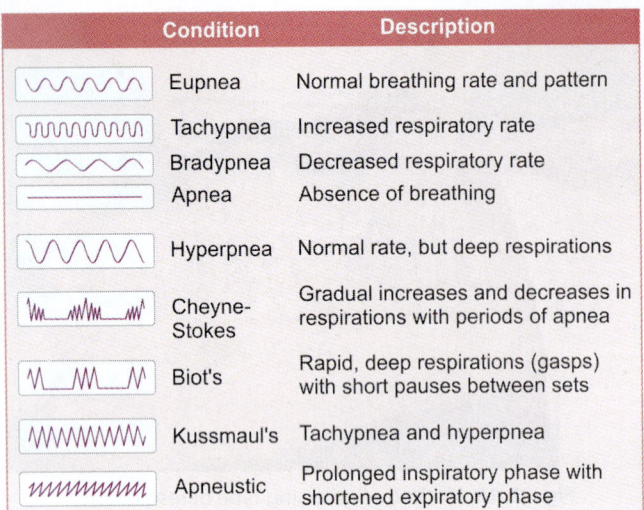

Fig. 2B.19: Different type of breathing patterns.

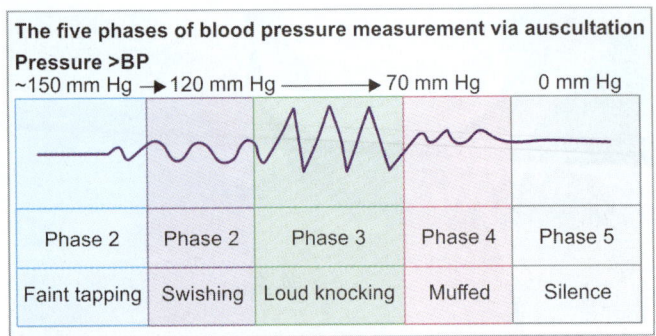

Types and Character of Korotkoff Sounds

AHA 2017 classification		
Blood pressure (BP) category	Systolic BP	Diastolic BP
Normal	<120 mm Hg And	<80 mm Hg
Elevated	120–129 mm Hg And	<80 mm Hg
Stage 1 hypertension	130–139 mm Hg Or	80–89 mm Hg
Stage 2 hypertension	≥140 mm Hg Or	≥90 mm Hg

Note: ESC guidelines 2018 and comparison table of JNC 7 and AHA 2017 are discussed in Annexures.

Airway Obstruction

- Upper airway obstruction—prolonged inspiration
- Lower airway obstruction—prolonged expiration.

BLOOD PRESSURE

Definition

Arterial blood pressure (BP) can be defined as the lateral pressure exerted by the moving column of blood on the walls of the arteries.

BP = Cardiac output × Peripheral resistance

Systolic blood pressure (SBP)	Diastolic blood pressure (DBP)
▪ Defined as the maximum BP in the arteries attainable during systole ▪ Normal: 120 + 20 mm Hg	▪ Defined as the minimum pressure that is obtained at the end of the ventricular diastole ▪ Normal range: 60–90 mm Hg
Pulse pressure (PP)	**Mean arterial pressure (MAP)**
▪ Denotes the difference between systolic and diastolic pressure ▪ PP = SBP – DBP = 40 mm Hg	▪ DBP + one-third pulse pressure ▪ Normal = 95 mm Hg

Korotkoff Sounds

KOROTKOFF SOUNDS	Systolic blood pressure (SBP)	120 mm Hg	Phase 1: A thud
		110 mm Hg	Phase 2: A blowing noise
		100 mm Hg	Phase 3: A softer thud
		90 mm Hg	Phase 4: A disappearing blowing noise (muffling)
	Diastolic blood pressure (DBP)	80 mm Hg	Phase 5: No Korotkoff sounds

Steps of examination blood pressure	
Key steps	Specific instructions
Step 1: Properly prepare the patient	▪ The patient should rest comfortably for 5 minutes prior to the measurement in the seated position with their back supported. The patient's legs should be uncrossed with feet flat on the floor **(Fig. 2B.20)** ▪ The patient should avoid caffeine, exercise, and smoking for at least 30 minutes before measurement ▪ Ensure that the patient has emptied his/her bladder ▪ Neither the patient nor the observer should talk before or during the measurement ▪ Measurements made while the patient is sitting or lying on an examining table do not fulfill these criteria
Step 2: Use proper technique for BP measurements	▪ Use a BP measurement device that has been validated, and ensure that the device is calibrated periodically ▪ The arm should be bare, supported and kept at heart level ▪ Position the middle of the cuff on the patient's upper arm at the level of the right atrium (the midpoint of the sternum) **(Fig. 2B.21)** ▪ Use a cuff with an appropriate bladder size: Bladder width should be close to 40% of the arm circumference and length should cover 80–100% of the arm circumference. The lower edge of the cuff should sit 3 cm above the elbow crease with the bladder centered over the brachial artery ▪ Either the stethoscope diaphragm or bell may be used for auscultatory readings

Contd...

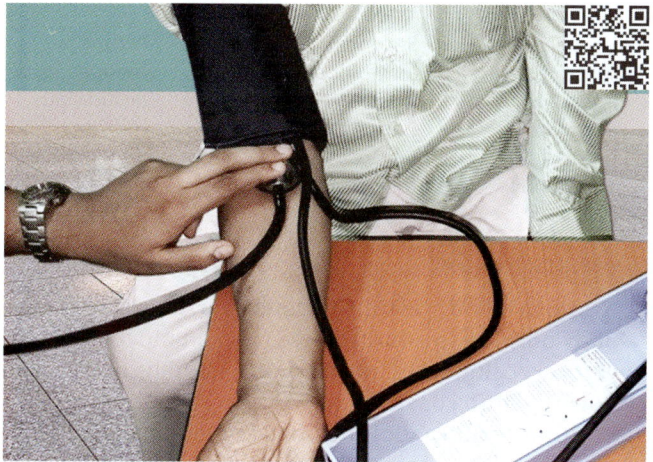

Fig. 2B.20: Demonstration of BP measurement.

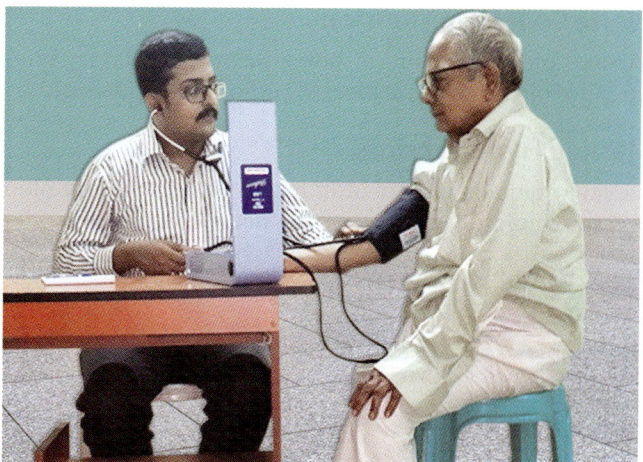

Fig. 2B.21: Demonstration of placement of BP cuff.

Contd...

Step 3: Take the proper measurements needed for diagnosis and treatment of elevated BP/hypertension	▪ At the first visit, record BP in both arms. Use the arm that gives the higher reading for subsequent readings ▪ Repeat blood pressure measurements should be taken 1–2 minutes apart ▪ Increase the pressure to 30 mm Hg above the level at which the radial pulse is extinguished ▪ Place the bell or diaphragm of the stethoscope over the brachial artery ▪ Open the control valve so that the rate of deflation of the cuff is 2 mm Hg per heartbeat ▪ Systolic blood pressure is the appearance of the first Korotkoff sound ▪ The diastolic blood pressure is the point at which the sound disappears (phase 5 Korotkoff) ▪ If Korotkoff sounds continue as the level approaches 0 mm Hg, listen for when the sound becomes muffled to indicate the diastolic blood pressure
Step 4: Properly document accurate BP readings	▪ Record BP to the closest 2 mm Hg on the sphygmomanometer, as well as the arm used and the position of the patient (supine, sitting or standing) ▪ Note the time of most recent BP medication taken before measurements
Step 5: Average the readings	▪ Use an average of ≥2 readings obtained on ≥2 occasions to estimate the individual's level of BP ▪ In presence of atrial fibrillation, minimum of 3 BP readings have to be estimated
Step 6: Provide BP readings to patient	▪ Provide patients the SBP/DBP readings both verbally and in writing

Selection Criteria for BP Cuff Size for Measurement of BP in Adults

Arm circumference	Usual cuff size
Usual cuff size	Small adult
27–34 cm	Adult
35–44 cm	Large adult
45–52 cm	Adult thigh

Auscultatory Gap (Fig. 2B.22)

An auscultatory gap also called as silent gap is the interval of pressure where Korotkoff sounds indicating true systolic pressure fade away and reappear at a lower pressure point during the manual measurement of blood pressure by auscultatory method. The auscultatory gap occurs when the first Korotkoff sound fades out for about 20–50 mm Hg only to return. It can result in following erroneous blood pressure reading:
1. Underestimation of systolic blood pressure
2. Overestimation of diastolic blood pressure

An auscultatory gap is common in elderly hypertensive patients. It occurs in some hypertensive patients only. Auscultatory gaps are related to carotid atherosclerosis and to increased arterial stiffness in hypertensive patients, independent of age.

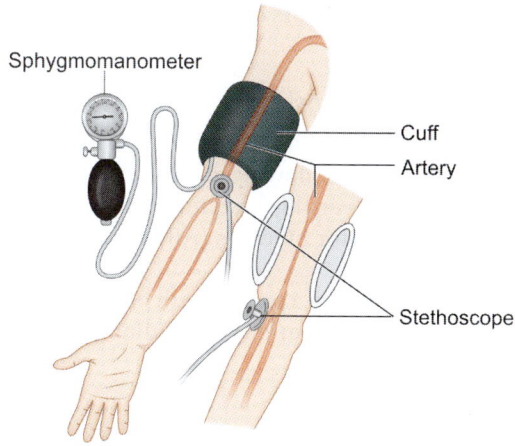

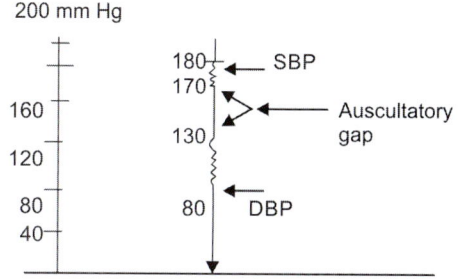

Fig. 2B.22: Auscultatory gap.

White Coat Hypertension

Normal blood pressure at home or on ambulatory blood pressure monitoring but elevated office blood pressure.

Masked Hypertension

Elevated blood pressure at home or on ambulatory blood pressure monitoring but normal office blood pressure.

Paroxysmal Hypertension

Episodic elevated BP.

- Pheochromocytoma
- Panic disorders
- Labile hypertension
- Carcinoid
- Clonidine withdrawal
- Renovascular hypertension
- Hypoglycemia
- Cheese reaction
- Anxiety
- Hyperthyroidism
- Coronary insufficiency
- Cluster or migraine headaches
- Seizure disorder
- CNS lesions (such as stroke, tumor, hemorrhage)
- Drugs—cocaine, lysergic acid diethylamide, amphetamine
- Baroreflex failure
- Factitious hypertension

Pseudo Hypertension

Defined as cuff diastolic blood pressure ≥15 mm Hg higher than simultaneously measured intra-arterial blood pressure. A palpable although pulseless, radial artery while the BP cuff is inflated above systolic pressure, is a positive **Osler sign**. Osler sign occurs due to Monckeberg's sclerosis of arteries.

Paradoxical Hypertension

On starting treatment with antihypertensives, the BP rises instead of falling in the following conditions.
1. Angiotensin-converting enzyme (ACE) inhibitors or angiotensin receptor blockers (ARBs) for a patient with renal artery stenosis
2. Beta-blockers given to a patient with pheochromocytoma
3. Beta-blockers in a patient with diabetic autonomic neuropathy.

Hypotension

Hypotension is defined as blood pressure that is lower than 90/60 mm Hg.

Reference: NIH

Cause of hypotension according to age group:

Younger adult	Any adult age group	Older adult
- Pregnancy - Vasovagal syncope	- Chronic liver disease - Diabetic autonomic neuropathy	- Parkinson's disease - Dysrhythmia

Contd...

Contd...

- Situational syncope - Primary amyloidosis - Primary autonomic failure	- Secondary amyloidosis - Addison's disease - Hypopituitarism - Severe hypothyroidism	- Micturition syncope - Carotid sinus syndrome - Vitamin B_{12} deficiency

Postural Hypotension/Orthostatic Hypotension

- A drop in blood pressure (hypotension) due to a change in body position (posture) when a person moves to a more vertical position, i.e., from sitting to standing or from lying down to sitting or standing.
- Postural (orthostatic) hypotension is diagnosed when, within 2–5 minutes of quiet standing (after a 5-minute period of supine rest), one or both of the following is present:
  - At least a 20 mm Hg fall in systolic pressure
  - At least a 10 mm Hg fall in diastolic pressure
- Many disorders can cause orthostatic hypotension, with the two major mechanisms being autonomic failure, which can be caused by multiple disorders, and severe volume depletion.

Autonomic failure	Volume depletion
- Diabetic neuropathy - Parkinson disease - Dementia with lewy bodies - MSA (Shy-Drager syndrome) - Spinal cord transection	- Acute or subacute volume depletion (due to diuretics, hyperglycemia, hemorrhage, or vomiting)
- Chronic kidney disease - Amyloidosis - Guillain-Barré syndrome - Paraneoplastic autonomic neuropathy - Familial dysautonomia (Riley-Day syndrome) - Primary autonomic failure (Bradbury-Eggleston syndrome)	- Chronic hypovolemia, a frequent feature of autonomic failure, exacerbates orthostatic symptoms

Postprandial Hypotension

In postprandial hypotension, blood pressure falls occur within one to two hours after a meal.

Nocturnal hypertension

The definition of nocturnal hypertension is night-time BP ≥120/70 mm Hg (>110/65 mm Hg by the new 2017 ACC/AHA guidelines). Clinic and morning home BP of <130/80 mm Hg is defined as masked nocturnal hypertension and as masked uncontrolled nocturnal hypertension under a medicated condition. The pattern of circadian rhythm of BP can be evaluated by ambulatory BP monitoring (ABPM).

In healthy subjects, night-time BP decreases by 10% to 20% of daytime BP (normal dipper pattern). This circadian rhythm of BP is determined partly by the intrinsic rhythm of central and peripheral clock genes, which regulate the neurohumoral factor and cardiovascular systems, and partly by the sleep–wake behavioral pattern.

Hypertensive patients without organ damage also exhibit the dipper pattern; however, those with organ damage tend

General Examination

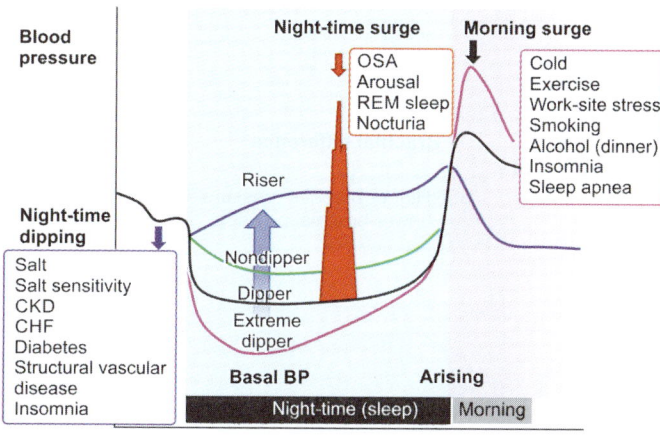

Fig. 2B.23: Nocturnal BP dipping patterns.

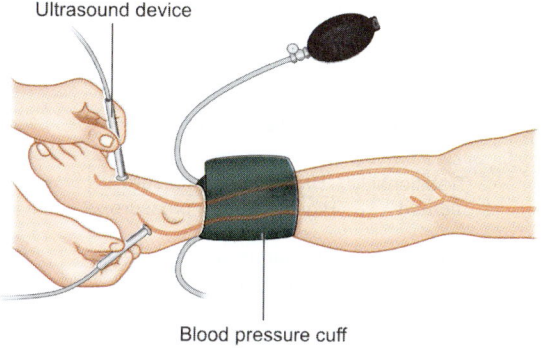

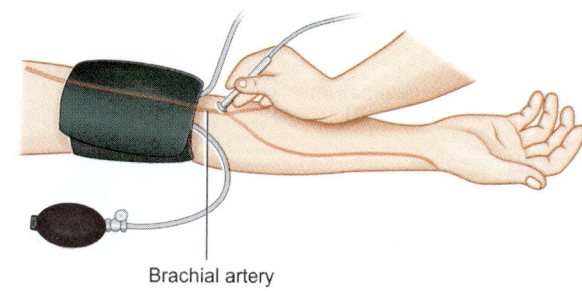

Fig. 2B.24: Measurement of ankle brachial index.

to exhibit nondipper patterns with diminished night-time BP fall.

Night-time BP dipping patterns are classified into 4 groups: dipper, nondipper, riser, and extreme dipper patterns **(Fig. 2B.23)**.

Ambulatory BP Monitoring (ABPM)

Thresholds for hypertension diagnosis based on ABPM	
24-h average	≥130/80 mm Hg
Awake (daytime) average	≥135/85 mm Hg
Asleep (night-time) average	≥120/70 mm Hg

Clinical Indications for ABPM
Identifying white-coat hypertension phenomena
False resistant hypertension in treated subjects
Identifying masked hypertension phenomena
• Masked hypertension in untreated subjects
• Masked uncontrolled hypertension in treated subjects
• Identifying abnormal 24-h blood pressure patterns
• Daytime hypertension
• Siesta dipping/postprandial hypotension
• Nocturnal hypertension
• Dipping status
◆ Morning hypertension and morning blood pressure surge
◆ Obstructive sleep apnea
◆ Increased blood pressure variability
Assessment of treatment
◆ Increased on-treatment blood pressure variability
◆ Assessing 24-h blood pressure control
◆ Identifying true resistant hypertension
Assessing hypertension in the elderly
Assessing hypertension in children and adolescents Assessing hypertension in pregnancy
Assessing hypertension in high-risk patients Identifying ambulatory hypotension
Identifying blood pressure patterns in Parkinson disease
Endocrine hypertension

ANKLE-BRACHIAL INDEX

- The ankle-brachial index (ABI) is the ratio of the systolic blood pressure (SBP) measured at the ankle to that measured at the brachial artery.

- Originally described by Winsor in 1950, this index was initially proposed for the noninvasive diagnosis of lower-extremity peripheral artery disease (PAD).
- Later, it was shown that the ABI is an indicator of atherosclerosis at other vascular sites and can serve as a prognostic marker for cardiovascular events and functional impairment, even in the absence of symptoms of PAD.
- The ABI is performed by measuring the systolic blood pressure from both brachial arteries and from both the dorsalis pedis and posterior tibial arteries after the patient has been at rest in the supine position for 10 minutes.
- The systolic pressures are recorded with a **handheld 5- or 10-mHz Doppler instrument (Fig. 2B.24)**.
- Calculating the ABI
  - An ABI is calculated for each leg. The ABI value is determined by taking the higher pressure of the 2 arteries at the ankle, divided by the brachial arterial systolic pressure. In calculating the ABI, the higher of the two brachial systolic pressure measurements is used. In normal individuals, there should be a minimal (less than 10 mm Hg) interarm systolic pressure gradient during a routine examination. A consistent difference in pressure between the arms greater than 10 mm Hg is suggestive of (and greater than 20 mm Hg is diagnostic of) subclavian or axillary arterial stenosis, which may be observed in individuals at risk for atherosclerosis **(Fig. 2B.25)**.
  - Calculated ABI values should be recorded to 2 decimal places.

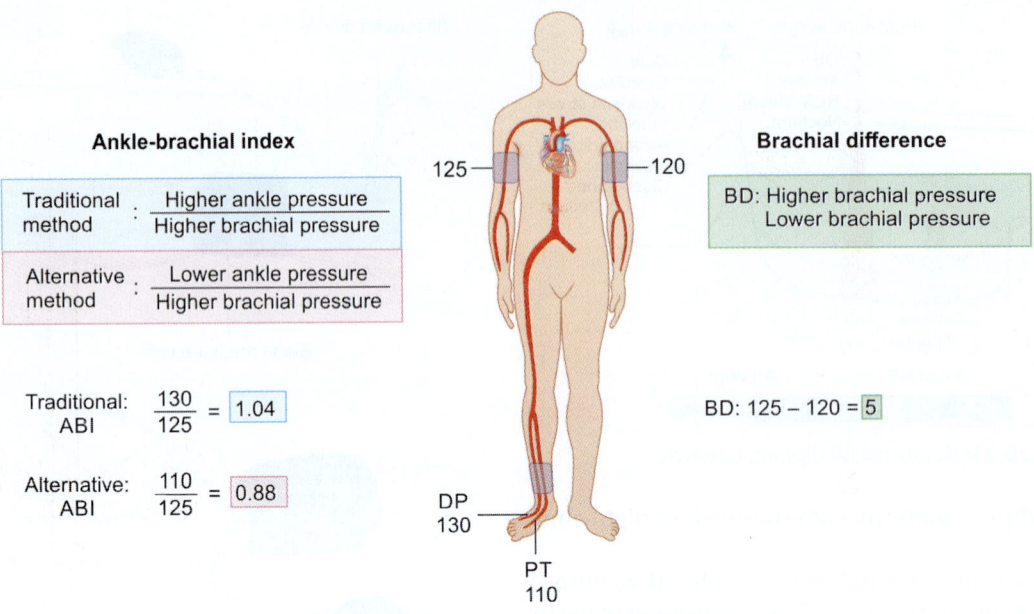

Fig. 2B.25: Calculating ankle brachial index.

ABI value	Interpretation
Greater than 1.4	Calcification/vessel hardening
1.0–1.4	Normal
0.9–1.0	Acceptable
0.8–0.9	Mild arterial disease
0.5–0.8	Moderate arterial disease
Less than 0.5	Severe arterial disease

JUGULAR VENOUS SYSTEM

Jugular Venous Pulse

It is defined as undulating top of oscillating column of blood in right internal jugular vein that faithfully represents the pressure and volumetric changes in the right side of heart which changes with various stages of cardiac cycle and respiration.

Why is the Right IJV Preferred?

- Right side internal jugular vein (IJV) is in direct connection (Fig. 2B.26).
- Straight line course through innominate vein to the SVC and right atrium
- IJV is less likely affected by extrinsic compression from other structures in neck
- Veins in the left side of the neck reach the heart by crossing the mediastinum, where they may be compressed by the normal aorta; causing the left jugular venous pressure to appear elevated even when the CVP and right atrial pressures are normal.

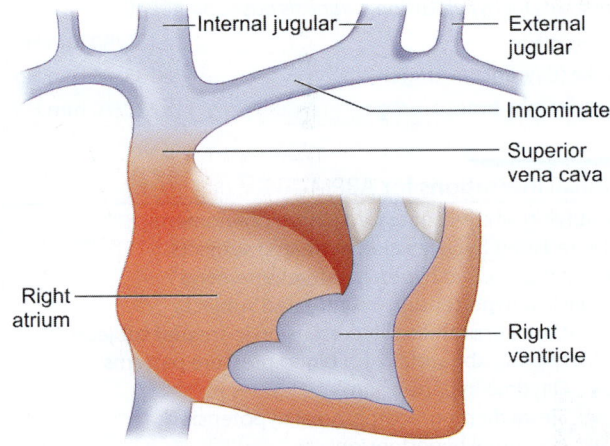

Fig. 2B.26: Anatomy of the right IJV.

Why internal jugular vein preferred over external jugular vein for JVP assessment?	
Internal jugular	External jugular
Straight communication with right atrium	Not in straight communication with right atrium
Less valves	More valves
Less influenced by fascial planes	More kinked by fascial planes
Less affected by sympathetic system	More affected by sympathetic system
	Vasoconstriction secondary to hypotension (in CCF) can make EJV small and barely visible

General Examination

Differences between carotid and JVP	
Carotid pulse	Jugular venous pulse
Better felt	Better seen
Cannot be obliterated	Can be obliterated (by pressure at root of neck)
One positive wave	Two positive and two negative waves
Medially seen	Laterally seen
Seen in lower part	Seen in upper part
Definite upper level absent	Definite upper-level present
Expansile impulse (outward)	Retractile impulse (inward). Descents >obvious than crests
Does not change with position	Changes with position
Does not change with respiration	Changes with respiration
Does not change with abdominal compression	Changes with abdominal compression

Steps of Examination of JVP (Figs. 2B.27 and 2B.28)

- Patient comfortably lying in semi reclined position (45° position).
- The patient's neck should be slightly turned towards the left side.
- Shining a light tangentially across the neck may help you see the waveform.

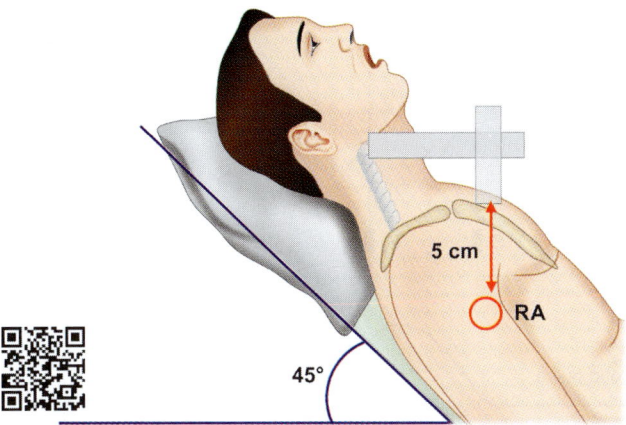

Fig. 2B.27: Method of measuring the JVP.

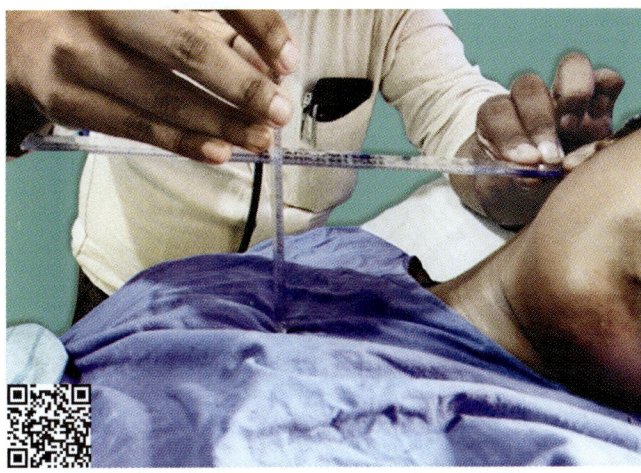

Fig. 2B.28: Examination of height of JVP.

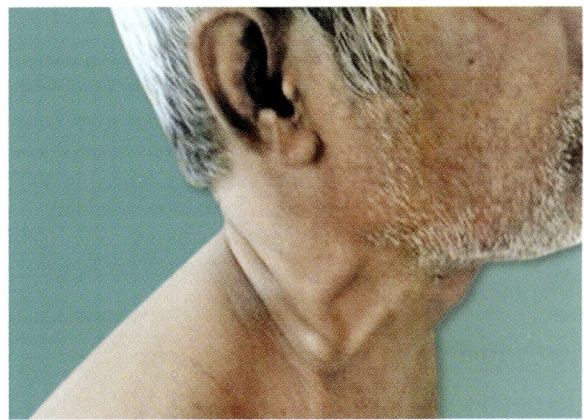

Fig. 2B.29: Image showing engorged neck veins.

- Observe for pulsation between two heads of sternocleidomastoid.
- Trace the pulsation and locate the upper level.
- Take two scales. Place one scale at the upper level of the JVP, parallel to the ground.
- Now place the second scale at the level of the sternal angle, perpendicular to the first scale.
- Measure the vertical height on the second scale.
- Express as _____ cm of water above sternal angle. Add 5 cm to this value to determine the right atrial pressure.
- Conversion: 1.36 cm of H_2O or blood = 1 mm Hg
- The normal JVP is **less than 4 cm** above the sternal angle; or is just visible above the clavicle in 45° position.
- Normal CVP is <7 mm of Hg or 9 cm H_2O.
- JVP is best measured at the end of expiration.

Note that the most common error in measuring JVP is underestimation. Measurement is also unreliable in patients with low CVP, those on mechanical ventilation, or those with short/thick necks.

Causes of Raised JVP

Engorged (Fig. 2B.29) and pulsatile neck vein	Engorged and nonpulsatile neck vein
Cardiac causes - Right heart failure - Congestive cardiac failure - Chronic constrictive pericarditis - Cardiac tamponade - Complete heart block - Restrictive cardiomyopathy - Superior vena cava (SVC) obstruction - Tricuspid stenosis	- Superior mediastinal syndrome - Valsalva maneuver - Chronic constrictive pericarditis (advanced stage)
Noncardiac causes - Pulmonary thromboembolism - Pulmonary hypertension - Acute nephritis - Pregnancy - Fluid overload status	

Waveforms of JVP (Figs. 2B.30 and 2B.31)

Component	Cardiac event responsible
A wave	Atrial contraction/systole
X wave (initial x descent)	Atrial relaxation

Contd...

Contd...

C wave	Closure of the tricuspid valve (some consider c wave is due to the impact of carotid pulsation)
X' wave (X descent following "C" wave)	Downward movement of the floor of the right atrium while the right ventricle contracts (called the 'descent of the base')
V wave	Atrial filling during ventricular systole
Y wave	RA emptying during ventricular diastole
H wave (Hirschfelder wave)	Seen in diastasis

"a" wave (most prominent of JVP)			
Absent	Atrial fibrillation		
Large/ giant "a" wave	Tricuspid stenosis (TS) Tricuspid atresia (TA) Right atrium (RA) myxomas	Right ventricular (RV) infarction RV cardiomyopathy	Pulmonary hypertension (PH) Pulmonary stenosis (PS) Pulmonary embolism (PE)
	Aortic stenosis (AS)* Hypertrophic cardiomyopathy (HCM)* (**Bernheim effect***)		

Contd...

Cannon "A" waves	Regular	Junctional rhythm Ventricular tachycardia (VT) (1:1 retrograde conduction)
	Irregular	Complete heart block (CHB) Atrioventricular (AV) dissociation
		Ventricular ectopics Ventricular tachycardia V pacing

*__Bernheim effect:__ Left-sided diseases causing prominent a wave, (i.e.) severe LVH with septal thickening interfere with RV filling resulting in prominent a wave.

"v" wave	
Diminished	Cause of diminished v wave is hypovolemia
Prominent	- Tricuspid regurgitation (TR)* - Atrial septal defect (ASD) - Ventricular septal defect (VSD), Gerbode defect—abnormal shunting between the left ventricle and the right atrium due to either a congenital defect or prior cardiac insults - Congestive heart failure (CHF) - Atrial fibrillation - Cor pulmonale

*In TR due to absent X and prominent V wave merging with C wave, it results in large positive systolic and regurgitant waves (CV wave) followed by a rapid deep 'y' descent. This may cause subtle motion of earlobe with each beat (LANSICI'S sign)

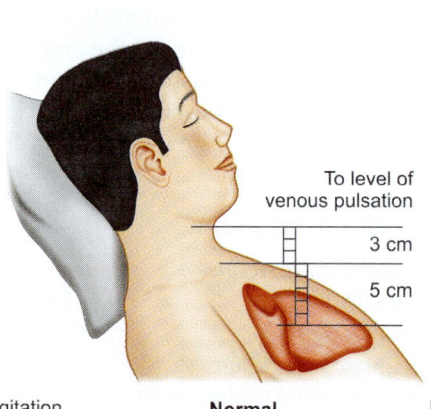

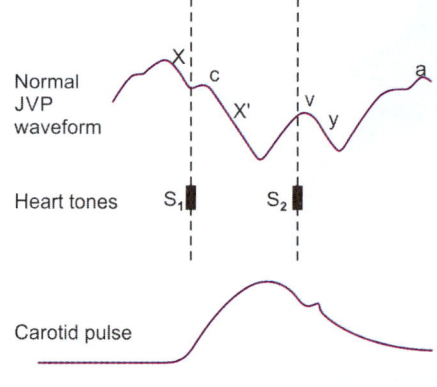

A. Tricuspid regurgitation

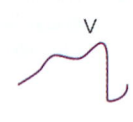

C. Constrictive pericarditis

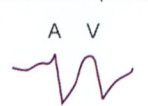

E. Atrial fibrillation

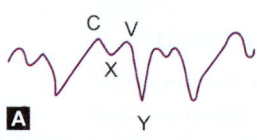

Normal

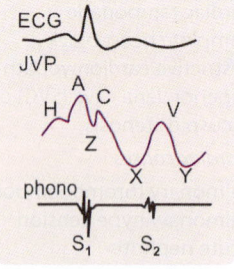

F. First degree AV block

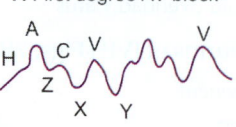

B. Tricuspid stenosis

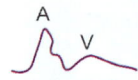

D. Atrial septal defect

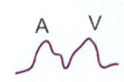

G. Complete AV block

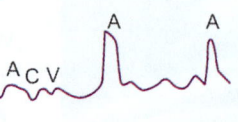

Figs. 2B.30A and B: (A) Jugular venous pulse demonstration: (B) Drawing demonstrating the proper technique to evaluate the venous pulse. Note the positioning of the penlight with respect to the patient's neck, as well as the placement of the right third finger over the left carotid artery.

Other Sites of JVP Estimation

Gaertner's Method

Normally, the superficial veins of dorsum of hand collapse when raised above the sternal angle. Persistent prominence is suggestive of raised central venous pressure (**Anthem sign**—when the same is tested by asking the patient to make a fist and raise the arm like an anthem pledge).

May's Sign

Visible engorged vein on the undersurface of tongue in sitting posture.

Abdominojugular Reflux (AJR) of Rundott (Previously Known as Hepatojugular Reflux)

Demonstration (Fig. 2B.33)

- The patient is placed in a 45° semi recumbent position and firm, consistent abdominal pressure 40 mm Hg is applied, preferably over the right hypochondrium (an inflated BP cuff may be used).
- Historically pressure was applied for 15 seconds; however, recent studies suggest 10 seconds is adequate.
- **Normal response:**
  - Transient rise of around 4 cm for about 4–5 cardiac cycles (approximately 5 sec)
- **Sustained response/positive response:**
  - Earliest sign of right heart failure (RHF), also seen in tricuspid regurgitation (TR)
- **Absent response/negative response:**
  - Obstruction/thrombosis of inferior vena cava (IVC) or hepatic veins as seen in Budd-Chiari syndrome.

Friederick's Sign of Constrictive Pericarditis

Friederick's sign describes a rapid fall and rise in the JVP. It occurs when stiff ventricles are unable to accommodate the rapid ventricular filling that should follow opening of the tricuspid valve in the presence of elevated atrial pressure.

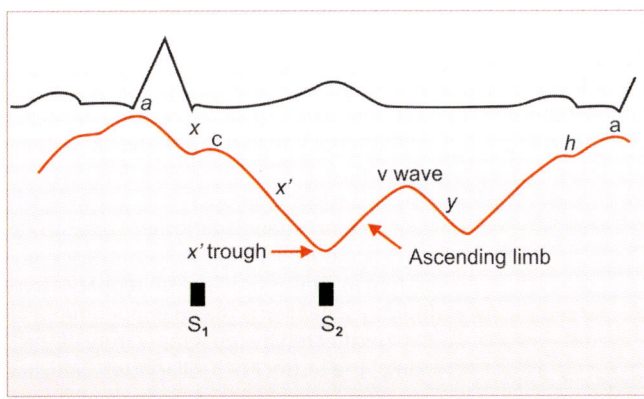

Fig. 2B.31: Jugular venous wave pattern JVP components and waveforms (Fig. 2B.30).

'X' descent (systolic collapse)	
Absent	Tricuspid regurgitation
Prominent	Tamponade Atrial septal defect (ASD) Pericarditis—constrictive

'Y' descent (diastolic collapse)	
Slow descent	Tamponade Tricuspid stenosis (TS), right atrial (RA) myxoma
Rapid descent	Constrictive pericarditis Severe tricuspid regurgitation (TR) Severe right ventricular (RV) failure

Differences between Constrictive Pericarditis and Cardiac Tamponade (Fig. 2B.32)

	X wave	Y wave
Pericarditis—constrictive	+	++ (prominent **Y**)
Tamponade	++ (prominent **X**)	--
TR	--	++

(Mnemonic: Prominent Y and X waves can be remembered with mnemonic **PaY TaX**)

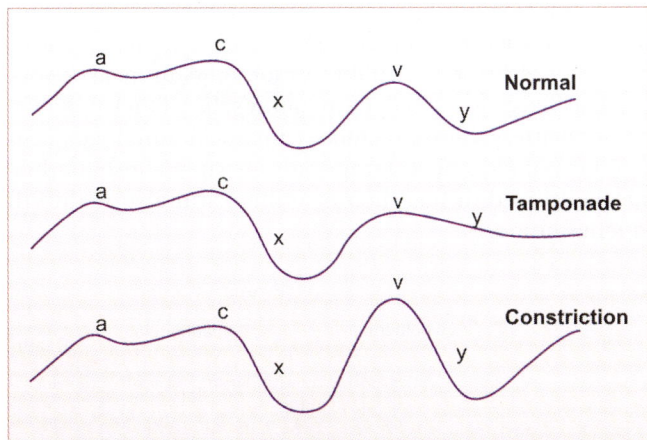

Fig. 2B.32: Waveforms of JVP in tamponade vs constrictive pericarditis.

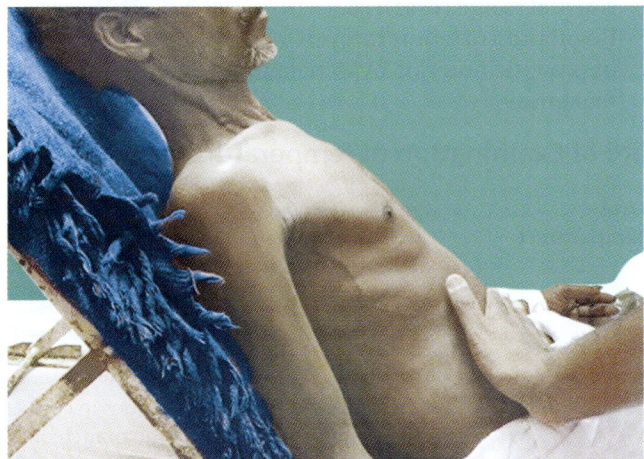

Fig. 2B.33: Demonstration of abdominojugular reflux.

Square Root Sign of JVP

Dip and plateau pattern of JVP seen in constrictive pericarditis.

Kussmaul Sign of JVP

Normally when the patient inspires, there is fall in the height of JVP due to increased negative intrathoracic pressure. Kussmaul sign is the paradoxical elevation of JVP during inspiration, Seen in:
- Constrictive pericarditis
- Severe heart failure
- Right ventricular infarction
- Restrictive cardiomyopathy.

M pattern in JVP		
Constrictive pericarditis	Due to prominent x and y waves	
ASD	Due to prominent A and V waves	

Raised jugular venous pressure with shock
- Congestive heart failure
- Cardiac tamponade
- Right ventricular infarction
- Tension pneumothorax
- Massive pulmonary embolism

BODY TEMPERATURE

Core Body Temperature

It usually refers to the temperature of the internal body core, measured under the tongue, in the ear canal or in the rectum.
- **Normal range (oral):** 36.8 ± 0.4°C (98.2 ± 0.7°F)
- **Regulation of temperature:** Under the control of neurons of preoptic anterior hypothalamus and posterior hypothalamus.

Site of Examination of Temperature

Oral temperature	- Probe placed under the tongue into the sublingual pockets and the lips closed around the instrument - The patient should not have recently smoked or ingested cold or hot food or drink - Usually tested for about 3 minutes - Oral temperature reflects changes in core body temperature through the branch of the external carotid artery which perfuses the posterior sublingual pockets
Rectal readings are 0.4–0.6°C higher than oral recordings	- Measured with a lubricated blunt-tipped glass thermometer inserted 4–5 cm (2.5 cm in children) into the anal canal at an angle 20° from the horizontal with the patient lying prone - Usually tested for about 3 minutes - Lags behind changes at other core sites as it is located far from the central nervous system as well as from the pulmonary artery - Indicates the deep visceral temperature. Can be affected by the temperature of the skin of the buttocks, the iliac artery and iliac vein
Tympanic temperature	- The scanning tip should be gently placed in the ear canal and then slowly inserted against the tympanic membrane snugly - Measures the infrared heat waves from the tympanic membrane - Close to hypothalamus and rapid measurement of core body temperature
Axillary readings lag behind oral temperature by 0.1–0.2°C	- Thermometer placed in the axilla and shoulder adducted - Convenient for patient - Core temperature cannot be assessed directly - Lags behind the changes in core body temperature
Temporal (forehead) measurement	- Placed on the skin of the forehead - An electronic thermometer that is fast and accurate - Less invasive than the tympanic thermometer and more reliable when used correctly

Thermometers (Fig. 2B.34)

- Glass thermometer and electric digital thermometer
- Glass thermometer bulbs contain an alloy called Galinstan.

Electric digital thermometers are more convenient than glass instruments because the probe cover is disposable, response time is quicker (allowing accurate measurements within 10–20 seconds), and there is a signal when the rate of change in temperature becomes insignificant.

The most common methods of temperature assessment that carry the least amount of risk for patient injury are the use of glass or electronic digital thermometers to measure oral, rectal, axillary, or vaginal temperatures; basal thermometers; temporal artery thermometers; tympanic thermometers; and liquid crystal forehead temperature strips. These methods can be utilized in healthcare settings and also within the patient's home.

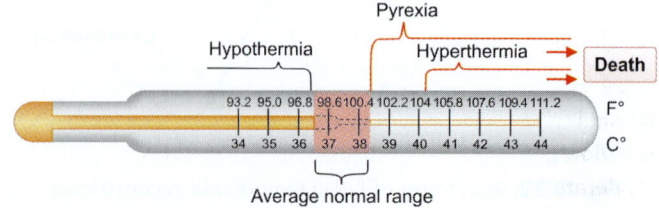

Fig. 2B.34: Thermometer showing marking in both Celsius and Fahrenheit.

Although the more invasive methods are more accurate, they carry a higher risk of potential complications, so they are not routinely utilized in areas outside of a critical care or surgical setting. Examples of invasive methods of temperature assessment are esophageal and rectal temperature probes, temperature-sensing indwelling urinary catheters, temperature-sensing pulmonary artery (PA) catheters, a cardiopulmonary bypass (CPB) machine, and extracorporeal membrane oxygenation (ECMO).

Circadian Variation of Temperature
- Circadian rhythm is governed by suprachiasmatic nuclei in anterior hypothalamus.
- Normal variation is 0.5–1.0°C over the day
- Lowest temperature is noted at 6:00 am and peaks at 4:00–6:00 PM.

Variation of Temperature During Menstrual Cycles
An abrupt increase of 0.3–0.5°C accompanies ovulation and may be useful as a fertility guide.

Fever
Fever is an elevation of body temperature that exceeds the normal daily variation and occurs in conjunction with an **increase in the hypothalamic set point**.

It can be defined as temperature of >37.2°C (98.9°F) at 6 AM or >37.7°C (99.9°F) at 4–6 PM.

When the hypothalamic set point is raised, the body is perceived to be cooler than the new set point. Shivering is initiated to generate heat. Blood is shunted from the periphery to the core to conserve heat and sweating is diminished.

The generated heat will raise the body temperature to match the elevated set point. When the hypothalamic set point is lowered, either as part of the normal diurnal fluctuations that occur during an infection or in response to antipyretic agents, heat is lost by evaporation (sweating) and radiation (cutaneous vasodilation).

Types of fever based on duration		
Acute fevers	<7 days	Infectious diseases such as malaria and viral-related upper respiratory tract infections
Subacute fevers	Usually not more than 2 weeks in duration	Typhoid fever and intra-abdominal abscess
Chronic or persistent fevers	>2 weeks duration	Chronic bacterial infections such as tuberculosis, viral infections like human immunodeficiency virus (HIV), cancers and connective tissue diseases

Grading of Fever Based on Body Temperature

Body temperature	°C	°F
Normal	37–38	98.6–100.4
Mild/low grade fever	38.1–39	100.5–102.2
Moderate grade fever	39.1–40	102.2–104.0
High grade fever	40.1–41.1	104.1–106.0
Hyperpyrexia	>41.1	>106.0

The conversion formula is:
1. T°F = 9/5 (T°C) + 32
2. T°C = 5/9 (T°F) – 32

Patterns of fever (Fig. 2B.35)		
Type of fever	*Description*	*Seen in*
Continuous or sustained fever	Defined as fever that does not fluctuate more than about 1°C (1.5°F) for 24 hours, but does not touch the baseline	Lobar and gram-negative pneumonia, typhoid, and acute bacterial meningitis
Remittent fever	Defined as fever with daily fluctuations exceeding 2°C but does not touch the baseline	Remittent fevers are often associated with infectious diseases such as infective endocarditis, rickettsia infections, and brucellosis
Intermittent fever	Defined as fever present only for several hours during the day	Malaria, pyogenic infections, tuberculosis (TB), schistosomiasis, lymphomas, leptospira, *Borrelia*, Kala-azar, or septicemia
Double quotidian fever (12 hours periodicity)		Kala-azar, gonococcal endocarditis. Adult-onset Still's disease
Quotidian fever (periodicity of 24 hours)		Mixed falciparum and vivax
Tertian fever (periodicity of 48 hours)		*Plasmodium falciparum*, ovale and vivax
Quartan fever (periodicity of 72 hours)		*Plasmodium malariae*
Pel-Ebstein's fever (intermittent low-grade fever characterized by 3–10 days of fever with subsequent afebrile periods of 3–10 days)		It is thought to be a typical but rare manifestation of Hodgkin's lymphoma
Relapsing fevers	Refer to those that are recurring and separated by periods with low-grade fever or no fever	Seen in malaria, lymphoma, *Borrelia*, cyclic neutropenia, and rat-bite fever

Fever with Night Sweats
It has been described in infectious diseases such as TB, *Nocardia*, brucellosis, liver or lung abscess, and subacute infective endocarditis, as well as in noninfectious diseases such as polyarteritis nodosa and cancers such as lymphomas.

Fever with Bradycardia
It is a feature of untreated typhoid, leishmaniasis, brucellosis, Legionnaire's disease and psittacosis, and yellow fever.

Fever with Unknown Origin
In 1961, pyrexia of unknown origin (PUO) was originally defined by Petersdorf and Beeson as an illness of more than 3 weeks duration, fever higher than 38.3°C (101°F) on several occasions and diagnosis uncertain after 1 week of study in hospital.

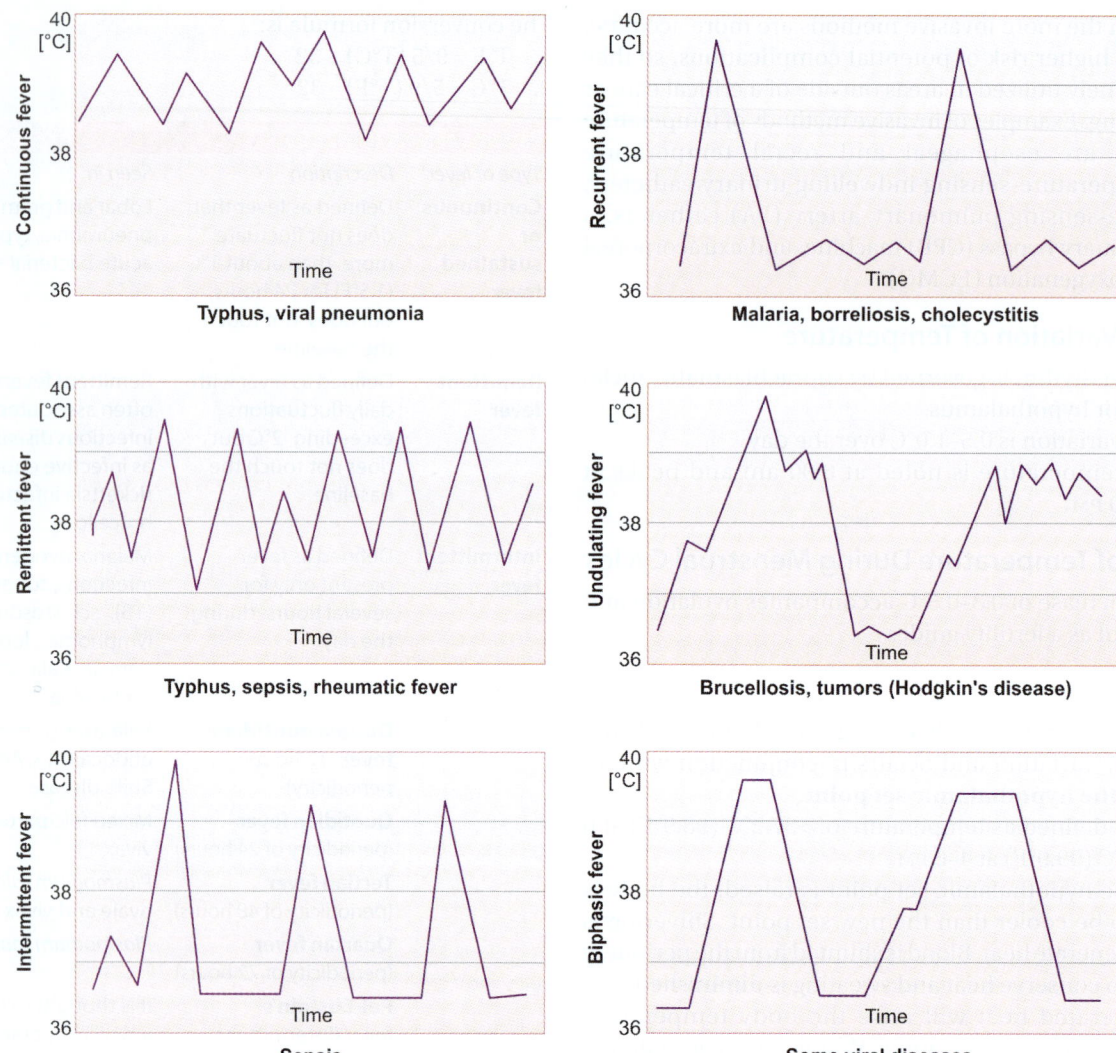

Fig. 2B.35: Clinical pattern of fevers.

This definition has been modified, removing the requirement that the evaluation must take place in the hospital and refined to include four different subgroups, each requiring different investigative strategies: Classical, nosocomial, neutropenic, and human immunodeficiency virus (HIV)-related.

Hyperpyrexia

(Body temperature >105°F)
Causes include:
- Pontine hemorrhage
- Rheumatic fever
- Meningococcal meningitis
- Cerebral malaria
- Septicemia
- Encephalitis
- Serotonin syndrome
- Thyroid storm
- Neuroleptic malignant syndrome.

Aseptic Fever

- Malignancies
- Acute myocardial infarction
- Sarcoidosis
- Chronic renal failure
- Collagen vascular diseases
- Drug fever
- Radiation sickness
- Postsurgical patients.

Drug Fever

It is a prolonged fever with relative bradycardia and hypotension. It persists 2–3 days even after drug is with drawn and is associated with rash and eosinophilia. For example, penicillin, procainamide, propylthiouracil, sulfonamides, anticonvulsant, etc.

Note: All drugs except digitalis can cause drug induced fever.

Nature of Defervescence

The **nature of fever defervescence** may also provide some diagnostic clues.

Defervescence by crisis (Fig. 2B.36)	Defervescence by lysis (Fig. 2B.37)
Within hours	Gradually over days
Example: Effective antimalarial therapy leads to fever deferevescence by crisis	Example: Typhoid fevers resolution occurs by lysis following effective antibiotics

General Examination

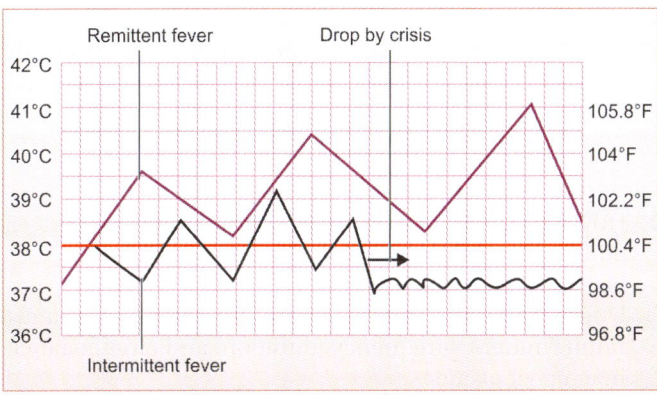

Fig. 2B.36: Defervescence by crisis.

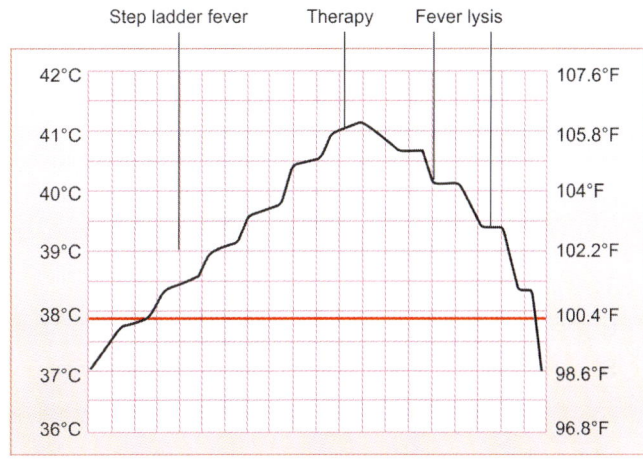

Fig. 2B.37: Defervescence by lysis in typhoid fever.

Disorders of increased body temperature	
Hyperpyrexia	The body's temperature regulation mechanism sets the body temperature above the normal temperature, then generates heat to achieve this temperature
Hyperthermia	Unchanged (normothermic) setting of the thermoregulatory center in conjunction with an uncontrolled increase in body temperature that exceeds the body's ability to lose heat
Heat stroke	Acute condition of hyperthermia that is caused by prolonged exposure to excessive heat/± humidity. The heat-regulating mechanisms of the body eventually become overwhelmed and unable to effectively deal with the heat, causing the body temperature to climb uncontrollably
Malignant hyperthermia	Occurs in individuals with an inherited abnormality of skeletal-muscle sarcoplasmic reticulum that causes a rapid increase in intracellular calcium levels in response to halothane and other inhalational anesthetics or to succinylcholine
Neuroleptic malignant syndrome (NMS)	Seen with neuroleptic use (antipsychotic phenothiazines, haloperidol, prochlorperazine, and metoclopramide) or the withdrawal of dopaminergic drugs. Characterized by "lead-pipe" muscle rigidity, extrapyramidal side effects, autonomic dysregulation, and hyperthermia

Hypothermia	
Hypothermia is defined as a core temperature below 35°C (95°F).	
Mild hypothermia	Core temperature 32–35°C (90–95°F)
Moderate hypothermia	Core temperature 28–32°C (82–90°F)
Severe hypothermia	Core temperature below 28°C (82°F)
Profound hypothermia	Core temperature <24°C (75°F) or <20°C (68°F)

Causes of Hypothermia

Decreased heat production	Increased heat loss
- Hypopituitarism - Hypoadrenalism - Hypothyroidism	- Burns - Cold immersion injuries - Vasodilatation from pharmacologic or toxicologic agents - Cold infusions - Overenthusiastic treatment of heatstroke

Contd...

Contd...

Impaired thermoregulation	Miscellaneous causes
- Central nervous system (CNS) trauma - Strokes - Toxicologic and metabolic derangements - Intracranial bleeding - Parkinson disease - CNS tumors - Wernicke disease - Multiple sclerosis	- Sepsis - Multiple trauma - Pancreatitis - Prolonged cardiac arrest - Uremia

Named fevers	Disease/organism
Glandular fever	Infectious mononucleosis (EBV)
Pappataci, 3 days, sandfly fever	Phlebotomus fever
Goal fever	*Rickettsia prowazekii*
Malta, undulating fever	Brucellosis
Relapsing fever	*Borrelia recurrentis* (louse) *B. duttoni* (Tick)
Rat bite fever	*Spirillum minus Streptobacillus moniliformis*
Trench or 5-day fever	*Bartonella quintana*
Oroya fever	*Bartonella bacilliformis*
Q fever	*Coxiella burnetti*
7-day fever	*Leptospira hebdomadis*
Pretibial fever	*L. atumnale*
Haverhill fever	*Streptobacillus moniliformis*
Pontiac fever	Legionella
Monkey fever	Kyasanur forest disease
Biphasic fever	Dengue Kala-azar Chikungunya Polio
Valley fever	Coccidioidomycosis
Dumdum/burdwan fever	Kala-azar
Brazilian purpuric fever	*H. aegyptius*

PAIN: THE FIFTH VITAL SIGN

Pain is recognized as the fifth vital sign. Assessment should include **(Fig. 2B.38)**:
- Location
- Intensity

	Pain assessment model	
S	Site	Where exactly is the pain?
O	Onset	What were they doing when the pain started?
C	Character	What does the pain feel like?
R	Radiates	Does the pain go anywhere else?
A	Associated symptoms	Nausea/vomiting
T	Time/duration	How long have they had the pain?
E	Exacerbating/relieving factors	Does anything make the pain better or worse?
S	Severity	Obtain an initial pain score

Fig. 2B.38: Pain assessment model.

- Character/quality
- Frequency
- Duration
- Pattern.

Location—determine as precisely as possible where the pain is felt. Indicate if the pain radiates or moves.

Intensity—a grade of how severe the pain is, using a pain assessment tool the resident finds easy to use, e.g., a numerical, verbal descriptor, faces, or behavioral.

Frequency
- The occurrence of the pain.
- How often the pain occurs?
- Is it breakthrough pain?

Quality—aching, annoying, cramping, exhausting, nauseating, pounding, sharp, throbbing, stabbing, agonizing, blowing, dull, fearful, nagging, penetrating, quivering, shooting, suffocating, numbness, tingling, weakness, spasm, burning, gnawing, pressure, squeezing, radiating, tingling, touch sensitive, etc.

Pain behaviors—facial (wrinkled forehead, tightly closed eyes, grimacing, and frowning), nonverbal behavior (bracing, rubbing, and guarding), and vocalizations (crying, yelling, groaning, and moaning).

Nonverbal indicators of discomfort—aggressive, crying, fearful, noisy respirations, pacing, repetitive, restless, rocking, confusion, irritability, increased activity, withdrawal, tense, calling out, grunting, knees pulled up, other change in usual activities, or behavior patterns/routine.

Duration
- How long does the pain last (minutes or hours)?
- Sudden or gradual onset.
- Is it consistent or persistent?
- Does it change over time or come and go (intermittent)? If intermittent—frequency, duration, and circumstances in which it occurs.

Pattern
- How does the pain start?
- What was being done when it started?
- What makes it better?
- What makes it worse?

Types of Pain
- Somatic pain (bone and muscle) is:
  - Relatively well localized, worse on movement
  - Tender to pressure over the area
  - Often accompanied by a dull background aching pain.
- Visceral pain is:
  - Often poorly localized, deep, and aching
  - Usually constant
  - Often referred (e.g., diaphragmatic irritation may be referred to the right shoulder; pelvic visceral pain is often referred to the sacral or perineal area).
- Neuropathic pain is:
  - A constant, superficial burning sensation, or a deeply aching quality that may be accompanied by some sudden, sharp, shooting, and lancinating (stabbing) pain.
  - In a relatively constant area of the body surface (dermatome), if caused by actual damage to a specific peripheral nerve, plexus, root, or spinal cord.

Pain Assessment Scales

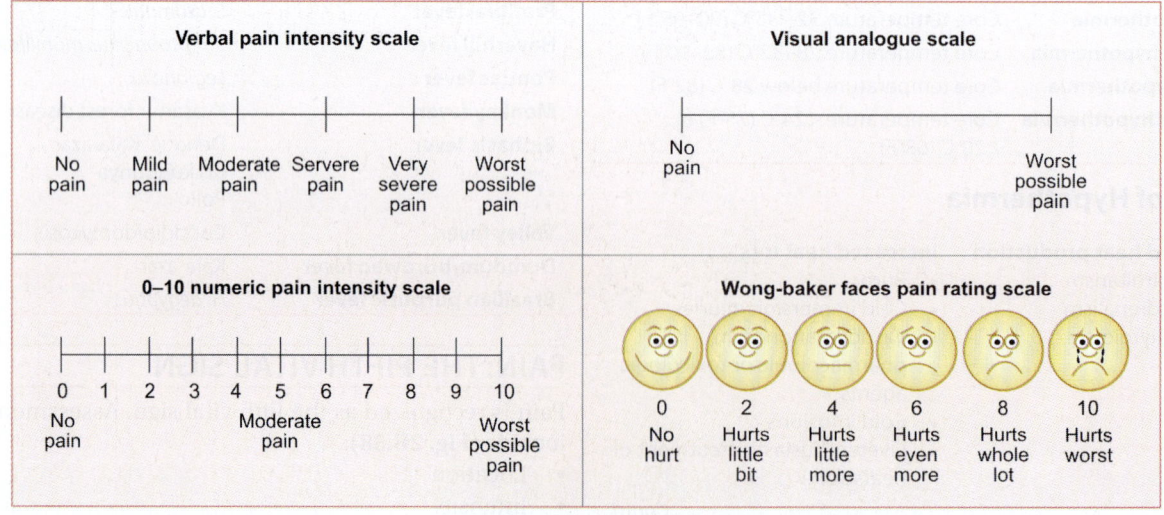

General Examination

C. PHYSICAL EXAMINATION

PALLOR

Definition
Paleness of skin and mucous membranes.

Sites of Examination
1. Conjunctiva **(Fig. 2C.1A)**
2. Tongue
3. Oral mucosa
4. Palmar crease **(Fig. 2C.2)**
5. Nail bed (Hb <8 g/dL).

After gently pulling down the patient's lower lid, we observe the lid's inner surface, comparing the color of the lid margin (its rim) with the conjunctival surface nearer to the globe.

In patients without anemia, there are two zones of color: a reddish color at the rim (due to its prominent vascular supply) and a contrasting paler color nearer to the globe (from prominent lymphoid tissue). In patients with anemia, the entire inner surface of the lower lid has a pale color **(conjunctival rim pallor, Fig. 2C.1B)**.

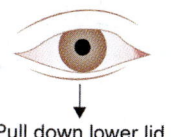
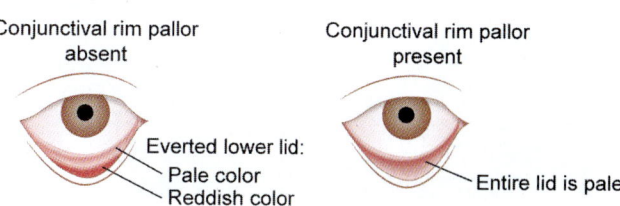

Fig. 2C.1B: Conjunctival rim pallor.

Grading of Pallor

Mild	Moderate	Severe
Cannot be detected clinically	Clinically visible	Clinically visible plus one of the following features • Palmar crease disappearance • Cervical venous hum (suggestive of chronic compensation)

Method of Elicitation of Cervical Venous Hum (Fig. 2C.3)

- Auscultate the root of the neck on the right side with bell of stethoscope, with patient in standing or sitting position.
- A continuous murmur will be heard.
- The cervical venous hum was first described by Pontain and hence called **Pontain's murmur.**
- The presence of a cervical venous hum indicates chronic compensated severe anemia.

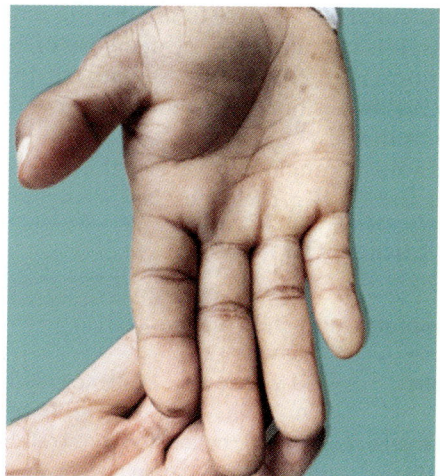

Fig. 2C.2: Demonstration of pallor in hands.

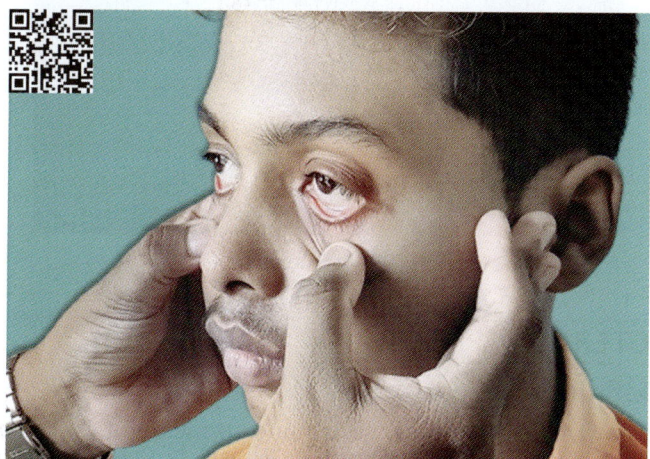

Fig. 2C.1A: Method of demonstration of pallor over conjunctiva.

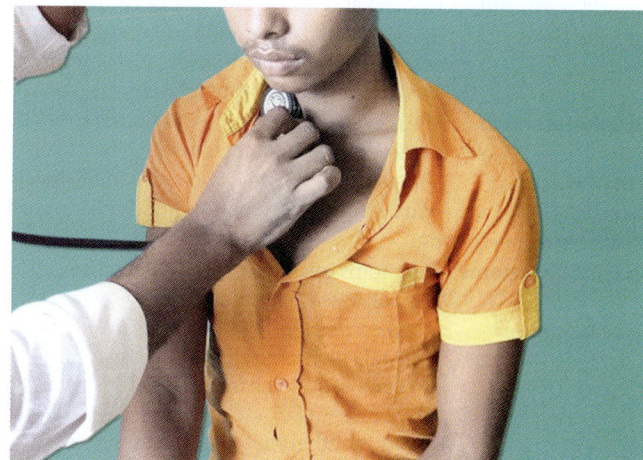

Fig. 2C.3: Demonstration of cervical venous hum.

Conditions Causing Pallor without Anemia
- Hypopituitarism
- Hypothyroidism
- Hypogonadism
- Shock
- Left heart failure.

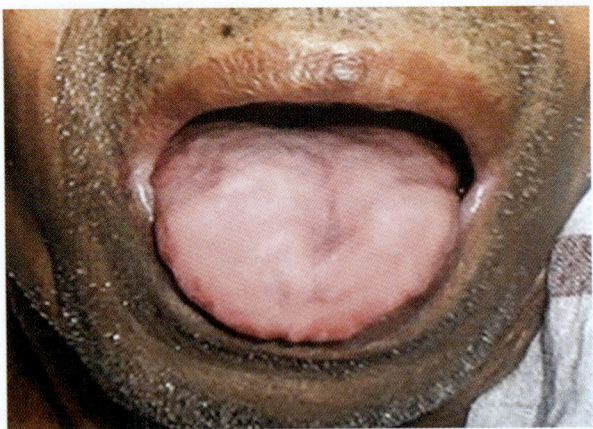

Fig. 2C.4: Bald tongue.

Definition of Anemia

Anemia is defined as decrease in circulating red blood cell (RBC) mass. It is characterized by decrease of hemoglobin concentration (Hb)/RBC count/hematocrit [packed-cell volume (PCV)] below normal for the patient's age, sex, and altitude of residence.

Normal adult hemoglobin level is in the range of 13–17 g/dL in males and 12–15 g/dL in females.

Clues for Etiology of Anemia

Iron deficiency anemia	
Specific symptoms	Pica, dysphagia, restless leg syndrome, and melena
Specific signs	Bald tongue **(Fig. 2C.4)**; Koilonychia **(Fig. 2C.5)**; Blue sclera **(Fig. 2C.6)**
Peripheral smear	Microcytic hypochromic red cells
Other specific investigation	Iron studies, BM staining for iron, stool/urine for occult blood, and endoscopy
Megaloblastic anemia	
Specific symptoms	Tingling and numbness Sensory ataxia
Specific signs	Glossitis, knuckle pigmentation **(Fig. 2C.7)**, absent deep tendon reflexes (DTRs), sensory loss, and positive Romberg's test
Peripheral smear	Macrocytic RBC's, hyper segmented neutrophils, and pancytopenia
Other specific investigation	Serum vitamin B_{12} levels, red cell folate levels, bone marrow examination, and Schillings test
Anemia of chronic disease	
Specific symptoms	Symptoms of chronic kidney, liver disease, and connective tissue disorders
Specific sign	• Hypertension, arteriovenous (AV) fistula—chronic kidney disease (CKD) • Signs of liver cell failure—chronic liver disease (CLD) • Signs of rheumatoid arthritis, systemic lupus erythematosus (SLE), etc.
Peripheral smear	Normocytic normochromic anemia ± pancytopenia
Other specific investigation	Renal function test, liver function tests, autoantibodies, and raised serum ferritin
Hemolytic anemia	
Specific symptoms	History of associated jaundice, developmental delay, family history positivity, recurrent blood transfusions, and gallstones

Contd...

Contd...

Specific signs	• Triad of anemia + jaundice + splenomegaly • Hemolytic (Chipmunk) facies **(Fig. 2C.8)** • Hyperpigmentation **(Fig. 2C.9)**, short stature, and leg ulcers
Peripheral smear	• Microcytic hypochromic (thalassemia) • Microspherocytes (hereditary spherocytosis) • Sickle cells • Reticulocytosis
Other specific investigation	Hemoglobin electrophoresis, Coombs test, sickling test, and osmotic fragility
Aplastic anemia	
Specific symptoms	Recurrent infections Bleeding manifestations
Specific signs	Signs of pancytopenia No organomegaly
Peripheral smear	Pancytopenia
Other specific investigation	• Bone marrow examination • Cytogenetics

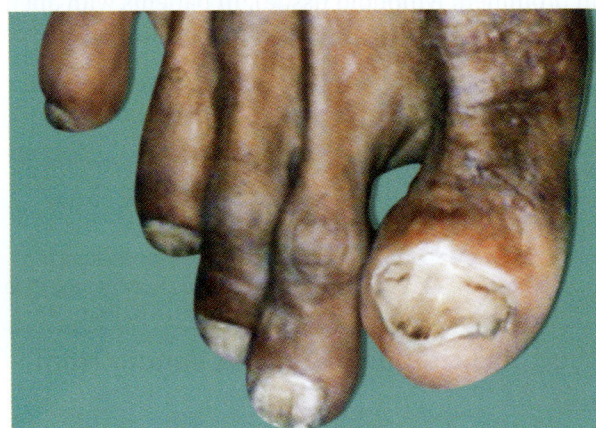

Fig. 2C.5: Koilonychia.

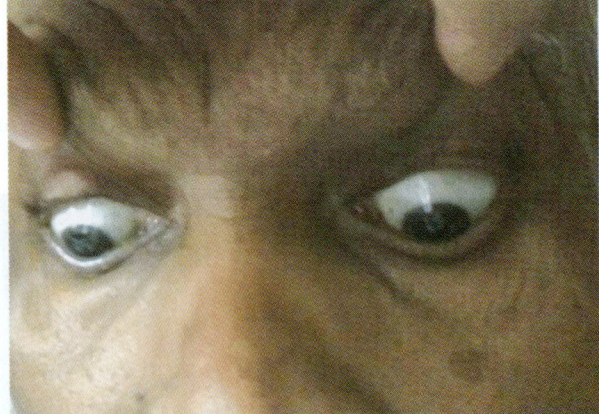

Fig. 2C.6: Blue sclera.

ICTERUS

Definition

Yellowish discoloration of skin, mucous membranes, sclera, and blood vessels secondary to increased bilirubin (bile pigments have affinity for elastin tissue).

General Examination

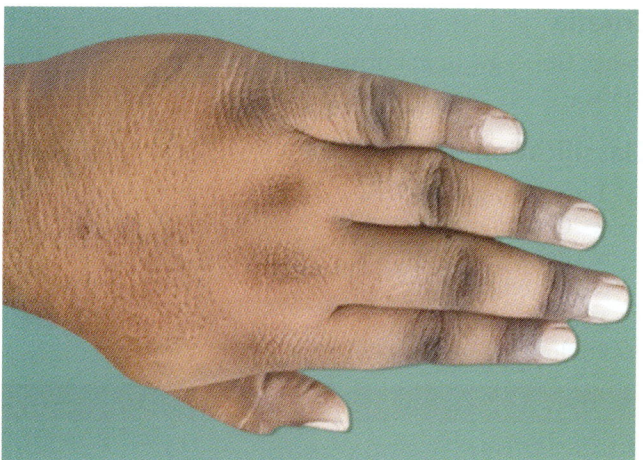

Fig. 2C.7: Knuckle pigmentation.

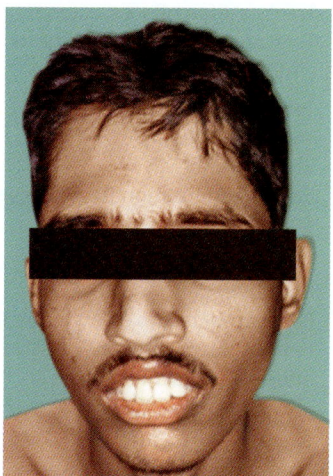

Fig. 2C.8: Chipmunk facies.

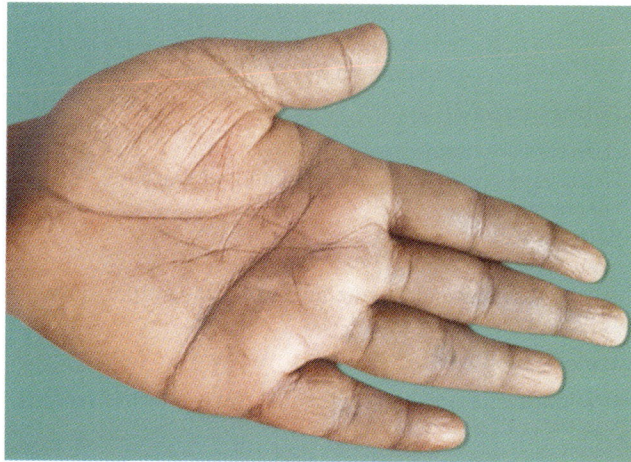

Fig 2C.9: Hyperpigmentation of palm.

Sites to Look for Jaundice
1. Sclera **(Fig. 2C.10)**
2. Sublingual mucosa
3. Oral cavity
4. Palms and soles
5. Skin.

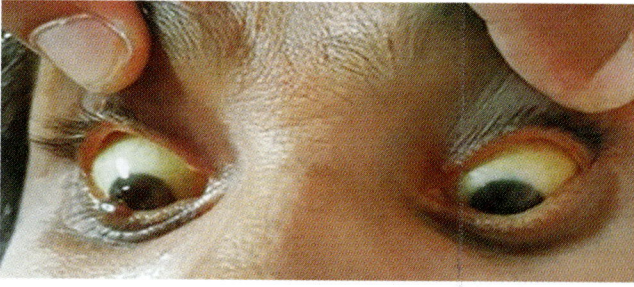

Fig. 2C.10: Demonstration of icterus.

Scleral icterus is a term commonly used but from a histopathologic perspective, it is a misnomer. Bilirubin has a high affinity for elastin, which is an abundant protein in the conjunctivae as well as the superficial, fibrovascular episclerae, but not the sclerae proper. One actually is observing icterus of the bulbar conjunctiva against the white background provided by sclera. Conjunctival icterus is often the first sign of hyperbilirubinemia. Hence, we recommended the use of term "conjunctival icterus" instead of "scleral icterus".

Why unexposed sclera/conjunctiva seen?
- When the sclera/conjunctiva is exposed to sunlight, bilirubin gets converted to its soluble form and hence exposed part of conjunctiva may not reveal mild jaundice.
- Yellowish discoloration can be normally seen in the exposed parts of sclera/conjunctiva which is called as muddy sclera/conjunctiva.

Serum Bilirubin Levels and Jaundice

0.3–1.2 mg/dL	Normal
1.2–2.5 mg/dL	Latent jaundice (generally not appreciated on clinical examination)
>2.5 mg/dL	Clinically appreciated

Yellowish discoloration without jaundice:
- Hypercarotenemia (here sclera is not affected)
- Hypothyroidism (due to decreased metabolism of carotene)
- Excessive exposure to phenols/nitric acid
- Use of drugs including quinacrine, sunitinib, and sorafenib.

Grading

No standard grading system is available; however, few examiners prefer the following:

Mild jaundice	Only sclera becomes yellow
Moderate jaundice	Skin also becomes yellow

Differentiating Type of Jaundice Based on Scleral Color

Lemon yellow	Most likely hemolytic jaundice
Dark yellow (Fig. 2C.11)	Obstructive jaundice
Greenish dark yellow	Longstanding obstructive jaundice due to oxidation of bilirubin to biliverdin

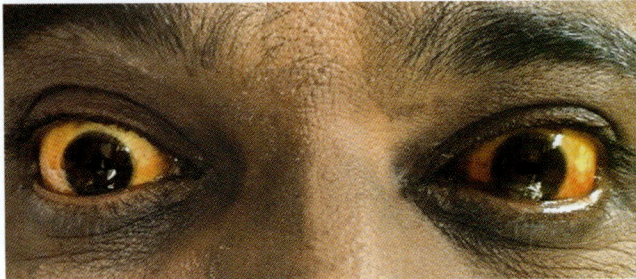

Fig. 2C.11: Dark yellow icterus.

Differentiating Jaundice Based on Clinical and Laboratory Findings

	Prehepatic (hemolytic)	Hepatic	Posthepatic (obstructive/ surgical)
History			
Urine	Normal	Yellow	Yellow
Stools	Normal	Normal	Pale clay like
Pruritus	–	±	++
Examination			
Bradycardia	–	–	+
Pallor	Present	Absent	Absent
Jaundice	Mild	Moderate	Severe
Splenomegaly	Present	Variable	Absent
Palpable gallbladder	±	–	++
Features of liver cell failure	Absent	+ (early feature)	± (late feature)
Laboratory data			
Serum bilirubin	UCB↑	UCB↑ + CB↑	CB↑
Serum enzymes	LDH↑	AST ↑ ALT ↑	ALP↑
Urine bilirubin	–	+	+
Urine urobilinogen	+	+	–
Examples			
Examples	Thalassemia Sickle cell anemia Sphero- cytosis Malaria Immune hemolytic anemias	Hepatitis (viral/ alcoholic/ drug induced) Infiltrative disorders Ischemic hepatitis	CBD stones Helminths in the CBD Carcinoma— head of pancreas Primary biliary cirrhosis Primary sclerosing cholangitis

(AST: aspartate aminotransferase; ALP: alkaline phosphatase; CB; conjugated bilirubin; CBD: common bile duct; LDH: lactate dehydrogenase; UCB: unconjugated bilirubin)

CYANOSIS

Definition
Bluish color of skin and mucous membranes resulting from an increased quantity of reduced hemoglobin (deoxygen- ated) or hemoglobin derivatives (methemoglobin or sulfhe- moglobin) in the small vessels of those tissues.

Criteria
Deoxy Hb >5 g% or abnormal Hb (metHb or sulfHb) ± SaO_2 <85%.

Classification
1. **True cyanosis:**
   a. Central cyanosis
   b. Peripheral cyanosis
   c. Mixed cyanosis.
2. **Pseudo cyanosis.**
   Etiology of Cyanosis

1. True cyanosis	
a. Central cyanosis	
Cardiac T T T T T E E	**Cyanotic heart diseases** • Truncus arteriosus • Transposition of great arteries • Total anomalous pulmonary venous connection (TAPVC) • Tetralogy of Fallot • Tricuspid atresia • Ebstein's anomaly • Eisenmengerization **(tardive cyanosis)**
Pulmonary	• Asthma • Chronic obstructive pulmonary disease (COPD) • Cor pulmonale • Respiratory failure of any cause like pneumonia, tension pneumothorax, massive pleural effusion, and acute pulmonary edema
Others	• High altitude • Polycythemia **Enterogenous or pigment cyanosis (replacement cyanosis)** • Methemoglobinemia (>1.5 g/dL) • Sulfhemoglobinemia (>0.5 g/dL) • Carboxyhemoglobin (produces cherry red discoloration)
b. Peripheral cyanosis	
• Low cardiac output • Local vasoconstriction (cold, frostbite, and Raynaud's phenomenon) • Arterial obstruction • Venous obstruction • Hyper viscosity conditions (multiple myeloma and polycythemia) • Cryoglobulinemia	
c. Mixed cyanosis	
Left ventricular failure (has both central and peripheral cyanosis)	
2. Pseudo cyanosis	

• Metals:
  ○ Gold
  ○ Silver
  ○ Mercury
  ○ Arsenic.
• Drugs:
  ○ Minocycline
  ○ Chloroquine
  ○ Chlorpromazine
  ○ Amiodarone.	

General Examination

Atypical presentation of cyanosis		
	Description	Example
Differential cyanosis	Cyanosis is seen in only lower limbs	PDA with eisenmengerization
Reverse differential cyanosis	Cyanosis is seen in only upper limbs	PDA with eisenmengerization and transposition of great arteries
Three by four cyanosis	In addition to lower limbs, the left upper limb may also be cyanosed	When the patent ductus opens proximal to the origin of left subclavian artery
Intermittent cyanosis		Seen in Ebstein's anomaly
Cyclical cyanosis		Bilateral choanal atresia
Orthocyanosis	Development of cyanosis only in upright position due to hypoxia occurring in erect posture	Seen in pulmonary arteriovenous malformation
Cyanosis absent despite of sufficient reduced hemoglobin		In severe anemia, carbon monoxide poisoning

Differences between central and peripheral cyanosis

Central cyanosis	Peripheral cyanosis
Due to inadequate oxygenation of systemic circulation	Due to sluggish peripheral circulation
It is a hypoxic hypoxia	It is a stagnant hypoxia
Site of examination: Tongue (**Fig. 2C.12**) Oral mucosa (**Fig. 2C.13**)	Site of examination: ■ Tip of nose ■ Ear lobule ■ Outer lips ■ Fingertips ■ Nail bed ■ Extremities

Extremities are warm	Extremities are cold
Do not improve on rewarming	Improves on rewarming
PaO_2 <85%	PaO_2 >85
Improves on oxygenation	Does not improve with oxygenation
Dyspnea and high-volume pulse seen	Usually absent
Exercise may worsen	Exercise may improve
May be associated with clubbing and polycythemia	

Note: Cyanosis is best appreciated in areas of the body, where the overlying epidermis is thin and the blood vessel supply abundant, such as the lips, malar prominences (nose and cheeks), ears, and oral mucous membranes (buccal and sublingual); it is better appreciated in fluorescent lighting.

Hyperoxia Test (Cardiac vs Pulmonary Cyanosis)

After giving 100% oxygen for 10 minutes, a repeat arterial blood gas (ABG) is done and if PaO_2 is <150 mm Hg then the cause is cardiac and if the PaO_2 improves to >200 mm Hg, the cause is respiratory.

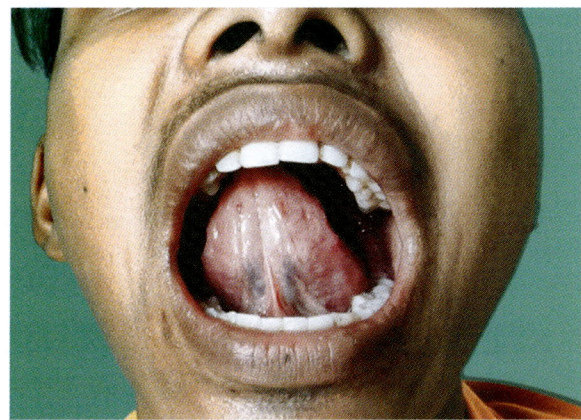

Fig. 2C.12: Demonstration of central cyanosis (in this patient mucosa is pink and lingual veins can be clearly demarcated, which is normal).

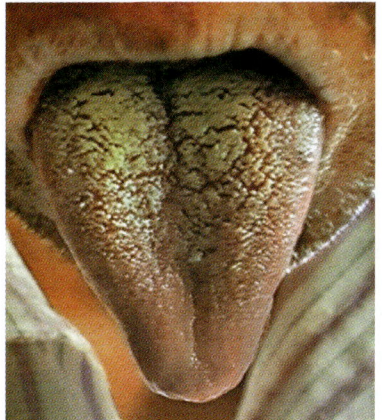

Fig. 2C.13: Bluish discoloration of tongue and oral mucosa suggestive of central cyanosis.

Iron Replete Cyanosis vs Iron Deplete Cyanosis

Iron replete cyanosis	Iron deplete cyanosis
It is compensated erythrocytosis which establishes equilibrium with hematocrit	It is decompensated erythrocytosis which fails to establish equilibrium with unstable, rising hematocrit
Iron replete cells are deformable	Iron deplete cells are less deformable
Hyper viscosity symptoms are rare	Hyper viscosity symptoms are frequent

Theories of Cyanosis

Admixture cyanosis	Secondary to shunts
Tardive cyanosis	Due to reversal of shunt (eisenmengerization)
Hypoxic cyanosis	Due to type 1 respiratory failure
Replacement cyanosis	Due to abnormal hemoglobins
Distributive cyanosis	Venous pooling of blood

CLUBBING (HIPPOCRATES FINGERS)

Definition

Selective bulbous enlargement of distal segment of digits with subsequent loss of normal angle between the nail and nail bed. Clubbing has three diagnostic features (**Fig. 2C.14**):

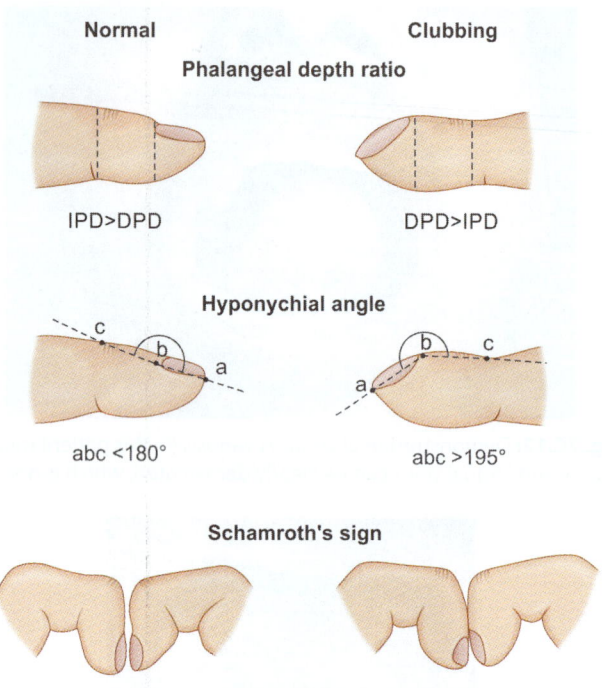

Fig. 2C.14: Demonstration of clubbing.

1. Loss of the hyponychial angle
2. Fluctuance of the nail
3. An abnormal phalangeal depth ratio

Theories of Clubbing

PDGF (role of platelet)	The megakaryocytes preferably lodge in the tips of the digits and locally release platelet derived growth factor (PDGF) and vascular endothelial growth factor (VEGF). These growth factors along with other mediators increase endothelial permeability and activate and cause proliferation of connective tissue cells (e.g., fibroblasts)
Neurogenic	Persistent vagal stimulation causes vasodilation and clubbing (e.g., lung carcinoma)
Hypoxic	Causes opening of deep arteriovenous fistula in fingers (e.g., tetralogy of Fallot)
• Ferritin • Prostaglandins • Bradykinin • Adenine nucleotides • 5-hydroxytryptamine	Circulating vasodilators, which are usually inactivated as blood passes through the lungs, bypass the inactivation process in the patients with right to left shunts

Grades of clubbing (Figs. 2C.15 to 2C.20)

Grade 1	Increased fluctuation of nail bed
Grade 2	• Loss of Lovibond angle/onychonychial angle (normal is <180°) • Profile sign • Schamroth sign
Grade 3	• Parrot beaking • Drumstick fingers (seen in severe cyanotic heart disease, bronchiectasis, and empyema)
Grade 4	• Pain along the distal ends of long bone due to subperiosteal new bone formation • Generally seen with bronchogenic carcinoma
Grade 5	Glossy changes in nails and adjacent skin with longitudinal striations (as proposed by Lung India)

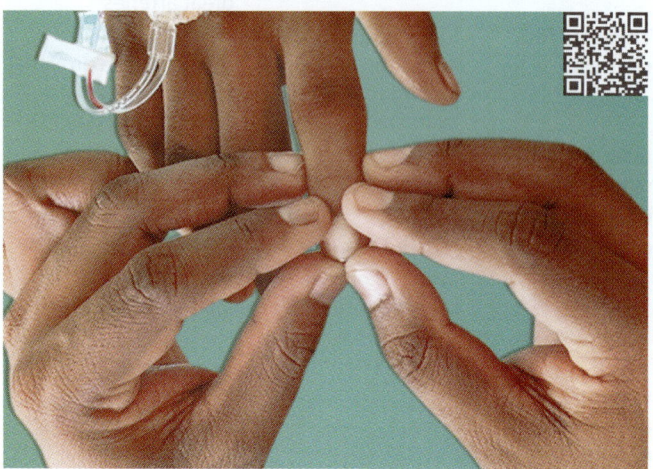

Fig. 2C.15: Demonstration of grade 1 clubbing.

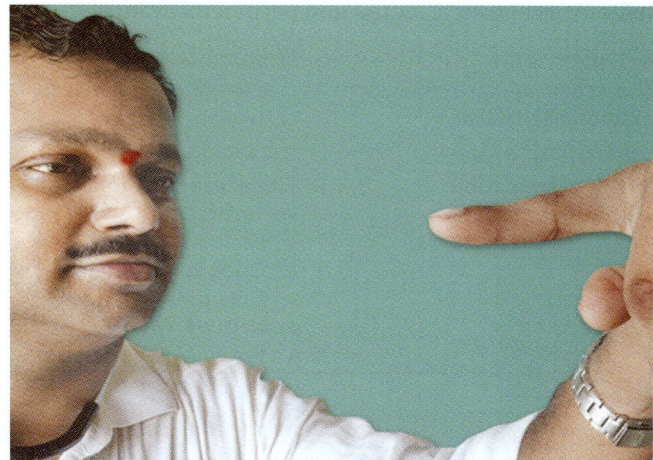

Fig. 2C.16: Demonstration of profile sign.

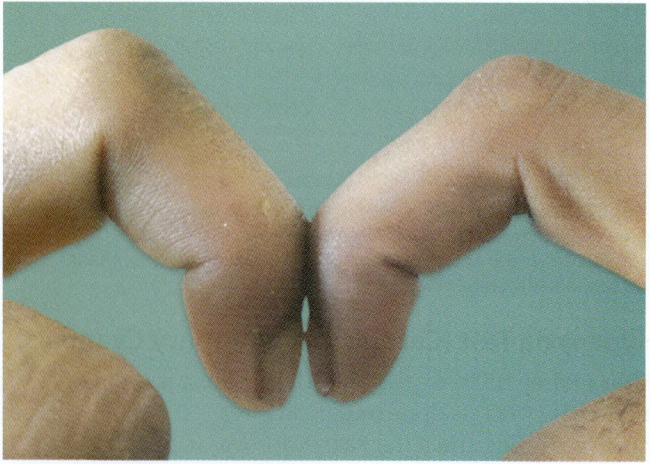

Fig. 2C.17: Demonstration of Schamroth's sign.

General Examination

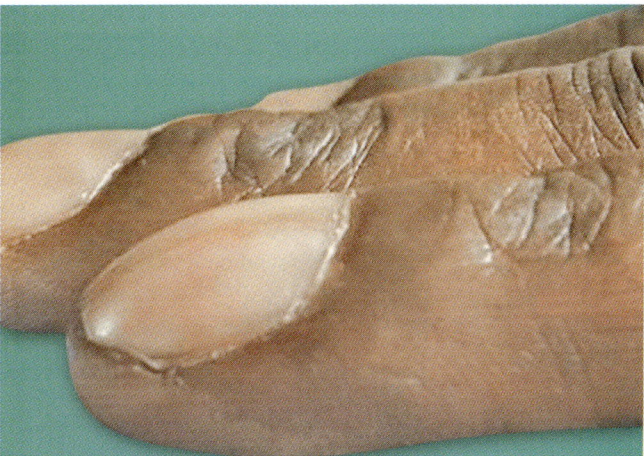

Fig. 2C.18: Demonstration of grade 3 clubbing.

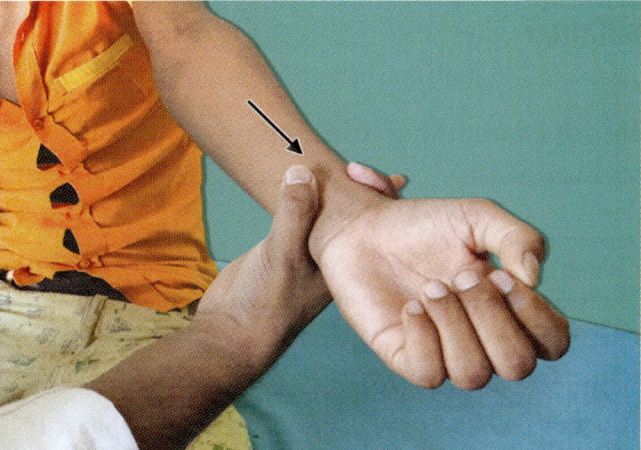

Fig. 2C.19: Demonstration of grade 4 clubbing.

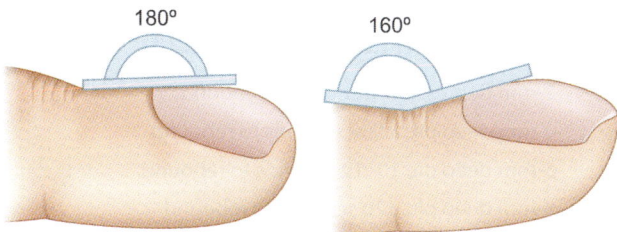

Lovibond's 'profile sign' Curth's modified profile sign

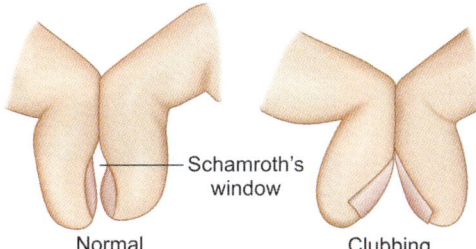

Schamroth's sign

Fig. 2C.20: Image depicting profile sign and Schamroth's sign.

Causes of clubbing	
Respiratory causes	
Malignancies	Bronchogenic carcinoma (30% cases) Mesothelioma
Suppurative diseases	Bronchiectasis Lung abscess Empyema
Interstitial lung disease (ILD) Pneumoconiosis	65% of cases
Tuberculosis	Seen in 30% cases as a sequela to complications
Sarcoidosis	Can be seen
Cardiac causes	
<ul><li>Subacute bacterial endocarditis</li><li>Atrial myxoma</li><li>Cyanotic heart disease</li><li>Acyanotic heart disease with eisenmengerization</li></ul>	
Gastrointestinal causes	
<ul><li>Inflammatory bowel disease (15–38%)</li><li>Ulcerative colitis</li><li>Crohn's disease</li><li>Primary biliary cirrhosis (24%)</li><li>Hepatocellular carcinoma</li><li>Chronic active hepatitis (29%)</li></ul>	
Neurological causes	
<ul><li>Syringomyelia</li><li>Median nerve injury</li><li>Hemiplegia</li></ul>	
Miscellaneous	
Pachydermoperiostosis (pan digital hereditary clubbing) Touraine-Solente-Gole syndrome	

Note: Chronic obstructive pulmonary disease (COPD) never causes clubbing.

Pachydermoperiostosis is associated with "spadelike" or "pawlike" enlargement of the hands and feet; joint effusions and skin changes (excessive sweating, generalized thickening (called pachyderma) and redundancy, especially over the forehead and scalp, leading to characteristic "bulldog" furrowing (cutis verticis gyrata) and leonine facies.

The "floating nail" sign: Normally, the root of the nail plate lies snugly against the bone of the distal phalanx; pressure on the root produces no movement. With clubbing, the root is separated from bone by connective tissue and edema; pressure upon the nail plate moves it toward the bone. The base of the nail becomes resilient and springy, and the nail feels as if it is floating on a cushion. As clubbing progresses, the nail becomes loosely attached, and the free edge of the nail plate may become visible or palpable as a horizontal ridge over the dorsal aspect of the finger.

Atypical presentation of clubbing	
Acute clubbing	<ul><li>Subacute bacterial endocarditis</li><li>Lung abscess</li><li>Empyema</li></ul>
Unilateral clubbing	<ul><li>Hemiplegia</li><li>Aneurysm of subclavian artery</li><li>Pancoast tumor</li></ul>

Contd...

Contd...

Pseudo clubbing	▪ Leprosy ▪ Leukemic infiltration ▪ Hyperparathyroidism ▪ Thyroid acropachy ▪ Sclerodactyly ▪ Exposure to vinyl chloride ▪ Subungual tumors or cysts
Painful clubbing	▪ Bronchogenic carcinoma ▪ Subacute bacterial endocarditis ▪ Lung abscess
Reversible clubbing	▪ Lung abscess ▪ Empyema
Unidigital clubbing	▪ Median nerve injury ▪ Trauma
Clubbing with cyanosis	▪ Cyanotic congenital heart diseases ▪ Interstitial lung disease
Differential clubbing: Upper limb (N) Lower limb (clubbing)	Patent ductus arteriosus (PDA) with reversal of shunt
Reverse differential clubbing: Upper limb (clubbing) Lower limb (N)	PDA + transposition of the great arteries (TGA) + reversal of shunt

Phalangeal Depth Ratio (Fig. 2C.21)

Ratio of distal phalangeal depth (DPD) with interphalangeal depth (IPD).
   <1 is normal, >1 is suggestive of clubbing.

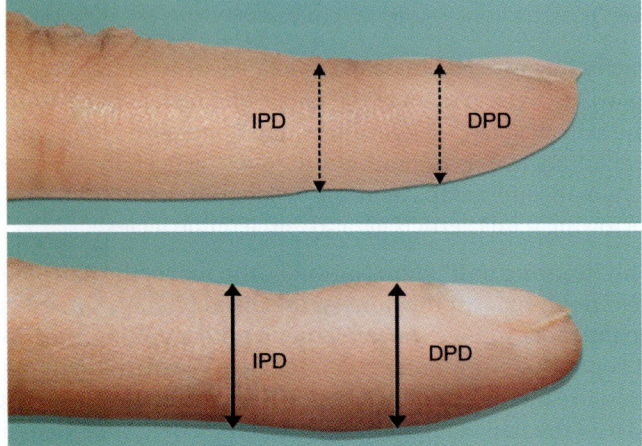

Fig. 2C.21: Picture depicting the phalangeal depth at proximal and distal interphalangeal joints.

Digital Index

Sum of phalangeal depth ratios of 10 fingers
   A digital index of 10.2 or higher is indicative of clubbing. Although, a phalangeal depth ratio of 1.0 or greater in any finger is suggestive of clubbing, digital index is more specific for clubbing.

Other Nail Changes

Nail changes	Causes
Koilonychia	▪ Iron deficiency anemia (IDA)–5.6% ▪ Hemochromatosis

Contd...

Contd...

Beaus' lines	▪ Measles ▪ Pneumonia ▪ Pulmonary infarction
Plummer nails	Seen in hyperthyroidism
Red nails	Congestive cardiac failure (CCF)
Blue nails	Copper or silver deposit
Black nails	▪ Peutz-Jegher's syndrome ▪ Cushing's disease ▪ Addison's disease
White nails	▪ Anemia ▪ Hypoalbuminemia ▪ Diabetes mellitus (DM) ▪ CCF ▪ Rheumatoid arthritis

EDEMA

Definition

Abnormal accumulation of fluid in the interstitium.

Sites of Examination of Edema

In mobile patient	Legs 2–3 cm above the medial malleolus
In bed ridden supine patient	▪ Sacrum ▪ Back over the scapula
To check for abdominal wall edema	Pinch the skin over the abdomen

Technique (Fig. 2C.22)

Press the skin and subcutaneous tissue for at least 15–20 seconds against a bony prominence (except for abdominal wall edema where we pinch the skin and subcutaneous tissue).

Grading of Pitting Edema (Fig. 2C.23)

1+	2-mm depression, immediate rebound
2+	4-mm deep pit, a few seconds to rebound
3+	6-mm deep pit, 10–12 seconds to rebound
4+	8-mm deep pit, >20 seconds to rebound

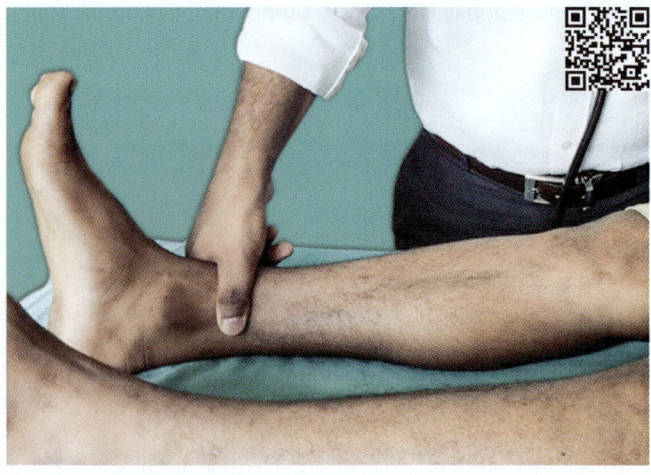

Fig. 2C.22: Method of eliciting pedal edema.

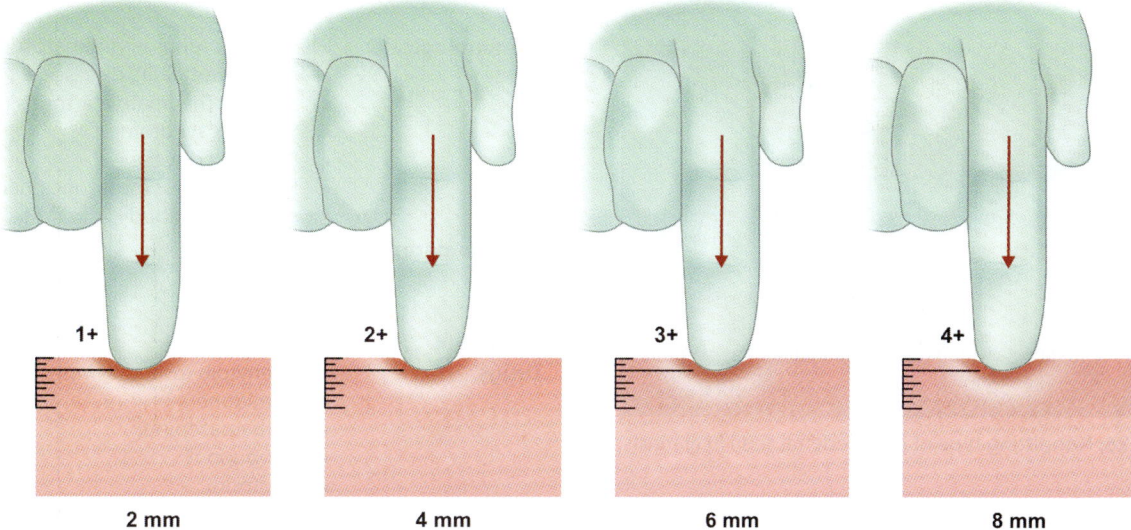

Fig. 2C.23: Grading of pitting edema.

Edema		
Pitting with rapid recovery	Pitting with slow recovery	Nonpitting (Brawny edema)
Recovers in <40 seconds	Recovery takes >40 seconds	▪ Does not pit or recover in few seconds ▪ Nontender ▪ Skin shows hyperkeratosis
Mechanism: ↑oncotic pressure Low serum protein	**Mechanism:** ↑hydrostatic pressure (N) serum protein	**Mechanism:** Lymphedema Lymphatic obstruction
Causes: **Increased protein loss** ▪ Burns ▪ Nephrotic syndrome ▪ Bowel disease **Decreased intake or synthesis** ▪ Kwashiorkor ▪ Malabsorption ▪ Liver disease	**Causes:** ▪ Systemic venous hypertension (HTN) ▪ Congestive heart failure (CHF) **(Fig. 2C.24)** ▪ Pericarditis ▪ Tricuspid valve diseases **Local venous HTN** ▪ Deep venous thrombosis (DVT) ▪ Inferior vena cava syndrome	**Causes:** Myxedema (Fig. 2C.25)—hypothyroidism **Pretibial myxedema**—Graves's disease **Upper limb** ▪ Breast cancer ▪ Radiation induced **Lower limb** ▪ Aplasia cutis ▪ Congenital (praecox, tarda, milroy's disease, and Meigs disease) ▪ Filariasis **(Fig. 2C.26)** ▪ Recurred streptococcal infection ▪ Malignancies
Facial edema: Trichinosis, hypothyroidism, allergies, nephrotic syndrome, and angioedema (Quincke's edema) **Neurogenic edema:** Secondary to autonomic dysfunction **Drug-induced edema:** Nifedipine, corticosteroids, estrogen, nonsteroidal anti-inflammatory drugs (NSAIDs), and insulin ▪ **May-Thurner syndrome**—chronic, unilateral, pitting edema due to compression of the left iliac vein by the right common iliac artery against the lumbar spine ▪ **Idiopathic edema**—chronic bilateral and pitting. Seen in females <50 age, more during menstrual cycles.		

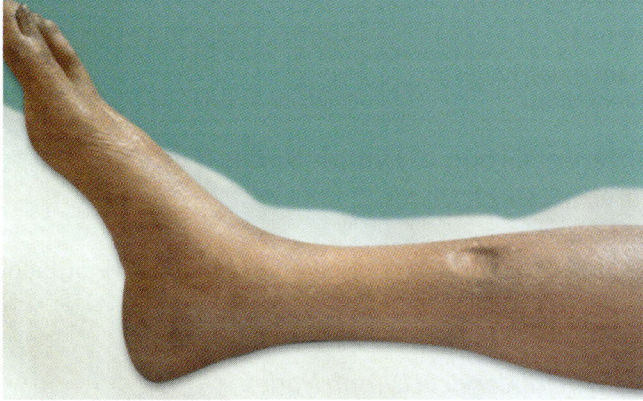

Fig. 2C.24: Pitting type of pedal edema seen in congestive cardiac failure.

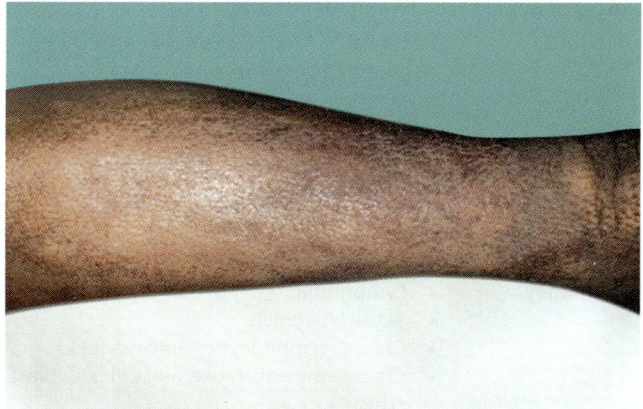

Fig. 2C.25: Nonpitting type of pedal edema seen in myxedema.

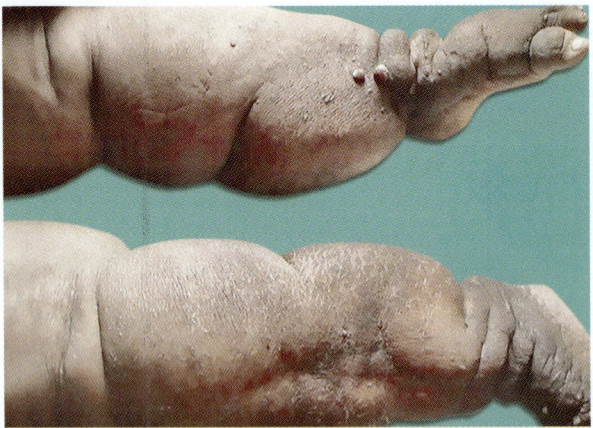

Fig. 2C.26: Nonpitting type of pedal edema seen in filariasis.

LYMPHADENOPATHY

Definitions

Generalized Lymphadenopathy

Generalized lymphadenopathy is defined as involvement of ≥2 noncontiguous lymph node groups and is typically indicative of systemic disease.

Significant lymphadenopathy (based on Size, Fixity and Consistency)

Size >2 cm in	Inguinal region
Size >1 cm in	Extrainguinal region
Any size	- Supraclavicular - Epitrochlear - Popliteal - Any lymph node with a lesion in the draining area
Based on fixity	- Fixed to each other (matting) - Fixed to underlying tissues - Fixed to skin
Based on consistency	- Hard/firm lymph nodes

Persistent Generalized Lymphadenopathy

It is defined as lymph nodes of more than **1** cm in size, in **2** or more areas persisting for **3** or more months (mnemonic **1-2-3**). Seen in human immunodeficiency virus/acquired immune deficiency syndrome (HIV/AIDS).

Causes of generalized lymphadenopathy		
Infections	Bacterial	- Disseminated TB - Secondary syphilis
	Viral	- HIV - Infectious mononucleosis
	Parasitic	- Toxoplasmosis
	Fungal	- Histoplasmosis - Coccidioidomycosis - Paracoccidioidomycosis
Malignancy		- Lymphomas - Acute leukemias - Chronic lymphocytic leukemia (CLL) - Chronic myeloid leukemia (CML) (in blast crisis)

Contd...

Immunological	- Systemic lupus erythematosus (SLE) - Adult-onset Still's disease - Juvenile rheumatoid arthritis (JRA) - Sjogren's syndrome - Kawasaki disease - Serum sickness (post zone phenomenon—excess of antibody)
Granulomatous	- Sarcoidosis - Amyloidosis - Histiocytosis X
Endocrine	Hyperthyroidism
Drugs	- Phenytoin (pseudolymphoma) - Primidone - Carbamazepine - Allopurinol - Captopril - Cotrimoxazole - Sulindac (NSAIDs) - Hydralazine - Beta-blockers
Syndromic lymphadenopathy	- Kikuchi-Fujimoto disease - Castleman's disease - Kimura disease - Rosai–Dorfman syndrome - Familial mediterranean fever
Miscellaneous	Niemann-Pick disease

Describing a Lymph Node

1. Size (significant or not)
2. Site
3. Number
4. Consistency
5. Overlying skin
6. Mobility
7. Tenderness
8. Draining area.

Consistency

Soft	Normal consistency
Hard	Malignancy
Indian rubber	Hodgkin's lymphoma
Shotty lymph node	Syphilis
Bubo (large node with central necrosis)	Lymphogranuloma venereum
Matted	Tuberculosis **(due to periadenitis)**
Hard lymph nodes in tuberculosis	Hyperplastic tuberculosis lymphadenopathy

Different Group of Lymph Nodes (Fig. 2C.27)

Cervical Lymph Nodes

Divided into:
- Superficial or deep (based on whether above or below deep cervical fascia)
- Vertical or horizontal

Superficial Cervical Lymph Nodes

They are superficial to deep cervical fascia. They include:

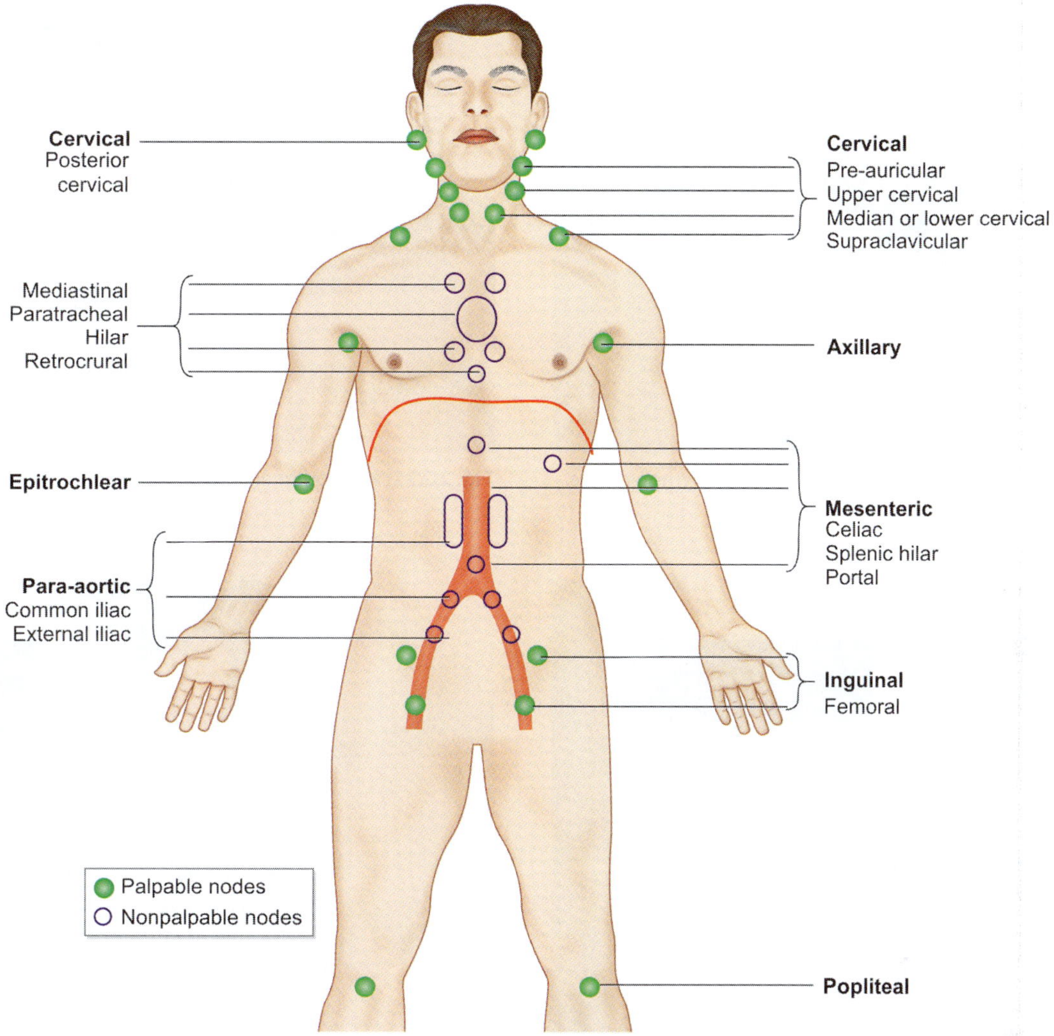

Fig. 2C.27: Image showing different groups of lymph nodes.

- External Waldeyer Ring
  - Submental
  - Submandibular bilateral
  - Preauricular bilateral
  - Postauricular bilateral
  - Occipital lymph nodes.
- Pretracheal
- Paratracheal
- Posterior triangle lymph nodes.

Deep Cervical Lymph Nodes
- **Horizontal:** Supraclavicular lymph nodes
- **Vertical:** Jugulodigastric and jugulo-omohyoid lymph nodes.

Examination of Cervical Lymph Nodes

Examination of anterior group of lymph nodes is done by standing behind the patient → flex the neck to relax the fascia → first feel for the submental group (using a single finger) **(Fig. 2C.28)** and then → bilateral submandibular **(Fig. 2C.29)** → bilateral preauricular **(Fig. 2C.30)** → jugulodigastric **(Fig. 2C.31)** → jugulo-omohyoid **(Fig. 2C.32)** → supraclavicular groups **(Fig. 2C.33)** (± pre- and paratracheal).

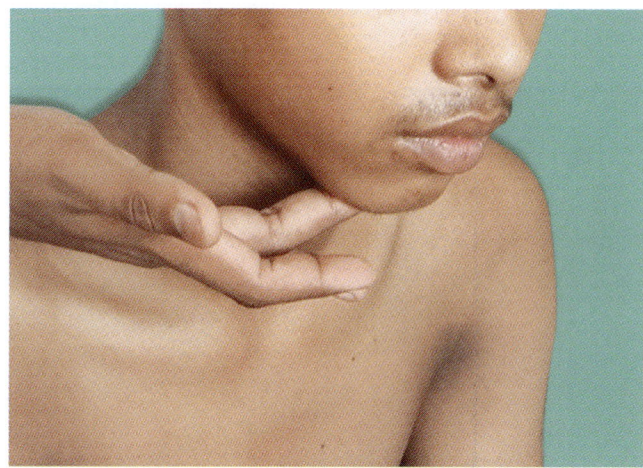

Fig. 2C.28: Method of examining submental group of lymph node.

Examination of posterior group of lymph nodes is done by standing in front of the patient → feel for the post auricular **(Fig. 2C.34)** → occipital **(Fig. 2C.35)** → posterior triangle group of lymph nodes **(Fig. 2C.36)**.

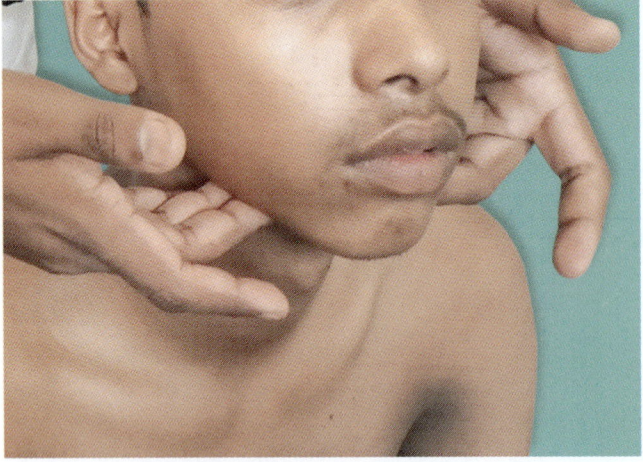

Fig. 2C.29: Method of examining submandibular lymph nodes.

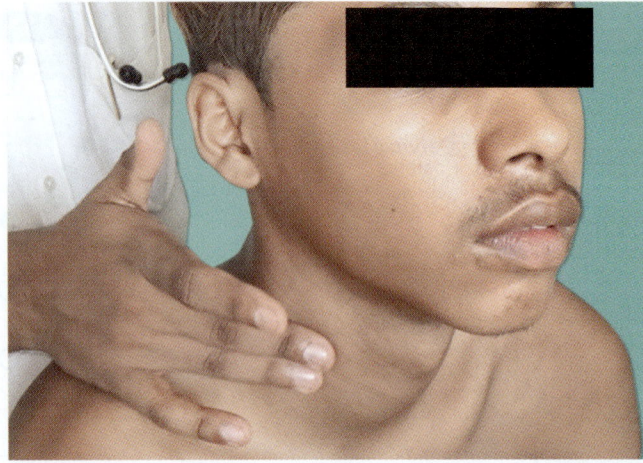

Fig. 2C.32: Method of examining jugulo-omohyoid lymph nodes.

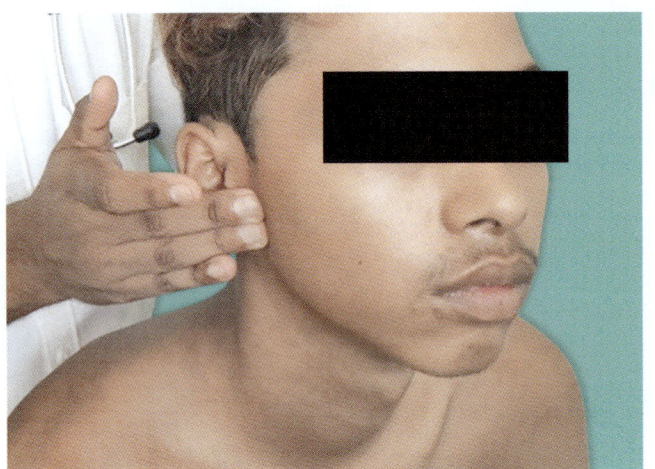

Fig. 2C.30: Method of examining preauricular lymph nodes.

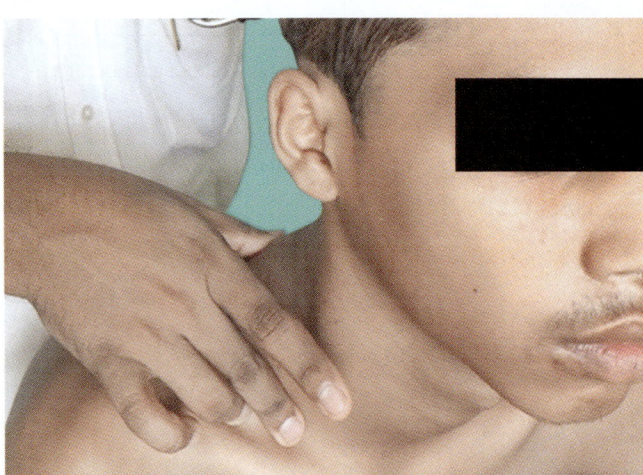

Fig. 2C.33: Method of examining supraclavicular lymph nodes.

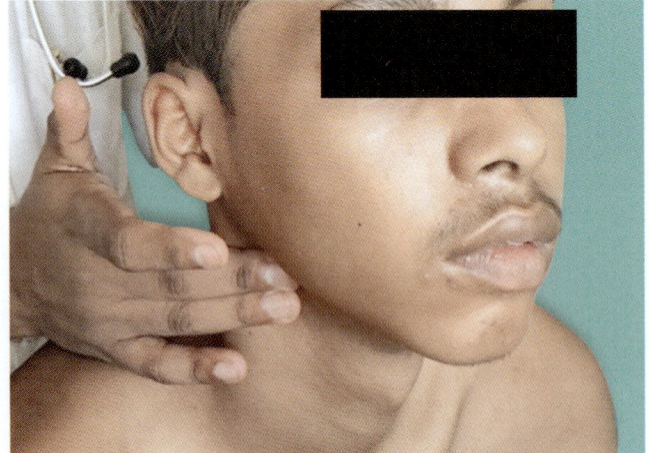

Fig. 2C.31: Method of examining jugulodigastric lymph nodes.

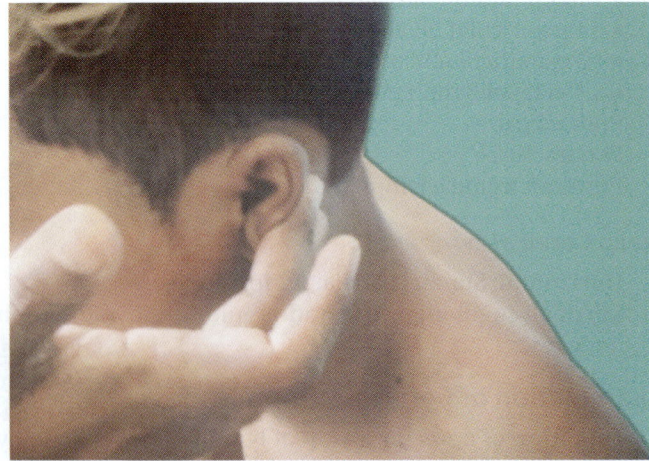

Fig. 2C.34: Method of examining postauricular lymph nodes.

General Examination

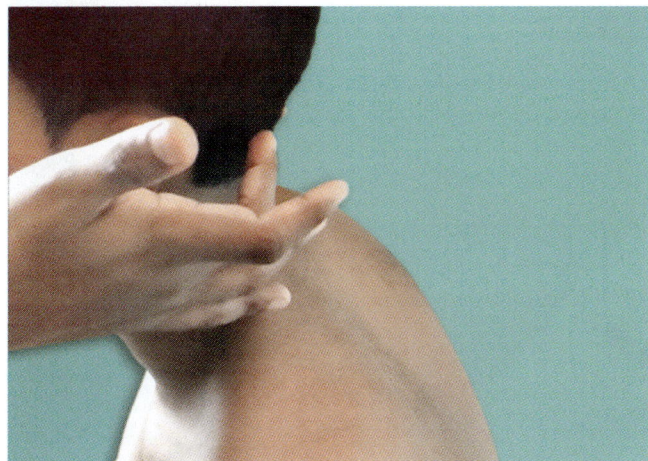

Fig. 2C.35: Method of examining occipital lymph nodes.

Other named lymph nodes	
Virchow node	Left supraclavicular node
Scalene node (Fig. 2C.37)	<ul><li>Sentinel node of bronchogenic carcinoma</li><li>Relax neck</li><li>Palpate (deep) between the two heads of SCM</li></ul>
Winterbottom sign	<ul><li>Posterior triangle lymph node enlargement</li><li>Seen in early phase of African trypanosomiasis</li></ul>
Causes of posterior triangle lymph node enlargement	<ul><li>Scalp infection</li><li>Measles</li><li>Rubella</li><li>Infectious mononucleosis</li><li>Trypanosomiasis</li></ul>
Node of Woods	Jugulodigastric lymph node enlargement seen in TB when spread via tonsils
Delphian node	Pretracheal node
External Waldeyer ring	Commonly seen to be enlarged in non-Hodgkin's lymphoma
Berry's node	Jugulo-omohyoid lymph nodes seen in thyroid malignancy

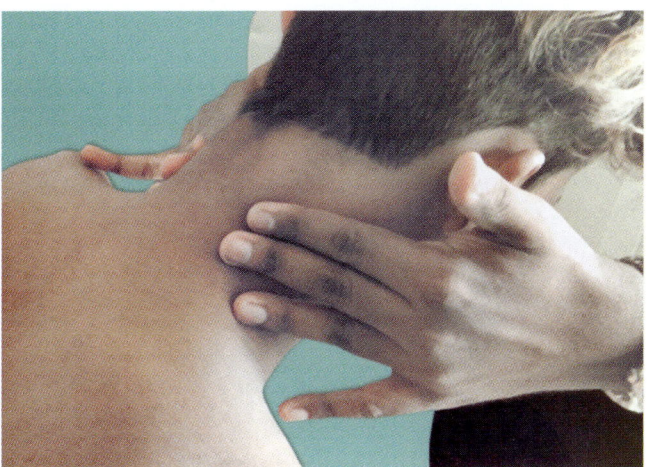

Fig. 2C.36: Method of examining posterior triangle lymph nodes.

Supraclavicular Lymph Nodes and Drainage

Right supraclavicular	Left supraclavicular
Right lung (all three lobes) Left lung lower lobe	Left lung upper lobe
	4 B's and Gonads: 1. Breast 2. Bronchus 3. Bowel 4. Bladder, and gonads (testis/ovaries)
Note: **Mechanism of left supraclavicular lymphadenopathy** in GI and other malignancies—reflux of tumor cells from the thoracic duct into left supraclavicular node at the junction of thoracic duct and left subclavian	
Trousseau sign of tetany: Carpopedal spasms **Trousseaus syndrome:** Migratory thrombophlebitis in malignancy **Troisier's sign:** Enlarged hard left supraclavicular lymph node (Virchow's node).	

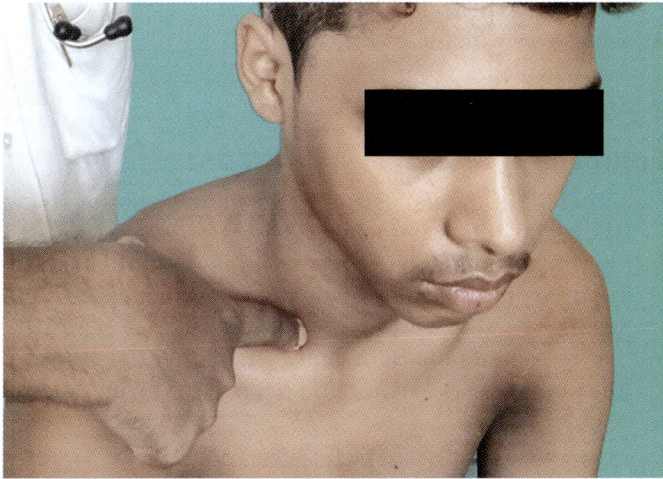

Fig. 2C.37: Method of examining scalene lymph nodes.

Axillary Group of Lymph Nodes

There are five axillary lymph node groups. Lymph nodes include:
1. Lateral (humeral)
2. Anterior (pectoral)
3. Posterior (subscapular)
4. Central
5. Apical nodes

Central and Apical Nodes

The apical nodes are the final common pathway for all of the axillary lymph nodes.

Note: Examine the right axillary lymph nodes with the left hand except for humeral (lateral) group (which is examined with right hand).

Examination of Right Axillary Lymph Nodes (Figs. 2C.38 to 2C.47)

```
Hyperabduct the right arm of patient
         ↓
Place the right forearm of patient on your left forearm
         ↓
Insinuate your left hand fingertips deep in axilla of patient
         ↓
Using your right hand to apply pressure over the patient's shoulder,
feel for the apical lymph nodes using your left hand
         ↓
Central group can be felt just below the apical group
         ↓
Anterior group can be felt on the anterior axillary fold
         ↓
Posterior group can be felt on the posterior axillary fold
         ↓
Lateral group is felt with examiner's right hand by palpating
over the patient's humerus
```

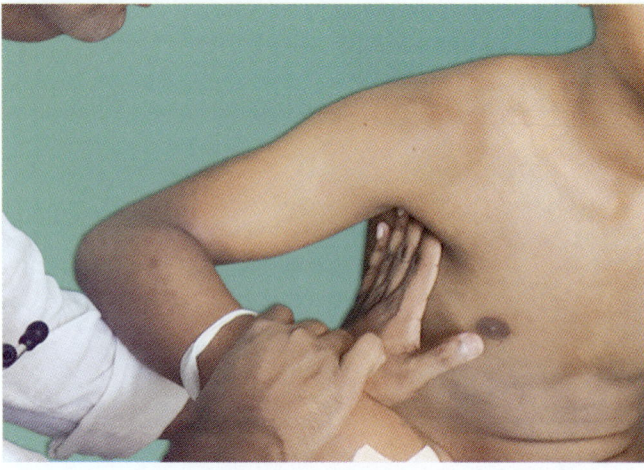

Fig. 2C.39: Method of examining right central group (axillary) lymph nodes.

Drainage areas of axillary lymph nodes:
1. Chest wall with breast
2. Parietal pleura
3. Upper limb.

Epitrochlear Group of Lymph Nodes

- Situated on medial aspect of the elbow, about 4–5 cm above the humeral trochlea.
- Epitrochlear station drains the lymph from the last two or three fingers and from the medial aspect of the hand itself.
- For examining the right elbow—rest the right elbow of the patient on the right-hand palm of the examiner and

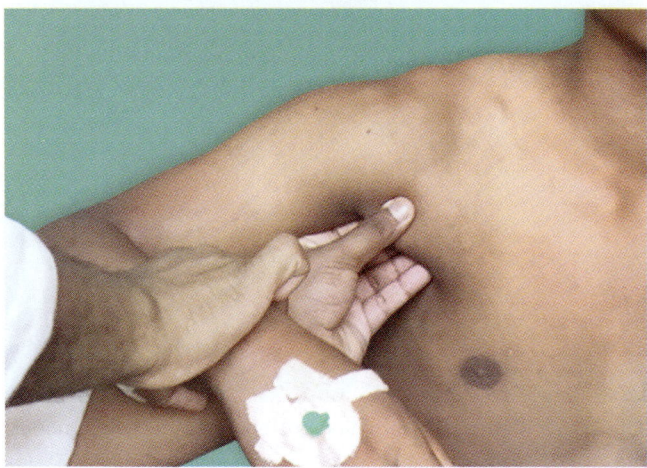

Fig. 2C.40: Method of examining right anterior group (axillary) lymph nodes.

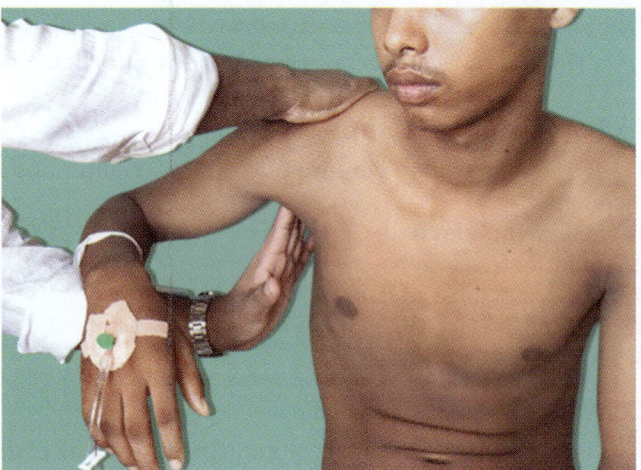

Fig. 2C.38: Method of examining right apical group (axillary) lymph nodes.

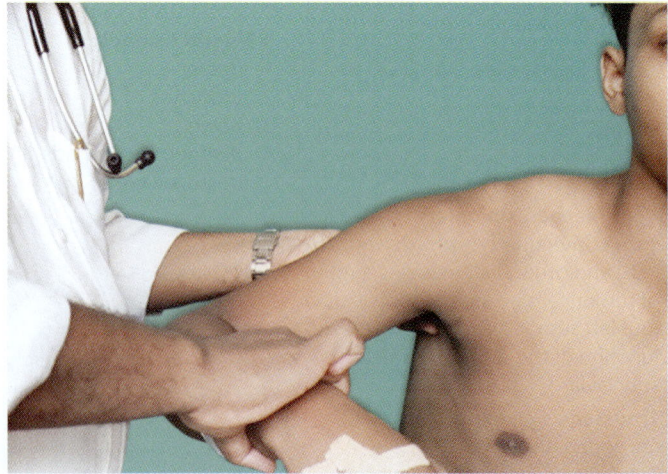

Fig. 2C.41: Methods of examining right posterior group (axillary) lymph nodes.

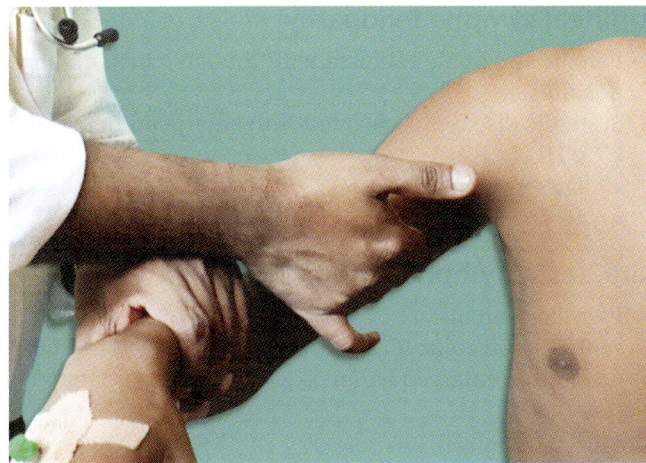

Fig. 2C.42: Method of examining right lateral group (axillary) lymph nodes.

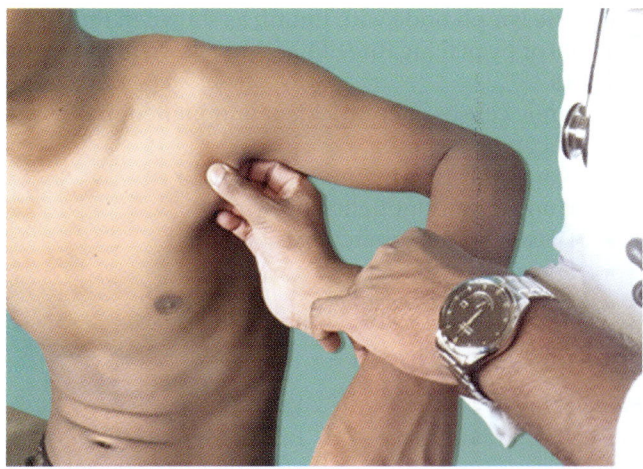

Fig. 2C.45: Method of examining left anterior group (axillary) lymph nodes.

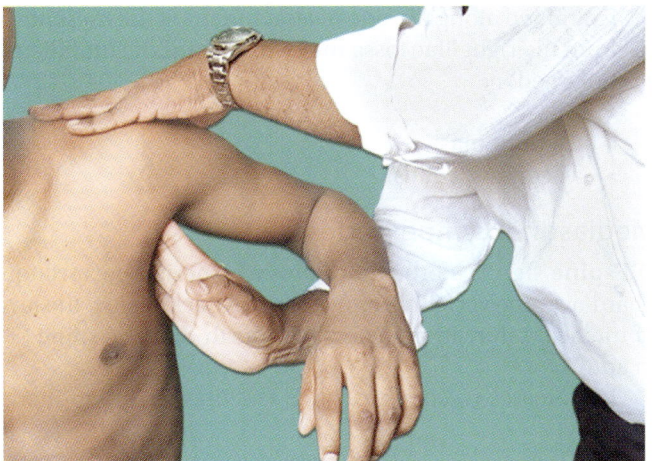

Fig. 2C.43: Method of examining left apical group (axillary) lymph nodes.

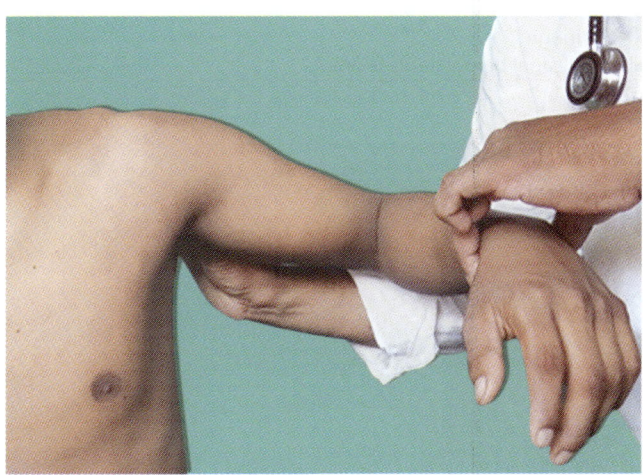

Fig. 2C.46: Method of examining left posterior group (axillary) lymph nodes.

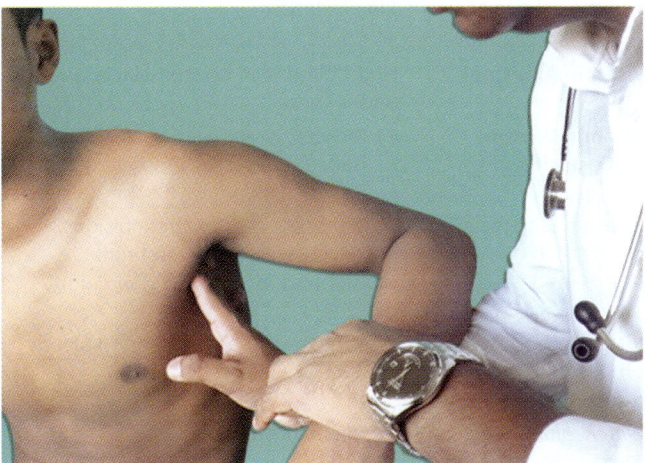

Fig. 2C.44: Method of examining left central group (axillary) lymph nodes.

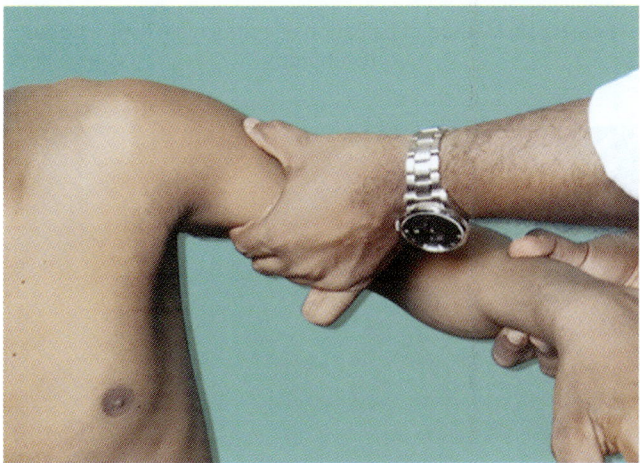

Fig. 2C.47: Method of examining left lateral group (axillary) lymph nodes.

feel the lymph node with thumb as shown in the **Figure 2C.48** or by placing three fingers as shown in the **Figure 2C.49**.

- Systemic causes of epitrochlear lymphadenopathy:
  - Secondary syphilis
  - Non-Hodgkin's lymphoma (NHL)
  - Human immunodeficiency virus
  - Disseminated tuberculosis
  - Sporotrichosis
  - Cat scratch disease.

Inguinal Lymph Nodes

Horizontal group	Vertical group
Palpated along the inguinal ligament	Palpated vertically downwards from the midpoint of inguinal ligament
Drains: • External genitalia • Scrotum • Perineum • Anal canal below dentate line	**Drains:** • Lower limb

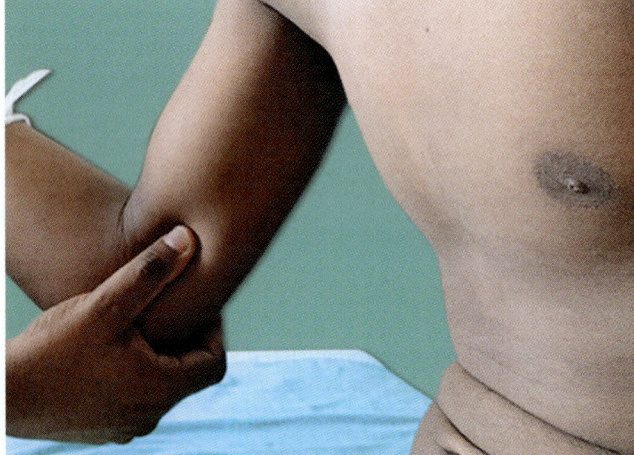

Fig. 2C.48: Method of palpation of epitrochlear lymph nodes (by thumb).

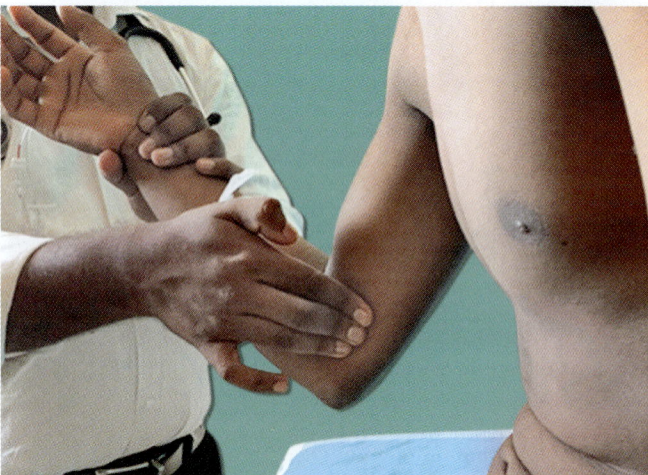

Fig. 2C.49: Method of palpation of epitrochlear lymph nodes (by three fingers).

Popliteal Lymphadenopathy

- Palpate the popliteal fossa with the knee in semi flexed position
- Systemic diseases associated with enlargement include:
  - NHL
  - Disseminated TB
  - HIV.

Para-aortic Lymphadenopathy

- Relax abdomen.
- With 2 hands placed over the epigastrium—one should feel for the enlarged lymph nodes by deep palpation.
- Enlarged in:
  - Lymphomas
  - Testicular malignancies
  - Tuberculosis.

Mesenteric Lymph Nodes

- Examined along the line of attachment of the mesentery, from the right iliac fossa medially toward the umbilicus.
- Enlarged in:
  - HIV
  - Lymphomas
  - Ulcerative colitis.

Mediastinal Lymph Nodes

D'Espine sign is a bronchophony/whispering pectoriloquy heard over the vertebral spines (on the back) below the level of tracheal bifurcation; below the fourth thoracic spine (T_4) in adults.

It indicates tracheobronchial (mediastinal) lymphadenopathy.

NUTRITIONAL ASSESSMENT

Nutritional deficiencies	
Vitamin deficiency	*Manifestation*
Fat-soluble vitamins	
Vitamin A, retinol	Night blindness, keratomalacia, and Bitot's spots
Vitamin D, ergo/cholecalciferol	• Rickets/osteomalacia • Bone pain, costochondral beading • Proximal myopathy
Vitamin E, tocopherol	Hemolysis, posterior column signs, ataxia, muscle wasting, retinitis pigmentosa-like changes, and night blindness
Vitamin K, phylloquinone, and other menaquinones	Bruising, purpura, nose, and GI bleeds
Water-soluble vitamin (B-complex and vitamin C)	
B_1 **(Thiamine)**	• Wernicke/Korsakoff • Beriberi • Nystagmus • Sixth cranial nerve palsy • Ataxia • Acidosis

Contd...

Contd...

	- Dementia - Paresthesiae - Neuropathy - Cardiac failure - Anemia
B$_2$ (Riboflavin)	- Ariboflavinosis - Angular stomatitis, glossitis, and magenta tongue
B$_3$ (Niacin)	- Pellagra - Dermatitis on sun-exposed areas - Dementia - Poor appetite, difficulty sleeping - Confusion, sore mouth
B$_4$ (Adenine)*	- Immune dysfunction - Aging
B$_5$ (Pantothenic acid)	- Nausea - Abdominal pain - Paresthesiae, burning feet
B$_6$ (Pyridoxine)	- Poor appetite - Lassitude - Oxaluria
B$_7$ (Biotin)	Dermatitis Depression, lassitude Muscle pains Electrocardiogram abnormalities, blepharitis
B$_8$ (Inositol)*	Depression and other psychiatric manifestations
B$_9$ (folic acid)	Macrocytic anemia Thrombocytopenia Megaloblastic bone marrow
B$_{10}$ (PABA)*	- Free radical damage - Sun burns and skin rashes
B$_{11}$ (salicylic acid)*	Works in tandem with vitamin B$_{12}$
B$_{12}$ (cobalamin)	- Subacute combined degeneration of spinal cord - Macrocytic anemia, icterus, knuckle pigmentation

Contd...

Contd...

Vitamin C (ascorbic acid)	- Scurvy - Poor wound healing, fatigue, limb pain, scorbutic rosary - Difficulty sleeping, gingivitis, perifollicular purpura - Hyperkeratosis
Minerals	
Iron	- Koilonychia - Smooth tongue - Anemia - Esophageal web
Copper	- Microcytic hypochromic anemia - Neutropenia - Scurvy-like bone lesions, osteoporosis
Minerals	
Zinc	- Acrodermatitis enteropathica - Peristomal/perinasal/perineal - Erythema, thin hair - Diarrhea, apathy, anorexia - Growth failure - Hypoglycemia - Distorted or diminished taste (hypogeusia)
Chromium	Peripheral neuropathy, hyperglycemia
Selenium	Cardiomyopathy
Iodine	Goiter
Others	
Protein deficiency	- Pitting edema - Hair: Thinning, easily pluck able with dyspigmentation or flag sign, and change in texture to silken, sparse hair - Dermatosis with desquamation of the so-called flaky-paint type with or without hyperpigmentation

*Vitamin B$_{4,8,10 \text{ and } 11}$ are no longer labeled as vitamins, as they do not fit the official definition of vitamin.

NAIL CHANGES

Various nail changes are shown in **Figure 2C.50**.

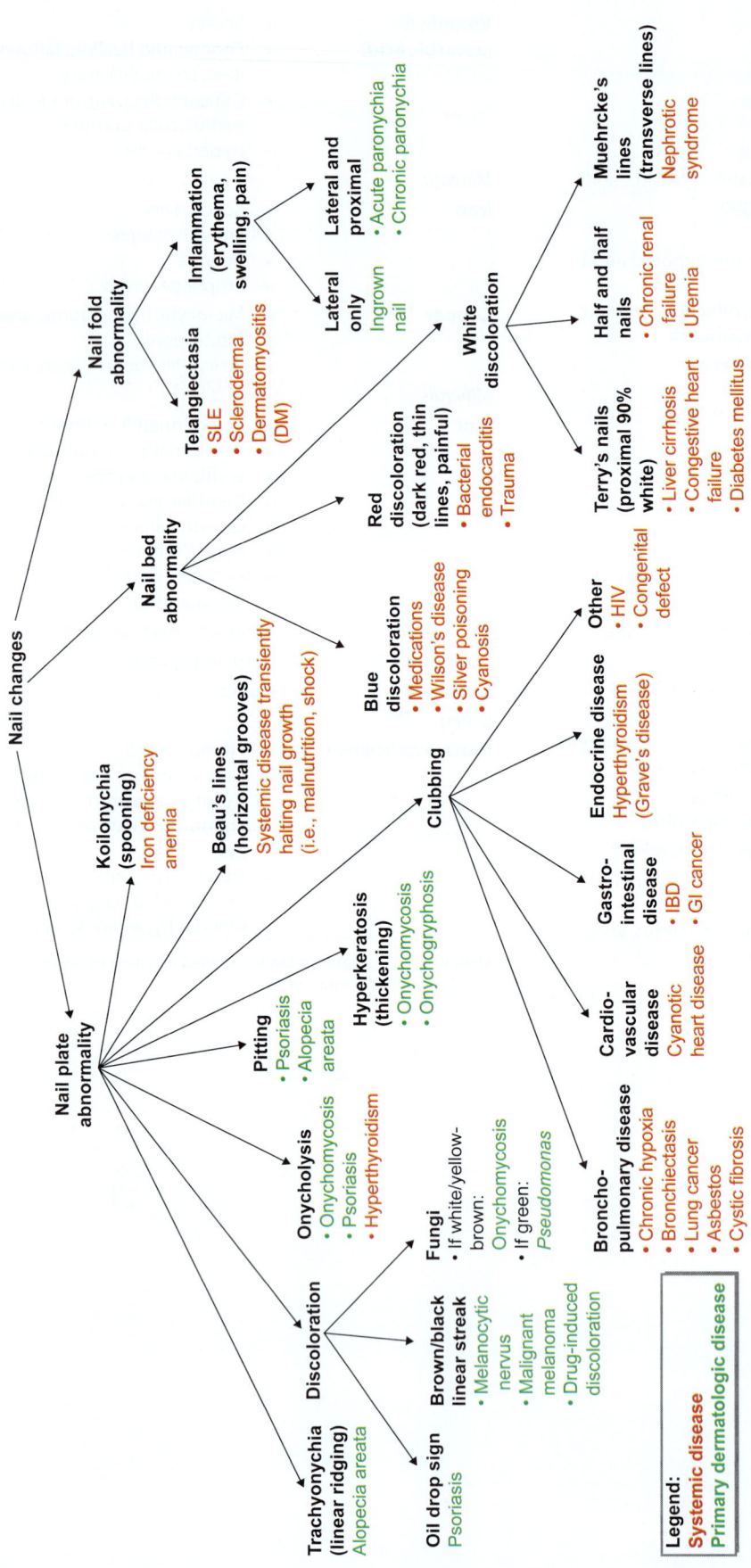

Fig. 2C.50: Common nail changes.

D. ANTHROPOMETRY

HEIGHT

Method of Measurement of Length/Height

- Recumbent length **(Fig. 2D.1)** is measured using an infantometer with a fixed head piece and horizontal backboard, and an adjustable foot piece. The **recorder supports the child's head** while the **examiner positions the feet** and ensures that the head lies in the Frankfort horizontal plane.
- Standing height **(Fig. 2D.2)** is an assessment of maximum vertical size. This stature measurement is collected on all sample persons (SPs) aged 2 years and older who are able to stand unassisted. Standing height is measured using a stadiometer with a fixed vertical backboard and an adjustable headpiece. Instruct the SP to stand with the **heels together and toes apart**. The toes should point slightly outward at approximately a 60°angle. Check that the back of the **head, shoulder blades, buttocks, and heels make contact with the backboard**.

Short Stature

Short stature is defined as a height that is below the 2.5th percentile or two or more standard deviations below the mean for age and gender for a given population. A growth velocity that is below the 5th percentile for age and gender is called growth deceleration (e.g., <5 cm/year after the age of 5 years). Dwarfism is defined as short stature for the age of the patient. Most common causes of dwarfism are familial short stature and constitutional delay of growth and puberty.

Cause of short stature	
Constitutional (hereditary)	- Gurkhas, African pygmies
Endocrine	- Cretin (ratio between upper and lower segments is ≤1 with mental retardation) - Pituitary dwarf (short limbed, normal intelligence but may be associated with infantilism) - Froehlich's syndrome (obese, diabetes insipidus, hypogonadism) - Cushing syndrome
Genetic	- Turner syndrome - Noonan syndrome - Hurler's syndrome - Morquio's syndrome - Multiple lentigines syndrome
Skeletal	- Ellis–Van Creveld syndrome (chondrodystrophic dysplasia, short arms, and legs) - Achondroplasia (short and bowed legs and arms, waddling gait) - Osteogenesis imperfecta
Acquired (in children)	- Rickets - Pott's spine

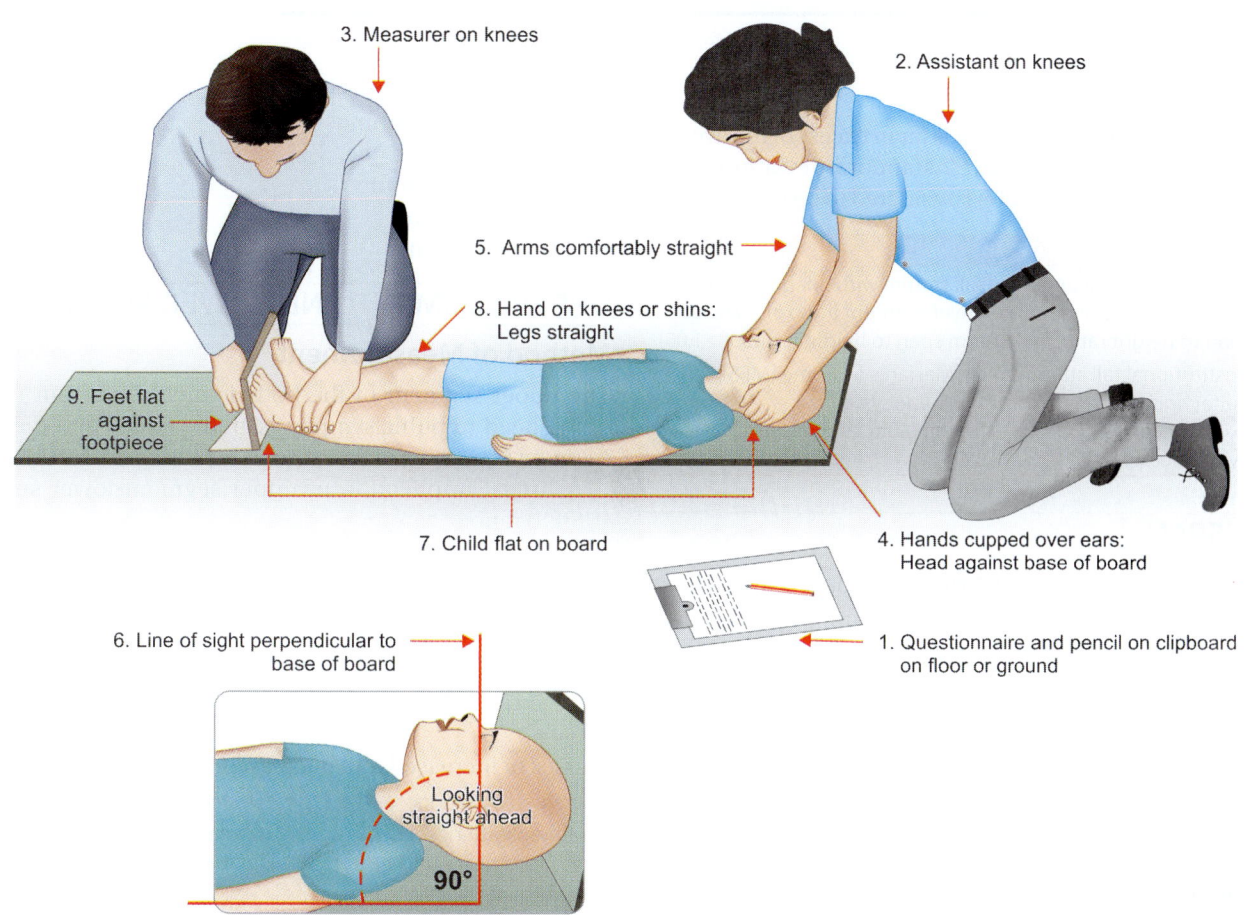

Fig. 2D.1: Measurement of recumbent length.

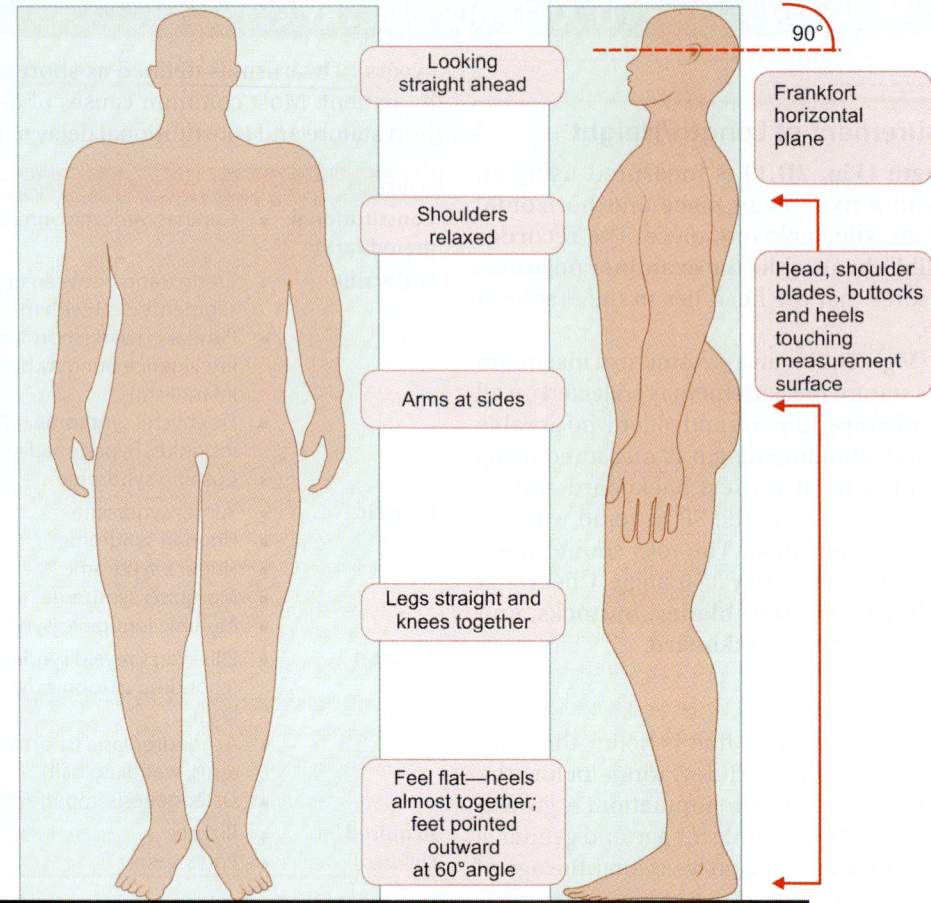

Fig. 2D.2: Measurement of vertical height.

Tall Stature

When the height of an individual is far in excess of the average normal for the age and race (≥2 standard deviation of the mean height), the individual is considered to be tall in stature.

Causes of tall stature	
Tall stature with equal upper and lower segments or equal arm span to height ratio	Tall stature with unequal upper to lower segment (ratio of ≤0.8) or arm span to height (ratio of ≥1.05)
<ul><li>Constitutional tall stature</li><li>Pituitary giants</li><li>Sexual precocity</li><li>Thyrotoxicosis</li></ul>	<ul><li>Marfan syndrome (MFS)</li><li>Homocystinuria</li><li>Klinefelter's syndrome</li></ul>

ARM SPAN

Method of Measurement of Arm Span

It is the distance between the tips of the middle fingers of one hand to the other when held abducted in horizontal plane. The arm span to height ratio is normally equal or ≤1.05.

Clinical implication of arm span vs height ratio:

Age	Ratio
At birth	The arm span is typically less than length (by at least 2.5 cm)
10 years of age in boys and 12 years of age in girls	The arm span exceeds height

Cause of increased arm span-height ratio:
- Klinefelter syndrome
- Homocystinuria
- Marfan's syndrome
- Sotos syndrome
- Hypogonadism

UPPER SEGMENT AND LOWER SEGMENT

Method of Measurement

The upper segment of the body is measured from the top of the head to pubic symphysis/pubic ramus and the lower segment is measured from the pubic ramus to the floor.

Clinical implication of upper segment-lower segment (US:LS) ratio:

Age	Ratio
Birth	1.7
3 years	1.33
5 years	1.17
10 years	1.0
>10 years	<1.0

Causes of increased and decreased US:LS ratio:

Increased US:LS ratio	Decreased US:LS ratio
Children with rickets, achondroplasia, and turner syndrome (because of decreased limb length)	Marfan syndrome (because of increased limb length)

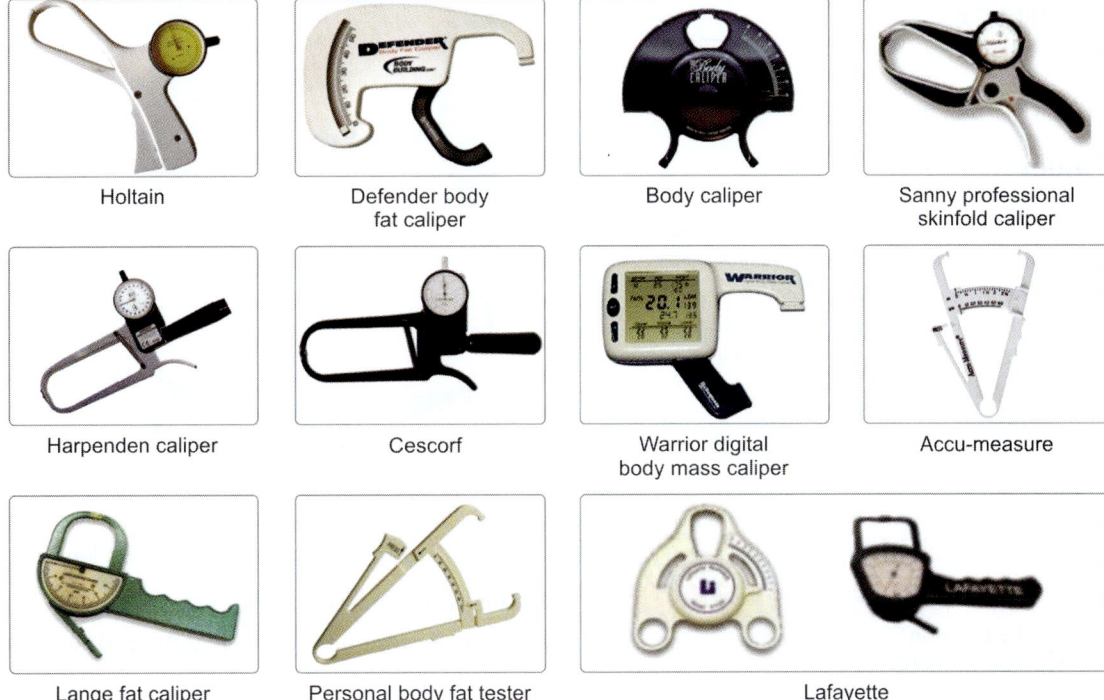

Fig. 2D.3: Different types of skinfold calipers.

SKINFOLD THICKNESS

Method of Measurement

- Approximately half of the total amount of fat tissue in the human body is located below the surface of the skin.
- This makes it possible to predict total body fat from skinfold thicknesses with a relative high degree of accuracy using a simple two-compartmental method.
- This accuracy is confirmed by CT scan as well as ultrasonic and radiographic techniques used to measure subcutaneous fat.
- In general, when measuring skinfold thickness. The assessor, using the forefinger and the thumb, grasps and lifts the subcutaneous tissue and skin from the underlying muscle.
- Places the pincers of the skinfold caliper (**Fig. 2D.3**) applying a constant pressure, 2 cm below the fingers at a depth of 1 cm.
- Holds this position for 3–4 seconds.
- Takes three measurements for accuracy.
- Provides the actual skinfold thickness in mm.

Triceps Skinfold (TSF) (Fig. 2D.4)

- A measure of subcutaneous fat stores taken at the midpoint of the posterior aspect of the humerus.
- Correlates closely with percentage of body fat and with total body fat.
- Triceps skinfold thickness varies between 6 mm and 12 mm in lean individuals and between 40 mm and 50 mm in obese individuals.
- Subject should be **standing** with **arms hanging loosely** at the sides.

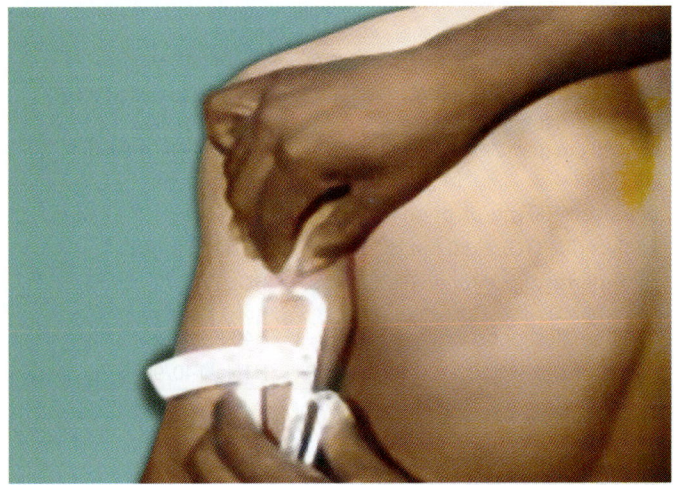

Fig. 2D.4: Triceps skinfold (TSF).

- Assessor to be positioned behind the subject.
- To locate the triceps skinfold site, **locate the site previously marked for the mid-arm circumference (MAC) measurement.**
- The triceps skinfold site is on the posterior surface of the arm, midway between the shoulder and the elbow.
- **Using the forefinger and the thumb** the assessor **grasps** and lifts the subcutaneous tissue and skin 2 cm above TSF site.
- Place the **pincers of the skinfold caliper** at the **TSF point at a depth of 1 cm**.
- Hold this position for 3–4 seconds.
- Take three measurements for accuracy.
- Provide the actual skinfold thickness in mm.

BODY MASS INDEX

Calculation

Formula is weight (kg)/height (m^2)

Body Mass Index

	World Health Organization (WHO)	Southeast Asian Countries (SEAC)
Underweight	<18.5	<18.5
Normal	**18.5–24.9**	**18.5–22.9**
Overweight	25–29.9	23–24.9
Preobese	—	25–29.9
Obese	≥30	≥30
Obese 1	30–40	30–40
Obese 2 (morbid)	40.1–50	40.1–50
Obese 3	>50	>50

Metabolic syndrome	
National Cholesterol Education Program Adult Treatment Panel III (NCEP ATP III) 2005*	**WHO 1999**
Essential criteria	
—	Insulin resistance
Additional criteria	
(≥3 of following)	(≥2 of following)
Waist circumference (WC) ▪ >90 cm (males) ▪ >80 cm (females)	**Waist-hip ratio (WHR)** ▪ 0.9 (males) ▪ >0.85 (females) ▪ BMI ≥30
Glucose ≥100 mg/dL or on Rx	
Triglyceride (TG) ≥150 mg/dL or on Rx	TG ≥150 mg/dL
High-density lipoprotein (HDL) <40 (males) <50 (females) or on Rx	HDL <35 (males) <40 (females)
Hypertension (HTN) ≥130/85 or on Rx	HTN ≥140/90

*Most commonly followed.

WAIST-HIP RATIO (FIG. 2D.5)

Method of Measurement

Waist Circumference

- Locate the narrowest point between ribs and iliac crests.
- Ensure that the tape measure is at the same height around the waist.
- Measure and state the measurement correctly to the nearest centimeter.
- **≥90 cm (adult male) and ≥80 cm (adult female) considered having abdominal obesity for south Asians.**
- **Differences in cut points abdominal obesity for south Asians and Europids.**

Abdominal obesity	South Asians	Europids
Men	WC ≥90 cm	WC ≥102 cm
Women	WC ≥80 cm	WC ≥88 cm

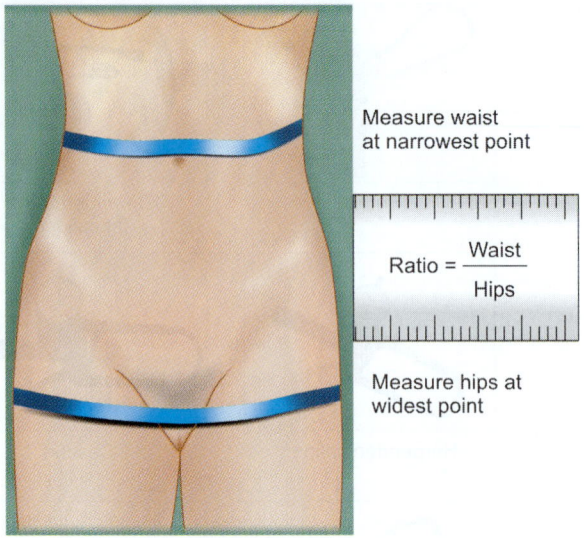

Fig. 2D.5: Examination of waist-hip ratio.

Hip Circumference

- Hip measurement is taken at the widest lateral extension of the hips.
- Ensure that the tape measure is horizontal.
- Measure and state the measurement correctly to the nearest centimeter.
- Calculate waist-hip ratio to two decimal places.

Clinical Implication

0.9 (males) or >0.85 (females) are criteria for metabolic syndrome.

MID-ARM CIRCUMFERENCE (FIGS. 2D.6 AND 2D.7)

- Locate the midpoint of the arm.
- Nondominant arm elbow flexed at 90° with palm facing upwards.
- Measurer stands behind the subject and locates the lateral tip of the acromion and the most distal point on the olecranon process.
- Place a tape measure so that it passes between these two landmarks and mark the midpoint.
- The subject stands erect with arms hanging freely at the sides and the palms facing the thighs.
- Place the tape measure perpendicular to the long axis of the arm at the marked midpoint and measure the circumference to the nearest mm (e.g., 18.1 cm).
- Provide the actual MAC in cm.

NECK CIRCUMFERENCE

- Neck circumference (NC) measurement, as a simple and time-saving screening measure, could be used to identify overweight and obese population.
- Measured on a plane as horizontal as possible, at a point just below the larynx (thyroid cartilage), and perpendicular to the long axis of the neck (the tape line in front of the neck should be placed at the same height as the tape line in the back of the neck).

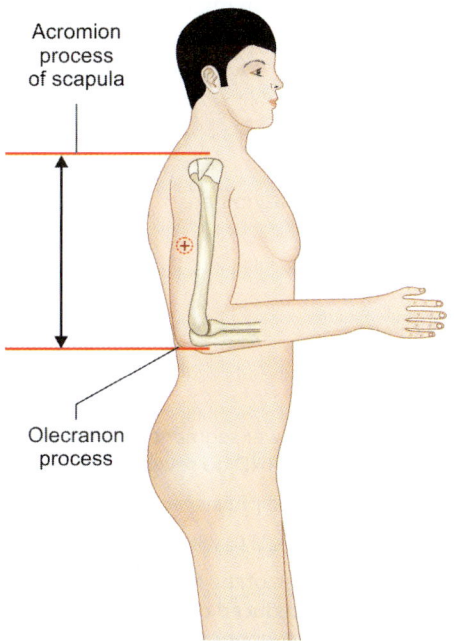

Fig. 2D.6: Method of marking midpoint for measuring mid-arm circumference.

- Varies based on population. Among South Asians, an NC of >34.9 cm for men and >31.25 cm for women were the best predictors for identifying metabolic syndrome.

NECK HEIGHT RATIO

- Neck length was measured as the linear distance between two easily recognizable and fixed bony points—the external occipital protuberance and the spinous process of C7 vertebra; with the patient standing upright and neck held in neutral position.
- Normal ratio of neck: height is 1:13 **(Bird index)**.
- Short neck is an important feature of conditions like Turner, Noonan, Klippel–Feil, and mucopolysaccharides.
- Neck height ratio (NHtR) has also been suggested to be a measure of upper body adiposity like NC.

MISCELLANEOUS TOPICS

Significant Weight Loss

- >10% of body weight × 6 months
- 5 kg or more × 1 month

Cachexia

Complex metabolic syndrome associated with underlying illness and is characterized by the loss of muscle with or without loss of fat mass.

Emaciation

Extreme weight loss and unnatural thinness due to a loss of the fatty, adipose tissue beneath the skin and muscle throughout body.

Weight for Age (W/A)

- General appreciation of nutritional status
- For growth monitoring.

Height for Age (H/A)

- Measure of linear growth deficit or **stunting**
- Slow progress
- Used for community diagnosis.

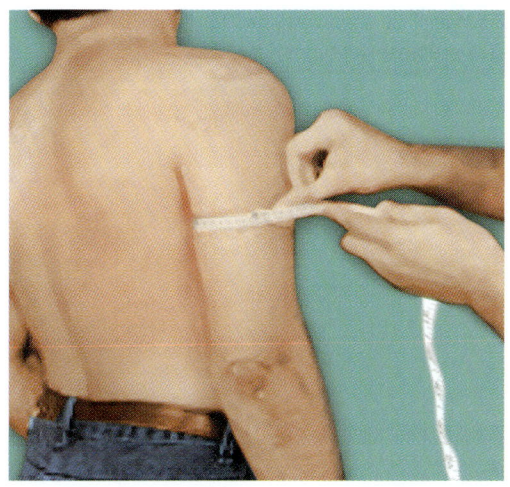

Fig. 2D.7: Method of measuring mid-arm circumference.

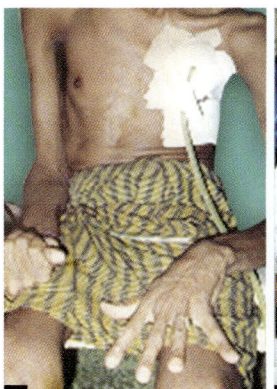
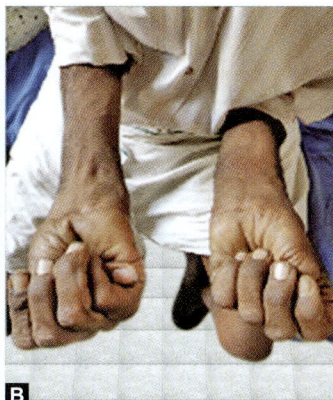
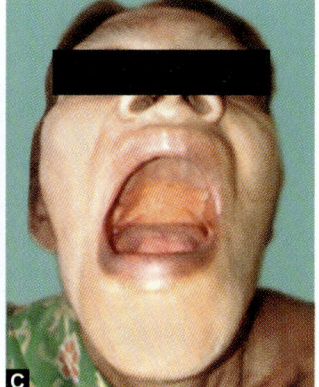
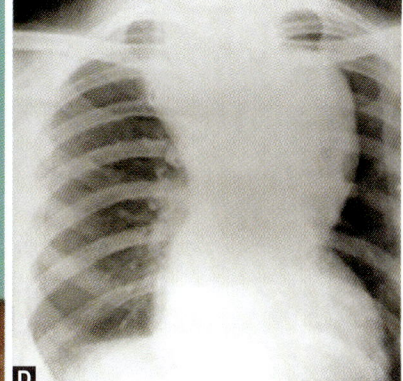

Figs. 2D.8A to D: Features of Marfan's syndrome. (A) Wrist sign; (B) Thumb sign; (C) High-arched palate; (D) Chest X-ray showing aortic root dilatation.

Weight for Height/Length (W/H)

- Measure of weight deficit according to length
- Measure of wasting
- Used for individual and community diagnosis.

MARFAN'S SYNDROME: DIAGNOSTIC CRITERIA AND FEATURES (FIGS. 2D.8A TO D)

Diagnostic criteria (modified Ghent criteria)	
In the **absence of family history** of MFS, the presence of one of any of the following criteria is diagnostic for MFS	In the **presence of family history** of MFS, the presence of one of any of the following criteria is diagnostic for MFS
1. Aortic criterion and ectopia lentis	1. Ectopia lentis
2. Aortic criterion and a causal FBN1 mutation	2. Systemic score ≥7 points
3. Aortic criterion and a systemic score ≥7	3. Aortic criterion
4. Ectopia lentis and a causal FBN1 mutation	

Aortic Criteria

Aortic diameter Z score ≥2 (above 20 years old), Z score ≥3 (below 20 years), or aortic root dissection.

Systemic Scoring

A systemic score ≥7 indicates major systemic involvement.

Calculate based on the following table:

Features	Points
Wrist **AND** thumb sign	3
Wrist **OR** thumb sign	1
Pectus carinatum deformity	2
Pectus excavatum or chest asymmetry	1
Hind-foot deformity	2
Plain pes planus	1
Pneumothorax	2
Dural ectasia	2
Protrusio acetabuli	2
Reduced upper segment/lower segment ratio **AND** increased arm span/height **AND** no severe scoliosis	1
Scoliosis or thoracolumbar kyphosis	1
Reduced elbow extension (≤170° with full extension)	1
Facial features [at least three of the following five features: dolichocephaly (reduced cephalic index or head width/length ratio), enophthalmos, down slanting palpebral fissures, malar hypoplasia, retrognathia]	1
Skin striae	1
Myopia >3 diopters	1
Mitral valve prolapse (all types)	1

CHAPTER 3

Respiratory System Examination

A. CASE SHEET FORMAT

HISTORY TAKING

Name:
Age:
Sex:
Residence:
Occupation:

Chief complaints:
1. _____ × days
2. _____ × days
3. _____ × days

History of presenting illness:

Cough:
- Duration
- Onset
- Progression
- Variation
  - Diurnal variation
  - Seasonal variation
  - Postural variation
- Aggravating factors
- Relieving factors

Expectoration:
- Duration
- Onset
- Progression
- Variation
  - Diurnal variation
  - Seasonal variation
  - Positional variation
- Aggravating and relieving factors
- Quantity of sputum (to be measured in mL)
- Color
- Smell
- Blood tinged
  - How often
  - Quantity
  - Fresh or altered

Dyspnea:
- Duration
- Onset
- Grade (MMRC grading is preferred)
- Progression
- Aggravating factors
- Relieving factors
- Orthopnea
- Trepopnea
- Platypnea
- Paroxysmal nocturnal dyspnea (PND)
- Any respiratory system complaints
  - Wheeze
  - Cough with expectoration

Chest pain:
- Duration
- Onset
- Site
- Type of pain/character of pain
- Radiation
- Diurnal variation (nocturnal angina)
- Variation with respiration
- Aggravating factors
- Relieving factors
- Associated symptoms
  - Nausea, vomiting, sweating
- Local tenderness

Wheeze:
- Duration
- Onset
- Progression
- Episodic or continuous
- Variation (diurnal or seasonal)
- Allergy
- Skin rashes
- Aggravating and relieving factors

Fever:
- Episodic or continuous
- Grade

- Chill and rigors
- Aggravating factors
- Relieving factors
- Variation
  - Diurnal variation

History of:
- Nasal discharge
- Recurrent cold/epistaxis
- Recurrent headaches
- Weight loss
- Anorexia
- Evening rise of temperature
- Smoking
- Belching
- Regurgitation of food
- Hoarseness of voice

Past history:
- Asthma
- Chronic obstructive airway disease
- Tuberculosis
- History of contact with tuberculosis
- Diabetes mellitus (DM)
- Hypertension (HTN)
- Ischemic heart disease (IHD)
- Seizure disorder

Family history: Respiratory diseases with a genetic component, e.g., cystic fibrosis, emphysema (alpha-1-antitrypsin deficiency).
(Draw pedigree chart representing three generations)

Personal history:
- Bowel habits
- Bladder habits
- Appetite
- Loss of weight
- Occupational exposure: Environmental inhalation is a significant cause of respiratory diseases. Coal miners ("black lung"), quarry workers (silicosis), insulation installers and shipyard workers (asbestosis), and cotton mill workers (byssinosis) represent notable COPD categories.
- Sleep
- Dietary habits and taboo
- Food allergies
- Smoking (in Smoking Index or Pack years)
- Alcohol history (___grams of alcohol/day or___units of alcohol/week)

Menstrual and obstetric history:
- G___P___L___A___
- Age of menarche___
- Menopause at___
- Flow—amenorrhea/oligomenorrhea/menorrhagia

Summarize:
Differential diagnosis:
1.
2.
3.

GENERAL EXAMINATION

Patient:
- Conscious
- Cooperative
- Obeying commands

Body mass index:
Weight (kg)/H^2 (m)
(Grading according to WHO for Southeast Asian countries)

Vitals:
- Pulse
  - Rate
  - Rhythm
  - Volume
  - Character
  - Vessel wall thickening
  - Radio-radial delay and radiofemoral delay
  - Peripheral pulses
- Blood pressure
- Respiratory rate
  - Regular
  - Abdominothoracic (male) or thoracoabdominal (female)
  - Usage of accessory muscles
- Jugular venous pulse
  - Waveform
- Jugular venous pressure
  - ____cm of blood above sternal angle (+ 5 cm water)
- Pulse oximetry
- Pain

On physical examination:
- Pallor:
- Icterus:
- Cyanosis:
- Clubbing:
- Lymphadenopathy:
- Edema:

Others:
- Use of accessory muscles of respiration
- Features suggesting type of respiratory failure
- External markers of tuberculosis if any
- External markers of malignancy if any

SYSTEMIC EXAMINATION

Upper Respiratory Tract Examination
- Nostrils:
- Nasal septum:
- Nasal polyps:
- Sinus tenderness:
- Tonsils:
- Postpharyngeal wall:

Lower Respiratory Tract Examination

Inspection
- Shape and symmetry:

- Supraclavicular hollowing/infraclavicular flattening
- Intercostal indrawing or rib crowding
- Spine:
- Sub costal angle:
- Trachea:
- Apex beat:
- Respiratory movements:

Area	Right	Left
Infraclavicular area—upper anterior chest		
Mammary area—lower anterior chest		
Supraclavicular area—upper posterior chest		
Inter- and infrascapular area—lower posterior chest		

- Visible pulsations/sinus/scars:

Palpation

Warm the palms by rubbing against each other before palpation:
- Spine: Position and tenderness
- Trachea:
- Apex:

Respiratory movements:

Area	Right	Left
Supraclavicular		
Infraclavicular		
Mammary		
Suprascapular		
Infrascapular		

Dimensions/measurements:

Transverse diameter	
Anteroposterior diameter	
Transverse/anteroposterior ratio	
Chest circumference	Expiration
	Inspiration
Right hemithorax	Expiration
	Inspiration
Left hemithorax	Expiration
	Inspiration
Chest expansion	Right hemithorax
	Left hemithorax
	Total
Spinoscapular distance	(Right side) and (left side)
Spinoacromial distance	(Right side) and (left side)

Vocal fremitus:

Areas	Right	Left
Supraclavicular		
Infraclavicular		

Contd...

Contd...

Mammary		
Axillary		
Infra-axillary		
Suprascapular		
Interscapular		
Infrascapular		

- Tactile fremitus:
- Friction fremitus:
- Tenderness:
- Subcutaneous emphysema:
- Rib crowding:
- Bony tenderness:

Percussion

Areas	Right	Left
Clavicular (direct percussion)		
Supraclavicular		
Infraclavicular		
Mammary		
Axillary		
Infra-axillary		
Suprascapular		
Interscapular		
Infrascapular		

- Shifting dullness:
- Tidal percussion:
- Traube's space:
- Kronig's isthmus:
- Liver dullness:
- Liver span:

Heart border:
- Right heart border:
- Left heart border:

Auscultation

Breath sounds:
- Vesicular/bronchovesicular/bronchial (tubular/cavernous/amphoric)
- Comment on intensity of breath sound—normal/increased/decreased

Areas	Right	Left
Supraclavicular		
Infraclavicular		
Mammary		
Axillary		
Infra-axillary		
Suprascapular		
Interscapular		
Infrascapular		

Vocal resonance:

Areas	Right	Left
Supraclavicular		
Infraclavicular		
Mammary		
Axillary		
Infra-axillary		
Suprascapular		
Interscapular		
Infrascapular		

Adventitious sounds (mention in specific areas):
- Crepitations (fine/coarse, inspiratory/expiratory)
- Rhonchi (inspiratory or expiratory/polyphonic or monophonic)
- Pleural rub

Additional tests (only in specific cases):
- Bronchophony:
- Egophony:
- Whispered pectoriloquy:
- Succussion splash:
- Post-tussive crepitations:
- Post-tussive suction
- Shifting dullness:
- Coin test:

Other Systems

Cardiovascular system:
- Inspection:
- Palpation:
- Percussion:
- Auscultation:

Gastrointestinal system:
- Inspection:
- Palpation:
- Percussion:
- Auscultation:

Nervous system:
- Higher mental functions:
- Cranial nerves:
- Sensory system:
- Motor system:
- Reflexes:
- Cerebellar system:
- Meningeal signs:

NOTES

B. DIAGNOSIS FORMAT

ANATOMICAL DIAGNOSIS
- Lung (right/left/bilateral) disease with (upper/middle/lower) lobe
- Pleural disease

PATHOLOGICAL DIAGNOSIS
Consolidation/fibrosis/collapse/obstructive lung disease/restrictive lung disease/effusion/pneumothorax.

ETIOLOGICAL DIAGNOSIS
Tuberculosis/bronchogenic carcinoma/smoking/occupation/trauma, etc.

COMPLICATIONS
Respiratory failure (type I or type II)/cor pulmonale.

EXAMPLES

Example 1
Right upper lobe fibrosis post-tubercular etiology, no evidence of respiratory failure or cor pulmonale.

Example 2
Bilateral obstructive lung disease—emphysema secondary to smoking with evidence of type 2 respiratory failure and cor pulmonale.

Example 3
Left-sided pleural effusion secondary to malignancy with no evidence of respiratory failure or cor pulmonale.

NOTES

Respiratory System Examination

C. DISCUSSION ON CARDINAL SYMPTOMS

Symptoms discussed include:
1. Cough
2. Expectoration
3. Hemoptysis
4. Dyspnea
5. Chest pain (with respect to respiratory system)
6. Others

COUGH

Definition: A sudden and variable expiratory thrust of air from the lungs through the air passages associated with phonation, which momentarily interrupts the physiological pattern of breathing.

Mechanism of cough production: Cough reflex initiated by chemical/mechanical stimuli **(Flowchart 3C.1)**. This is carried by the afferents which are type C and type 1 fibers and innervate pharynx, larynx, large airways, terminal bronchiole and lung parenchyma. Afferents travel via vagus and superior laryngeal nerve. Nucleus tractus solitarius (NTS) in brainstem is the cough center. Efferents travel via vagus, phrenic, spinal motor nerves to the larynx, trachea, bronchi, diaphragm producing cough.

Mechanical events during cough production: The mechanical events involved in a typical cough are rapid successions of **(Figs. 3C.1A to C)**:
1. Inspiratory phase: A fairly deep initial inspiration (2.5–3 L)
2. Compressive phase: The tight closure of the glottis, reinforced by the supraglottic structures
3. Expiratory phase: The quick and forceful contraction of the expiratory muscles → the sudden opening of the glottis while the contraction of the expiratory muscles continues.

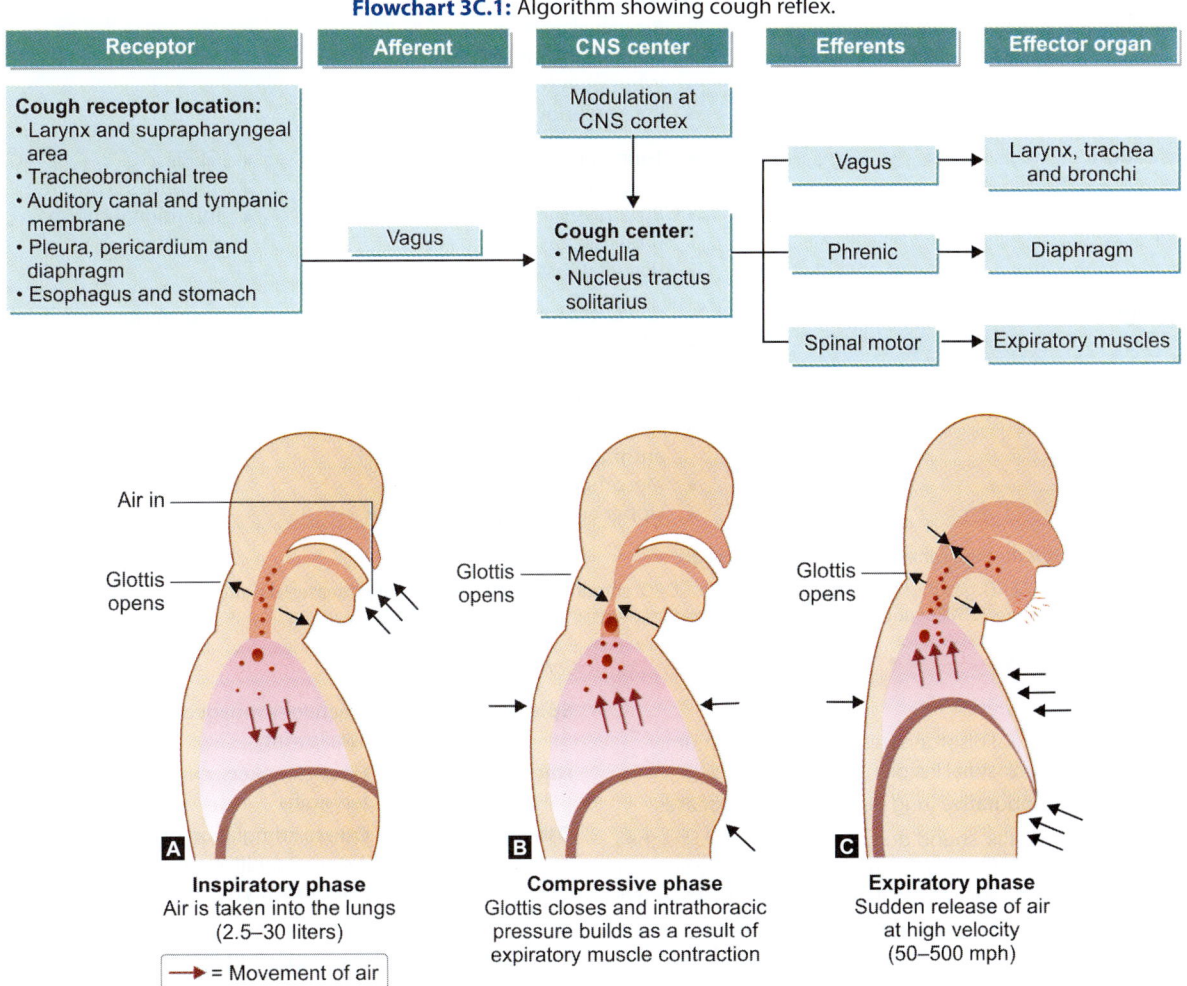

Flowchart 3C.1: Algorithm showing cough reflex.

Figs. 3C.1A to C: Mechanical events during cough production: (A) Inspiratory phase; (B) Compressive phase; (C) Expiratory phase.

Classification:
- **Based on etiology:** The etiology can be classified into respiratory causes and nonrespiratory causes.
- **Based on duration of cough:** Cough has been classified into acute (less than 3 weeks), subacute (3–8 weeks), and chronic (more than 8 weeks; **Box 3C.1**).
- **Based on expectoration:** It is also classified into productive or dry cough depending on the presence or absence of expectoration, respectively **(Table 3C.1)**. Different types of coughs are summarized in **Table 3C.2**.

> **Box 3C.1: Chronic cough with normal chest X-ray.**
> - Cough variant asthma
> - Tropical eosinophilia
> - Upper airway cough syndrome
> - Aspiration
> - Habitual cough
> - Foreign body
> - Drugs, angiotensin converting enzyme inhibitors
> - Chronic bronchitis
> - Chronic idiopathic cough

TABLE 3C.1: Classification of cough based on etiology.

Cough	Duration	Respiratory causes	Nonrespiratory causes
Acute cough	Less than 3 weeks	- Tracheobronchitis - Upper respiratory tract infections (URTI) - Bronchopneumonia - Viral pneumonia - Acute-on-chronic bronchitis - Pulmonary embolism **Sudden onset:** - Bronchial asthma - Asthmatic bronchitis - Whooping cough - Foreign body	- LVF - GERD
Subacute cough	3–8 weeks	- Tuberculosis, pneumonia (bacterial, viral, fungal) - *B. pertussis* - Bronchiectasis - Postviral tussive syndrome	- GERD - Tourette's syndrome - Intentional cough
Chronic cough*	Lasting for more than 8 weeks	- COPD, asthma - ILD - Tuberculosis - Lung cancer - Pneumoconiosis (asbestosis, silicosis, anthracosis, etc.) - Mesothelioma of lung - Upper airway cough syndrome	- Drug induced (ACE inhibitors, beta blockers, NSAIDs) - Habit cough syndrome

*Chronic cigarette smoking is the most common cause of chronic cough.
(LVF: left ventricular failure; GERD: gastroesophageal reflux disease; COPD: chronic obstructive pulmonary disease; ILD: interstitial lung disease; ACE: angiotensin converting enzyme; NSAIDs: nonsteroidal anti-inflammatory drugs)

TABLE 3C.2: Different types of cough.

Types	Features
Dry cough	Pleural disorders, diseases of interstitium, mediastinal lesions
Productive cough	Suppurative lung disease, airway diseases
Brassy/Gander cough	Metallic sound due to compression of trachea by intrathoracic space occupying lesions or aortic aneurysms also known as leopards growl
Bovine cough	Loss of expulsive nature as in a tumor pressing on the recurrent laryngeal nerve
Paroxysmal cough	Whooping cough, chronic bronchitis, foreign body, bronchial asthma
Barking cough	Involvement of epiglottis, croup (laryngotracheobronchitis), hysteria
Spluttering cough	Tracheoesophageal fistula, cough while swallowing
Hacking cough	Heavy smokers, chronic pharyngitis or laryngitis
Otogenic cough	Due to stimulation of Arnold's nerve in the external auditory meatus (impacted wax/foreign body)

EXPECTORATION/SPUTUM

Sputum can be described under the following headings:
- Quantity
- Quality
- Odor

Quantity	
Normal	10–15 mL/24 hours
Bronchorrhea	- Production of more than 100 mL/20 teaspoons in 24 hours - Bronchiectasis - Lung abscess - Bronchoalveolar carcinoma - Organophosphorus poisoning - Pulmonary alveolar proteinosis
Quality	
Mucoid	Chronic bronchitis, bronchial asthma
Mucopurulent	Infections
Purulent	Lung abscess, bronchiectasis
Rust-colored purulent sputum	Pneumococcal pneumonia
Currant-jelly and sticky sputum	*Klebsiella pneumoniae*
Blood-tinged foamy sputum	Pulmonary edema (pink frothy)
Greenish	*Pseudomonas*
Granules—yellow/black	Actinomycosis
Anchovy sauce (brown)	Amebic abscess rupturing into lung
Black (melanoptysis)	Carbon particles discolor the sputum gray (as in cigarette smokers) or black (as in coal miners or with smoke inhalation)
Odor	
Foul smelling sputum	Anaerobic infection seen in lung abscess, bronchiectasis

Special Points

- Chronic expectoration of large amounts of purulent and foul-smelling sputum is strongly suggestive of bronchiectasis.
- Sudden production of such sputum in a febrile patient
- Indicates a lung abscess.
- **Three-layer sputum** consisting of a foamy upper layer, mucous middle layer, and viscous purulent bottom layer is pathognomonic of bronchiectasis.
- **Postural variation** in sputum: Bronchiectasis, lung abscess.

TABLE 3C.3: Causes of hemoptysis.

Structure involved	Common causes	Uncommon causes
Bronchial disease	Bronchial carcinoma, bronchiectasis, acute and chronic bronchitis	Bronchial adenoma, foreign body
Parenchymal disease of lung	Pulmonary tuberculosis (Rasmussen's aneurysm—dilation of a pulmonary artery in a tuberculous cavity), lung abscess, pneumonia (particularly *Klebsiella*), fungal infections	Parasites (e.g. hydatid disease, flukes), trauma, actinomycosis, mycetoma

Contd...

Contd...

		(aspergilloma and invasive aspergillosis), pulmonary contusion/laceration (traumatic)
Vascular diseases of the lung	Pulmonary infarction	Goodpasture's syndrome, polyarteritis nodosa, idiopathic pulmonary hemosiderosis, primary pulmonary hypertension
Cardiovascular disease	Acute left ventricular failure	Mitral stenosis, aortic aneurysm, pulmonary thromboembolism
Hematological disorders		Leukemia, hemophilia, anticoagulants, hemorrhagic diathesis

HEMOPTYSIS

Definition: Hemoptysis is defined as coughing of blood originating from below the vocal cords. Hemoptysis can range from blood-streaking of sputum to the presence of gross blood in the absence of any accompanying sputum. The different causes of hemoptysis are given in **Table 3C.3**.

The clinical clues of hemoptysis, differences between true and false hemoptysis and differences between hemoptysis and hematemesis are described in **Tables 3C.4 to 3C.6**, respectively.

TABLE 3C.4: Clinical clues of hemoptysis.

Clinical clues	Suggested diagnosis
Anticoagulant use	**Medication effect, coagulation disorder**
Tobacco use	**Acute bronchitis, chronic bronchitis, pneumonia, lung cancer**
Dyspnea on exertion, fatigue, orthopnea, paroxysmal nocturnal dyspnea, frothy pink sputum	**Congestive heart failure, left ventricular failure and mitral stenosis**
Fever, productive cough	**Upper respiratory tract infection, acute bronchitis, pneumonia, lung abscess**
History of cancer (e.g., breast, colon, or kidney)	**Endobronchial metastasis from carcinoma**
History of chronic lung disease, recurrent lower respiratory tract infection, cough with copious purulent sputum	**Bronchiectasis, lung abscess**
Pleuritic chest pain, calf tenderness	**Pulmonary embolism or infarction**
Toxic symptoms	**Tuberculosis**

Contd...

Contd...	
Weight loss	**Emphysema, lung cancer, tuberculosis, bronchiectasis, lung abscess**
Melena, alcoholism, chronic use of nonsteroidal anti-inflammatory drugs (NSAIDs)	**Gastritis, gastric or peptic ulcer, esophageal varices**
Association with menses	**Catamenial hemoptysis**
Cachexia, clubbing, hoarseness	**Lung cancer, small cell carcinoma**
Clubbing	**Lung cancer, bronchiectasis, lung abscess**
Dullness to percussion, fever, crepitations	**Pneumonia**

TABLE 3C.5: Differences between true and false hemoptysis.

True hemoptysis	False hemoptysis/pseudo-hemoptysis
Below vocal cords	Above vocal cords (gum bleeding/upper airway (nasopharyngeal) bleeding
Persists as blood tinged sputum	Does not persist
May be mixed with sputum	Not mixed with sputum
History of cardiopulmonary disease	Obvious by ENT examination
Chest X-ray may be abnormal	Normal chest X-ray

TABLE 3C.6: Differences between hemoptysis and hematemesis.

Hemoptysis	Hematemesis
Coughing of blood. Cough precedes hemoptysis	Vomiting of blood. Nausea and vomiting precedes hematemesis
History of cardiopulmonary disease	History of gastrointestinal disease
Bright red in color	Dark brown/coffee brown in color
Sputum remains blood stained after the attack for few days	Usually followed by melena
Mixed with sputum	Mixed with gastric contents
Blood is frothy due to admixture of air	Airless and not frothy
Alkaline	Acidic
Sputum contains hemosiderin laden macrophages	No
Melena absent	Melena present

Massive hemoptysis: Life-threatening (or) massive hemoptysis is defined as coughing of blood >150 mL/episode (or) >600 mL/24 hours. Only 5% of hemoptysis is massive but mortality is 80%. Clinical definition of massive hemoptysis is any bleeding that result in a threat to life because of airway or hemodynamic compromise due to bleeding. The different causes of massive hemoptysis are given in **Box 3C.2**.

Box 3C.2: Causes of massive hemoptysis.
- Pulmonary tuberculosis
- Pulmonary infarction
- Bronchiectasis
- Bronchogenic carcinoma
- Massive pulmonary embolism
- Cystic fibrosis
- Lung abscess
- Necrotizing pneumonia
- Mitral stenosis
- Pulmonary arteriovenous malformation

DYSPNEA

Definition

"Dyspnea" is a term used to characterize a subjective experience of breathing discomfort that is comprised of qualitatively distinct sensations that vary in intensity (undue awareness of unpleasant breathing).

Mechanism of Dyspnea

Chemoreceptors	
Peripheral	Carotid and aortic bodies (sensitive to changes pO_2, pCO_2 and H^+)
Central	Medulla (sensitive only to changes in pCO_2, not pO_2, change in pH of cerebrospinal fluid)
Increased work of breathing	
Airflow obstruction	Bronchial asthma, chronic obstructive pulmonary disease (COPD), tracheal obstruction
Decreased pulmonary compliance	Pulmonary edema, fibrosis, allergic alveolitis
Restricted chest expansion	Ankylosing spondylitis, respiratory paralysis, kyphoscoliosis
Increased ventilatory drive	
Increased physiological dead space (V/Q mismatch)	Consolidation, collapse, pleural effusion (PE), pulmonary edema
Hyperventilation due to receptor stimulation	
Chemoreceptors	Acidosis, hypoxia (shock, pneumonia), hypercapnia
J receptors at alveolocapillary junction	Pulmonary edema, pulmonary embolism, pulmonary congestion (activates Hering-Breuer reflex which terminates inspiratory effort before full inspiration is achieved—rapid and shallow)
Muscle spindles in intercostal muscles	Tension-length disparity
Central	Exertion, anxiety, thyrotoxicosis, pheochromocytoma
Impaired respiratory muscle function	
Diseases with impaired muscle function	Poliomyelitis, Guillain-Barre syndrome (GBS), myasthenia gravis

Respiratory System Examination

TABLE 3C.7: Differences between paroxysmal nocturnal dyspnea (PND) orthopnea.

	Paroxysmal nocturnal dyspnea	Orthopnea
Definition	Episode of sudden onset of dyspnea 2–2.5 hours after sleep	Dyspnea in recumbent posture
Timing	Patient wakes up from rapid eye movement (REM) sleep	Occurs soon after lying down
Method of relief	Sits up with legs hanging down, stands up, air hunger, self-ventilates of comfort	Gets up, uses more pillows, sleeps in erect posture
Mechanism	Depressed respiratory center. Sympathetic overactivity during REM→ catecholamine surge resulting in tachycardia → interstitial pulmonary congestion → respiratory center lags behind → perceived as acute dyspnea. There is sudden transient increase in PCWP	Shifting of venous blood (>400 mL) into pulmonary circulation, V/Q mismatch, compression of diaphragm, postural diastolic dysfunction. There is a slow sustained rise in pulmonary capillary wedge pressure (PCWP)
Associated symptoms	Angina, perspiration, palpitation, rarely hemoptysis	All the symptoms of congestive cardiac failure (CCF)
Oxygen saturation	Transient hypoxia	Normal
Differential diagnosis	Night mares/panic attacks/nocturnal hypoglycemia/obstructive sleep apnea (OSA)	COPD/gross obesity/acute asthma/gross ascites

Orthopnea

Dyspnea develops in recumbent position and is relieved by sitting up or by elevation of the head with pillows.

The severity can be graded by the number of pillow used at night, e.g., three pillow orthopnea.

Pathophysiology of Orthopnea
- Pulmonary congestion during recumbency (cannot be pumped out of LV) seen in congestive heart failure (CHF), chronic obstructive pulmonary disease (COPD) and bronchial asthma.
- Increased venous return.
- Diaphragm elevation leading to decreased vital capacity.

Conditions Associated with Orthopnea
Orthopnea is classically seen in left heart failure but can also occur in constrictive pericarditis, COPD, bilateral diaphragmatic palsy, asthma triggered by gastric reflux, and gross ascites.

Paroxysmal Nocturnal Dyspnea

Attacks of dyspnea occur at night and awaken the patient from sleep. The important differences between orthopnea and PND are given in **Table 3C.7**.

Mechanism (Fig. 3C.2)
- It is due to decreased responsiveness of respiratory center in brain during sleep and pulmonary congestion (due to increased sympathetic activity during REM sleep), that occurs 2–3 hours after onset of sleep.
- Absorption of edema fluid with increase in right ventricular output causing over filling of the lungs.
- Takes 10–30 minutes for recovery after upright posture.
- Specific sign of LV dysfunction and includes ischemic heart disease, aortic valve disease, hypertension, cardiomyopathy.
- It has low sensitivity (<30%) but 75% specificity to diagnose heart disease.

Differential Diagnosis for Paroxysmal Nocturnal Dyspnea
- Left heart failure
- Nocturnal episodes of asthma
- Postnasal discharge with attendant severe cough
- Sleep apnea with arousal

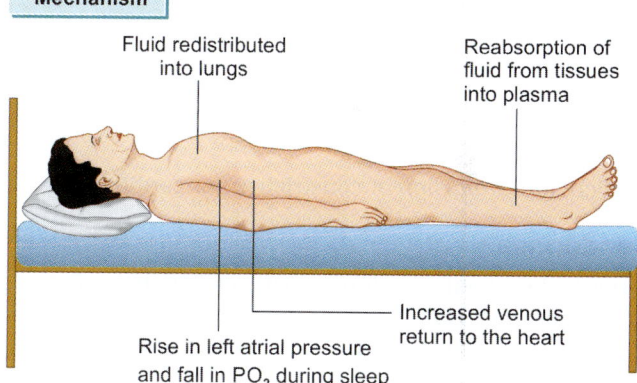

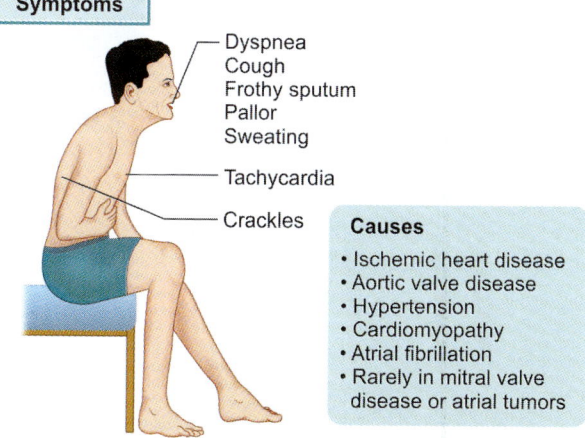

Fig. 3C.2: Mechanism of paroxysmal nocturnal dyspnea (PND).

- Nightmares
- Nocturnal angina with dyspnea (angina equivalent)
- Nocturnal aspiration in gastroesophageal reflux disease
- Nocturnal episodes of recurrent minute pulmonary emboli
- Nocturnal hypoglycemia.

Trepopnea

Aggravation of dyspnea when lying on one side and relieved by lying on opposite side.

Causes

- **Unilateral lung disease:** Uninvolved normal lung receives more blood supply due to gravity.
- **Congestive heart failure:** Lying on right side enhances venous return and sympathetic activity.
- **Lung tumor:** Gravity-induced compression of blood vessels or lung.
- **Pleural effusion:** Dyspnea is seen when lying on unaffected side due to compression of healthy lung.

Platypnea

Dyspnea on sitting or standing and relieved by supine position.

Causes

- Venous to arterial shunting (lung bases)
- Intracardiac shunts (ASD, pneumonectomy)
- Intrapulmonary right to left shunt [hepatopulmonary syndrome, pulmonary embolism (PE), COPD]
- Acute respiratory distress syndrome (ARDS)
- Straight back syndrome
- Pericardial effusion or constrictive pericarditis.

Bendopnea

A newly described symptom in patients with heart failure is mediated via a further increase in ventricular filling pressures during bending in subjects whose sitting ventricular filling pressures are already high, particularly in patients with low cardiac index **(Fig. 3C.3)**.

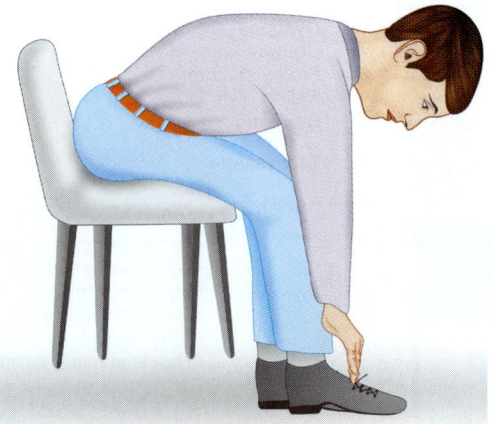

Fig. 3C.3: A patient sits in a chair, bends at the waist, and touches his or her feet. Bendopnea is considered present if dyspnea occurs within 30 seconds of bending.

Causes of acute severe breathlessness is shown in **Box 3C.3**.

Box 3C.3: Acute severe breathlessness.
- Pulmonary edema
- Massive pulmonary embolism
- Acute severe asthma
- Acute exacerbation of COPD
- Severe pneumonia
- Tension pneumothorax
- Foreign body/mucous plug
- Epiglottitis (children)
- Metabolic acidosis
- Psychogenic

Approach to Dyspnea

Onset and duration	
Minutes to hours (rapid onset)	Pneumothorax, acute asthma, pulmonary embolism (PE), pulmonary edema, foreign body
Hours to days (gradual onset)	Pneumonia, pleural effusion, anemia, Guillain–Barre syndrome (GBS)
Months to years (slow onset)	Pulmonary tuberculosis (PTB), COPD, carcinoma, fibrosing alveolitis
Severity	
Medical Research Council (MRC) (Table 3C.8)	Discussed below
Modified Medical Research Council (mMRC) (Table 3C.9)	
New York Heart Association (NYHA) (Table 3C.10)	

Aggravating and relieving factors	
Improves on weekend/holidays	Occupational asthma, extrinsic alveolitis
Recumbency/sleep	Orthopnea/paroxysmal nocturnal dyspnea (PND)
Associated symptoms (Table 3C.11)	
Pleuritic chest pain	Pneumonia, pulmonary infarction, rib fracture, pneumothorax
Central nonpleuritic chest pain	Myocardial infarction, massive pulmonary embolism
Cough or wheeze	Asthma, pulmonary embolism, pneumothorax

TABLE 3C.8: Medical Research Council (MRC) grading of breathlessness.

1. Note troubled by breathlessness except on strenuous exertion
2. Short of breath when hurrying on level ground or walking up slight hill
3. Walks slower than people of same age or stops after 15 minutes when walking at own pace on level
4. Stops after 100 yards (90 m) or after few minutes in level ground
5. Too breathless to leave house, dress or undress

Respiratory System Examination

TABLE 3C.9: Modified Medical Research Council (MMRC) grading of breathlessness.

Grade	Description of breathlessness
Grade 0	I only get breathless with strenuous exercise
Grade 1	I get short of breath when hurrying on level ground or walking up a slight hill
Grade 2	On level ground, I walk slower than people of the same age because of breathlessness, or I have to stop for breath when walking at my own pace on the level
Grade 3	I stop for breath after walking about 100 yards or after a few minutes on level ground
Grade 4	I am too breathless to leave the house or I am breathless when dressing

TABLE 3C.10: New York Heart Association (NYHA) classification of breathlessness.

NYHA Class	Patients with cardiac disease (description of heart failure related symptoms)
Class I (Mild)	Patients with cardiac disease but without resulting in limitation of physical activity. Ordinary physical activity does not cause undue fatigue, palpitation, dyspnea or anginal pain
Class II (Mild)	Patients with cardiac disease resulting in **slight limitation** of physical activity. They are comfortable at rest. Ordinary physical activity results in fatigue, palpitation, dyspnea, or anginal pain
Class III (Moderate)	Patients with cardiac disease resulting in **marked limitation** of physical activity. They are comfortable at rest. Less than ordinary activity causes fatigue, palpitation, dyspnea or anginal pain
Class IV (Severe)	Patients with cardiac disease resulting in the inability to carry on any physical activity without discomfort. Symptoms of heart failure or the anginal syndrome may be present even at rest. If any physical activity is undertaken, discomfort is increased

Note: NYHA classification system is subjective and poorly reproducible.

TABLE 3C.11: Causes of acute and chronic dyspnea.

Acute dyspnea	Chronic dyspnea
Cardiovascular system	
Cardiogenic acute pulmonary edema	Chronic heart failure, myocardial ischemia
Respiratory system	
- Acute severe bronchial asthma - Acute exacerbation of COPD - Spontaneous pneumothorax - Pneumonia - Acute pulmonary embolism - Acute respiratory distress syndrome - Inhaled foreign body (especially in children) - Lobar collapse - Laryngeal edema (e.g., anaphylaxis) or obstruction	- Chronic obstructive pulmonary disease (COPD) - Chronic bronchial asthma - Bronchial carcinoma - Interstitial lung disease (e.g., sarcoidosis, fibrosing alveolitis, extrinsic allergic alveolitis, pneumoconiosis) - Chronic pulmonary thromboembolism - Lymphatic carcinomatosis - Large pleural effusion(s) - Severe anemia - Obesity - Deconditioning

Contd...

Contd...

Nonrespiratory, noncardiac causes	
Metabolic acidosis (e.g., diabetic ketoacidosis, lactic acidosis, uremia, overdose of salicylates, ethylene glycol poisoning)	Psychogenic hyperventilation (anxiety or panic-related)

Pitfalls of mMRC Grading

- The mMRC dyspnea scale quantifies disability attributable to breathlessness, and is useful for characterizing baseline dyspnea in patients with respiratory diseases.
- It describes baseline dyspnea, but does not accurately quantify response to treatment of COPD.

TIMING OF DYSPNEA

The timing and pattern of respiration helps to determine the structure most likely responsible for the dyspnea. Dyspnea may occur during inspiration, expiration or both (mixed). Clinically inspiratory dyspnea implies a lesion in the respiratory tract outside the thorax, whereas expiratory and mixed dyspnea occur in patients with thoracic or metabolic disease. Expiratory dyspnea should be further classified as obstructive or restrictive.

Causes of inspiratory dyspnea	Causes of obstructive expiratory dyspnea
- Stenotic nares - Gross deviated nasal septum - Nasal polyps - Rhinosinusitis - Enlarge adenoids in young children - Foreign body aspiration - Laryngotracheal trauma - Tonsillar hypertrophy - Peritonsillar abscess - Retropharyngeal abscess - Vocal cord/vocal fold palsy - Acute laryngotracheitis - Epiglottitis - Pertussis - Spasmodic croup	- Tracheal collapse - Tracheobronchitis - Foreign body - Neoplasia - Enlarged lymph nodes - Enlarged left atrium - Asthma - COPD
Causes of noisy restrictive dyspnea	*Causes of silent restrictive expiratory dyspnea*
- Pulmonary edema - Pneumonia - Pulmonary fibrosis - Neoplasia - Pulmonary infarction - Pulmonary embolism - Ascites - Pregnancy - Organomegaly - Gastric dilatation—volvulus - Neoplasia	- Pneumothorax - Pleural effusion - Thickened pleura - Diaphragmatic hernia - Chest tumors

CHEST PAIN

Chest pain discussed in detail under Chapter 4.

Respiratory Causes
- Upper sternal—tracheitis
- Pleuritic—associated with breathing
- Neurologic—invasion of nerves.

Pleuritic chest pain is characterized by sudden and intense sharp, stabbing, or burning pain in the chest when inhaling and exhaling. It is exacerbated by deep breathing, coughing, sneezing, or laughing. When pleuritic inflammation occurs near the diaphragm, pain can be referred to the neck or shoulder. Pleuritic chest pain is caused by inflammation of the parietal pleura (dry pleurisy) and can be triggered by a variety of causes.

Pulmonary embolism, myocardial infarction, pericarditis, aortic dissection, pneumonia, and pneumothorax are the six serious conditions that cause pleuritic pain.
- Chest tightness also known as chest pressure. It is combination of dull chest pain as well as chest discomfortness. Common causes of chest tightness are high blood pressure, asthma, COPD and gastroesophageal reflux disease (GERD).

OTHER SYMPTOMS

Noisy breathing (partial obstruction of airway):

Laryngeal level	Stridor (inspiratory sound)
Oropharyngeal level	Stertor
Tracheal level	Rattling
Bronchial level	Wheezing (inspiratory/expiratory)

Hoarseness of voice:
- Inflammatory: Acute and chronic laryngitis
- Smoke inhalation
- Neoplastic: Carcinoma/laryngeal papillomatosis
- Recurrent laryngeal nerve damage: Post-thyroidectomy carcinoma of lung/breast
- Neurological: Myasthenia gravis, hypothyroidism
- Rheumatoid arthritis: Involvement of cricoarytenoid joint
- Habitual dysphonia
- Reinke's dysphonia
- Singer's nodules/vocal cord polyps
- Gastroesophageal reflux disease (GERD).

Hiccoughs
Respiratory causes include basal pneumonia and pleurisy.

Snoring
Feature of obstructive sleep apnea.

NOTES

D. DISCUSSION ON EXAMINATION

GENERAL EXAMINATION

Built and Nourishment
Body mass index (BMI), anthropometry has been discussed in detail in Chapter 2D of general examination.

Respiratory diseases associated with emaciation:
1. Respiratory diseases associated with HIV
2. Pulmonary tuberculosis
3. Malignancy.

Pickwickian syndrome (obesity hypoventilation syndrome):
1. Obesity
2. Hypoxia
3. Pulmonary HTN.

Vital Examination (with Respect to Respiratory System)

Pulse:
- Rate—tachycardia (any pneumonia, febrile illness, hypoxia)
- Irregular pulse seen in multifocal atrial tachycardia, atrial fibrillation
- Bounding pulse—CO_2 retention
- Pulsus paradoxus—acute exacerbation of COPD/asthma.

Respiratory rate:
(For details on respiratory rate refer chapter on vitals examination).

Blood pressure:
- Wide pulse pressure—in hypercapnia
- Low blood pressure—seen with hypoxia, acute respiratory distress
- Postural hypotension—Addison's disease, paraneoplastic.

Jugular venous pressure:
- Elevated: In cor pulmonale, tricuspid regurgitation. Pulmonary hypertension
- Nonpulsatile jugular venous pressure (JVP): Superior vena cava (SVC) obstruction.

Temperature:
- Evening rise of temperature: Tuberculosis
- High spiking fevers: Lung abscess, empyema, pneumonias.
- Temperature fall by crisis: Pneumonias.

Pallor:
- Tuberculosis
- Malignancy
- Any cause of massive hemoptysis.

Polycythemia:
Chronic respiratory diseases with underlying hypoxia are usually associated with polycythemia.
So, if patient with COPD has anemia look for other causes like GI bleed, CKD or coexistent malignancy.

Icterus:
- Hepatitis secondary to antitubercular (ATT) drugs
- Atypical pneumonias (hemolytic jaundice)
- Cor pulmonale—congestive hepatomegaly
- As a part of multiple organ dysfunction syndrome (MODS)
- Rarely metastasis to liver.

Edema:
- Cor pulmonale
- Bronchiectasis leading to hypoproteinemia (due to loss of protein in the sputum and nephrotic syndrome secondary to amyloidosis)—100 mL of sputum can cause 3–4 g of protein loss.
- Hypercapnia-induced dilation of the precapillary sphincters.
- Reduced renal blood flow with relatively preserved glomerular filtration rate and elevated levels of renin, aldosterone, arginine vasopressin and atrial natriuretic peptide.

Cyanosis, clubbing, and lymphadenopathy described in detail in the Chapter 2D of general examination.

Lymphatic drainage of lung	
Most of the lung (right upper lobe, right middle lobe, right lower lobe, left lower lobe)	Right tracheobronchial → right bronchomediastinal → right supraclavicular lymph node
Left upper lobe	Left tracheobronchial → left bronchomediastinal → left supraclavicular lymph node

Lymphatic drainage of pleura (Fig. 3D.1)	
Cervical pleura	Axillary lymph nodes
Parietal pleura	- Anterior: Internal mammary nodes - Posterior: Extrapleural nodes
Diaphragmatic pleura	- Internal mammary nodes, cardiophrenic nodes - Para-aortic, intercostal and posterior mediastinal nodes
Mediastinal pleura	Internal mammary nodes

Oral Cavity Examination
- Halitosis seen in suppurative lung diseases
- Tobacco staining of the teeth
- Poor oral hygiene
- Oral markers of malignancy—leukoplakia, erythroplakia, submucous fibrosis.
- Cyanosis or polycythemia.
- Oral candidiasis—due to inhaled steroids.
- Posterior pharyngeal wall/tonsils—infection.

External markers of tuberculosis:
- Matted lymph nodes
- Erythema nodosum

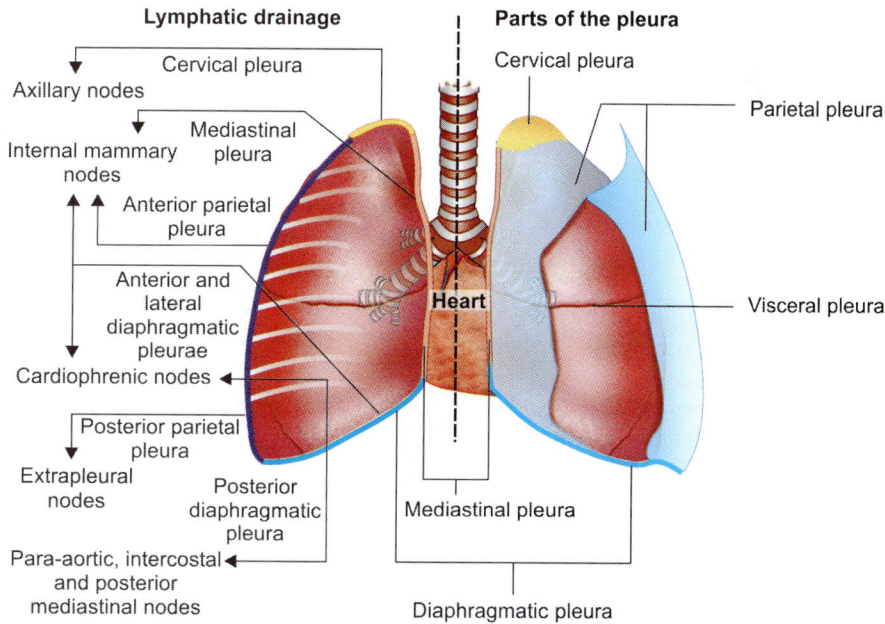

Fig. 3D.1: Parts of pleura with corresponding lymphatic drainage.

- Phlyctenular conjunctivitis
- Choroid tubercle
- Discharging sinuses
- Scrofuloderma
- Lupus vulgaris, tuberculids
- Beaded vas deferens
- Positive Mantoux test
- Generalized tinea versicolor
- Uveitis.

External markers of malignancy:
- Cachexia
- Grade IV clubbing (HPOA)
- Hard lymph nodes
- Acanthosis nigricans
- Horner's syndrome
- Superior vena cava (SVC) obstruction features—non-pulsatile, dilated jugular venous pressure (JVP), facial flushing and edema, conjunctival suffusion, papilledema, dilated veins on the chest wall.

Features of respiratory failure:

	Type 1	Type 2
Definition	Hypoxemic respiratory failure (type 1) is characterized by an arterial oxygen tension (PaO_2) lower than 60 mm Hg with a normal or low arterial carbon dioxide tension ($PaCO_2$)	Hypercapnic respiratory failure (type 2) is characterized by a $PaCO_2$ higher than 50 mm Hg
Sensorium	Anxious agitated	Drowsy to comatose
Peripheries	Cold	Warm
Pulse	Feeble	Bounding
Blood pressure	Low	Wide pulse pressure
Cyanosis	+	–
Asterixis	–	+
Respiratory rate	Tachypneic	Normal to low
Papilledema	–	+
Cause	<ul><li>ARDS</li><li>Pneumonia</li><li>Acute severe asthma</li><li>Tension pneumothorax</li></ul>	<ul><li>COPD</li><li>Obesity</li><li>Respiratory muscle paralysis</li></ul>

Type 3 (perioperative): Functional residual capacity falls below closing volume as a result of atelectasis in postoperative patients. This is generally a subset of type 1 failure but is sometimes considered separately because it is common

Type 4 (shock): Secondary to cardiovascular instability like in severe septic shock, causing hypoperfusion of respiratory muscles leading to hypercapnia and hypoxia

Features of Cor Pulmonale

Right ventricular dilatation:
- Parasternal heave
- Epigastric pulsation.

Right ventricular failure:
- Raised JVP
- Pedal edema
- Tender hepatomegaly
- Ascites
- Sustained abdominojugular reflux is first sign of RVF.

EXAMINATION OF RESPIRATORY SYSTEM

Examination of Upper Respiratory Tract

Demarcation of upper and lower respiratory tract:
- Externally: Demarcated by cricoid cartilage
- Internally: Demarcated by glottis.

Nose
- Deviated nasal septum
- Nasal flaring (outward inspiratory motion of the nares) is a valuable sign of respiratory distress
- Nasal polyps may be seen in:
  - Asthma (atopic variety)
  - Allergic bronchopulmonary aspergillosis (ABPA)
  - Cystic fibrosis
  - Wegener's granulomatosis
- Color of nasal mucosa
  - Pale and moist mucosa found in allergic rhinitis
  - Swollen and red mucosa found in chronic rhinitis
- Nasal discharge
  - Bilateral
    - Mucoid nasal discharge found in allergic rhinitis
    - Watery nasal discharge found in vasomotor rhinitis
    - Purulent nasal discharge found in bacterial infection, such as after common cold, in localized sinus infection and rhinosinusitis.
  - Unilateral
    - Purulent discharge found when there is a foreign body in the nose.
    - New onset, unilateral, crystal clear discharge following head injury suggests a cerebrospinal fluid leak.
- Epistaxis
  - Trauma, rhinitis, hypertension, impaired coagulation from disease, drug induced, i.e., anticoagulants, nonsteroidal anti-inflammatory drugs and alcohol excess.

Throat (Oropharynx)
Postnasal drip resembles like cobblestone: Caused by various medical conditions including sinusitis (inflammation of the sinuses), viral infections such as the common cold, rhinitis (a runny nose that may be acute or chronic), allergies, or bacterial infections, reflux, or gastroesophageal reflux disease.

Significant findings in the upper respiratory tract:
- Nasal turbinate hypertrophy or polyps causing airway obstruction
- Sinus tenderness suggestive of sinusitis
- Kartagener's syndrome:
  - Recurrent sinusitis with ciliary dyskinesia
  - Bronchiectasis
  - Situs inversus
  - Male infertility
- Granulomatosis with polyangitis (GPA)
  - Necrotizing granulomas of the upper airway
- Samter's triad
  - Aspirin sensitivity
  - Bronchial asthma
  - Ethmoidal polyps
- Young's syndrome
  - Sinopulmonary disease
  - Azoospermia
- Eosinophilic granulomatosis with polyangiitis (EGPA)
  - Asthma/allergic rhinitis
  - Eosinophilia
  - Vasculitis
  - Granuloma

Inspection (Lower Respiratory Tract)

Surface marking of lung:

Right side 3 lobes	Left side 2 lobes
1. Right upper lobe (RUL)	1. Left upper lobe (LUL)
2. Right middle lobe (RML)	2. Left lower lobe (LLL)
3. Right lower lobe (RLL)	

Demarcating lower lobe of either side (Figs. 3D.2 to 3D.5): Lower lobe of either lungs can be demarcated from other lobes by drawing a curvilinear line (major interlobar fissure/oblique fissure) joining three bony points:
1. Starting from T2/T3 spinous process, curvilinear line along the medial border of scapula
2. Crossing the 5th rib in the midaxillary line
3. Reaching the 6th rib in midclavicular line part of lung below this line is lower lobe.

Marking right middle lobe:
Draw a straight line (minor interlobar fissure/horizontal fissure) from the 4th rib at right sternal border towards the midaxillary line cutting the major interlobar fissure at 5th rib. The triangular area represents RML.

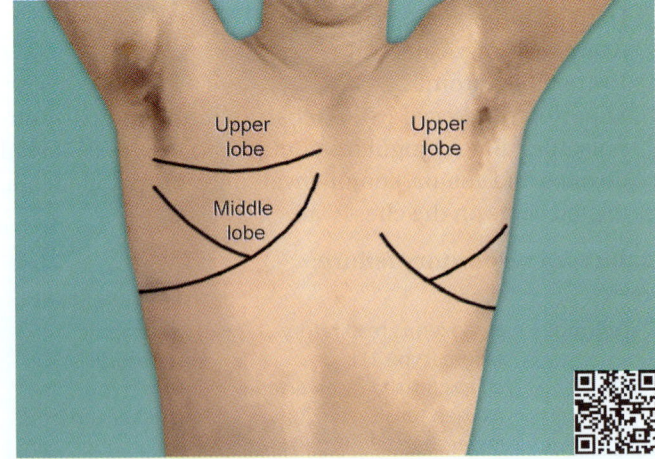

Fig. 3D.2: Anterior view of chest showing surface marking of lung fissures and lobes.

Respiratory System Examination

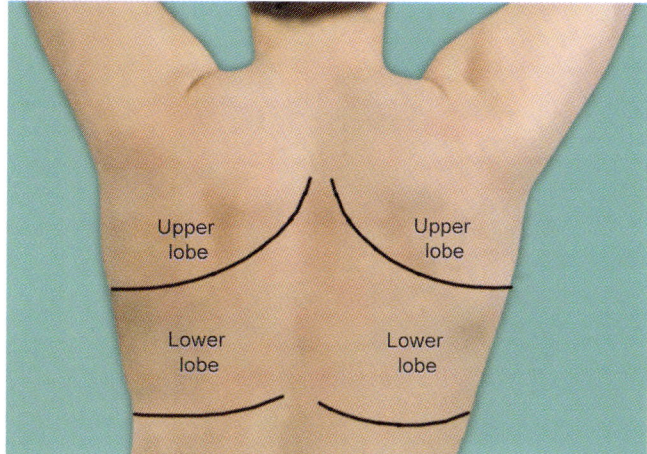

Fig. 3D.3: Posterior view of chest showing surface marking of lung fissures and lobes.

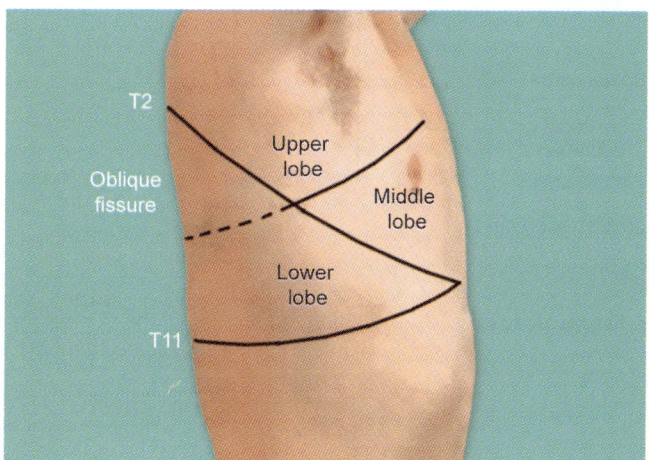

Fig. 3D.4: Right lateral view of chest showing right major interlobar (IL) fissure and right minor IL fissure.

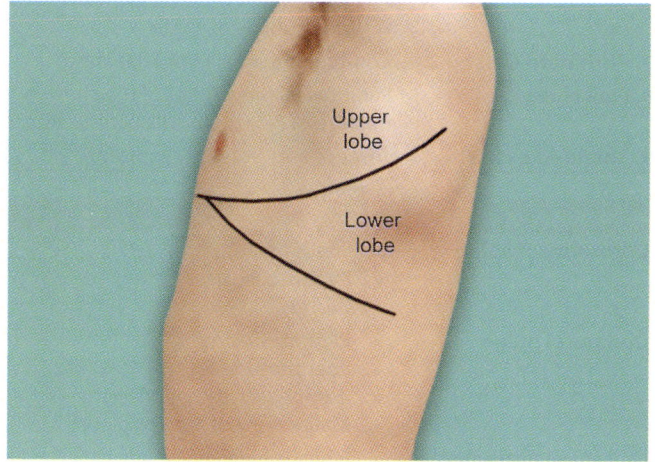

Fig. 3D.5: Left lateral view of chest showing left major interlobar fissure.

Level of lower border	Midclavicular line	Midaxillary line	Scapular
Lung (Figs. 3D.6 and 3D.7)	6th rib	8th rib	10th rib
Pleura	8th rib	10th rib	12th rib

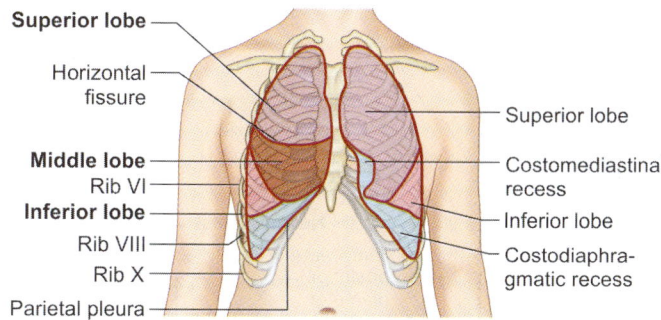

Fig. 3D.6: Lower margin of lung in midclavicular line and midaxillary line.

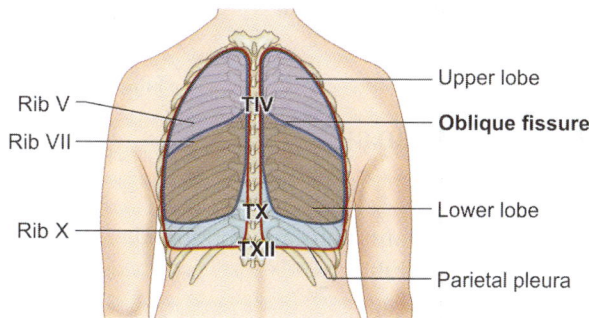

Fig. 3D.7: Lower margin of lung in scapular line.

Examination of chest:

Front examination	Back examination	Axillary examination
Predominantly to look for upper and middle lobe	Predominantly to look for lower lobe pathology	All three lobes can be assessed
Examined with patient in upright sitting position with hand by the side	Examined with patient in sitting upright with hands placed on the opposite shoulder and neck flexed	Examined with patient in the sitting position with hands raised above the shoulder and placed on the occiput

Position of patient during examination can be:
- Sitting—most of the examination is done in this position
- Standing—spine and shoulder droop
- Supine—shifting dullness.

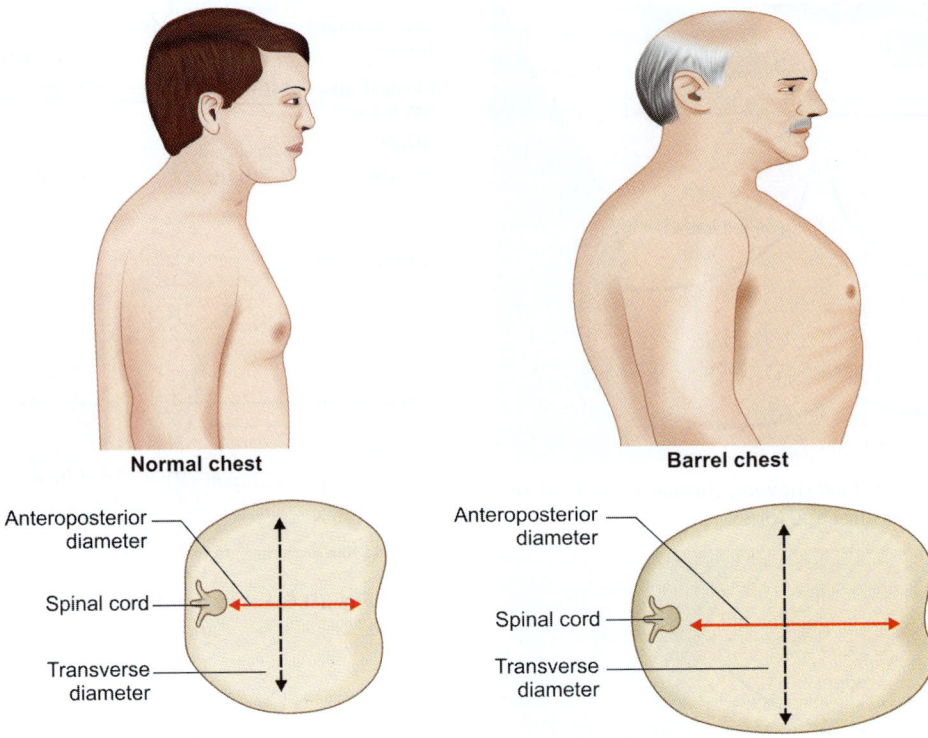

Fig. 3D.8: Normal- and barrel-shaped chest.

Normal chest (Fig. 3D.8):
- Spine—central
- Shape
  - Circular—infants and early childhood
  - Elliptical—adults
  - Circular—old age
- Vertical length > transverse diameter > AP diameter
- Transverse: AP = 7:5 (called as **Hutchinson's index**)
- Subcostal angle ≤90 (more acute in males).

Deformities of chest	
1. Flat chest (alar chest)	Anteroposterior ratio is 2:1
2. Pectus carinatum (Fig. 3D.9) (pigeon chest/keel chest)	Forward protrusion of sternum seen in rickets and childhood respiratory disease like asthma. Can also be seen in Marfan syndrome
3. Pectus excavatum (Fig. 3D.9) (funnel chest, cobbler's chest)	Funnel like depression at the lower end of the chest, seen in Marfan syndrome. Displaces the heart to the left. Ventilation capacity of the lung is restricted
4. Rachitic chest	<ul><li>Funnel shaped</li><li>Keel breast</li><li>Harrison sulci (horizontal groove where the diaphragm attaches to the ribs—seen in rickets, chronic asthma and COPD)</li><li>Vertical grooves on either side of sternum</li><li>Rachitic rosary (bead like enlargement of costochondral junction especially 4/5/6 ribs)—painless and seen in vitamin D deficiency</li></ul>
5. Scorbutic rosary	<ul><li>Sharp angulation of the ribs arising due to backward displacement of sternum</li><li>Painful and seen in vitamin C deficiency</li></ul>
6. Barrel-shaped chest (Fig. 3D.8)	COPD—emphysema<ul><li>Anteroposterior: Transverse diameter is 1:1</li><li>Exaggerated thoracic kyphosis</li><li>Wide subcostal angle</li></ul>
7. Phthinoid chest	Combination of alar and flat chest
8. Flail chest	Paradoxical movement of the chest in fracture of 3 or more consecutive ribs
9. Shield-like chest	Turner's and Noonan syndrome

Asymmetry of chest	
Deformity of spine	<ul><li>Scoliosis</li><li>Kyphoscoliosis</li><li>Gibbus</li></ul>
Unilateral bulge	<ul><li>Pleural effusion</li><li>Pneumothorax</li><li>Compensatory hypertrophy</li><li>Malignancy of lung or pleura</li></ul>
Unilateral flattening	<ul><li>Fibrosis</li><li>Collapse</li><li>Fibrothorax</li><li>Pneumonectomy</li><li>Agenesis of one lung (McLeod's syndrome/Swyer–James syndrome)</li><li>Mastectomy</li><li>Absent pectoralis major (Poland's syndrome)</li></ul>

Contd...

Local bulging (fullness)	▪ Supraclavicular fullness (pancoast tumor/lymphadenopathy/massive pleural effusion/tension pneumothorax) ▪ Empyema necessitans (cough impulse present) ▪ Aortic aneurysm ▪ Malignant infiltration ▪ Pericardial effusion ▪ Surgical emphysema
Local retraction	▪ Apical tuberculosis (**Morenheims** fossa/infraclavicular fossa) ▪ Lung fibrosis

Trachea:
Normally central or slightly deviated to right.

Trail sign (Fig. 3D.10):
In the presence of tracheal deviation, there is prominence of the clavicular head of sternocleidomastoid of same side. The investing layer of cervical fascia splits to enclose the sternocleidomastoid and then falls back and continues as the pretracheal fascia. When there is tracheal shift to one side, the fascia covering the ipsilateral sternocleidomastoid relaxes. The sternocleidomastoid goes into a state of contraction making the clavicular head prominent.

- Clinical implication of tracheal shift: It suggests upper mediastinal shift.
- Indicates upper lobe fibrosis or collapse.

Apical impulse:
- Normally 10 cm from sternal margin or ½ inch medial to Mid clavicular line.
- Clinical implication: Suggests lower mediastinal shift.

Examination of drooping of shoulder (Fig. 3D.11):
Examine the standing patient from behind to look for position of shoulder. Drooping of shoulder indicates volume loss on that side (collapse/fibrosis/fibrothorax/pneumonectomy). Rarely, it can be seen with paralysis of trapezius.

Associated features include:
- Prominent medial border of scapula on the affected side
- Space between medial border of scapula and spine is decreased
- Inferior angle of scapula is at the lower level (normally it is at level of T7 vertebra).

Examination of spine:
- Look for position of spine
- Look for scoliosis/kyphosis/lordosis/gibbus (**Figs. 3D.12A and B**)
- In emphysema there is exaggerated thoracic kyphosis.

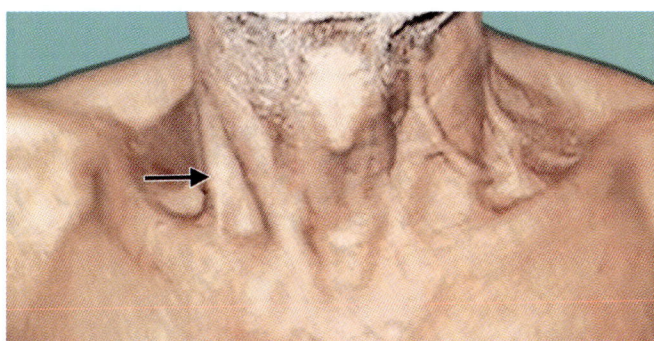

Fig. 3D.10: Trail sign showing undue prominence of sternocleidomastoid on the right side due to tracheal shift to right.

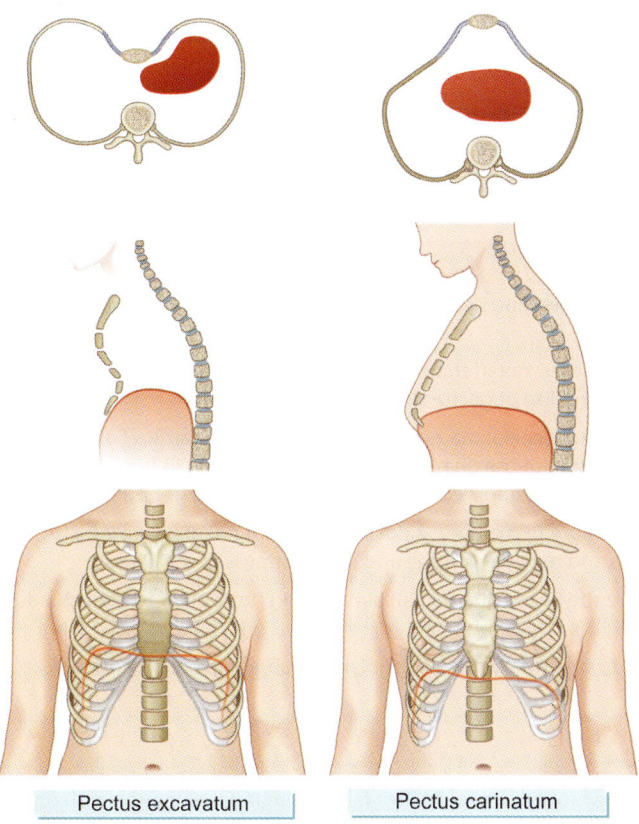

Fig. 3D.9: Pectus excavatum and pectus carinatum.

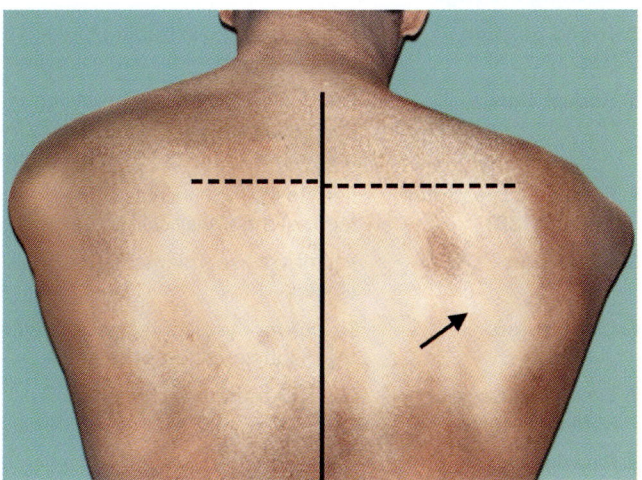

Fig. 3D.11: Shoulder drooping on right side.

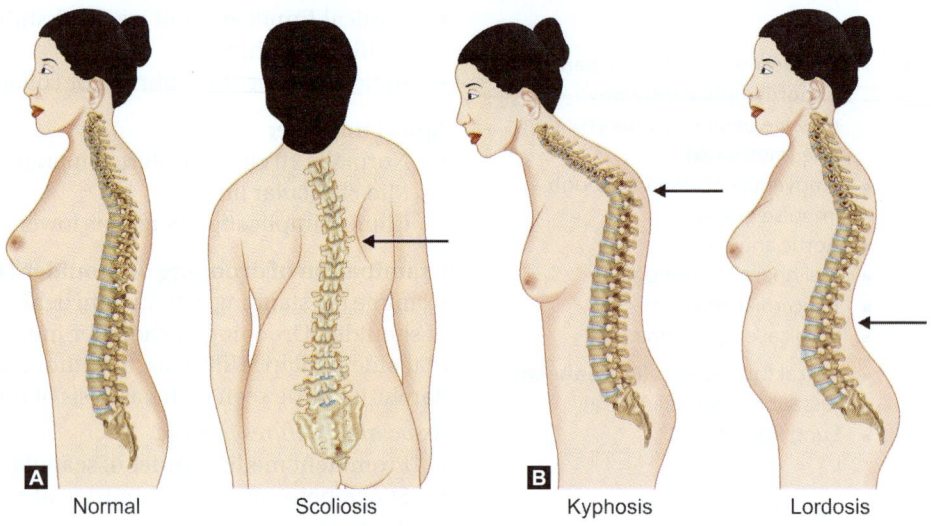

Figs. 3D.12A and B: Spine deformities.

Causes of scoliosis	
Neuromuscular causes	- Spina bifida - Marfan syndrome - Cerebral palsy - Friedreich's ataxia - Spinocerebellar degeneration - Charcot-Marie-Tooth disease - Syringomyelia - Poliomyelitis - Muscular dystrophy (Duchenne's, facioscapulohumeral, myotonic dystrophy)
Degenerative	- Osteoporosis - Postspine surgery

Contd...

Contd...	
Osteopathic	Klippel Feil syndrome
Congenital scoliosis	- Down's syndrome - Prader-Willi syndrome
Respiratory diseases	- Fibrosis - Fibrothorax
Idiopathic	—

Differentiation of congenital versus acquired scoliosis: On bending forwards acquired scoliosis disappears but congenital scoliosis persists.

Respiratory movements: (describe as equal/diminished in a particular area).

Abnormal signs in respiratory system	
1. Sitting up and catching the edge	Described in COPD where the patient sits up and fixes shoulders to use latissimus dorsi for expiration
2. Tripod position (Fig. 3D.13A)	Patient is sitting in leading forward posture with their outstretched hands on their knees. This position fixes and lifts the shoulder girdle and improves the function of pectoralis major and minor
3. Hoover sign	Paradoxical inspiratory indrawing of lateral rib cage (costal margin). It is a sign of chronic airflow obstruction. Pulmonary hyperinflation leads to loss of apposition of the diaphragmatic fibers resulting in horizontal orientation of fibers. When these horizontally oriented fibers contract, the costal margins get pulled inwards
4. Pursed lip breathing (Fig. 3D.13B)	Seen in COPD to increase the intra-alveolar pressure to maintain a positive intraluminal pressure which reduces the airway collapse, airway resistance and residual volume and hence improves ventilation
5. Dahl's sign	Patches of hyperpigmentation/bruising above the knees due to constant tenting position of the hands and elbows
6. Litten's sign	To look for the diaphragmatic movement, sit to one side of the patient lying in supine position and look at the diaphragmatic movements
7. Excessive usage of SCM and scalene	COPD or asthma
8. Paradoxical respiration	Indrawing of abdominal wall when the rib cage moves outwards. Best felt by bimanual palpation with one hand over the patient's chest and other on the abdomen. Indicates respiratory muscle weakness

Respiratory System Examination

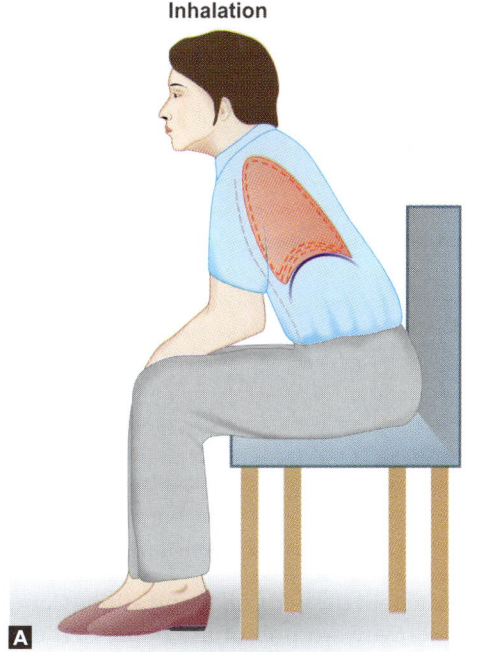
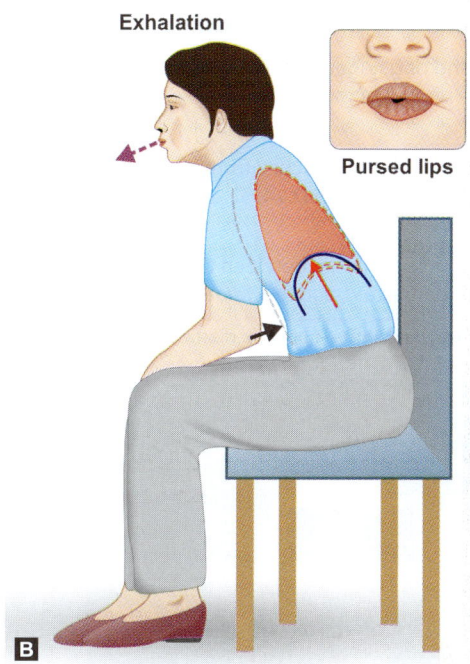

Figs. 3D.13A and B: Tripod position with pursed lip breathing.

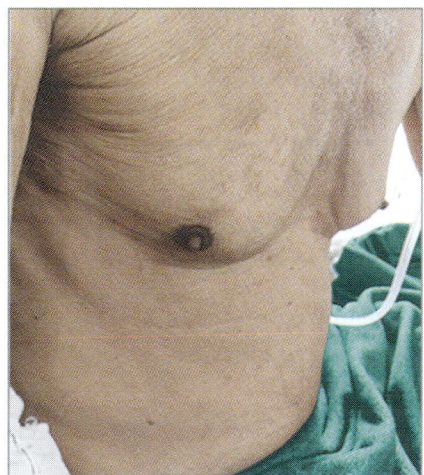

Fig. 3D.13C: Intercostal retractions.

Inspiratory intercostal retraction (Fig. 3D.13C):
Mild degree of intercostal retraction in the lower chest is normal. Bilateral lower intercostal retractions is seen in COPD.

Unilateral intercostal retraction	Bilateral intercostal retraction
▪ Collapse ▪ Fibrosis ▪ Adherent pericarditis (**Broadbent's sign**—indrawing of lower anterior chest wall with each ventricular systole)	▪ Indicates upper airway obstruction (adenoids/foreign body) ▪ Hyperinflation of chest (COPD)

Visible pulsations/scars/sinuses:

Visible pulsation or vessels	
Collaterals around scapula	Coarctation of aorta (**Suzman's sign**)
Engorged veins over the anterior part of chest	SVC obstruction seen in ▪ Bronchogenic carcinoma ▪ Mediastinal growth ▪ Mediastinal lymph nodes ▪ Aortic aneurysm ▪ Chronic mediastinal fibrosis
Pulsatile swelling in anterior chest wall	Aortic aneurysm
Visible scars	
▪ Previous surgery (lobectomy) ▪ Pleural fluid aspiration site ▪ Lymph node biopsy site	
Sinuses	
▪ Abscess draining points ▪ Empyema thoracis (usually in tuberculosis/actinomycosis)	

Palpation (Lower Respiratory Tract)

Trachea:
- Normal length: 4–5 cm above suprasternal notch
- Normal cricoid to suprasternal notch distance is 3–4 finger breadth (decreased in COPD due to hyperinflation).

Method of palpation for tracheal position:

Keep the index and ring finger of the right hand on medial ends of the clavicle
↓
With middle finger trace the trachea from above downwards **(Fig. 3D.14)**
↓
Then, insinuate the middle finger between the trachea and sternal head of sternocleidomastoid, and feel for resistance **(Fig. 3D.15)**

Note: **Implication of tracheal shift**—upper mediastinal shift

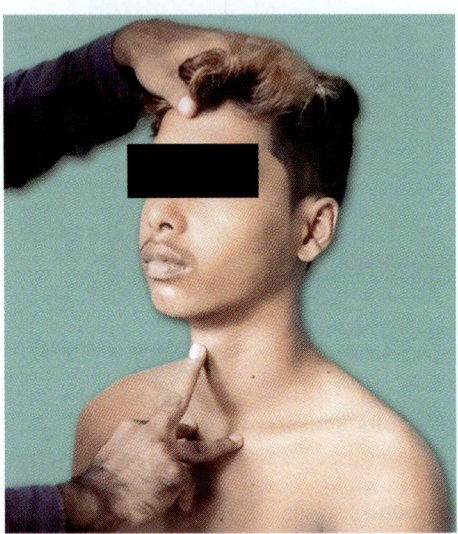

Fig. 3D.14: Tracing the trachea down with the middle finger.

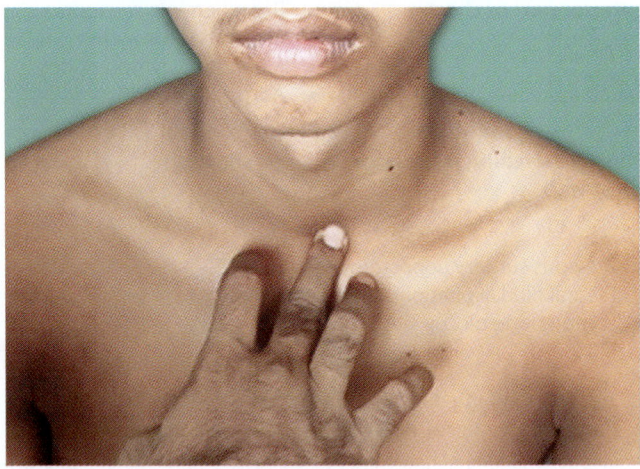

Fig. 3D.15: Insinuate the middle finger between the trachea and sternal head of sternocleidomastoid, and feel for resistance.

Oliver's sign (tracheal tug sign) (Fig. 3D.16):
Stand behind patient and hold cricoid cartilage give a slight upward thrust.

Positive test	Downward pull with each heart beat suggestive of aortic aneurysm
Negative test	Normal
False positive	Mediastinal tumor attached to abdominal aorta
False negative	Thrombosed aortic aneurysm

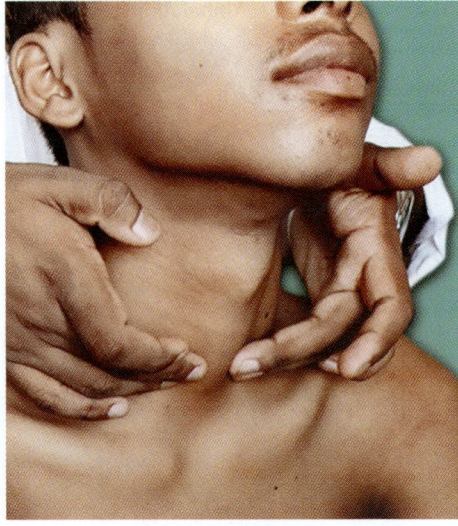

Fig. 3D.16: Demonstration of Oliver's sign.

- **Tracheal descent on inspiration (Campbell sign):** Due to downward pull of the depressed diaphragm in long standing hyperinflation of lung.
- **Laryngeal fixation:** Increased pressure on cricoid cartilage due to inflammatory or neoplastic lesion in mediastinum.

Apical impulse:
- Confirm the position of apex
- Comment on character
- Watch for thrills and other palpable heart sounds
- **Implication of apical impulse shift:** It suggests lower mediastinal shift.

Apex not felt/seen in respiratory diseases:
1. Emphysema
2. Left-sided pleural effusion
3. Left-sided pneumothorax.

Mediastinal shift with respect to respiratory diseases	
Shift to same side	▪ Fibrosis ▪ Collapse ▪ Pneumonectomy/lobectomy
Shift to opposite side	▪ Pleural effusion ▪ Pneumothorax ▪ Tumor or mass
No shift of mediastinum	Unilateral disease ▪ Pneumonia Bilateral disease ▪ COPD ▪ Asthma ▪ Bronchiectasis ▪ Interstitial lung disease

Examination of respiratory movements	
Upper anterior chest (Figs. 3D.17A and B)	▪ Examined by placing the palms in the infraclavicular areas ▪ Look for superior anterior movement of the palms ▪ This examines the **pump handle** movement of the upper lobes

Contd...

Contd...

Lower anterior chest (Figs. 3D.18A and B)	• Grasp the sides of the chest and approximate the tips of the thumbs in the mammary area with loose fold of skin in between • Watch for separation of the thumbs and compare the movements with each respiration • It demonstrates the **bucket handle** movements of the lower chest
Upper posterior chest (Fig. 3D.19)	• Examine from the back by placing hand in the supraclavicular fossa and watch for movements superiorly • This demonstrates the movement of the apical segment
Lower posterior chest (Fig. 3D.20)	• Grasp the sides of the chest and approximate the tips of the thumbs in the infrascapular area with loose fold of skin in between • Watch for separation of the thumbs and compare the movements with each respiration • This demonstrate the lower lobe movements

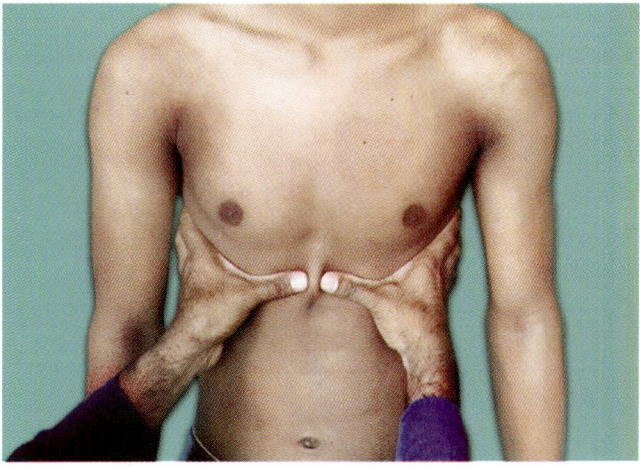

Fig. 3D.18A: Examination of respiratory movements of lower anterior chest.

Elevation of ribs

↓

Increase in lateral diameter of thoracic cavity

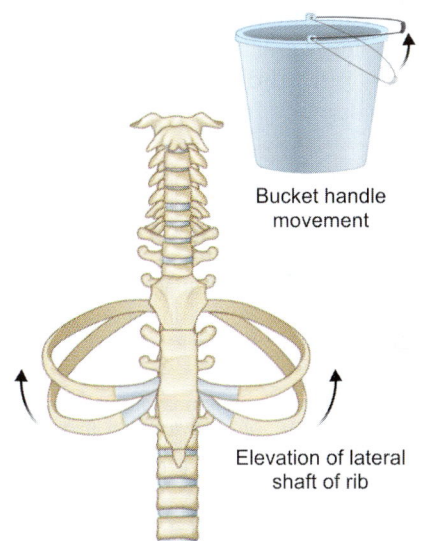

Fig. 3D.18B: Bucket handle movement.

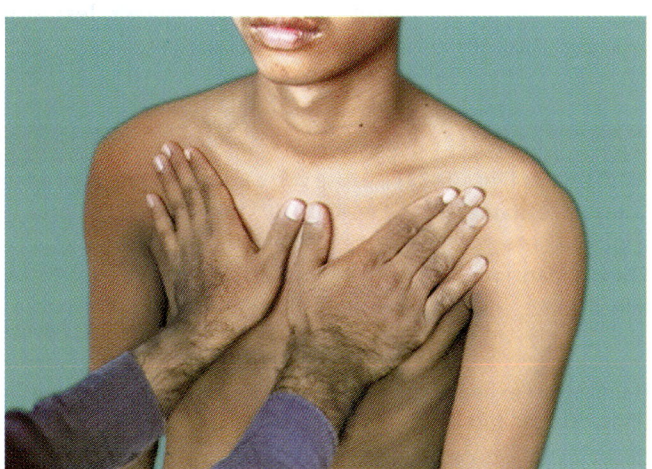

Fig. 3D.17A: Examination of respiratory movements of upper anterior chest.

Elevation of ribs

Increase in anteroposterior diameter of thoracic cavity

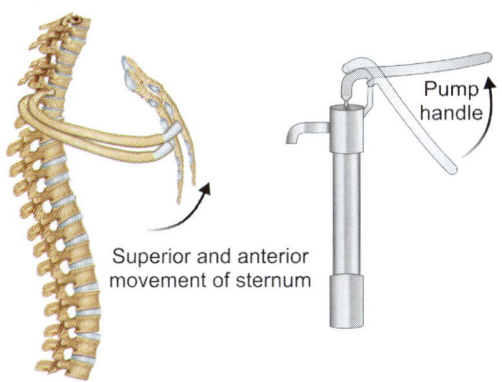

Fig. 3D.17B: Pump handle movement.

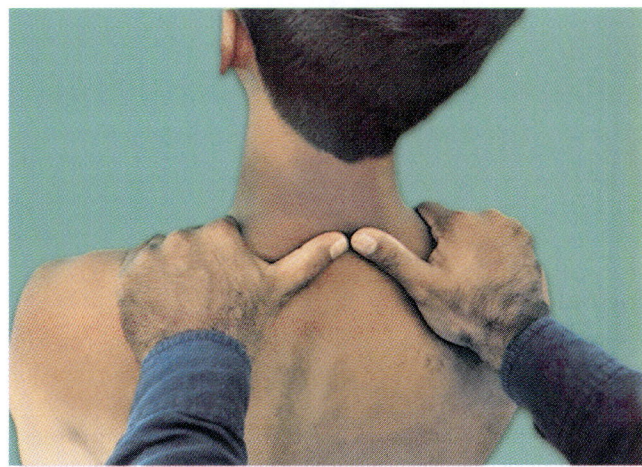

Fig. 3D.19: Examination of respiratory movements of upper posterior chest.

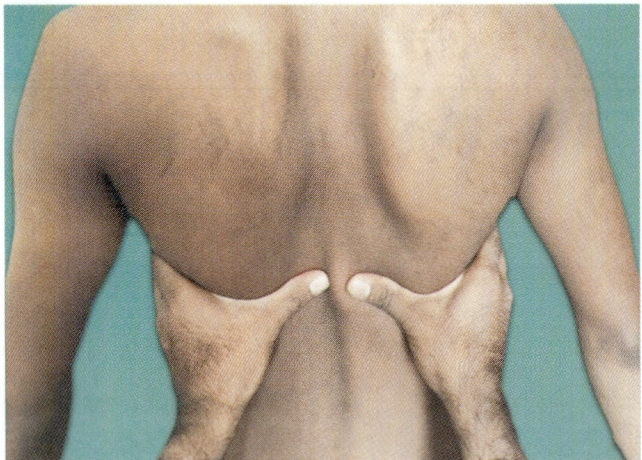

Fig. 3D.20: Examination of respiratory movements of lower posterior chest.

Diaphragmatic movements:
- Place one hand on chest and other hand on the abdomen (Fig. 3D.21)
- Normally—both hands are lifted during inspiration
- If chest rises but abdomen remains static—suggests an abdominal pathology which is fixing the abdomen
- If chest rises but abdomen retracts—suggests diaphragmatic palsy.

Causes of decreased chest movements	
Unilateral	Bilateral
• Pleural effusion	• COPD
• Empyema	• Asthma
• Pneumothorax	• Interstitial lung disease
• Fibrosis	• Ankylosing spondylitis
• Collapse	• Systemic sclerosis

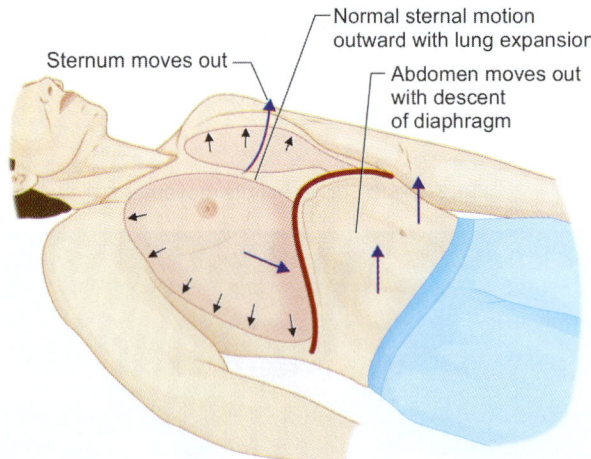

Normal Inspiration

Descent of the diaphragm raises intra-abdominal pressure moving the abdomen outwards along with chest expansion. The sternum moves outward.

In the hyperinflated patient with obstructive lung diseases the flattened diaphragm pulls in the lower ribs at end-inspiration (Hoover's sign). The sternum is pulled cephalad by the action of the strap muscles of the neck. The abdomen may be retracted by the passive transmission of intrathoracic pressure across the dysfunctional diaphragm.

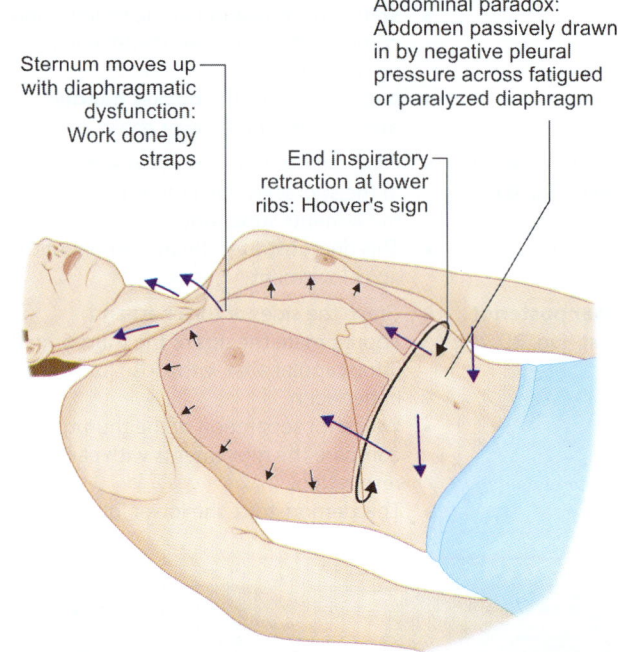

Measurements of chest diameters	
AP diameter (Fig. 3D.22)	Use two cardboards and place as shown in **Figure 3D.22**.
Transverse diameter (Fig. 3D.23)	Normal ratio of AP:T = 5:7
Chest expansion (Fig. 3D.24)	Normal = 5–8 cm (adult), decreases with age (e.g., 60 years ≥3 cm is considered normal) COPD/ILD expansion is <1.5 cm
Hemithorax expansion (Figs. 3D.25A and B)	Stand on side and place the tape from spine to midsternal as shown in **Figures 3D.25A and B**.

Note: Chest expansion should be assessed as the difference of measurement between deep inspiration to deep expiration.

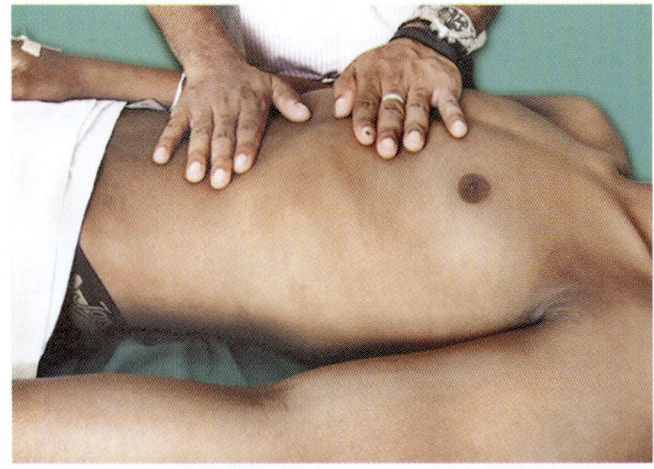

Fig. 3D.21: Examination of diaphragmatic movements.

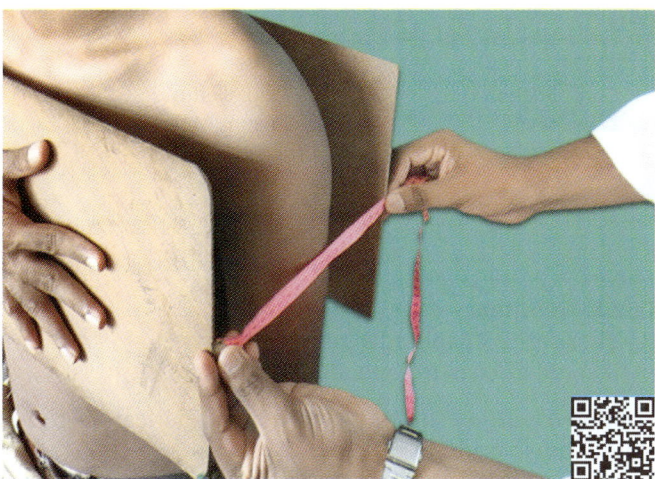

Fig. 3D.22: Examination of anteroposterior diameter.

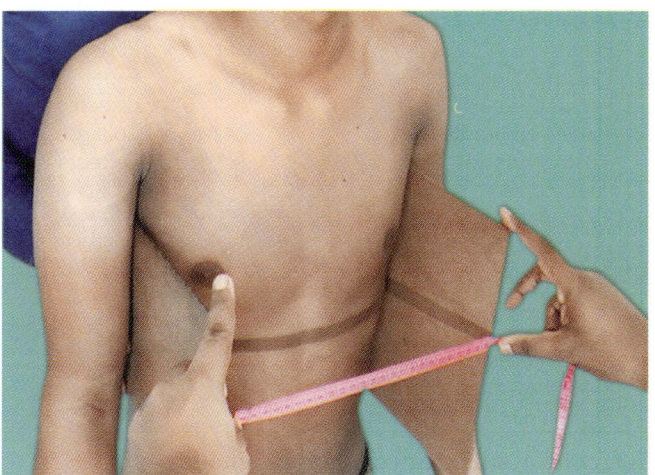

Fig. 3D.23: Examination of transverse diameter.

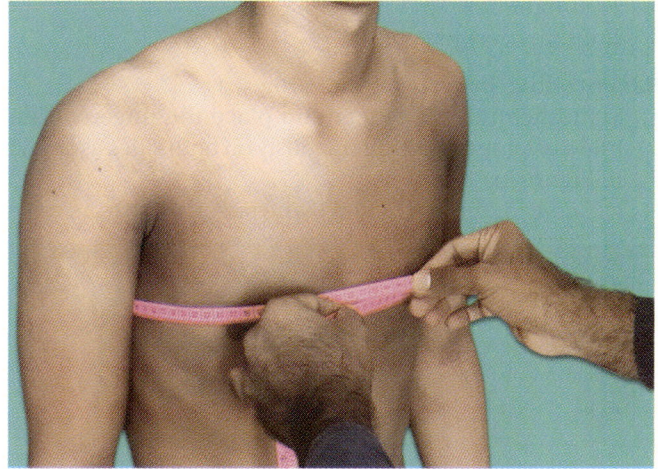

Fig. 3D.24: Examination of chest expansion (crossed tape).

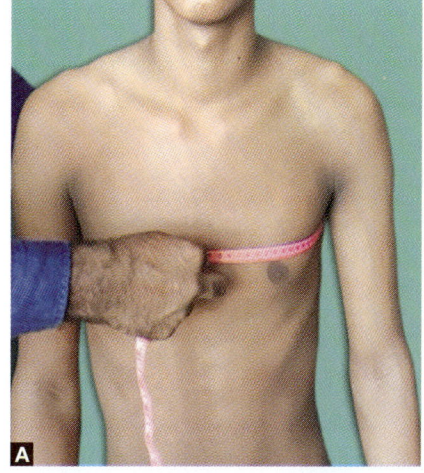

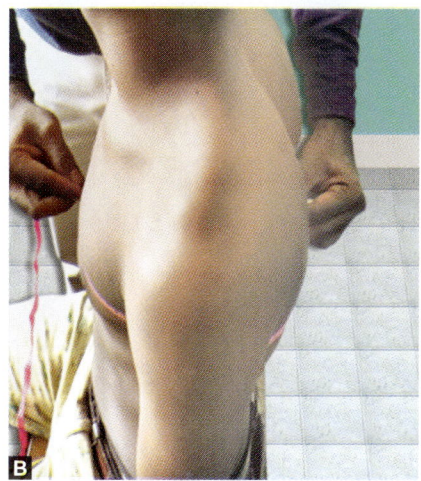

Figs. 3D.25A and B: Examination of hemithorax circumference.

THE MOST IMPORTANT EXAMINATION FINDING IS TO CHECK FOR HEMITHORAX EXPANSION AND HEMITHORAX MEASUREMENT

Remember: "The side that moves less is the site of disease."

Increased hemithorax size with decreased hemithorax movement	Decreased hemithorax size with decreased hemithorax movement	Normal hemithorax size with decreased hemithorax movement
▪ Pleural effusion ▪ Pneumothorax	▪ Fibrosis ▪ Collapse	Consolidation

Examination of spinoscapular distance (Fig. 3D.26): It is the distance between the spine and the scapular line (scapular line is the vertical line passing through the inferior angle of scapula).

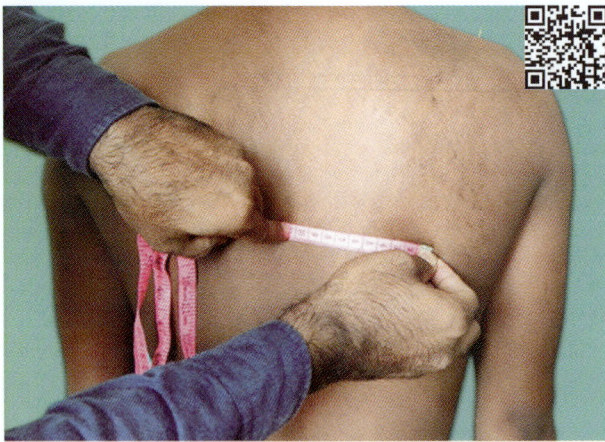

Fig. 3D.26: Examination of spinoscapular distance.

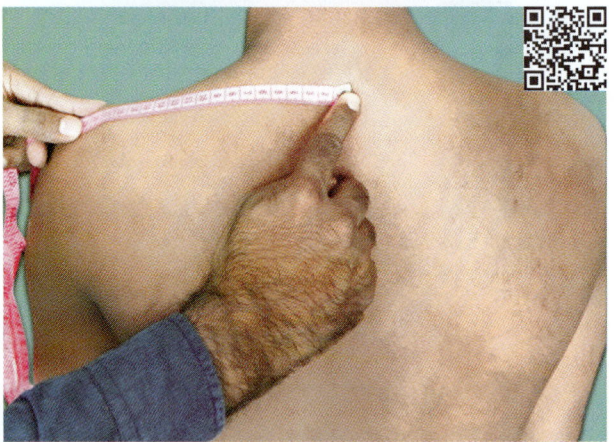

Fig. 3D.27: Examination of spinoacromion distance.

Examination of spinoacromion distance (Fig. 3D.27): It is the distance measured between the spine and the tip of acromion process.

Vocal fremitus:
- The sounds produced by vocal cords are transmitted along the tracheobronchial tree and heard/felt over the chest wall.
- Place the ulnar border of the hands on identical areas on both sides of the chest **(Fig. 3D.28)**.
- Ask the patient to repeat "one-one-one-"

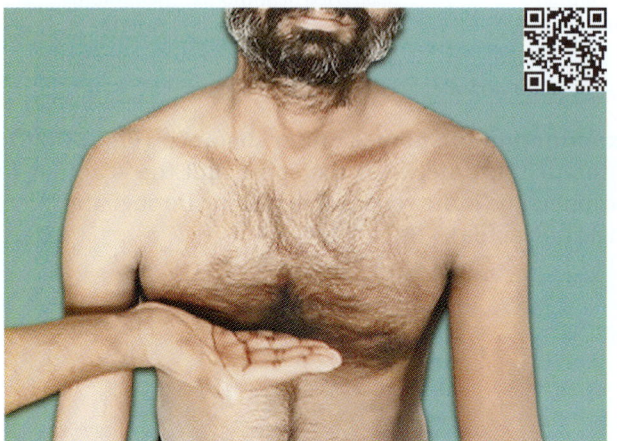

Fig. 3D.28: Demonstration of vocal fremitus.

Vocal fremitus	
Increased	*Decreased*
▪ Consolidation ▪ Large cavity ▪ Bronchopleural fistula	▪ Pleural effusion ▪ Pneumothorax ▪ Fibrosis ▪ Collapse ▪ Asthma ▪ Emphysema ▪ Thick pleura

Tactile fremitus:
- These are palpable adventitious sounds
- It could be coarse crepitations or rhonchi.

Friction fremitus: These include palpable pericardial rub or pleural rub (e.g., dry pleurisy).

Tenderness:

Over intercostal spaces	*Over ribs*	*Over spines*
▪ Empyema ▪ Pleurisy ▪ Malignant mesothelioma ▪ Pneumothorax ▪ Tietze's syndrome (costochondritis) ▪ Pneumonia ▪ Pulmonary abscess ▪ Hepatic abscess ▪ Pulmonary embolism ▪ Pulmonary infarction ▪ Herpes zoster before appearance of eruption ▪ Intercostal muscle pain ▪ Recent injury to the chest	▪ Rib fracture ▪ Malignant deposits in the ribs	▪ Spinal injury ▪ Potts disease ▪ Paget's disease ▪ Collapse vertebra *Over sternum* Due to leukemia/ infiltration

Detection of subcutaneous emphysema:
Spongy crepitant feeling on palpation
1. Injury to chest wall or airway
2. Pneumothorax
3. Rupture of esophagus

Rib crowding/intercostal widening:
- Stand behind the patient and place the fingers in the intercostal spaces simultaneously on both sides as shown in **Figure 3D.29**.
- Observe for the separation of the fingers

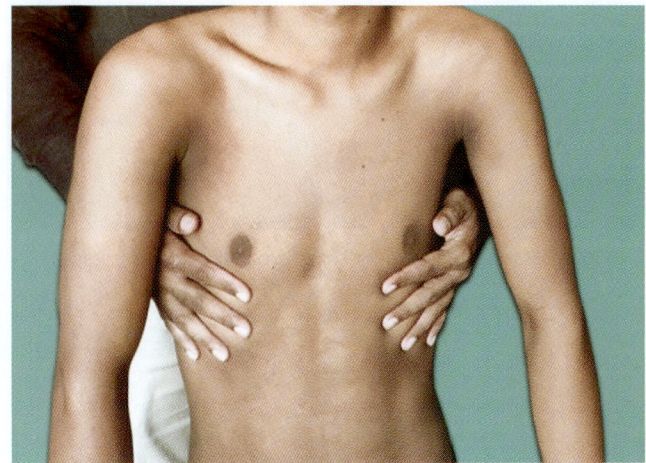

Fig. 3D.29: Examination of rib crowding.

Respiratory System Examination

Rib crowding		Intercostal widening	
Unilateral	*Bilateral*	*Unilateral*	*Bilateral*
▪ Atelectasis ▪ Collapse ▪ Fibrosis ▪ Pneumonectomy	▪ Interstitial lung disease ▪ Fibrosis (bilateral)	▪ Pneumothorax ▪ Pleural effusion	Emphysema

Percussion (Lower Respiratory Tract)

Preferably done in sitting position, supine position is needed for demonstrating shifting dullness.

Position of patient for percussion:
- **Anterior chest (Fig. 3D.30):** Sits up straight with hands by his side
- **Axilla (Fig. 3D.31):** Raise the arm over the head and place over the back of head
- **Posterior of chest (Fig. 3D.32):** Sits up with hands crossed and placed over the opposite shoulders.

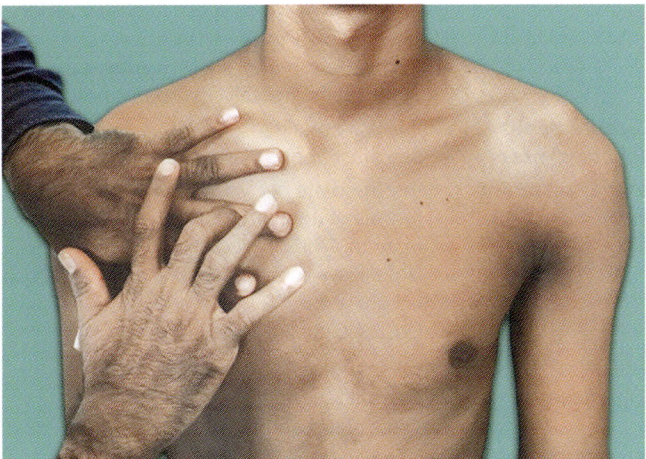

Fig. 3D.30: Demonstration of percussion of anterior chest.

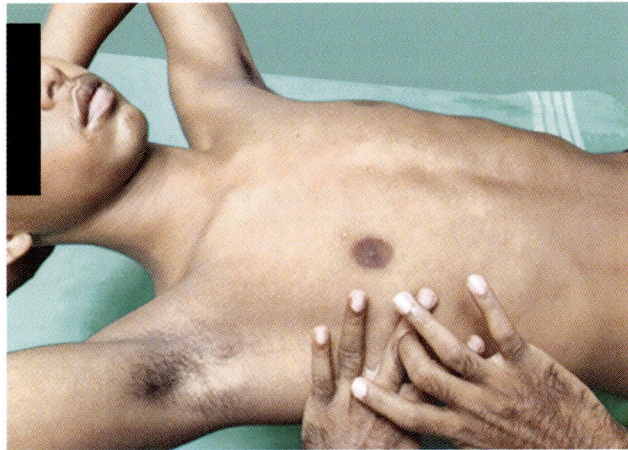

Fig. 3D.31: Demonstration of percussion of axillary area.

Rules of Percussion

1. **Direction of percussion:** Always percuss from resonant to nonresonant area.
2. **Pleximeter** is usually the middle phalanx of middle finger of left/nondominant hand and is firmly placed on the surface while rest of fingers are slightly lifted off.

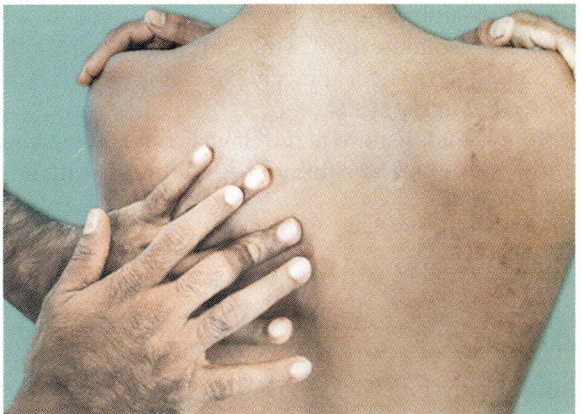

Fig. 3D.32: Demonstration of percussion over the posterior chest.

3. **Plexor/plessor** (percussing finger) is middle finger of the right/dominant hand.
4. The movement of the plexor hand should be sudden and originating from the wrist.
5. The pleximeter must be kept parallel to the border to be percussed.
6. Percuss around 2–3 times over each area.
7. Percussion has to be heard as well as felt.
8. Always percuss the identical areas of chest for comparison.
9. The distance between the pleximeter finger and the ear should preferably be maintained.
10. Normal location of percussion notes (**Fig. 3D.33**).

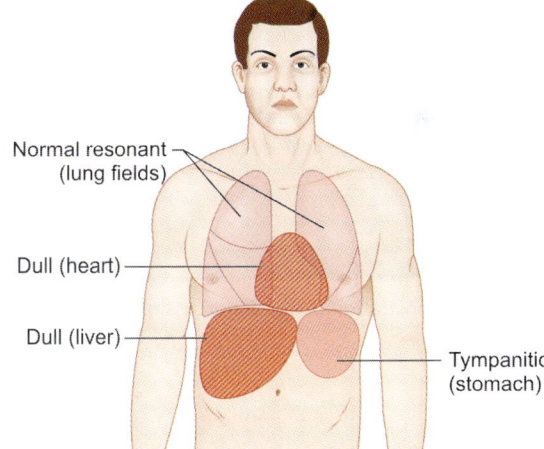

Fig. 3D.33: Normal location of percussion notes.

Types of Percussion

Heavy percussion	Light percussion
Posterior part of chest	Anterior part of chest and abdomen

Direct percussion	Indirect percussion	Auscultatory percussion
Directly over the bony structures like clavicle and sternum	By percussing over the pleximeter finger with the plexor/plessor	Was first described by Laennec and used to delineate the size of organs by placing the stethoscope directly above the structure to be outlined, followed by percussion from the periphery towards the organ of interest

Direct percussion (Fig. 3D.34):
- Percuss the middle third of the clavicle with plexor finger.
- Stretch the skin over the clavicle using the left hand as shown in **Figure 3D.34**.
- Normally middle third of the clavicle is resonant whereas the medial and lateral thirds are dull (because of muscles attached).

Impaired note	Heard in apical fibrosis
Dull note	Mass lesion like pancoast tumor
Widening of zone of resonance	Heard in pneumothorax or emphysema

Flicking percussion: Flicking using thumb and finger—done for percussion of the abdomen, cardiac border and to check for metallic note of pneumothorax.

Guarino's method of auscultatory percussion:
- Examined with patient sitting up and examiner facing the back of the patient.
- Place the stethoscope around 3 cm below the last rib in the scapular line as shown in **Figure 3D.35**.
- Now percuss with the free hand (by finger flicking or with pulp of the finger) along 3 or more parallel lines from the apex of each hemithorax perpendicularly downward towards the base to note the dullness.

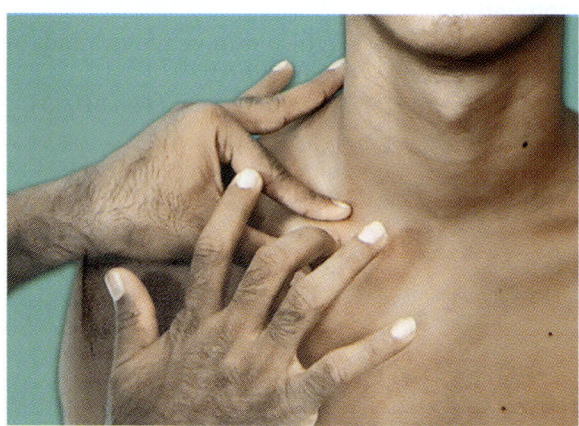

Fig. 3D.34: Demonstration of direct percussion over the clavicle.

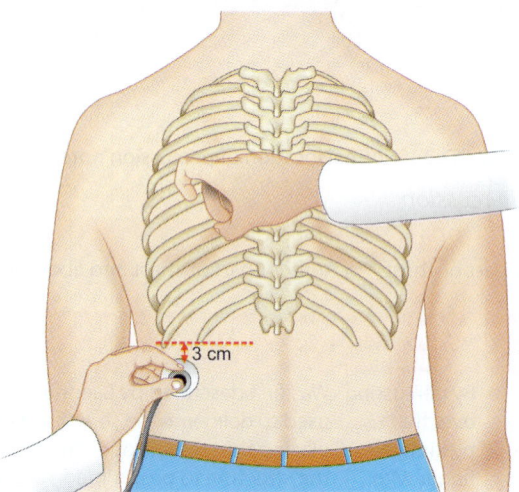

Fig. 3D.35: Guarino's method of auscultatory percussion in pleural effusion.

Lung Resonance

Normal:
- Vesicular resonance
- Front of chest more resonant
- Lesion >5 cm from chest wall or <2–3 cm in size will not alter the percussion note.

Abnormal types of percussion notes	
Quantitative	*Qualitative*
▪ Tympanic note	▪ Crackpot
▪ Subtympanic note	▪ Amphoric
▪ Hyper-resonant note	▪ Bell tympany
▪ Impaired note	
▪ Dull/woody dull note	
▪ Stony dull note	

Quantitative types	
Tympanic note	▪ It is a drum-like note ▪ Normally seen over the stomach, intestine—Traube's space (any percussion over hollow viscus) ▪ In chest—superficial cavity, subcutaneous emphysema (metallic tympanic note)
Subtympanic (skodaic) note	▪ It is Boxy quality ▪ Seen just above pleural effusion
Hyper-resonant note	▪ Intermediate between normal and tympanic note ▪ Bilateral—emphysema ▪ Unilateral—pneumothorax, compensatory emphysema ▪ Large bullae
Impaired note	▪ Airless areas (fibrosis, collapse)
Dull note	▪ Consolidation ▪ Thick pleura (fibrothorax)
Flat dull/Woody dull	▪ Can be elicited by percussing over the thigh ▪ Seen in pleural effusion
Stony dullness	▪ Pain over the pleximeter finger with resistance felt by plexor ▪ Large pleural effusion ▪ Large solid tumor

Qualitative types	
Cracked pot resonance	▪ Normally seen in chest of infants or child during the act of crying ▪ Pathological lung cavity with communication with bronchus due to sudden expulsion of air form the cavity to bronchus ▪ Artificially imitated by beating clasped hands over the knee
Amphoric	▪ Low pitched hollow note ▪ Normally seen in trachea and cheek distended with air ▪ Pathologically seen in pneumothorax and large cavity
Bell tympany	▪ High pitched metallic or tympanic note ▪ Seen in massive pneumothorax ▪ Place coin on affected side of chest and percuss with another coin while simultaneously auscultating the back

Respiratory System Examination

Dullness in presence of fluid in lung	
Straight line dullness/shifting dullness	Hydropneumothorax
S-shaped curve of Ellis	Pleural effusion

5-7-9 rule:
The upper border of liver dullness is at 5th intercostal space (ICS) in midclavicular line, 7th ICS in the midaxillary line and 9th ICS in the scapular line.

Topographical Percussion of Lung
Apical percussion:
- **Kronig's isthmus:** It is a band of resonance in the supraclavicular area bounded anteriorly by the posterior border of the clavicle, medially by the neck muscles, posteriorly by the anterior border of trapezius, extended laterally till the acromioclavicular joint.
- Stand behind the patient, place the pleximeter finger over the neck and percuss from lateral to medial as shown in **Figure 3D.36**.
- On percussion there is dull zone medially and laterally, and only middle part is resonant.
- Dullness in this area suggests apical tuberculosis, Pancoast tumor or apical fibrosis.
- The zone of resonance may be widened in emphysema or apical pneumothorax.

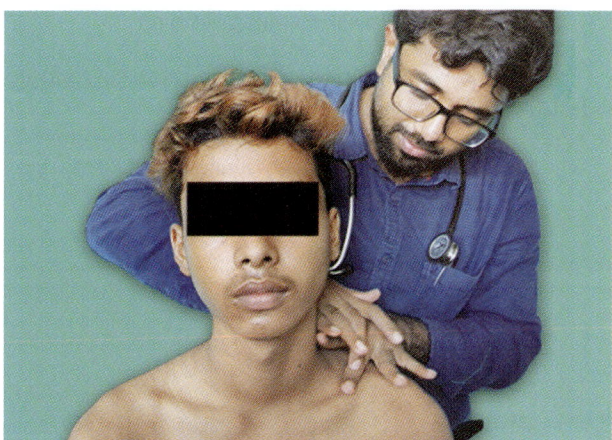

Fig. 3D.36: Percussion of apical area (Kronig's isthmus).

Tidal percussion:
- Tidal percussion is a measure of diaphragmatic excursion
- It is used to differentiate whether the causes of dullness are above the diaphragm (subpulmonic effusion) or below (subphrenic collections)
- With patient in, percuss the right side of the chest from above downwards till you get the liver dullness. Normally, it is in 5th intercostal space.
- Ask the patient to take a deep inspiration and hold his breath.
- Now percuss the same area
- Normally, dullness moves down by 1–2 intercostal spaces as shown in **Figure 3D.35**.
- Tidal percussion is negative in right-sided subpulmonic effusion, diaphragmatic paralysis.
- In emphysema, since the lung is already fully expanded tidal percussion will be negative **(Figs. 3D.37A and B)**.

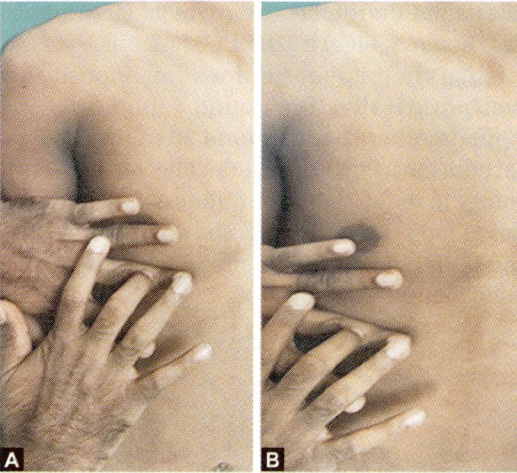

Figs. 3D.37A and B: Demonstration of tidal percussion: (A) Expiration; (B) Inspiration (Note the change in liver dullness from expiration to inspiration).

Percussion of Traube's space (Fig. 3D.38):
It is a semilunar space in the left anterior chest bounded by:
- Above by 6th rib
- Below by left costal margin
- Laterally by anterior axillary line.

Normal Traube's space percussion	Tympanic note
Obliteration of Traube's space	<ul><li>Left sided pleural effusion</li><li>Pericardial effusion</li><li>Massive splenomegaly</li><li>Enlarged left lobe of the liver</li><li>Full stomach or fundic mass</li></ul>
Upward shift of Traube's space	<ul><li>Left diaphragmatic paralysis</li><li>Left lower lobe collapse or fibrosis</li></ul>

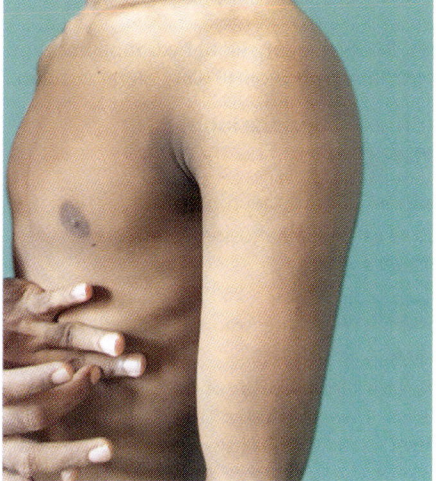

Fig. 3D.38: Percussion of Traube's space.

Shifting dullness:
It is classically described for hydropneumothorax. It can also be demonstrated in pleural effusion.

Steps:
- Percuss the anterior chest in sitting position, from above downward to get upper border of dullness. You will get a

level of straight-line dullness perpendicular to long axis of body as shown in **Figure 3D.39A**. Mark this level.
- Now, make the patient lie down in opposite lateral position/normal side (for around 5 minutes in case of hydropneumothorax and around 30 minutes in case of pleural effusion). Percuss over the affected side and note the change in the straight-line dullness which will now be parallel to long axis of body as shown in **Figure 3D.38B**. Shifting dullness may be absent in case of empyema or loculated pleural effusion.

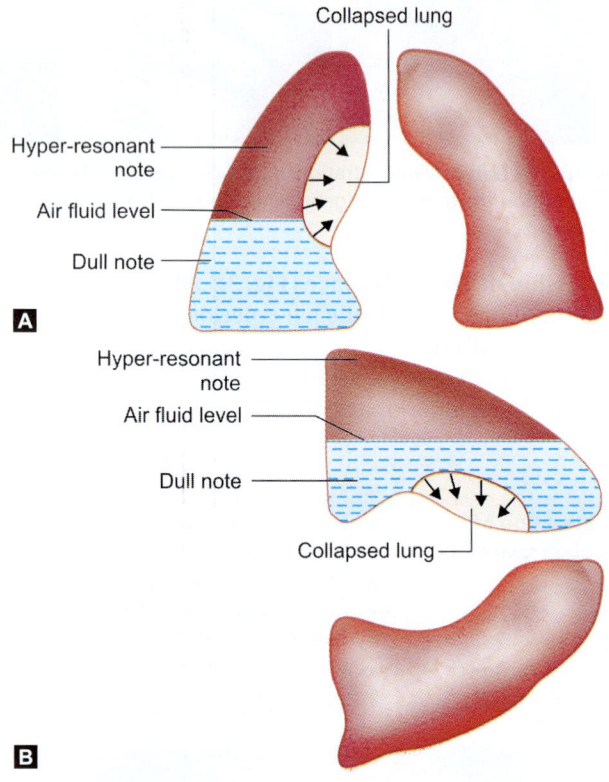

Figs. 3D.39A and B: Right hydropneumothorax: (A) Sitting position; (B) Left lateral position.

Special findings in percussion:

Special finding	Clinical condition
Shifting dullness	Hydropneumothorax
S-shaped curve of Ellis (Damoiseau's curve)	Pleural effusion (moderate)
Obliteration of Traube's space	Pleural effusion (left sided)
Grocco's triangle (Fig. 3D.39) (Paravertebral triangle of dullness)	**Boundaries of Grocco's triangle:** - **Medially:** The mid-spinal line from the level of the effusion to the level of the tenth dorsal vertebra - **Below:** A horizontal line extending outwards from the tenth dorsal vertebra along the lower limit of lung resonance - **Laterally:** A curved line connecting these two lines **Clinical condition:** Seen over the back of the chest, on the opposite side of effusion in moderate to massive pleural effusions

Contd...

Contd...

Garland's triangle (Fig. 3D.40)	- Small area of resonance next to the spine found in patients with large unilateral pleural effusions - Lower relaxed part of the lung in moderate or large pleural effusion is tympanic or subtympanic
William's tracheal resonance	**Description:** - Area of tympany over the first or second intercostal space, close to sternum **Seen in:** - Patch of consolidation or fibrosis interposed between the trachea or a major bronchus and the chest wall - Referred to as **"pulled trachea syndrome"** in fibrotic apical tuberculosis
Wintrich's sign	**Description:** - Percussion note over an area during inspiration appears clearer and higher-pitched with the mouth open than with it closed **Seen in:** - Lung cavity communicating with a bronchus, pneumothorax or mediastinal tumor
Gerhardt's sign	**Description:** - Percussion note over an area appears lower pitched with the patient recumbent than with him standing or sitting **Seen in:** - Lung cavity containing both fluid and air
Friedreich's sign	**Description:** - Percussion note over an area becomes higher in pitch during forced inspiration than during expiration **Seen in:** - Lung cavity

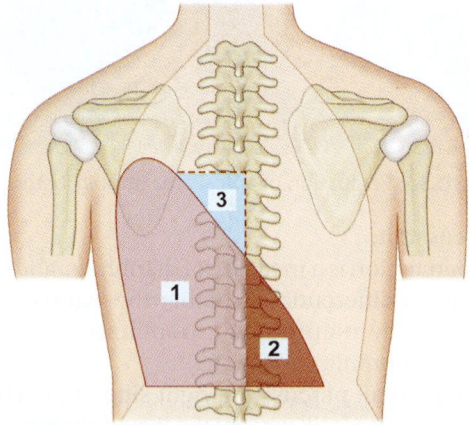

Fig. 3D.40: Special findings in percussion: (1) Effusion, (2) Rauchfuss-Grocco triangle, (3) Garland triangle.

Auscultation (Lower Respiratory Tract)

Position of patient:

In upright position	Front	Sitting or standing
	Back	Preferably sitting and leaning forward with neck flexed and arms crossed in front
In recumbent position	Back	Turn the patient sideways or slip the steth underneath the patient

Respiratory System Examination

Breathing advice:
Ask the patient to breathe through the mouth. If not cooperating ask the patient to count numbers or cough successively and then observe during deep inspiration.

A quiet room and a stethoscope are needed when examining the patient with the intent of auscultating their breath sounds.

The diaphragm of the stethoscope should be used for the assessment

The examination should not be conducted over clothing of any kind, regardless of how thin that clothing may be; it should be done in such a manner that the stethoscope has direct contact with the skin.

Normal physiology of breath sounds:

Mechanism of sound production	
In larger airways (pharynx, large airways of trachea and lung)	*In smaller airways*
Sounds are generated due to turbulence	Higher frequencies are lost due to dampening when they travel from higher to smaller airways
They are the source of sound	They are just filter sounds and not the source of sound
Sound frequencies are of range 200–2,000 Hz	Sound frequencies are of range 200–400 Hz
Heard over the upper sternum	Heard over most other areas of lung

Grading of breath sound intensity	
0	Absent breath sounds
1	Barely audible breath sound
2	Faint but definitely audible breath sound
3	Normal breath sound
4	Louder than normal breath sound

Graphical representation of breath sounds	
Upstroke	Inspiratory element
Downstroke	Expiratory element
Length	Duration or timing
Thickness	Loudness or intensity
Angle between upstroke and downstroke made with a vertical line	Pitch of respiratory sound Lower the angle higher is the pitch

Types of normal breathing	
Vesicular breathing	Most areas of chest
Tracheal/bronchial breathing	- Larynx - Trachea - Between C7 and T3
Bronchovesicular	- Anteriorly 1st and 2nd intercostal space - Posteriorly between the scapula

Vesicular breath sounds	
Characteristics	- Rustling or breezy quality - Longer duration of inspiratory phase (which includes both tubular and alveolar phase) - Higher pitch of inspiratory sound - I:E = 2–3:1 - Absence of pause between I and E
Distribution	Most of chest

Contd...

Contd...

Intensity	- Louder: Infraclavicular, axillary and infrascapular areas - Diminished: Lower margins of lung and over the scapular areas
Mode of production	Distension and separation of alveolar walls by the in rushing current of air
Graphical representation	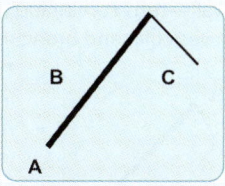

a. Tubular phase of inspiration
b. Alveolar phase of inspiration
c. Expiration

Tracheal (bronchial) breath sounds	
Characteristics	- Character is aspirate or guttural - Expiration in longer - Expiration is louder - Expiration has high pitch - I:E = 1:1 - There is a pause between inspiration and expiration (due to **absence of alveolar phase**)
Distribution	- Larynx - Trachea
Mode of production	Due to in and out movement of air through narrow aperture of glottis
Graphical representation	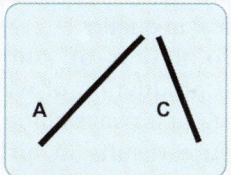

a. Tubular phase of inspiration
b. ABSENT
c. Expiration

Type of bronchial breathing		
Tubular	*Amphoric*	*Cavernous*
High-pitched sounds at the bronchioles are conducted to the chest wall without modification, e.g. - Consolidation - Above the level of pleural effusion - Massive pericardial effusion (Ewart's sign)	Low-pitched bronchial breathing with high-pitched overtones producing a metallic quality, e.g. - Open pneumothorax due to bronchopleural fistula - Large communicating cavity	Low-pitched sound with a peculiar hollow quality, e.g., cavity

Bronchovesicular breath sounds (also known as vesicular breath sounds with prolonged expiration)	
Characteristics	- Intermediate in character between vesicular and bronchial breath sounds - Expiratory phase is louder, longer, higher pitched than inspiratory, or hollow character, but there is no gap between expiration and inspiration

Contd...

Contd...

Distribution	• Upper part of sternum • Up to 3rd/4th dorsal spines between scapula • At times over the lung apices particularly on right side
Mode of production	Usually seen when air containing lung tissue is interposed between a large bronchus and the chest wall—thus combining the characteristics of both vesicular and bronchial breath sounds
Graphical representation	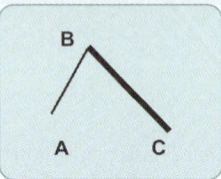 • Tubular phase of inspiration • Alveolar phase of inspiration • Expiration

It is the hallmark auscultatory finding of obstructive lung disease like chronic obstructive pulmonary disease and asthma

Diminished intensity of breath sounds	
Defect in production	Defect in transmission
• Bronchial obstruction • Emphysema • Respiratory muscle paralysis	• Pleural effusion • Pneumothorax • Thickened pleura • Thick chest wall • Fibrosis

Adventitious Sounds (Flowchart 3D.1)

Continuous adventitious sounds:
- Lasts for more than 250 ms
- Sinusoidal and musical in quality
- Mechanism of production of sound: Important prerequisite for the production of wheeze is airflow limitation. Narrowing of airways along with increased intrathoracic pressure results in airflow limitation producing sinusoidal oscillations.
- For example: Wheeze and rhonchi.

Wheeze	Rhonchi
High-pitched sounds	Low-pitched sounds
400 Hz	150–200 Hz
Hissing/shrill quality (sibilant)	Snoring quality (sonorous)
Predominantly arise from small airways obstruction	Usually produced when air moves through tracheobronchial passages in the presence of mucus or respiratory secretions

Classification of wheezes/rhonchi:
1. Monophonic or polyphonic
2. Inspiratory or expiratory

Monophonic	Polyphonic
Single tones	Diffuse, multiple tones, both phases
Due to local pathology producing bronchial (large airway) obstruction 1. Tumor 2. Foreign body aspiration 3. Bronchostenosis 4. Mucous plug 5. Lymph node compression	Due to dynamic compression 1. COPD 2. Bronchial asthma 3. Tropical pulmonary eosinophilia 4. Hypersensitivity pneumonitis 5. Eosinophilic pneumonia 6. Churg-Strauss syndrome

Sequential inspiratory wheeze:
- Series of sequential but not overlapping inspiratory sounds or occasionally a single sound, resulting from opening of airways which had become abnormally apposed during previous expiration.
- Occur in deflated areas of lung and are heard in lung fibrosis, mainly fibrosing alveolitis.

Discontinuous Adventitious Sounds (Rales/Crepitations/Crackles)

- These are discontinuous/intermittent, explosive, nonmusical and harsh in quality
- Mainly inspiratory (can be in expiratory or both).

Mechanism of crepitation:
1. Bubbling sounds produced by passage of air through accumulated secretions.
2. Sudden snapping opening of successive small airways when airflow is through it.

Fine crepitations	Coarse crepitations
Due to snapping opening of successive small airways as air enters the airways during inspiration	Due to bubbling sounds produced by passage of air through accumulated secretions
High pitched (soft)	Low-pitched (loud)
Smaller airways	Larger airways
Heard during inspiration	Heard during inspiration and expiration
Not modified by coughing	Modified by coughing
Not palpable	May be palpable
For example 1. Indux crepitations (initial stages of pneumonia) 2. Pulmonary edema (early phase) 3. Interstitial lung disease 4. Asbestosis 5. Hypersensitivity pneumonitis 6. Sarcoidosis	For example 1. Redux crepitations (resolution phase of pneumonia) 2. Pulmonary edema (late phase) 3. Bronchiectasis 4. Lung abscess 5. Bronchitis

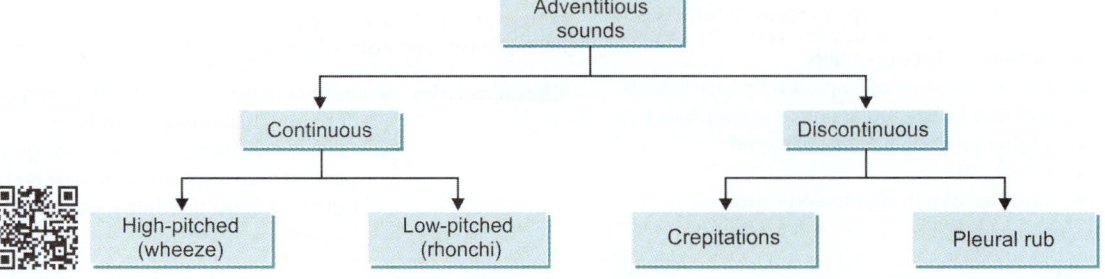

Flowchart 3D.1: Algorithm showing adventitious sounds.

Inspiratory crepitations		Expiratory crepitations
Early	Acute bronchitis Chronic bronchitis	**R**edux crepitations (**R**esolution phase of pneumonia) Pulmonary edema (late phase) Bronchiectasis Lung abscess Bronchitis
Mid	Bronchiectasis Resolving phase of Pneumonia	
Late	Interstitial lung disease Asbestosis Early pneumonia Pulmonary edema	

Few named crepitations	
Coarse leathery crepitations	Bronchiectasis
Velcro crepitations	Interstitial lung disease
Posture induced crackles	Appearance of fine crackles while changing of posture (sitting to supine or supine with passive leg elevation). Auscultate in the posterior axillary line in the 8th, 9th and 10th intercostal spaces after 3 minutes of supine position. It indicates ischemic heart disease with heart failure
Post-tussive crepitations	Crepitations which are not present normally but appear after a bout of cough. Seen in early pneumonia, early tuberculosis and lung abscess
Tracheal Rales (Death Rattle)	Usually heard over the trachea or lungs in seriously ill patients who are unable to cough out their respiratory secretions

Stridor:
- High-pitched whistling or grating sound which is produced by upper airway obstruction.
- It is louder over the neck than the chest wall.
- Indicates extrathoracic upper airway obstruction (like foreign body, acute epiglottitis, supraglottic malignancies, etc.)
- It usually seen during inspiration, however, can be seen in expiration in intrathoracic tracheobronchial obstruction.

Pleural rub:
- It is harsh discontinuous, localized, nonmusical, superficial grating sound due to rubbing of the inflamed pleural surfaces against each other.
- It is heard in both phases of respiration and disappears on holding the breath.

Causes:
- Dry pleurisy
- Consolidation
- Infarction

Differences between pleural rub and crepitations:

Pleural rub	Crepitations
Both inspiratory and expiratory phases	Inspiratory/expiratory or both
Localized to small area	Widespread
No change after coughing	May clear after coughing
Pressure on stethoscope increases the sound	No effect
Associated with pleuritic chest pain and local tenderness	No pain or tenderness

Vocal resonance:
- Make the patient sit
- Place the stethoscope firmly on the chest wall
- Ask the patient to speak "one-one-one" or "ninety-nine" repeatedly
- Compare corresponding areas anteriorly, in axilla and posteriorly.
- Increased vocal resonance

Vocal resonance	
Increased	*Decreased*
Consolidation Large cavity Bronchopleural fistula	Pleural effusion Pneumothorax Fibrosis Collapse Asthma Emphysema Thick pleura

Note: In upper lobe fibrosis, VR is increased due to the pulled trachea.

Variations of vocal resonance	
Bronchophony	Increase in loudness as well as clarity of the sound **Seen in:** - Consolidation - Just above level of pleural effusion - On spine up to T4
Aegophony	Selected amplification of high frequency sounds. "E" is heard as "A" **Seen in:** - Consolidation (it is the auscultatory sign of consolidation) *Mode of production:* - Due to interposition of a thin layer of fluid between the lung and chest wall, allowing transmission of overtones but damping off lower fundamental tones, or - Due to partial compression of lung tissue underneath the upper part of effusion, altering the normal relationship between bronchi and lung parenchyma and thus reinforcing high-pitched nasal sounds
Whispering pectoriloquy	When the whispered sound in the chest wall is heard clearly and distinguishably as if uttered directly into the external ear **Seen in:** - Fairly large cavity in the lung communicating with the bronchus - Massive or diffuse consolidation of lung tissue overlying or adjacent to a bronchus

Other Auscultatory Features

Post-tussive suction: It is a sign of superficial collapsible cavity seen in active tuberculosis. When you auscultate a cavernous bronchial breathing (which indicates a cavity), ask the patient to cough. A suction sound will be heard if the cavity collapses.

Prerequisites for post-tussive suction:
- Superficial cavity
- Thin-walled cavity
- Has to be communicating with bronchus
- Surrounding lung should be normal.

Succussion splash (hippocrates succussion):
- It is seen in hydropneumothorax
- First percuss and get the air fluid level in hydropneumothorax
- Keep the diaphragm at the air-fluid level
- Hold the opposite shoulder of the patient and shake vigorously as shown in **Figure 3D.41**.
- Tinkling or splashing sound will be heard.
- Other conditions like large cavity with fluid, diaphragmatic hernia can also produce succussion splash.

Coin test:
- High-pitched metallic or tympanic note
- Place one coin flat on affected side of chest (posteriorly/anteriorly) and percuss with another coin perpendicularly on it, while simultaneously auscultating from the opposite direction of the same affected side as shown in **Figure 3D.42**.
- Seen in massive pneumothorax/hydropneumothorax.

Scratch sign:
- Used for diagnosis of pneumothorax
- Patient sitting, place the diaphragm of the stethoscope in the midpoint of sternum or spine
- Scratch the chest wall from mid axillary line towards the sternum on either side.
- Sound will be louder on the side of pneumothorax.

Hamman's mediastinal crunch:
- Loud cracking or clicking sound heard in the 3rd to 5th intercostal spaces near the left sternal border synchronous with the heartbeat.
- It is the sign of mediastinal emphysema (pneumomediastinum) or can also be seen in left-sided pneumothorax.

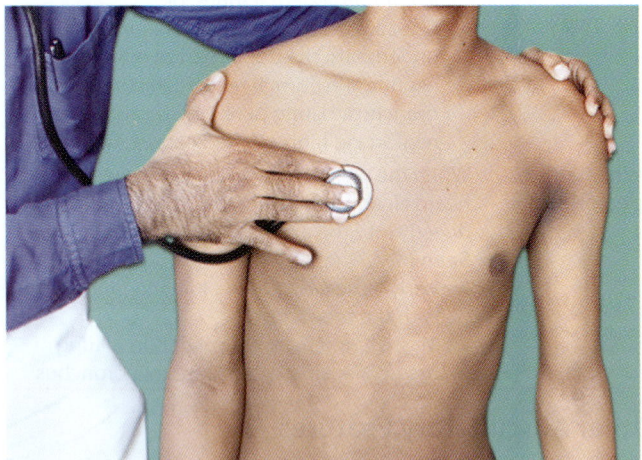

Fig. 3D.41: Demonstration of succussion splash.

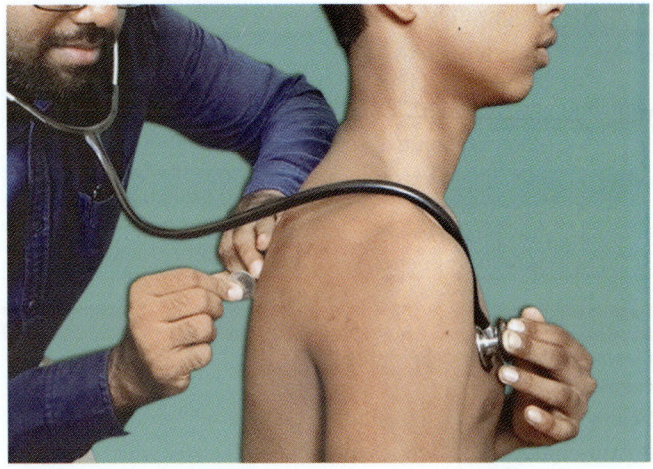

Fig. 3D.42: Demonstration of coin test.

Forced expiratory time (FET):
- It is a simple inexpensive and sensitive bedside test to detect airflow obstruction.
- Instruct the patient to inhale up to the total lung capacity and then blow it as fast and complete as possible.
- Place the bell of stethoscope in suprasternal notch and time the audible expiration.
- A value less than 5 seconds indicates FEV1/FVC more than 60%, whereas FET more than 6 seconds indicates FEV1/FVC less than 50%.

Summary of findings in pleural effusion based on the severity				
Finding	Mild effusion (<300 mL)	Moderate effusion (300–1,500 mL)	Massive effusion (>1,500 mL)
Tachypnea	No	Present	Significant
Chest expansion	Normal	Decreased on the effected side	Significantly decreased on the effected side
Tactile fremitus	Normal	Decreased	Absent
Breath sounds	Vesicular	Decreased	Absent or bronchial
Contralateral tracheal or mediastinal shift	Absent	Absent	Present
Bulging intercostal spaces	No	Sometimes	Present
Egophony	No	Yes	Yes

E. RESPIRATORY SYSTEM: SUMMARY OF FINDINGS IN COMMON RESPIRATORY DISEASES

	Findings	Fibrosis	Collapse	Pleural effusion	Pneumothorax	Hydropneumothorax	Consolidation	Cavity	Emphysema	ILD
Inspection	Trachea/mediastinum	Pulled to same side	Pulled to same side	Pushed to opposite side	Pushed to opposite side	Pushed to opposite side	Central	Central	Central	Central
Inspection	Retraction/bulge	Retraction on the affected side	Retraction on the affected side	Bulging/fullness on the affected side	Bulging/fullness on the affected side	Bulging/fullness on the affected side	—	—	Barrel-shaped chest	Bilaterally diminished movements
Palpation	Chest expansion	Reduced on the effected side	Reduced on the effected side	Reduced on the effected side	Reduced on the effected side	Reduced on the effected side	Reduced on the effected side	Reduced on the effected side	Reduced bilaterally	Reduced bilaterally
Palpation	Hemithorax dimension	Reduced on the effected side	Reduced on the effected side	Increased on the effected side	Increased on the effected side	Increased on the effected side	Normal dimensions	Normal dimensions	Bilaterally inflated lungs with AP:T diameter = 1:1	Decreased or normal chest dimensions
Palpation	Vocal fremitus	Reduced	Reduced	Reduced	Reduced	Reduced	Increased	Increased in the presence of communication with bronchus	Bilaterally equal	Bilaterally equal
Percussion	Percussion note	Impaired note over fibrosed lung	Dull note over the collapsed lung	Stony dull note over the pleural effusion and skodiac resonance at the level of pleural effusion	Hyper-resonant note over the pneumothorax	Hyper-resonant note above the air fluid level and dull note below the air fluid level	Woody Dull note over the consolidation	Large cavity gives resonant note	Hyper-resonant note over bilateral lung fields	Resonant note heard over bilateral lung fields
Percussion	Special findings	William's tracheal resonance	—	• Ellis curve pattern of upper level of effusion • Grocco's triangle • Obliteration of Traube's space • Garland's triangle	Bell tympany can be appreciated (Coin test positive)	Shifting dullness, straight line dullness, succussion splash, Bell tympany can be appreciated (Coin test positive)		• Wintrich's sign (cavity communicating with bronchus) • Friedreich's sign • Gerhardt's sign	• Liver dullness is pushed down • Negative for tidal percussion	
Auscultation	Breath sounds	Diminished breath sounds	Absent breath sounds	Absent breath sounds	Absent breath sounds	Absent breath sounds	Tubular breath sounds	Cavernous breath sounds	Vesicular breath sounds with prolonged expiration	Vesicular breath sounds
Auscultation	Adventitious sounds/ special findings	Fine crepitations	—	—	Bell tympany can be appreciated (Coin test positive)	Bell tympany can be appreciated (Coin test positive)	Crepitations heard	Post-tussive suction (in superficial cavity)	Rhonchi heard over the bilateral lung fields	Fine Velcro crepitations
Auscultation	Vocal resonance	Reduced	Reduced	Reduced	Reduced	Reduced	Increased bronchophony, egophony, whispering pectoriloquy)	Increased in the presence of communication with bronchus	Bilaterally equal	Bilaterally equal

NOTES

CHAPTER 4: Cardiovascular System Examination

A. CASE SHEET FORMAT

HISTORY TAKING

Name:

Age:

Sex:

Residence:

Occupation:

Chief complaints (describe in chronological order):
1. _____ × days/month/year
2. _____ × days
3. _____ × days

Dyspnea:
- Duration
- Onset
- Grade
- Progression
- Aggravating factors
- Relieving factors
- Diurnal variation
- Orthopnea
- Trepopnea
- Platypnea
- Bendopnea
- Paroxysmal nocturnal dyspnea
- Associated symptoms
  - Wheeze
  - Cough with expectoration

Chest pain:
- Duration
- Onset
- Site
- Type of pain
- Radiation
- Diurnal variation (nocturnal angina)
- Aggravating factors
- Relieving factors
- Associated symptoms
  - Nausea, vomiting, sweating
- Dyspepsia
- Local tenderness
- Angina equivalents.
  - Dyspnea
  - Diaphoresis
  - Discomfort in lower jaw
  - Dyspeptic symptoms
  - Fatigue

Palpitations:
- Duration
- Onset and offset
- Fast or slow
- Regular or irregular
- Precipitating factors
- Associated symptoms
  - Stoke Adams
  - Shortness of breath/syncope/presyncope/chest pain
- Postpalpitation diuresis

Syncope:
- Duration
- Onset
- Frequency of attacks and last attack
- Awareness
- Precipitating factors
- Associated symptoms

Pedal edema:
- Duration
- Onset
- Progression
- Aggravating factors
- Relieving factors
- Is it preceded by facial puffiness or followed by facial puffiness?
- Associated symptoms: Abdominal distension

Other symptoms:
- Hemoptysis

- Bleeding manifestations
- Recurrent LRTI
- Cyanosis
- Decreased urine output
- Gastrointestinal symptoms
- Right hypochondrial pain
- Fatigability
- Fever
- Rheumatic fever history
- Infective endocarditis
- Cyanotic spells
- Squatting after exertion
- Limb weakness/slurred speech/altered sensorium/involuntary movements/seizures

Pasthistory:
- Asthma
- Chronic obstructive airway disease
- Tuberculosis
- History of contact with tuberculosis
- Diabetes mellitus
- Hypertension
- Ischemic heart disease (IHD)
- Seizure disorder
- Thyroid disorder
- History of sudden cardiac death

Family history:
Three generation pedigree chart to be drawn

Personal history:
- Bowel habits
- Bladder habits
- Appetite
- Loss of weight
- Occupational exposure
- Sleep
- Dietary habits and taboo
- Food allergies
- Smoking Index or Pack years
- Alcohol history (if yes mention in grams of alcohol)

Treatment history:
- Drugs using
- Frequency of drug (e.g., drug taken 5 times a week most likely to be digoxin)
- Duration of usage
- Any blood test to be monitored (e.g., INR for warfarin)
- Any intramuscular injections (once in 3 weeks IM injection most likely to be benzathine penicillin for rheumatic heart disease prophylaxis)
- Medications that cause increased urine output and relieve breathlessness(Likely to be diuretic)

Menstrual and obstetric history:
- Parity, live births, abortions (PLA)
- Age of menarche
- Age of menopause
- Duration of menstrual cycle
- Associated dysmenorrhea/menorrhagia

Summarize:

Differential diagnosis:

1.

2.

3.

GENERAL EXAMINATION

Patient
- Conscious
- Coherent
- Cooperative
- Obeying commands

Body Mass Index (BMI)
- Weight (kg)/Height^2 (meters)
- Grading according to WHO for Southeast Asian countries
- Arm span
- Upper segment: Lower segment ratio

Vitals Examination
- Pulse
    - Rate
    - Rhythm
    - Volume
    - Character
    - Vessel wall thickening
    - Radioradial delay and radiofemoral delay
    - Peripheral pulses
    - Apex-pulse deficit if patient is in AF
- Blood pressure
    - Right arm
    - Left arm
    - Leg—right and left
    - Postural drop in BP
    - Mean of three recordings if patient is in AF
- Respiratory rate
    - Regular/irregular
    - Abdominothoracic (male) or thoracoabdominal (female)
    - Usage of accessory muscles
- Jugular venous pressure
    - Centimeter (cm) of water (blood) above sternal angle (+ 5 cm from the right atria)
    - Jugular venous pulse waveform
    - Abdominojugular reflux
- Pulse oximetry saturation

Physical Examination
- Pallor:
- Icterus:
- Cyanosis:
- Clubbing:
- Lymphadenopathy:
- Edema:

Others
- Signs of infective endocarditis
- Signs of rheumatic fever
- Any dysmorphic facies/stigmata od congenital heart disease
- Fundus

SYSTEMIC EXAMINATION

Inspection
- Chest shape and symmetry
- Breast abnormalities
- Spine deformity
- Precordial bulge
- Parasternal heave
- Cardiovascular pulsations
  - Apical impulse
  - Pulsation in aortic and pulmonary area
  - Sternoclavicular joint pulsations
  - Left parasternal pulsations
  - Epigastric pulsations
  - Ectopic pulsations
- Distended veins/scars/sinuses

Palpation
- Confirmation of shape and symmetry
- Palpation of precordium
- Palpation for sounds, thrills
- Tracheal tug

Percussion
- Right heart border
- Left heart border
- Left 2nd IC space
- Sternal percussion

Auscultation
- **Apex (mitral area)**
  - S1
  - S2
  - S3, S4
  - OS/clicks
  - Murmur
    1. Timing
    2. Grade
    3. Quality
    4. Pitch
    5. Configuration
    6. Radiation
    7. Best heard with diaphragm or bell
    8. Patient position
    9. With breath held in inspiration or expiration
    10. Dynamic auscultation

Scan QR code for dynamic auscultation video

- **Tricuspid area**
  - S1
  - S2
  - S3, S4
  - OS/clicks
  - Murmur
    1. Timing
    2. Grade
    3. Quality
    4. Pitch
    5. Configuration
    6. Radiation
    7. Best heard with diaphragm or bell
    8. Patient position
    9. With breath held in inspiration or expiration
    10. Dynamic auscultation
- **Erb's neoaortic area**
  - S1
  - S2
  - S3, S4
  - Clicks
  - Murmur
    1. Timing
    2. Grade
    3. Quality
    4. Pitch
    5. Configuration
    6. Radiation
    7. Best heard with diaphragm or bell
    8. Patient position
    9. With breath held in inspiration or expiration
    10. Dynamic auscultation.
- **(R) 2nd intercostal space (aortic area)**
  - S1
  - S2
  - S3, S4
  - Clicks
  - Murmur
    1. Timing
    2. Grade
    3. Quality
    4. Pitch
    5. Configuration
    6. Radiation
    7. Best heard with diaphragm or bell
    8. Patient position
    9. With breath held in inspiration or expiration
    10. Dynamic auscultation.
- **(L) 2nd intercostal space (pulmonary area)**
  - S1
  - S2
  - S3, S4
  - Clicks
  - Murmur
    1. Timing
    2. Grade
    3. Quality
    4. Pitch
    5. Configuration
    6. Radiation

7. Best heard with diaphragm or bell
8. Patient position
9. With breath held in inspiration or expiration
10. Dynamic auscultation.

- **Other areas**
  - Axilla
  - Epigastrium
  - Clavicle
  - Carotid
  - Back (interscapular area)

OTHER SYSTEM EXAMINATION

Respiratory:
- Inspection:
- Palpation:
- Percussion:
- Auscultation:

Gastrointestinal system:
- Inspection:
- Palpation:
- Percussion:
- Auscultation:

Nervous system:
- Higher mental functions:
- Cranial nerves:
- Sensory system:
- Motor system:
- Reflexes:
- Cerebellar system:
- Meningeal signs:

B. DIAGNOSIS FORMAT

ACQUIRED/CONGENITAL HEART DISEASE

For Acquired Heart Disease
- Acquired heart disease possible etiology (rheumatic/ischemic/cardiomyopathy/degenerative/BAV)
- Valvular involvement (MS/MR/AS/AR/others) with severity grading
- With/without evidence of pulmonary artery hypertension (grading)
- Patient in or not in atrial fibrillation (if AF present look for signs of thromboembolism)
- With or without evidence of heart failure (right/left/congestive)
- With or without signs of infective endocarditis
- With or without signs of active rheumatic carditis
- Patient is in New York Heart Association (NYHA) class (I/II/III/IV)

Example: Acquired valvular heart disease, possibly rheumatic etiology, with severe mitral stenosis and moderate mitral regurgitation, with severe pulmonary artery hypertension, patient in atrial fibrillation and congestive cardiac failure, with no signs of infective endocarditis, thromboembolism or active rheumatic carditis. Patient is in NYHA class III.

For Congenital Heart Disease
- Congenital cyanotic (if cyanotic-mention, if it is increased/decreased pulmonary blood flow)/acyanotic heart disease
- Type of defect (shunt)
- With/without evidence of pulmonary artery hypertension (grading)
- Patient in or not in atrial fibrillation (if AF present look for signs of thromboembolism)
- With or without evidence of heart failure (right/left/congestive)
- With or without signs of infective endocarditis
- Patient is in NYHA class (I/II/III/IV).

Note: Mention if any features of dysmorphic facies or syndromes.

Example: Congenital acyanotic heart disease, atrial septal defect with pulmonary artery hypertension, with left to right shunt, patient not in atrial fibrillation, no evidence of heart failure or infective endocarditis. Patient in NYHA class II. Patient has features of Holt–Oram syndrome.

=== NOTES ===

C. DISCUSSION ON CARDIAC CYCLE

SYSTOLE AND DIASTOLE

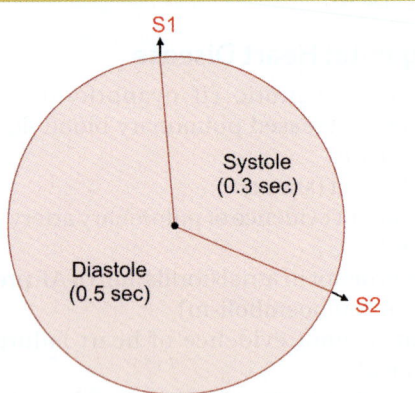

Fig. 4C.1: Systole and diastole.

Systole is represented by S1 to S2 in clockwise direction and diastole is represented by S2 to S1 in clockwise direction. And these events continuously repeat.

EVENTS OF CARDIAC CYCLE

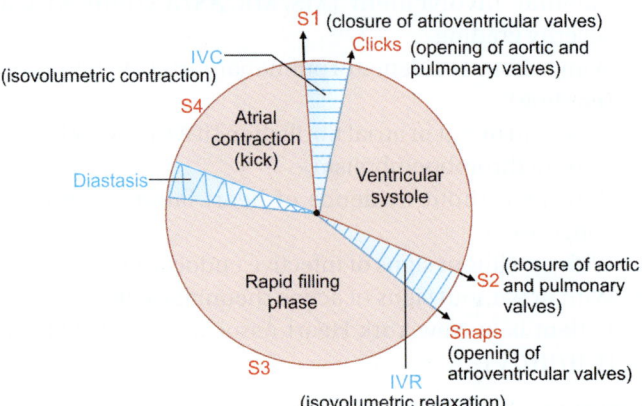

Fig. 4C.2: Major events during cardiac cycle.

In **Figure 4C.1**, cardiac cycle is represented as cyclical events beginning from S1 and ending back at S1 in clockwise fashion. Assuming the heart rate of 72 beats/min, each cardiac cycle is of 0.8 seconds duration. 0.3 seconds is ventricular systole and 0.5 seconds is ventricular diastole.

Let us describe the cardiac events in clockwise fashion beginning from S1 (See **Figure 4C.2** also)

S1	S1 marks the closure of the atrioventricular valves (mitral and tricuspid valves)
Isovolumetric contraction	Next, the ventricles begin to contract; however, the aortic and pulmonary valves are not yet open. This phase of ventricular contraction where both AV valves and aortic/pulmonary valves are closed is called as **isovolumetric contraction** as depicted in **Figure 4C.2**
Clicks	Opening of aortic and pulmonary valves causes sounds called clicks
Ventricular systole	Immediately after opening of aortic and pulmonary valves, blood in the ventricles is ejected out
S2	Next, the semilunar valves (aortic and pulmonary) close producing heart sound S2
Isovolumetric relaxation	The ventricles begin to relax but the atrioventricular valves are yet to open. This phase where ventricles relax but both atrioventricular valves and aortic/pulmonary valves are closed is called as **isovolumetric relaxation**
Snaps	Opening of atrioventricular valves causes diastolic sounds called "Snaps"
Rapid filling phase of ventricular diastole—S3	Opening of AV valves is followed by rapid filling of ventricle due to pressure difference
Diastasis	The pressure difference gradually reduces and the flow between the atria and ventricles minimizes. This phase of cardiac cycle where the blood flow between atria and ventricles is minimum is called the **"diastasis"**
Atrial contraction (KICK)—S4	Diastasis is followed by atrial contraction/atrial kick which is responsible for pumping the additional blood from atrium into the ventricles. At the end of atrial contraction, the atrioventricular valves close producing heart sound S1 and cycle repeats

Jugular Venous Pressure Waveform—Timing with Other Cardiac Events

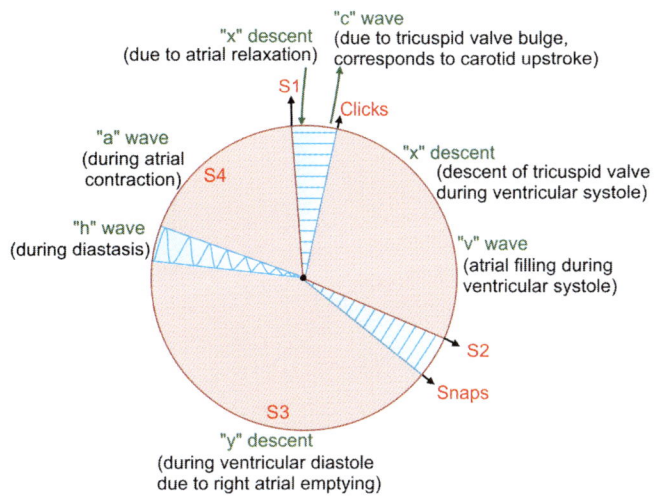

Fig. 4C.3: Timing of JVP with cardiac events.

"a" wave	- It coincides with atrial contraction - It is seen in diastole and - It precedes S1
X wave (initial x descent)	- It is due to atrial relaxation - It is seen in systole - It follows S1
C wave	- It is due to bulge of tricuspid valve into the right atrium - It is seen in systole - Coincides with carotid upstroke - Absent in humans
X' wave (x descent following 'c' wave)	- It is due to descent in floor of RA with downward pull of TV with continued ventricular contraction - It is seen in systole - It follows clicks (if audible)
V wave	- It is due to atrial filling during ventricular systole - Seen in late systole extends up to early diastole - It precedes S2
Y wave	- It is due to RA emptying during ventricular diastole - Seen in diastole (after IVR phase) - It follows opening snap (if audible)
h wave (Hirschfelder wave)	- It is brief positive wave during the diastasis - Seen in diastole just before a-wave - Not clinically appreciable - Referred as z point by Paul wood

Now, let us superimpose waves of jugular venous pressure (JVP) onto the cardiac cycle. JVP has the following waves, starting from a, x, c, x', v, y, and h which repeat in a cyclical fashion. Clinically appreciable waves are four, two in systole (i.e., "x" descent and "v" wave) and two in diastole (i.e., "y" descent and "a" wave). The timing of JVP with respect to cardiac cycle has been depicted in **Figure 4C.3**. The waves in JVP include:

CARDIAC MURMURS—TIMING WITH OTHER CARDIAC EVENTS (FIG. 4C.4)

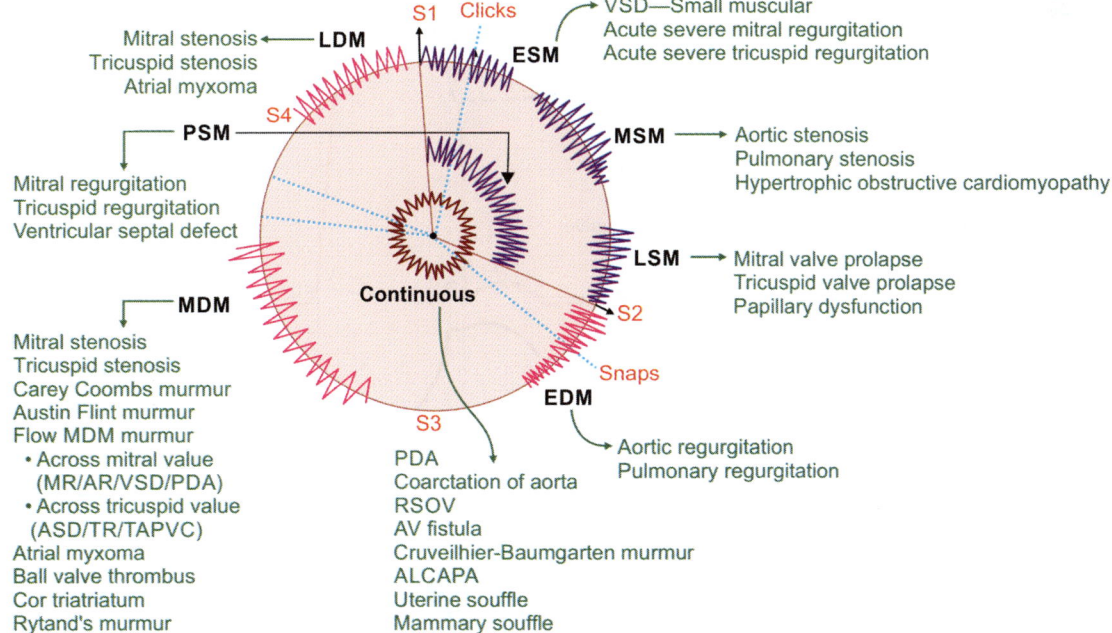

Fig. 4C.4: Timing of cardiac murmurs and pictorial representation on the diagram of cardiac cycle.

To remember murmurs:
Note 1: **ESM/PSM**—due to valve abnormalities of mitral and tricuspid valve (regurgitant lesions); **MSM**—due to valve abnormalities of aortic and pulmonary valve (stenotic lesions); **LSM**—due to prolapse of mitral and tricuspid valve; **EDM**—due to valve abnormalities of aortic and pulmonary valve (regurgitant lesions); **MDM**—due to valve abnormalities of mitral and tricuspid valve; **LDM**—atrial myxomas.
Note 2: **Early murmurs** are regurgitant lesions; **Mid murmurs** are stenotic lesions; **Late murmurs** are prolapse/papillary dysfunction/myxomas

ECG WAVEFORM—TIMING WITH OTHER CARDIAC EVENTS (FIG. 4C.5)

- Atrial contraction follows the **P wave** of the ECG.
- Isovolumetric contraction and systole follows the **QRS wave** of the ECG.
- Diastole follows the **T wave** of ECG.

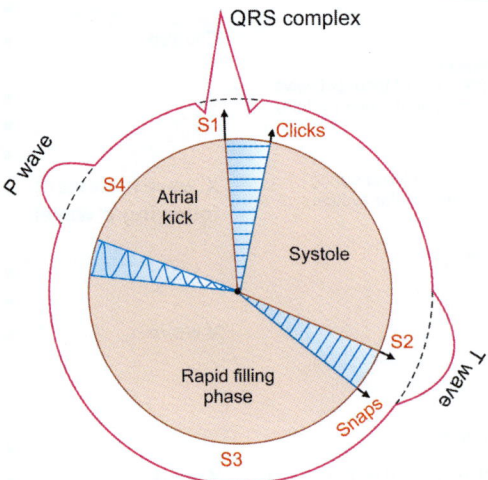

Fig. 4C.5: Timing of waves of ECG and pictorial representation on the diagram of cardiac cycle.

STANDARD REPRESENTATION OF ALL CARDIAC EVENTS IN CARDIAC CYCLE (FIG. 4C.6 AND TABLE 4C.1)

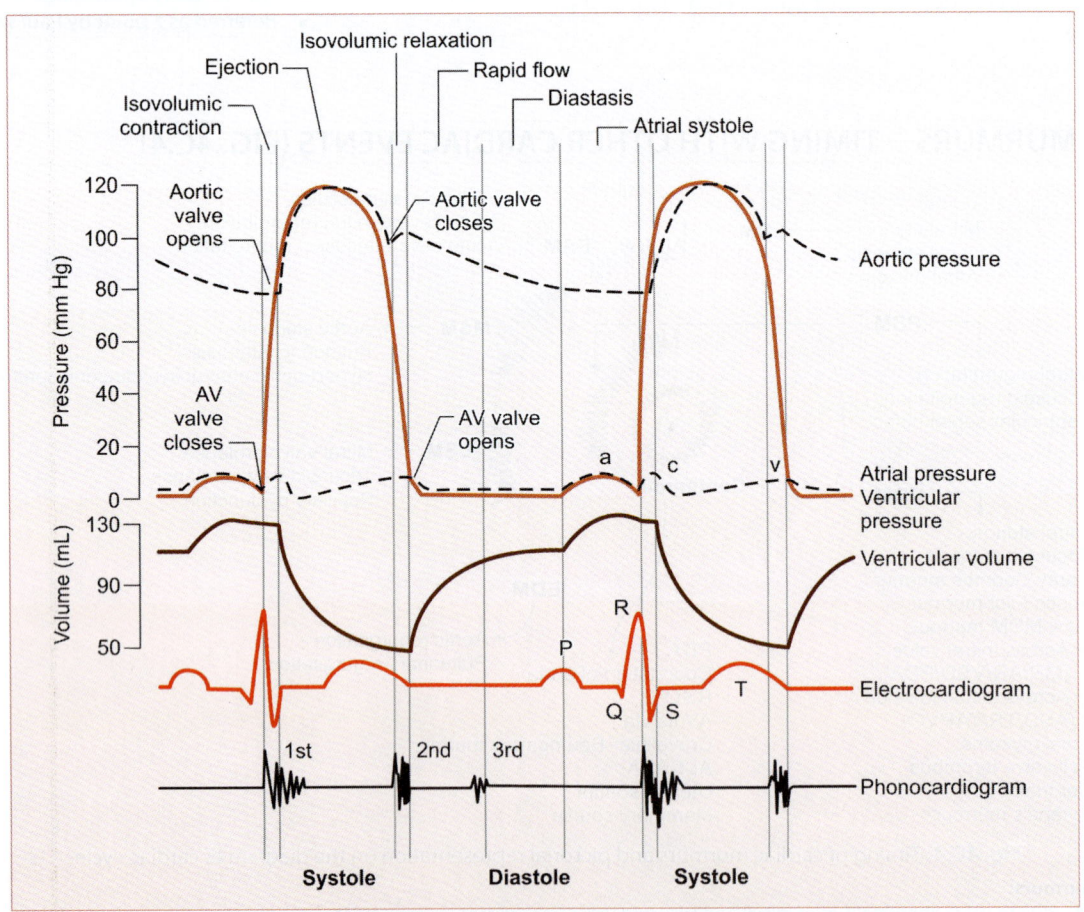

Fig. 4C.6: Wiggers diagram—events of cardiac cycle during systole and diastole (phonogram, electrocardiogram, volumes and pressure changes).

TABLE 4C.1: Pressure changes during cardiac cycle.

Pressures (mm Hg)			
Right atrium		Left atrium	
Mean	3	Mean	8
a wave	6	a wave	10
v wave	5	v wave	12
Right ventricle		Left ventricle	
Peak systolic	25	Peak systolic	130
End-diastolic	4	End-diastolic	8
Pulmonary artery		Aorta	
Mean	15	Mean	85
Peak systolic	25	Peak systolic	130
End-diastolic	9	End-diastolic	70
Pulmonary capillaries		Systemic capillaries	
Mean	9	Mean	25

NOTES

D. DISCUSSION ON CARDINAL SYMPTOMS

CHEST PAIN

Chest pain is a common symptom of cardiac disease. It can be due to noncardiac causes such as anxiety or diseases involving the respiratory, musculoskeletal or gastrointestinal systems. It can be acute, ongoing or episodic in nature. Episodic is most common type and classified into typical, atypical and noncardiac chest pain based on the presence or absence of three features:

1. Precipitated by exertion or emotional stress
2. Quality—retrosternal heaviness or squeezing
3. Relieved by rest or with nitrates

Typical—all three criteria are met

Atypical—only two criteria are met

Noncardiac chest pain—meet only one criteria

Causes of Chest Pain (Fig. 4D.1)

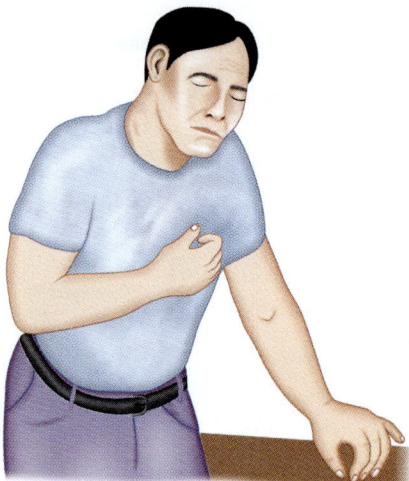

Fig. 4D.1: Causes of chest pain.

Cardiac
1. Coronary artery disease
   - Angina pectoris
   - Myocardial infarction
2. Valvular disease
   - Mitral valve prolapse
   - Aortic stenosis/regurgitation
3. Pericarditis
4. Hypertrophic cardiomyopathy

Vascular
Dissection of aorta

Pulmonary
1. Pleuritis
2. Pneumothorax
3. Pulmonary embolism
4. Pneumonia

Gastrointestinal
1. Reflux esophagitis
2. Diffuse esophageal spasm
3. Hiatus hernia
4. Peptic ulcer disease
5. Cholecystitis
6. Pancreatitis

Musculoskeletal
1. Costochondritis
2. Arthritis
3. Muscle spasm
4. Bone tumor

Neural
Shingles/herpes zoster

Emotional
1. Anxiety
2. Depression

Differential Diagnosis of Chest Pain (Table 4D.1)

TABLE 4D.1: Differential diagnosis of chest pain.

Potentially life-threatening causes	Common nonlife-threatening causes

• Acute coronary syndromes: Acute myocardial infarction (MI), ST-segment elevation MI, non-ST-segment elevation MI
• Unstable angina
• Pulmonary embolism
• Aortic dissection
• Myocarditis
• Tension pneumothorax
• Acute chest syndrome/crisis in sickle cell anemia
• Pericarditis
• Boerhaave's syndrome (perforated esophagus)
• Gastrointestinal: Perforated peptic ulcer, acute pancreatitis, acute cholecystitis
	• Gastrointestinal
	  • Biliary colic
	  • Gastroesophageal reflux disease
	  • Peptic ulcer disease
	• Pulmonary
	  • Pneumonia
	  • Pleuritis
	• Musculoskeletal pain: Costochondritis (Tietze's syndrome), intercostal myalgia/neuralgia, fracture of the ribs (cough, trauma), secondaries in the ribs, Bornholm disease
	• Thoracic radiculopathy: Texidor's twinge (precordial catch syndrome)
	• Emotional: Anxiety
	• Neural: Shingles/herpes zoster

Differential Features of Ischemic Cardiac and Noncardiac Pain (Table 4D.2)

TABLE 4D.2: Differential features of ischemic cardiac and noncardiac pain.

Features	Ischemic cardiac pain	Noncardiac pain
Site	Central, diffuse	Peripheral, localized
Character of pain	Tight, squeezing, dull, constricting, choking or 'heavy'	Sharp, stabbing, catching
Precipitation/provocation	Exertion, emotion, cold weather or postprandial	Spontaneous, not related to exertion and reproducible with palpation
Radiation	Jaw/neck/shoulder	Usually, no radiation
Relieving factors	Rest (in less than 5 minutes), nitrates **Note:** Patients with UA can have characteristic angina that does not relieve with rest or nitrates completely—s/o ongoing ischemia	Not relieved by rest or by nitrates
Associated features	Breathlessness, diaphoresis, nausea and vomiting (features s/o autonomic system activation)	Depends on the cause

Differentiating Features of the Common Causes of Chest Pain (Table 4D.3)

TABLE 4D.3: Differentiating features of the common causes of chest pain.

Disease	Description	Location	Radiation	Associations
Acute coronary syndromes	Crushing, tightening, squeezing, or pressure like	Retrosternal, left anterior chest or epigastric	Right (R) or left (L) shoulder, R or L arm/hand/jaw	Dyspnea, diaphoresis, nausea
Pulmonary embolism	Heaviness, tightness	Whole chest (massive) or focal chest (segmental)	None	Dyspnea, unstable vital signs, feeling of impending doom if massive or just tachycardia, tachypnea if segmental
Aortic dissection	Ripping, tearing	Midline, substernal	Interscapular area of back	Secondary arterial occlusion of aortic branches (e.g., paraplegia-subclavian artery involvement)
Pericarditis/cardiac tamponade	Sharp, constant or pleuritic	Substernal	None	Fever, dyspnea, pericardial friction rub
Pneumothorax	Sudden, sharp, lancinating, pleuritic	One side of chest	Shoulder, back	Dyspnea
Perforated esophagus	Sudden, sharp, after forceful vomiting	Substernal	Back	Dyspnea, diaphoresis, signs of sepsis

Types of angina	
Angina	Angina is a symptom of myocardial ischemia that is recognized clinically by its character, its location and its relation to provocative stimuli
Stable angina	Angina is typical in character that occurs on exertion or emotion or postprandially or during cold weather lasting for less than 5 minutes and does not have increasing severity. Relieves with rest or sublingual nitrates
Unstable angina	This is a form of acute coronary syndrome. It has at least one of these three features: 1. It occurs at rest (or with minimal exertion), usually lasting more than 10 minutes 2. It is severe and of new onset (i.e., within the prior 4–6 weeks) 3. It occurs with a crescendo pattern (i.e., distinctly more severe, prolonged, or frequent than before)
Variant angina/prinzmetal angina	Caused due to epicardial coronary artery vasospasm; most common in middle-aged females
Microvascular angina/cardiac syndrome X	Angina-like chest pain in the context of normal epicardial coronary arteries on angiography with microvascular endothelial dysfunction; unresponsive to nitrates
Episodic angina	This syndrome is one in which pains having the characters of effort angina occurring at longer or shorter intervals independent of effort
Nocturnal angina	Seen in severe aortic regurgitation. Proposed mechanisms are: 1. Bradycardia at night prolongs diastole duration. Regurgitation time is prolonged and coronary perfusion is decreased. 2. Increased LVEDP decrease coronary perfusion in chronic AR [coronary perfusion pressure (CPP) = DBP – LVEDP] 3. Dilated left ventricular (LV), increased LV mass, increased demand (demand supply mismatch) 4. Diastolic coronary stealing, Venturi effect of AR jet
Angina decubitus	It is angina that occurs when a person is lying down (not necessarily only at night) without any apparent cause. Occurs because gravity redistributes fluids in the body; difficult to differentiate from nocturnal angina
Angina of stooping	Angina occurring while bending or stooping due to altered hemodynamics in deficient coronary circulation are exaggerated and produce anginal pain
Second wind, or warm up, angina	Describes patients with ischemic heart disease and exertional angina that forces them to stop; after the first bout of angina, they are able to continue with minor, or even without any, further symptoms. Ischemic preconditioning and collateral recruitment are proposed mechanisms
Linked angina	It is associated with: 1. Gastroesophageal and duodenal disorders and diseases 2. Gallbladder disease 3. Cervical spondylitis
Refractory angina	Angina that cannot be controlled with optimal medical therapy and where revascularization is not feasible
Status anginosus	It is a clinical term denoting periods of frequently recurring anginal pain at rest, indistinguishable from the pain of cardiac infarction or from its prodromal manifestation, but without the electrocardiographic and laboratory evidences of classical cardiac infarction
Vincent's angina	Fusospirochetal infection of the pharynx and palatine tonsils, causing "ulceromembranous pharyngitis and tonsillitis"

Contd...

Contd...

Ludwig's angina	Severe diffuse cellulitis that presents as an acute onset and spreads rapidly, bilaterally affecting the submandibular, sublingual, and submental spaces
Abdominal angina	Postprandial pain that occurs in the mesenteric vascular occlusive disease; most commonly associated with significant CAD
Angina sine dolore	A painless episode of coronary insufficiency. It is associated with diabetes mellitus and also called silent ischemia

The modified Medical Research Council (mMRC) scale and the New York Heart Association (NYHA) scale

Response category	mMRC	NYHA
0	Breathlessness only with strenuous exercise	
1	Breathlessness when hurrying on the level or up a slight hill	No limitation in ordinary physical activity
2	Breathlessness when walking at own pace on the level	Mild breathlessness and fatigue, slight limitation during ordinary activity
3	Breathlessness when walking 100 yards or for a few minutes	Marked limitation of physical activity due to breathlessness and fatigue even during less-than-ordinary activity
4	Breathless when taking a bath or breathless while dressing/undressing	Experience symptoms even while at rest

Canadian Cardiovascular Society (CSS) functional classification of angina	
Class I	Ordinary activity (e.g., walking, climbing stairs at own pace) does not bring on angina. Angina occurs only with strenuous, rapid, or prolonged exertion at work or during recreation
Class II	Slight limitation of ordinary activity. Symptoms occur when walking or climbing stairs rapidly, walking up a hill, walking upstairs after a meal, in cold weather, in wind, or when under emotional stress, or only a few hours after waking, and climbing more than one flight of ordinary stairs at a normal pace and in normal conditions
Class III	Marked limitation of ordinary activity. Symptoms occur after walking 50–100 yards on the level, or climbing more than one flight of ordinary stairs in normal conditions
Class IV	Inability to carry on any physical activity without discomfort. Angina may be present at rest

Angina Equivalents

These are commonly seen in elderly and diabetics (with autonomic neuropathy) where ischemic angina is absent and they present with:
- Shortness of breath
- Perspiration/diaphoresis
- Syncope
- Gastrointestinal (GI) symptoms—upper abdominal pain, nausea, and vomiting
- Fatigue

PALPITATIONS

Definition

Palpitation is the term used to describe an uncomfortable increased awareness of one's own heartbeat or the sensation of slow, rapid or irregular heart rhythms.
- Palpitations do not always indicate the presence of arrhythmia and conversely, an arrhythmia can occur without palpitations.
- Palpitations are usually noted when the patient is quietly resting.
- Palpitation can be either intermittent or sustained and either regular or irregular.
- A change in the rate, rhythm or force of contraction can produce palpitations.
- Associated with neck pulsations **(frog's sign in SVT)**
- Associated with worsening shortness of breath/angina
- History of postpalpitation diuresis
- Differentiate volume overload palpitations from arrhythmic palpitations

Causes of Palpitations (Table 4D.4)

TABLE 4D.4: Causes of palpitations.

Cardiac causes	Drug induced
■ **Cardiac arrhythmias** • Premature atrial and ventricular contractions • Supraventricular and ventricular arrhythmias ■ **Structural heart diseases** • Atrial myxoma, valvular heart disease • Congenital heart disease, cardiomyopathy • Mitral valve prolapse	■ Alcohol (use or withdrawal) ■ Atropine ■ Amphetamines ■ Caffeine, nicotine ■ Cocaine ■ Beta agonists, theophylline
Psychosomatic disorders	**Endocrine**
■ Generalized anxiety, major depression, panic disorder	■ Hyperthyroidism, hypoglycemia, pheochromocytoma
High output states	**Miscellaneous and idiopathic**
■ Anemia, beriberi, fever, pregnancy, thyrotoxicosis	■ Emotional stress, hyperventilation, premenstrual syndrome, strenuous physical activity

Duration and Frequency of Palpitations

- Duration may be either short-lasting or persistent.
- Note the onset and offset of palpitations.
- Frequency: It may occur daily, weekly, monthly, or yearly.

Types of palpitations	
Extrasystolic palpitations	Ectopic beats, usually produce feelings of "missing/skipping a beat" and/or a "sinking of the heart" interspersed with periods during which the heart beats normally. Patients report that the heart seems to stop and then start again. It can often even be seen in young individuals, usually without any disease of the heart, and generally benign
Tachycardiac palpitations	These are the rapid fluctuation like "beating wings" in the chest. It may be regular (e.g., in atrioventricular tachycardia, atrial flutter, or ventricular tachycardia) or irregular or arrhythmic (e.g., in atrial fibrillation)
Anxiety-related palpitations	They are usually associated with anxiety episodes. They begin and end gradually

Associated Symptoms and Circumstances

- Palpitations developing after sudden changes in posture are usually due to orthostatic intolerance or to episodes of atrioventricular nodal re-entrant tachycardia.
- Occurrence of syncope or other symptoms, such as severe fatigue, dyspnea, or angina, in addition to palpitations, is more common with structural heart disease.
- Hypersecretion of natriuretic hormone results in polyuria/postpalpitation diuresis in atrial fibrillation.
- Palpitations associated with anxiety or during panic attacks are usually due to sinus tachycardia secondary to the mental disturbance.
- Palpitations may be produced by an increase in the sympathetic drive during physical exercise.

Typical descriptions of palpitations	
Flip-flopping in the chest	Palpitations are sensed as the heart seeming to stop and then start again, producing a pounding or flip-flopping sensation. This type of palpitation is generally caused by supraventricular or ventricular premature contractions
Rapid fluttering in the chest	It is due to a sustained ventricular or supraventricular arrhythmia, including sinus tachycardia
Pounding in the neck	An irregular pounding feeling in the neck is caused by atrioventricular dissociation, with independent contraction of the atria and ventricles, resulting in occasional atrial contraction against a closed tricuspid and mitral valve. This produces cannon A waves, which are intermittent increases in the "A" wave of the jugular venous pulse. **Cannon A** waves may be seen with ventricular premature contractions, third degree or complete heart block, or ventricular tachycardia (VT)

DYSPNEA

Discussed in detail in section of symptomatology, Chapter 3C.

SYNCOPE

Definition

Syncope is defined as a transient loss of consciousness due to inadequate cerebral blood flow with loss of postural tone. It is associated with spontaneous return to baseline neurologic function without any resuscitative efforts.

- **Presyncope** is the term used for lightheadedness in which the individual thinks he/she may black out.
- **Classical vasovagal syncope:** Syncope triggered by emotional or orthostatic stress such as venipuncture (experienced or witnessed), painful or noxious stimuli, fear of bodily injury, prolonged standing, heat exposure, or exertion.

Mechanism

- Global hypoperfusion of cerebral cortices or focal hypoperfusion of the reticular activating system.
- About one-third of individuals may develop a syncopal episode during their lifetime.
- Its incidence increases with age (sharp rise at age 70 years).
- Cardiac syncope has a high incidence (about 24%) of subsequent cardiac arrest.

Causes of True Syncope (Table 4D.5)

TABLE 4D.5: Causes of true syncope.

Cardiac causes	Noncardiac causes
■ **Cardiac arrhythmias:** Ventricular tachycardia, paroxysmal supraventricular tachycardia, long QT syndrome, Brugada syndrome, bradycardia (Mobitz type II or 3rd degree heart block, sick sinus syndrome) ■ **Structural cardiac or cardiopulmonary disease:** Valvular heart disease (AS, MS, PS), obstructive cardiomyopathy, atrial myxoma, acute aortic dissection, pericardial disease/tamponade, massive or submassive pulmonary embolus/severe pulmonary hypertension, acute myocardial infarction/ischemia	■ **Neurocardiogenic syncope' vasovagal or vasodepressor syncope':** Classical vasovagal syncope, situational syncope, carotid sinus syncope, glossopharyngeal neuralgia, micturition syncope ■ **Orthostatic hypotension:** Autonomic failure which may be primary (e.g., pure autonomic failure, multiple system atrophy, Parkinson's disease with autonomic failure) or secondary (e.g., diabetic neuropathy) ■ **Neurovascular syncope:** Vascular steal syndromes

Classification of Syncope

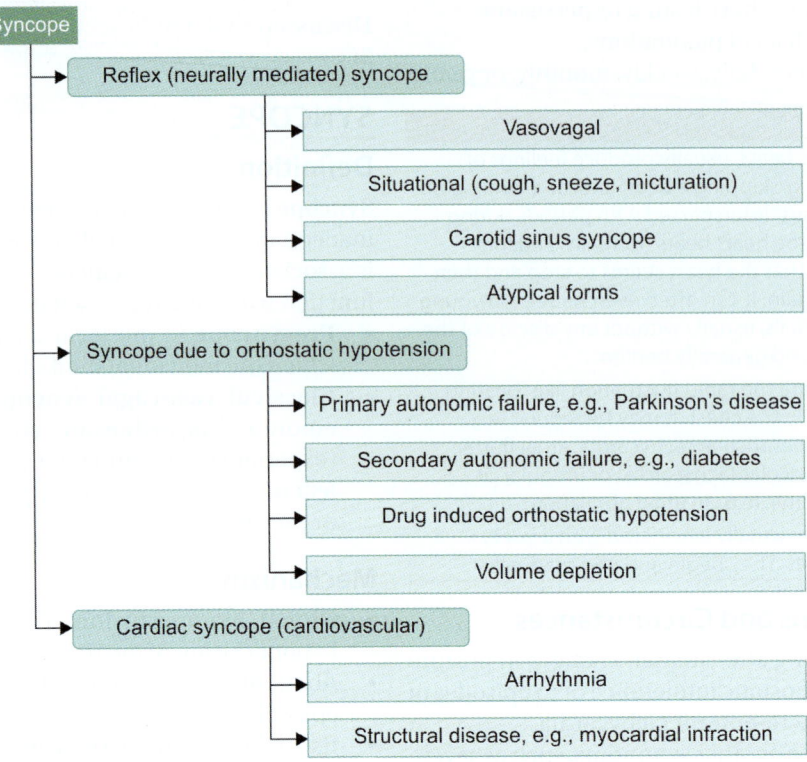

Causes of Pseudosyncope (Box 4D.1)

Box 4D.1: Causes of pseudosyncope.
• Seizures • Metabolic or toxic abnormalities: Hypoglycemia and other encephalopathy • Neurologic syncope: Subarachnoid hemorrhage, transient ischemic attack, complex migraine headache • Psychogenic syncope • Drug-induced loss of consciousness: Drugs of abuse and alcohol

PEDAL EDEMA

Definition

Pedal edema is a sign and is defined as the abnormal fluid accumulation in the interstitial space that exceeds the capacity of physiological lymphatic drainage. Pedal edema as a common presentation as swelling of lower limbs is manifestation of various systemic and nonsystemic diseases.

Approach to pedal edema (Flowchart 4D.1)	
Site and distribution	Whether the pedal edema is unilateral or bilateral: ▪ Unilateral edema results mainly due to local causes like deep vein thrombosis (DVT), cellulitis, compartment syndrome, and filarial lymphatic obstruction ▪ Bilateral pedal edema is mainly due to systemic causes like congestive cardiac failure, anemia, chronic kidney disease, and chronic liver disease
Duration of illness	Short duration of the illness indicates an acute cause like cellulitis, DVT, compartment syndrome, etc., which usually occurs in 72 hours
Association with pain	▪ **Painless:** Edema due to heart failure, hypoproteinemia, and lymphedema ▪ **Painful:** Deep vein thrombosis and cellulitis. *A dull aching type of pain is seen in chronic venous insufficiency*
Variability of edema	▪ Venous edema due to congestive cardiac failure and venous insufficiency is aggravated by standing and improves with overnight limb elevation during sleep ▪ *Idiopathic edema* which is seen in females and increases throughout the day due to upright posture
History of systemic illness	▪ Symptoms of systemic diseases like exertional dyspnea, orthopnea, paroxysmal nocturnal dyspnea, and chest pain point to cardiac failure ▪ History of oliguria and puffiness of face suggest renal etiology ▪ Long-term alcohol consumption, yellowish discoloration of eyes and urine, and abdominal distension points to cirrhosis of liver ▪ Symptoms of endocrine disorders like hypothyroidism are often missed ▪ Similar history about all other systemic causes of pedal edema should be elicited in detail ▪ Patients who are bedridden for a prolonged period of time have dependent edema over the sacral area

Contd...

Contd...

History of drug intake	Drugs like calcium channel blockers, nonsteroidal anti-inflammatory drugs (NSAIDs) and steroids
History of trauma and radiation	Trauma and radiation can cause cellulitis and compartment syndrome leading to pedal edema
Miscellaneous causes	Obstructive sleep apnea can also cause pedal edema due to right ventricular failure

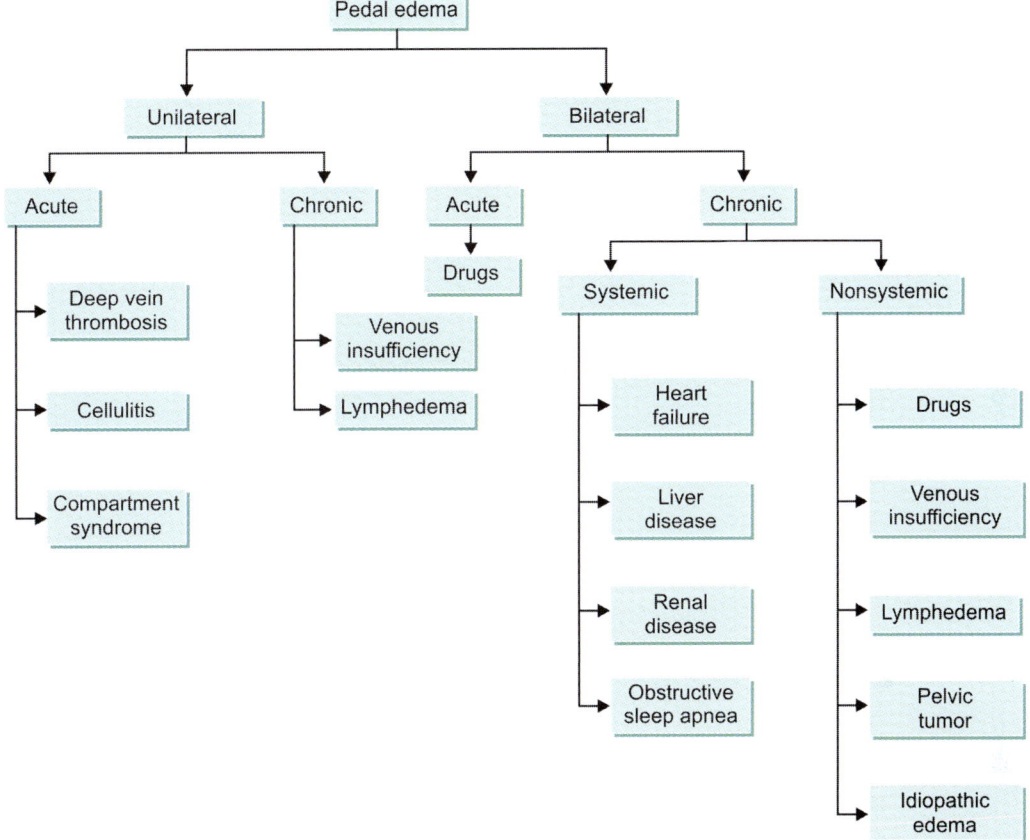

Flowchart 4D.1: Algorithm for approach to pedal edema.

Other Symptoms

- **Symptoms of low cardiac output**: Fatigue, dizziness, and syncope
- **Symptoms of pulmonary hypertension:** Exertional fatigue, angina (secondary to RV subendocardial ischemia) and exertional dyspnea
- **Fever:** Rheumatic fever and infective endocarditis
- **Symptoms of heart failure**: Fatigue, anorexia, weight gain, leg swelling, exertional fatigue, decreased urine output, perspiration, confusion, cough, hemoptysis, and wheezing.

NOTES

E. DISCUSSION ON EXAMINATION

GENERAL EXAMINATION

Vitals

Pulse, blood pressure and jugular venous pressure: Discussed in detail in Chapter 2B.

Anthropometry: Discussed in the Chapter 2D.

PHYSICAL EXAMINATION

Signs of infective endocarditis (Figs. 4E.1A to F):
- Fever
- Pallor
- Clubbing
- Splinter hemorrhages under nail beds
- Mucosal petechiae
- Janeway lesions
- Osler's nodes
- Roth spots on fundus.

Signs of rheumatic fever:
- Fever
- Arthritis
- Erythema marginatum
- Subcutaneous nodules
- Tachycardia.

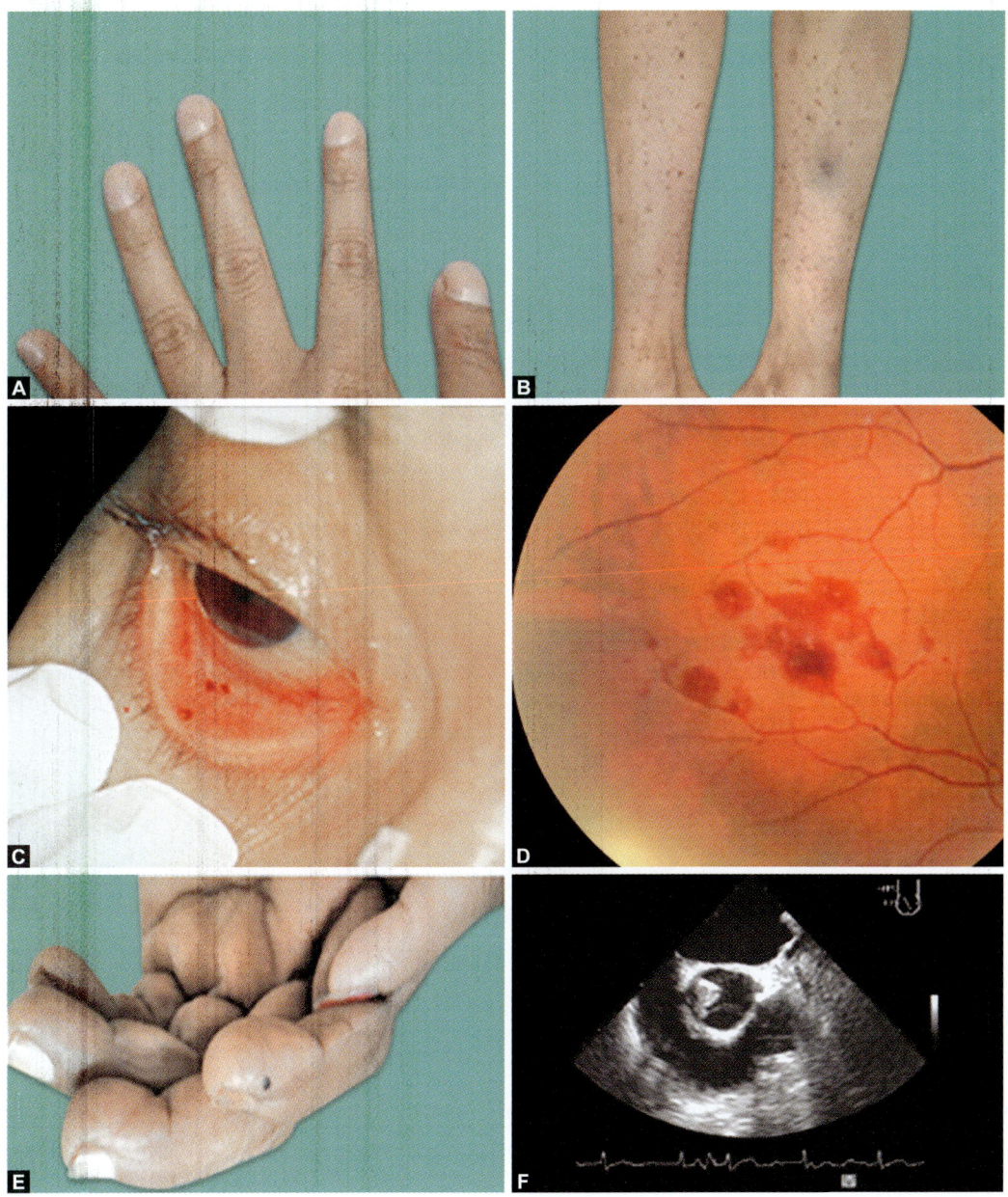

Figs. 4E.1A to F: Signs of infective endocarditis: (A) Clubbing; (B) Petechiae; (C) Subconjunctival hemorrhage; (D) Roth spots; (E) Osler's nodes; (F) Echocardiography showing vegetation.

Stigmata of congenital heart disease

Syndrome	Cardiac defects	Other features
Down syndrome (trisomy 21) (CHILD HAS MANY PROBLEM) (Fig. 4E.2)	ECD, VSD	- **C**ataract - **H**ypotonia - **H**ypothyroidism - **I**ncreased gap between 1st and 2nd toe (sandal gap) - **L**eukemia - **D**uodenal atresia - **H**irschsprung's disease - **A**lzheimer's disease - **S**imian crease - **M**ental retardation - **M**icrognathia - **A**tlantoaxial instability - **Ny**stagmus - **P**rotruding tongue - **P**oor hearing - **R**ound face - **R**espiratory infections - **O**cciput is flat - **O**blique palpebral fissure - **B**rushfield spots - **B**rachycephaly - **L**ow nasal bridge - **L**anguage problem - **E**picanthic fold - **E**ar folded - **M**ongolian slant - **M**yoclonus
Marfan syndrome	Aortic aneurysm, aortic and AML prolapse with MVP and MR	Arachnodactyly with hyperextensibility, subluxation of lens and other joint deformities
William's syndrome	- Supravalvular AS - PA stenosis (peripheral PS most common)	Varying degrees of mental retardation, so-called elfin facies (consisting of some of the following: Upturned nose, flat nasal bridge, long philtrum, flat malar area, wide mouth, full lips, widely spaced teeth, periorbital fullness), hypercalcemia of infancy
Rubella syndrome	PDA and pulmonary stenosis (peripheral PS most common)	**Triad of the syndrome:** Deafness, cataract, and CHDs Others include Intrauterine growth retardation, microcephaly, microphthalmia, hepatitis, neonatal thrombocytopenic purpura
Noonan's syndrome (Turner-like syndrome)	PS (dystrophic pulmonary valve), LVH (or anterior septal hypertrophy)	Similar to Turner's syndrome but may occur in phenotypic male and without chromosomal abnormality
LEOPARD syndrome (multiple lentigines syndrome)	PS, HOCM, long PR interval	Lentiginous skin lesion, ocular hypertelorism, pulmonary stenosis, abnormal genitalia, retarded growth, deafness
Holt-Oram syndrome (cardiac-limb syndrome)	ASD, VSD	Defects or absence of thumb or radius
Ellis–van Creveld syndrome (chondroectodermal dysplasia)	ASD, single atrium	Short stature of prenatal onset, short distal extremities, narrow thorax with short ribs, polydactyly, nail hypoplasia, neonatal teeth
DiGeorge syndrome	Interrupted aortic arch, truncus arteriosus, VSD, PDA, TOF	Hypertelorism, short philtrum, down slanting eyes, hypoplasia or absence of thymus and parathyroid, hypocalcemia, deficient cell-mediated immunity
Cornelia de Lange's (de Lange's) syndrome	VSD	Hirsutism, prenatal growth retardation, microcephaly, anteverted nares, downturned mouth, mental retardation
CHARGE syndrome	TOF, truncus arteriosus, aortic arch anomalies (e.g., vascular ring, interrupted aortic arch)	Coloboma, choanal atresia, growth or mental retardation, genitourinary anomalies, ear anomalies, genital hypoplasia
Ehlers Danlos syndrome	TOF, ASD, great vessel aneurysms	Joint hypermobility, easy bruisability, hernia, kyphoscoliosis

(AS: aortic stenosis; ASD: atrial septal defect; ECD: endocardial cushion defect; HOCM: hypertrophic obstructive cardiomyopathy; LVH: left ventricular hypertrophy; PA: pulmonary artery; PS: pulmonary stenosis; TOF: tetralogy of Fallot; VSD: ventricular septal defect; CHDs: congenital heart diseases; PDA: patent ductus arteriosus)

Cardiovascular System Examination

Features of Down Syndrome (Fig. 4E.2)

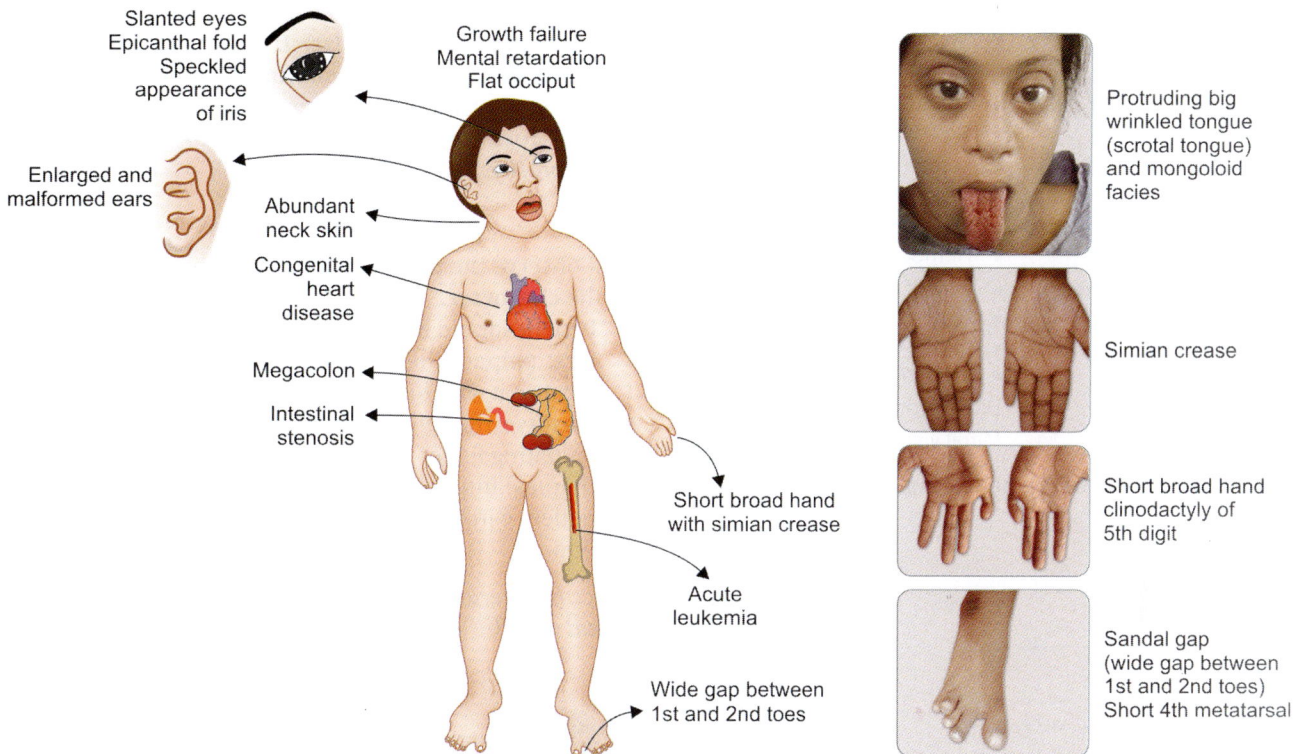

Fig. 4E.2: Features of Down syndrome.

Features of Turner Syndrome (Fig. 4E.3)

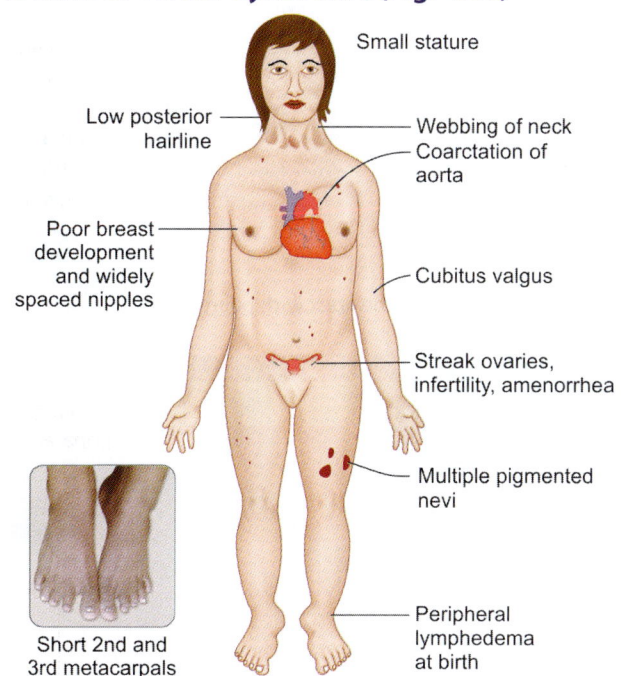

Fig. 4E.3: Features of Turner syndrome.

SYSTEMIC EXAMINATION

All cardiovascular examination must be simultaneously timed with carotid pulse. Findings synchronous with carotid upstroke is systolic and if it is asynchronous, it is diastolic.

Inspection and Palpation of Heart

Palpation of CVS (Fig. 4E.4)

Tips of fingers	For localizing the pulsations
Metacarpal heads	For appreciating the thrills
Heel of hand	For appreciating the heave

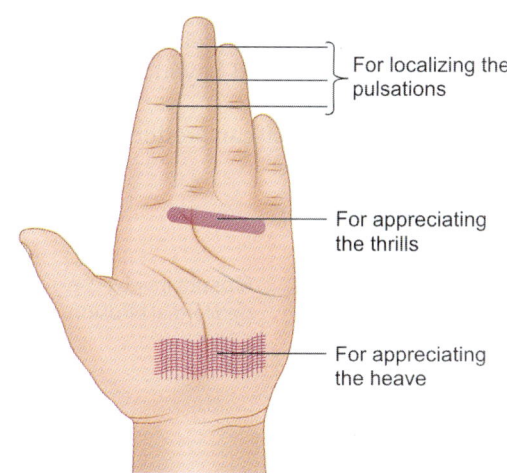

Fig. 4E.4: Showing sites of hand for palpation of pulses, thrills and heave.

Chest deformity and associated clinical diseases:

Chest deformity	Associated diseases
Barrel shaped	Chronic obstructive pulmonary disease and cor pulmonale
Broad shield like chest	- Turner syndrome - Noonan syndrome
Pectus carinatum	- Marfan's syndrome - Noonan syndrome
Pectus excavatum	- Marfan's syndrome - Homocystinuria
Straight back syndrome	- Loss of normal kyphosis - Expiratory splitting of S2 - Midsystolic murmur - Prominent pulmonary artery
Male gynecomastia	Digitalis or spironolactone
Female hypomastia	Mitral valve prolapse (MVP)

Topographical areas of the heart (Fig. 4E.5):

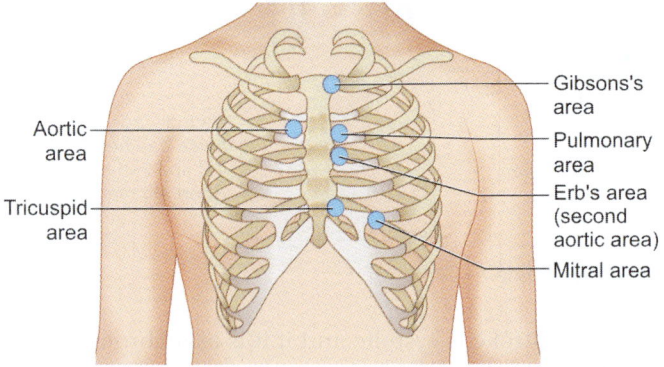

Fig. 4E.5: Illustration of areas of auscultation.

Precordial Bulge

- Patient in supine position, stand at the foot end of the bed and look for precordial bulge
- If present, indicates right ventricular dilatation in childhood
- ***Classically seen only with congenital heart diseases like atrial septal defect (ASD)***
- Costal cartilage fuses by 16 years of age, so cardiac diseases which are acquired beyond 16 years may not have a precordial bulge
- Acquired heart disease that can produce precordial bulge is juvenile mitral stenosis.

Causes of precordial bulge:

Cardiovascular causes	
Ribs involved, e.g., cardiac enlargement of long duration	Ribs not involved, e.g., pericardial effusion
Noncardiovascular causes	
- Skeletal deformity - Bronchogenic carcinoma - Mediastinal growth	

Apical Impulse

Definition

It is the **outermost** and **lowermost** point of **definite** cardiac impulse which imparts a perpendicular gentle thrust to a palpating finger in early systole followed by a slight medial retraction in mid to late systole.

Point of maximal impulse: It need not necessarily be the apex beat, since the maximal precordial pulsation may be produced by an enlarged or hypertrophied RV, a dilated aorta or pulmonary artery, or a LV wall motion abnormality.

Method of Examination of Apical Impulse

First observe the **position** of apical impulse, then comment on the **character**.
- Patient should be in supine position
- First palpate the apex with the palm **(Fig. 4E.6)**, then localize it with fingertip **(Fig. 4E.7)**
- Observe the amplitude and duration of the lift of the palpating finger
- If apical impulse is not palpable in supine position, the patient can be put in left lateral position and examination done.

Note: In lateral position—do not comment on position of apical impulse.

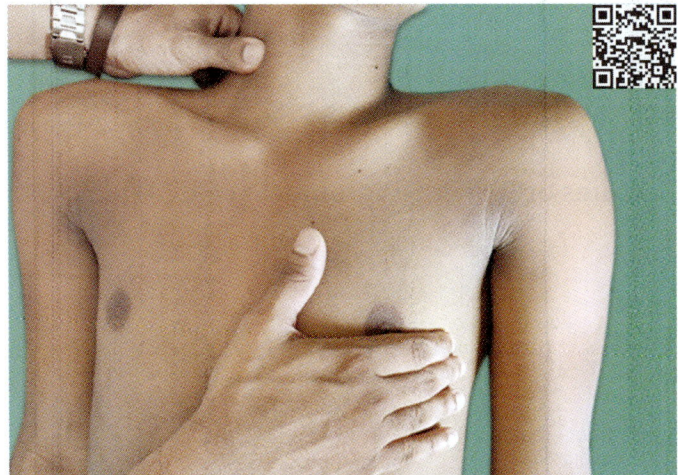

Fig. 4E.6: Palpating the apex with palm flat on the chest.

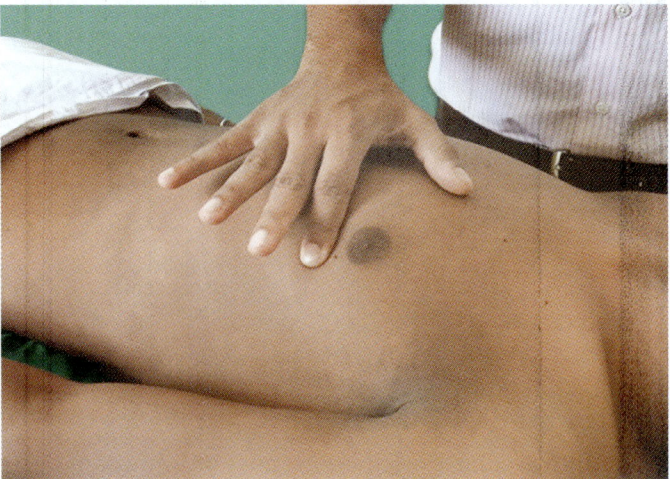

Fig. 4E.7: Localizing the apex with the fingertip.

Cardiovascular System Examination

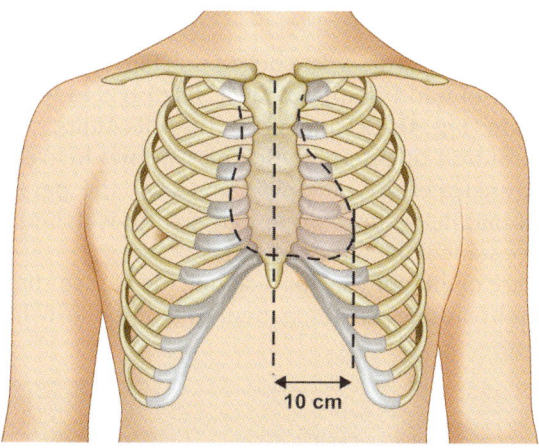

Fig. 4E.8: Location of cardiac impulse.

Features of normal cardiac impulse:

Location	Left 5th ICS, 1–2 cm medial to MCL (or) ≤10 cm from the midsternal line (**Fig. 4E.8**)
Extent	<2.4 cm or one ICS
Duration	<50% of systole

(ICS: intercostal space; MCL: midclavicular line)

Mechanism of normal apical impulse:
Anterior and counterclockwise rotation of left ventricle (LV) due to isovolumic contraction during early systole and medial retraction due to clockwise rotation of the LV during late systole.

Abnormalities of apex (Figs. 4E.9 and 4E.10)	
Absent (not seen nor felt)	**Cardiovascular causes** ■ Pericardial effusion ■ Dextrocardia **Noncardiac causes** ■ Behind rib ■ Obesity or thick chest wall ■ COPD/emphysema ■ Left-sided pleural effusion ■ Left-sided pneumothorax
Tapping	Mitral stenosis (palpable S1—**closing snap**)
Hyperdynamic	■ Increased in amplitude ■ Duration is >1/3–<2/3 of systole ■ Occupies more than one intercostal space (hence called **diffuse apex**) Occurs in LV **volume overload** conditions **Physiological** ■ Thin chest ■ Pectus excavatum ■ High output states **Pathological** ■ AR ■ MR ■ VSD ■ PDA ■ AV fistula
Heaving	■ Increase in amplitude ■ Duration is >2/3 of systole ■ Confined to one intercostal space

Contd...

Contd...

	Occurs in LV **pressure overload** ■ AS ■ Systemic hypertension ■ HCM ■ Coarctation of aorta
Double apical impulse	■ HOCM ■ LV aneurysm ■ LV dyssynergy
Triple or quadruple or wavy impulse	HOCM
Retractile	Severe TR
See-saw apex	LV aneurysm
Systolic retraction followed by diastolic expansion	Constrictive pericarditis

(AR: aortic regurgitation; AS: aortic stenosis; AV fistula: arteriovenous fistula; COPD: chronic obstructive pulmonary disease; HOCM: hypertrophic obstructive cardiomyopathy; LVH: left ventricular hypertrophy; MR: mitral regurgitation; PDA: patent ductus arteriosus; VSD: ventricular septal defect; LV: left ventricular; TR: tricuspid regurgitation)

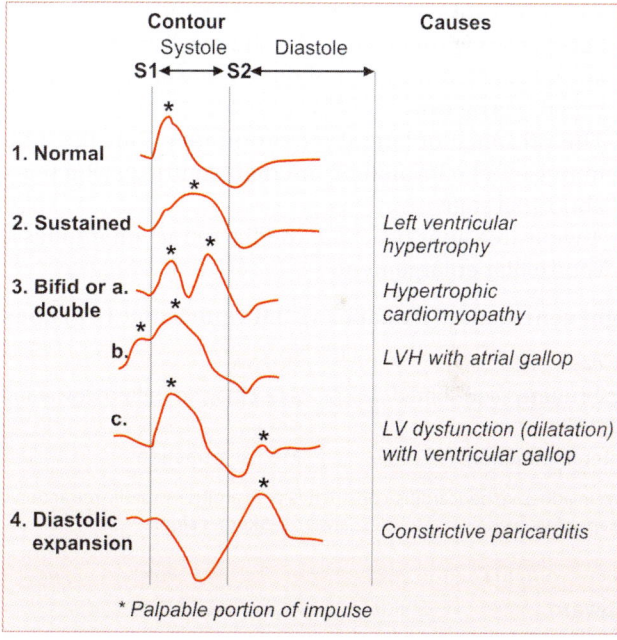

Fig. 4E.9: Apicogram showing different types of cardiac apex.

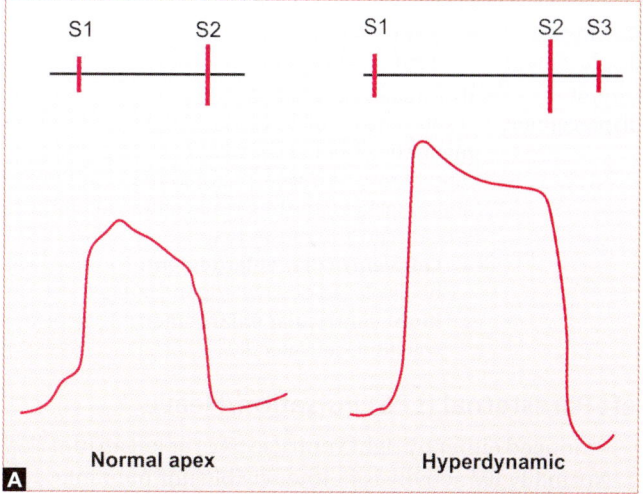

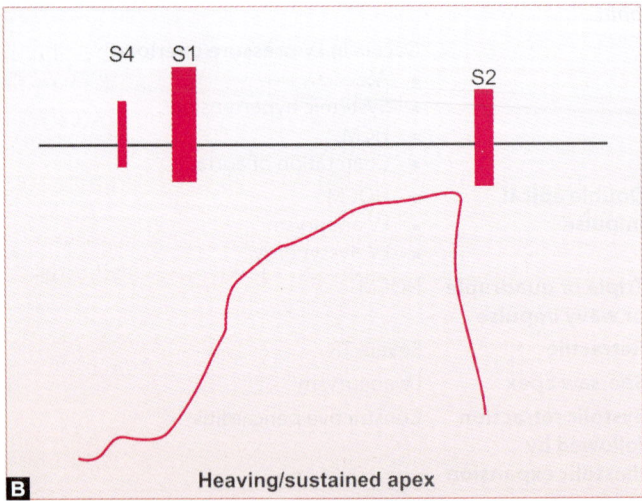

Figs. 4E.10A and B: Co-relation of apex with heart sounds.

Which Ventricle is Causing the Apical Impulse?

- The heart during systole, becoming smaller, generally withdraws from the chest wall except for the apex. The effect of this withdrawal on the chest wall can be observed as an inward movement of the chest wall during systole called "**retraction**".
- The presence of lateral retraction identifies the apical impulse to be formed by the right ventricle, which is an abnormal state.
- A wide area apex beat with medial retraction implies left ventricular enlargement.

Right ventricular (RV) apex vs left ventricular (LV) apex:

RV apex	LV apex
Apex rotated and shifted laterally	Apex may be shifted down and out
Lateral retraction	Medial retraction

Note: In adhesive pericarditis/constrictive pericarditis—systolic retraction of the apex followed by diastolic expansion—**Skoda's sign.**

Displacement of apex	
Upward displacement	■ Children ■ Ascites ■ Abdominal tumor ■ Pericardial effusion
Downward displacement	■ Mediastinal growth ■ Aortic aneurysm
Lateral displacement	If trachea is also shifted along with the displacement of apex beat, then it is due to mediastinal shift as a result of conditions such as lung fibrosis, collapse, pneumothorax or skeletal abnormalities If the trachea is central but the apex is displaced, the causes may be: ■ **Left ventricular enlargement:** The apex will be displaced downwards and laterally ■ **Right ventricular enlargement:** The apex will displaced laterally

Left Parasternal (LPS) Pulsation/Heave

- Produced either by right ventricle (RV) or left atrium (LA).
- Normally RV activity is neither visible nor palpable.

Examination of LPS Area

- Heel of hand with wrist cocked up **(Fig. 4E.11)** or ulnar border of hand is applied over 3/4/5 ICS in left sternal margin **(Fig. 4E.12)** and felt for the pulsations.
- In children or thin patients, parasternal heave can be demonstrated by placing a pen over the parasternal area parallel to the sternal margin and watched for the movement of the tip of the pen.
- In case of difficulty in appreciating the parasternal heave from breathing, ask the patient to momentarily hold the breath.

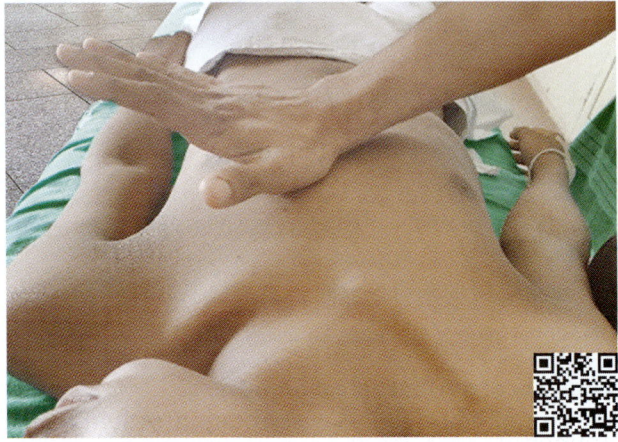

Fig. 4E.11: Examination of parasternal heave (with heel of the hand in cocked up position).

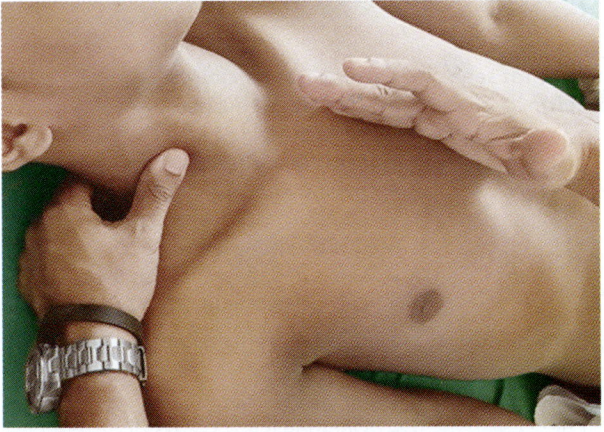

Fig. 4E.12: Examination of parasternal heave (by placing ulnar border).

All India Institute of Medical Science (AIIMS) Grading of Parasternal Heave

Grade I	Grade II	Grade III
■ Visible ■ Not palpable	■ Visible ■ Palpable ■ Obliterable	■ Visible ■ Palpable ■ Not obliterable
Ill-sustained	>50% of systole	Full systole

How to differentiate RV and LA parasternal heave?

RV parasternal heave	LA parasternal heave
■ Synchronous with apex ■ Early systole	■ Not synchronous with apex ■ Late systole ■ Seen in severe MR

Conditions where LPS pulsations are seen	
Physiological	- Children - Reduced AP diameter
Right ventricular hypertrophy associated	**Pressure overload** - Pulmonary HTN - Pulmonary stenosis **Volume overload** - TR - ASD - VSD
Normal RV	- **Moderate to severe MR** (jet or squid effect)—regurgitant jet of blood into LA pushes the RV anteriorly - **Regional wall motion abnormality (RWMA) of LV**—dyskinetic motion of LV septum pushes RV forwards during the systole

Note:
1. There is no parasternal heave in TOF
2. In MS with MR there is both LAE and RVH, hence very prominent parasternal heave is seen

(AP: anteroposterior; ASD: atrial septal defect; HTN: hypertension; LAE: left atrial enlargement; LV: left ventricular; MR: mitral regurgitation; RVH: right ventricular hypertrophy; TR: tricuspid regurgitation; VSD: ventricular septal defect; LA: left atrium; RV: right ventricular)

Aortic and Pulmonary Pulsations (Base of the Heart)

Examined in sitting and leaning forward position with breath held in expiration (**Erb's maneuver**—described in auscultation section).

Aortic area	Pulmonary area
Right 2nd ICS area	Left 2nd ICS area
Visible pulsations	
- Aneurysm of aorta - Chronic AR	- Pulmonary HTN - Pulmonary artery dilatation - Pulmonary artery aneurysm - Hyperdynamic pulmonary artery circulation
Palpable heart sounds	
- A2 (sHTN) - Ejection click (bicuspid aortic valve)	- P2 (pHTN)—**diastolic shock** - Ejection click (valvular pulmonary stenosis of doming type)
Palpable murmurs	
- AS - AR (dilated root—AR)	- PS - PDA (Gibsons area—left 1st ICS) - Graham steel murmur

(AR: aortic regurgitation; AS: aortic stenosis; HTN: hypertension; pHTN: pulmonary hypertension; sHTN: systemic hypertension; ICS: intercostal space PDA: patent ductus arteriosus; PS: pulmonary stenosis)

Sternoclavicular Pulsations

Suprasternal pulsations	- Aneurysm of arch of aorta - Thyroidea ima artery
Right sternoclavicular joint	- Aortic dissection - Aneurysm of aorta - Aortic regurgitation - Right aortic arch - Blalock-Taussig shunt

Epigastric Pulsations

- The subxiphoid region should be palpated by placing the thumb/index finger/palm of the hand over the epigastrium with the fingertip pointing towards the patient's head (**Fig. 4E.13**).
- Gentle pressure is applied downward (posteriorly) and upward towards the head.
- The patient should be asked to take a deep inspiration in order to move the diaphragm down. This facilitates the palpation of the right ventricle.
- If the impulse were palpable pushing the tip of the thumb/fingertips downward (toward the feet), it would indicate a palpable right ventricular impulse.
- Transmitted abdominal aortic pulsations will cause the impulse to strike the pulp/palmar aspect of the thumb/hand.
- Transmitted hepatic pulsations are felt from the right side onto lateral surface of the examining finger.

Causes of epigastric pulsations	
Cardiac causes	RVH (due to any cause)
Aortic causes	- Thin build - Aneurysm of descending aorta - Aortic regurgitation
Hepatic causes	- Presystolic/diastolic: TS - Systolic: TR

(RVH: right ventricular hypertrophy; TR: tricuspid regurgitation; TS: tricuspid stenosis)

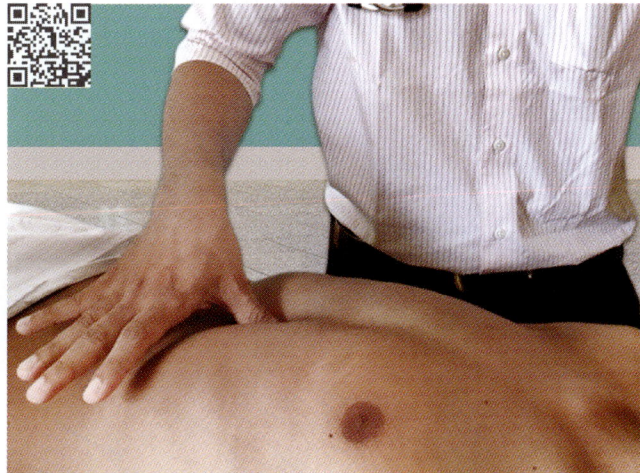

Fig. 4E.13: Demonstration of epigastric pulsations.

Other Pulsations

At back	- **Suzman's sign** in coarctation of aorta - Pulmonary arteriovenous fistula
At neck	- Aortic regurgitation - Carotid aneurysm - Subclavian artery aneurysm

Thrills

- Thrills are palpable murmurs (grade IV or more intensity).
- It is described as *purring of the cat*.
- Best felt with head of the metacarpal bones.
- Can be systolic, diastolic or continuous.

Area	Timing	Cause
Mitral (apex)	- Systolic - Diastolic	- Severe MR - MS
Left sternal border	- Systolic	- VSD
Pulmonary area	- Systolic	- PS
Aortic area	- Systolic - Diastolic	- AS - Acute severe AR
Left 1st ICS	- Continuous	- PDA or rupture of sinus of Valsalva

Note: As a rule, thrills in the apex of heart are diastolic and thrills in the base of the heart are systolic (exceptions are systolic thrill of severe MR and diastolic thrill of severe AR).

(AR: aortic regurgitation; AS: aortic stenosis; ICS: intercostal space; MR: mitral regurgitation; MS: mitral stenosis; PDA: patent ductus arteriosus; PS: pulmonary stenosis; VSD: ventricular septal defect)

Other Sounds Palpable at Apex

Low frequency sounds	
LV S3	LVF, MR
LV S4 (LVEDP >15–18 mm Hg)	- AS - HCM - MR/AR - CAD
Pericardial knock	Constrictive pericarditis
High frequency sounds	
S1	Tapping apex of MS
OS	Early diastolic sound in MS
Ejection systolic click	AS (congenital—bicuspid aortic valve)
Tumor PLOP	LA/RA myxoma
Murmurs (thrills)	
Systolic	- MR - AS - VSD
Diastolic	MS

(AR: aortic regurgitation; AS: aortic stenosis; CAD: coronary artery disease; HCM: hypertrophic cardiomyopathy; LA: left atrial; LV: left ventricular; LVF: left ventricular failure; MR: mitral regurgitation; MS: mitral stenosis; PDA: patent ductus arteriosus; RA: right atrial; VSD: ventricular septal defect)

Other Palpable Sounds in Parasternal Area

Low frequency sounds	
RV S3 (increased flow to ventricles)	- RV failure - Chronic TR - ASD
RV S4 (against increased pressures of ventricle)	- PS - Decreased RV compliance
High frequency sounds	
OS	TS
Murmurs (thrills)	
Systolic	TR
Diastolic	TS

(ASD: atrial septal defect; OS: opening snap; PS: pulmonary stenosis; RV: right ventricular; TR: tricuspid regurgitation; TS: tricuspid stenosis)

Note:

Palpable S1	Tapping apex
Palpable S2	Diastolic shock (palpable P2)
Constrictive pericarditis	Diastolic knock or pericardial knock

Dilated vessels:
1. Dilated veins: Caudal flow [superior vena cava (SVC) obstruction]; cranial flow [inferior vena cava (IVC) obstruction]
2. Collaterals are seen with coarctation of the aorta (COA) For example, **Suzman's sign**—seen in COA where **collaterals** are seen in interscapular and infrascapular region.

Scars (Fig. 4E.14)

Median sternotomy (Generally done when there is need for connecting a heart lung machine)	Coronary artery bypass grafting (CABG)
Lateral thoracotomy	All valve replacement surgeries Patent ductus arteriosus (PDA) surgery scar

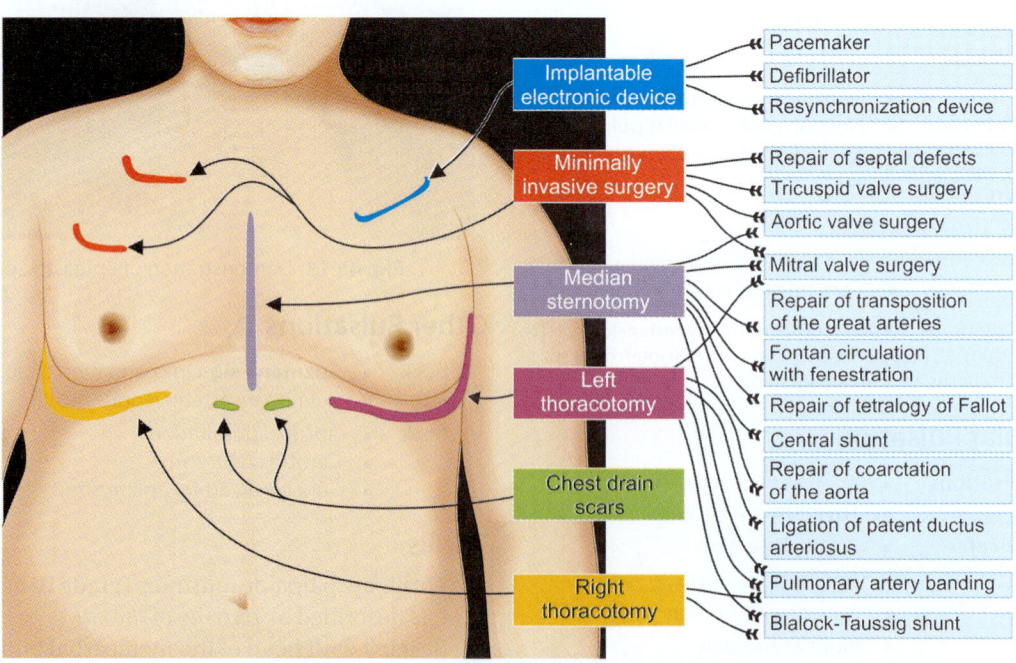

Fig. 4E.14: Image showing different surgical scars for cardiac disease.

Tracheal Tug (Oliver's Sign)

Raise the chin of patient and apply the upward pressure on two sides of cricoid cartilage **(Fig. 4E.15)**.

Positive	Downward pull with each heartbeat	Aortic aneurysm
False positive		Due to mediastinal mass
False negative	Do not move with heartbeat	Thrombosed aortic aneurysm

Percussion

Determination of Heart Border

Right heart border:
- Percuss from above downward in midclavicular line up to the liver dullness **(Fig. 4E.16)**.
- Start percussing one space above the liver dullness **(Fig. 4E.17)**, from the right midclavicular line to the sternum keeping the pleximeter finger parallel to the sternal edge **(Figs. 4E.18A and B)**.
- Repeat this in two more consecutive spaces above.

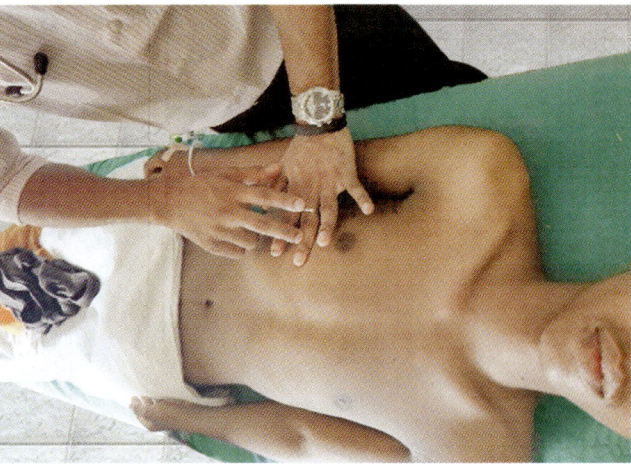

Fig. 4E.16: Percuss from above downward in midclavicular line up to the liver dullness.

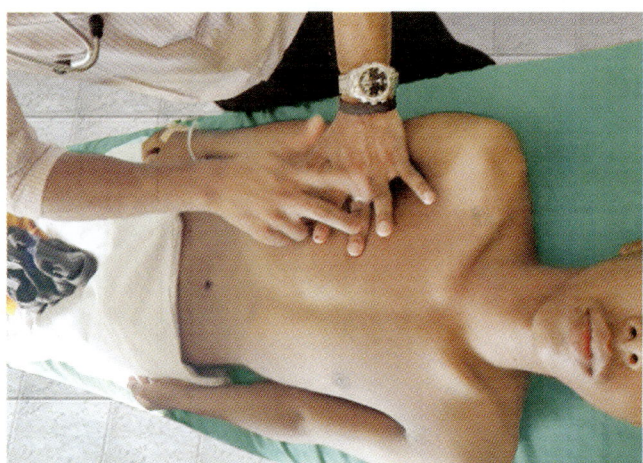

Fig. 4E.17: Now, go one space above the liver dullness.

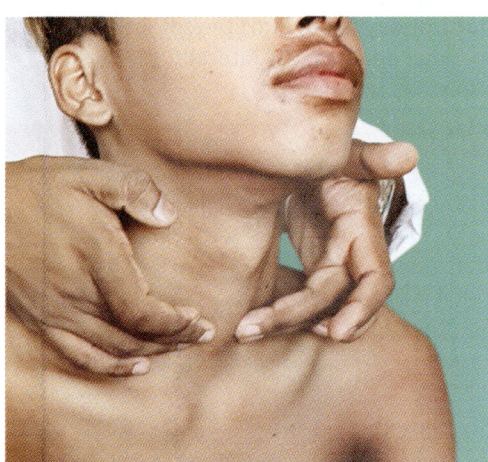

Fig. 4E.15: Demonstration of Oliver's sign.

Dullness corresponding to right sternal margin	Normal
Dullness outside the right sternal edge	• Pericardial effusion • Dextrocardia • Cardiac enlargement • Right atrial enlargement • Mediastinal mass • Lung pathology

Left heart border:
- Palpate the apex.
- In same ICS go to the midaxillary line and start percussing medially.
- Direction of percussion should be parallel to the apparent left heart border **(Figs. 4E.19A and B)**.

Normally	Corresponds to the apex
Dullness outside apex seen in	• Large pericardial effusion • Left ventricular aneurysm

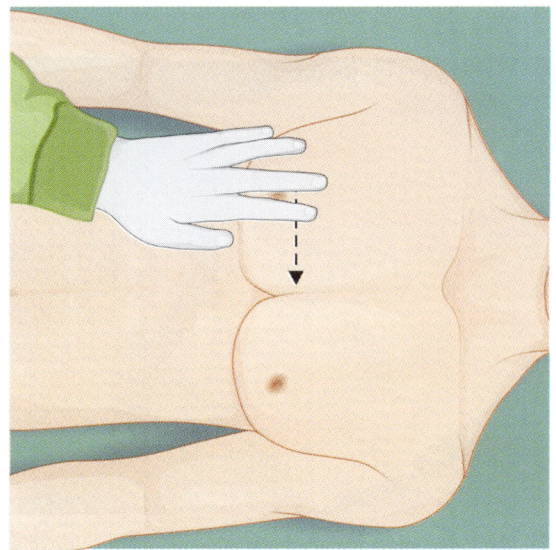

Fig. 4E.18A: Illustration showing direction of percussion of right heart border.

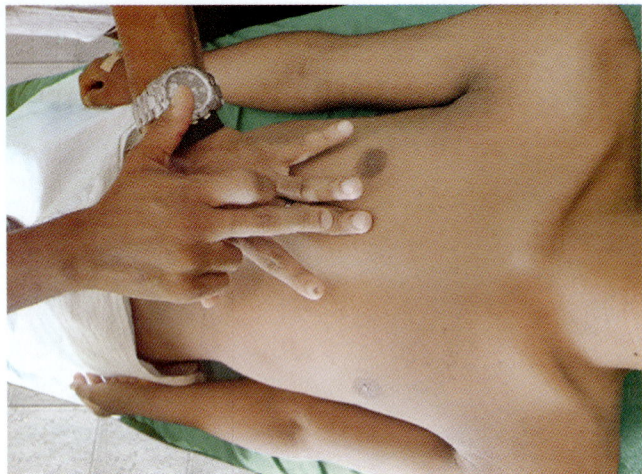

Fig. 4E.18B: Change the direction of percussing finger parallel to heart border and move medially till you get dullness (due to right heart border).

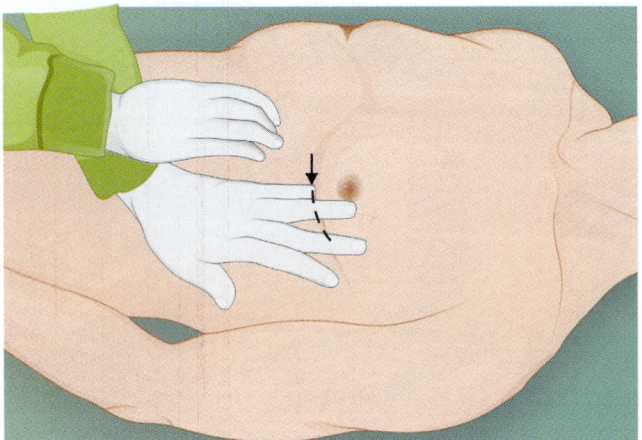

Fig. 4E.19A: Illustration showing direction of percussion of left heart border.

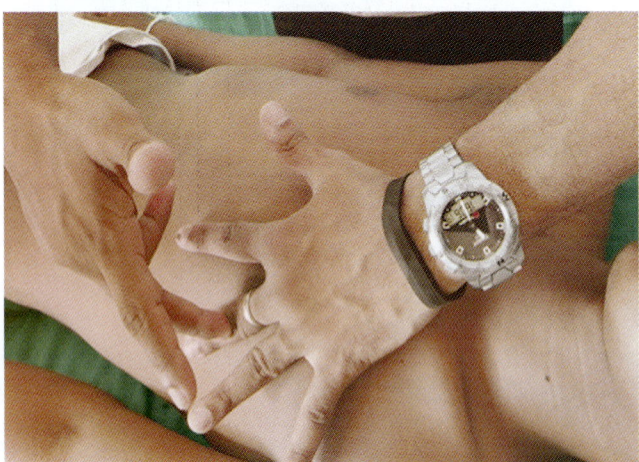

Fig. 4E.19B: Percussion for left heart border from midaxillary line and start percussing medially with percussing finger parallel to the apparent heart border.

Note: Position of pleximeter while percussing the heart border showing should be always parallel to the presumed borders of heart as showed in **Figure 4E.20**.

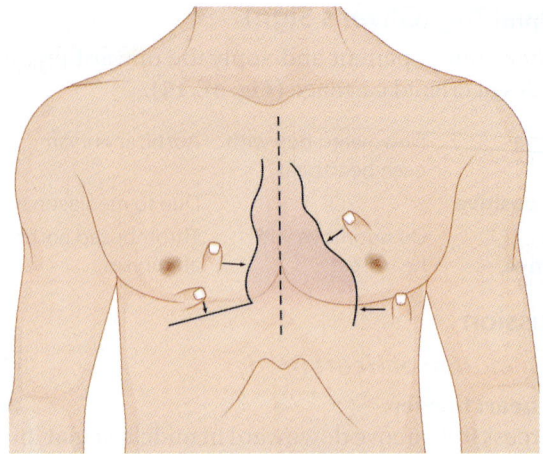

Fig. 4E.20: Illustration showing placement of pleximeter finger during percussion of heart borders.

Percussion of Aortic and Pulmonary Areas

- **For aortic area:** Start percussing parallel to the right sternal edge and percuss laterally.
- **For pulmonary area:** Start percussing parallel to the left sternal edge and percuss laterally.
- Normally it is resonant.

Aortic area	Pulmonary area (Fig. 4E.21)
Resonant (normal)	*Resonant (normal)*
Dullness	Dullness
▪ Dilated aorta	▪ Dilated PA
▪ Aortic aneurysm	▪ PAH
▪ Superior mediastinal mass	▪ PDA
	▪ Levoposed aorta

(PA: pulmonary artery; PAH: pulmonary arterial hypertension; PDA: patent ductus arteriosus)

Note:
***Rotch sign**—seen with moderate to large pericardial effusion causing obliteration of cardiohepatic angle.

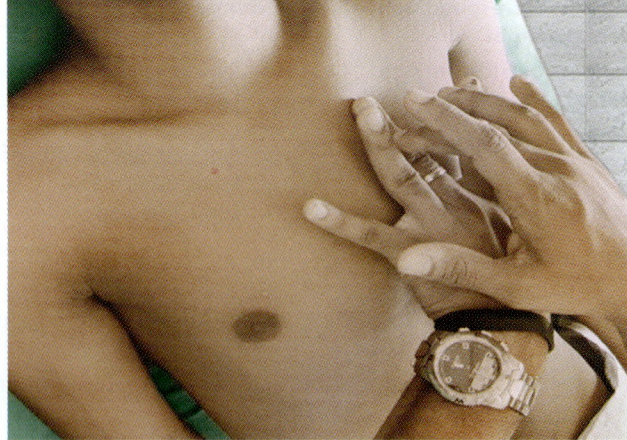

Fig. 4E.21: Percussion of left 2nd intercostal space.

Auscultation

Hearing of human beings:
- Capability is 20–20,000 Hz
- Sensitivity is 1,000–5,000 Hz

- Minimum time gap to differentiate two sounds by human ear is 20 ms.

Characters of cardiac sounds:
- **Loudness:** Implies amplitude or intensity.
- **Pitch:** Implies frequency.

Difference between low and high frequency heart sounds	
Low frequency	High frequency
<125 Hz	>300 Hz
Low pitch	High pitch
Rough rumbling	Soft blowing
For example: S3, S4, pericardial knock MDM (TS/MS)	For example: S1, S2, ESC, OS Systolic murmur of (MR, AR)
Better appreciated with **bell** of stethoscope by applying low pressure over the chest	Better appreciated with **diaphragm** of stethoscope by applying firm pressure over the chest piece

(AR: aortic regurgitation; ESC: early systolic click; OS: opening snap; MDM: mid-diastolic murmur; MR: mitral regurgitation; MS: mitral stenosis; TS: tricuspid stenosis)

Topographical areas of heart (Fig. 4E.22)	
Mitral area	Corresponds to apex (normally in left 5th ICS 1–2 cm medial to mid clavicular line
Tricuspid area	Lower left sternal edge corresponding to 5th ICS
Aortic area	Right 2nd ICS
Neoarotic area (Erb's neo aortic area)	Left 3rd ICS
Pulmonary area	Left 2nd ICS

Other areas	
Axilla	PSM of MR
Epigastrium	PSM of TR
Carotid artery	• Conduction of AS murmur • Carotid bruit
Gibson's area	• Left 1st ICS (PDA)
Roger's area	• Left 4th ICS (VSD)
Interscapular area	• Coarctation of aorta • Aneurysm of descending aorta
Subclavian artery (supraclavicular area)	Bruit over this area heard in aortoarteritis
Femoral artery	Durozier's murmur of AR

(AR: aortic regurgitation; AS: aortic stenosis; ICS: intercostal space; MR: mitral regurgitation; PDA: patent ductus arteriosus; PSM: pansystolic murmur; TR: tricuspid regurgitation; VSD: ventricular septal defect)

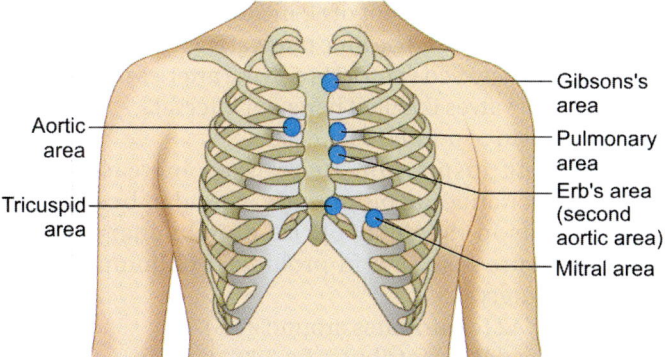

Fig. 4E.22: Illustration of areas of auscultation.

Sequence of Auscultation

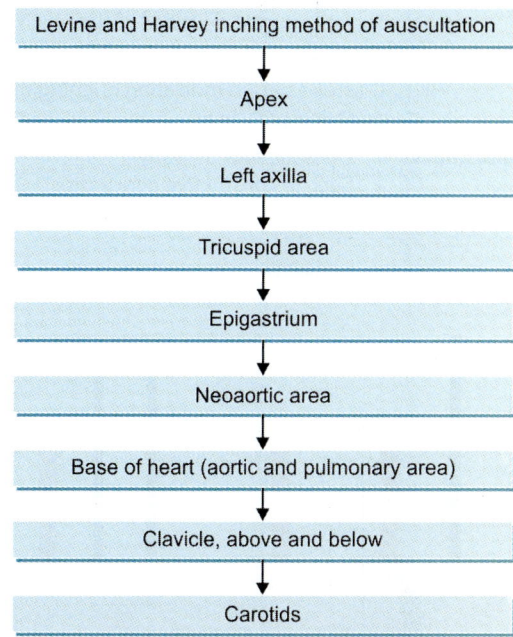

Position of patient during auscultation	
Left lateral decubitus	Mitral area
Supine	Tricuspid area
Sitting and leaning forward (Erb's maneuver)	Aortic or pulmonary area

CARDIAC CYCLE AND HEART SOUNDS

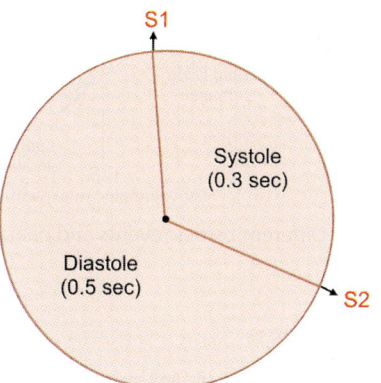

Fig. 4E.23: Cardiac cycle.

Cardiac Cycle Duration (Fig. 4E.23)

Assuming heart rate of 72, each heartbeat is approximately 0.8 seconds in which 0.5 seconds is diastole and 0.3 seconds is systole.

Heart sounds (Figs. 4E.24A and B)	
S1	• Closing of mitral and tricuspid valves • Marks the onset of ventricular systole
S2	Closing of aortic and pulmonary valves
S3	Rapid filling phase of ventricle
S4	Filling of ventricle due to atrial contraction

Cardiovascular System Examination

Others	
Clicks	Systolic sounds are called clicks which can be either ejection click or nonejection clicks
Snaps	Diastolic sounds indicating opening of mitral and tricuspid valves
Pericardial knock	• Diastolic sounds (early) • Seen in constrictive pericarditis

- Increased ionotropic activity of heart (directly proportional)
- Loss of isovolumetric contraction leads to soft S1 (MR, AR, VSD)
- Thoracic cavity and chest wall (high frequency murmurs are more attenuated with soft tissues).

Variations of S1		
Loud	*Soft*	*Variable*
• MS (mild to moderate), TS • ASD (loud T1) • Tachycardia • Short PR interval • Hyperdynamic circulation • Thin people	• Muffled in pan-systolic murmurs—MR, TR (here valves are wide and do not coaptate) • MS (severe calcific) • AR (increased LV filling and premature closure of mitral valve) • Bradycardia • Long PR, heart blocks • Obesity, emphysema, effusion	• Atrial fibrillation • Ventricular tachycardia (AV dissociation) • Complete heart blocks (cannon sound)

When do you say loud S1?
When S1 is heard with the same intensity as that of mitral area in the base of heart (aortic and pulmonary areas)

Splitting of S1

Wide splitting	Reverse splitting (T1 → M1)
• Ebstein's anomaly • ASD • Complete RBBB • LV pacing	• Ectopics • Severe MS • Complete LBBB • RV pacing

Note: In Ebstein's anomaly one can hear S1 split, S2 split, OS, S4 and pulmonary ejection click.

(AR: aortic regurgitation; ASD: atrial septal defect; AV: atrioventricular; LV: left ventricular; MR: mitral regurgitation; TR: tricuspid regurgitation; MR: mitral regurgitation; MS: mitral regurgitation; MS: mitral stenosis; TS: tricuspid stenosis; RBBB: right bundle branch block; LBBB: left bundle branch block)

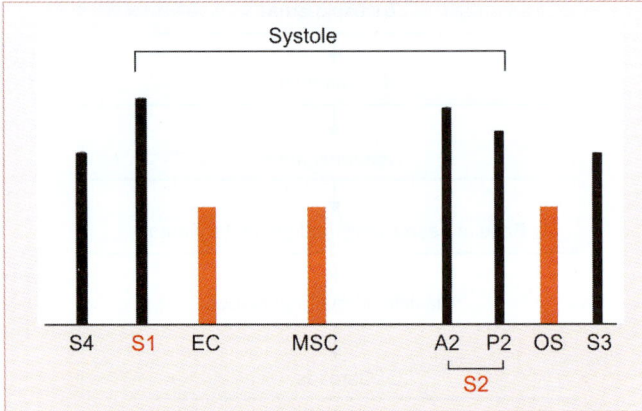

Fig. 4E.24A: Image showing different heart sounds.
(EC: ejection click; MSC: midsystolic click; OS: opening snap)

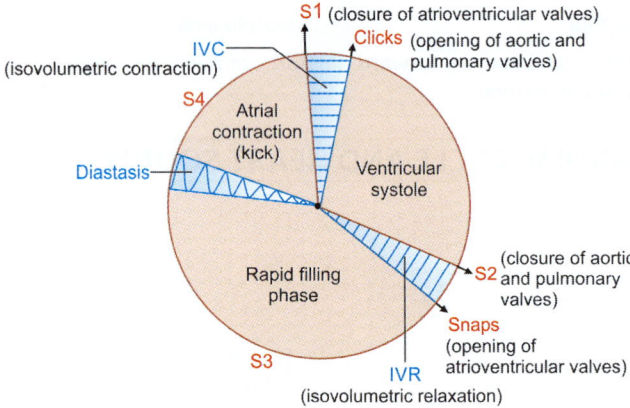

Fig. 4E.24B: Different cardiac events and heart sounds.

Heart Sounds

First Heart Sound (S1)

- Two audible components (M1 and T1)
- Two inaudible components (muscular in origin coinciding with beginning of LV contraction and opening with semilunar valves respectively)
- Order of appearance (1st inaudible component → M1 → T1 → 2nd inaudible component)
- M1–T1 interval = 20 ms
- It is loudest at apex
- Coincides with carotid upstroke
- Determinants of S1
  - Structural integrity of valve
  - Position of the valve at the onset of ventricular systole
  - PR interval (inversely proportional)

Second Heart Sound (S2)

- Two components (A2 and P2)
- A2 → P2
- A2–P2 time interval is <30 ms (expiration) and 40–50 ms (inspiration).
- Heard best in base of the heart (pulmonary and aortic areas).
- The loudest component of S2 in pulmonary area is A2.
- The loudest component of S2 in aortic area is A2.
- **Hang out interval**: The time interval from the crossover of pressures between ventricles and the arteries to the actual closure of valves is called hang out interval.
- Mechanism of normal split of S2:
  - During inspiration there is an increase in the capacitance of pulmonary vascular bed → this results in the delay of rise of pulmonary arterial pressure resulting in prolonged pulmonary hang out interval.
  - Early A2 (contributes around 27%).
  - Delayed P2 (contributes for 73%).

- Physiological split is inspiratory and disappears on standing, due to decreased venous return (while pathological split persists on standing).

Variations of S2 (Fig. 4E.25)

A2	
Loud	Soft
- Hyperdynamic state, sHTN - Aneurysm of aorta - Aortic root dilatation (e.g., syphilis, ankylosing spondylosis) - TGA - Pulmonary atresia	- AS: Rheumatic/Degenerative - AR - Aortic sclerosis (elderly) - Thick chest wall, obesity, emphysema

When do you say loud A2?
Normally A2 is loudest at the base (aortic and pulmonary area). A2 is considered to be loud if the intensity in the mitral area is same as the base of the heart

P2	
Loud	Soft
- Hyperkinetic states - pHTN - Dilation of pulmonary trunk - Aneurysm of pulmonary artery - Thin chest wall - Condition with L → R shunt	- PS - Dysplastic pulmonary valve - Thick chest wall, obesity, emphysema

When do you say loud P2?
Normally A2 is louder than P2 even in pulmonary area but if P2 is as loud as A2 in pulmonary area, it is considered as loud P2

Single S2
- Severe AS, aortic atresia
- Severe PS, pulmonary atresia
- Fallot's tetralogy (A2 becomes loud and P2 disappears)

(AR: aortic regurgitation; AS: aortic stenosis; pHTN: pulmonary hypertension; PS: pulmonary stenosis; sHTN: systemic hypertension; TGA: transposition of the great arteries)

Splitting of 2nd heart sound

Narrow split	Wide and variable split	Wide and fixed split
Severe pHTN	- **Chest deformity:** Funnel chest and straight back syndrome - **Due to early A2:** MR, VSD - **Due to late P2:** RBBB, LV pacing, ectopics from LV	- ASD - Severe RV failure - Acute pulmonary embolism

Note:
Why do you get wide fixed split in ASD?

Wide split is due to	Fixed split is due to
- Increased RV ejection time - Prolonged pulmonary hangout interval - RBBB	- Free communication between two atria has similar degree of stroke volume across PA and aorta during both inspiration and expiration - Already prolonged pulmonary hangout interval cannot be further prolonged

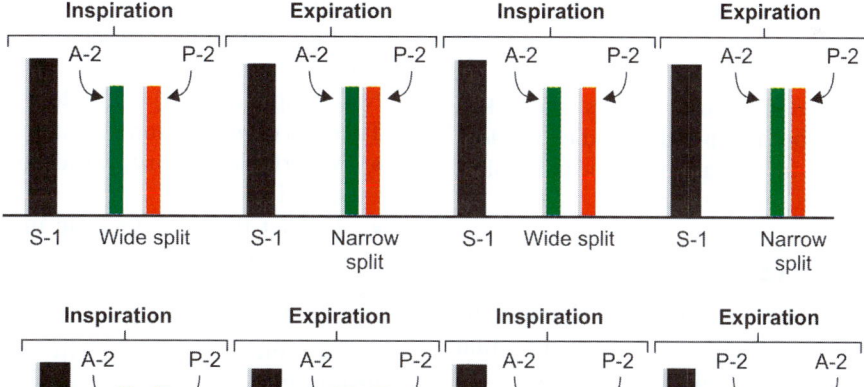

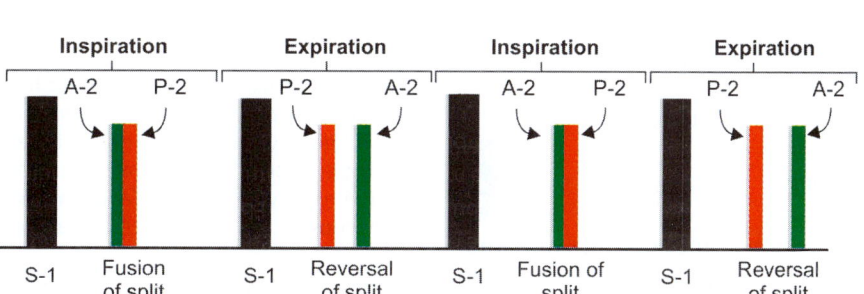

Fig. 4E.25: Variations of 2nd heart sound.

Paradoxical split (reverse split)	
▪ P2 comes before A2 ▪ Split is prominent and wider during expiration, while it narrows during inspiration ▪ Causes due to either early P2 or late A2	
Early P2	*Late A2*
▪ Complete LBBB ▪ RV pacing ▪ PVCs of RV	▪ Severe AS ▪ Severe sHTN ▪ HCM

(AS: aortic stenosis; ASD: atrial septal defect; HCM: hypertrophic cardiomyopathy; LBBB: left bundle branch block; LV: left ventricular; MR: mitral regurgitation; pHTN: pulmonary hypertension; PVCs: premature ventricular contractions; RBBB: right bundle branch block; RV: right ventricular; sHTN: systemic hypertension; VSD: ventricular septal defect)

Valvular diseases and S2	
MS	▪ Mild to moderate → normal ▪ Severe MS with pHTN → loud P2
MR	▪ Mild to moderate → normal ▪ Severe → wide and variable ▪ MR + CAD/HOCM → reverse split
AS	Severe AS → reverse split (severe AS)
AR	▪ Root pathology → A2 loud—tambor ▪ Valvular pathology → A2 soft

(AR: aortic regurgitation; AS: aortic stenosis; CAD: coronary artery disease; HOCM: hypertrophic obstructive cardiomyopathy; MR: mitral regurgitation; MS: mitral stenosis; pHTN: pulmonary hypertension)

Second Heart Sound in Pulmonary Hypertension
- P2 heard at apex in the absence of ASD or other RV forming apex suggests pulmonary hypertension (PH). Note that normally P2 is heard only at 2nd left intercostal space.
- P2 palpable in the 2nd left intercostal space suggests PH. It should be palpable in both inspiration and expiration. It is likely that sometimes in expiration may be palpable if both A2 and P2 become fused in expiration.

THIRD HEART SOUND (S3)

- Third heart sound (S3) is a low-pitched early diastolic sound best heard with the bell. Also called as ventricular sound or protodiastolic sound/gallop.
- It coincides with rapid ventricular filling immediately after opening of the atrioventricular valves and is therefore heard after the second sound as 'lub-dub-dum.'
- It is almost never heard at the base of heart (aortic and pulmonary area).
- Less palpable than S4.
- S3 occurs 0.13–0.18 seconds after A2 and coincides with the latter portion of the descending limb of the "V" wave of the JVP
- It is sign of ventricular systolic dysfunction.
- Prerequisite
  ▪ Nonobstructed AV valve.
- Best head with bell
  ▪ LVS3—left lateral position at apex during expiration.
  ▪ RVS3—left sternal edge in supine position during inspiration.

Causes of S3		
Physiological and hyperdynamic states	*Pathological LV S3*	*Pathological RV S3*
▪ Children ▪ Under 40 years ▪ Athletes ▪ Pregnancy ▪ Other hyperdynamic states	▪ Left ventricular failure ▪ Aortic regurgitation ▪ Mitral regurgitation ▪ Ischemic heart disease ▪ Cardiomyopathy	▪ Right ventricular failure ▪ Endomyocardial fibrosis

PERICARDIAL KNOCK

- Cause—sudden cessation of ventricular filling
- Seen in—**constrictive pericarditis**
- Timing—comes earlier than S3
- Frequency—higher than S3.
- **Diastolic knock** is a palpable pericardial knock in constrictive pericarditis.
- Correlate with other clinical findings like:
  ▪ Rapid 'y' descent
  ▪ Kussmaul's sign
  ▪ Systolic retraction of apex (Broadbent's sign)
  ▪ Congestive hepatomegaly with ascites.

FOURTH HEART SOUND (S4)

- It is a low frequency late diastolic or presystolic sound heard during atrial contraction.
- It is also called as a presystolic or an atrial diastolic gallop (even though it is ventricular in origin).

Prerequisites:
- Healthy contracting atrium.
- Nonobstructive AV valve.
- Noncompliant (stiff) ventricle.
- Theories of production of S4:
  ▪ Ventricular theory (rapid deceleration of incoming blood).
  ▪ Impact theory (dynamic impact of the heart with chest wall).
- Best head with bell.
- LVS4—left lateral position at apex during expiration.
- RVS4—left sternal edge in supine position during inspiration.
- S4 may be confused with split S1. Firm pressure by the diaphragm of stethoscope eliminates S4 but not split S1.

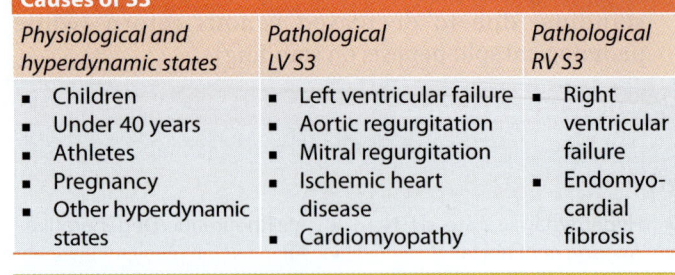

Causes of S4:
- Physiological: >60 years
- Pathological:

Pathological S4	
RV S4	*LV S4*
Right ventricular hypertrophy due to: ▪ Pulmonary hypertension ▪ Pulmonary stenosis	▪ Systemic hypertension ▪ Hypertrophic cardiomyopathy ▪ Ischemic heart disease (especially acute myocardial infarction) ▪ Acute mitral regurgitation ▪ Anemia, thyrotoxicosis and AV fistula

Note:
1. Triple gallop rhythm: S1, S2, S3 (or S4) with HR >100
2. Summation rhythm: S1, S2, S3, S4 with HR >100

CLICKS AND SNAPS

Clicks	Snaps
High-pitched systolic sounds	High-pitched diastolic sounds
Produced by aortic and pulmonary valve opening	Produced by mitral and tricuspid valve opening

Clicks

Clicks	Ejection clicks		Nonejection clicks
Timing	Early systolic		Mid to late systolic
Pathology	Vascular (dilated vessel)	Valvular (diseased valve)	Valve prolapse
Left sided causes	Systemic hypertension Aneurysm of aortic root	Bicuspid aortic valve	Mitral valve prolapse
Right sided causes	Dilated pulmonary artery (idiopathic or secondary to pulmonary arterial hypertension)	Congenital pulmonary stenosis	Tricuspid valve prolapse

Note: Pulmonary valvular ejection click seen in congenital pulmonary stenosis is the only event occurring in the right side of the heart which is better heard on expiration. This is phasic click.

Opening Snaps

- High pitched diastolic sound occurring 0.04–0.12 seconds after A2 (S3 occurs 0.12 seconds after A2) due to opening of mitral or tricuspid valves.
- Occurs after S2 and before S3.
- **Mechanism of opening snap (OS):**
  - Stenotic anterior mitral/tricuspid valve leaflet suddenly bulging downward into the ventricular cavity like a dome, with a snapping sound when the valve is rapidly opened during diastole. So, OS is heard only if leaflets are mobile.
  - OS occurs when movement of valve suddenly stops, at point when ventricular pressure drops below that of atrial pressure.

In mitral stenosis (MS):
- It is the most important auscultatory sign of valvular involvement in MS (pathognomonic sign).
- Absent OS indicates the calcification of body of the mitral leaflets.
- The time interval between A2 and OS is inversely proportional to the severity of the MS.
- **Best heard:** During expiration, just medial to the cardiac apex with the diaphragm of the stethoscope.

Other conditions with OS:
- Mitral regurgitation (10%)
- Tricuspid stenosis
- Atrial septal defect.

Differences between OS, split S2 and S3:

	Opening snap (OS)	S2 split	S3
Area	Medial to apex	Base of heart	At the apex
On standing	A2-OS increases	A2-P2 decreases	Disappears
Pitch	High	High	Low
Best heard	Diaphragm	Diaphragm	Bell

Other sounds:

Tumor PLOP	Seen in myxomas
Prosthetic valve sounds	- Metallic S1 heard with mechanical mitral valve - Metallic S2 heard with mechanical aortic valve

Note: Bioprosthetic valves heart sounds are normal.

PERICARDIAL RUB

It is the sound produced due to sliding (apposition) of the two inflamed layers (visceral and parietal pericardium) of the pericardium.

- **Phases:** It is triphasic
  - Systolic (because of ventricular contraction),
  - Diastolic (due to ventricular relaxation and expansion during diastole), and
  - Atrial systolic (secondary to atrial contraction at the end of diastole)
- **Character:** It is scratchy, grating, leathery or creaking in character. Its intensity varies over time, and with the position of the patient.
- **Best heard:** With diaphragm of stethoscope on the left sternal border (3rd and 4th intercostal space) leaning forward at the end of expiration. It may be audible over any part of the precordium but is often localized. It can be better appreciated with patient in knee elbow position.
- Pericardial friction rubs always tend to accentuate on inspiration because the pericardium is distorted and pulled by the inspiratory expansion of the lungs and the descent of the diaphragm (this is a point that can be used to differentiate it from usual left-sided murmurs which will not increase on inspiration).
- A pleuropericardial rub is a similar sound that occurs in time with the cardiac cycle but is also influenced by respiration and is pleural in origin. Pleural disappear if patient holds the breath.

SUMMARY OF AUSCULTATION OF HEART SOUNDS

Physical finding	Associated cardiac condition(s)
First heart sound (S1)	
Loud S1	Mitral stenosis, tricuspid stenosis, Lown-Ganong-Levine syndrome, tachycardia
Soft S1	Mitral regurgitation, severe congestive heart failure, calcified mitral valve, left bundle branch block, long PR interval (1st degree atrioventricular block)
Widely split S1	Right bundle branch block, Ebstein's anomaly, right atrial myxoma
Reversed splitting of S1	Severe mitral stenosis, left atrial myxoma, left bundle branch block
Variable intensity S1	Atrial fibrillation
Second heart sound (S2)	
Aortic valve closure (A2) and pulmonary closure (P2)	
Soft/absent A2	Severe aortic stenosis (scan QR code for heart sound)
Loud S2—loud A2	Systemic hypertension
Loud S2—loud P2	Pulmonary hypertension
Reduced splitting of S2	Pulmonary hypertension
Increased splitting of S2—early A2	Mitral regurgitation
Increased splitting of late P2—electrical delay of P2	Right bundle branch block
Increased splitting of late P2—mechanical delay of P2	Pulmonary stenosis, ventricular septal defect, obstruction right ventricle, right ventricular failure, mitral regurgitation (with pulmonary hypertension)
Fixed splitting of S2	Atrial septal defect
Paradoxically split S2—electrical delay of A2	Left bundle branch block, right ventricular pacing, right ventricular ectopic beat (delayed excitation of left ventricular systole)
Paradoxically split S2—mechanical delay of A2	Severe aortic outflow obstruction (aortic stenosis), systolic hypertension, large aorta-to-pulmonary artery shunt, ischemic heart disease, cardiomyopathy, aortic coarctation, patent ductus arteriosus
Single S2 (absence of physiological splitting)	Tetralogy, truncus arteriosus, tricuspid atresia
Muffled heart sounds	Pericardial effusion
Third heart sound (S3)	
S3 present, 0.14–0.16 seconds after S2	Ventricular septal defect, atrial septal defect, aortic regurgitation, mitral regurgitation, tricuspid regurgitation, patent ductus arteriosus, pregnancy, congestive heart failure, hyperdynamic circulation (fever, anemia, atrioventricular fistula, thiamine deficiency, hyperthyroidism, infection, Paget's disease, pregnancy), physiological <40 years old
Fourth heart sound (S4)	
S4 present, 0.08–0.12 seconds before S1	Hypertension (systemic or pulmonary), hypertrophic cardiomyopathy, acute myocardial infarction, coronary artery disease, congestive heart failure, aortic stenosis, pulmonary stenosis
Early systolic clicks (ejection sounds)	
High frequency systolic ejection clicks, 0.09–0.14 seconds after first heart sound (S1)	Aortic stenosis (bicuspid aortic valve), pulmonary stenosis, pulmonary hypertension, dilated pulmonary artery, left ventricular outflow obstruction
Midsystolic clicks (nonejection sounds)	
Medium-to-high frequency clicks, 0.17–0.27 seconds after S1	Mitral valve prolapse (and associated late systolic murmur), tricuspid valve prolapse, nonmyxomatous mitral valve disease, adhesive pericarditis, atrial myxoma, atrial septal aneurysms, left ventricular aneurysm
Early diastolic opening snap (OS)	
High-frequency sound, 0.04–0.12 seconds after second heart sound (S2)	Mitral stenosis, tricuspid stenosis
Early mid-diastolic tumor plops	
Low frequency sound, 0.04–0.12 seconds after S2	Atrial myxoma
Early mid-diastolic pericardial knocks	
Pericardial knock, 0.06–0.14 seconds after S2	Constrictive pericarditis

MURMURS

Sudden deceleration of blood produces heart sounds while heart murmurs are produced by turbulent flow (Reynold's number >2,000) across an abnormal valve, septal defect or outflow obstruction, or by increased volume or velocity of flow through a normal valve.

Mechanism

- Increased blood velocity
- Decreased blood viscosity
- Valve—narrowed or incompetent; organic or relative
- Abnormal connection
- Vibration of loose structure
- Diameter of vessel increased or decreased.

Rushmer RF postulated 6 mechanism of production of murmurs:

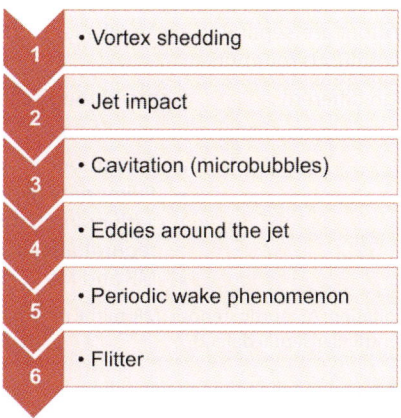

1. Vortex shedding
2. Jet impact
3. Cavitation (microbubbles)
4. Eddies around the jet
5. Periodic wake phenomenon
6. Flitter

Murmurs are described under the following headings:
1. Timing
2. Grade
3. Quality
4. Pitch
5. Configuration
6. Radiation/conduction
7. Best heard with diaphragm or bell
8. Patient position
9. With breath held in inspiration or expiration
10. Variation with other maneuvers
11. Location of maximum intensity

Timing (Fig. 4E.26)

Timing refers to the portion of the cardiac cycle that the murmur occupies. Murmurs may be systolic, diastolic, or continuous. Systolic murmurs may be:
- Early systolic murmurs
- Midsystolic murmurs
- Late systolic murmurs
- Pansystolic murmurs.

Systolic Murmurs

Murmur and description	Example
Early systolic murmurs (begin with the first heart sound and extend to middle or late systole)	- VSD (small muscular VSD/large VSD with pulmonary hypertension) - Acute severe MR - Acute severe TR
Midsystolic/ejection systolic murmurs (begin following a murmur-free interval in early systole and end with a murmur-free interval (of variable duration) in late systole	- Aortic stenosis - Pulmonary stenosis - HOCM
Late systolic murmurs (begin during the last half of systole and may or may not extend to the second heart sound)	- Mitral valve prolapse - Tricuspid valve prolapse - Papillary muscle dysfunction
Pansystolic murmurs (begin with the first heart sound and extend to or through entire systole, muffling S1. They are sometimes called **holosystolic murmur** but in holosystolic murmur and S1 is distinct (e.g., VSD)	- Mitral regurgitation - Tricuspid regurgitation - Ventricular septal defect - Rare—early PDA/PDA with Eisenmenger

(HOCM: hypertrophic obstructive cardiomyopathy; MR: mitral regurgitation; PDA: patent ductus arteriosus; TR: tricuspid regurgitation; VSD: ventricular septal defect)

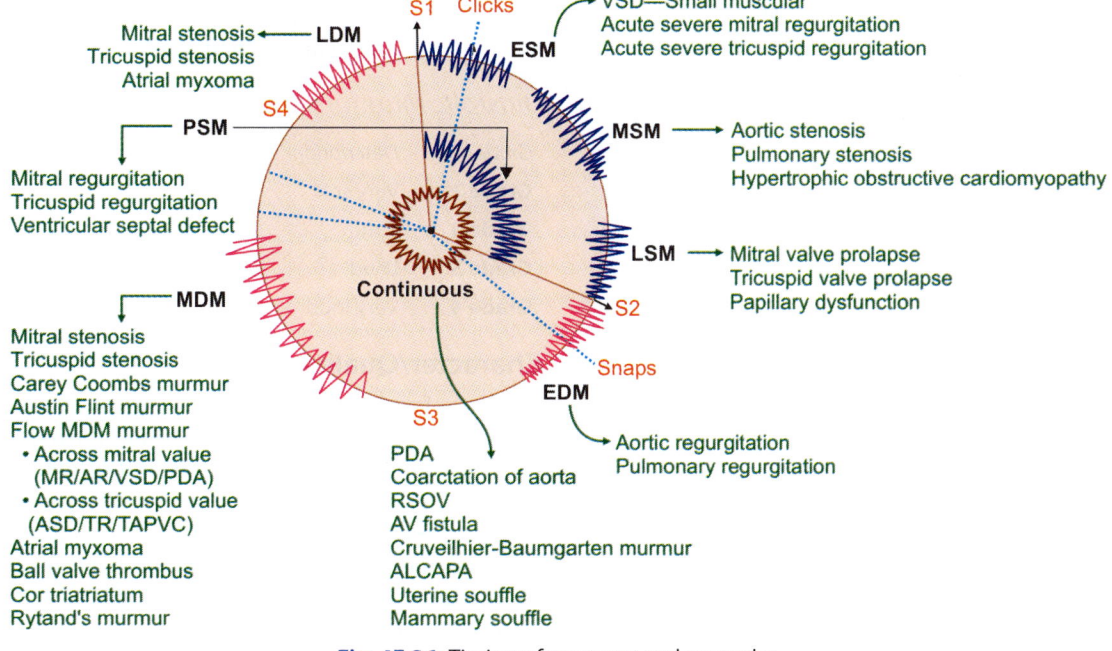

Fig. 4E.26: Timing of murmurs and examples.

Diastolic murmurs may be:
- Early diastolic
- Mid-diastolic
- Late diastolic/presystolic

Diastolic Murmur

Murmur	Example
Early diastolic murmur	1. Aortic regurgitation 2. Pulmonary regurgitation

Mid-diastolic murmur	1. Mitral stenosis 2. Tricuspid stenosis
	3. Carey Coombs murmur of acute rheumatic fever
	4. Austin Flint murmur of chronic aortic regurgitation
	5. Flow MDM murmur:
	  a. Across mitral valve: MR, AR, VSD, PDA
	  b. Across tricuspid valve: ASD, TR, TAPVC
	6. Atrial myxoma
	7. Ball valve thrombus
	8. Cor triatriatum
	9. Rytand's murmur of complete heart block

Late diastolic murmurs/presystolic murmur	1. Mitral stenosis 2. Tricuspid stenosis 3. Myxoma

(AR: aortic regurgitation; MDM: mid-diastolic murmur; MR: mitral regurgitation; PDA: patent ductus arteriosus; TAPVC: total anomalous pulmonary venous connection; TR: tricuspid regurgitation; VSD: ventricular septal defect)

Continuous Murmurs

The continuous murmur is the murmur that begins in systole and continues without interruption, *encompassing the second sound,* throughout diastole or part of diastole.

Continuous murmurs
A. Systemic to pulmonary communication 1. Patent ductus arteriosus 2. Aortopulmonary window 3. Anomalous origin of left coronary artery from pulmonary artery (ALCAPA) 4. Tricuspid atresia 5. Truncus arteriosus 6. Shunts for tetralogy of Fallot (TOF) surgery—Waterson, Potts, or Blalock-Taussig shunt
B. Systemic to right heart connection 1. Coronary AV fistula 2. Rupture sinus of Valsalva
C. Left atrium to right atrium connection 1. Lutembacher syndrome
D. Arteriovenous fistula 1. Systemic 2. Pulmonary
E. Normal flow through constricted arteries 1. Coarctation of aorta 2. Peripheral pulmonary stenosis 3. Renal artery stenosis

F. Increased flow through normal vessels
1. Venous
  a. Cervical venous hum
  b. Cruveilhier–Baumgarten murmur

Contd...

Contd...

2. Arterial
  a. Mammary soufflé
  b. Uterine soufflé
  c. Thyrotoxicosis
  d. Tumors—hepatoma, hypernephroma

Differential Diagnosis of Continuous Murmur

Systolic-diastolic murmurs	To and fro murmurs
Murmur in systolic and murmur in diastolic but S2 is heard distinctly. The two murmurs are separated by small silence differentiating them from continuous murmurs.	
Occurs through different orifices	Occurs through same orifice
VSD with AR	- AS with AR - Pulmonary hypertension with pulmonary regurgitation - MR and MS

(AR: aortic regurgitation; AS: aortic stenosis; MR: mitral regurgitation; MS: mitral stenosis; VSD: ventricular septal defect)

Grading of Murmurs

Systolic Murmurs

Levine and Freeman grading of systolic murmurs		
Grade	Description	Thrill
Grade 1	Murmur so faint that it can be heard only with special effort	Absent
Grade 2	Murmur is faint but is immediately audible	
Grade 3	Murmur that is moderately loud	
Grade 4	Murmur that is very loud	
Grade 5	A murmur that is extremely loud and is audible with one edge of the stethoscope touching the chest wall	Present
Grade 6	A murmur that is so loud that it is audible with the stethoscope just removed from contact with the chest wall	

Diastolic Murmurs (by AIIMS)

Grade	Description	Thrill
Grade 1	Very soft	Absent
Grade 2	Soft	
Grade 3	Loud	Present
Grade 4	Very loud	

Character/Quality

Quality refers to the tonal effect of the murmurs. Frequently used descriptors are *blowing, musical, squeaking, whooping, honking, harsh, rasping, grunting, and rumbling.*

Frequency or Pitch

- Relates to the velocity of the blood at the site of origin of the murmur and is designated as high, medium, or low. In general, the higher the velocity, the higher the pitch of the murmur.

- Murmurs that emanate from areas of stenosis where velocity is lower are typically low to medium pitched.

Configuration (Figs. 4E.27 to 4E.29)

Configuration of a murmur refers to its shape.
- To a large degree it is a function of intensity and duration.
- Crescendo murmurs progressively increase in intensity.
- Decrescendo murmurs progressively decrease in intensity.
- With crescendo-decrescendo murmurs (diamond or kite-shaped murmurs), a progressive increase in intensity is followed by a progressive decrease in intensity.
- Plateau murmurs maintain a relatively constant intensity.

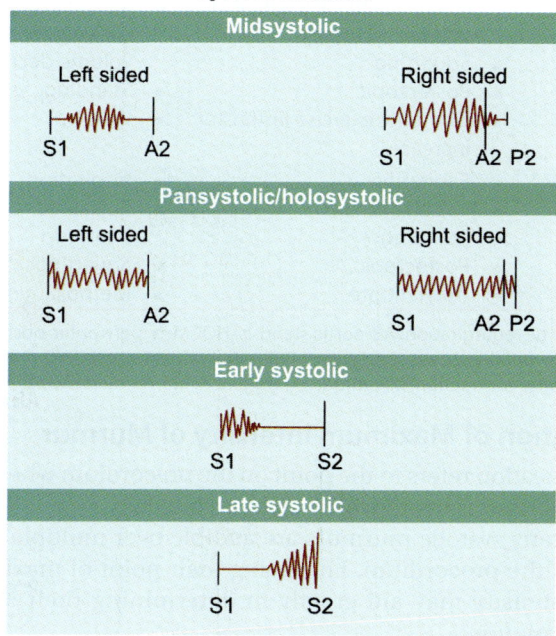

Fig. 4E.27: Configuration of systolic murmurs.

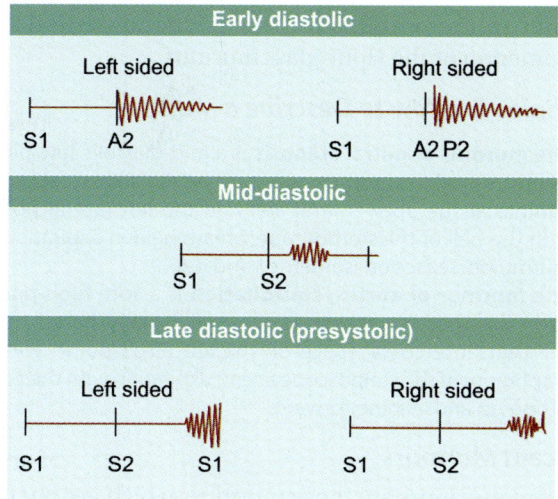

Fig. 4E.28: Configuration of diastolic murmurs.

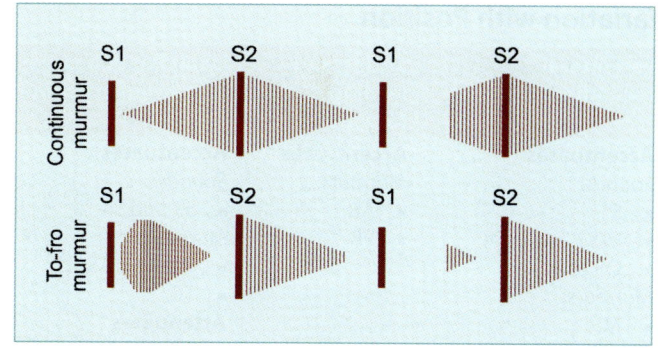

Fig. 4E.29: Configuration of continuous and to-fro murmurs.

Radiation/Conduction (Fig. 4E.30)

Reflects the intensity of the murmur and the direction of blood flow.

Radiation	Conduction
It is through noncardiac structures	It is through anatomical continuity
Intensity decreases with distance	Intensity remains same or decreases with distance
Mitral regurgitation murmur (PSM) radiates to axilla. Tricuspid regurgitation radiates to epigastrium	Aortic stenosis murmur (ESM) conducts to the carotid

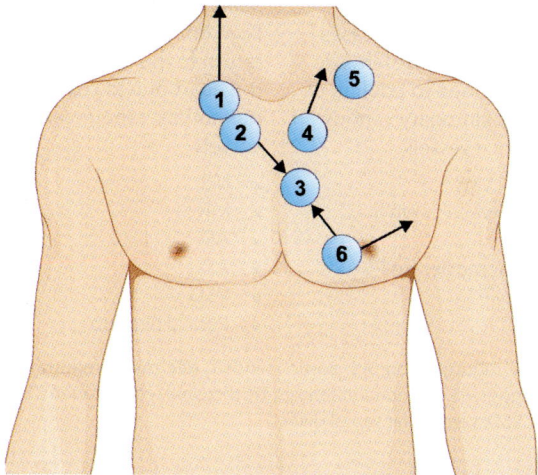

Fig. 4E.30: Radiation of murmurs: (1) ESM of AS conducting to carotids; (2) EDM of AR in right 2nd ICS radiating to left 3rd ICS; (3) PSM of TR radiating to upper left sternal border; (4) ESM of PS conducting towards clavicle; (5) Murmur of PDA at infraclavicular area radiates to back; (6) PSM of MR radiating to axilla or base of heart.

Best Heard with Bell or Diaphragm

Best heard with bell	Best heard with diaphragm
MDM of MS and TS (other sounds: S3, S4, pericardial knock)	Systolic murmur of MR, TR, AS and diastolic murmur of AR (other sounds: S1, S2, ESC, OS)

(AR: aortic regurgitation; AS: aortic stenosis; MDM: mid-diastolic murmur; MR: mitral regurgitation; MS: mitral stenosis; TR: tricuspid regurgitation; TS: tricuspid stenosis)

Variation with Position

Left lateral recumbent position	Sitting and leaning forward	Lying flat or passive leg raising in supine position
Accentuates *Sounds:* - S1 - LVS3 and LVS4 - OS of MS *Murmurs:* - MS - MR - Click and murmur of MVP - Austin Flint murmur	**Accentuates** *Murmurs:* - AR - PR	**Accentuates** *Sounds:* - S3 and S4 *Murmurs:* - Valvular AS/PS - TR **Attenuates** - EDM of AR - Murmur of HOCM - MVP murmur and click are delayed

(AR: aortic regurgitation; AS: aortic stenosis; EDM: early diastolic murmur; HOCM: hypertrophic obstructive cardiomyopathy; MR: mitral regurgitation; MS: mitral stenosis; MVP: mitral valve prolapse; OS: opening snap; TR: tricuspid regurgitation; TS: tricuspid stenosis)

Variation with Respiration

Breathing produces a greater effect on the right side of the heart than the left side.

Right-sided murmurs increase on inspiration	Left-sided murmurs increase on expiration
Inspiration increases venous return to the right side of the heart by increasing flow in the vena cava but decreases venous return to the left side of the heart due to pooling of blood in pulmonary venous capacitance vessels	Expiration decreases venous return to the right side of the heart by reducing vena cava flow, but increases venous return to the left side of the heart due to collapse of pulmonary venous capacitance vessels
- TS - TR (Carvallo's sign*) - PR - Mild or moderate PS - Severe PS	- MS - MR - AS - AR - VSD - Pericardial rub

(AR: aortic regurgitation; AS: aortic stenosis; MR: mitral regurgitation; MS: mitral stenosis; PS: pulmonary stenosis; TR: tricuspid regurgitation; TS: tricuspid stenosis; VSD: ventricular septal defect)

Note:
1. **Rivero-Carvallo sign***: When the murmur of tricuspid valve regurgitation gets louder with deep inspiration.
2. The effects of inspiration on systolic murmurs can be accentuated by employing Müller's maneuver (forced inspiration on a closed glottis).
3. Reversed Rivero-Carvallo sign: Inspiratory reduction in murmur intensity—reported in patients with right sided hypertrophic obstructive cardiomyopathy and straight back syndrome.

Variation with Other Maneuvers

- The physiologic maneuvers are breathing, standing, sudden squatting, isometric hand grip exercise, Valsalva maneuver (described at the end), passive leg raising, and attention to the beat following a postextrasystolic pause.
- The pharmacological interventions used most commonly in clinical practice are amyl nitrite administration and intravenous infusion of alpha-adrenergic agonists (phenylephrine or methoxamine).

Valvular disease	Accentuated by	Attenuated by
MS	- Expiration - Exercise, squatting, amyl nitrate, isometric hand grip	- Inspiration, sudden standing
MR	- Expiration - Squatting - Isometric exercise	- Sudden standing - Valsalva - Amyl nitrate
AS	- Expiration - Post-PVC beat - Squatting - Lying flat from standing	- Valsalva - Standing - Handgrip
AR	- Expiration - Sitting up and leaning forward - Squatting - Isometric exercise - Vasopressors	- Amyl nitrate - Valsalva
MVP	- Murmur and click later if LV volume increases - Squatting - Postectopic - Isometric exercise (intensity increases)	- Murmur and click earlier if LV volume decreases - Standing - Valsalva
HOCM	- Expiration - Valsalva strain - Standing - Postectopic - Amyl nitrate	- Inspiration - Sustained handgrip - Squatting - Methoxamine

(AR: aortic regurgitation; AS: aortic stenosis; HOCM: hypertrophic obstructive cardiomyopathy; LV: left ventricular; MVP: mitral valve prolapse; PVC: premature ventricular contraction; MR: mitral regurgitation; MS: mitral stenosis)

Location of Maximum Intensity of Murmur

- Location refers to the point on the precordium where the murmur is heard with maximum intensity.
- Many systolic murmurs are audible over multiple areas of the precordium. Localizing their point of maximum intensity may aid greatly in determining their site of evolution.

Example: In aortic stenosis—gallavardin phenomenon seen. Two distinct systolic murmurs are heard; one high pitched murmur in the aortic area and the other musical systolic murmur in the mitral area. This is due to periodic wake phenomenon or the Hour-glass murmur.

Examples for How to Describe a Murmur

- **The murmur of mitral stenosis** is a mid-diastolic low-pitched rough rumbling murmur with presystolic accentuation best audible at the apex (mitral area), in the left lateral position with the bell of the stethoscope, breath held in expiration. The murmur increases on isometric hand grip.
- **The murmur of aortic regurgitation** is a soft, high-pitched, early diastolic, decrescendo murmur usually heard best at the third intercostal space on the left (Erb's point) with the diaphragm of the stethoscope at end expiration with the patient sitting up and leaning forward.

Innocent Murmurs

Innocent murmurs are those murmurs which are not due to recognizable lesions of the heart or blood vessels. They are most common in children and adolescents.

Cardiovascular System Examination

	Venous return/preload		Afterload		Drugs	
	Increase (Leg raise/Squat)	Decrease (Valsalva/Standing)	Increase (Handgrip)	Decrease (Amyl nitrate)	Diuretic	ACEIs
MS, AS	↑	↓	↓(AS) / Negligible effect in (MS)	↑(AS)	Yes, but better AS (Replace) / MS (Ballon)	✗
MR, AR	↑	↓	↑	↓	✓	✓
VSD	↑	↓	↑	↓	✓	✓
HOCM	↓	↑	↓	↑	✗	✗
MVP	↓	↑	↓	↑	✗	✗

The Seven S's of innocent murmurs:

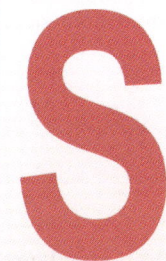

1. Sensitive (changes with child's position or with respiration)
2. Short duration (not holosystolic)
3. Single (no associated clicks or gallops)
4. Small (murmur limited to a small area and nonradiating)
5. Soft (low amplitude)
6. Sweet (not harsh sounding)
7. Systolic (occurs during and is limited to systole)

Examples of innocent murmurs:

Systolic
1. Vibratory systolic murmur (Still's murmur)
2. Pulmonic systolic murmur (pulmonary trunk)
3. Mammary soufflé
4. Peripheral pulmonic systolic murmur (pulmonary branches)
5. Supraclavicular or brachiocephalic systolic murmur
6. Aortic systolic murmur

Diastolic All diastolic murmurs are pathological (not innocent)

Continuous
1. Venous hum
2. Continuous mammary soufflé

Named murmurs	
Carey Coombs murmur	Mid-diastolic murmur, in rheumatic fever
Austin Flint murmur	Mid-late diastolic murmur, in aortic regurgitation (AR)
Graham-Steel murmur	High pitched, diastolic, in pulmonary regurgitation
Rytand's murmur	Mid-diastolic atypical murmur, in complete heart block
Docks murmur	Diastolic murmur, left anterior descending (LAD) artery stenosis
Mill wheel murmur	Due to air in right ventricle (RV) cavity following cardiac catheterization
Stills murmur	Inferior aspect of lower left sternal border, systolic ejection sound, vibratory/musical quality in subaortic stenosis, small ventricular septal defect
Gibson's murmur	Continuous machinery murmur of patent ductus arteriosus (PDA)
Key–Hodgkin murmur	Diastolic murmur of aortic regurgitation. Hodgkin correlated this diastolic murmur with retroversion of the aortic valve leaflets, seen in syphilitic aortic regurgitation
Cabot–Locke murmur	Diastolic murmur heard best at the left sternal border. Heard in anemic patients. The murmur resolves with treatment of anemia
Roger's murmur	It is the loud pansystolic murmur which is heard maximally at the left sternal border in small ventricular septal defect (VSD)
Pontains murmur	Cervical venous hum in severe anemia
Cole-Cecil murmur	AR murmur in left axilla due to higher position of apex
Cruveilhier-Baumgarten venous hum	It is diagnostic of portal venous hypertension

Auscultation for Mitral Stenosis (Fig. 4E.31)

- Patient in left lateral position
- Breath held in expiration
- Using bell of stethoscope
- Time the murmur with carotid.

Auscultation of Tricuspid Area (Fig. 4E.32)

- Patient in supine position
- Breath held in inspiration
- Using diaphragm of stethoscope
- Murmur increases on hepatic compression or passive leg raise.

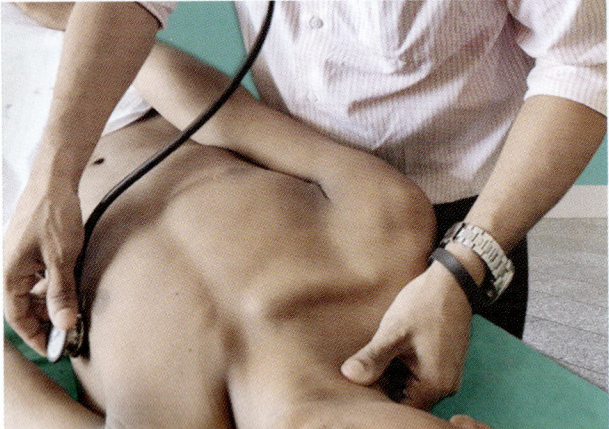

Fig. 4E.31: Auscultation of mitral area—mid-diastolic murmur of mitral stenosis.

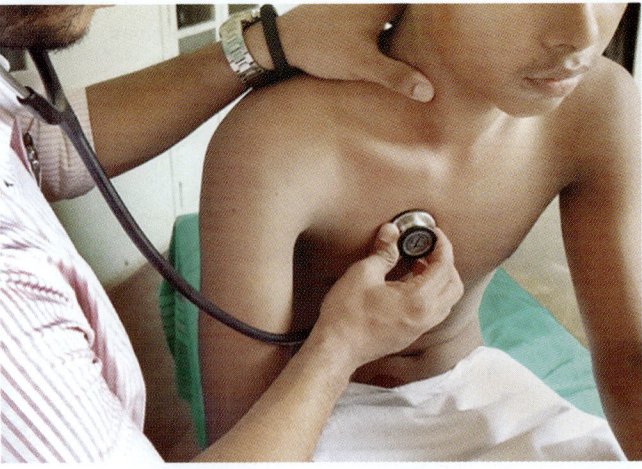

Fig. 4E.33: Auscultation of aortic area (Erb's maneuver).

Changing murmurs
Murmurs which change in character or intensity from moment to moment: • Carey Coombs murmur • Infective endocarditis • Atrial thrombus • Atrial myxomas

Gallivardian Phenomenon

- Aortic systolic murmur spreads to the mitral area, sounding longer but softer, mimicking a pansystolic murmur.
- This phenomenon is characterized by a harsh and rough-sounding murmur at the right upper sternal border (aortic area) that takes on a more musical or high-pitched quality when listened to at the apex of the heart (mitral area), which can be mistaken for mitral regurgitation.
- Perform inch-by-inch auscultation along the sash line to detect changes
- The sash line is an imaginary line passing through the right carotid, aortic area, second aortic area, and mitral area.

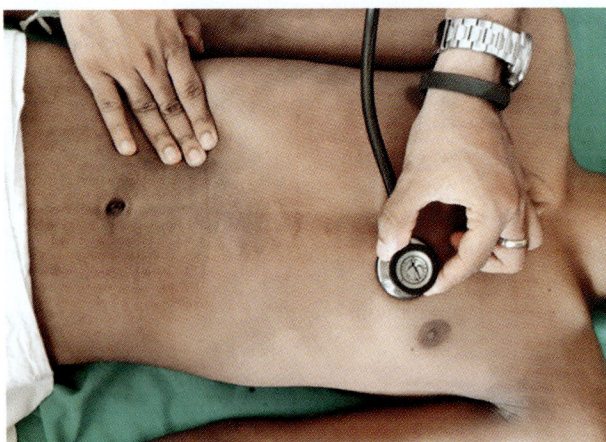

Fig. 4E.32: Auscultation of tricuspid regurgitation.

Auscultation of Aortic Area (Fig. 4E.33)

- Patient in sitting up and leaning forward position
- Breath held in expiration
- Using diaphragm of stethoscope
- Time the murmur with carotid.

SUMMARY OF HEART MURMURS

Physical finding	Associated cardiac condition(s)
Timing	
Early systolic	Ventricular septal defect, acute mitral regurgitation, acute tricuspid regurgitation
Holosystolic (pansystolic)	Mitral regurgitation, tricuspid regurgitation, ventricular septal defect
Midsystolic (ejection systolic)	Aortic stenosis, pulmonary stenosis, hypertrophic obstructive cardiomyopathy, atrial septal defect, aortic coarctation, pregnancy, mammary soufflé, innocent murmur
Late systolic	Myocardial infarction, ischemia, diffuse myocardial disease, mitral regurgitation from mitral valve prolapse
Early diastolic	Aortic regurgitation, pulmonary regurgitation (± Graham Steell murmur)
Mid-diastolic	Mitral stenosis, tricuspid stenosis, atrial myxoma (right or left), acute severe aortic regurgitation (Austin-Flint murmur), acute rheumatic fever (Carey Coombs murmur)
Presystolic (late diastolic)	Tricuspid stenosis, mitral stenosis, atrial myxoma (right or left), acute severe aortic regurgitation (Austin-Flint murmur)
Continuous	Patent ductus arteriosus, cervical venous hum, mammary soufflé, congenital or acquired arteriovenous shunt (e.g., coronary arteriovenous fistula, ruptured aneurysm of aortic sinus of Valsalva into a right heart chamber, anomalous left coronary artery, intercostal arteriovenous fistula), small atrial septal defect with a high left atrial pressure, proximal coronary artery stenosis, pulmonary artery branch stenosis, bronchial collateral circulation, aortic coarctation
Modulation (shape)	
Diamond (crescendo-decrescendo)	Aortic stenosis, pulmonary stenosis, hypertrophic obstructive cardiomyopathy
Decrescendo	Aortic regurgitation, pulmonary regurgitation
Plateau	Mitral regurgitation, tricuspid regurgitation
Location	
5th intercostal space midclavicular line/apical	Mitral stenosis/regurgitation, hypertrophic obstructive cardiomyopathy
Right 5th interspace	Tricuspid stenosis/regurgitation
Right 2nd interspace base	Aortic stenosis/regurgitation
Right 1st interspace or higher	Supravalvular aortic stenosis
Right supraclavicular fossa	Cervical venous hum
Left 2nd interspace/upper sternal border	Pulmonic stenosis/regurgitation, patent ductus arteriosus
Left 3–4th interspace	Tricuspid regurgitation, hypertrophic obstructive cardiomyopathy
Left and right of sternum, 4–6th interspace	Ventricular septal defect
Back/interscapular	Patent ductus arteriosus, aortic coarctation
Intensity	
1	Faint, must tune in
2	Easily heard
3	Moderately loud
4	Palpable thrill and loud
5	Very loud
6	Heard with stethoscope off chest
Frequency (pitch)	
High	Mitral regurgitation, acquired pulmonary regurgitation, aortic regurgitation
Low	Mitral stenosis (rumble), tricuspid stenosis, congenital pulmonary regurgitation, acute severe aortic regurgitation
Radiation	
Axillary	Mitral regurgitation (anterior or laterally directed jet)
Back/subscapular	Mitral regurgitation (posteriorly directed jet), patent ductus arteriosus, aortic coarctation
Neck (carotids)	Aortic stenosis, hypertrophic obstructive cardiomyopathy, supravalvular aortic stenosis (louder in right neck)
Quality	
Blowing	Mitral regurgitation
Varying throughout cycle	Pericarditis (pericardial friction rub)

Contd...

Contd...

Maneuver	Murmur that becomes louder
Squatting, raising legs i.e., increase venous return (left ventricular volume)	Aortic stenosis, aortic regurgitation, mitral stenosis, mitral regurgitation, ventricular septal defect, patent ductus arteriosus
Valsalva, inhalation of amyl nitrate, sitting up, standing, i.e., decrease left ventricular volume	Mitral valve prolapse (and lengthens murmur), hypertrophic obstructive cardiomyopathy
Handgrip, phenylephrine, or transient arterial occlusion by inflation of bilateral arm cuffs to 20 mm Hg above systolic blood pressure for 5 seconds (increases systemic arterial resistance)	Mitral regurgitation, aortic regurgitation, ventricular septal defect
Holosystolic louder in inspiration	Tricuspid regurgitation (Carvallo's sign), pulmonary stenosis, pulmonary regurgitation
Following a premature beat or a long RR interval	Aortic stenosis, pulmonary stenosis

OTHER SYSTEM EXAMINATION

Respiratory system	• Hoarseness of voice (enlarged left atrium—Ortner's syndrome) • Hemoptysis • Left lower lobe collapse or consolidation (pericardial effusion) • Basal crepitations [left ventricular failure (LVF)] • Pleural effusion (LVF) • Rhonchi (pulmonary edema)
Gastrointestinal tract	• Tender hepatomegaly (right heart failure) • Splenomegaly (infective endocarditis) • Ascites (right heart failure) • Dysphagia (due to large left atrium)
Nervous system	Stroke (hemiplegia/Horner's syndrome, cranial nerve palsies)

PULSATILE LIVER

Examination of Pulsatile Liver

- Patient in 45° recumbent position
- Two methods are described:
    1. **Bimanual palpation (Fig. 4E.34):** Place one palm over the anterior surface of the right lower chest and other palm on the posterolateral surface of the right lower chest. Pulsations of the liver are felt between the two palms.
    2. **Make fist of the** right hand and placing the knuckles and fingers in the right lower intercostal spaces and feel for the pulsatile liver as shown in **Figure 4E.35**.

Systolic pulsation	Diastolic pulsations (presystolic)
• TR • AR	TS

(AR: aortic regurgitation; TR: tricuspid regurgitation; TS: tricuspid stenosis)

Valsalva Maneuver

The Valsalva maneuver is a forceful attempted exhalation against a closed glottis.

Instruction:
Take a deep breath, close your mouth and pinch your nose with the thumb and index finger and attempt to breathe out gently, keeping your cheek muscles tight, not allowing the air to escape by keeping the lips pursed.

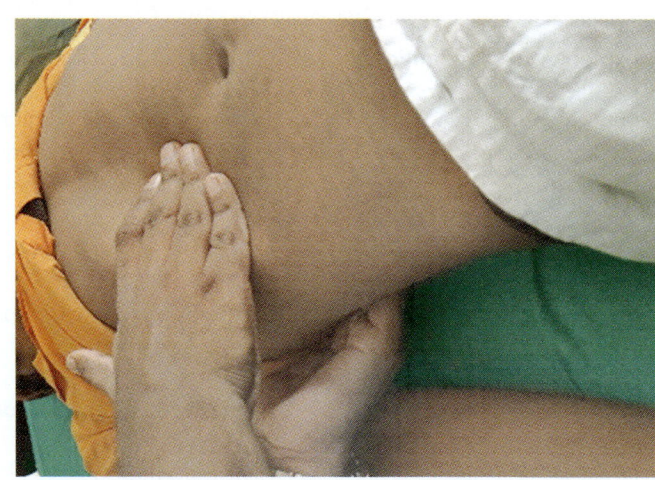

Fig. 4E.34: Bimanual method of palpation of pulsatile liver.

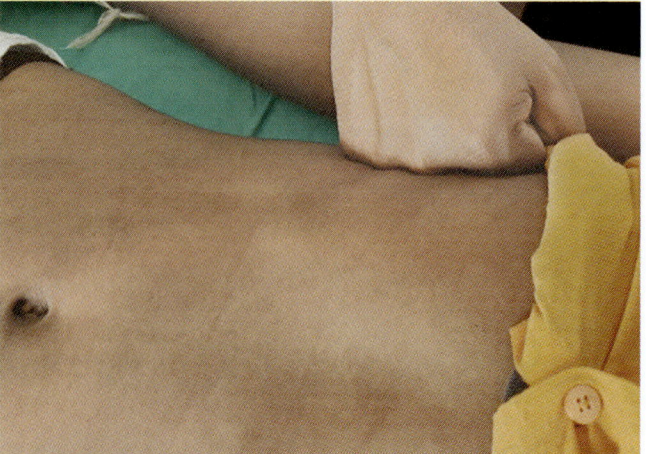

Fig. 4E.35: Examining the pulsatile liver by making fist and placing the knuckles and fingers in the intercostal spaces.

"Standard" or "quantitative":
Blowing out with an open glottis into a tube of a sphygmomanometer against the pressure of 40 mm Hg.

Phases of Valsalva Maneuver

Physiological effects on blood pressure, heart rate and phases of Valsalva maneuver are presented in **Figure 4E.36**.

Phases of Valsalva maneuver	
Phase 1	• The onset of blowing. • The pressure within the chest and abdomen increases and presses upon the arteries in the chest, which results in an increase in mean arterial blood pressure **(Fig. 4E.36)**. This activates the baroreceptor reflex, which results in an increase in parasympathetic (vagal) activity and hence in a drop in heart rate • The increased intrathoracic pressure also reduces the amount of blood that comes into the right atrium (decreased venous return or preload)
Phase 2	A decrease of venous return results in a lower amount of blood that is ejected from the heart, which results in a decrease of central venous pressure and consequently in a decrease of mean arterial blood pressure. This activates the baroreflex, which results in a decrease of the parasympathetic (vagal) activity and consequent increase of the heart rate, and in an increase in sympathetic activity, which constrict the arteries (an increase of peripheral resistance) and results in a slight rise of the blood pressure at the end of phase 2 (2b)
Phase 3	Relaxation—the end of the maneuver. The intrathoracic pressure decreases, so the intrathoracic arteries widen, which results in a brief drop in blood pressure. At the same time, the venous blood fills the heart
Phase 4	The heart ejects the blood into the arterial system against increased peripheral resistance (which has developed in phase 2), so the blood pressure rises again (blood pressure overshoot). This activates the baroreflex, which results in a drop in heart rate (bradycardia). Eventually, both the blood pressure and heart rate normalize

Uses

- Eustachian tube dysfunction
- Heart murmurs: Valsalva increases murmurs in hypertrophic cardiomyopathy and mitral valve prolapse and decreases them in atrial septal defects and aortic stenosis.
- Congestive heart failure: Valsalva responses lost.
- Function of the autonomous nervous system:
  - An abnormal blood pressure response (for example, an absence of the blood pressure rise in phase 4) suggests an abnormality of the sympathetic system.
  - An abnormal heart rate response suggests an abnormality of the parasympathetic system. Valsalva maneuver that can be used as a provocative test to check for neurogenic orthostatic hypotension, Chiari malformation, the Valsalva maneuver (coughing) triggers a headache at the back of the head.
- Diagnosis of inguinal hernia, prolapse of the uterus, bladder or vagina, varicocele and intrinsic sphincter deficiency in stress urinary incontinence system.
- Valsalva maneuver can help: Equalize the pressure between the middle ear and the ambient pressure during scuba diving, driving from a steep hill, elevator descending, parachuting or plane landing or in individuals with Eustachian tube dysfunction.

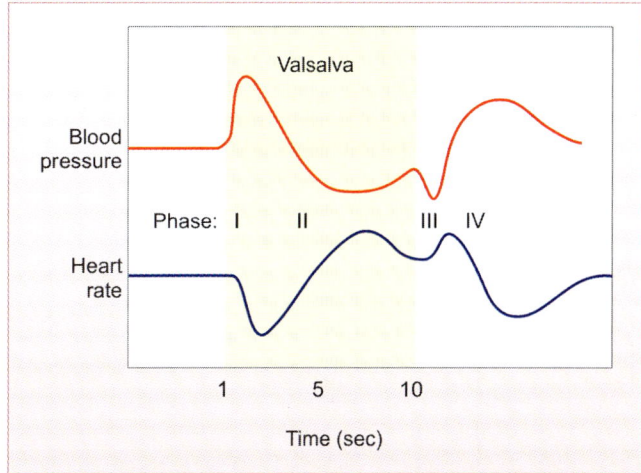

Fig. 4E.36: Mean arterial blood pressure and heart rate changes during the Valsalva maneuver.

Modified Valsalva Maneuver

Modified Valsalva maneuver is used to terminate an attack of supraventricular tachycardia (SVT); it includes blowing against a closed glottis followed by lying down face up and raising legs with the help of an assistant, may be effective in 19–54% of cases.

Various Phases of Valsalva Maneuver and its Associated Changes

Phase	1	2a	2b	3	4
Intrathoracic pressure	↑	↑	↑	N	N
Mean arterial blood pressure	↑	↓	↑	↓	↑
Heart rate	↓	↑	↓	↑	↓
Sympathetic activity	↓	↓	↑	↑	↑
Parasympathetic (vagal) activity	↑	↑	↓	↓	↑

Reversed Valsalva—Müller's Maneuver

Müller's maneuver is the opposite of the Valsalva maneuver and includes forced exhalation followed by an attempted forceful inhalation with a closed mouth and nose or just with a closed glottis. The test can be used to evaluate weakness of the soft palate and throat walls in individuals with obstructive sleep apnea.

F. SUMMARY OF FINDINGS IN COMMON CARDIOVASCULAR DISEASES

Findings	MS	MR	AS	AR	TR	ASD	VSD	PDA
Pulse	• Low volume • Irregularly irregular (if associated with AF)	• High volume, Irregularly irregular (if associated with AF)	• Low volume, **Pulsus parvus et tardus** • Anacrotic pulse • Apicocarotid delay—severe AS	• High volume, **collapsing pulse** • **Water hammer pulse** • **Pulsus bisferiens**	Normal	• Normal • Irregularly irregular (if associated with AF)	High volume	High volume, collapsing
Blood pressure	• Low BP • Mean of 3 readings to be taken if atrial fibrillation is present	• Wide pulse pressure • Mean of 3 readings to be taken if atrial fibrillation is present	• Low BP • Systolic decapitation • **Coanda effect:** Right upper limb BP >left upper limb BP (supravalvular AS)	• Wide pulse pressure • **Hills sign**—lower limb BP >20 mm of upper limb BP	Normal	Normal	Wide pulse pressure	Wide pulse pressure
JVP	• Raised in heart failure **Prominent a waves**—pulmonary hypertension without atrial fibrillation • **Absence of a wave**—atrial fibrillation • **Prominent v waves** (c-v waves) and rapid y descent → tricuspid regurgitation	• Raised in heart failure **Prominent a waves**—pulmonary hypertension without atrial fibrillation • **Absence of a wave**—atrial fibrillation • **Prominent v waves** (c-v waves) and rapid y descent → tricuspid regurgitation	• Usually normal • Raised in heart failure • Rarely prominent a wave—Bernheim effect	• Usually normal • Raised in heart failure	• Raised with most prominent 'giant' v wave in the jugular venous pulse (a **c-v wave** replaces the normal x descent) • **Earlobe pulsations** (Lancisi's sign)	"M" pattern—a and v waves have equal height, a wave becomes taller when pulmonary hypertension develops or associated mitral stenosis (MS)	Raised in heart failure	Raised in heart failure
Apex	**Tapping** apex	**Hyperdynamic** Down and out apex	Heaving	**Hyperdynamic** down and out apex	Normal	Normal	Mild displaced down and out	Hyperdynamic down and out apex
Parasternal heave	Present (RVH or left atrial enlargement)	Present (RVH or left atrial enlargement)	No	No		Present	Present	+/−

Findings		MS	MR	AS	AR	TR	ASD	VSD	PDA
Thrills		Diastolic thrill at apex	Systolic thrill at apex in acute or severe MR	Systolic thrill over the aortic and carotid area	Diastolic thrill in aortic/neoarotic area	Systolic thrill in left lower sternal edge	Nil	Left 4–5 ICS parasternal area	Continuous thrill at the upper-left sternal edge
Heart sounds	S1	Loud	Soft	Normal	Soft	Soft	Loud	Soft	Loud
	S2	• Loud P2 (pulmonary hypertension) • Narrow split (pulmonary hypertension)	• Loud P2 (pulmonary hypertension) • Narrow split (pulmonary hypertension)	• Soft A2 (valvular AS) • Loud A2 (bicuspid aortic valve) • Paradoxical split (severe AS)	• Normal • Tambor A2 in syphilitic AR	Loud P2 with narrow split (pulmonary hypertension)	• P2 loud • Wide fixed split	P2 loud	• P2 loud • Paradoxical split
	S3	RVS3 (present in failure)	RV/LVS3 (present in failure)	LVS3 in failure	LVS3 in severe AR	RVS3	RVS3	+/−	+/−
	S4	Never	Present in acute MR	Present. Indicates severe AS	+/−	—	RVS4 (Eisenmenger's)	RVS4 (Eisenmenger's)	RVS4 (Eisenmenger's)
	Others	Opening snap	OS in 10%	AEC in bicuspid aortic valve	—	—	PEC (Eisenmenger's)	PEC (Eisenmenger's)	PEC (Eisenmenger's)
Murmurs		• MDM at mitral area • PSM at tricuspid area • ESM at pulmonary area • EDM (Graham Steel) at pulmonary area	• PSM in mitral area radiation to axilla/base • Flow MDM at mitral area • PSM at tricuspid area • ESM at pulmonary area • EDM (Graham Steel) at pulmonary area	• ESM in aortic area conducting to carotid • Systolic murmur at mitral area Gallavardin phenomenon	• EDM in aortic/neoarotic area • Flow ESM in aortic area • MDM at mitral area (Austin Flint) • Diastolic murmur in left axilla (Cole-Cecil murmur)	Blowing PSM: At the lower-left sternal border that is increased during inspiration and reduced during expiration (de-Carvallo's sign).	ESM in pulmonary area and MDM in tricuspid area. Once Eisenmenger's—EDM in pulmonary area and PSM in tricuspid area	PSM heard best at the left sternal edge (3rd, 4th and 5th intercostal space)	Continuous harsh "machinery-like"/ Gibson's murmur heard with late systolic accentuation in the first left intercostal space below the clavicle
Other features		Palpable P2 (diastolic shock)	Palpable P2 (diastolic shock)	—	Peripheral signs	Pulsatile liver	Precordial bulge	Aortic insufficiency in approximately 5%	Differential cyanosis and clubbing when Eisenmenger's develops

(AR: aortic regurgitation; AS: aortic stenosis; ASD: atrial septal defect; EDM: early diastolic murmur; ESM: ejection-systolic murmur; MDM: mid-diastolic murmur; MR: mitral regurgitation; MS: mitral stenosis; PS: pulmonary stenosis; PDA: patent ductus arteriosus; PSM: pansystolic murmur; TR: tricuspid regurgitation; VSD: ventricular septal defect)

QR codes represent sounds heard on auscultation.

CHAPTER 5: Gastrointestinal System

A. CASE SHEET FORMAT

HISTORY TAKING

Name:

Age:

Sex:

Residence:

Occupation:

Chief Complaints

1. _____ × days
2. _____ × days
3. _____ × days

History of presenting illness

Abdominal Distension
- Duration
- Onset
- Progression
- Aggravating factors
- Relieving factors
- Associated symptoms
- Is it preceded by pedal edema or followed by it?

Pedal edema:
- Duration
- Onset
- Progression
- Aggravating factors
- Relieving factors
- Is it preceded by facial puffiness or followed by it?

Abdominal pain:
- Onset
- Site
- Type of pain
- Radiation
- Aggravating factors
- Relieving factors
- Associated symptoms

Nausea and vomiting:
- Episodes
- Contents
- Blood tinged or not
- How many hours after consumption of food associated with pain abdomen?
- Conditions with nausea and vomiting but not associated with pain abdomen:
  - Metabolic
  - Neurologic
  - Drug induced
  - Psychogenic

Other symptoms:
- Heart burn, flatulence, and waterbrash
- Hematemesis and melena
- Dysphagia
- Constipation and diarrhea

Altered bowel habit:
- Stool color
- Stool odor
- Stool frequency
- Blood tinged or melena

Jaundice—itching and high colored urine

Other symptoms:
- Fever
- Weight loss
- Pain in oral cavity
- Halitosis
- Hiccups
- Other relevant history

Past History
- Asthma
- Chronic obstructive airway disease
- Tuberculosis
- History of contact with tuberculosis
- Diabetes mellitus (DM)
- Hypertension (HTN)

- Ischemic heart disease (IHD)
- Seizure disorder

Family History
Draw a three generations pedigree chart

Personal History
- Bowel habits
- Bladder habits
- Appetite
- Loss of weight
- Occupational exposure
- Sleep
- Dietary habits and taboo
- Food allergies
- Smoking index or pack years
- Alcohol history

Menstrual and Obstetric History
- G P L A
- Age of menarche
- Menopause at
- Flow—ameno/oligo/menorrhagia

Summarize
Differential diagnosis:
1.
2.
3.

GENERAL EXAMINATION

Patient
- Conscious
- Coherent
- Cooperative
- Obeying commands

Body Mass Index (BMI)
- Weight (kg)/Height^2 (meters)
- Grading according to WHO for Southeast Asian countries

Vitals
- **Pulse**
  - Rate:
  - Rhythm:
  - Volume:
  - Character:
  - Vessel wall thickening:
  - Radio-radial delay and radio-femoral delay:
  - Peripheral pulses:
- **Blood pressure**
- **Respiratory rate**
  - Regular/irregular
  - Abdominothoracic/thoracoabdominal
  - Usage of accessory muscles:
- **Jugular venous pressure**
  - cm of blood above sternal angle (+ 5 cm water from right atrium)
- **Jugular venous pulse**
  - Waveform (describe waves)

On Physical Examination
- Pallor:
- Icterus:
- Cyanosis:
- Clubbing:
- Lymphadenopathy:
- Edema:

Other Head to Toe Signs of Liver Cell Failure
1. Alopecia
2. Fetor hepaticus
3. Jaundice
4. Parotid swelling
5. Gynecomastia
6. Testicular atrophy
7. Loss of secondary sexual characters
8. Spider nevi
9. Palmar erythema
10. Dupuytren's contracture
11. Asterixis
12. Xanthelasma
13. Signs of chronic cholestasis (scratch marks due to pruritus).

SYSTEMIC EXAMINATION

The order of examination of abdomen is preferably done—Inspection → Auscultation → Palpation → Percussion (as the auscultatory findings might change post-palpation and percussion).

Inspection
- Shape/distension (localized/generalized) and flanks (free/full)
- Skin over the abdomen
- Symmetry
- Umbilicus
- Movement of corresponding quadrants with respiration
- Dilated veins
- Visible mass
- Visible pulsations
- Visible peristalsis
- Scars or sinuses
- Divarication of recti

Palpation
- Superficial palpation
  - Warmth
  - Tenderness
  - Guarding
  - Rigidity

- Deep palpation
  - Liver
    - Size
    - Shape
    - Border or edge
    - Surface
    - Tenderness
    - Consistency
    - Movement with respiration
    - Pulsation
  - Spleen
    - Location
    - Size
    - Shape
    - Consistency
    - Surface
    - Edge
    - Tenderness
    - Movement with respiration
  - Gallbladder
  - Other palpable mass
- Bimanual palpation
  - Kidneys
    - Location
    - Size
    - Shape
    - Consistency
    - Surface
    - Edge
    - Tenderness
    - Movement with respiration
- Dipping method (in case of large ascites)
- Hernia orifices
- Direction of flow in veins (if dilated veins present)
- Abdominal girth measurement
- Spino-umbilical distance
- Xiphisternum to umbilicus distance (x) in cm
- Umbilicus to pubic symphysis distance in cm (y)
  - Ratio of x/y

Percussion
- Liver
- Spleen
- Traube's space
- Fluid
  - Shifting dullness
  - Fluid thrill
  - Puddle sign

Auscultation
- Bowel sounds
- Succussion splash
- Bruit
- Venous hum
- Friction rub

Examination of
- Scrotum
- Spine
- Supraclavicular fossa

Per Rectal Examination

Per Vaginal Examination

NOTES

B. DIAGNOSIS FORMAT

CIRRHOSIS/LIVER DISEASE
- Acute hepatitis <4 weeks
  or
  Subacute hepatitis
  or
  Chronic (cirrhosis/hepatitis >6 months)
  or
  Acute on chronic liver disease (ACLD)
- Compensated or decompensated
- Possible etiology—alcohol/post viral/toxin/nonalcoholic steatohepatitis (NASH)
- With complications—portal hypertension with or without gastrointestinal (GI) bleed/hepatic encephalopathy (preferable to mention stage)/spontaneous bacterial peritonitis/hepatocellular carcinoma/hepatorenal syndrome/others.

EXAMPLE
Decompensated chronic liver disease—cirrhosis secondary to alcohol, with portal hypertension, with upper gastrointestinal (UGI) bleed, patient in stage 2 hepatic encephalopathy with no evidence of spontaneous bacterial peritonitis or other complications.

NOTES

C. DISCUSSION ON CARDINAL SYMPTOMS

ABDOMINAL SWELLING

Abdominal swelling is a manifestation of numerous diseases. Patients may complain of bloating or abdominal fullness. Patients with abdominal distension from *ascites* may report the new onset of an inguinal or umbilical hernia. Dyspnea may result from pressure against the diaphragm.

Causes

The causes of abdominal swelling can be remembered conveniently as the *seven Fs*: **flatus, fat, fluid, fetus, feces, full bladder, or a "fatal growth"/neoplasm.**

Flatus	■ The normal small intestine contains ~200 mL of gas made up of nitrogen, oxygen, carbon dioxide, hydrogen, and methane ■ *Aerophagia*, the swallowing of air, can result in increased amounts of oxygen and nitrogen in the small intestine and lead to abdominal swelling ■ Increased intestinal gas is the consequence of bacterial metabolism of excess fermentable substances such as lactose and other oligosaccharides, which can lead to production of hydrogen, carbon dioxide, or methane
Fat	■ Weight gain with an increase in abdominal fat can result in an increase in abdominal girth ■ Visceral obesity is associated with metabolic syndrome, insulin resistance, and cardiovascular disease ■ It can also be a manifestation of certain diseases, such as Cushing's syndrome
Fluid	The accumulation of fluid within the abdominal cavity (ascites) often results in abdominal distension
Fetus	Pregnancy results in increased abdominal girth. Typically, an increase in abdominal size is first noted at 12–14 weeks of gestation when the uterus moves from the pelvis into the abdomen
Feces	In the setting of severe constipation or intestinal obstruction, increased stool in the colon leads to increased abdominal girth. These conditions are often accompanied by abdominal discomfort or pain, nausea, and vomiting and can be diagnosed by imaging studies
Fatal growth/ neoplasm	An abdominal mass can result in abdominal swelling. Neoplasms, abscesses, or cysts can grow to sizes that lead to increased abdominal girth. Enlargement of the intra-abdominal organs, specifically the liver (hepatomegaly) or spleen (splenomegaly), or an abdominal aortic aneurysm can result in abdominal distension
Full bladder	Bladder distension may also result in lower abdominal swelling. It will be associated with anuria

JAUNDICE

Discussed in detail in Chapter 2C: Physical Examination.

GASTROINTESTINAL BLEEDING

Gastrointestinal bleeding (GIB) presents as either overt or occult bleeding.

Overt GIB	Occult GIB
Overt GIB is manifested by *hematemesis*, vomitus of red blood, or "coffee-grounds" material; *melena*, black, tarry stool; and/or *hematochezia*, passage of red or maroon blood from the rectum	**Occult GIB** may present with *symptoms of blood loss or anemia*, such as lightheadedness, syncope, angina, or dyspnea; or with iron deficiency anemia or a positive fecal occult blood test on routine testing

GIB is also categorized by the site of bleeding as:
1. UGIB (esophagus, stomach, and duodenum)
2. LGIB (colonic), small intestinal, or obscure GIB (if the source is unclear)

Hematemesis is the vomiting of blood, which may be obviously red or have an appearance similar to coffee grounds.

Melena is the passage of black, tarry stools due to altered blood. It usually means bleeding episodes from sites above the ligament of Treitz. However, even up to middle of transverse colon can produce melena. It takes 50 mL or more of blood in the stomach to turn stools black. One to two liters of blood administered orally will cause bloody or tarry stools for up to 5 days, the first such stool usually appearing within 4 to 20 hours after ingestion.

Hematochezia is the passage of fresh blood per anus, usually in or with stools. Usually seen in lower GI bleeding.

Note: *Hematochezia can occur due to upper GI bleeding if the volume of blood is so large that gastric and intestinal secretions are unable to convert hemoglobin to acid hematin.*

Causes of upper gastrointestinal bleeding is shown in **Figure 5C.1**.

Upper Gastrointestinal Sources of Bleeding

Causes		
Esophageal causes	*Gastric causes*	*Duodenal causes*
■ Esophageal varices ■ Esophagitis ■ Esophageal cancer ■ Esophageal ulcers ■ Mallory–Weiss tear	■ Gastric ulcer ■ Gastric cancer ■ Gastritis ■ Gastric varices ■ Dieulafoy's lesions ■ Gastric antral vascular ectasia ■ Portal hypertensive gastropathy	■ Duodenal ulcer ■ Vascular malformations including aortoenteric fistulae ■ Hemobilia or bleeding from biliary tree ■ Hemosuccus pancreaticus or bleeding from the pancreatic duct ■ Severe superior mesenteric artery syndrome

Gastrointestinal System

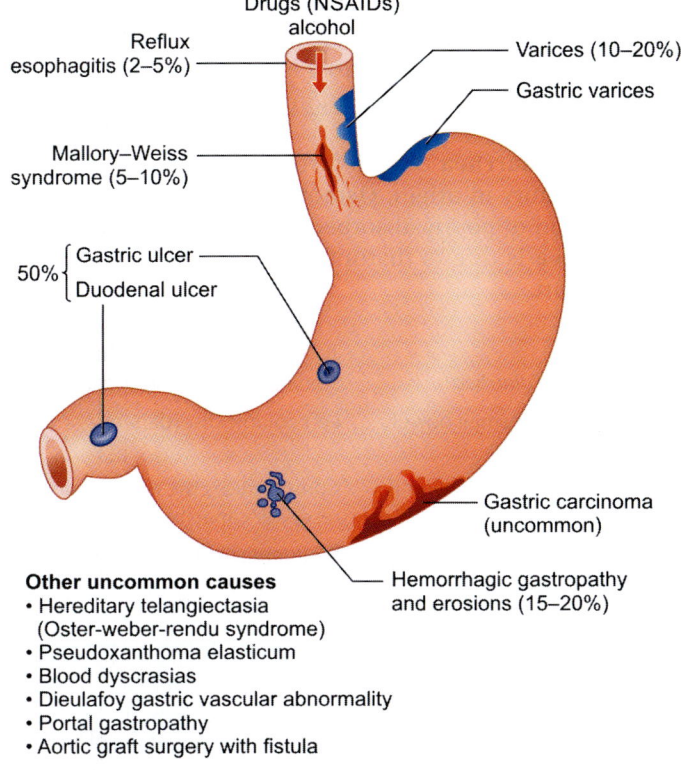

Fig. 5C.1: Causes of upper gastrointestinal bleeding.

Contd...	
Neoplasia (polyp, ulcerated lesions)	Neoplasia (polyp, ulcerated lesions)
Inflammatory bowel disease	Radiation
Infectious colitis	
Angiodysplasia	Meckel's diverticulum
Radiation colitis/proctitis	Aortoenteric fistula
	Mesenteric ischemia

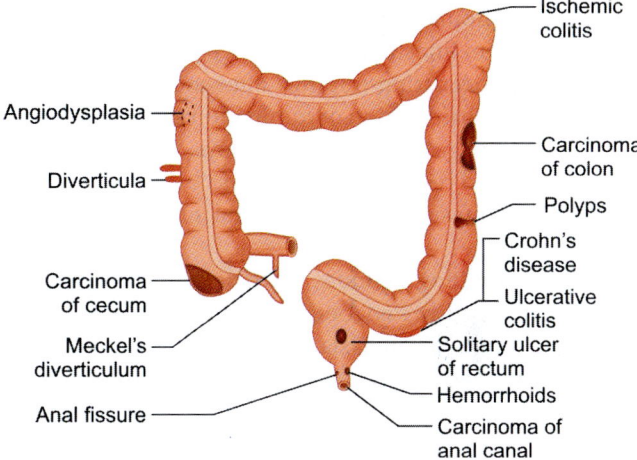

Fig. 5C.2: Lower gastrointestinal bleeding.

Lower Gastrointestinal Bleeding (Fig. 5C.2)

Causes of LGI bleeding	
Colonic bleeding (95%)	*Small intestinal bleeding (5%)*
Diverticular disease	Angiodysplasia
Anorectal disease (hemorrhoid, anal fissure, fistula in ano, solitary rectal ulcer, etc.)	Crohn's disease and infectious disease

Contd...

NAUSEA AND VOMITING (TABLE 5C.1)

Definitions

Nausea is the subjective feeling of a need to vomit. *Vomiting* (emesis) is the oral expulsion of gastrointestinal contents due to gut and thoracoabdominal wall contractions.

TABLE 5C.1: Causes of nausea and vomiting.		
Intraperitoneal	*Extraperitoneal*	*Medications/metabolic disorders*
Obstructing disorders - Pyloric obstruction - Small bowel obstruction - Colonic obstruction - Superior mesenteric artery syndrome **Enteric infections** - Viral - Bacterial **Inflammatory diseases** - Cholecystitis - Pancreatitis - Appendicitis - Hepatitis **Altered sensorimotor functions** - Gastroparesis - Intestinal pseudo-obstruction - Gastroesophageal reflux - Chronic nausea vomiting syndrome - Cannabinoid hyperemesis syndrome - Rumination syndrome **Biliary colic** **Abdominal irradiation**	**Cardiopulmonary disease** - Cardiomyopathy - Myocardial infarction **Labyrinthine disease** - Motion sickness - Labyrinthitis **Intracerebral disorders** - Malignancy - Hemorrhage - Abscess - Hydrocephalus **Psychiatric illness** - Anorexia and bulimia nervosa - Depression **Postoperative vomiting**	**Drugs** - Cancer chemotherapy - Antibiotics - Antiarrhythmic drugs - Digoxin - Oral hypoglycemic agents - Oral contraceptives - Antidepressants - Anti-Parkinson's agents - Smoking cessation agents **Endocrine/metabolic disease** - Pregnancy - Uremia - Ketoacidosis - Thyroid and parathyroid disease - Adrenal insufficiency **Toxins** - Ethanol

Mechanism of Initiation of Emesis

Brainstem nuclei—including the nucleus tractus solitarius; dorsal vagal and phrenic nuclei; medullary nuclei regulating respiration; and nuclei that control pharyngeal, facial, and tongue movements—coordinate initiation of emesis involving neurokinin NK1, serotonin 5-HT3, and vasopressin pathways.

Clinical Clues for Diagnosis

1. Gastroparesis and pyloric obstruction elicit vomiting within an hour of eating.
2. Emesis from intestinal blockage occurs later.
3. Vomiting occurring minutes after meal consumption prompts consideration of rumination syndrome.
4. With severe gastric emptying delays, the vomitus may contain food residue ingested days before.
5. Feculent emesis is noted with distal intestinal or colonic obstruction.
6. Bilious vomiting excludes gastric obstruction, whereas emesis of undigested food is consistent with a Zenker's diverticulum or achalasia.
7. Vomiting can relieve abdominal pain from a bowel obstruction, but has no effect in pancreatitis or cholecystitis.
8. Profound weight loss raises concern about malignancy or obstruction.
9. An intracranial source is considered if there are headaches or visual field changes.
10. Vertigo or tinnitus indicates labyrinthine disease.

Projectile vomiting is a type of severe **vomiting** in which stomach contents are forcefully propelled several feet away from the patient and is usually not associated with nausea. It is a classical feature of **raised intracranial tension**.

DIARRHEA

Definitions

Diarrhea is loosely defined as passage of abnormally liquid or unformed stools at an increased frequency. For adults on a typical Western diet, stool weight >200 g/days can generally be considered as diarrhea.

Diarrhea may be further defined as *acute* if <2 weeks, *persistent* if 2–4 weeks, and *chronic* if >4 weeks in duration.

Types of Diarrhea

1. **Inflammatory diarrhea** is characterized by frequent, small-volume, bloody stools and may be accompanied by tenesmus, fever, or severe abdominal pain. Inflammatory diarrhea is suspected with the demonstration of leukocytes or leukocyte proteins (e.g., calprotectin or lactoferrin) on stool examination.
2. **Fatty stools** are suggested by a history of weight loss, greasy or bulky stools that are difficult to flush, and oil in the toilet bowl that requires a brush to remove. Floating stools indicate gas production by colonic bacteria, not steatorrhea.
3. **Watery diarrhea** can be further classified as osmotic or secretory in origin. **Osmotic diarrhea** is due to the ingestion of poorly absorbed ions or sugars. **Secretory diarrhea** is due to disruption of epithelial electrolyte transport.

Large-volume versus small-volume diarrhea	
Large-volume diarrhea	*Small-volume diarrhea*
Right colonic or small bowel disorders	Left colonic disorders
The rectosigmoid reservoir is intact	Compromises the rectosigmoid reservoir capacity
Individual bowel movements are less frequent and larger	Frequent small-volume bowel movements

Normal rectosigmoid colon functions as a storage reservoir.

Acute diarrhea	*Chronic diarrhea*
More than 90% of cases of acute diarrhea are caused by infectious agents; these cases are often accompanied by vomiting, fever, and abdominal pain. The remaining 10% are caused by medications, toxic ingestions, ischemia, food indiscretions, and other conditions (Table 5C.2)	Diarrhea lasting >4 weeks warrants evaluation to exclude serious underlying pathology. In contrast to acute diarrhea, most of the causes of chronic diarrhea are noninfectious (Table 5C.3)

TABLE 5C.2: Causes of acute diarrhea.	
Viral infection	Viral gastroenteritis; Norovirus or rotavirus
Bacterial infection	*Campylobacter, Escherichia coli, Salmonella* or *Shigella*
Parasitic infection	*Cryptosporidium, Entamoeba histolytica* or *Giardia*
Traveler's diarrhea	Consuming food or drinks contaminated with bacteria, parasites or viruses
Medication	Antibiotics and long-term use of proton pump inhibitors, increased risk of *Clostridium difficile* infections
Food allergy or intolerance	Cow's milk, egg, seafood, soy or fructose or lactose intolerance
Digestive disorder	Celiac disease, Crohn's disease, irritable bowel syndrome or ulcerative colitis
Artificial sweetener	Mannitol, sorbitol, or xylitol found in sugar-free candies or gums

TABLE 5C.3: Causes of chronic diarrhea.	
Fatty diarrhea	*Watery diarrhea*

- *Malabsorption syndromes*:
  • Mucosal diseases (e.g., celiac disease, Whipple's disease)
  • Mesenteric ischemia
  • Short bowel syndrome
  • Small intestinal bacterial growth
- *Maldigestion*:
  • Inadequate luminal bile acid concentration
  • Pancreatic exocrine insufficiency
Inflammatory diarrhea
- Diverticulitis
- Infectious diseases:
  • Invasive bacterial infections (e.g., tuberculosis and yersiniosis)
  • Invasive parasitic infections (e.g., amebiasis and strongyloidiasis)
  • Pseudomembranous colitis (*Clostridium difficile* infection)
  • Ulcerating viral infections (cytomegalovirus, herpes simplex virus)
- Inflammatory bowel diseases: Crohn's disease, ulcerative colitis
- Ischemic colitis
- Neoplasia: Carcinoma of colon, lymphoma
- Radiation colitis
	- Osmotic diarrhea:
	  • Carbohydrate malabsorption
	  • Osmotic laxatives
	- Secretory diarrhea
	- Bacterial toxins
	- Congenital syndromes (e.g., congenital chloride diarrhea
	- Disordered motility, regulation:
	  • Diabetic autonomic neuropathy
	  • Irritable bowel syndrome
	  • Post sympathectomy diarrhea
	  • Post vagotomy diarrhea
	- Diverticulitis
	- Endocrinopathies: Addison's disease, carcinoid syndrome, gastrinoma, hyperthyroidism, mastocytosis, medullary carcinoma of thyroid, pheochromocytoma, somatostatinoma, and VIPoma
	- Laxative abuse (stimulant laxatives)
	- Medication and toxins

Mimics of Diarrhea

Pseudo diarrhea, or the frequent passage of small volumes of stool, is often associated with rectal urgency, tenesmus, or a feeling of incomplete evacuation, and accompanies irritable bowel syndrome (IBS) or proctitis.

Fecal incontinence is the involuntary discharge of rectal contents and is most often caused by neuromuscular disorders or structural anorectal problems.

Overflow diarrhea may occur in nursing home patients due to fecal impaction that is readily detectable by rectal examination.

CONSTIPATION

Definition

Constipation refers to bowel movements that are infrequent or hard to pass.

Obstipation is intractable constipation that has become refractory to cure or control. There is an inability to pass any feces or flatus.

Tenesmus is stated by patients as the unpleasant symptom that there remains something to evacuate from the rectum despite passing a stool. It is often painful. It indicates rectal inflammation.

Etiology of constipation	
Functional (nonorganic) or retentive	Includes constipation due to fecal withholding behaviors and when all organic causes have been ruled out
Anatomic causes	Include anal stenosis or atresia, anteriorly displaced anus, imperforate anus, intestinal stricture, and anal stricture
Abnormal musculature	Related causes include prune belly syndrome, gastroschisis, Down syndrome, and muscular dystrophy
Intestinal nerve abnormality	Related causes include Hirschsprung disease, pseudo-obstruction, intestinal neuronal dysplasia, spinal cord defects, tethered cord, and spina bifida
Drugs	Like anticholinergics, narcotics, antidepressants, lead, and vitamin D intoxication
Metabolic and endocrine causes	Like hypokalemia, hypercalcemia, hypothyroidism, diabetes mellitus (DM), or diabetes insipidus
Other causes	Include celiac disease, cystic fibrosis, cow milk protein allergy, inflammatory bowel disease, scleroderma among others

DYSPEPSIA

Definition

Rome III criteria for dyspepsia
≥1 of the following: 1. Postprandial fullness 2. Early satiation (inability to finish a normal-sized meal) 3. Epigastric pain or burning

Causes of dyspepsia are summarized in **Table 5C.4**.

TABLE 5C.4: Causes of dyspepsia.
Luminal gastrointestinal tract
- Chronic gastric or intestinal ischemia - Food intolerance - Functional dyspepsia - Gastroesophageal reflux disease - Gastric or esophageal neoplasms - Gastric infections (e.g., cytomegalovirus, fungus, tuberculosis, and syphilis) - Gastroparesis (e.g., diabetes mellitus, postvagotomy, scleroderma, chronic intestinal pseudo-obstruction, postviral, and idiopathic) - Irritable bowel syndrome - Peptic ulcer disease - Parasites (e.g., *Giardia lamblia*, *Strongyloides stercoralis*)
Medications
Acarbose, aspirin, other nonsteroidal anti-inflammatory drugs (including cyclooxygenase-2 selective agents), colchicine, digitalis preparations, estrogens, ethanol, glucocorticoids, iron, levodopa, niacin, narcotics, nitrates, orlistat, potassium chloride, quinidine, sildenafil, and theophylline

Contd...

Contd...

Pancreaticobiliary disorders
- Biliary pain: Cholelithiasis, choledocholithiasis, and sphincter of Oddi dysfunction
- Chronic pancreatitis
- Pancreatic neoplasms

Systemic conditions
Adrenal insufficiency, congestive heart failure, diabetes mellitus, hyperparathyroidism, myocardial ischemia, pregnancy, renal insufficiency, and thyroid disease

DYSPHAGIA

Definition

Dysphagia, from the Greek *dys* (difficulty, disordered) and *phagia* (to eat), refers to the sensation that food is hindered in its passage from the mouth to the stomach. Causes of oropharyngeal and esophageal dysphagia are listed in **Tables 5C.5 and 5C.6,** respectively.

TABLE 5C.5: Causes of oropharyngeal dysphagia.

Neuromuscular causes	Structural causes
- Amyotrophic lateral sclerosis (ALS) - Multiple sclerosis - Muscular dystrophy - Myasthenia gravis - Parkinson's disease - Polymyositis or dermatomyositis - Stroke - Thyroid dysfunction	- Carcinoma - Infections of pharynx or neck - Osteophytes or other spinal disorders - Prior surgery or radiation therapy - Proximal esophageal web - Plummer–Vinson syndrome - Thyromegaly - Zenker's diverticulum

TABLE 5C.6: Common causes of esophageal dysphagia.

Motility (neuromuscular) disorders	Structural (mechanical) disorders
***Primary disorders*:** - Achalasia - Diffuse esophageal spasm - Hypertonic lower esophageal sphincter (LES) - Ineffective esophageal motility - Nutcracker (high-pressure esophagus)	***Intrinsic factors*:** - Carcinoma and benign tumors - Diverticula - Eosinophilic esophagitis - Esophageal rings and webs (except Schatzki ring) - Foreign body - Lower esophageal (Schatzki) ring - Medication-induced stricture - Peptic stricture
***Secondary disorders*:** - Chagas disease - Reflux-related dysmotility - Scleroderma and other rheumatological disorders	***Extrinsic factors*:** - Mediastinal mass - Spinal osteophytes - Vascular compression

ODYNOPHAGIA

Definition

Odynophagia, or painful swallowing, is a specific feature for esophageal involvement. It usually reflects an inflammatory process in the esophageal mucosa. Causes of odynophagia are listed in **Table 5C.7**.

TABLE 5C.7: Causes of odynophagia.

Caustic ingestion: Acid, alkali

Pill-induced injury:
- Alendronate and other bisphosphonates
- Aspirin and other NSAIDs
- Iron preparations
- Potassium chloride (especially slow-release form)
- Tetracycline and its derivatives
- Quinidine
- Zidovudine

Infectious esophagitis:
- *Viral*: Cytomegalovirus, Epstein–Barr virus, herpes simplex virus, and human immunodeficiency virus
- *Bacteria*: Mycobacteria (tuberculosis or *Mycobacterium avium* complex)
- *Fungal*: *Candida albicans*, histoplasmosis
- *Protozoan*: *Cryptosporidium*, *Pneumocystis*

Severe reflux esophagitis

Esophageal carcinoma

PAIN IN ABDOMEN

The history of a patient with abdominal pain includes determining whether the pain is acute or chronic and a detailed description of the pain and associated symptoms, which should be interpreted with other aspects of the medical history.

Acute versus Chronic Pain

There is no strict time period that will classify the differential diagnosis unfailingly. A clinical judgment must be made that considers whether this is an accelerating process, one that has reached a plateau, or one that is long-standing but intermittent. Patients with chronic abdominal pain may present with an acute exacerbation of a chronic problem or a new and unrelated problem. Pain of less than a few days' duration that has worsened progressively until the time of presentation is clearly "acute". Pain that has remained unchanged for months or years can be safely classified as chronic. Pain that does not clearly fit either category might be called subacute and requires consideration of a broader differential than acute and chronic pain.

Description of Pain

Pain is discussed under the following headings:
1. **Location and radiation:** The location of abdominal pain helps narrow the differential diagnosis as different pain syndromes typically have characteristic locations (described in the tables below). For example, pain involving the liver or biliary tree is generally located in the right upper quadrant, but it may radiate to the back or epigastrium. Because hepatic pain only results when the capsule of the liver is "stretched", most pain in the right upper quadrant is related to the biliary tree. Pain radiation is also important: the pain of pancreatitis classically bores to the back, while renal colic radiates to the groin.

2. **Temporal elements:** The onset, frequency, and duration of the pain are helpful features. The pain of pancreatitis may be gradual and steady, while perforation and resultant peritonitis begins suddenly and is maximal from the onset.
3. **Quality:** The quality of the pain includes determining whether the pain is burning or gnawing, as is typical of gastroesophageal reflux and peptic ulcer disease, or colicky, as in the cramping pain of gastroenteritis or intestinal obstruction.
4. **Severity:** The severity of the pain generally is related to the severity of the disorder, especially if acute in onset. For example, the pain of biliary or renal colic or acute mesenteric ischemia is of high intensity, while the pain of gastroenteritis is less marked. Age and general health may affect the patient's clinical presentation. A patient taking corticosteroids may have significant masking of pain, and older adult patients often present with less intense pain.
5. **Precipitants or palliation:** Determining what precipitates or palliates the pain can help narrow the differential. The pain of chronic mesenteric ischemia usually starts within one hour of eating, while the pain of duodenal ulcers may be relieved by eating and recur several hours after a meal.
6. **Position/posture:** The pain of pancreatitis is classically relieved by sitting up and leaning forward. Peritonitis often causes patients to lie motionless on their backs because any motion causes pain. Obtaining a history of pain occurring in relationship to eating lactose- or gluten-containing foods may be helpful in identifying sensitivities to these food constituents. Patients with foodborne illness may become ill after eating certain foods.

Associated Symptoms

- **Other gastrointestinal symptoms:** We ask about associated nausea, vomiting, diarrhea, constipation, hematochezia, melena, and changes in stool (e.g., change in caliber). For patients with right upper quadrant pain or concern for liver disease, we also ask about jaundice and changes in the color of urine and stool. The bowel habit is an important part of the history for chronic abdominal pain. While many organic lesions can result in chronic diarrhea, IBS often presents with swings between diarrhea and constipation, a pattern that is much less likely with organic disease.
- **Genitourinary symptoms:** Patients with symptoms, such as dysuria, frequency, and hematuria are more likely to have a genitourinary cause for their abdominal pain.
- **Constitutional symptoms:** Symptoms, such as fever, chills, fatigue, weight loss, and anorexia would be concerning for infection, malignancy, or systemic illnesses [e.g., inflammatory bowel disease (IBD)].
- **Cardiopulmonary symptoms:** Symptoms, such as cough, shortness of breath, orthopnea, and exertional dyspnea suggest a pulmonary or cardiac etiology. Orthostatic hypotension may indicate early shock or be associated with adrenal insufficiency.
- **Other:** Patients with diabetic ketoacidosis will have symptoms of polyuria and thirst. Patients with suspected IBD should be asked about extraintestinal manifestations.

Other Medical History

- **Specific questions for women:** Women should be screened for sexually transmitted diseases and risks for pelvic inflammatory disease (e.g., new or multiple partners). Premenopausal women should be asked about their menstrual history (last menstrual period, last normal menstrual period, and cycle length) and use of contraception. They should also be asked about vaginal discharge or bleeding, dyspareunia, or dysmenorrhea, as these symptoms suggest a pelvic pathology.
- **Past medical history:** A history of surgeries and procedures should be obtained to assess risk for differing etiologies (e.g., a history of abdominal surgery is a risk factor for obstruction). A history of cardiovascular disease (CVD) or multiple risk factors for CVD in a patient with epigastric pain raises concern for a myocardial ischemia.
- **Medications:** A comprehensive medication list should be elicited as this can inform the differential. For example, patients taking high doses of nonsteroidal anti-inflammatory drugs (NSAIDs) are at risk for gastropathy and peptic ulcer disease. Patients with recent antibiotic use or hospitalization are at risk for *Clostridioides* (formerly *Clostridium*) *difficile*. Patients on chronic steroids are at risk for adrenal insufficiency and may be immunosuppressed with atypical presentations of abdominal pain.
- **Other history:** Alcohol—it is important to ask about alcohol intake to assess for the possibility of liver disease and pancreatitis.
- **Family history:** Family history should be asked as appropriate based on other history. For example, patients with history concerning for IBD or cancer should also be asked about family history.
- **Travel history:** A travel history is important to elicit in patients with symptoms consistent with gastroenteritis or colitis (e.g., nausea, vomiting, and diarrhea) to consider infectious etiologies.
- **Sick contacts:** Often patients are in contact with someone with gastroenteritis before having similar symptoms. Patients with foodborne illness may also have close contact with similar illness.

Site of Pain and Possible Etiology

Causes of right upper quadrant (RUQ) abdominal pain.

RUQ	Clinical features
Biliary	
Biliary colic	Intense dull discomfort located in the RUQ or epigastrium. Associated with nausea, vomiting, and diaphoresis. Generally, lasts at least 30 minutes plateauing within 1 hour. Benign on abdominal examination
Acute cholecystitis	Prolonged (>4–6 hours), RUQ or epigastric pain, fever. Patients will have abdominal guarding and Murphy's sign
Acute cholangitis	Fever, jaundice, and RUQ pain
Sphincter of Oddi dysfunction	RUQ pain similar to other biliary pain
Hepatic	
Acute hepatitis	RUQ pain with fatigue, malaise, nausea, vomiting, and anorexia. Patients may also have jaundice, dark urine, and light-colored stools
Perihepatitis (Fitz-Hugh-Curtis syndrome)	RUQ pain with a pleuritic component. Pain is sometimes referred to the right shoulder
Liver abscess	Fever and abdominal pain are the most common symptoms
Budd–Chiari syndrome	Symptoms include fever, abdominal pain, abdominal distension (from ascites), lower extremity edema, jaundice, gastrointestinal bleeding, and/or hepatic encephalopathy
Portal vein thrombosis	Symptoms include abdominal pain, dyspepsia, or gastrointestinal bleeding

Causes of epigastric abdominal pain

Epigastric	Clinical features
Acute myocardial infarction	May be associated with shortness of breath and exertional symptoms
Acute pancreatitis	Acute onset, persistent upper abdominal pain radiating to the back
Chronic pancreatitis	Epigastric pain radiating to the back
Peptic ulcer disease	Epigastric pain or discomfort is the most prominent symptom
Gastroesophageal reflux disease	Associated with heartburn, regurgitation, and dysphagia
Gastritis/gastropathy	Abdominal discomfort/pain, heartburn, nausea, vomiting, and hematemesis
Functional dyspepsia	The presence of one or more of the following: postprandial fullness, early satiation, epigastric pain, or burning
Gastroparesis	Nausea, vomiting, abdominal pain, early satiety, postprandial fullness, and bloating

Causes of left upper quadrant (LUQ) abdominal pain

LUQ	Clinical features
Splenomegaly	Pain or discomfort in LUQ, left shoulder pain, and/or early satiety
Splenic infarct	Severe LUQ pain
Splenic abscess	Associated with fever or LUQ tenderness
Splenic rupture	May complain of LUQ, left chest wall, or left shoulder pain that worsens with inspiration

Causes of lower abdominal pain

Lower abdomen	Localization	Clinical features
Appendicitis	Generally right lower quadrant	Periumbilical pain initially that radiates to the right lower quadrant. Associated with anorexia, nausea, and vomiting
Diverticulitis	Generally left lower quadrant, right lower quadrant more common in Asian patients	Pain usually constant and present for several days prior to presentation. May have associated nausea and vomiting
Nephrolithiasis	Either	Pain most common symptom, varies from mild-to-severe. Generally flank pain but may have back or abdominal pain
Pyelonephritis	Either	Associated with dysuria, frequency, urgency, hematuria, fever, chills, flank pain, and costovertebral angle tenderness
Acute urinary retention	Suprapubic	Present with lower abdominal pain and discomfort, inability to urinate
Cystitis	Suprapubic	Associated with dysuria, frequency, urgency, and hematuria
Infectious colitis	Either	Diarrhea is the predominant symptom, but may also have associated abdominal pain which may be severe

Causes of diffuse abdominal pain

Diffuse/poorly characterized	Clinical features
Bowel obstruction	- Most common symptoms are nausea, vomiting, crampy abdominal pain, and obstipation - Distended tympanic abdomen with high-pitched or absent bowel sounds
Perforation of the gastrointestinal tract	Severe abdominal pain, particularly following procedures
Acute mesenteric ischemia	Acute and severe onset of diffuse and persistent abdominal pain often described as pain out of proportion to examination
Chronic mesenteric ischemia	Abdominal pain after eating ("intestinal angina"), weight loss, nausea, vomiting, and diarrhea
Inflammatory bowel disease (ulcerative colitis/Crohn's disease)	Associated with bloody diarrhea, urgency, tenesmus, bowel incontinence, weight loss, and fever
Viral gastroenteritis	Diarrhea accompanied by nausea, vomiting, and abdominal pain
Spontaneous bacterial peritonitis	Fever, abdominal pain, and/or altered mental status
Dialysis-related peritonitis	Abdominal pain and cloudy peritoneal effluent. Other symptoms and signs include fever, nausea, diarrhea, abdominal tenderness, and rebound tenderness
Colorectal cancer	Variable presentation, including obstruction and perforation
Celiac disease	Abdominal pain in addition to diarrhea with bulky, foul smelling, floating stools due to steatorrhea and flatulence
Ketoacidosis	Diffuse abdominal pain, nausea and vomiting
Adrenal insufficiency	Diffuse abdominal pain, nausea and vomiting
Foodborne illness	Mixture of nausea, vomiting, fever, abdominal pain, and diarrhea
Irritable bowel syndrome	Chronic abdominal pain with altered bowel habits
Constipation	Diffuse abdominal pain
Diverticulosis	May have symptoms of abdominal pain and constipation
Lactose intolerance	Associated with abdominal pain, bloating, flatulence, and diarrhea. Abdominal pain may be cramping in nature

Common sites for referred pain is shown in **Figure 5C.3**.

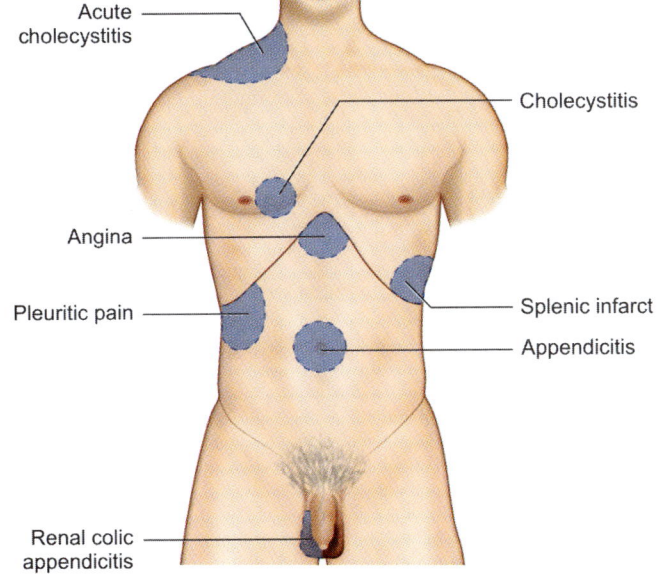

Fig. 5C.3: Common sites for referred pain.

Maneuvers for Ameliorating Abdominal Pain

Maneuver	Affected organ	Clinical example
Belching	Stomach	Gastric distension
Eating	Stomach, duodenum	Peptic ulcer
Vomiting	Stomach, duodenum	Pyloric obstruction
Leaning forward	Retroperitoneal structures	- Pancreatic cancer - Pancreatitis
Flexion of knees	Peritoneum	Peritonitis
Flexion of right thigh	Right psoas muscle	Appendicitis
Flexion of left thigh	Left psoas muscle	Diverticulitis

NOTES

D. DISCUSSION ON EXAMINATION

GENERAL EXAMINATION

General Physical Examination in Gastroenterology and Hepatobiliary System

Pulse
- Tachycardia—anemia, hypovolemia
- Bradycardia—obstructive jaundice
- High volume pulse—cirrhosis of liver
- Low volume pulse—sepsis, gastrointestinal (GI) bleed

Blood pressure
- Wide pulse pressure—cirrhosis
- Low blood pressure—sepsis, upper gastrointestinal (UGI) bleed

Fever
- Spontaneous bacterial peritonitis (SBP)
- Hepatoma
- Cirrhosis
- Hepatitis
- Abscess
- Pancreatitis
- Inflammatory bowel disease

Pallor
- GI bleed
- Anemia of chronic disease
- Macrocytic anemia—liver disease, B_{12} and folate deficiencies

Icterus
- Hepatic/posthepatic causes

Cyanosis
- Hepatopulmonary syndrome
- Pleural effusion

Clubbing
- Primary biliary cirrhosis
- Inflammatory bowel disease
- Hepatocellular carcinoma (HCC)

Lymphadenopathy
- Tuberculosis
- HIV
- Lymphoma

Pedal edema
- Cirrhosis
- Nephrotic syndrome
- Chronic kidney disease (CKD)

Peripheral Signs of Chronic Liver Disease

Skin, nail and hands
1. Spider nevi (telangiectatic superficial blood vessels with central feeding vessel)
2. Clubbing of hands (especially biliary cirrhosis and hepatocellular carcinoma)
3. Leukonychia
4. Palmar erythema (blotchy appearance over the thenar and hypothenar eminence)
5. Bruising
6. Dupuytren's contracture (sign of alcoholism)
7. Scratch marks (cholestatic jaundice)
8. Pyoderma gangrenosum—associated IBD, primary biliary cirrhosis (PBC) or autoimmune cirrhosis

Endocrine—due to estrogen excess
1. Gynecomastia
2. Atrophy of testis
3. Loss of axillary and pubic hair

Others
1. Parotid and lacrimal gland swelling (sign of alcoholism)
2. Fetor hepaticus (characteristic sweet-smelling breath)
3. Asterixis

Signs of Cirrhosis of Liver

Jaundice
- Jaundice is not a common feature of cirrhosis, its more common with acute diseases.
- Mechanisms of jaundice in cirrhosis:
  - Failure to excrete bilirubin (mainly)
  - Intrahepatic cholestasis (superadded hepatitis/tumor)
  - Hemolysis due to hypersplenism (not a major contributor).
- If in cirrhosis patient has jaundice suspect superadded hepatitis, HCC or specific type of cirrhosis like PBC.

Hepatomegaly
- **Early stages:** Liver is enlarged, firm to hard, irregular, and nontender. Hepatomegaly is not common in cirrhosis but common when the cirrhosis is due to **alcoholic liver disease, nonalcoholic steatohepatitis (NASH) and hemochromatosis.** Hepatomegaly may indicate transformation into HCC.
- **Late stages:** Liver decreases in size and nonpalpable due to progressive destruction of liver cells and accompanying fibrosis.

Ascites
- Ascites due to liver failure and portal hypertension.
- It signifies advanced disease.
  (Discussed in detail later)

Spider Naevi

Spider nevi (Fig. 5D.1) (Spider telangiectasia; vascular spiders; spider angiomas; arterial spiders, and nevus araneus)	
Description	Consists of a central arteriole from which numerous small vessels radiate peripherally-resembling spider's legs. Whole spider disappears when central arteriole is compressed with a pinhead. When compression is released filling occurs from center to periphery Spider angioma has three features: a body, legs, and surrounding erythema Spider nevi may also be associated with numerous small vessels scattered randomly through the skin on the upper arms (**paper money skin**)
Pathophysiology	Due to arteriolar changes induced by hyperestrogenism
Location	Usually found only in the necklace area, i.e., above the nipples, territory drained by the superior vena cava, such as: head and neck, upper limbs, front and back of upper chest Rare below the diaphragm (possibly due to higher vasomotor gradient)
Size	Vary from pinhead to 0.5 mm in diameter
Clinical demonstration	Applying pressure over the body of spiders with a glass slide (diascopy) (**Fig. 5D.2**), or pinhead (**Fig. 5D.3**) leading to pallor with refilling following the release of pressure
Significance	They are a strong indicator of liver disease but can be found in other conditions
Causes	*Liver disorders* / *Others*
	<ul><li>Viral hepatitis</li><li>Alcoholic hepatitis</li><li>Hepatocellular carcinoma</li><li>Treatment with sorafenib</li></ul> / <ul><li>Third trimester of pregnancy</li><li>Rheumatoid arthritis</li><li>Thyrotoxicosis</li><li>Also normally seen in 2% of healthy population</li></ul>
Differential diagnosis	<ul><li>Venous star, Campbell de Morgan spots, petechiae, insect/mosquito bites and hereditary hemorrhagic telangiectasias (Osler–Weber-Rendu syndrome)</li><li>Differentiating features of venous star:<ul><li>Blood flows from the periphery of the star centrally and thence into the collecting vein; the direction of flow is the exact opposite of that in the arterial spider</li><li>The pattern, shape and size are much more variable than in the arterial spider</li><li>Color frequently is blue</li><li>Are common on the dorsum of the feet, around the ankle and the lower legs both front and back, and above the knee on the medial aspect of the thigh</li><li>Histologically they are dilated veins</li></ul></li></ul>

Contd...

Contd...

Clinical significance in liver disease	<ul><li>Spider nevi correspond with a higher risk of mortality among patients with the alcoholic liver disease. They also suggest a high likelihood of esophageal varices and are indicative of the extent of hepatic fibrosis</li><li>Size more than 15 mm—80% chances of variceal bleed</li><li>*Florid spider telangiectasia, gynecomastia, and parotid enlargement are most common in **alcoholic hepatitis***</li><li>*Florid spiders and new onset clubbing in a patient with cirrhosis indicates **hepatopulmonary syndrome***</li></ul>

Palmar Erythema (Liver Palm)

- Can be seen early but is of limited diagnostic value, as it occurs in many conditions associated with a hyperdynamic circulation (e.g., normal pregnancy).

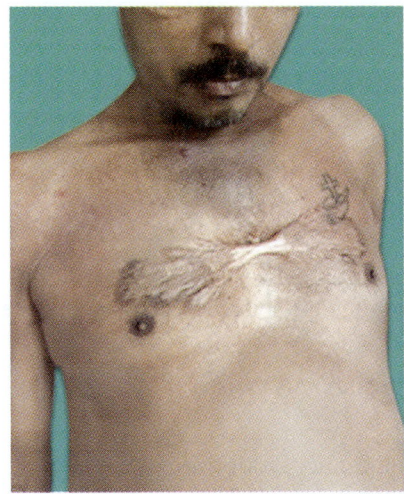

Fig. 5D.1: Cirrhosis of liver with ascites and spider nevi. Patient in addition has tattoo and keloid—which may suggest viral hepatitis as the cause of cirrhosis.

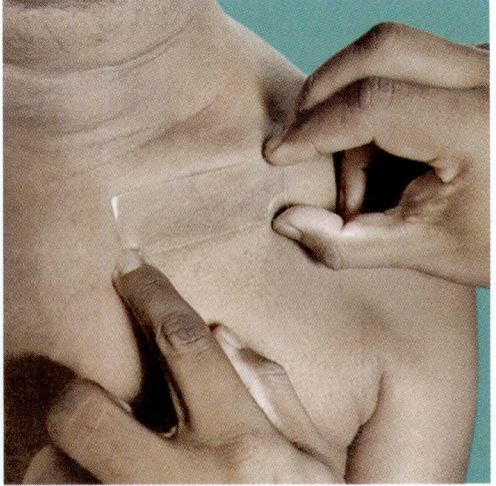

Fig. 5D.2: Demonstration of spider naevi (glass slide method).

Gastrointestinal System

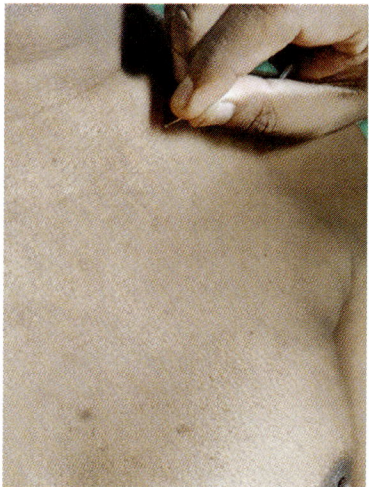

Fig. 5D.3: Demonstration of spider nevi (pinhead method).

- **Cause:** Develops due to increased peripheral blood flow. In cirrhosis, circulatory changes results in increased peripheral blood flow and decreased visceral blood flow (especially to the kidneys).
- **Sites involved:** Prominent in the thenar and hypothenar eminences of palm. Spares the central portion of the palm. May be seen on the sole.

Endocrine Changes

- **Diminished body hair and loss of hair:** Seen mainly in males with loss of male hair distribution. Alopecia affects usually the face, axilla and chest and is due to hyperestrogenism. *Causes of hyperestrogenism:* Due to increased peripheral formation of estrogen resulting from diminished hepatic clearance of the precursor, androstenedione. *Effects of hyperestrogenism:* Alopecia, gynecomastia, and testicular atrophy.
- **Hyperglycemia**: 80% of cirrhotics have impaired glucose tolerance, 20% develop diabetes.
- **Gynecomastia (Fig. 5D.4):** Found in males (atrophy of breasts in females).
    - **Cause**: Due to increased estradiol/free testosterone ratio.
    - **Examination (Fig. 5D.5):** Appear as palpable nodule (2 cm or greater, subareolar).
    - **Microscopy**: Proliferation of glandular tissue of breast.

Pseudo gynecomastia is accumulation of subareolar fat tissue without palpable nodule. Seen in obesity and Cushing's syndrome:

Causes of gynecomastia
▪ Cirrhosis of liver
▪ Drugs:
• Spironolactone
• Cimetidine

Contd...

Contd...
- • Digoxin
- • Ketoconazole
- • Estrogens
- • Isoniazid
- • Antiandrogens—flutamide, finasteride
- ▪ Physiological (puberty/aging)
- ▪ Klinefelter's syndrome
- ▪ Hypogonadism
- ▪ Tumor:
  - • Testes
  - • Lung

Testicular Atrophy

Due to hyperestrogenic state, it is characterized by a small size compared with Prader's orchidometer **(Fig. 5D.6)**, soft testes with loss of testicular sensation (sickening sensation in epigastrium on squeezing the testes). The dimensions of the average adult testicle is 4.5 × 3.5 × 2.5 cm, and the volume is 15–25 mL.

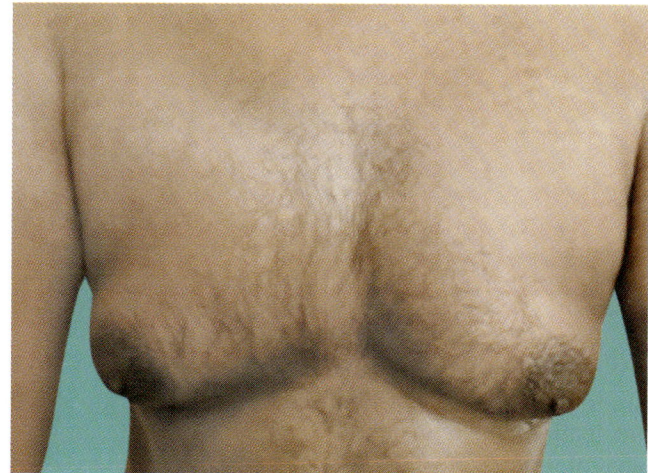

Fig. 5D.4: Gynecomastia.

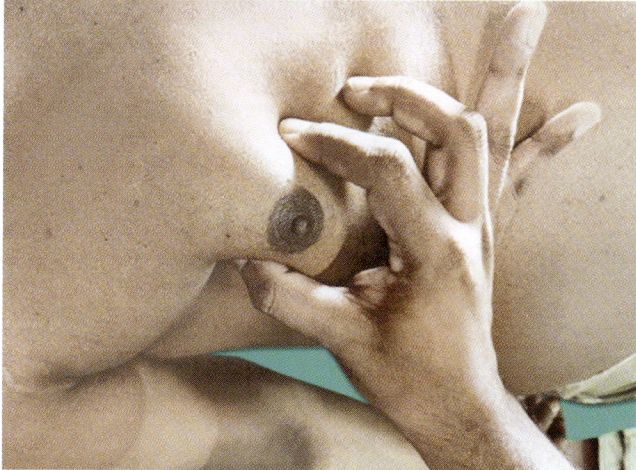

Fig. 5D.5: Palpation breast bud in gynecomastia.

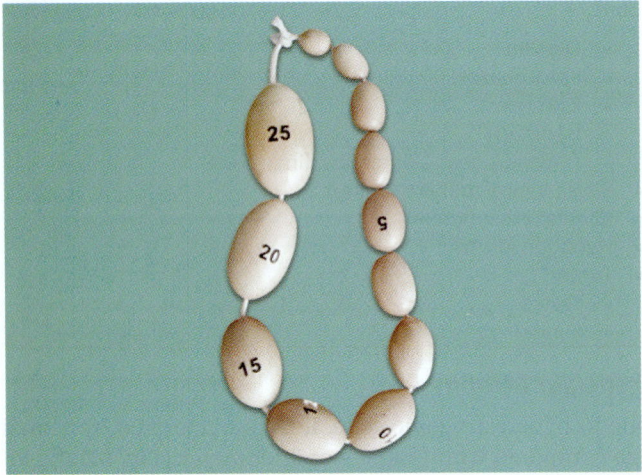

Fig. 5D.6: Prader's orchidometer.

Endocrine changes in females:
Irregular menses, amenorrhea, and atrophy of breast.

Dupuytren's Contracture (It is a Sign of Alcoholism)

Pathophysiology	Fibrosis of palmar aponeurosis probably caused by local microvessel ischemia. Platelet and fibroblast-derived growth factors promote fibrosis
Sites involved	Flexion contracture of the fingers (Fig. 5D.7) (especially ring and little fingers)
Other causes of Dupuytren's contracture	Diabetes mellitus, rheumatoid arthritis, and manual labor (workers exposed to repetitive handling tasks or vibration)

Clubbing and Central Cyanosis

Due to development of pulmonary arteriovenous shunts that leading to hypoxemia (Orthodeoxia—platypnea in hepatopulmonary syndrome).

Nail Changes
- **White (Terry's)** chalky and brittle nails **(Fig. 5D.8)** can be easily demonstrated on comparison with normal person nails when placed side by side **(Fig. 5D.9)**.

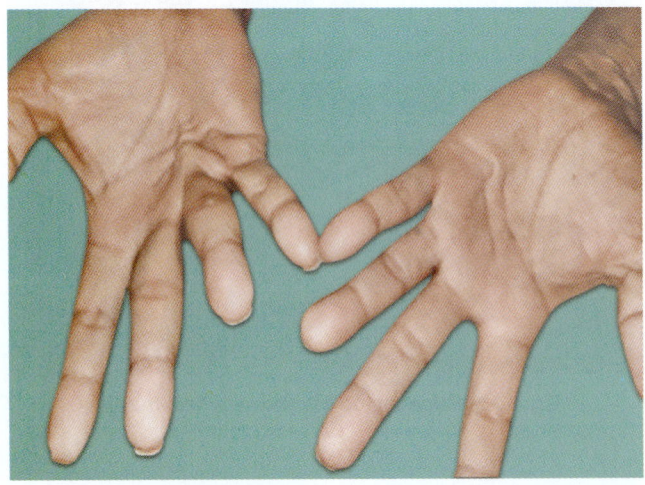

Fig. 5D.7: Dupuytren's contracture.

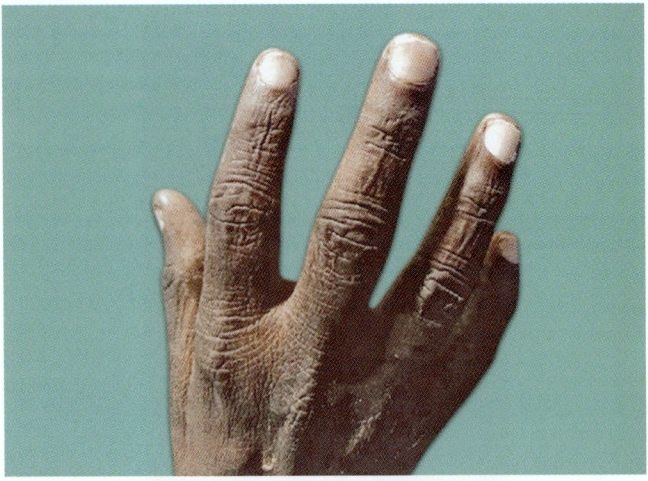

Fig. 5D.8: White nails.

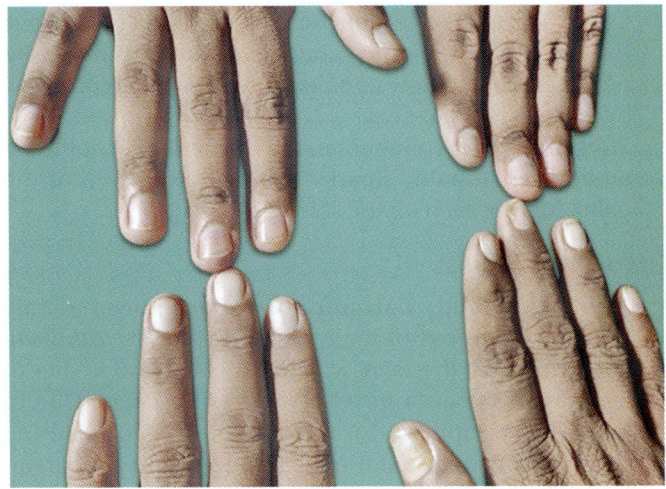

Fig. 5D.9: Leukonychia—compare with nails of normal person (preferably hands to be placed side by side).

- **Muehrcke's nails:** Characterized by transverse white lines that disappear on applying pressure and these lines do not move with growth of nail.
- **Clubbing** is present in primary biliary cirrhosis or hepatoma.

Parotid and Lacrimal Gland Enlargement (Fig. 5D.10)

Observed commonly in alcoholic cirrhosis due to associated autonomic dysfunction.

Anemia
It can be due to various causes:
- Acute and chronic blood loss from varices
- Nutritional deficiency of vitamin B_{12} and folate
- Hypersplenism
- Bone marrow suppression by alcohol
- Hemolysis
- **Zieve's syndrome:** Alcohol-induced hemolytic anemia with hypercholesterolemia.

Gastrointestinal System

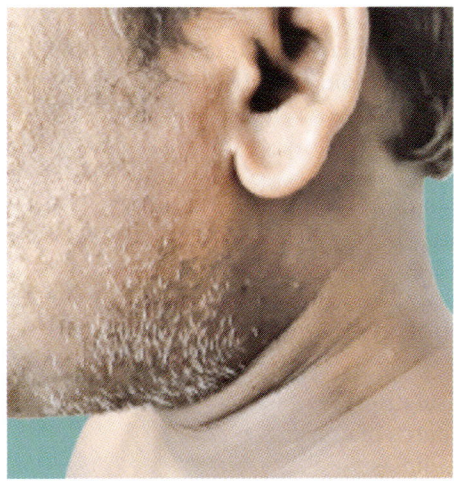

Fig. 5D.10: Diminished facial hair with parotid enlargement.

Fetor Hepaticus
- Sweet, pungent smell
- It is due to volatile **dimethyl sulfide**, especially in portosystemic shunting and liver failure and hepatic encephalopathy.

Asterixis/Flapping Tremor
- Asterixis is a disorder of motor control characterized by an inability to actively maintain a position and consequent irregular myoclonic lapses of posture affecting various parts of the body independently.
- It is a type of negative myoclonus characterized by a brief loss of muscle tone in agonist muscles followed by a compensatory jerk of the antagonistic muscles.
- **Demonstration of asterixis of hand (Fig. 5D.11):** Asterixis is tested by extending the arms, dorsiflexing the wrists, and spreading the fingers to observe for the "flap" at the wrist. The flap is due to irregular myoclonic lapses of posture caused by involuntary 50–200 ms silent periods appearing in tonically active muscles.

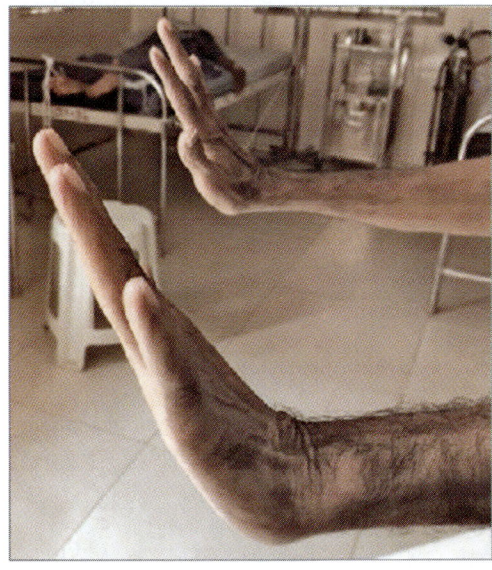

Fig. 5D.11: Demonstration of asterixis in hands.

- **Demonstration of asterixis of leg (Fig. 5D.12):** Testing asterixis at the hip joint involves keeping the patient in a supine position with knees bent and feet flat on the table, leaving the legs to fall to the sides. Negative myoclonus of the lower limbs at the hip joints repetitively occurs and is appreciated by looking at the knees.

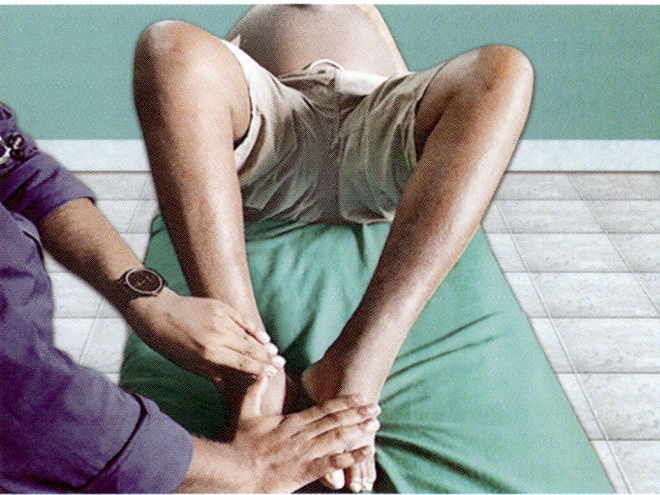

Fig. 5D.12: Demonstration of flapping tremors in legs—on leaving the legs to fall apart a negative myoclonus can be noticed by observing the knee.

Causes of asterixis (flapping tremor)

Bilateral asterixis	Unilateral asterixis
Metabolic: Liver failure, azotemia, respiratory failure	**Focal brain lesions at:**
Sedatives: Benzodiazepines, barbiturates	- Thalamus
Anticonvulsants: Phenytoin (phenytoin flap), carbamazepine, valproic acid, gabapentin	- Corona radiata
Antipsychotics: Lithium	- Anterior cerebral artery territory
Antibiotics: Ceftazidime	- Primary motor cortex
Others: Metoclopramide	- Parietal lobe
Dyselectrolytemia: Hypomagnesemia, hypokalemia	- Cerebellum
Bilateral structural brain lesions	- Midbrain
	- Pons

Signs Pointing the Etiology of Cirrhosis

Signs	Etiology of cirrhosis
Parotid enlargement, Dupuytren's contracture	**Alcohol**
Tattoo marks, jaundice	**Hepatitis B/C**
Metabolic syndrome	**NASH**
Xanthoma, xanthelasma, obstructive jaundice	**Primary biliary cirrhosis**
Skin hyperpigmentation, organomegaly, diabetes	**Hemochromatosis**
Emphysema and cirrhosis	**Alpha-1 antitrypsin deficiency**
Long-standing heart failure	**Cardiac cirrhosis**

Contd...

Contd...

Tender liver with absent abdominojugular reflux	**Budd–Chiari syndrome**
Arthritis, skin changes, nephritis	**Autoimmune**
Deforming arthritis on treatment	**Methotrexate induced**
Kayser–Fleischer (KF) ring on cornea	**Wilson's disease**

Signs of Chronic Alcoholism
- Parotid swelling
- Dupuytren's contracture

ORAL CAVITY EXAMINATION

A torch, tongue depressor, and gloves (for palpation) are needed.

Lips
- Angular stomatitis, cheilitis—iron deficiency, riboflavin deficiency
- Herpes labialis
- Circumoral pigmentation: Addison's disease.

Teeth
- Caries
- Color/staining—tobacco, tetracycline (yellow), fluorosis (chalk white), red/erythrodontia (porphyria)
- Shape of teeth—peg-shaped incisors and moon molars in congenital syphilis, widely spaced teeth in acromegaly.

Gums
- Gingivitis
- Gum bleeding—scurvy, vitamin K deficiency, acute leukemia, thrombocytopenia, coagulopathies, gingivitis
- **Gum hypertrophy**
    - Drugs—phenytoin, nifedipine, cyclosporine
    - Pregnancy
    - Acute myeloid leukemia (AML)—M4, M5
    - Chronic gingivitis
    - Tumors—epulis
- Ulcers and pyorrhea

Tongue
- Macroglossia—acromegaly, myxedema, amyloidosis, Down syndrome
- Coated tongue—typhoid, candidiasis
- Color of tongue
- Pale—anemia
- Red beefy—B_{12} deficiency
    - Magenta—B_2 deficiency
    - Bluish—cyanosis
    - Yellowish—jaundice
    - Strawberry—scarlet fever
- Dry tongue—dehydration, anticholinergics, diabetes
- Leukoplakia, hairy leukoplakia
- Fissuring
- Geographic tongue—desquamated epithelium
- Median rhomboid glossitis

Buccal Mucosa
- Ulcers
- Pigmentation
- Candidiasis
- Koplik spots

Palate/Pharynx
- Ulcers
- Postnasal drip
- White patch of tonsil:
    - Candidiasis
    - Diphtheria
    - Agranulocytosis
    - Infectious mononucleosis
    - Follicular tonsillitis
    - Vincents angina
    - Malignancy
    - Tonsillolith

Causes of oral ulcers	
Aphthous ulcer	
Infections	**Gastrointestinal disease**
- Herpetic stomatitis - Chickenpox - Hand, foot, and mouth disease - Herpangina - Infectious mononucleosis - Human immunodeficiency virus (HIV) - Acute necrotizing gingivitis - Tuberculosis - Syphilis - Candida	- Celiac disease - Crohn's disease - Ulcerative colitis **Connective tissue disorders** - Lupus erythematosus - Behçet's syndrome - Reiter's disease
Dermatological disorders	**Malignancy Drugs**—cytotoxic agents, antibiotics **Radiation** **Trauma**
- Lichen planus - Pemphigus - Pemphigoid - Erythema multiforme - Dermatitis herpetiformis - Linear immunoglobulin A (IgA) disease - Epidermolysis bullosa	

Pigmentation of oral mucosa
- Addison's disease - Peutz–Jeghers syndrome - Hemochromatosis - Heavy metal—lead (Burtonian line) - Acanthosis - Drugs like hormones, oral contraceptives, cyclophosphamide, busulfan, bleomycin, clofazimine, chloroquine - Pregnancy - Laugier–Hunziker syndrome - Nevi - Malignant melanoma

Gastrointestinal System

SYSTEMIC EXAMINATION

The order of examination of abdomen is preferably done—Inspection → Auscultation → Palpation and Percussion. (*As the auscultatory findings might change post-palpation and percussion*)

Inspection

Position of patient:
- Most of the gastrointestinal tract (GIT) examination (inspection) is done in supine position (standing position is adapted for examination of dilated veins).
- Expose from chest to mid-thigh preferably.
- Relax abdominal wall muscles by flexing the thigh with arms by the side of the patient.

Shape of abdomen (Fig. 5D.13):

Shape	Condition seen
Scaphoid	Normal
Generalized abdominal distension [The 7 F's]	1. Fluid 2. Fat 3. Flatus 4. Feces 5. Fetus 6. Full bladder 7. Fatal neoplasm
Localized abdominal distension	Indicates an organomegaly or mass
Fullness of flanks indicates	Free fluid

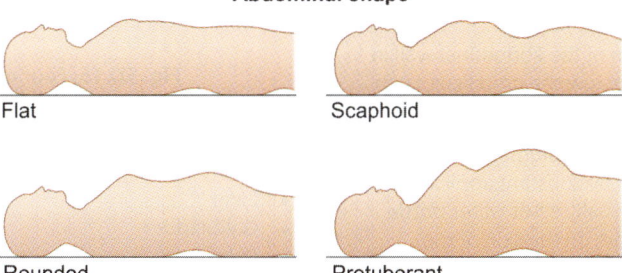

Abdominal shape

Flat | Scaphoid
Rounded | Protuberant

Fat
Fat is the most common cause of a protuberant abdomen and is associated with generalized obesity. The abdominal wall is thick. Fat in the mesentery and omentum also contributes to abdominal size. The umbilicus may appear sunken. The percussion note is normal. An apron of fatty tissue may extend below the inguinal ligaments. Lift it to look for inflammation in the skin fold or even for a hidden hernia.

Gas
Gaseous distension may be localized, as shown, or generalized. It causes a tympanitic percussion note. Increased intestinal gas production due to certain foods may cause mild distension. More serious are intestinal obstruction and adynamic (paralytic) ileus. Note the location of the distension. Distension becomes more marked in colonic than in small bowel obstruction.

Tumor
A large, solid tumor, usually rising out of the pelvis, is dull to percussion. Air-filled bowel is displaced to the periphery. Causes include ovarian tumors and uterine myomata.
Occasionally, a markedly distended bladder may be mistaken for such a tumor.

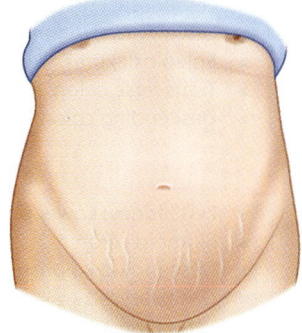
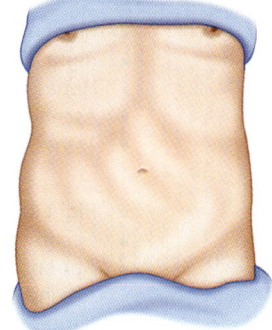
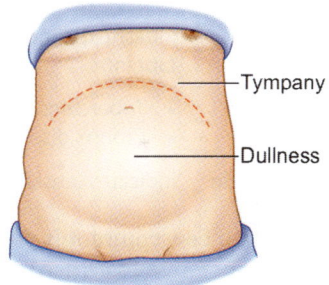

Pregnancy
Pregnancy is common cause of a pelvic "tumor." Listen for the fetal heart.

Ascitic fluid
Ascitic fluid seeks the lowest point in the abdomen, producing bulging flanks that are dull to percussion. The umbilicus may protrude. Turn the patient onto one side to detect the shift in position of the fluid level (shifting dullness).

Fig. 5D.13: Shape of abdomen.

Skin over the abdomen:

Findings	Seen in
Discoloration	**Pancreatitis** • **Cullen's sign**—discoloration around umbilicus • **Grey Turner's sign**—discoloration over the flanks
Ecchymosis or purpura	Coagulopathy
Striae atrophica or gravidarum (white or pink wrinkled linear marks)	• Recent change in size of the abdomen • Pregnancy • Ascites • Wasting diseases • Severe dieting
Purple striae	Cushing's syndrome (pigmented)
Linea nigra	Pigmentation of the abdominal wall in the midline below the umbilicus, seen in pregnancy
Erythema ab igne	• Brown mottled pigmentation produced by constant application of heat, usually a hot water bottle or heat pad, on the skin of the abdominal wall • It is a **sign of chronic pain** as in chronic pancreatitis
Paracentesis marks	Indicate diagnostic/therapeutic ascitic tapping
Sinuses	• Tuberculosis • Crohn's disease
Stretched shiny skin	Indicates tense ascites

Scars (Fig. 5D.14): Few commonly employed incisions over the abdomen as shown in **Figure 5D.14**.

Quadrants of abdomen (Fig. 5D.15): Abdomen can be grossly divided into four quadrants as shown in **Figure 5D.15** with help of transumbilical plane and median plane.

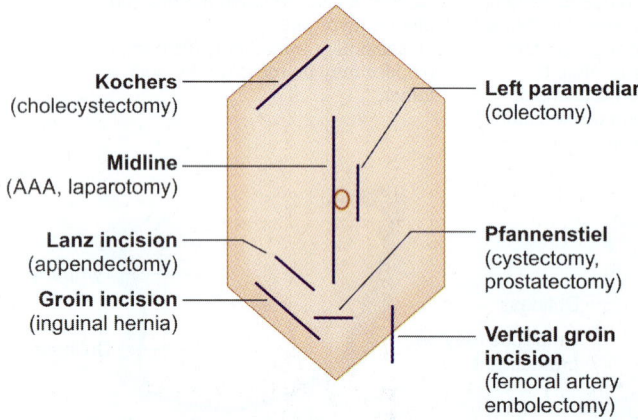

Fig. 5D.14: Surgical incisions commonly employed.

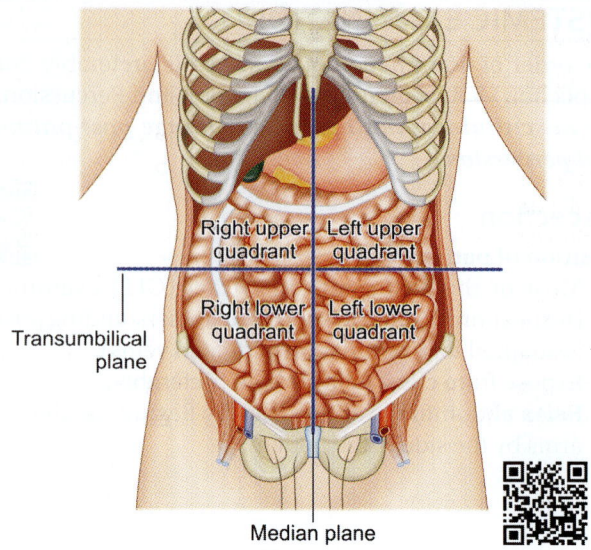

Fig. 5D.15: Four quadrants of the abdomen.

Abdominal Structures by Quadrants

Right upper quadrant	Left upper quadrant
• Liver • Gallbladder • Pylorus • Duodenum • Pancreas: Head • Right adrenal gland • Right kidney: Upper pole • Hepatic flexure • Ascending colon: Portion • Transverse colon: Portion	• Liver, left lobe • Spleen • Stomach • Pancreas: Body • Left adrenal gland • Left kidney: Upper pole • Splenic flexure • Transverse colon: Portion • Descending colon: Portion
Right lower quadrant	**Left lower quadrant**
• Right kidney: Lower pole • Cecum • Appendix • Ascending colon: Portion • Right ovary • Right fallopian tube • Right ureter • Right spermatic cord • Uterus (if enlarged) • Bladder (if enlarged)	• Left kidney: Lower pole • Sigmoid colon • Descending colon: Portion • Left ovary • Left fallopian tube • Left ureter • Left spermatic cord • Uterus (if enlarged) • Bladder (if enlarged)

Regions of abdomen (Fig. 5D.16): Abdomen can also be divided into nine regions with the help of right and left midclavicular line, transtubercular plane, and subcostal plane as shown in **Figure 5D.16**.

Umbilicus:

Finding	Seen in
Slightly retracted and inverted	Normal
Everted	Suggestive of tense ascites
Umbilical hernia	Indicate lax abdominal wall with gross ascites
Umbilical node	Sister Mary Joseph node seen in metastasis from GIT cancers

Contd...

Contd...

Normally,

$$\frac{\text{Distance between xiphisternum and umbilicus}}{\text{Distance between umbilicus and pubis symphysis}} = 1.6$$

Ratio decreased— umbilicus is displaced up (smiling umbilicus)	• Pelvic mass • Ovarian tumors
Ratio increased— umbilicus displaced down (weeping umbilicus)	• Upper abdominal mass • Ascites
Spinoumbilical distance (distance between ASIS to umbilicus)	• Normally equidistant • Shift of umbilicus to one side indicates tumors/mass originating from other side

Movement with Respiration

Method of examination: Shine a light, across the patient's abdomen, and watch for the abdominal wall movements.

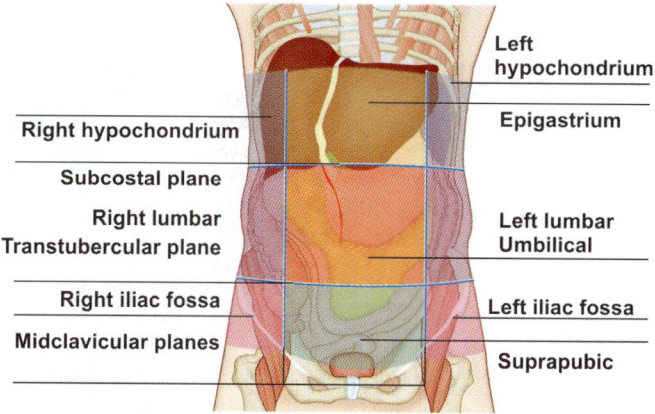

Fig. 5D.16: Planes and nine areas of the abdomen.

Finding	Seen in
Normal	• Gentle rise in the abdominal wall during inspiration and a fall during expiration • Corresponding areas move equally on both sides
Diminished or absent movements	Generalized peritonitis (the still, silent abdomen)

Visible Peristalsis

Site of obstruction	Direction of peristalsis
Obstruction at the pylorus	Peristalsis from the left costal margin to right
Obstruction in the distal small bowel	• Right to left (or) • Irregular pattern

Note: Visible peristalsis may be a normal finding in very thin elderly patients with lax abdominal muscles.

Visible mass: Figure 5D.17 demonstrates the underlying intra-abdominal structures with respect to the regions.

Divarication of recti (diastasis of recti): It is a gap between the rectus abdominis muscle which becomes prominent on straining **(Fig. 5D.18)**. Make the patient lie supine and tense the abdominal muscles by lifting the head **(Fig. 5D.19)**, a midline defect can be seen and felt. It is common after postpartum and also can be seen with tense ascites.

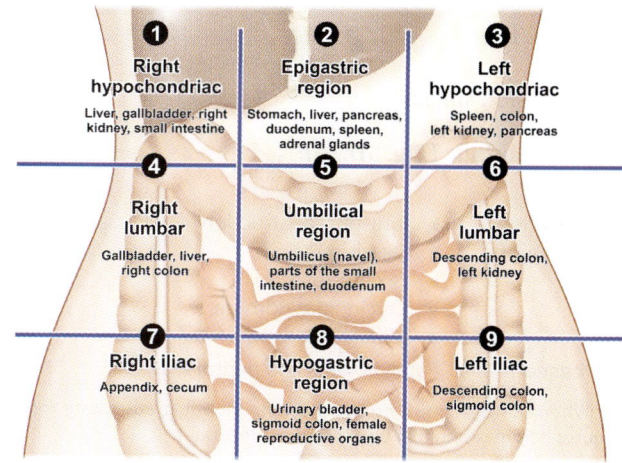

Fig. 5D.17: Pictorial representation of corresponding areas and underlying structures.

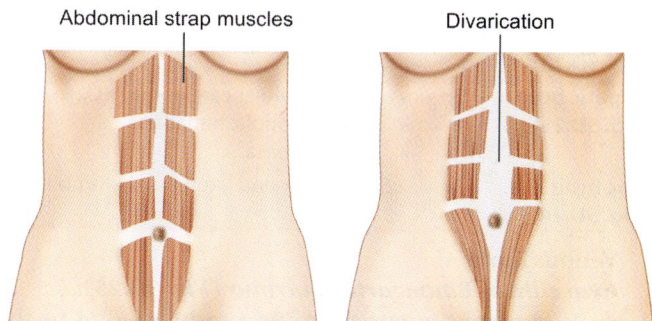

Fig. 5D.18: Divarication of recti.

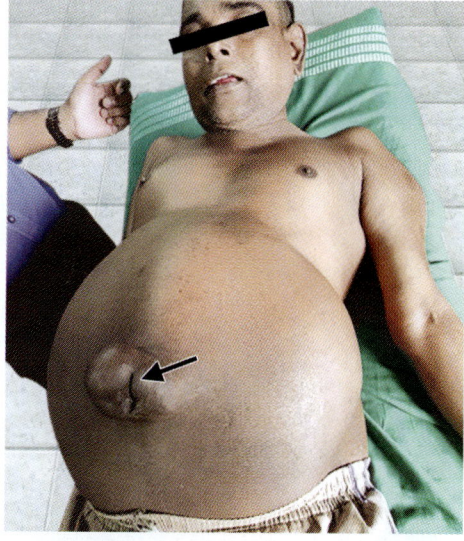

Fig. 5D.19: Midline defect suggestive of divarication of recti, on asking the patient to raise the head off the bed. Also, patient has umbilical hernia.

AUSCULTATION

Note that the abdomen should be auscultated prior to palpation. Auscultate in all four quadrants of the abdomen.
1. Bowel sounds
2. Bruits
3. Venous hum
4. Rubs
5. Succussion splash

1. **Bowel sounds (Fig. 5D.20):**

Normal	7–35 per minute
Increased (borborygmi)	<ul><li>Intestinal obstruction</li><li>Diarrhea</li><li>Laxative use</li><li>Carcinoid syndrome</li><li>Massive GI bleed</li></ul>
Decreased	Paralytic ileus and peritonitis

Note: When bowel sounds are not present, one must auscultate for a full 3 minutes before saying that bowel sounds are absent.

2. **Bruits:**

Renal artery bruit (Fig. 5D.21)	<ul><li>2.5 cm above and lateral to the umbilicus in transpyloric plane</li><li>Indicates partial renal artery stenosis</li></ul>
Abdominal aorta (Fig. 5D.22)	Epigastrium in aortic aneurysm or aortoarteritis
Hepatic bruit (Fig. 5D.23)	<ul><li>Hepatocellular carcinoma (HCC)</li><li>Acute alcoholic hepatitis</li><li>Hemangioma</li></ul>
Iliac bruit (Fig. 5D.24)	2.5 cm below and lateral to the umbilicus

3. **Venous hum:**
    Cruveilhier–Baumgarten murmur (Fig. 5D.25):
    - It is a continuous murmur, produced due to the opening of the paraumbilical vein in the falciform ligament.
    - It is heard midway between the xiphisternum and umbilicus on the right side of the epigastrium.

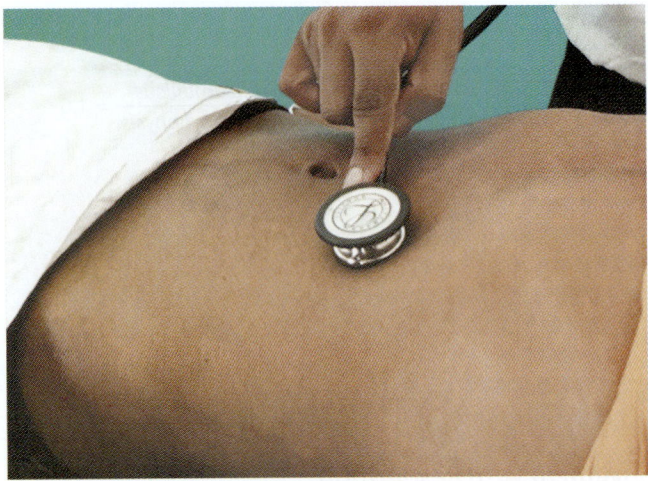

Fig. 5D.21: Renal artery bruit—2.5 cm above and later to umbilicus in transpyloric plane.

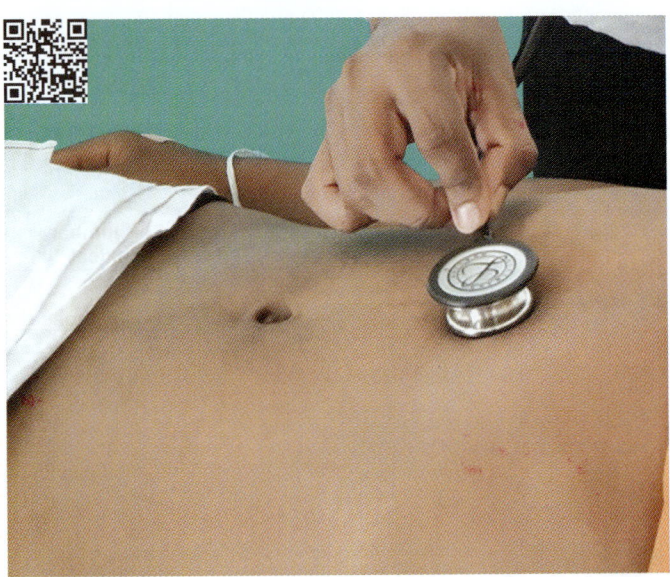

Fig. 5D.22: Abdominal aorta bruit in the epigastrium in the midline.

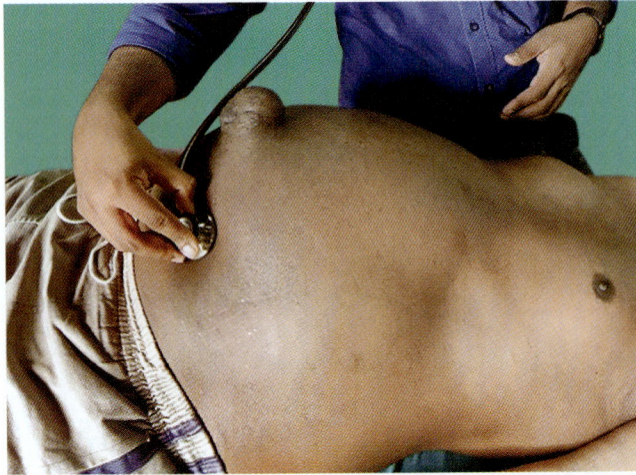

Fig. 5D.20: Auscultation of bowel sounds.

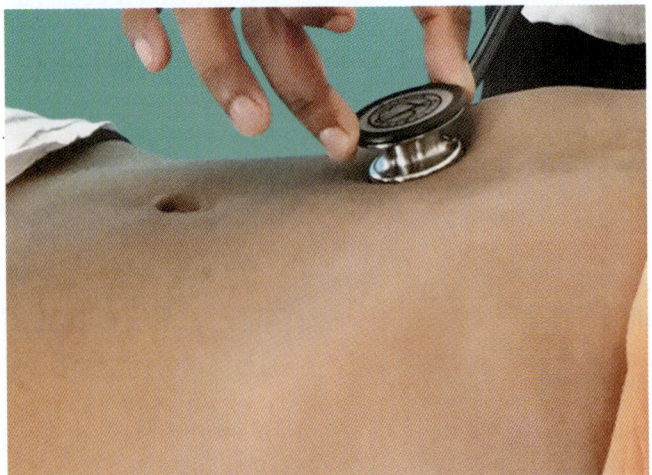

Fig. 5D.23: Hepatic bruit.

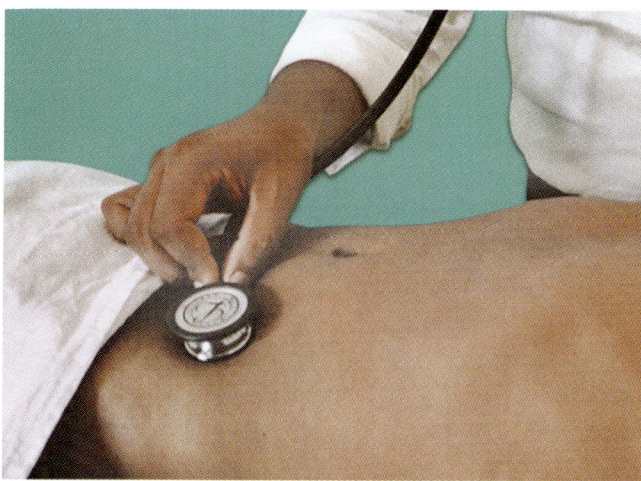

Fig. 5D.24: Iliac bruit—2.5 cm below and lateral to umbilicus.

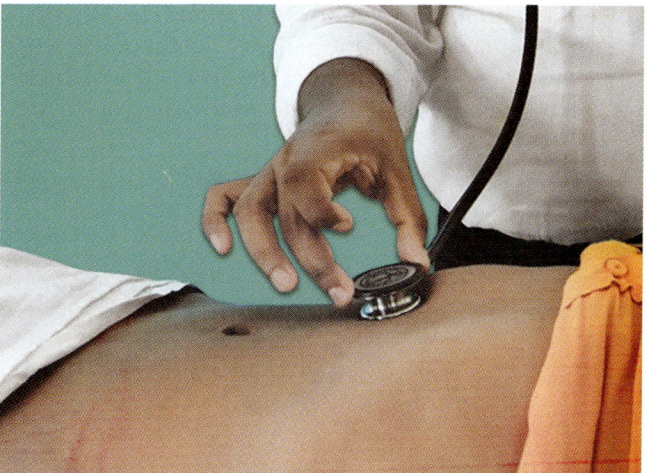

Fig. 5D.25: Cruveilhier–Baumgarten murmur heard midway between the xiphisternum and umbilicus on the right side of the epigastrium.

- A patent umbilical vein excludes an extrahepatic cause of portal hypertension because the umbilical vein arises from the intrahepatic portion of the left portal vein.

4. **Rubs:**
   - **Hepatic friction rub** is a superficial, scratchy sound heard on the liver.
     Commonly seen with:
     - HCC
     - Post-liver biopsy
     - Hepatic infarcts
     - Gonococcal peritonitis (Fitz-Hugh-Curtis syndrome)
   - **Splenic rub** is a coarse, scratching sound coinciding with inspiration over the left upper quadrant due to splenic infarct.
     Commonly seen with:
     - Subacute bacterial endocarditis
     - Chronic myeloid leukemia
     - Sickle cell anemia

- After splenic puncture (e.g., in diagnosis of chronic kala-azar).

5. **Succussion splash:**
   - When you auscultate the patient's epigastrium/left upper quadrant and then shake the patient a "splash-like" noise is heard.
   - If heard several hours after eating, it suggests delayed gastric emptying which may be due to gastric outlet obstruction.
   - Thoracic succussion splash has been described in achalasia cardia, hydropneumothorax, and large hiatal hernia.

PALPATION AND PERCUSSION OF THE ABDOMEN

The following scheme is suggested for palpating the abdomen:
- Start in left lower quadrant of abdomen and repeat in all quadrants as described below.
   - Palpate lightly initially, followed by deep palpation.
   - Feel for left kidney → spleen → right kidney → liver → aorta and para-aortic glands → common femoral vessels → urinary bladder → both groins → external genitalia.

EXAMINATION OF INDIVIDUAL ORGANS

Examination of Liver

Location
- Right hypochondriac region
- Epigastric region
- Left hypochondriac region

Extent
- Upper border—6th rib anteriorly
- Inferior border—crosses midline at the level of transpyloric plane (at the level of L1 vertebrae).

INSPECTION
- Watch for the fullness in the right hypochondrium and epigastrium (epigastrium usually represents left lobe).
- Direction of enlargement is towards the right iliac fossa.

Palpation
The following methods of palpation have been discussed:
1. Traditional method/conventional method
2. Preferred method
3. Alternate method
4. Hooking method
5. Dipping method

1. **Traditional method/conventional method (Fig. 5D.26):**
   - Place right hand on the right iliac fossa, parallel to the costal margin.
   - Keep the hand steady during inspiration and feel for the liver edge as it descends with each inspiration.

- If the edge is not felt, move the hand upwards towards the costal margin by 1 cm during expiration.
- Repeat the procedure till the liver border is felt.

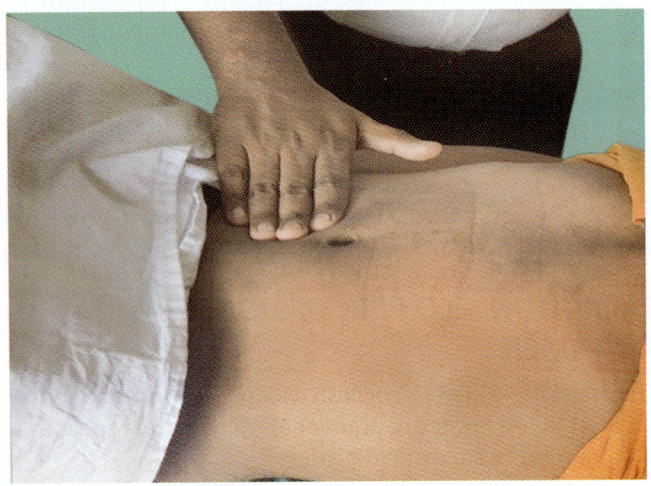

Fig. 5D.26: Traditional method of palpation of liver.

2. **Preferred method (Fig. 5D.27):**
   - Sit on the right side the patient facing the head end of the patient.
   - Now place both hands side-by-side flat on the abdomen in the right subcostal region lateral to the rectus with the fingers pointing towards the ribs.

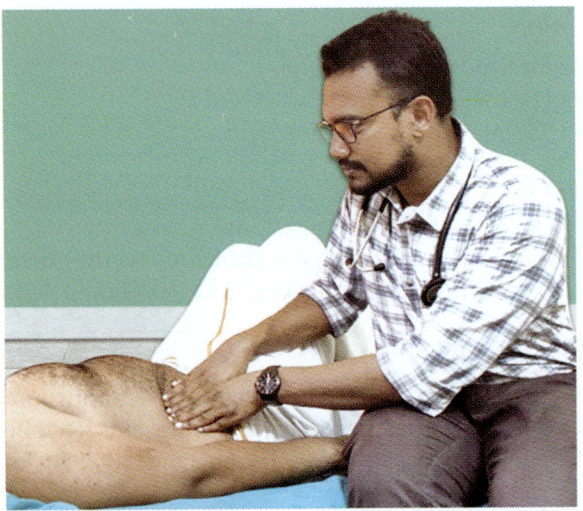

Fig. 5D.27: Preferred method of palpation of liver.

   - If resistance is felt, move the hands further down until resistance disappears.
   - Exert gentle pressure and ask the patient to inspire deeply.
   - The border of the liver can be felt on the tips of the fingers.
   - This procedure can be repeated from lateral to medial to trace the entire edge of the liver.

3. **Alternate method (Fig. 5D.28):**
   - Place the right hand below and parallel to the right subcostal margin.
   - The liver edge will then be felt against the radial border of the index finger.

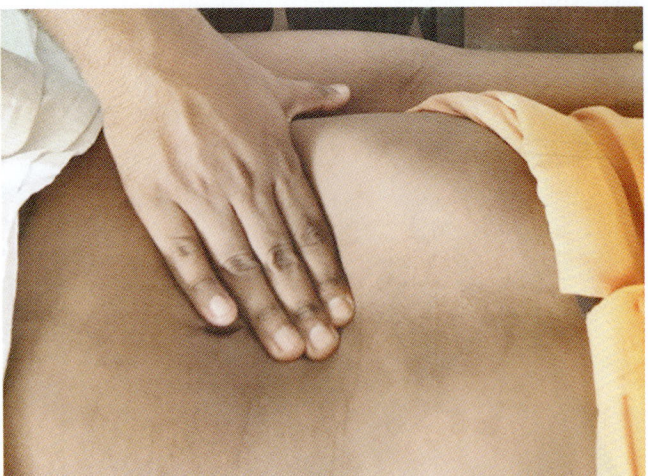

Fig. 5D.28: Alternate method of palpation of liver.

4. **Hooking method of liver examination (Fig. 5D.29):**
   - Examiner stands at the patient's right shoulder, facing the foot end and examines the lower edge of the liver by curling the fingertips under the right costal margin.

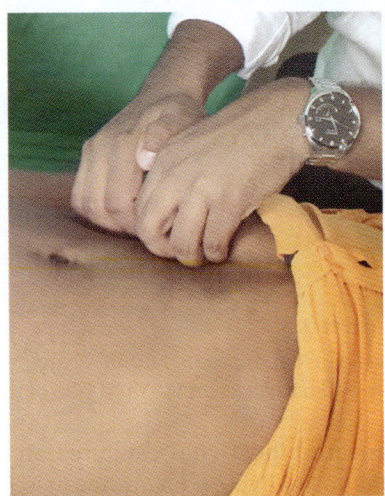

Fig. 5D.29: Hooking method of palpation of liver.

5. **Dipping method of liver palpation in ascites (Fig. 5D.30):**
   - Place both hands one over the other, over the area to be palpated.
   - Rapidly flex your metacarpophalangeal joints, so that your fingers suddenly dip into the patient's abdomen.
   - This displaces the fluid, enhancing the palpation of underlying organ.

Liver Span

- The liver span is the distance in centimeters between the upper border of the liver in the right midclavicular line, as determined by percussion (i.e., where lung resonance changes to liver dullness), and the lower border, as determined by either percussion or palpation **(Figs. 5D.31 to 5D.33)**.
- The upper border of the liver is assessed using a heavy percussion technique. Light percussion is used to locate

Gastrointestinal System

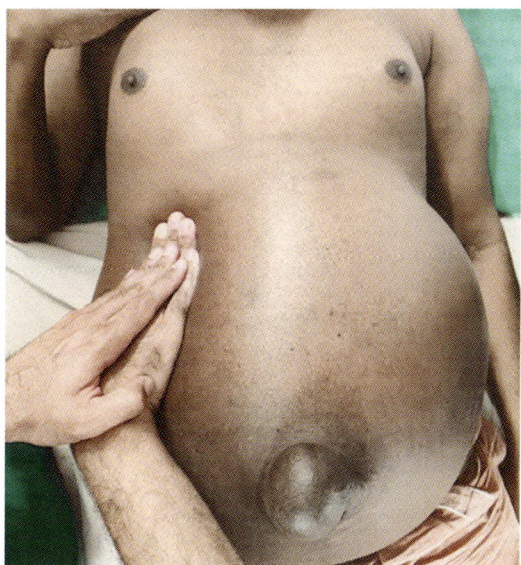

Fig. 5D.30: Dipping method of palpation of liver.

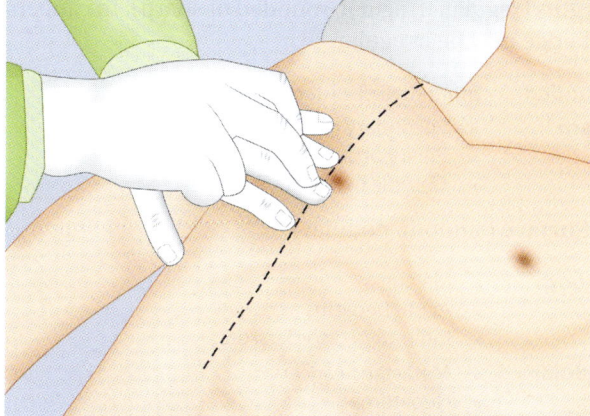

Fig. 5D.32: Percuss along the midclavicular line.

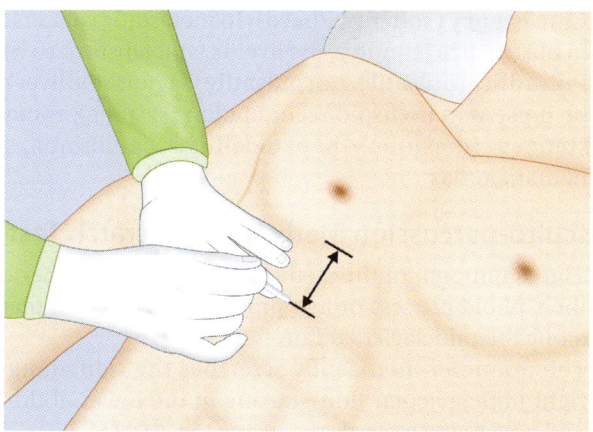

Fig. 5D.33: Mark the upper and lower border of dullness.

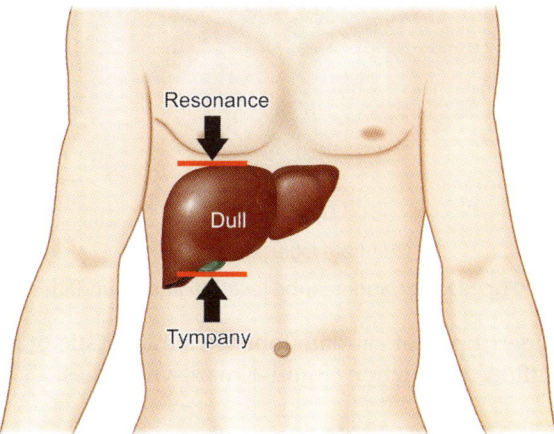

Fig. 5D.31: Liver span.

the lower edge of the liver. Light percussion is required because heavy percussion may underestimate the lower extent of the liver border.
- The normal liver span is <13 cm.
- In midclavicular line: Normally 6–12 cm.
- In midsternal line (left lobe): Normally 4–8 cm.
- The clinical estimate of the liver span is usually an underestimation of the actual liver size by about 2–5 cm.
- There are several problems with predicting liver size by percussion.
- If ascites is present, the examiner can only speculate about the correct size of the liver.

A more common cause of overestimating liver size (false-positive measurement) is some form of chronic obstructive lung disease. This makes percussion of the upper border of the liver difficult.

Obesity in a patient can cause problems in both percussion and palpation. Distension of the colon may obscure the lower liver dullness. This may result in underestimating the size of the liver (false-negative measurement).

Liver span	Condition seen
Increased	Hepatomegaly
Decreased	Shrunken liver as in cirrhosis
False positive for enlarged liver	▪ Right-sided pleural effusion ▪ Right lower lobe consolidation

Note: In conditions like emphysema of the lung, the liver may be pushed down. The edge may be palpable, leading the examiner to believe that the patient has hepatomegaly when the real problem is a hyperinflated lung. Percussion will reveal that the upper border is lower than expected.

If the liver is enlarged and palpable, assess the following:
- **Location of the edge in cm below the costal margin in the midclavicular or anterior axillary line.**
- **Span (in cm)**
- **Tenderness** (tender/nontender)

Tender hepatomegaly	Painless hepatomegaly
▪ Right heart failure ▪ Acute hepatitis (viral/alcoholic/drug induced) ▪ Liver abscess (amoebic/pyogenic) ▪ Hepatoma ▪ Infarcts ▪ Actinomycosis ▪ Acute Budd–Chiari syndrome	▪ Fatty liver ▪ Infiltrative and storage disorders ▪ Malaria ▪ Leukemia ▪ Lymphoma

Margins (regular, irregular, rounded or sharp). In cancers the liver edge may be irregular.

Rounded	Infiltrative disorders
Sharp	<ul><li>Secondary metastases, acute hepatitis</li><li>Biliary obstruction</li><li>Chronic hepatitis</li></ul>

- **Surface** (smooth, nodular).

Smooth	<ul><li>Malaria</li><li>Acute hepatitis</li><li>Infiltrative disorders, etc.</li></ul>
Nodular	<ul><li>Metastatic cancers</li><li>Hepatoma</li><li>Alcoholic cirrhosis (micronodular)</li><li>Posthepatic cirrhosis (macronodular)</li></ul>

- **Consistency (soft/firm/hard):** In metastatic cancers and in obstructive jaundice, the liver is typically firm to hard.
- **Pulsatility (pulsatile/not pulsatile):** A pulsatile liver may be present in tricuspid regurgitation (systolic), tricuspid stenosis (diastolic), hepatocellular carcinoma, and hemangiomas.

Ausculto-percussion Method (The Scratch Test)

- The diaphragm of the stethoscope is placed either over the xiphoid process or just superior to the costal margin along the midclavicular line.
- The examiner then gently scratches the skin along the right midclavicular line, starting in the lower abdomen and advancing towards the head **(Fig. 5D.34)**.
- The sound produced by the scratching changes in quality and intensity when over the liver, as sounds are much more easily transmitted through the solid organ.

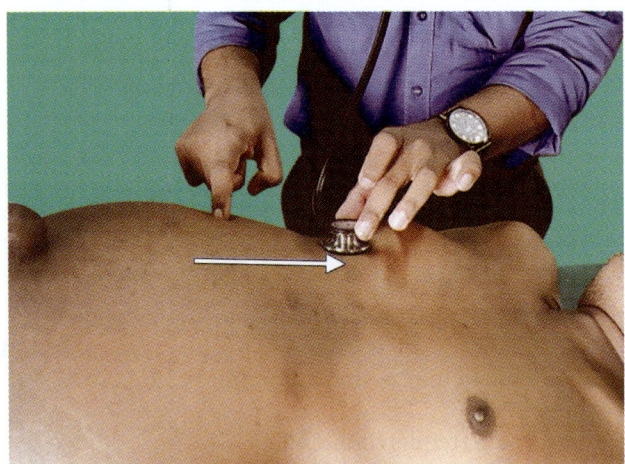

Fig. 5D.34: Demonstration of ausculto-percussion method.

Causes of Hepatomegaly (Fig. 5D.35)

Causes of hepatomegaly can be grossly grouped under the headings of infections, malignancies, infiltrative disorders, hematological disorders, and vascular disorders as shown in **Figure 5D.35**. Massive hepatomegaly (>10 cm) seen with hepatoma.

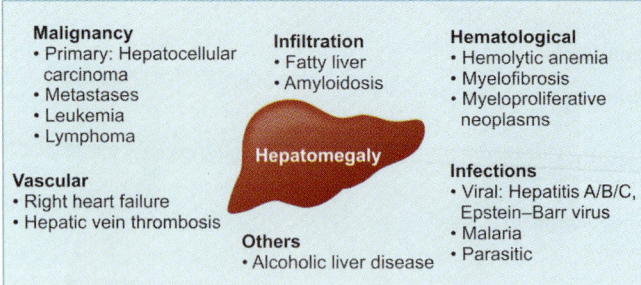

Fig. 5D.35: Causes of hepatomegaly.

Caudate Lobe (Fig. 5D.36)

- Arises from the right lobe of the liver, on the postero-superior surface.

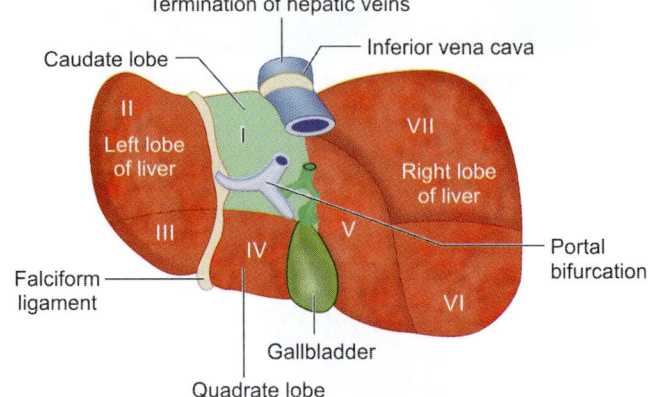

Fig. 5D.36: Caudate lobe location and boundaries.

- Hypertrophy of caudate lobe is characteristic of hepatic outflow obstruction (Budd–Chiari syndrome).

Riedel's Lobe (Fig. 5D.37)

- Congenital variant projecting from the right lobe of the liver.
- May be mistaken for gallbladder or right kidney.

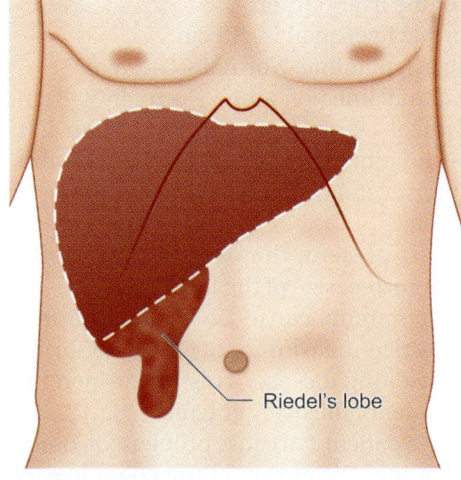

Fig. 5D.37: Anomalous lobe of the liver projecting from right lobe.

Examination of Spleen

Normal characteristics:

Dimensions	▪ 12 cm length, 7 cm width ▪ 13 cm craniocaudal diameter
Weight	<250 g
Location (Fig. 5D.38)	▪ Along—9th, 10th, 11th ribs midaxillary line ▪ Along the long axis of 10th rib
Extent	▪ **Anteriorly** (lower pole): Up to midaxillary line ▪ **Posteriorly:** The superior angle of spleen is 4 cm lateral to T10 spine
Margin	There is a **notch** on the inferolateral border, and this may be palpated when the spleen is enlarged

Normal spleen is not palpable clinically except in following scenarios:
- Only occasionally palpable in 1–3% of New Guinea population.
- Tip may be palpable in newborn up to 3 months of age.

Splenic enlargement:
- Before becoming clinically palpable—spleen enlarges in superior and posterior direction.
- It has to enlarge two to three times of normal to become palpable.

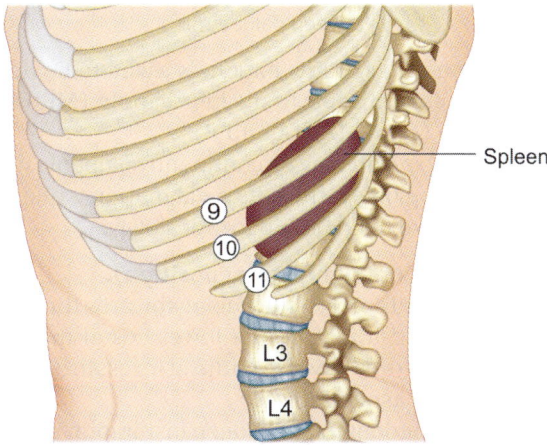

Fig. 5D.38: Surface marking of spleen.

- Once palpable, it appears (felt) below tip of 10th rib (beneath/under the left costal margin) and further enlarges downwards, medially (inwards), and forwards towards umbilicus (LHC to RIF).

Grading of enlargement/splenomegaly:

Based on largest dimension	
Moderate splenomegaly	*Severe splenomegaly*
11–20 cm	>20 cm

Based on distance from costal margin (Fig. 5D.39)		
Mild (tip) enlargement	Moderate enlargement	Severe (marked) enlargement
1–2 cm (<3 cm)	**3–7 cm** (3–8 cm) Between costal margin and umbilicus	**7+ cm** >8 cm below left costal margin >1,000 g dry weight. Crossing midline

Note: Size of the spleen is measured from the left costal margin to the tip along the long axis of spleen.

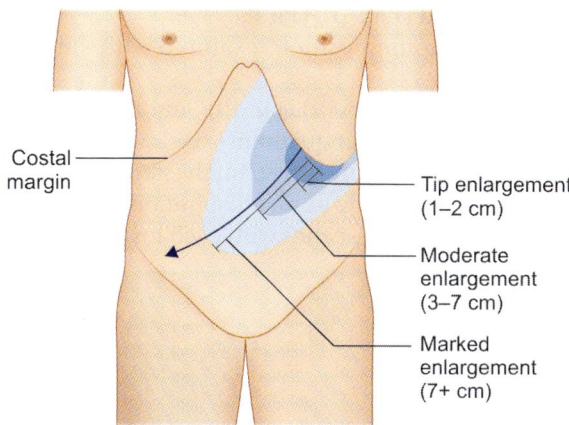

Fig. 5D.39: Grading of splenomegaly.

Hackett's grading system for palpable splenomegaly (Fig. 5D.40):

Grade	Description
Grade 0	Normal impalpable spleen
Grade 1	Spleen palpable only in deep inspiration
Grade 2	Spleen palpable on midclavicular line halfway between umbilicus and costal margin
Grade 3	Spleen expands towards the umbilicus
Grade 4	Spleen goes past the umbilicus
Grade 5	Spleen expands towards pubic symphysis

Inspection: Fullness may be seen emerging from the left upper quadrant extending diagonally towards the right lower quadrant (RLQ).

Palpation: Following methods of palpation have been discussed:
1. Classical method
2. Bimanual method
   a. In supine position
   b. In right lateral position
3. Hooking method
   a. In supine position
   b. In right lateral position
4. Middleton's maneuver
5. Dipping method

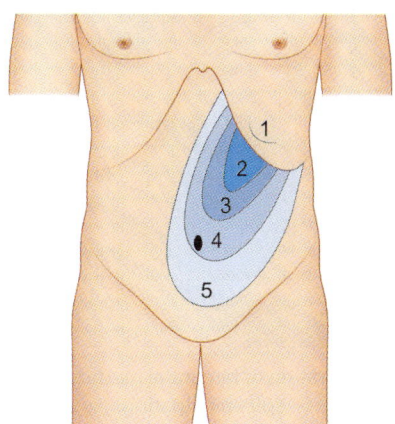

Fig. 5D.40: Hackett's grading system for palpable splenomegaly.

Classical method (Fig. 5D.41):
- Patient in supine position, examine with single hand (right).
- Place the hand in the RLQ in RIF and move diagonally towards the left upper quadrant.
- Hand should be firmly placed on the abdominal wall.
- Keep the hand steady during inspiration and feel for the splenic edge as it descends with each inspiration.

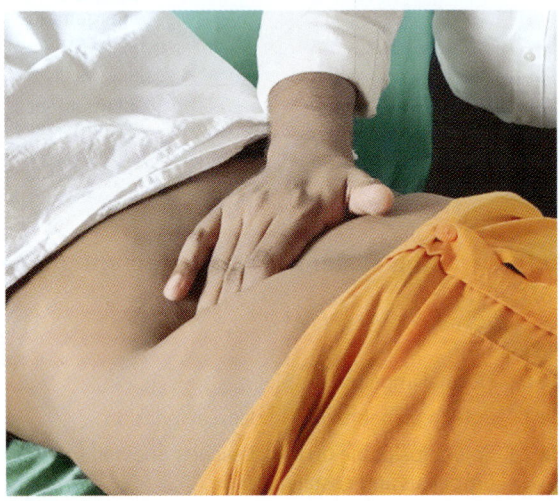

Fig. 5D.41: Demonstration of classical method of spleen palpation.

- If edge is not felt move the hand diagonally towards LUQ by 1 cm during expiration.
- Repeat the procedure.
- Tip of the fingers are used to feel the splenic tip.

Bimanual (supine position) (Fig. 5D.42):
- Place palm of left hand over the left lowermost rib cage posterolaterally, restricting the expansion of left lower ribs on inspiration.
- While applying firm pressure with the left hand, ask the patient to take deep inspiration.
- Insinuate the right hand beneath the left costal margin and feel for the splenic edge.

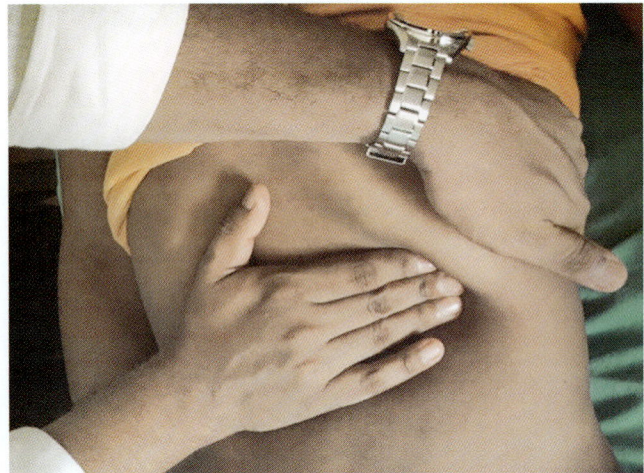

Fig. 5D.42: Demonstration of bimanual method (supine position) of spleen palpation.

Bimanual (right lateral position):
- Done with patient lying in right lateral position with the left hip and knee flexed.
- Rest of maneuver is similar to above.

Hooking method (supine position) (Fig. 5D.43):
- The physician hooks his fingers beneath the left costal margin as the patient inspires.

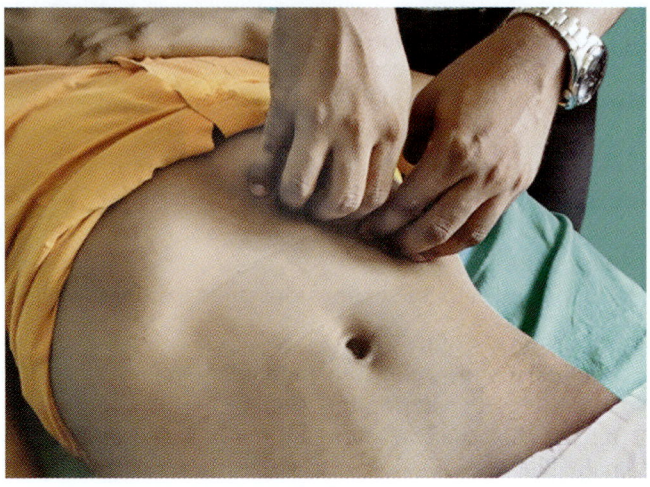

Fig. 5D.43: Demonstration of hooking method (supine position) of spleen palpation.

- For better appreciability, patient is asked to lie down on his left fist just inferior to his left scapula **(Middleton's maneuver) (Figs. 5D.44A and B)**
- From above, spleen may be continently palpable with two hands arching below the left costal margin while patient is asked to take deep breath in/out slowly.

Hooking maneuver (right lateral position):
- Examiner stands on left side facing towards the foot end
- With one hand hook the left lower costal margin and with other hand, give a counter-pressure from the posterolateral aspect.
- Now ask the patient to take a deep inspiration and feel for the tip of the spleen, by hooking the fingers.

Dipping method:
- It is done in marked ascites
- Similar to dipping method of liver (as described below under the palpation of liver).

The following methods of percussion have been discussed:
1. Castell's method
2. Traube's space percussion
3. Nixon's method of percussion

1. **Percussion by Castell's method (spleen percussion sign)**
   - With patient in supine position, percuss in the lowest left intercostal (IC) space in the anterior axillary line **(Figs. 5D.45 and 5D.48)** (usually the 8th or 9th IC space—Castell's point)
   - This space should remain resonant during full inspiration.

Gastrointestinal System

	Full inspiration	Full expiration
Normal	Resonant	Resonant
Mild splenomegaly*	Dull	Resonant
Moderate/severe splenomegaly	Dull	Dull

*Percussion sign is considered positive, when a change in percussion note is observed between full expiration and full inspiration.

2. **Percussion of Traube's (semilunar) space**
   - It is a semilunar space in the left anterior chest bounded by:
     - Above by 6th rib
     - Below by left costal margin
     - Laterally by anterior axillary line
   - With patient supine, percuss inferior to lung resonance from medial to lateral (**Figs. 5D.46 and 5D.48**) (as described by **Barkun**). Normally, a tympanic note heard due to gastric air bubble.

Obliteration of Traube's space	<ul><li>Massive splenomegaly</li><li>Left-sided pleural effusion</li><li>Pericardial effusion</li><li>Enlarged left lobe of the liver</li><li>Full stomach or fundic mass</li></ul>
Upward shift of Traube's space	<ul><li>Left diaphragmatic paralysis</li><li>Left lower lobe collapse or fibrosis</li></ul>

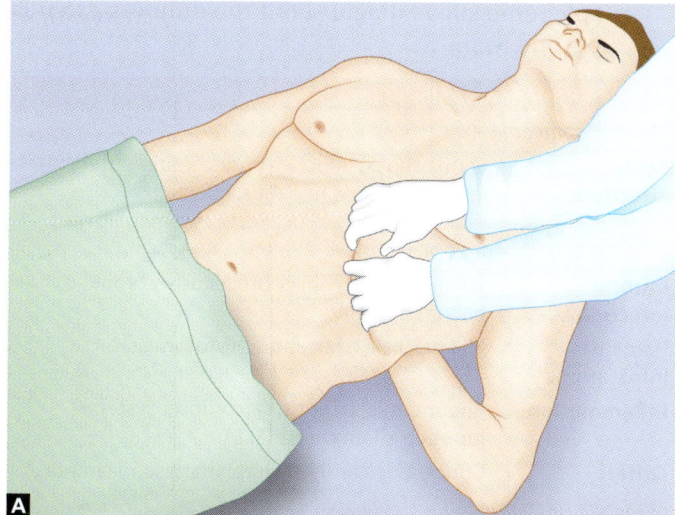
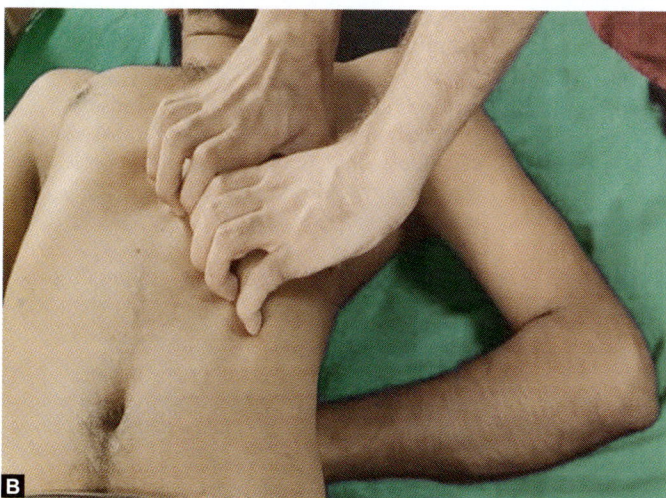

Figs. 5D.44A and B: Demonstration of hooking method with Middleton's maneuver percussion.

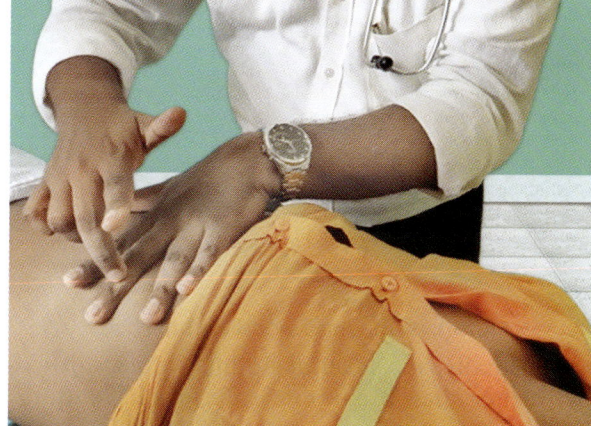

Fig. 5D.46: Percussion of Traube's space.

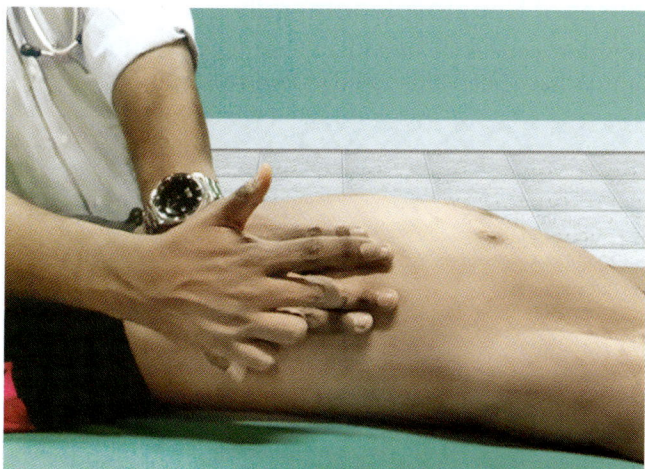

Fig. 5D.45: Percussing the lowest left intercostal space in anterior axillary line—Castell's method of splenic percussion.

- Dullness on full inspiration indicates possible splenic enlargement (a positive Castell's sign).
- Most sensitive of all clinical signs with sensitivity 82% and specificity 83%.

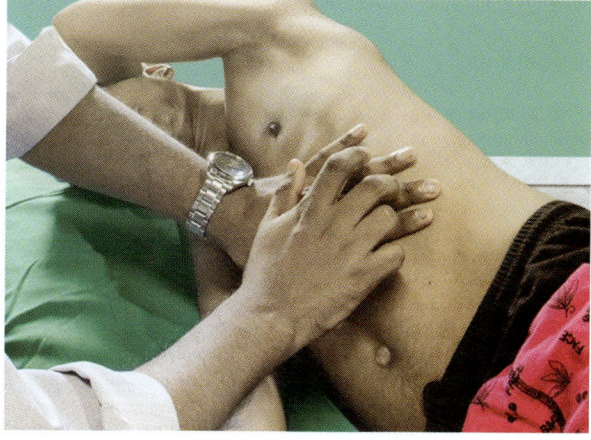

Fig. 5D.47: Percussing the posterior axillary line in right lateral position (Nixon's method).

splenomegaly is diagnosed if the dullness extends beyond 8 cm.

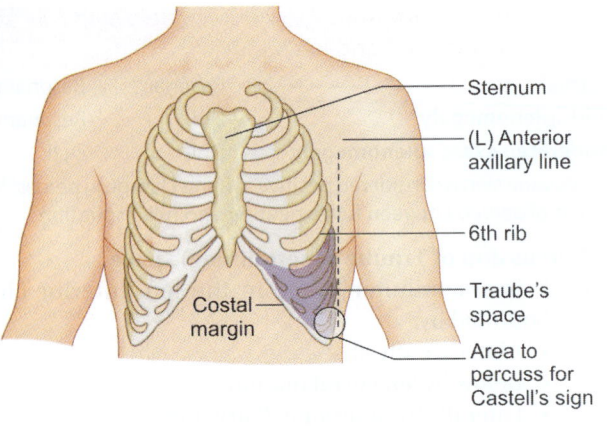

Fig. 5D.48: Landmarks of Traube's space and Castell's sign.

3. **Percussion by Nixon's method**
   - Patient is first placed in the right lateral decubitus position.
   - Percussion starts at the midpoint of the left costal margin and is continued upward perpendicular to the left costal margin (**Figs. 5D.47 and 5D.49**).

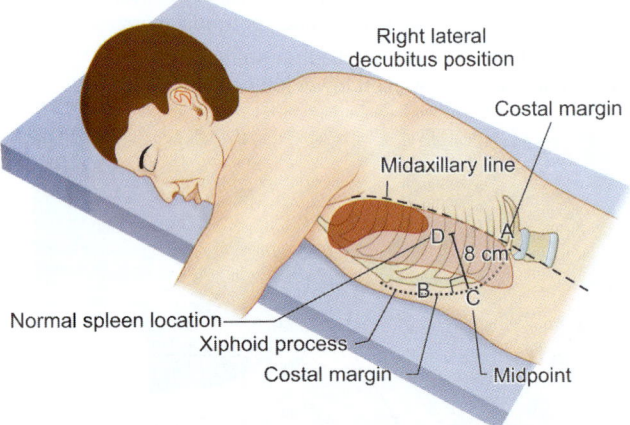

Fig. 5D.49: Landmarks for Nixon's method.

- Normally, the level of dullness does not extend further than 8 cm above the costal margin and

Causes of splenomegaly	
Mild splenomegaly	
Acute infections	Septic shock, infective endocarditis, enteric fever, infectious hepatitis, infectious mononucleosis, brucellosis, cytomegalovirus, toxoplasmosis
Chronic infections	Tuberculosis, syphilis, brucellosis, chronic bacteremia, HIV
Parasitic infestations	Malaria, kala-azar, and schistosomiasis
Inflammation	Rheumatoid arthritis, sarcoidosis, systemic lupus erythematosus (SLE)
Others	Congestive cardiac failure, thalassemia minor
Moderate splenomegaly	
Neoplastic	Lymphomas, acute leukemias, chronic lymphocytic leukemia, chronic myeloid leukemia
Non-neoplastic	Cirrhosis of liver (with portal hypertension), chronic hemolytic anemia, malaria, kala-azar, sarcoidosis, infectious mononucleosis, splenic abscess, amyloidosis, hemochromatosis, polycythemia vera
Severe (massive) splenomegaly	
Common causes	Chronic myeloid leukemia, myelofibrosis, kala-azar, primary splenic lymphomas (hairy cell, mantle cell, marginal B cell), portal hypertension (extrahepatic portal vein thrombosis), hyper-reactive malarial splenomegaly (tropical splenomegaly)
Uncommon causes	Gaucher's disease, Niemann–Pick disease, thalassemia major, splenic cysts and tumors of spleen, *Mycobacterium avium* complex (MAC) infection in HIV patients

Causes of Hepatosplenomegaly

Common causes of hepatosplenomegaly and associated features have been illustrated in **Figure 5D.50**.

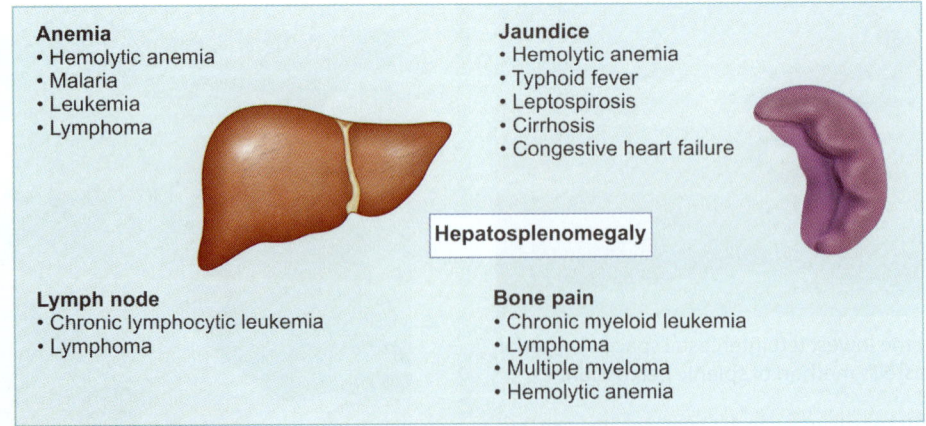

Fig. 5D.50: Causes of hepatosplenomegaly.

Examination of Gallbladder

- Location: Lateral edge of rectus abdominis near the tip of right 9th costal margin
- Moves with respiration
- Upper border continues with liver
- Causes of enlarged gallbladder:
    - Carcinoma head of pancreas
    - Common bile duct (CBD) obstruction
    - Mucocele of gallbladder
    - Carcinoma of gallbladder
- **Murphy's sign**: In acute cholecystitis, at the height of inspiration, patient stops breathing with a gasp as a mass is felt.
- **Courvoisier's law:** In a jaundiced patient, if the gallbladder is palpable, it is unlikely to be due to a CBD gallstone obstruction.
    - A gallbladder containing stones is likely to have been chronically diseased and subject to repeated, although possibly subclinical, episodes of cholecystitis. This results in extensive fibrosis of the gallbladder wall which is then unable to distend when obstructed.
    - The converse of this law is not true; the cause of jaundice in nonpalpable gallbladder is not necessarily gallstones as 50% of dilated gallbladders are not palpable.
    - Exceptions of Courvoisier's law
        1. Double impaction: Stones, simultaneously occluding the cystic duct and the distal CBD. The stone in the CBD causes obstructive jaundice and a synchronous stone in the cystic duct leads to mucocele or empyema of gallbladder
        2. Pancreatic calculus obstructing the ampulla of Vater
        3. Oriental cholangiohepatitis (ductal stones formed secondary to liver fluke infestation)
        4. Periampullary carcinoma in patients with cholecystectomy
        5. Mirizzi syndrome: A stone is lodged in Hartman's pouch causing intense inflammation in the region of Calot's triangle and compressing the common hepatic duct, while also obstructing the gallbladder; this causes the gallbladder to distend.

Examination of Kidney

Examination of Left Kidney

- The right hand is placed anteriorly in the left lumbar region while the left hand is placed posteriorly in the left loin **(Fig. 5D.51)**.
- Ask the patient to take a deep breath in, press the left hand forward and the right hand backward, upward and inward.
- Left kidney is usually not palpable (except when low lying or enlarged).
- If palpable, it is described as bimanually palpable and ballotable.
- **Bimanually palpable:** As it can be felt as a swelling between both right and left hands.
- **Ballotable:** It can be pushed from one hand to the other. It is due to perinephric fat which allows the free movement of the kidney in the retroperitoneum.

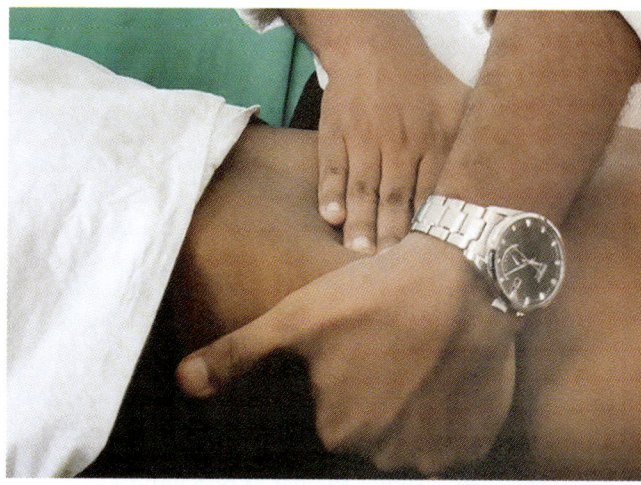

Fig. 5D.51: Palpation of left kidney.

Palpation of Right Kidney

- Place the right hand horizontally in the right lumbar region anteriorly with the left hand placed posteriorly in the right loin **(Fig. 5D.52)**.
- Push forwards with the left hand, press the right hand inward and upward and ask the patient to take a deep breath in.
- The lower pole of the right kidney, unlike the left, is commonly palpable in thin patients and is felt as a smooth, rounded swelling which descends on inspiration.
- It is also bimanually palpable and ballotable.

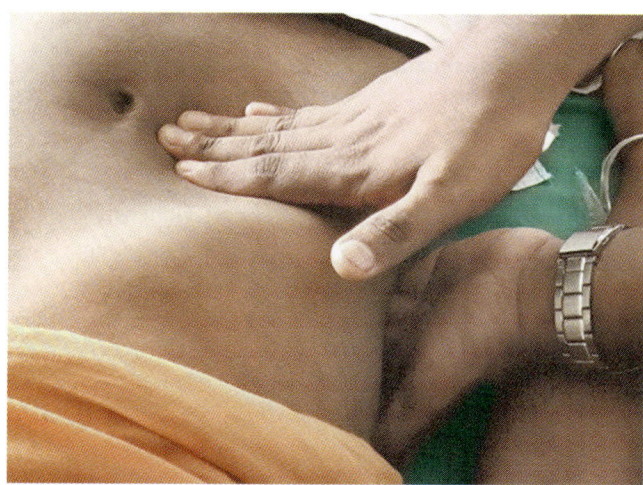

Fig. 5D.52: Palpation of right kidney.

Causes of unilateral and bilateral kidney enlargement:

Unilateral kidney enlargement	Bilateral kidney enlargement
▪ Renal cell carcinoma	▪ Polycystic kidneys
▪ Hydronephrosis	▪ Bilateral hydronephrosis

RENAL ANGLE (FIG. 5D.53)
- An area located on either side of the human back between the lateral borders of the erector spinae muscles and inferior borders of the 12th rib.
- Overlies the lower part of kidney.

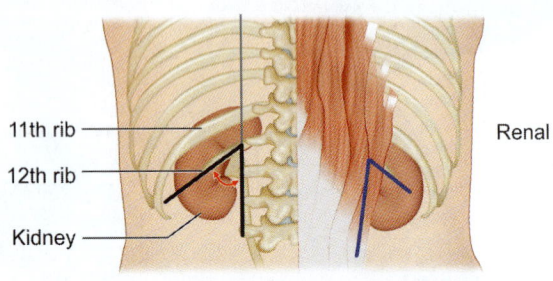

Fig. 5D.53: Renal angle.

MURPHY'S KIDNEY PUNCH (COSTOVERTEBRAL ANGLE TENDERNESS)

It is performed by striking the fist of one hand against the dorsal surface of the other hand, which is placed flat along the posterior costovertebral angle (CVA) margin. Normally, percussion in CVA should not elicit tenderness.

Causes of Costovertebral Angle Tenderness (Fig. 5D.54)
- Acute pyelonephritis
- Calculi
- Perinephric abscess

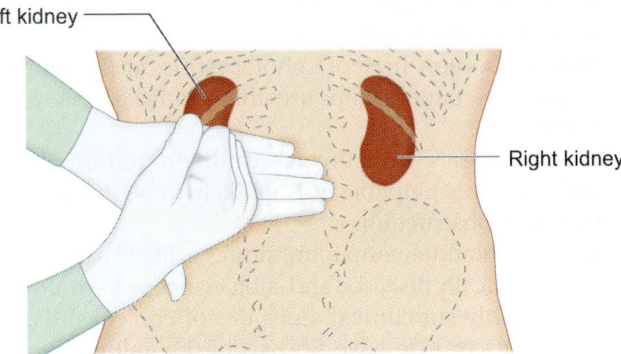

Fig. 5D.54: Costovertebral angle.

Differences between spleen and left kidney		
Characteristics	Spleen	Left kidney
Location	Left hypochondrium	Left lumbar
Direction of enlargement	Towards RIF	Towards left hypochondrium and LIF
Movement with respiration	+	–
Insinuation between left costal margin and organ	Not possible	Possible
Bimanual palpation	–	+
Ballotability	–	+
Crossing midline	Can cross midline	Never cross midline
Notch	+	–
Band of colonic resonance	–	+

Differences points between liver versus spleen versus kidney			
Features	Liver	Spleen	Kidney
Location	Right hypochondrium	Left hypochondrium	Lumbar
Direction of enlargement	Towards RIF	Towards RIF	Towards hypochondrium and iliac fossa
Movement with respiration	+	+	–
Insinuation of fingers between the costal margin and organ	Not possible	Not possible	Possible
Bimanually palpable	–	–	+
Ballotability	–	–	+
Anterior percussion	Dull	Dull	Tympanic

Examination of Free Fluid in Abdomen

Ascites

Definition:
Ascites is defined as the accumulation of free fluid in the peritoneal cavity. The peritoneal cavity can accumulate as much as 60 L of fluid.

Massive ascites and tense ascites are the clinical terms and are described later.

Etiology of ascites			
Nonperitoneal causes		Peritoneal causes	
Intrahepatic portal hypertension	▪ Cirrhosis ▪ Fulminant hepatic failure ▪ Veno-occlusive disease	Granulomatous peritonitis	▪ Tuberculous peritonitis ▪ Fungal and parasitic infections ▪ Sarcoidosis ▪ Foreign bodies (cotton, starch, barium)
Extrahepatic portal hypertension	▪ Hepatic vein obstruction (i.e., Budd–Chiari syndrome) ▪ Congestive heart failure	Malignant ascites	▪ Primary peritoneal mesothelioma ▪ Secondary peritoneal carcinomitosis
Hypoalbuminemia	▪ Nephrotic syndrome ▪ Protein-losing enteropathy ▪ Malnutrition	Vasculitis	▪ Systemic lupus erythematosus ▪ Henoch–Schönlein purpura
Miscellaneous disorders	▪ Myxedema ▪ Ovarian tumors ▪ Pancreatic and biliary ascites	Miscellaneous disorders	▪ Eosinophilic gastroenteritis ▪ Whipple disease ▪ Endometriosis
Chylous	Secondary to malignancy, trauma		

Serum-ascites albumin gradient (SAAG):
- SAAG = (serum albumin) – (albumin level of ascitic fluid)
- The SAAG is a better discriminant than older measures (transudate versus exudate) for the causes of ascites.
- The presence of a gradient ≥1.1 g/dL (≥11 g/L) predicts that the patient has portal hypertension with 97% accuracy.

High albumin gradient (SAAG ≥1.1 g/dL)	Low albumin gradient (SAAG <1.1 g/dL)
▪ Cirrhosis ▪ Alcoholic hepatitis ▪ Heart failure ▪ Massive hepatic metastases ▪ Heart failure/constrictive pericarditis ▪ Budd–Chiari syndrome ▪ Portal vein thrombosis ▪ Idiopathic portal fibrosis	▪ Peritoneal carcinomatosis ▪ Peritoneal tuberculosis ▪ Pancreatitis ▪ Serositis ▪ Nephrotic syndrome ▪ Biliary ascites ▪ Bowel obstruction ▪ Bowel infarction

Ascites praecox: It is defined as appearance of **ascites** before the generalized edema. It is usually associated with chronic constrictive pericarditis.

Causes of ascites without significant edema:
- Chronic constrictive pericarditis
- Tuberculous peritonitis
- Malignant peritonitis
- Pancreatic ascites
- Acute Budd–Chiari syndrome

Grading systems of ascites		
The International Ascites Club grading (2003)		Traditional system
Grade 1	Mild ascites detectable only by ultrasonography	1+ is minimal and barely detectable 2+ is moderate 3+ is massive but not tense 4+ is massive and tense
Grade 2	Moderate ascites manifested by moderate symmetrical abdominal distension	
Grade 3	Large or gross ascites with marked abdominal distension	

The following methods have been discussed of demonstration of ascites:
1. Fullness of flank
2. Horseshoe dullness
3. Shifting dullness
4. Fluid wave/fluid thrill
5. Puddle sign
6. Auscultatory percussion sign of Guarino

1. **Bulging flanks/fullness of flanks/horseshoe dullness**
   - Occurs when the weight of abdominal free fluid is sufficient to push the flanks outward **(Fig. 5D.55)**.

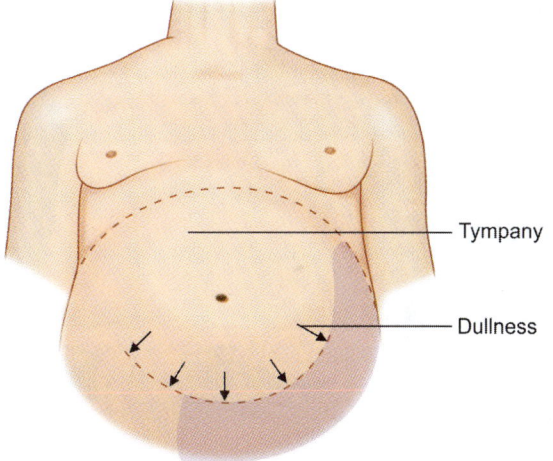

Fig. 5D.55: Horseshoe dullness.

- On inspection, it can be seen as fullness of flanks or bulging of flanks.
- Bulging of flanks can be caused by ascites or by obesity.
- One method for discriminating between the two is to test for flank dullness.
- With the patient recumbent, gas-filled loops of bowel will characteristically float on top of ascites, making the percussion note tympanic at the umbilicus and dull beyond the fluid meniscus into the flanks—horseshoe dullness.

2. **Shifting dullness (Fig. 5D.56):**
   - Presence of shifting dullness indicates at least 1.5 L of free fluid in the peritoneal space.

   Examination (Figs. 5D.57A to K):
   - Patient in supine position, start percussion from above downwards in the midline, till below the umbilicus you get dullness.

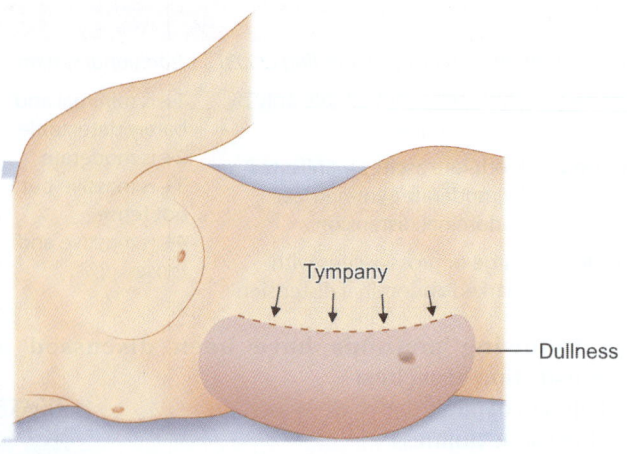

Fig. 5D.56: Shift of dullness on lying in lateral decubitus position.

- This dullness could be due to distended urinary bladder, hence repeat this after making the patient empty the bladder.
- Now, begin by percussing at the umbilicus and moving toward the flanks.
- The transition from air to fluid can be identified when the percussion note changes from tympanic to dull.
- Mark the dullness-tympany transition point.
- Turn the patient to opposite lateral side and wait for 30–60 seconds.
- Now percuss the area again.
- The area of tympany will shift towards the top and the area of dullness shifts towards the bottom.
- Repeat the same maneuver on the opposite side.

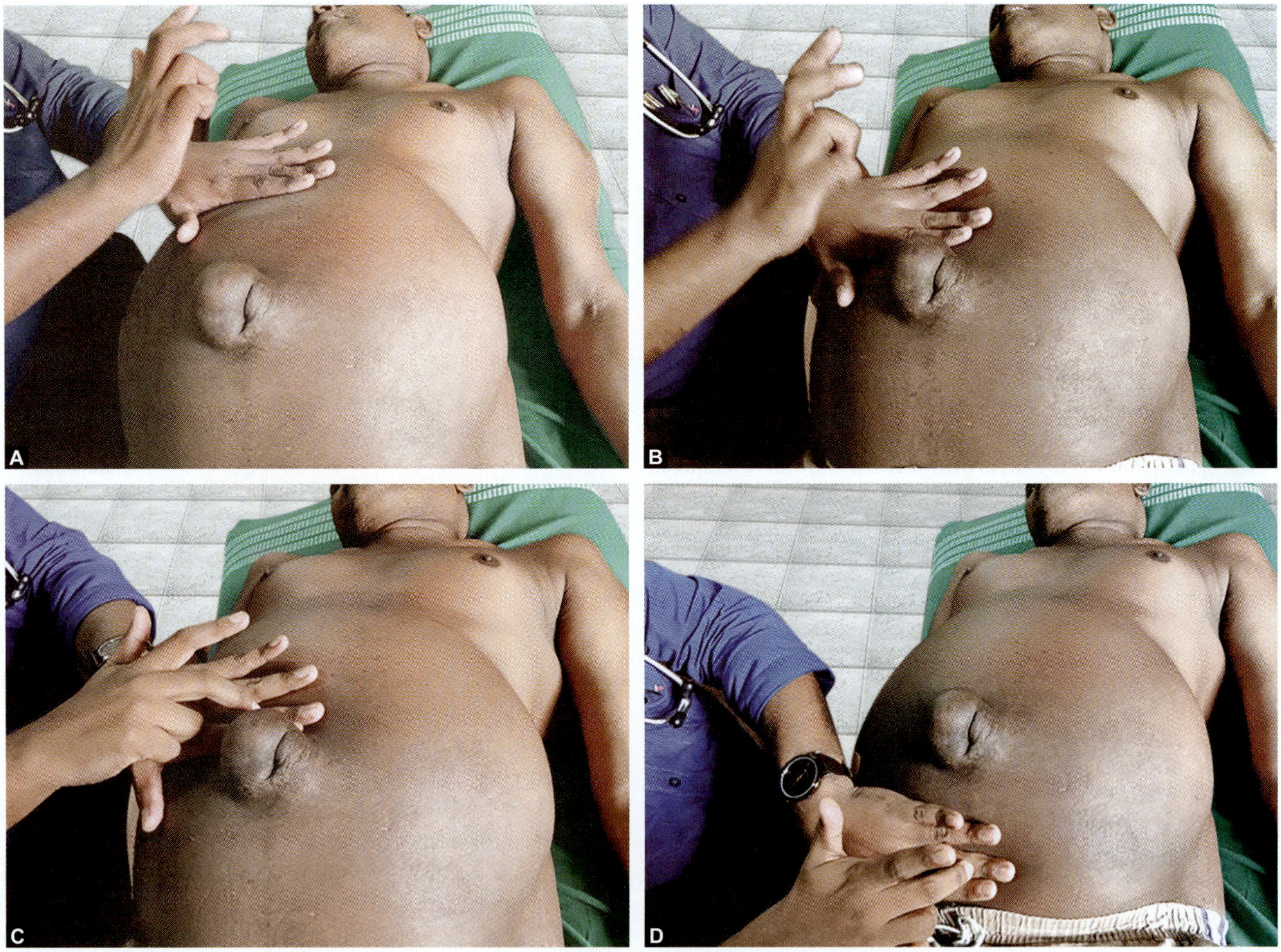

Figs. 5D.57A to D

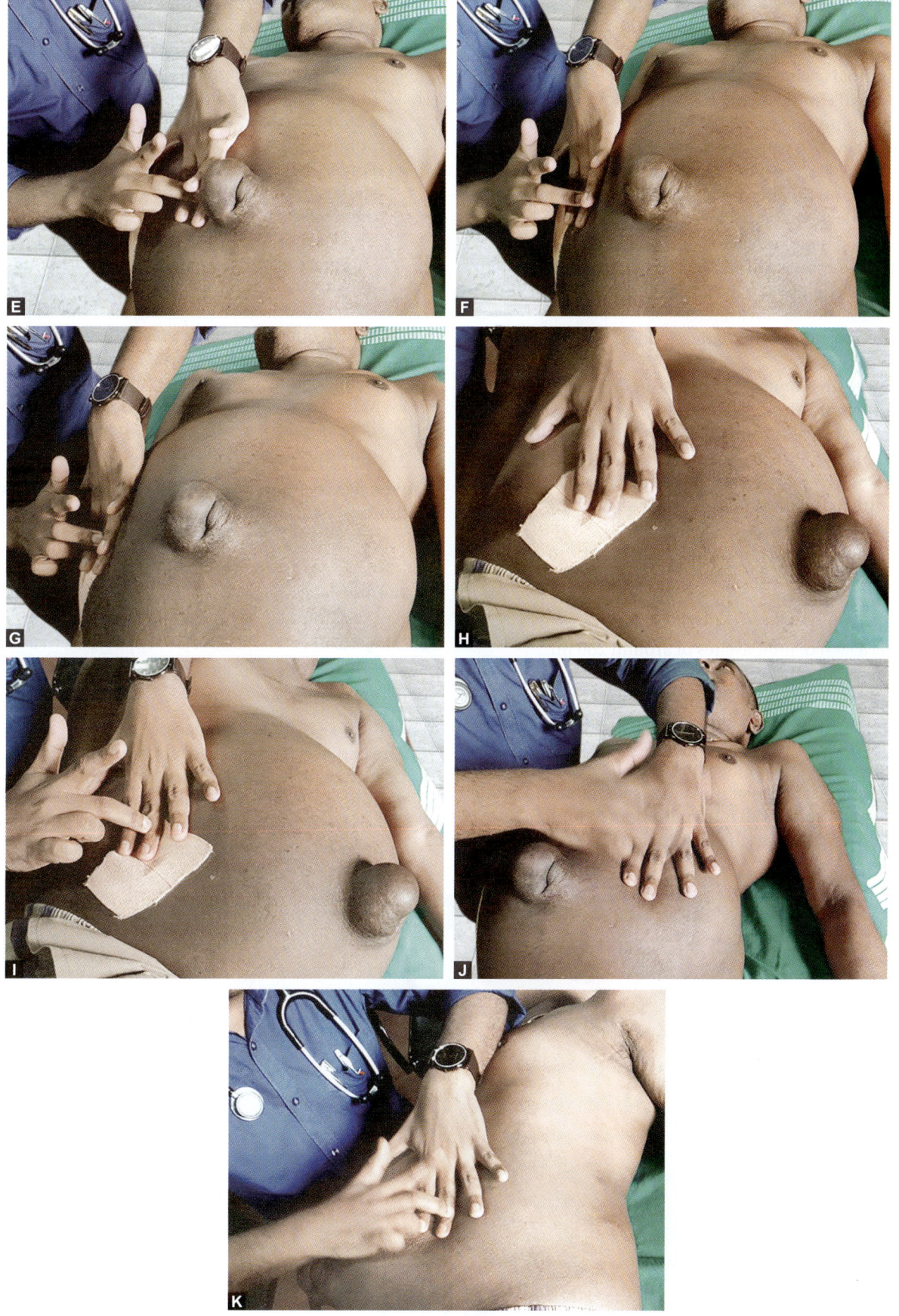

Figs. 5D.57E to K
Figs. 5D.57A to K: Demonstration of shifting dullness.

Causes of ascites without shifting dullness:
1. Massive ascites
2. Loculated ascites
3. Minimal ascites

3. **Fluid thrill (fluid wave) assessment for ascites:**
    - In supine position, ask the patient or an assistant to place the ulnar surface of one hand above the umbilicus, pressing firmly (so the subcutaneous tissue and fat does not jiggle) with the hand pointing towards the patient's toes **(Fig. 5D.58)**.
    - Use one hand to palpate and one hand to percuss.
    - Place a hand on the lateral aspect of the patient's abdomen between the costal margin and the ilium in the anterior axillary line.
    - Tap one side of the patients flank sharply with your fingertips.
    - Feel on the opposite flank for an impulse transmitted through the fluid.
    - Repeat procedure by flicking on the other side.
    - Results:
        - **Positive**: An easily palpable impulse is felt on the opposite side of tapping suggesting ascites of around more than 2 liters.
        - **Negative**: No impulse is felt.
        - **False positive**: Can be felt over large ovarian cyst or large hydatid cyst or large hydronephrosis.

4. **Puddle sign (Fig. 5D.60):**
    - It is a sign of mild ascites of around 250 mL.
    - Not frequently done.
    - Patient is prone for 3–5 minutes and then examined in knee-elbow position as shown in the **Figure 5D.58**.
    - Diaphragm of the stethoscope is placed over the most dependent area of the abdomen. Place diaphragm of the stethoscope over the umbilical region and scratch the abdominal wall from periphery to umbilicus.
    - Sudden change in the note is a positive sign.
    - Signs can be false positive in case of massive splenomegaly or a distended urinary bladder.

5. **Auscultatory percussion (described by Guarino):**
    - After voiding, the patient sits or stands so that free fluid gravitates to the pelvis, and the examiner places a stethoscope in the midline, immediately above the pubic crest.
    - Finger-flicking percussion is performed along radial spokes from the subcostal margin downward toward the pelvis.
    - The percussion note is initially dull but changes sharply to a loud note at the border of increased pelvic density.
    - In the absence of ascites, the border is approximately 4.5 cm above the pelvic crest (the pelvic baseline).
    - In patients with ascites, free fluid raises the demarcating border clearly above the pelvic baseline.
    - When the patient is supine, this clear line of demarcation is obliterated because the free fluid gravitates to the flanks.

The sensitivity, specificity, and likelihood ratio of different methods of examination of ascites:

Method	Amount of fluid	LR+	LR-	Sn	Sp
Fullness of flanks		2.0	0.3	0.81	0.59
Horseshoe dullness		2.0	0.3	0.84	0.59
Shifting dullness	1.5 liters	2.7	0.3	0.77	0.72
Fluid thrill	>2 liters	6.0	0.4	0.62	0.9
Puddle sign	250 mL	1.6	0.8	0.45	0.73

What is tense ascites and massive ascites?
- The earliest clinical sign of ascites is puddle sign which is positive with as low as 250 mL of ascitic fluid.
- Shifting dullness is a specific sign of ascites which occurs due to the floating of the bowel loops in ascitic fluid. This appears when the fluid accumulation is around 1.2 L.

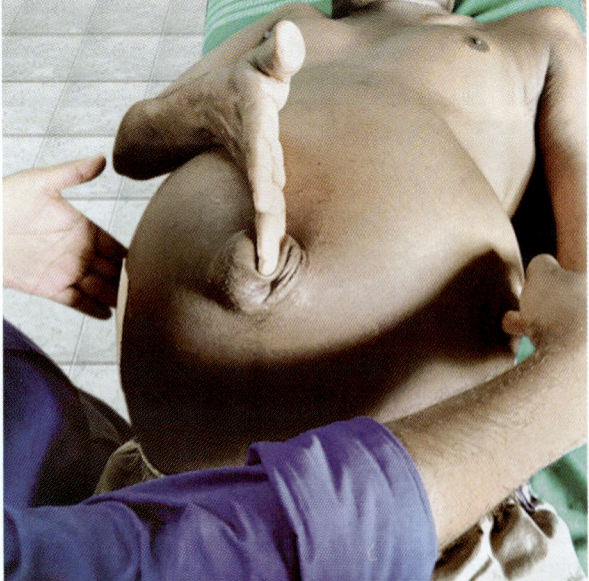
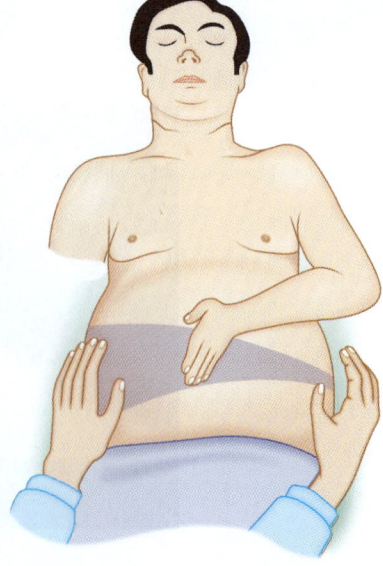

Fig. 5D.58: Demonstration of fluid thrill.

- As the fluids accumulate further, fluid thrill appears (at around 2 L). Appearance of fluid thrill makes the ascites tense.
- As the ascitic fluid fills, the mesentery is stretched and bowel loops float in the ascitic fluid. As the mesentery can only stretch up to a limit, further fluid accumulation results in the submersion of bowel loops. At this stage, shifting dullness disappears; however, fluid thrill persists **(Fig. 5D.59)**. This condition is called as massive ascites.

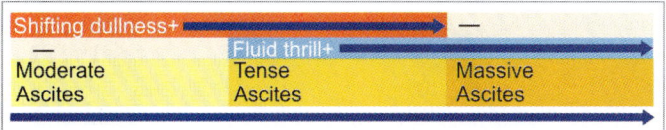

Fig. 5D.59: Schematic representation showing the relationship between shifting dullness and fluid thrill with respect to increasing ascites.

Diagrammatic representation of signs of ascites is shown in Figure 5D.60.

Examination of Dilated Veins

Position of Patient

Make the patient stand and examine the anterior abdominal wall, the flanks, and back for dilated veins. Dilated tortuous veins are significant.

Steps of examination (Harvey's sign) (Figs. 5D.61A to D):
- The direction of blood flow in the veins is examined by placing the tips of the index fingers together and compressing the vein.
- Then, the fingertips are slid apart producing an empty segment of the vein between the fingers **(Fig. 5D.62A)**.
- Then, one finger is removed, and filling of the vein is observed **(Fig. 5D.62B)**.
- The procedure is repeated but now the opposite finger is removed, and filling is observed **(Fig. 5D.62C)**.
- The direction of flow of the veins is the direction in which the filling was rapid and more.

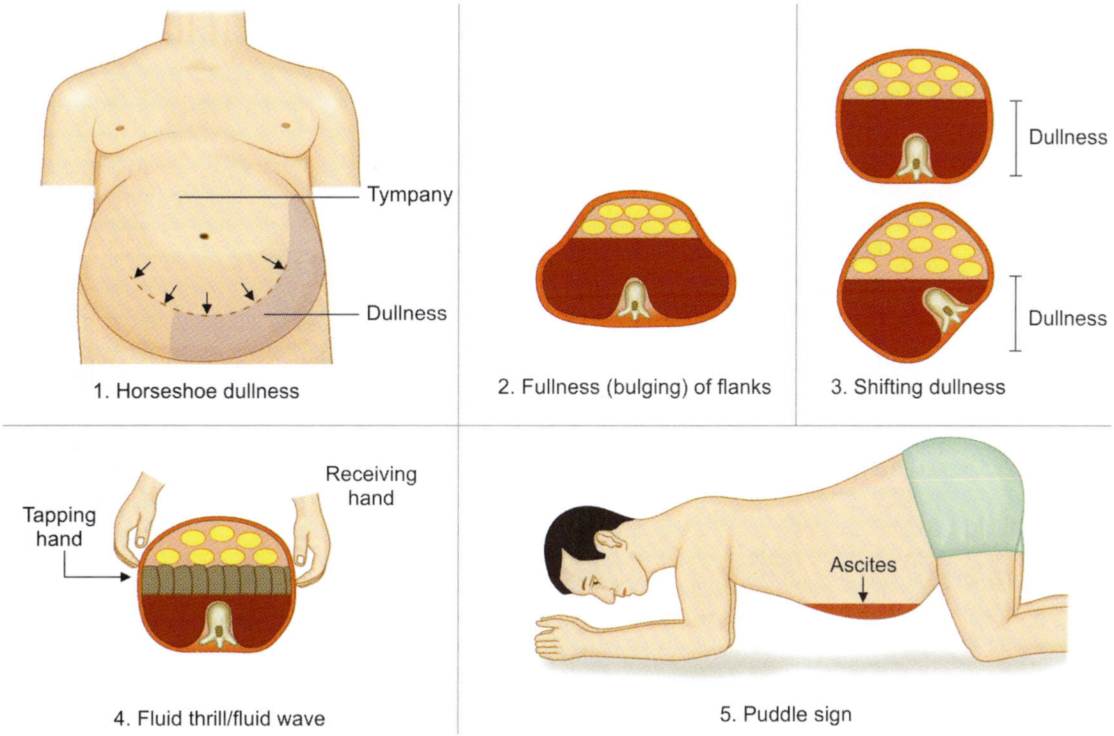

1. Horseshoe dullness
2. Fullness (bulging) of flanks
3. Shifting dullness
4. Fluid thrill/fluid wave
5. Puddle sign

Fig. 5D.60: Signs of ascites.

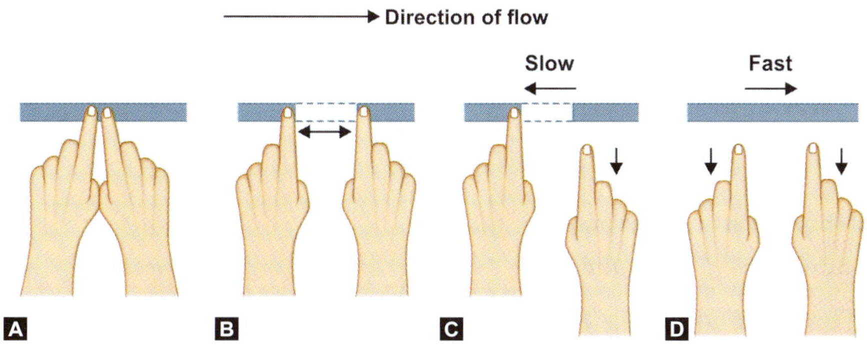

Scan QR code for procedure of ascites tap

Figs. 5D.61A to D: Harvey's sign.

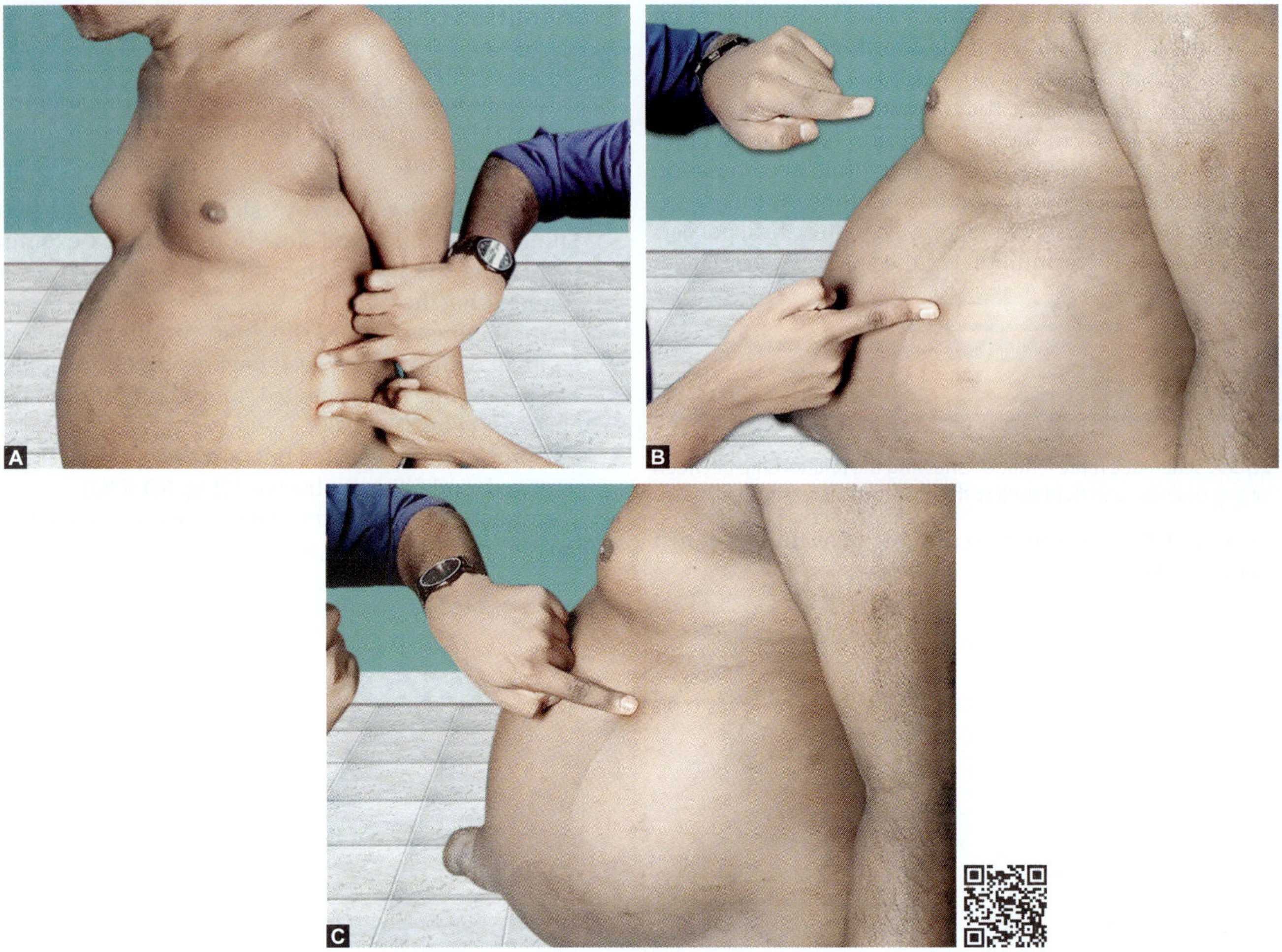

Figs. 5D.62A to C: (A) The fingertips are slid apart producing an empty segment of the vein between the fingers; (B) One finger is removed and filling of the vein is observed; (C) Procedure is repeated but, now the opposite finger is removed, and filling is observed.

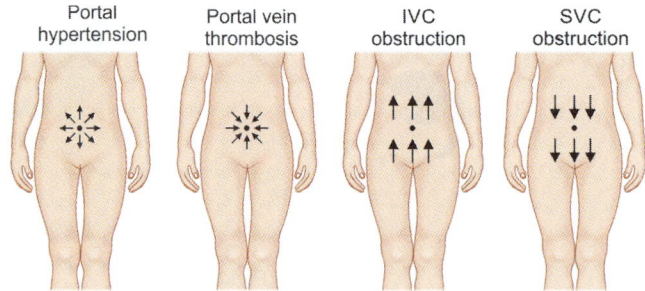

Fig. 5D.63: Direction of flow of veins.

Condition (Fig. 5D.63)	Direction of flow in veins above umbilicus	Direction of flow in veins below umbilicus
Normal (veins not visible)	Upwards	Downwards
Portal hypertension (veins are visible and tortuous)	Upwards	Downwards
Portal vein thrombosis	Downwards	Upwards
Superior vena cava (SVC) obstruction	Downwards	Downwards
Inferior vena cava (IVC) obstruction	Upwards	Upwards

Note: Caput Medusa: Dilated tortuous veins around the umbilicus resembling the head of Medusa.

Per-rectal Examination

Rectal examination consists of:
- Visual inspection of the perianal skin
- Digital palpation of the rectum
- Assessment of neuromuscular function of the perineum

Preferred position of examination:
The *lateral decubitus*, or *Sims position*, provides optimal examination. The patient lies on the left side with the buttocks near the edge of the examining table or bedside with the right knee and hip in slight flexion.

The rectal examination involves both inspection and palpation. First, using a gloved hand, the examiner inspects the buttocks for fistulous tracts, the skin tags, excoriations, blood, fissures in patients with inflammatory bowel disease, rectal prolapse, and superficial ulcers.

Palpation of the rectum can reveal ulcers and masses. Tenderness may be felt with prostatitis, pelvic inflammatory disease, tubo-ovarian abscesses, ovarian cysts, ectopic pregnancy, and inflammatory bowel disease.

Also note the consistency, color, and presence of frank or occult blood in the stool (melena). Black stools result from degraded blood (melena), iron, licorice, bismuth, rhubarb, or overindulgence in chocolate cookies. Red-colored stools may be due to brisk bleeding known as hematochezia (usually distal to the ligament of Treitz).

Hemorrhoids are usually not felt unless thrombosed. Proctoscopy is the best way to look for hemorrhoids.

Others

Per vaginal/per speculum examination:
- In female patients with ascites, ovarian neoplasms, pelvic tumor, per vaginal mass/bleeding can be detected.
- GIT examination is incomplete without examination of the **three S's; Scrotum, Spine, and Supraclavicular Fossa**
- **Scrotum**—hydrocele, hernia, testicular atrophy, and testicular tumors
- **Spine**—metastasis and Pott's spine
- **Supraclavicular fossa**—metastasis to left scalene node

COMPLICATIONS OF CIRRHOSIS

Table 5D.1 represents complications of cirrhosis.

TABLE 5D.1: Complications of cirrhosis.

Portal hypertension and its sequelae	Hepatic encephalopathy	Hepatocellular carcinoma
Ascites	Portal gastropathy	Bleeding manifestations and coagulopathy
Spontaneous bacterial peritonitis	Hepatorenal syndrome	Cirrhotic cardiomyopathy
Portopulmonary hypertension	Hepatopulmonary syndrome	Hepatic hydrothorax
Coagulopathy, thrombocytopenia, hyponatremia	Endocrine dysfunction—adrenal insufficiency, gonadal dysfunction, and thyroid dysfunction	Cirrhotic osteodystrophy

Hepatic Encephalopathy

Types of Hepatic Encephalopathy (Fig. 5D.64)

West Haven criteria clinical grade of hepatic encephalopathy			
Grade	New classification	Description	Asterixis
Grade 0/Minimal HE	COVERT	Lack of detectable changes in personality or behavior	Absent
Grade 1		Trivial lack of awareness, euphoria or anxiety, shortened attention span, impaired performance of addition	May be present
Grade 2	OVERT	Lethargy or apathy, minimal disorientation for time or place, subtle personality change, inappropriate behavior, slurred speech, impaired performance of subtraction	Present
Grade 3		Somnolence to semi-stupor, but responsive to verbal stimuli, confusion, gross disorientation	Usually, absent
Grade 4		Coma (unresponsive to verbal or noxious stimuli)	–

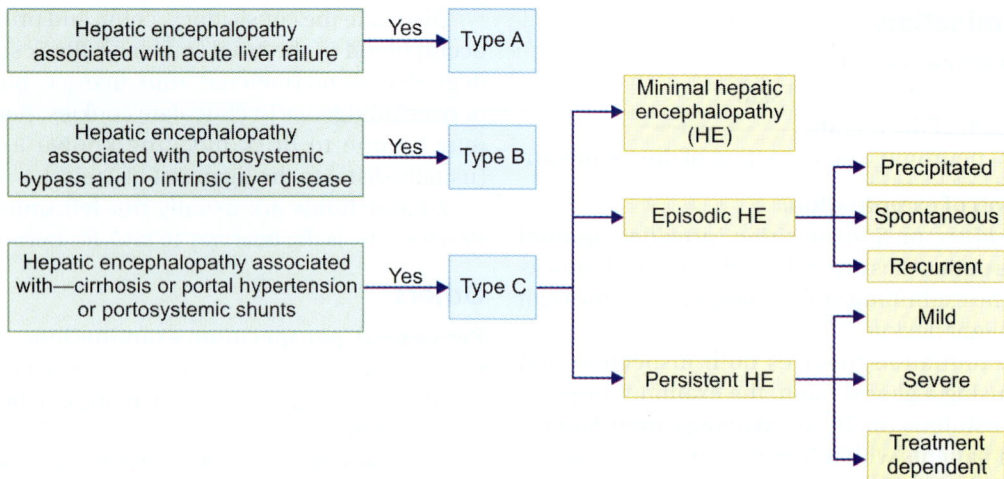

Fig. 5D.64: Types of hepatic encephalopathy.

Asterixis:
Described earlier in signs of liver cell failure.

Diagnosis of Minimal Hepatic Encephalopathy
It is currently based on neuropsychometric tests, including the number connection test, digit symbol test, and the block design test.

Reitan's number-connection test (Fig. 5D.65):
There are 25 numbered circles which can normally be joined together within 30 seconds.

Hepatorenal Syndrome

Diagnostic criteria for hepatorenal syndrome
All of the following must be present for the diagnosis of hepatorenal syndrome (HRS)
- Cirrhosis with ascites - Serum creatinine >1.5 mg/dL - No improvement of serum creatinine (decrease to a level of 1.5 mg/dL or less) after at least 2 days of diuretic withdrawal and volume expansion with albumin - Absence of shock - No current or recent treatment with nephrotoxic drugs - Absence of parenchymal kidney disease as indicated by proteinuria >500 mg/day, microhematuria (>50 red blood cells per high power field), and/or abnormal renal ultrasonography

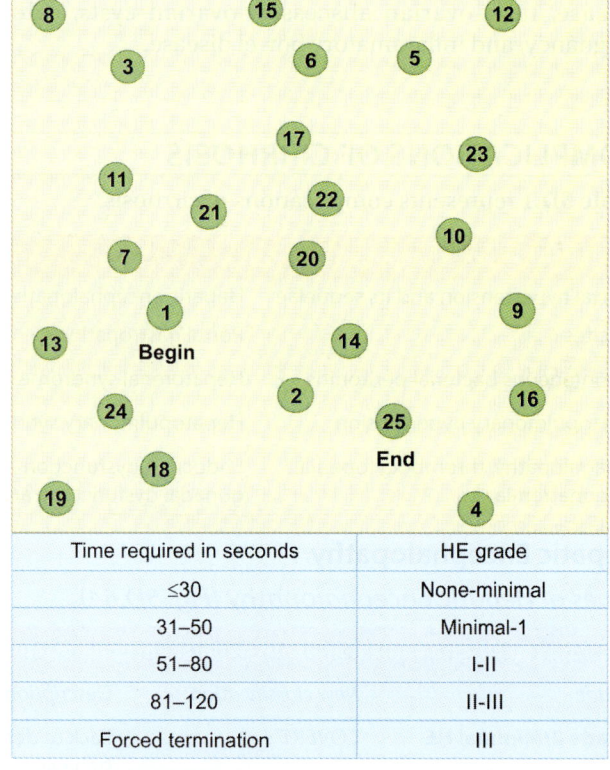

Time required in seconds	HE grade
≤30	None-minimal
31–50	Minimal-1
51–80	I-II
81–120	II-III
Forced termination	III

Fig. 5D.65: Reitan's number-connection test.

Types of hepatorenal syndromes (HRS)	
Acute kidney injury (AKI) type of HRS (HRS-AKI) Type 1 hepatorenal syndrome	*Non-AKI type of HRS (HRS-NAKI) Type 2 hepatorenal syndrome (further classified as HRS-AKD and HRS-CKD)*
- It is characterized by progressive oliguria, a rapid rise of the serum creatinine to above 2.5 mg/dL and has a very poor prognosis - Usually precipitated by spontaneous bacterial peritonitis - Without treatment, median survival is less than 1 month, and almost all patients die within 10 weeks after the onset of renal failure	- It is characterized by a reduction in glomerular filtration, moderate and stable increase in serum creatinine (>1.5 mg/dL), but it is fairly stable and has a better prognosis than type 1 HRS - Usually occurs in patients with refractory ascites (resistant to diuretics) - Median survival is 3–6 months

Precipitating factors for hepatorenal syndrome	
- Gastrointestinal bleeding - Aggressive paracentesis - Diuretic therapy	- Sepsis including spontaneous bacterial peritonitis - Diarrhea

SITES OF PORTOSYSTEMIC ANASTOMOSIS (FIG. 5D.66)

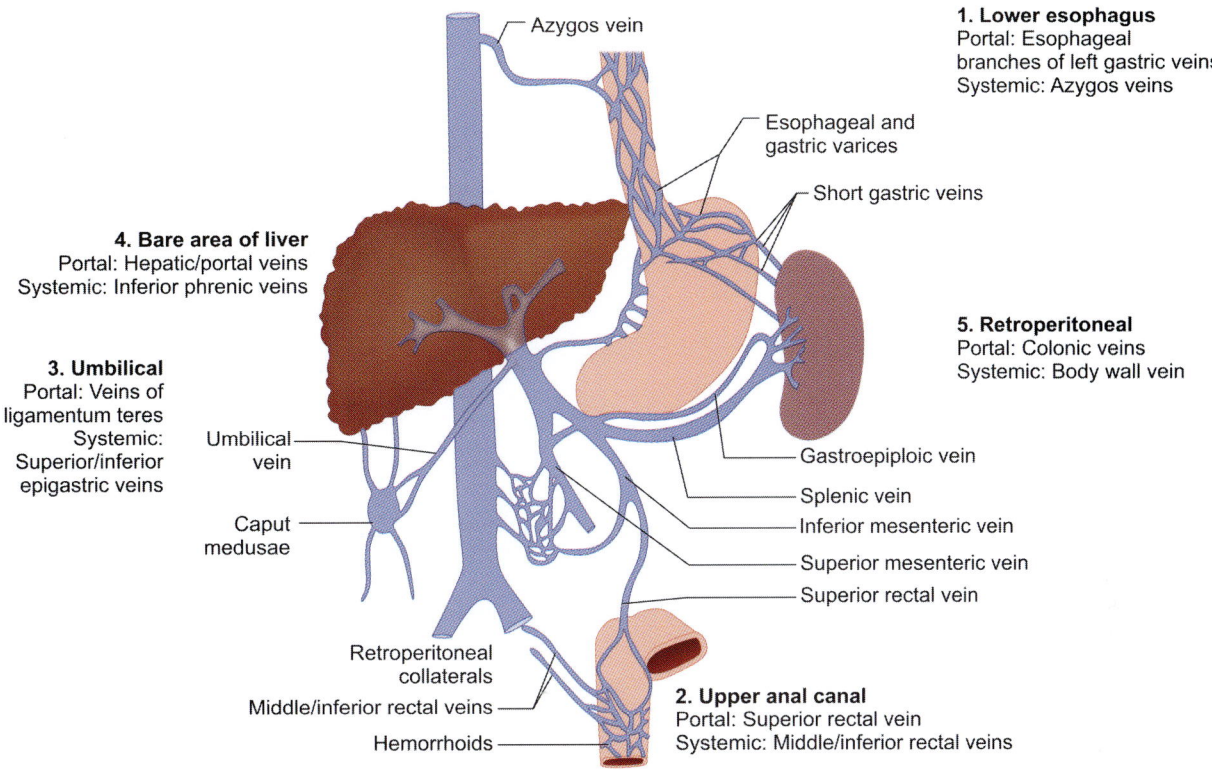

Fig. 5D.66: Sites of portosystemic anastomosis in cirrhosis.

CLASSIFICATION OF PORTAL HYPERTENSION (FIG. 5D.67)

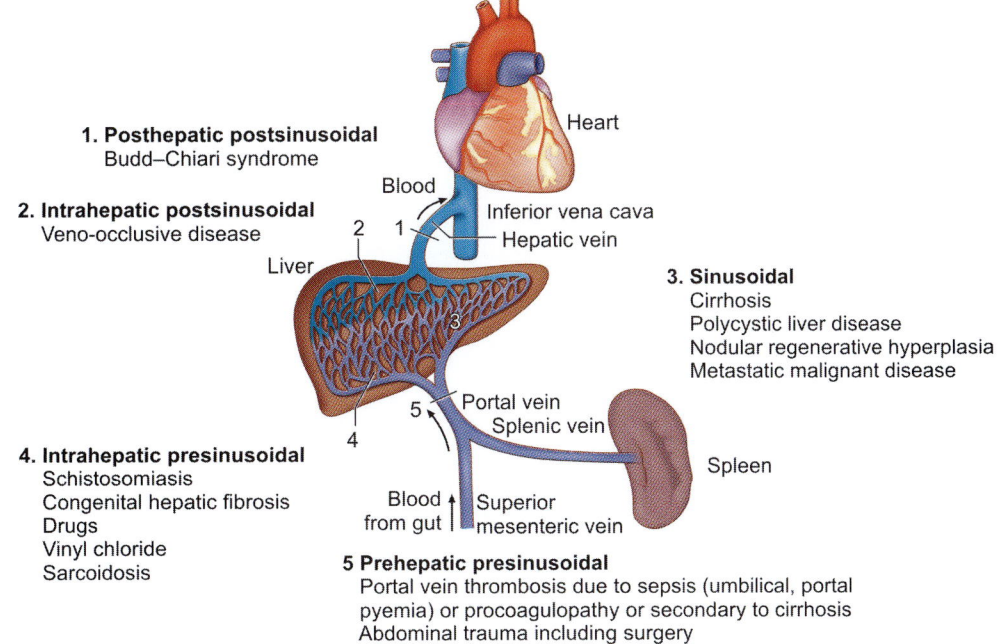

Fig. 5D.67: Classification of portal hypertension according to site of vascular obstruction.

NOTES

Chapter 6: Nervous System

A. CASE SHEET FORMAT

HISTORY TAKING

Name:
Age:
Sex:
Residence:
Occupation:

Chief complaints:
1. _____ × days
2. _____ × days
3. _____ × days

History of presenting illness:

HIGHER MENTAL FUNCTION

Altered state of consciousness:
- Onset
- Any seizures and blackouts
- Any fall/head injuries
- Any ear or nose bleed
- Any ear pain or discharge
- Fever
- Drug history
- Any addictions.

Mental state and cognition:
- State of alertness and drowsiness
- Memory disturbances
- Language disturbances
- Changes in the mood and affect (loss of spontaneity)
- Loss of spatial orientation
- Diminished ability to carry out routine activities of daily living.

Other higher mental functions:
- Speech difficulty
- Difficulty to recognize people or objects
- Inappropriate crying or laughter
- Lack of interest
- Social disinhibition
- Delusions/hallucinations.

CRANIAL NERVE DYSFUNCTION

Ask about:
- Alterations in smell, vision, and taste
- Double vision/visual symptoms
- Alteration in facial sensation
- Facial asymmetry
- Difficulty in swallowing and chewing
- Speech alterations
- Vertigo/hearing abnormalities/ringing sensation in the ears
- Hoarseness of voice, nasal regurgitation, and nasal intonation of speech
- Pain/difficulty in neck movements.

MOTOR DYSFUNCTION

Weakness

Distribution of weakness:
- Is it symmetrical/asymmetrical
- Complete or partial weakness
- Limbs involved: Ipsilateral or contralateral
- Patterned weakness.

Onset and progression:
- *Acute, subacute, or chronic.*

Progression of the weakness:
- *Ascending weakness or descending weakness*
- *Ellsberg phenomenon*
- *Variation throughout the day*
- *Muscles/limb(s) involved.*

Proximal upper limb—shoulder/arm	Difficulty in combing hair, reaching overhead objects, winging of scapula
Distal upper limb—forearm/hand	Finger/wrist drop, poor hand grip, cannot open jar, difficulty in buttoning/unbuttoning
Proximal lower limb—pelvic/thigh	Cannot rise from chair or squatting position, waddling gait
Distal upper limbs—leg/foot	Difficulty in gripping *chappals*, cannot walk on heels/toes, foot drop
Neck muscles	Dropped head/broken neck
Trunk	Inability to roll on the bed, sit up from lying position

Example
Guillain–Barré syndrome (GBS): History of preceding gastrointestinal (GI) infection followed by acute onset difficulty in getting up from squatting position, difficulty walking, progressing to involve upper limbs (difficulty combing hair), and neck muscle weakness. No sensory symptoms.

Wasting/Loss of Muscle Bulk
- Wasting—present/absent
- Fasciculations—present/absent

Stiffness of Limbs
- Stiffness—present/absent
- Heaviness—present/absent

Gait Abnormalities
- Limp or dragging foot
- Criss-cross walking (scissoring)/swinging leg in semicircles (circumduction)

Involuntary Movements
- Type
- Symmetrical/Asymmetrical
- Part of the body involved
- Present at rest
- Functional disability.

SENSORY DYSFUNCTION
- Numbness/loss of feeling
- Altered sensations
  - Paresthesia (tingling and pin-needles)
  - Spontaneous pain
  - With stimulus
- Pattern of sensory loss.

CEREBELLAR HISTORY
- Swaying to one side
- Tremors while reaching objects
- Lack of coordination of activities
- Overshooting acts
- Abnormal involuntary eye movements (oscillopsia/nystagmus).

HISTORY SUGGESTING MENINGITIS/RAISED INTRACRANIAL PRESSURE
- Headache
- Neck pain
- Projectile vomiting
- Blurring of vision
- Seizures
- Photophobia.

HISTORY SUGGESTING AUTONOMIC DYSFUNCTION
- Dryness of skin
- Palpitations
- Excessive perspiration
- Syncopal attacks/postural giddiness
- Bladder dysfunction:
  - Urinary retention
  - Loss of awareness of bladder control
  - Frequency, urgency
  - Urge/overflow incontinence.

REVIEW OF COMMON NEUROLOGICAL SYMPTOMS

Headaches
- Onset and duration of headache
- Location of headache, unilateral versus bilateral
- Severity
- Frequency
- Radiation
- Quality of headache (dull and diffuse)
- Types:
  a. Continuous
  b. Pulsating
  c. Stabbing
  d. Sharp
  e. Throbbing
  f. Dull
  g. Thunderclap
- Alleviating factors
- Triggers for the headache/aggravating factors
- Temporal association
- Association with nausea/vomiting/tearing of eyes/redness of eyes
- Vision changes before or during headache
- Precipitating factors:
  - Stress
  - Variation with menstrual cycle
  - Allergens
  - Sleep deprivation
  - Coughing
  - Straining
  - Bending forwards
- Associated motor/sensory symptoms: Weakness, numbness, and tingling in upper or lower extremities

- Photophobia/phonophobia
- Systemic symptoms—weight loss, low energy, and anorexia
- Fever and neck stiffness
- History of head trauma
- History of migraine
- Family history of migraines
- Effect on daily activities
- Use of oral contraceptive pills
- Caffeine intake
- Smoking and alcohol history
- Other substance abuse history.

Example
Classical migraine: Visual aura followed by insidious onset, unilateral, severe pulsating type of heading lasting for >4 hours associated with nausea and photophobia. Repeated such attacks every month with a history of some identifiable precipitating factors and a positive family history of migraine.

Seizures
- Age at onset/duration of illness
- Duration of each episode
- Frequency
- Factors which precipitate these episodes
- Injuries sustained as a result of the seizure
- Postictal symptoms: Confusion
- Associated sensory deficits
- Associated motor deficits
- Associated cognitive deficits
- Muscle spasms
- Anatomical progression of motor involvement (e.g., Jacksonian March)
- Symptoms suggesting aura
- Associated incontinence
- Tongue biting and salivation
- Automatisms associated with these episodes
- History of head trauma
- Perinatal infection
- Drug history
- History of seizure disorder in the past/childhood
- Family history of seizure disorders
- Effect on daily activities.

Example
Generalized tonic-clonic seizure (GTCS): Abrupt onset tonic-clonic contraction of muscle associated with tongue bite and urinary incontinence. Patients generally regain consciousness within few minutes with postictal confusion and headache.

Past history:
- Asthma
- Chronic obstructive airway disease
- Tuberculosis
- History of contact with tuberculosis
- Diabetes mellitus (DM)
- Hypertension (HTN)
- Ischemic heart disease (IHD)
- Seizure disorder and drugs used (in detail)
- Neurological interventions/surgeries.

Family history:
(Draw pedigree chart representing three generations)

Personal history:
- Bowel habits
- Bladder habits
- Appetite
- Loss of weight
- Occupational exposure
- Sleep
- Dietary habits and taboo
- Food allergies
- Smoking (in smoking Index or Pack years)
- Alcohol history (_____grams of alcohol/day or_____ units of alcohol/week).

Menstrual and obstetric history:
- G__P__L__A__
- Age of menarche____
- Menopause at____
- Flow—amenorrhea/oligomenorrhea/menorrhagia.

Summarize:
Differential diagnosis:
1.
2.
3.

GENERAL EXAMINATION
Patient
- Conscious
- Coherent
- Cooperative
- Obeying commands

Body Mass Index (BMI)
- Wt (kg)/Ht^2 (meters)
- Grading according to WHO for Southeast Asian countries.

Vitals
- **Pulse**
  - Rate
  - Rhythm
  - Volume
  - Character
  - Vessel wall thickening
  - Radio-radial delay and radio-femoral delay
  - Peripheral pulses
- **Carotid and vertebral bruit**
- **Blood pressure**
  - Right arm
  - Left arm
  - Leg—right/left
- **Respiratory rate**
  - Regular
  - Abdominothoracic (male) or thoracoabdominal (female)
  - Usage of accessory muscles

- **Jugular venous pulse**
  - Waveform
- **Jugular venous pressure**
  - __ cm of blood above sternal angle (+5 cm water)

On Physical Examination
- Pallor
- Icterus
- Cyanosis
- Clubbing
- Lymphadenopathy
- Edema

Others Head to Toe
- Nerve thickening
- Neurocutaneous markers
- External markers of atherosclerosis
- Signs of nutritional deficiency, alcoholism, etc.
- Any other general examination finding

NERVOUS SYSTEM EXAMINATION
- Right/left-handed person
- Education

HIGHER MENTAL FUNCTIONS
- Consciousness—if impaired document using Glasgow coma scale
- Orientation to time/place/person
- Memory:
  - Immediate (repetition—30 seconds)
  - Recent (up to 5 minutes—recall)
  - Remote (>5 minutes)
- Intelligence
- Mood/emotion
- Concentration and calculation (subtract seven from 100)
- Speech:
  - comprehension
  - Fluency/Word output
  - Repetition
  - Reading
  - Writing
  - Naming objects
  - Phonation
  - Aphasia
  - Dysarthria
- Apraxia—present/absent
- Hemineglect—present/absent
- Hallucinations and delusions—present/absent

Cranial nerves	R	L

Olfactory—I nerve:
Sense of smell (peppermint, soap, coffee, lemon peel or vanilla)
*Both eyes shut, one nostril checked at a time
Appreciate smell ± identify it

Contd...

Contd...

Optic—II nerve:
Visual acuity (perception of light/hand movements and finger counting/Snellen's chart at 6 meters/Jaeger's chart at 14 inches)
Visual field (confrontation method/menace reflex)—mention defects, if any
Color vision (Ishihara's test)
Fundus

Oculomotor, trochlear, abducens—III, IV, VI nerves:
Eyelids (any ptosis)
Position of eyeballs at rest (any deviation, exophthalmos, enophthalmos) Extraocular movements:
I. Binocular movements
   - Saccadic:
   - Pursuit:
   - Reflex (doll's eye, caloric stimulation)
II. Uniocular movements
   (#Comment on ophthalmoplegia, if present—supranuclear, internuclear, individual nerves, or muscles)
Pupil
- Size (in mm)
- Shape
- Reaction
- Direct light reflex
- Consensual light reflex
- Accommodation reflex
Nystagmus
(Describe whether spontaneous or provoked type—horizontal, vertical, rotatory or pendular)

Trigeminal nerve—V nerve:
- **Sensory:**
  - Touch
  - Pain
  - Temperature
  - (To be checked on all three divisions around the jawline, on the cheek, and on the forehead)
- **Motor:**
  - Jaw deviation
  - Hollowing above and below zygoma
  - Clenching teeth (feel temporalis and masseter)
  - Open mouth against resistance
  - Side to side movement of jaw (pterygoid)
- **Reflexes:**
  - Corneal—present/absent (superficial reflex, 5th nerve afferent, 7th nerve efferent)
  - Jaw jerk—present/absent/exaggerated (deep reflex, afferent and efferent, both 5th nerve, center mid-pons)

Facial nerve—VII nerve:
Facial asymmetry (look for absence of wrinkling, drooping of corner of mouth, obliteration of nasolabial fold, widened palpebral fissures)

Contd...

Contd...
- **Motor:**
  - Frontalis (raise the eyebrows)
  - Orbicularis oculi (shut the eyes tight)
  - Buccinator (show teeth, smile, blow check, whistle)
  - Orbicularis oris (close lips, pronounce labials "p","#"b","#"m")
  - Platysma (pull down the corners of mouth)
  (## Look for Bell's phenomenon)
- **Sensory:**
  - Anterior 2/3rd tongue taste (sugar, lime, salt, quinine)

Lacrimation hyperacusis—present/absent
Emotional fibers checking—emotions preserved or not

Vestibulocochlear nerve—VIII nerve:
The ability to hear the sound produced by rubbing the thumb and forefinger together is then tested for each ear at distances up to a few centimeters
- Rinne's test—air conduction/bone conduction (AC/BC)
- Weber's test—lateralized/centralized
- Caloric test [Irrigates one external auditory canal with cool (about 30°C) or warm (40°C) water. Normally, cool water in one ear produces nystagmus on the opposite side. Warm water produces it on the same side]

Glossopharyngeal, vagus IX, X nerve: Note the patient's ability to drink water and eat solid food and also see the character, volume and sound of the patient's voice.
- Position of uvula at rest
- Movement of uvula on saying "ah"— any deviation
- Gag reflex—present/absent/exaggerated
- Taste over the posterior third of the tongue and can be tested

Spinal accessory—XI nerve:
- Sternocleidomastoid (instruct the patient to rotate head against resistance applied to the side of the chin to tests the function of the opposite sternocleidomastoid muscle. To test both sternocleidomastoid muscles together, the patient flexes the head forward against resistance placed under the chin)
- Trapezius (shrugging a shoulder against resistance)

Hypoglossal nerve—XII:
Inspection:
- Size of tongue
- Symmetry/any wasting
- Fasciculation (inside mouth)
- Deviation—side (on protrusion)
- Tremors

Palpation:
- Tone
- Power

MOTOR SYSTEM

Attitude
- Upper limb
- Lower limb

Bulk
Inspection: Symmetry, generalized wasting comment on small muscle wasting, deformities, claw hand, foot drop, if any.

Measurement in cm	R	L
Arm (10 cm above olecranon)		
Forearm (10 cm below olecranon)		
Thigh (18 cm above the superior border of patella)		
Leg (10 cm below the tibial tuberosity)		

Note: Bilateral similar distance from fixed bony points till the maximum bulk of muscle.

Tone

	R	L
Upper limb		
Lower limb		

Note: Comment whether normal, hypotonia or hypertonia (spasticity/rigidity).

Power
Fix the proximal portion of a limb when the movements of the distal portion are being examined.

0	Complete paralysis
1	A flicker of contraction only
2	Power detectable only when gravity is excluded by postural adjustment
3	Limb can be held against gravity but not resistance
4	Limb can be held against gravity and some resistance
5	Normal power

Muscle	R	L

Neck
- **Flexors** (SCM, platysma, scalene, suprahyoid, infrahyoid, longus colli and capitis, rectus capitis)
- **Extensors** (trapezius and paravertebral muscles—splenius, erector spinae, transversospinalis, interspinal intertransverse)
- *Note:* Avoid active movement checking if cervical cord injury suspected.

Shoulder
- **Abduction** (0–15°—supraspinatus, 15–90°—middle fibers of deltoid, above 90°—trapezius and serratus anterior)
- **Adduction** (pectoralis major, latissimus dorsi and teres major)
- **Flexion** (biceps brachii (both heads), pectoralis major, anterior deltoid, and coracobrachialis)

Contd...

Contd...

- **Extension** (posterior deltoid, latissimus dorsi, and teres major)

Elbow
- Flexion (biceps brachii)
- Extension (triceps brachii)

Wrist
- Flexion (FCR, FCU)
- Extension (ECRL, ECRB, ECU)

Hand grip (long flexors)

Small muscles of hand

Trunk (rectus abdominis, transversus abdominis, oblique, pyramidalis)
- Elevation of head or leg in supine position
- Beevor's sign if present
- Abdominal breathing with epigastric bulging s/o intercostal muscle weakness
- Increased excursion of coastal margins, inability to sniff s/o diaphragmatic weakness

Scan QR code for Beevor's sign

Hip
- Flexion (iliopsoas)
- Extension (gluteus maximus)
- Abduction (gluteus medius and minimus, tensor fascia lata)
- Adduction (adductor longus, brevis, and magnus)

Knee
- Flexion (hamstrings—biceps femoris, semimembranosus and semitendinosus)
- Extension (quadriceps)

Ankle
- Plantar flexion (gastrocnemius, soleus)—stand on tip toe
- Dorsiflexion (tibialis anterior)—stand on heels
- Inversion (tibialis anterior and tibialis posterior)
- Eversion (peroneus longus, brevis and tertius)

Small muscles of foot, EHL (if needed)

REFLEXES

Superficial reflexes	R	L
Corneal (cranial nerve V and VII)		
Abdominal: - Epigastric (T6–T9) - Mid-abdominal (T9–T11) - Hypogastric (T11–L1)		
Cremasteric (L1, L2)		
Anal reflex (S2, S3)		
Plantar: - Reflexogenic zone—S1 - Afferent nerve—tibial nerve - SC segments—L4, L5, S1, S2		
Chaddock's (lateral aspect of foot from below up), Gordon's (calf), Oppenheim's (anterior tibia), Schaffer's (Achilles tendon), Gonda's (press down 4th toe), Stransky's (adduct little toe), Bing's (pinprick on dorsolateral foot)		

Deep tendon reflexes	R	L
Jaw jerk (afferent and efferent both 5th nerve and center mid-pons)		
Biceps (C5, C6)		

Contd...

Contd...

Brachioradial/supinator/radial periosteal (C5, C6)		
Triceps (C6, C7, C8)		
Knee jerk/quadriceps/patellar reflex (L2, L3, L4)		
Ankle jerk (L5, S1, S2)		
Clonus—present/absent - Patellar - Ankle		

Latent reflexes (suggest pyramidal lesion if present unilaterally) Tromner's/finger flexor reflex/Hoffmann's sign Wartenberg's sign

By convention the deep tendon reflexes are graded as follows:
- 0 = no response; always abnormal
- 1+ = a slight but definitely present response; may or may not be normal
- 2+ = a brisk response; normal
- 3+ = a very brisk response; may or may not be normal
- 4+ = a tap elicits a repeating reflex (clonus); always abnormal

Please do reinforcement maneuvers before saying DTR's are absent

Primitive reflexes
- Glabellar tap
- Palmomental (both sides)
- Sucking
- Rooting
- Pout and snout
- Grasp

Involuntary movements (describe in detail)
Coordination (described later under cerebellum)

SENSORY SYSTEM

Primary sensation	R	L
Touch		
Pain		
Temperature		
Vibration		
Joint position sense		
*Any sensory level		
*Pattern of sensory loss (graded/dissociative/crossed/hemi)		

Cortical sensation (to be tested only in the presence of intact primary sensation)	R	L
Tactile localization (topognosis)		
Two point discrimination		
Stereognosis		
Graphesthesia (figure identification)		
Sensory extinction		

Romberg's test:

CEREBELLAR SIGNS

Upper extremity	R	L
Limb ataxia: - Outstretched arm test - Finger nose test - Nose-finger-nose test - Finger-finger test		

Contd...

Contd...

Rapid alternating movements:
- Rapid hand tapping
- Pronation-supination
- Thigh slapping

Pointing and past pointing

Writing (macrographia)

Rebound phenomenon (arm)

Tremors (intention)

Lower limbs	R	L
Heel knee test		
Pendular knee jerk		
Finger toe test		
Rapid alternating movements—foot tapping		
General		
Titubation		
Nystagmus		
Tremors(intention)		
Hypotonia		
Truncal ataxia		
Tandem walking		
Gait		

GAIT

- Base—wide or narrow
- Slow/rapid
- Falling to sides
- Look which part of foot touches ground first (toe/heel)
- How high foot lifted above ground?
- Hand swing
- Turning around
- Position of hip, sound produced while foot touches ground.

Signs of Involvement of Autonomic Nervous System

- Dryness of skin/excessive sweating/spoon test
- Postural hypotension
- Heart rate—baseline, on respiration, on standing
- Palpable bladder
- Pupillary reactions
- Valsalva maneuver.

Signs of Meningeal Irritation

- Neck stiffness
- Kernig's sign
- Brudzinski's sign—neck, leg, and pubis.

Skull and Spine

- Deformities
- Tenderness
- Short neck.

SOFT NEUROLOGICAL SIGNS

- ***Pyramidal/pronator drift*** describes a tendency for the hand to move upward and supinate if the hands are held outstretched in a pronated position (palms downward), or to pronate downward if the hands are held in supination.
- ***Cerebellar drift*** is generally outward and slightly upward
- ***Parietal drift*** is an updrift due to loss of position sense
- ***Nonorganic—downward drift without pronation***
- ***Pseudo drift—slight pronation without downward drift***

OTHER SYSTEMS

Respiratory system:
- Inspection:
- Palpation:
- Percussion:
- Auscultation:

Cardiovascular system:
- Inspection:
- Palpation:
- Percussion:
- Auscultation:

Gastrointestinal system:
- Inspection:
- Palpation:
- Percussion:
- Auscultation:

B. DIAGNOSIS FORMAT

GENERAL FORMAT

Nature of Disease

- Onset: Sudden/acute/subacute/chronic (sudden—vascular, acute—demyelinating, subacute—infections/space occupying lesions, chronic—degenerative)
- Deficit: Monoplegia/hemiplegia/quadriplegia/paraplegia/nerve palsies/ataxia/sensory disturbance/movement disorders.

Site of Involvement of Nervous System

- Upper motor neuron disease—intracranial (brain or cerebellum) or extracranial (spinal cord)
- Lower motor neuron disease—anterior horn cell disease, radiculopathies, neuropathies, neuromuscular junction diseases, and myopathies.

FOR CEREBROVASCULAR ACCIDENT

Sudden onset, right-sided dense hemiplegia with right upper motor neuron (UMN) facial palsy due to cerebrovascular accident possible thrombotic in etiology with site of lesion being left internal capsule, possibly involving the lenticulostriate branch of middle cerebral artery (MCA). Patient is in state of neuronal shock. Patient has following risk factors _____.

FOR NEUROPATHY

Acute onset of symmetrical flaccid quadriplegia (ascending) with no evidence of sensory, bowel, bladder involvement with bilateral lower motor neuron (LMN) facial palsy, possible site of lesion in the peripheral nerve, pathology being demyelination—acute inflammatory demyelinating polyneuropathy (AIDP).

FOR SPINAL CORD DISEASE

Subacute onset of symmetrical spastic paraplegia with involvement of sensory, bladder, and bowel; with no involvement of cranial nerves with vertebral tenderness at T4-5, possible site of lesion is spinal cord, the disease being compressive myelopathy.
- Horizontal level
  - Extradural extramedullary
- Vertical level
  - Motor level: Above T10
  - Sensory level: At T8
  - Autonomic level: Above T12
  - Reflex level: Above T10
  - Spinal level: T8
  - Vertebral level: T5.

Possible etiology: Tuberculosis—Pott's spine.

FOR EXTRAPYRAMIDAL (PARKINSON'S DISEASE)

Insidious onset, slowly progressive, degenerative disease involving the motor system (in the form of rigidity and tremors) with no evidence of sensory, cranial nerves or bowel, bladder, we would consider involvement of extrapyramidal system probably parkinsonism with no evidence of secondary causes, no signs or symptoms of Parkinson's plus syndromes, functional status—Stage III (Hoehn and Yahr staging system).

FOR ATAXIA

Insidious onset, slowly progressive, symmetrical ataxia and cerebellar signs of trunk and limbs with no evidence of sensory, cranial nerve or autonomic involvement. I would like to consider the possibility of degenerative cerebellar ataxia possibly inherited (family history +ve).

C. CENTRAL NERVOUS SYSTEM: DISCUSSION ON CARDINAL SYMPTOMS

DISCUSSION ON CARDINAL SYMPTOMS

Taking a Neurological History

The neurological history should be a focused, goal-directed exercise that seeks to answer the following questions:
1. Which part of the nervous system is affected by "a pathological process" and is causing the symptoms (where is the lesion)? Is it a single lesion or are there multiple diffuse lesions? Alternatively, is there a diffuse problem affecting many neurological systems?
2. What is the underlying pathological process (e.g., vascular, inflammatory, degenerative)?
3. Is this a purely neurological problem or a neurological manifestation of a systemic disease?

Note:
- Ask the patient to tell their story in their own words
- Explore each symptom in detail, evaluating the evolution and the way the symptoms affect the ability to function
- Ask for an eyewitness account when cognition or consciousness is involved
- If you cannot make a neurological diagnosis, take the history again before arranging investigations.

Pathology of neurological diseases		
Acute	Subacute	Chronic
Vascular-stroke Demyelination Metabolic	Infection Space occupying lesions Metabolic	Degeneration

HIGHER MENTAL FUNCTION

Altered State of Consciousness
- Onset
- Any seizures, blackouts
- Any fall/injuries
- Any ear or nose bleed
- Fever
- Any ear pain or discharge
- Drug history
- Any addictions.

Other Higher Mental Functions
- Speech difficulty
- Difficulty to recognize people or objects
- Memory defects
- Inappropriate crying or laughter
- Lack of interest
- Social disinhibition
- Delusions/hallucinations.

Mental State and Cognition
- Changes in the memory
- State of alertness and drowsiness
- Changes in the mood and affect (loss of spontaneity)
- Language changes
- Loss of spatial orientation
- Diminished ability to carry out routine activities of daily living.

CRANIAL NERVE DYSFUNCTION

Ask about:

CN	Symptoms
1	Smell disturbance
2, 3, 4, 6	Diplopia, blurred vision, blindness, difficulty in opening eyelid (CN3)
5	Difficulty in chewing, loss of sensations over face
7	Deviation of angle of mouth, accumulation of food at one side of the mouth, dribbling of saliva, loss of taste sensation, hyperacusis
8	Tinnitus, hearing loss, dizziness, loss of balance
9, 10	Nasal intonation, nasal regurgitation of food, dysphagia, difficulty in speech, hoarseness of voice
11	Difficulty in neck/shoulder movements
12	Difficulty in mixing food in the mouth, difficulty in speech

For example: *Left LMN 7th nerve palsy—history of retroauricular pain followed by abrupt onset deviation of angle of mouth to right with slurring of speech and difficulty in left eye closure with history of hyperacusis.*

MOTOR DYSFUNCTION

Weakness

Distribution of Weakness
- Is it symmetrical/asymmetrical?
- Plegia—complete loss of power—0/5 versus paresis—incomplete loss of power
- One limb: Monoparesis
- Two limbs, same side: Hemiparesis
- Both lower limbs: Paraparesis
- All four limbs: Quadriparesis (or tetraparesis)
- **Pentaplegia** is a spinal cord injury at or above C4 level, resulting in complete loss of motor functions below the injury level and paralysis of respiratory muscles.
- **Diplegia/triplegia:** Two (contralateral to each other) or three limbs (upper and lower limbs), e.g., right upper limb and left lower limb or left arm and both legs, both arms and one leg.
- Patterned weakness: The pattern of pyramidal weakness is weakness of upper limbs extensors and lower limbs flexors.

For example: *Right MCA territory embolic infarct—history of sudden onset, complete loss of power in left upper limb, lower limb associated with left UMN facial palsy. Weakness—maximum at onset, nonprogressive.*

Causes of monoplegia affecting the lower limb	Causes of monoplegia affecting the upper limb
1. Stroke, affecting anterior cerebral artery territory. 2. Cerebral venous sinus thrombosis affecting superior sagittal sinus. 3. Trauma, head injury, with contusion in the frontal lobe. 4. Infection, such as granuloma affecting frontal lobe. 5. Trauma to the lumbosacral plexus, diabetic lumbosacral plexopathy. 6. Functional or psychogenic.	1. Stroke, affecting superior division of contralateral middle cerebral artery territory, affecting parietal lobe, or unpaired anterior cerebral artery. 2. Head injury, with contusion in the parietal lobe. 3. Trauma to the brachial plexus. 4. Injury to multiple cervical nerve roots. 5. Functional or psychogenic.

Causes of hemiplegia

1. Ischemic or hemorrhagic stroke, affecting contralateral cerebral hemisphere, internal capsule, brainstem or ipsilateral upper cervical cord.
2. Cerebral venous sinus thrombosis with venous infarction of contralateral cerebral hemisphere.
3. Acute central nervous system infection, such as meningitis or encephalitis, brain abscess, granulomatous infections.
4. Head injury causing contusion/bleeding in the contralateral cerebral hemisphere, internal capsule, basal ganglia, or brainstem.
5. Tumor affecting cerebral hemisphere, internal capsule, basal ganglia, brainstem or cervical cord.
6. Bleeding into a brain tumor on the contralateral side.
7. Demyelinating illness, such as acute disseminated encephalomyelitis (ADEM) or multiple sclerosis (MS).
8. Todd's paresis.
9. Mill's hemiplegic variant of motor neuron disease (MND).

Causes of Quadriplegia (Table 6C.1)

TABLE 6C.1: Causes of quadriplegia.

UMN causes	LMN causes
- Cerebral palsy - Bilateral brainstem lesion (glioma) - Craniovertebral junction anomaly - High cervical cord compression - Multiple sclerosis - Motor neuron disease	- Acute anterior poliomyelitis - GB syndrome - Peripheral neuropathy - Myopathy or polymyositis - Myasthenia gravis - Periodic paralysis - Snake bite, organophosphorus poisoning, etc.

Causes of Paraplegia

Causes of Flaccid Paraplegia (LMN type)

- **UMN lesion in shock stage,** i.e., sudden onset or history of long duration as in extradural transverse myelitis and spinal injury **(Table 6C.2)**
- **Lesion involving anterior horn cells:**
  - Acute anterior poliomyelitis
  - Progressive muscular atrophy (a variety of motor neuron disease)
- **Diseases affecting nerve root:** Tabes dorsalis, radiculitis, GB syndrome
- **Diseases affecting peripheral nerves:**
  - Acute inflammatory demyelinating polyradiculoneuropathy (GB syndrome)
  - High cauda equina syndrome

Contd...

Contd...

- Disease of peripheral nerves involving both the lower limbs
- Lumbar plexus injury (psoas abscess or hematoma)
- **Diseases affecting myoneural junction:**
  - Myasthenia gravis, Lambert-Eaton syndrome
  - Periodic paralysis due to hypo- or hyperkalemia
- **Diseases affecting muscles:** Myopathy.

Onset and Progression

- Onset—acute, subacute, or chronic.
- Progression—reversible, stable nonreversible, fluctuating, stuttering or step-ladder, or progressive.
- **Ascending weakness**—first lower limbs → upper limbs (GB syndrome, extramedullary compressive myelopathy)
- **Descending weakness**—first upper limbs → lower limbs (Miller Fisher variant of GB syndrome, intramedullary compressive myelopathy).
- **Ellsberg phenomenon**—compressive lesions near the high cervical cord produce weakness of the ipsilateral shoulder and arm followed by weakness of the ipsilateral leg, then the contralateral leg, and finally the contralateral arm, an "anticlock-wise" pattern that may begin in any of the four limbs.

TABLE 6C.2: Causes of spastic paraplegia [upper motor neuron (UMN) type lesion].

A. Gradual onset	B. Sudden onset
Cerebral causes	
- Parasagittal meningioma - Hydrocephalus	- Thrombosis of unpaired anterior cerebral artery or superior sagittal sinus
Spinal causes	
Compressive or transverse lesion in the spinal cord: Cord compression **Noncompressive or longitudinal lesion** or systemic disease of the spinal cord - Motor neuron disease (MND), e.g., amyotrophic lateral sclerosis - Multiple sclerosis, Friedreich's ataxia - Subacute combined degeneration (i.e., from vitamin B_{12} deficiency) - Lathyrism, Syringomyelia, Erb's spastic paraplegia, Tropical spastic paraplegia - Radiation myelopathy	**Compressive causes** - Injury to the spinal cord (fracture-dislocation or collapse of the vertebra) - Intervertebral disc prolapse - Spinal epidural abscess or hematoma **Noncompressive causes** - Acute transverse myelitis - Thrombosis of anterior spinal artery - Hematomyelia (from arteriovenous malformation, angiomas, or endarteritis)

Muscles/Limb(s) Involved

Proximal upper limb—shoulder/arm:	Difficulties combing hair, reaching for high objects, winging of scapula
Distal upper limb—forearm/hand:	Finger/wrist drop, poor hand grip, cannot open jar, difficulty in buttoning/unbuttoning

Contd...

Contd...

Proximal lower limb—pelvic/thigh:	Cannot rise from chair or squatting position, waddling gait
Distal lower limbs—leg/foot:	Difficulty in gripping chappals, cannot walk on heels/toes, foot drop
Neck muscles	Dropped head/broken neck
Trunk	Inability to roll on the bed

Variation throughout day—fatigability: In postsynaptic neuromuscular junction disorders like myasthenia gravis the weakness worsens on exertion.
- **Wasting/loss of muscle bulk**—wasting is a feature of LMN disease. Florid wasting is seen in motor neuron disease. Usually associated with fasciculations. In late stages of UMN disease, disuse atrophy may be seen. Wasting of muscles also results in undue prominence of underlying bones.
- **Stiffness of limbs**—increased tone of the limbs resulting in stiffness and heaviness of limbs is a characteristic feature of UMN disease. Patients may complain that the limbs are heavy as log of wood in spasticity, while they may say that the limbs are floppy in LMN diseases.
- **Gait abnormalities:** It may aid in the diagnosis.
  - Limp or dragging foot—might suggest LMN disease/foot drop
  - Scissoring/circumduction may suggest UMN disease.
- **Involuntary movements:**
  - Type
  - Symmetrical/asymmetrical
  - Part of the body involved
  - Present at rest
  - Functional disability.

SENSORY DYSFUNCTION

- Numbness/loss of feeling
- Altered feeling:
  - Paresthesia
  - Dysesthesias (tingling, pin-needles)
  - Spontaneous pain
- Pattern of sensory loss:

Pattern of sensory loss	Site of the lesion
Hemisensory loss—same side face and body	Internal capsule/thalamus
Crossed sensory—one side face, opposite side body	Lateral medulla
Ascending sensory loss—lower limbs → upper limb	Extramedullary compressive myelopathy
Descending sensory loss—upper limbs → lower limb	Intramedullary compressive myelopathy
Dissociative sensory loss (only pain and temperature lost, posterior column sensations preserved)	Intramedullary compressive myelopathy (syringomyelia) Lateral medullary syndrome Anterior cord syndrome
Definite sensory level (below which all sensations lost)	Suggestive of spinal cord disease
Graded sensory loss—glove and stocking	Suggestive of peripheral neuropathy

Positive and Negative Symptoms

Abnormal sensory symptoms can be divided into two categories: Positive and negative.

Positive Symptoms

- Altered sensation that are described as pricking, bandlike, lightning-like, shooting aching, knife piercing or stabbing (lancination), burning, scarring, electrical. Such symptoms are often painful.
- Positive phenomena usually result from trains of impulses generated at sites of lowered threshold or heightened excitability along a peripheral or central sensory pathway.
- Because positive phenomena represent excessive activity in sensory pathways, they may or may not be associated with a sensory deficit (loss) on examination.

Negative Symptoms

- Represent loss of sensory function and are characterized by diminished or absent feeling that often is experienced as numbness and by abnormal findings on sensory examination.
- It is estimated that at least one-half of the afferent axons innervating a particular site are lost or functionless before a sensory deficit can be demonstrated by clinical examinations.
- Subclinical degrees of sensory dysfunction may be revealed by sensory nerve conduction studies.
- Sensory symptoms may be either positive or negative but sensory signs on examination are always a measure of negative phenomena.

Sense	Test device	Endings activated	Fiber size mediating
Pain	Pin prick	Cutaneous nociceptors	Small
Temperature (heat)	Warm metal object	Cutaneous thermoreceptors for hot	Small
Temperature (cold)	Cold metal object	Cutaneous thermoreceptors for cold	Small
Touch	Cotton wisp, fine brush	Cutaneous mechanoreceptors, also naked endings	Large and small
Vibration	Tuning fork, 128 Hz	Mechanoreceptors, especially (Pacinian corpuscles)	Large
Joint position	Passive movements of specific joints	Ruffini endings in Joint capsule, muscle spindles	Large

CEREBELLAR EXAMINATION

Coordination and Balance

1. Difficulty in walking
2. Unsteadiness
3. Falls
4. Staggering
5. Loss of balance in dark.

AUTONOMIC DYSFUNCTION

Bladder Dysfunction (Table 6C.3)
- History of:
  - Urinary retention
  - Loss of awareness of bladder control
  - Frequency, urgency, urge and overflow maintenance.

MENINGEAL SIGNS
- Headache
- Projectile vomiting
- Photophobia
- Neck pain

OTHERS
Dizziness, vertigo, blackouts, and fatigue

Dizziness: It covers many complaints, from a vague feeling of unsteadiness to severe, acute vertigo. It is frequently used to describe lightheadedness felt in panic and anxiety, during palpitations, and in syncope or chronic ill-health. The real nature of this symptom must be determined.

Vertigo: An illusion of movement—is more definite. It is a sensation of rotation, or tipping. The patient feels that the surroundings are spinning or moving. It is distinctly unpleasant and often accompanied by nausea or vomiting and fear of fall.

Blackout like dizziness, is a descriptive term implying either altered consciousness, visual disturbance or falling. Epilepsy, syncope, hypoglycemia, anemia must be considered. However, commonly no sinister cause is found. A careful history from an eyewitness is essential.

Fatigue is another common symptom of neurological disorders.

TABLE 6C.3: Various causes of neurogenic bladder.

Type	Uninhibited bladder/ detrusor hyperreflexia	Automatic bladder/ detrusor sphincteric dyssynergia	Autonomous bladder/detrusor areflexia	Sensory atonic bladder	Motor atonic bladder
Site of lesion	Suprapontine neurologic disorder, mostly frontal lobe	UMN disorder of the suprasacral spinal cord	LMN lesion at the sacral cord	LMN lesion—peripheral nerve	
Causes	Frontal tumors, parasagittal meningioma, ACA aneurysm, NPH	Spinal cord trauma, compressive myelopathy, myelitis	Cauda equina syndrome, conus medullaris lesion, spinal shock	Diabetes mellitus, amyloidosis, tabes dorsalis	Lumbosacral meningomyelocele, tethered cord syndrome, lumbar canal stenosis
Bladder sensation	Preserved	Interrupted	Absent	Absent	Intact
Size of bladder	Normal	Small	Large	Large	Large
Ability to initiate voiding	Present	Absent	Absent	Present	Lost
Type of incontinence	Urge/social disinhibition	Urge	Overflow	Overflow	Overflow
Residual urine	Nil	Small	Large amount	Large	Large
Anal sphincter tone	Normal	Normal	Lost	Normal	Lost
Perianal sensation	Normal	Normal	Absent	Absent	Preserved
Bulbocavernous/ anal reflex	Normal	Normal	Absent	Absent	Preserved
Treatment	Anticholinergic medication	Self-intermittent catheterization	Continuous catheterization		

NECK PAIN

Deformities: Infantile torticollis	**Infections of bone:** TB of cervical spine. Pyogenic infection of cervical spine.	**Tumors:** Benign and malignant tumors in relation to cervical spine and nerve roots.
Arthritis of spinal joints: Rheumatoid arthritis-ankylosing spondylitis (RA-AS) Cervical spondylosis	**Mechanical derangement:** ■ Prolapsed cervical disc ■ Cervical spondylolisthesis ■ Whiplash injury ■ Cervical spine fracture ■ Neck muscle strain ■ Neck sprain	**Referred pain:** ■ Ear ■ Throat ■ Brachial plexus ■ Angina (pain extends to neck) ■ Aortic aneurysm ■ Meningismus

BACKACHE

Musculoskeletal	Infectious
- Nonspecific musculoskeletal backpain - Spondylolysis/spondylolisthesis - Scoliosis - Scheuermann disease - Disc degeneration and/or prolapsed	- Discitis - Vertebral osteomyelitis including tuberculosis (Pott disease) - Epidural abscess - Sacroiliac joint infection
Others	Nonspinal infection
- Intervertebral disc calcification - Congenital absence of pedicle - Vertebral apophyseal fracture - Aneurysmal bone cyst - Sacroiliac joint stress reaction - Idiopathic juvenile osteoporosis	- Paraspinous muscle abscess - Pyelonephritis - Pneumonia - Pelvic inflammatory disease - Endocarditis - Viral myalgias
Inflammatory	Neoplastic
- Ankylosing spondylitis - Psoriatic arthritis - Inflammatory bowel disease-associated arthritis - Reactive arthritis	- Osteoid osteoma - Leukemia or lymphoma - Solid malignancy, primary or metastatic - Other benign tumor: Neurofibroma, vascular malformation
Others	
- Appendicitis - Sickle cell pain crisis - Syringomyelia - Cholecystitis - Pancreatitis	- Chronic recurrent multifocal osteomyelitis - Psychosomatic illness - Nephrolithiasis - Ureteropelvic junction obstruction

RED FLAGS FOR ACUTE LOW BACK PAIN

History
- Cancer
- Unexplained weight loss
- Immunosuppression
- Prolonged use of steroids
- Intravenous drug use
- Urinary tract infection
- Pain worse at night or when supine
- Fever
- Significant trauma related to age
- Bladder or bowel incontinence
- Urinary retention (with overflow incontinence)

Physical examination
- Saddle anesthesia
- Loss of anal sphincter tone
- Major motor weakness in lower extremities
- Fever
- Vertebral tenderness
- Limited spinal range of motion
- Neurologic findings persisting beyond 1 month

NOTES

D(i). GENERAL EXAMINATION IN NEUROLOGY

GENERAL PHYSICAL EXAMINATION IN NERVOUS SYSTEM

Pulse
- Decreased pulse rate—increased intracranial pressure (ICP)—Cushing reflex
- Resting tachycardia autonomic dysfunction
- Irregularly irregular—atrial fibrillation (AF)
- Feeble pulse, carotid bruit–atherosclerosis.

Blood Pressure
- Increased BP—intracranial (IC) bleed—reactionary hypertension
- Cushing's reflex.
- Orthostatic hypotension

Jugular Venous Pressure
Increased in high output states.

Fever
- Meningitis
- Encephalitis
- CVA
- Brain abscess
- Epidural abscess
- Vasculitis
- ADEM
- seizures
- Hypothalamic dysfunction.

Pallor
- Vitamin B_{12} deficiency
- Pica, restless leg syndrome—iron deficiency
- Chronic liver disease (CLD), chronic kidney disease (CKD)—encephalopathy.

Icterus
- Hepatic encephalopathy
- Kernicterus.

Clubbing
- Syringomyelia
- Chronic hemiplegia
- Median nerve injury.

Lymphadenopathy
- Lymphoma—neuropathy, cerebellar ataxia, intracranial metastasis
- Paraneoplastic syndrome:
  - Lung carcinoma—Lambert-Eaton myasthenic syndrome
  - Lymphoma.
- Drug induced pseudo lymphoma—phenytoin.
- HIV
- Mononucleosis

Pedal Edema
- Chronic liver disease
- Chronic kidney disease
- Autonomic dysfunction.

Signs of Nutritional Deficiency
Discussed earlier.

NEUROCUTANEOUS SYNDROMES/ PHAKOMATOSES

The neurocutaneous syndromes include a heterogeneous group of disorders characterized by abnormalities of both the integument and central nervous system (CNS).

Most disorders are familial and believed to arise from a defect in differentiation of the primitive ectoderm.

Common neurocutaneous syndromes	
▪ Neurofibromatosis I and II ▪ Tuberous sclerosis ▪ Von Hippel–Lindau disease ▪ Ataxia-telangiectasia (Louis–Bar syndrome ▪ Sturge–Weber syndrome ▪ Klippel–Trenaunay–Weber syndrome ▪ Osler–Weber–Rendu syndrome ▪ PHACE syndrome ▪ Wyburn–Mason syndrome ▪ Linear nevus sebaceous syndrome ▪ Neurocutaneous melanosis ▪ Waardenburg syndrome type 1 and 2 ▪ Fabry's disease	▪ Lentiginosis, deafness, cardiopathy syndrome ▪ Hypomelanosis of Ito ▪ Xeroderma pigmentosum ▪ Cockayne's syndrome ▪ Rothmund-Thomson syndrome ▪ Sjögren-Larsson syndrome ▪ Neuroichthyosis ▪ Werner syndrome and progeria ▪ Incontinentia pigmenti ▪ Neurocutaneous melanosis ▪ Retinal—neurocutaneous cavernous hemangioma syndrome (Weskamp-Cotlier syndrome)

Neurofibromatosis [Fig. 6D(i).1]
Two types of neurofibromatosis (type 1 and type 2).

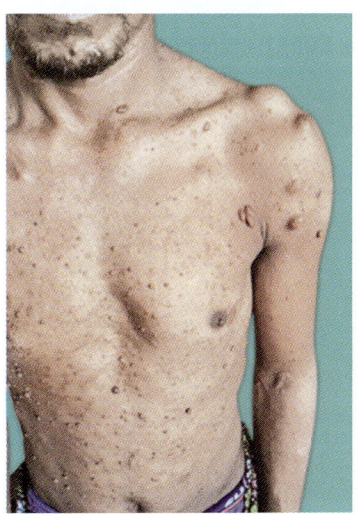

Fig. 6D(i).1: Neurofibromas.

Neurofibromatosis 1

Synonyms: von Recklinghausen disease and Watson disease. Most prevalent neurocutaneous syndrome.
- Autosomal dominant
- The *NF1* gene on chromosome region 17q11.2 encodes a protein also known as neurofibromin. Neurofibromin acts as an inhibitor of the oncogene Ras.

Diagnostic Criteria

Two out of the following seven signs
1. Six or more café-au-lait macules over 5 mm in greatest diameter in prepubertal individuals and over 15 mm in greatest diameter in postpubertal individuals.
2. Axillary or inguinal freckling.
3. Two or more iris Lisch nodules [**Fig. 6D(i).2**].
4. Two or more neurofibromas or one plexiform neurofibroma.
5. A distinctive osseous lesion, such as sphenoid dysplasia (which may cause pulsating exophthalmos) Or cortical thinning of long bones with or without pseudarthrosis.
6. Optic gliomas.
7. A first-degree relative with NF1 whose diagnosis was based on aforementioned criteria.

Conditions with Café-au-lait Macules [Fig. 6D(i).3]
- Neurofibromatosis type 1 and 2
- McCune–Albright syndrome
- Ataxia telangiectasia
- Bloom's syndrome
- Familial café-au-lait macules.

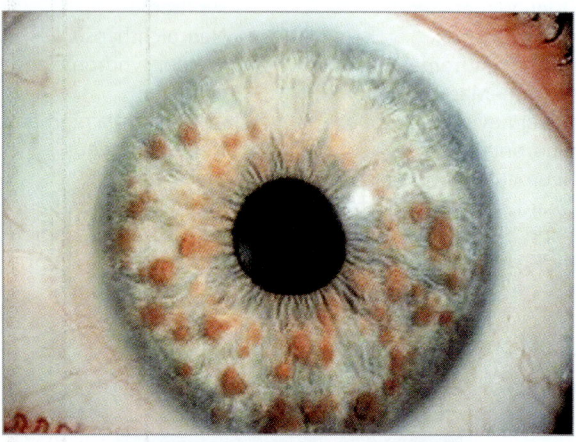

Fig. 6D(i).2: Iris nodules (Lisch nodules).

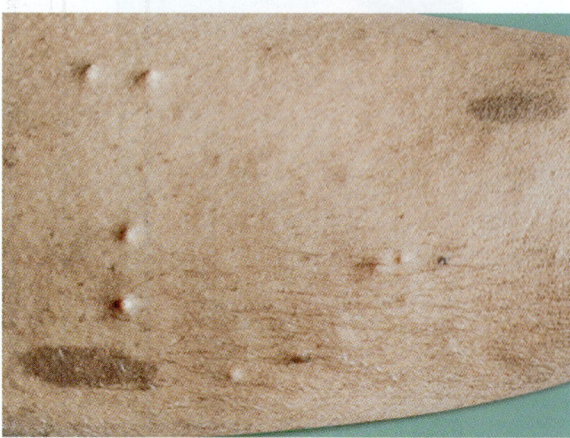

Fig. 6D(i).3: Café-au-lait macules (CALM).

Neurofibromatosis 2

The *NF2* gene (also known as merlin or schwannomin) is located on chromosome 22q1.11.

Diagnostic Criteria for Neurofibromatosis 2

One of the following three features is present
1. Bilateral vestibular schwannomas
2. A parent, sibling, or child with NF2 and either unilateral vestibular schwannoma or any two of the following: Meningioma, schwannoma, glioma, neurofibroma(ependymoma), or posterior subcapsular lenticular opacities
3. Multiple meningiomas (two or more) and unilateral vestibular schwannoma or any two of the following: Schwannoma, glioma, neurofibroma, or cataract.

Tuberous Sclerosis [Table 6D(i).1]
- Also called Bourneville disease
- Autosomal dominant
    - Widespread hamartomas—brain, eyes, skin, kidneys, liver, heart, and lungs.
    - Clinical triad described by Vogt:
      EPI-LOI-A
        - Epilepsy
        - Low intelligence
        - Adenoma sebaceum [**Figs. 6D(i).4A to C**].

TABLE 6D(i).1: Diagnostic criteria for tuberous sclerosis complex (TSC).

Major features	Minor features
Facial angiofibromas or forehead plaque	Multiple randomly distributed pits in dental enamel
Nontraumatic ungual or periungual fibroma (Koenen's tumour)	Hamartomatous rectal polyps
Shagreen patch (connective tissue nevus) **(Fig. 6D(i).4A)**	Bone cysts
Hypomelanotic macules (more than three) **(Fig. 6D(i).4B)**	Cerebral white matter migration lines
Multiple retinal nodular hamartomas	Gingival fibromas
Cortical tuber	Nonrenal hamartoma
Subependymal nodule	Retinal achronic patch
Subependymal giant cell astrocytoma	"Confetti" skin lesions
Cardiac rhabdomyoma, single or multiple	Multiple renal cysts
Lymphangiomyomatosis	
Renal angiomyolipoma	

Definite TSC: Either two major features or one major feature with two minor features
Probable TSC: One major feature and one minor feature
Possible TSC: Either one major feature or two or more minor features

Sturge–Weber Syndrome [Fig. 6D(i).5]
- Results from anomalous development of the primordial vascular bed in the early stages of cerebral vascularization.
- As a result, brain becomes atrophic and calcified, particularly in the molecular layer of the cortex.

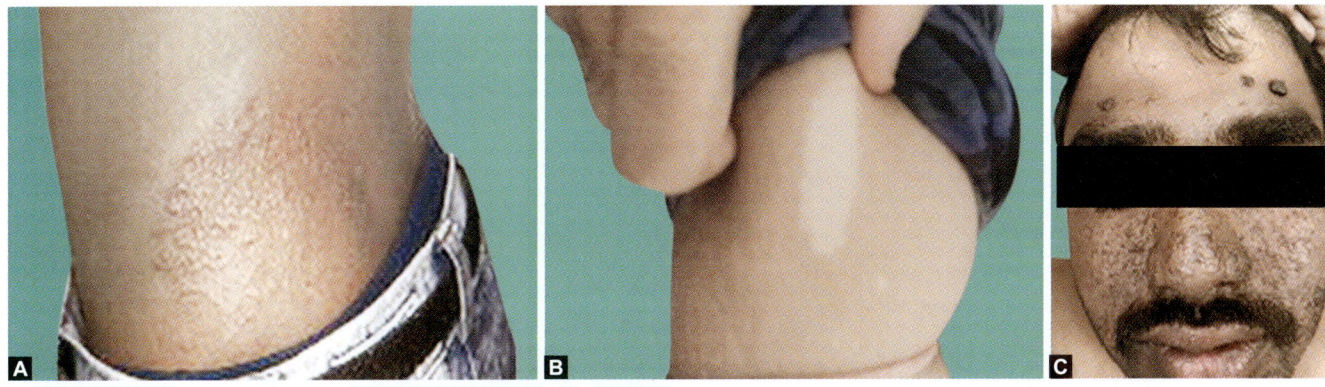

Figs. 6D(i).4A to C: (A) Shagreen patch; (B) Ash leaf-shaped macule is a hypopigmented macule oval at one end and pointed at the opposite end; (C) Adenoma sebaceum.

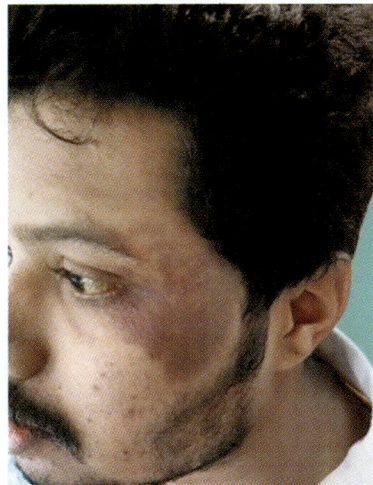

Fig. 6D(i).5: Sturge–Weber syndrome.

Clinical Manifestations

- Facial capillary malformation—port-wine stain
- Unilateral facial nevus
- Buphthalmos and glaucoma of the ipsilateral eye
- Seizures in the 1st year of life in most patients.

Skull Radiograph

Serpentine or railroad track intracranial calcification in the occipitoparietal region.

Von Hippel–Lindau Disease

- Autosomal dominant trait
- von Hippel–Lindau (VHL) tumor suppressor gene located on 3p25-26.

Clinical Features

- Cerebellar hemangioblastoma
- Retinal angioma
- Cystic lesions of the kidneys, pancreas, liver, and epididymis
- Pheochromocytoma.

Phace Syndrome

- Posterior fossa malformation
- Hemangiomas ipsilateral to the aortic arch
- Arterial anomalies
- Coarctation of the aorta, aplasia or hypoplasia of carotid arteries, aneurysmal carotid dilatation, aberrant left subclavian artery
- Eye abnormalities—glaucoma, cataracts, microphthalmia, and optic nerve hypoplasia.

Ataxia Telangiectasia

- Autosomal recessive
- Chromosome 11
- Cerebellar atrophy
- Telangiectasia appears on bulbar conjunctiva and skin
- Sinopulmonary infections
- Lymphoreticular malignancies
- Immune deficiency.

NERVE THICKENING

Detecting enlargement of accessible nerves is very helpful in assessing patients with peripheral nerve disorders, as only a few types of neuropathy lead to nerve thickening. Clinical landmarks and sites of palpable nerves are given in **Table 6D(i).2** and **Figure 6D(i).6**.

TABLE 6D(i).2: Clinical landmarks of palpable nerves.		
Nerve	Anatomical site	Palpated against
Supraorbital [Fig. 6D(i).7]	Forehead	Orbital ridge of frontal bone
Infraorbital	Cheek	Zygomatic bone
Greater auricular [Figs. 6D(i).8 and 6D(i).9]	Neck, anterior branch across the sternocleidomastoid, posterior branch over the sternocleidomastoid	Sternocleidomastoid
Ulnar [Fig. 6D(i).10]	Elbow joint	Behind medial epicondyle in olecranon groove
Superficial radial	Above wrist joint	Against lateral border of radius
Median	Near wrist joint, proximal to the flexor retinaculum	Against carpal bones
Common peroneal [Fig. 6.D(i).11]	Knee joint	Against fibular head

Contd...

Contd...

Posterior tibial	Ankle joint, below and behind medial malleolus	Against calcaneus
Sural	Lateral side of lower third of leg	Fibula

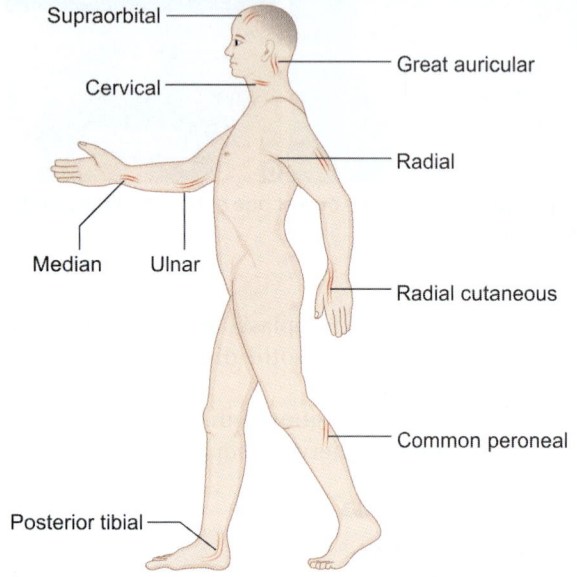

Fig. 6D(i).6: Sites of palpable nerves.

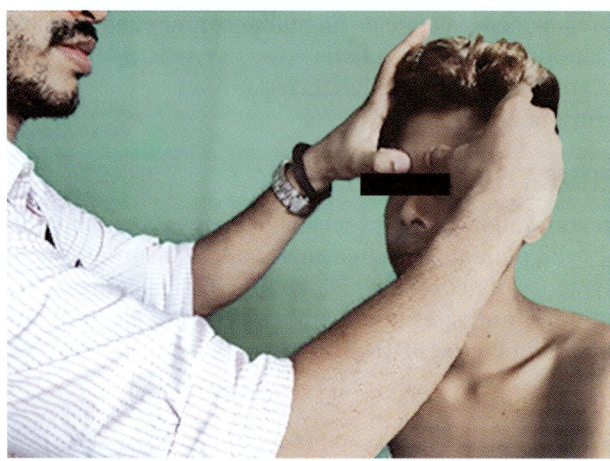

Fig. 6D(i).7: Supraorbital nerve.

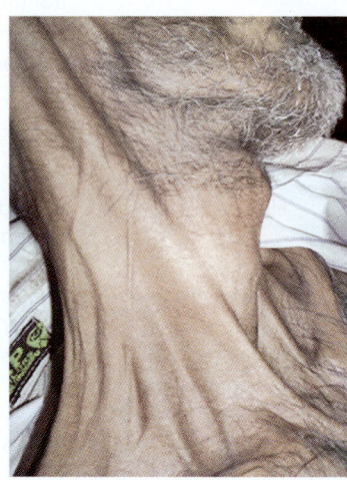

Fig. 6D(i).8: Greater auricular nerve.

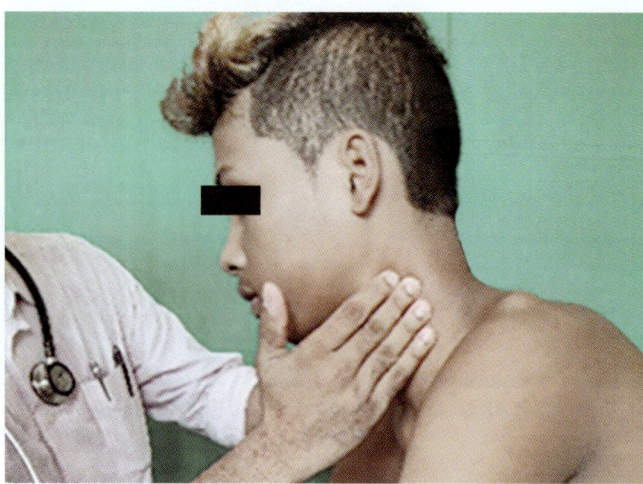

Fig. 6D(i).9: Greater auricular nerve of neck.

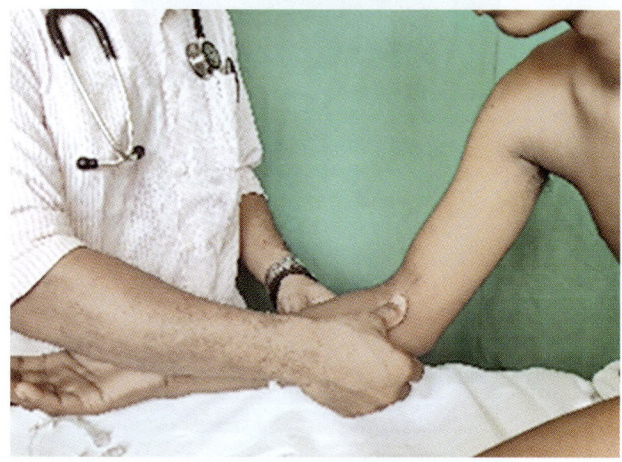

Fig. 6D(i).10: Ulnar nerve.

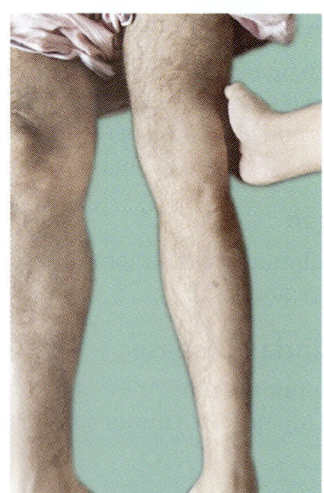

Fig. 6D(i).11: Common peroneal nerve.

Causes of Nerve Thickening

Infective Leprosy

Hereditary

- Hereditary motor and sensory neuropathy types 1 and 3 (Charcot–Marie–Tooth neuropathy, Dejerine–Sottas syndrome)
- Refsum's disease.

Acquired immune mediated:
- Chronic inflammatory demyelinating polyradiculoneuropathy (CIDP)
- Chronic inflammatory sensory polyradiculopathy (CISP)
- Multifocal acquired demyelinating sensory and motor polyneuropathy (MADSAM)
- Relapsing Guillian-Barre syndrome (GBS).

Tumors of nerves or nerve sheath:
- Localized hypertrophic neuropathy
- Schwannoma
- Neurofibromatosis 1 and 2.

Nerve infiltrations:
- Neurolymphomatosis
- Acromegaly
- Amyloidosis
- Sarcoidosis.

NOTES

D(ii). HIGHER MENTAL FUNCTIONS

NERVOUS SYSTEM EXAMINATION

Handedness

Handedness	
Right-handed (90–95%)	Left-handed (5–10%)
99% have—left dominant Hemisphere	60–70% have—left dominant Hemisphere
1% have—right dominant Hemisphere	15–20% have—right dominant Hemisphere
	15–20% have—mixed dominance

Examination

Any of the following methods can be adopted:
- Ask the patient to kick a football, normally the dominant side leg is used.
- Ask the patient to peep through a keyhole, normally the dominant side eye is used.
- Ask the patient to fold the arms in front one over the other, the dominant hand is the one which lies anteriorly.
- Ask the patient to "stand at ease" position, the dominant hand is the one which lies posteriorly.

Clinical Implications

1. Handedness is important for rehabilitation of the patient (right-handed individuals—dominant left hemisphere needs to be aggressively rehabilitated so as to have minimal residual deficit).
2. Degenerative diseases like Huntington's disease have been postulated to be more common in individuals with right dominant cortex.
3. Failure to develop clear hemispheric dominance has been implicated in dyslexia, stuttering, mirror writing, learning disability, and general clumsiness.

Education

- Formal education up to standard.
- It is important for testing components of higher mental functions like calculation, reading, and writing.

CONSCIOUSNESS

The ascending reticular activating system (RAS) arising from the reticular formation of the brainstem, primarily the paramedian tegmentum of the upper pons and midbrain, and projects to the paramedian, parafascicular, centromedian, and intralaminar nuclei of the thalamus. This is the primary control of consciousness.

The hypothalamus is also important for consciousness; arousal can be produced by stimulation of the posterior hypothalamic region.

Coma	- It is a state of complete loss of consciousness from which the patient cannot be aroused by ordinary stimuli.

Contd...

Contd...

	- There is complete unresponsiveness to self and the environment. - The patient in coma has no awareness of themselves, makes no voluntary movements and has no sleep-wake cycles.
Stupor	- It is a state of partial or relative loss of response to the environment in which the patient's consciousness may be impaired to varying degrees. - The patient can be aroused only with vigorous or unpleasant stimuli (e.g., sharp pressure or pinch, or rolling a pencil across the nail bed). - No significant voluntary verbal or motor responses. - Mass movement responses may be observed in response to painful stimuli or loud noises. **For example:** - Bilateral cerebral hemisphere disease - Upper brainstem diseases
Lethargy/ drowsiness	Patient can usually be aroused or awakened and may then appear to be in complete possession of their senses, but promptly falls asleep when left alone. It resembles normal sleepiness. **For example:** High brainstem disturbances
Obtundation	Refers to moderate reduction in the patient's level of awareness such that stimuli of mild-to-moderate intensity fail to arouse; when arousal does occur, the patient is slow to respond.
Vegetative state	- Return of irregular sleep-wake cycles and normalization of the so-called vegetative functions—respiration, digestion, and blood pressure control. - The patient may be aroused, but remains unaware of his or her environment. There is no purposeful attention or cognitive responsiveness. - It is a result of bilateral hemispheric damage with a spared and intact brainstem.
Persistent vegetative state	Individuals who remain in a vegetative state 1 year or longer after traumatic brain injur (TBI) and 3 months or more after anoxic brain injury. Minimally conscious state–those who do not meet diagnostic criteria for coma or PVS
Confusional state	Patients may appear alert, but are confused and disoriented. It is usually tested in three dimensions: 1. Time 2. Place 3. Person.
Delirium	It is an acute organic mental disorder characterized by confusion, restlessness, incoherence, inattention, anxiety, or hallucinations which may be reversible with treatment. **For example:** - Toxicity (alcohol) - Infections

Contd...

Contd...

Catatonia	- Symptom of psychotic state in which the patient is otherwise normal.
	- He does not follow movements, does not appear to pay attention to surroundings and will often have a plastic rigidity of limbs which may remain in any position in which they are placed (however bizarre the position may be).

It is preferable to describe the patient's state of responsiveness or use an objective and well-defined scheme, such as the Glasgow Coma Scale (GCS).

Glasgow Coma Scale					
Eye opening		*Best verbal response*		*Best motor response*	
				Obeys commands	6
		Oriented and converses	5	Localizes pain	5
Open spontaneously	4	Converses, but disoriented, confused	4	Exhibits flexion withdrawal	4
Open only to verbal stimuli	3	Uses inappropriate words	3	Decorticate rigidity	3
Open only to pain	2	Makes incomprehensible sounds	2	Decerebrate rigidity	2
Never open	1	No verbal response	1	No motor response	1

Maximum score = **15**
Minimum score = **3**
Coma is equal to GCS of **8 or less**.

Mnemonic (GCS → EVM = 4, 5, and 6)

Note: In intubated patients, verbal response is denoted as V_T.

Glasgow coma scale–pupils score

- The Glasgow coma scale-pupils score (GCS-P) was described in 2018 as a strategy to combine the two key indicators of the severity of traumatic brain injury into a single simple index
- Calculation of the GCS-P is by subtracting the pupil reactivity score (PRS) from the Glasgow coma scale (GCS) total score:
  GCS-P = GCS–PRS
- The pupil reactivity score is calculated as follows:

Pupils unreactive to light	Pupil reactivity score
Both pupils	2
One pupils	1
Neither pupils	0

- The GCS-P score can range from 1 and 15 and extends the range over which early severity can be shown to relate to outcomes of either mortality or independent recovery.

ORIENTATION

Time	Ask for year, season, month, date, and time
Place	Ask for country, state, city, hospital name, and floor/ward
Person	What is your name? How old are you? Where were you born? What is the name of your wife/husband?

Findings are documented in the medical record as follows: Patient is alert and oriented × 3 (time, person, and place) or × 2 (person, place) depending on the domains correctly identified.

An additional domain that can be examined is **circumstance.**

(What happened to you? What kind of a place is this? Why do people come here?)

APPEARANCE/BEHAVIOR

- Mood and affect
- Thought and perception

These have been discussed under Chapter 9—Approach to Psychiatric Illness.

MEMORY

Classification of Memory

Explicit memory (declarative memory)	Implicit memory
Involves conscious recall and requires integrity of various cortical regions	Does not require conscious recall. Involves basal ganglia and cerebellum
Can be tested bedside	Cannot be tested bedside
It includes:	It includes:
- Immediate (prefrontal cortex) - Recent (medial temporal structures) - Remote (widespread neocortical areas)	- Procedural memory (basal ganglia)—like riding a car - Classical conditioning (cerebellum) - Probabilistic classification learning (basal ganglia)

Examination of Explicit Memory

Types of memory	Description and testing	Areas in brain
Immediate (working memory)	- Digit span is a test of immediate memory, a very short-term function - Ask patient to repeat series of random digits forward and backward - Normal digit span is 7 ± 2	Dorsolateral frontal lobe, prefrontal cortex, and perisylvian cortex
Recent (short-term)	- Recent, or short-term memory is tested by giving the patient items (pen, phone, and bottle) to recall - After ensuring the patient has registered the items, proceed with other testing. After approximately 5 minutes, ask the patient to recall the items.	- Mammillothalamic tract - Hippocampus - Parahippocamal cortex (spatial memory) - Amygdala (emotional aspects) - Perirhinal cortex (for visual) - Medial temporal structures a and connections.

Contd...

Contd...

Remote (long-term)	A patient's fund of information reflects their remote memory. The fund of information includes schooling details, famous personalities, major events in history, etc.	- Widespread - Neocortical areas

Episodic memory refers to the system involved in remembering particular episodes or experiences, such as the movie you saw last weekend or the meeting you attended yesterday. **Semantic memory** refers to the type of long-term memory concerned with factual details outside of personal details

Budson and price concept of memory systems: The frontal lobe can be considered as filing clerk, deciding which information has to be filed or retrieved. The medial temporal lobes are the actual filing cabinets for recent memories and the neocortical regions are filing cabinets for remote memories

Wernicke's encephalopathy—**G**lobal confusion, **O**phthalmoplegia and **A**taxia (mneumonic—GOA).

Korsakoff's psychosis: Recent memory loss + confabulation (anteromedial thalamus)

Amnesia

Anterograde amnesia	Impaired registration and recall of new information
Retrograde amnesia	Impaired recall of information registered within a certain interval before the disease onset

ATTENTION

- Attention is the directing of consciousness to a person, thing, perception, or thought.
- It depends on the capacity of the brain to process information from the environment or from long-term memory.
- To examine selective attention the doctor asks the patient to repeat a short list of numbers forward or backward (digit span test).
- Normally, individuals can recall seven forward and five backward numbers.
- **Sustained attention (or vigilance)** is examined by determining how long the patient is able to maintain attention on a particular task (time on task).
- **Alternating attention (attention flexibility)** is examined by requesting the patient to alternate back and forth between two different tasks (e.g., add the first two pairs of numbers, then subtract the next two pairs of numbers).
- Requesting the patient to perform two tasks simultaneously determines divided attention.
- For example, the patient talks while walking (Walkie–Talkie test).

INTELLIGENCE/CALCULATION

Serial sevens, or spelling of any word backward.

COGNITION ASSESSMENT TOOL

- Mini Mental Status Examination (MMSE)—Folstein's

O	Orientation	Place Time	10
R	Registration	Name 3 objects	3
A	Attention and calculation	Serial 7/word backward	5
R	Registration recall	Recall previously named 3 objects	3
L	Language	3 stage command Name two objects, Read and follow, Draw a pentagon, Repetition, Write a sentence	9

- MMSE total score:
    - 21–24: Mild cognitive dysfunction
    - 10–20: Moderate
    - Less than 10: Severe.
- Montreal cognitive assessment (MoCA)
- Cognitive state test (COST)
- Addenbrooke's cognitive examination (ACE)
- Cambridge cognitive examination (CAMCOG)
- Brief cognitive assessment tool (BCAT), and
- Short test of mental status (STMS).

SPEECH

Definitions

Phonation	It is defined as the production of vocal sounds without word formation; it is entirely a function of the larynx
Vocalization	It is the sound made by the vibration of the vocal folds, modified by working of the vocal tract
Speech	It consists of words which are articulate vocal sounds that symbolize and communicate ideas
Articulation	It is the enunciation of words and phrases; it is a function of organs and muscles innervated by the brainstem
Language [Fig. 6D(ii).1]	It is a mechanism for expressing thoughts and ideas as follows: - By speech (auditory symbols) - By writing (graphic symbols), or - By gestures and pantomime (motor symbols) - Language may be regarded as any means of expressing or communicating feeling or thought using a system of symbols. - It is a function of the cerebral cortex
Aphasia	Aphasia is an acquired disorder with loss or defective language content of speech resulting from damage to the speech centers within the dominant (usually left in 97%) hemisphere
Paraphasia	Substitution in the components of speech, e.g., foon for spoon
Neologism	Use of words which are nonexistent. Classically seen with Wernicke's aphasia
Jargon	Completely meaningless speech containing neologisms and paraphasias. Described in Wernicke's aphasia
Echolalia	Continuous repetition of heard words or sentences. Seen with transcortical sensory and transcortical mixed aphasias

Contd...

Nervous System

Contd...

Alexia	It is the impairment of visual word recognition, in the context of intact auditory word recognition and writing ability
Agraphia	It is the inability to write, as a language disorder resulting from brain damage
Anomia	In this, word approximates the correct answer but it phonetically inaccurate (plentil for pencil)—phonemic paraphasia. When the patient cannot say the appropriate name when an object is shown but can point the object when the name is provided, it is known as one way or retrieval- based naming deficit
Mutism	Unable to speak or make sound
Aphonia	Unable to produce sound
Aphemia	Loss of speech

Genesis of speech is shown in Figure 6D(ii).2.

Slurred speech can be because of aphasia or dysarthria:

Aphasia	Dysarthria
Aphasia is a disorder of language	Dysarthria is a disorder of the motor production or articulation of speech
Usually due to cerebral dysfunction/lesions	Dysarthria is defective articulation of sounds or words of neurologic origin (usually brainstem)
Aphasia usually affects other language functions, such as reading and writing	In dysarthria, there are often other accompanying bulbar abnormalities, such as dysphagia

Contd...

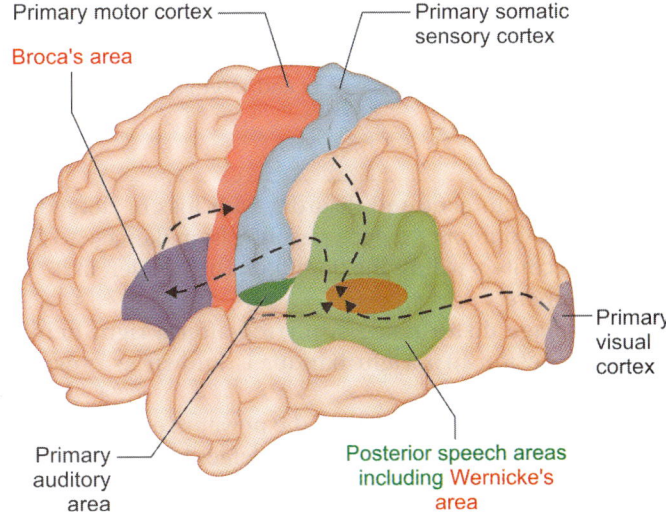

Fig. 6D(ii).1: Language and the brain.

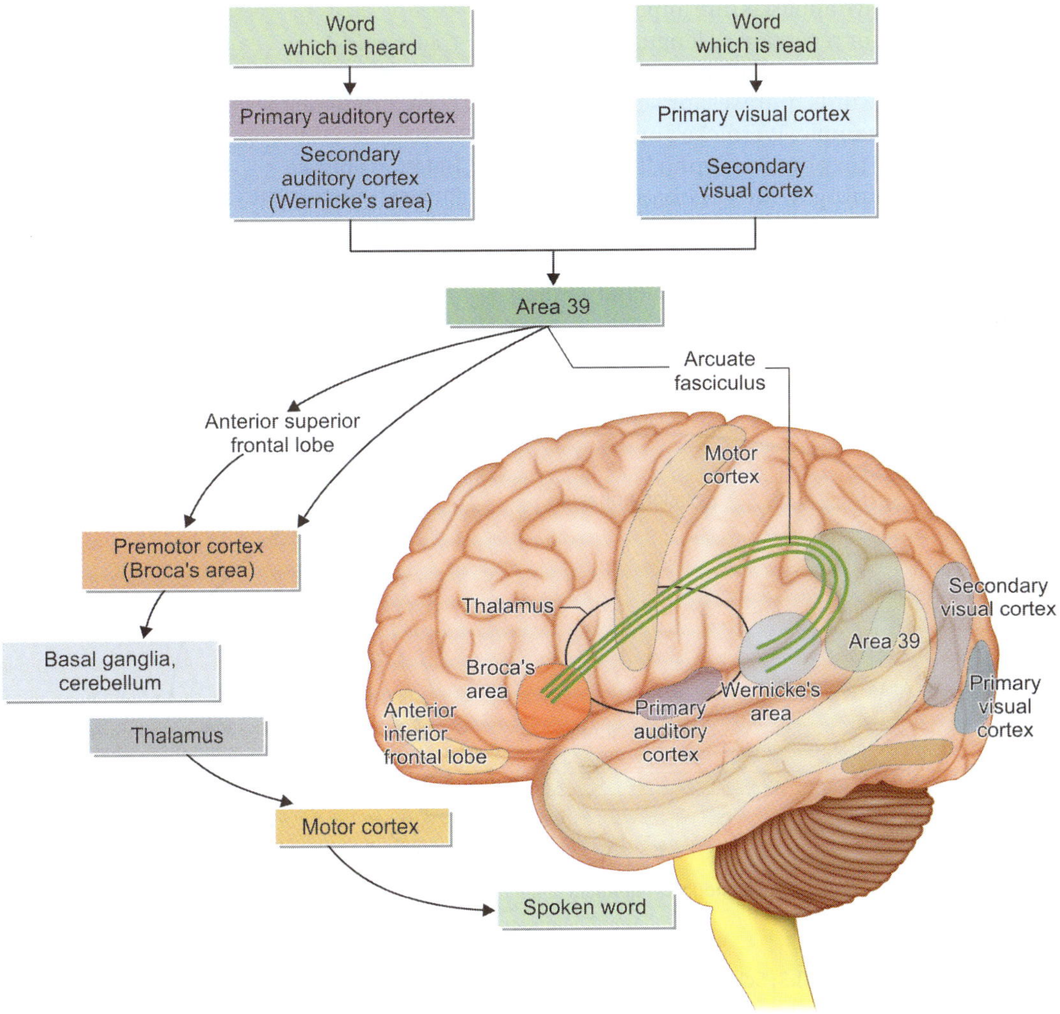

Fig. 6D(ii).2: Genesis of speech.

Wernicke's area (area 22)	Arcuate fasciculus	Broca's area (area 44)
Decoding of sounds into language information (comprehension)	Communication between the Broca's and Wernicke's area. Needed for speech repetition	Responsible for spontaneous speech output (i.e., fluency). Approximate number words produced per minute is 100/min for males and 150/min for females

APHASIAS

- Aphasia is an acquired disorder with loss or defective language content of speech resulting from damage to the speech centers within the dominant (usually left in 97%) hemisphere.
- A language disturbance occurring after a right hemisphere lesion in a right hander is known as crossed aphasia.
- It includes defect in or loss of the power of expression by speech, writing, or gestures or a defect in or loss of the ability to comprehend spoken or written language or to interpret gestures.
- Aphasia may be categorized according to whether the speech output is fluent or nonfluent.
    - **Fluent aphasias** (receptive aphasias) are impairments mostly due to the input or reception of language with difficulties either in auditory verbal comprehension or in the repetition of words, phrases, or sentences spoken by others. For example, Wernicke's aphasia.
    - **Nonfluent aphasias** (expressive aphasias) are difficulties in articulating with relatively good auditory, verbal comprehension. For example, Broca's aphasia [Fig. 6D(ii).3].
- **Normal fluency** 100–150 words/min, sentence length >7 words.
- Reduced fluency in Broca's aphasia, transcortical motor aphasia, global aphasia, and primary progressive aphasia.

Domains of Language

1. Spontaneous speech/fluency
2. Comprehension
3. Repetition
4. Reading
5. Writing
6. Naming.

C—Comprehension (requires intact Wernicke's and transcortical sensory area)
R—Repetition (requires intact Wernicke's, arcuate fibers, and Broca's area)
F—Fluency (requires intact Broca's and transcortical motor area) [Flowchart 6D(ii).1].

	Aphasia	Site of lesion	C	R	F
1.	Wernicke's—sensory/receptive/posterior	Infarction of inferior division of middle cerebral artery	–	–	+
2.	Broca's—motor/expressive/anterior	Infarction of superior frontal branch of middle cerebral artery	+	–	–
3.	Conduction/arcuate	Arcuate fasciculus	+	–	+
4.	Transcortical sensory	Posterior watershed zone	–	+	+
5.	Transcortical motor	Anterior watershed zone	+	+	–
6.	Isolation aphasia (mixed transcortical aphasia)	Both anterior and posterior watershed areas	–	+	–
7	Global aphasia	Dominant frontal, parietal and superior temporal lobe	–	–	–

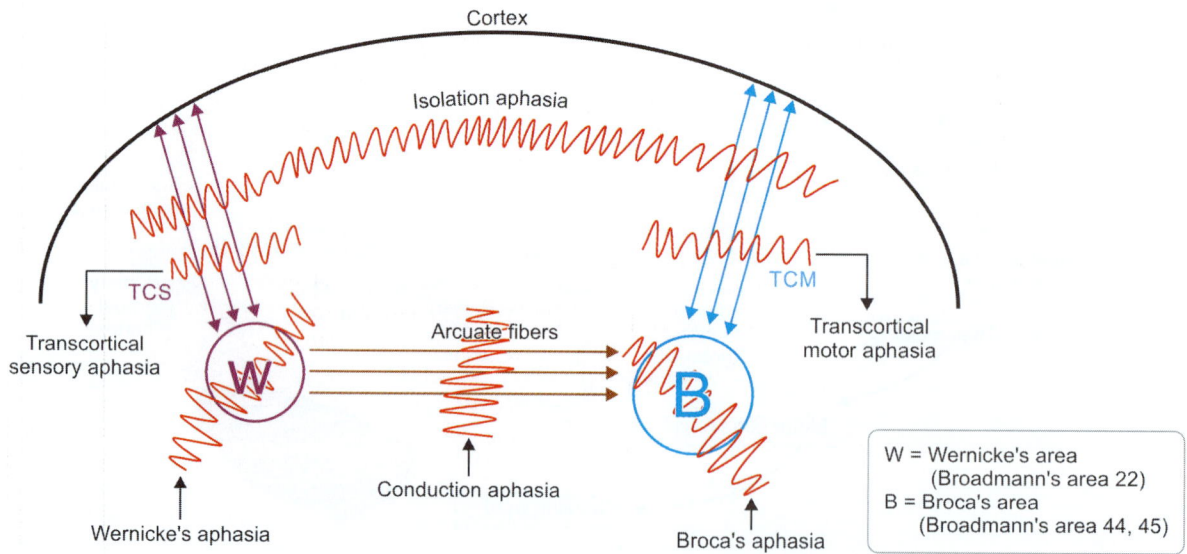

Fig. 6D(ii).3: Schematic representation of aphasias and associated lesions.

Flowchart 6D(ii).1: Approach for aphasias.

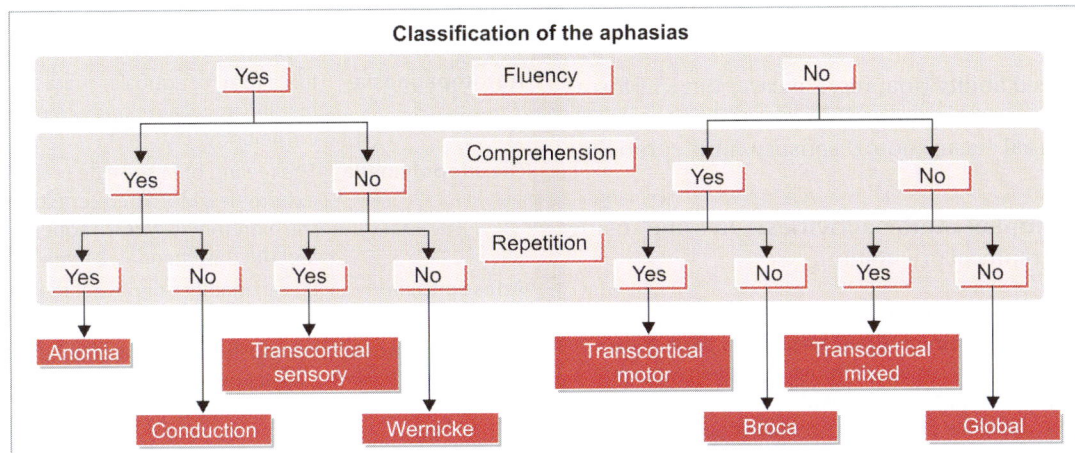

Note:
C—Comprehension
R—Repetition
F—Fluency

Once the comprehension, repetition, and fluency are intact, we look for Reading, Writing, and Naming disorders associated with reading, writing, and naming.

		R	W	N
Alexia without agraphia	Occipitotemporal region	–	+	+
Alexia with agraphia	Left angular gyrus	–	–	+
Nominal/anomic/amnesic	Temporoparietal	+	+	–

- Lesions in the anterior limb of internal capsule/basal ganglia can produce Broca's like aphasia.
- Lesions in the thalamus can produce Wernicke's like aphasia.
- Most common type of aphasia seen in stroke: Broca's aphasia.
- Overall most common type of aphasia is anomic aphasia.

DYSARTHRIAS

Production of sounds requires:
1. Normal respiration
2. Muscles of articulation (labial, lingual, and palatal muscles)
3. Phonation (by larynx)
4. Resonance (by nasopharynx).

Articulated Sounds

Articulated labials (b, p, m, and w) are formed principally by the lips.
Modified labials (o and u, and to a lesser extent i, e, and a) are altered by lip contraction.
Labiodentals (f and v) are formed by placing the teeth against the lower lip.
Linguals are sounds formed with tongue action.
t, d, l, r, and n are tongue point, or alveolar sounds formed by touching the tip of the tongue to the upper alveolar ridge.
S, z, sh, zh, ch, and j are dentals, or tongue blade sounds. **To hear distorted linguals**, place the tip of your tongue against the back of your bottom teeth, hold it there and say "top dog," "go jump", and "train".
To hear distorted labials, hold your upper lip between the thumb and forefinger of one hand and your bottom lip similarly with the other and say "my baby".
Gutturals (velars, or tongue back sounds, such as k, g, and ng) are articulated between the back of the tongue and the soft palate.
Palatals (German ch and g, and the French gn) are formed when the dorsum of the tongue approximates the hard palate.

Types of dysarthrias		
Types	Description	Cause
Flaccid (lingual, buccal, and guttural)	LMN weakness of facial, lingual, or pharyngeal muscles ■ **Facial paralysis** causes difficulty with labials, such as b, p, m, and w ■ **Tongue paralysis** affects a large number of sounds, particularly l, d, n, s, t, and x ■ **Palatal paralysis** produces a nasal twang in speech	Cerebrovascular accidents (especially brainstem lesions)
Spastic (hot potato voice)	Strained, slurred hot potato-like voice	UMN weakness (bilateral), e.g., pseudobulbar palsy
Ataxic speech	**Scanning speech:** Undue separation of syllables (monosyllable speech)	Cerebellar diseases
	Staccato speech: Explosive type of speech with emphasis on syllables	
Hypokinetic	Slow monotonous, low voice with inappropriate silence	Extrapyramidal (parkinsonism)
Hyperkinetic dysarthria	Distorted speech with continuous change in articulation	Chorea, athetosis, and dyskinesias
Myasthenic dysarthria	Voice is normal in the beginning but becomes weak as sentences progress	Myasthenia gravis

APRAXIA

Definition

Apraxia is impaired ability (inability) to carry out (perform) skilled, complex, and organized motor activities in the presence of normal basic motor, sensory, and cerebellar functions.

Examples of complex motor activities: Dressing, using cutlery, and geographical orientation.

Types of apraxia	
Ideomotor apraxia	Most common. It is the inability to perform a specific motor command/act (e.g., cough, lighting a cigarette with a matchstick) in the absence of motor weakness, incoordination, and sensory loss or aphasia. Site of lesion is bilateral parietal lobe. Buccofacial apraxia involves apraxic deficits in movements of the face and mouth. Limb apraxia encompasses apraxic deficits in movements of the arms and legs
Dressing apraxia	Site of lesion is nondominant parietal lobe. It is inability to wear his/her dress
Constructional apraxia	It is inability to copy simple diagrams or build simple blocks. Site of lesion is nondominant parietal lobe
Ideational apraxia	It is a deficit in the execution of a goal-directed sequence of movements even with real object (e.g., asked to pick up a pen and write, the sequence of uncapping the pen, and placing the cap at the opposite end). This is commonly associated with confusion and dementia rather than focal lesions associated with aphasic conditions
Gait apraxia (Bruns ataxia)	Seen in normal pressure hydrocephalus (NPH)
Gaze apraxia	Part of Balint syndrome
Other apraxia	Speech apraxia, conceptual apraxia, and conduction apraxia

AGNOSIA

Definition

Agnosia is failure to recognize objects (e.g., places, clothing, persons, sounds, shapes, or smells), despite the presence of intact sensory system.
Site of lesion: Contralateral parietal lobe.

Types of agnosia	
Visual agnosia	Failure to recognize what is seen with eyes despite the presence of intact visual pathways. The individual can describe the shape, color, and size without naming it. Site of lesion is in the posterior occipital or temporal lobes
Prosopagnosia	A type of visual agnosia in which patient cannot identify familiar faces, sometimes the reflection of his or her own face in the mirror even including their own. Site of lesion is parieto-occipital lobe

Contd...

Contd...

Simultanagnosia	It is inability to perceive more than one object at a time
Autotopagnosia	It is a form of agnosia, characterized by an inability to localize and orient different parts of the body
Pseudopolymelia	The feeling of false—the feeling of false extremities. More frequent, the patients feel the extremities. More frequent, the patients feel the third hand
Anosognosia	It is an inability or refusal to recognize a defect or disorder that is clinically evident
Auditory agnosia	It consists of the loss of ability to know objects on sounds characteristic for them (clock—on ticking)

DELUSIONS

Definition

Delusion is a belief held with strong conviction despite superior evidence to the contrary (strongly held false beliefs). It is a disorder of content of thought.

Types of delusion (based on their content)	
Persecutory delusions	Conviction that others are out to get me
Grandiose delusions	Belief that one has special powers or status
Nihilistic delusions	Conviction that "my head is missing/rotting", "I have no body", and "I am dead"
Erotomanic delusions	Believing a movie star loves them
Somatic delusions	Believing head is filled with air/worms
Delusions of reference	Believing story in a book is referring to them
Delusions of control/passivity	Believing one's thoughts and movements are controlled by aliens
Other delusions are	Delusions of misinterpretation, hypochondrial delusions, fantastic/bizarre delusions, delusions of passivity, delusions of jealousy

HALLUCINATIONS

Definition

Hallucinations are perceptions without external stimuli *(wakeful sensory experiences of content that is not actually present)*. They can occur in any sensory modality, most common being **visual or auditory**.

For example, hearing voices when no one else is present, or seeing "visions". Other types include tactile (cocaine bug), olfactory, gustatory, command kinesthetic/psychomotor, and lilliputian and complex hallucinations.

Pseudohallucinations

These are hallucinations that are perceived as originating in the external world, not in the patient's own mind.

Hypnagogic and Hypnopompic Hallucinations

In narcolepsy 2, specific hallucinations are seen. **Hypnagogic:** They occur when falling asleep. **Hypnopompic:** They occur on waking up from sleep. (mnemonic—hypno**GO**gic hallucinations are perceived while **GO**ing to sleep).

Hallucinations	Illusions
Perceptions without external stimuli	Misperceptions of real external stimuli
For example, hallucinating that someone is talking to them when there is no actual stimulus	For example, mistaking a rope for snake

Functions and effects of damage to various lobes of cerebral hemispheres are listed in Table 6D(ii).1 and Figure 6D(ii).4:

TABLE 6D(ii).1: Functions and effects of damage to various lobes of cerebral hemispheres.

Lobe	Function	Cognitive/behavioral effects of damage
Frontal **P**lease **SMILE** (MNEMONIC)	**P**ersonality	
	Social behavior	Antisocial behavior
	Micturition	Incontinence
	Intelligence	
	Language	Expressive dysphasia
	Emotional response	Disinhibition
Parietal: Dominant side	Language	Dysphasia, dyslexia
	Calculation	Acalculia
	Others	Apraxia, agnosia
Parietal: Nondominant side	Spatial orientation	Spatial disorientation, neglect of contralateral side
	Constructional skills	Constructional apraxia, dressing apraxia
Temporal: Dominant side	Auditory perception	Receptive aphasia
	Language	Dyslexia
	Verbal memory	Impaired verbal memory
	Smell	
	Balance	
Temporal: Nondominant side	Auditory perception	Impaired nonverbal memory
	Melody/pitch perception	Impaired musical skills (tonal perception)
	Nonverbal memory	
	Smell	
	Balance	
Occipital	Visual processing	Visual inattention, visual loss, visual agnosia (Anton–Babinski syndrome)

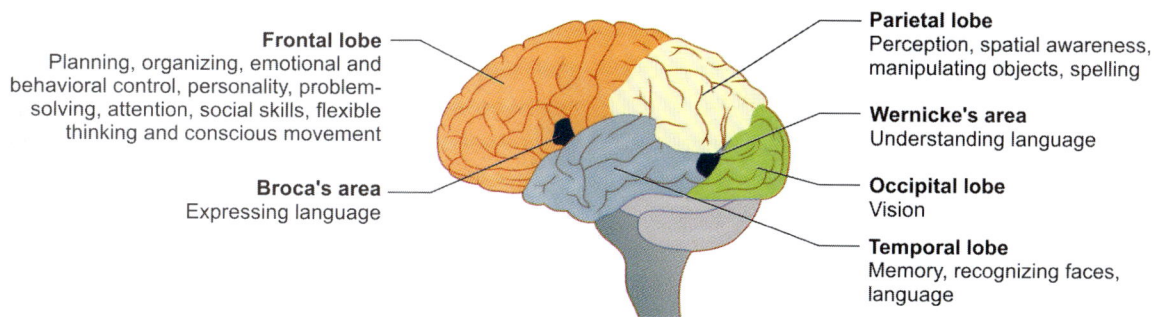

Fig. 6D(ii).4: Various lobes of cerebral hemispheres.

LESIONS OF NONDOMINANT (RIGHT) HEMISPHERE
Neglect
Definition → directed inattention, or a relative lack of attention, paid to one hemisphere; patients are less aware (or completely unaware) of objections or actions in one side of the world (usually the left).

Diagnosis
- *Severe forms* → patients completely ignore left side, denying that, such as side even exists; they may leave their left side ungroomed, unshaven, and undressed; may leave food on left side of plate uneaten; may deny they have a left hand, and when confronted with it, may claim that it is actually the examiner's.

Contd...

Contd...

- *Milder forms* → may perform actions with their left side only with encouragement or after repeated prodding.
- *Most sensitive sign* → extinction to double simultaneous stimulation; sensory stimuli applied singly to either side are properly felt, but when both sides are stimulated simultaneously, only the non-neglected side is felt; extinction may exist with tactile, visual, or auditory stimulation.
- *Etiology* → lesions in right hemisphere (frontal or parietal lobe), most commonly an acute finding after stroke.
  - *Frontal lobe* lesion → more of a motor neglect in which patient has tendency to not use left side for motor actions
  - *Parietal lobe* lesion → more of a sensory neglect in which stimuli from the left side tend to be ignored.

Others

- **Prosody** → while semantic elements of language (pure meaning) reside in dominant hemisphere, some other elements of successful oral communication (e.g., proper voice inflection) reside in nondominant hemisphere.
- **Anosognosia** → tendency to be unaware of one's deficits in some patient's with right hemispheric lesions
  - For example, patient with complete left hemiplegia may insist on immediate discharge from hospital because he feels nothing is wrong
  - For example, patient with dense left hemianopia may wonder why she keeps bumping into others since she notices nothing wrong with her vision.

NOTES

D(iii). CRANIAL NERVES

CRANIAL NERVE I—OLFACTORY NERVE

Prerequisites for Examination
- Rule out nose blocks
- Close eyes while examining
- Test each nostril separately.

Substances Which Can be Used for Testing
- Peppermint
- Soap
- Coffee beans
- Lemon peel
- Vanilla.

Note: **Avoid** irritants like ammonia as they directly stimulate the trigeminal nerve endings.

Method of Examination
- Examine each nostril separately while occluding the other **[Fig. 6D(iii).1]**.
- With the patient's eyes closed and one nostril occluded, bring the test substance near the open one.
- Instruct the patient to sniff (*sniffing creates a better airflow pattern for reaching olfactory endings*) repetitively and to tell you when an odor is detected, identifying the odor, if recognized.
- Bring the test odor up to within 30 cm or less of the nose.
- Repeat for the other nostril and compare the two sides.

Note: The side that might be abnormal should be examined first.

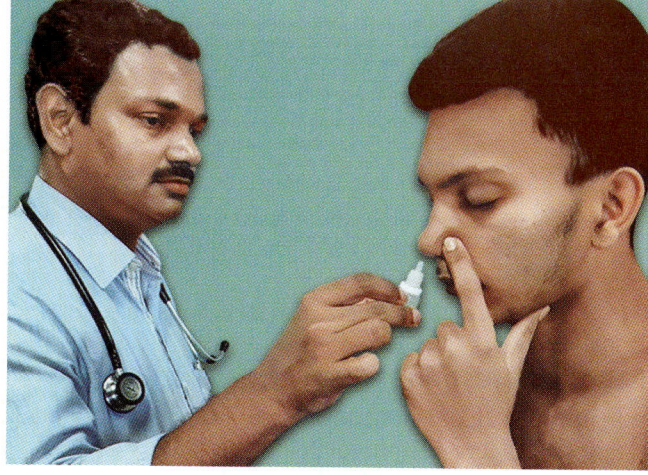

Fig. 6D(iii).1: Method of examination of olfactory nerve.

Interpretation
- Patient able to detect smell, recognize, and name
- Patient able to detect smell, recognize but not name
- Patient able to detect, but not recognize or name.

Olfactory pathway
The **1st order neurons** of the olfactory system are bipolar sensory cells that lie in the olfactory epithelium, which occupies a small area on the superior nasal concha, upper nasal septum, and roof of the nose
↓
Peripheral and central processes
↓
Olfactory axons
↓
Pierce the cribriform plate
↓
Olfactory bulb
↓
Within the olfactory bulbs, axons of incoming fibers synapse on dendrites of mitral and tufted cells in the olfactory glomeruli. The mitral and tufted cells are the output cells of the olfactory bulb
↓
2nd order neurons (predominantly mitral cells)
↓
Pass through the anterior perforating substance

Medial striae	Lateral striae
Carry axons across the medial plane of anterior commissure where they meet the olfactory bulb of opposite side	Primary olfactory cortex (pyriform cortex, amygdala, olfactory tubules, and secondary olfactory cortex)

Note:
- The olfactory nerves are the **unmyelinated filaments** that pass through the cribriform plate.

Disturbances in olfaction
Anosmia/Persistent loss of smell

Physiological:
- Normal aging
- Pregnancy

Local causes:
- Acute rhinitis (most common cause)
- Sinusitis
- Heavy smoking
- Atrophy of bulb
- Dental trauma

Systemic causes:
- Postviral illness
- Parkinson's disease
- Alzheimer's disease
- Meningitis
- Head trauma
- Intracranial tumors
- Vitamin B_{12} deficiency
- Refsum's disease
- Substance abuse—cocaine, amphetamine
- Chemotherapeutic agents
- Multiple sclerosis
- Korsakoff syndrome
- Anterior cerebral artery diseases
- Psychiatric conditions

Contd...

Contd...
- Endocrine diseases:
  - Diabetes mellitus
  - Hypothyroidism
- Chronic kidney diseases.

Syndromes associated:
- **Foster–Kennedy syndrome** (anosmia, optic atrophy of one eye, and contralateral eye papilledema due to tumor in brain)
- **Pseudo-Foster-Kennedy syndrome** (above features in absence of tumor)
- **Kallmann syndrome**
- **Turner syndrome**

Impaired smell

K: Korsakoff
B: Basilar meningitis
C: Chorea Huntington's
A: Anterior cerebral artery diseases
S: Spinocerebellar ataxia
H: Hydrocephalus

Other miscellaneous points
- Anosmia is commonly associated with hypogeusia/ageusia
- Olfactory hallucinations: Usually of unpleasant odors like burned rubber, can occur in temporal lobe epilepsy, migraine and schizophrenia
- Hyperosmia: May be seen with Addison's disease, cystic fibrosis or pituitary tumors
- Merciful anosmia—atrophic rhinitis.
- UPSIT is a quantitative smell and taste test, helps to identify malingering.
- Unilateral anosmia—unaware of any impairment.

Notes:
- Olfactory is the only nerve which does not process through thalamus.
- Olfactory and optic are the two nerves which do not pass through brainstem.
- Loss of smell is usually associated with loss of taste sensation (Aguesia/hypogeusia).

CRANIAL NERVE II—OPTIC NERVE

*The optic nerve is the only cranial nerve that can be visualized directly. The intracranial subarachnoid space continues along the vaginal sheaths of meninges, transmitting the raised ICP causing papilledema.

1. Visual acuity
2. Visual field
3. Color vision
4. Fundus examination.

Visual Acuity

Assessment of visual acuity is usually done by asking the patient to read the specific charts as described below. Each eye is examined individually. The least possible distance with best vision is considered as the viewing distance.

Visual acuity	
For far vision	*For near vision*
Snellen chart [**Fig. 6D(iii).2**]	Jaeger chart [**Fig. 6D(iii).3**]
Examined at 6 m	Examined at 30 cm
Described as x/y → x (numerator—suggests the viewing distance of patient) and y (denominator—viewing distance of normal person)	• Describes as J1, J2, etc. • Normal range of near vision is J1 to J4

Note: In absence of Snellen's chart finger counting can be done.

Defects in visual acuity may be due to:
- Refractive errors (improves with pinhole)
- Cataract (may worsen with pinhole)
- Vitreous opacity, etc.
- Optic nerve or chiasmal lesions

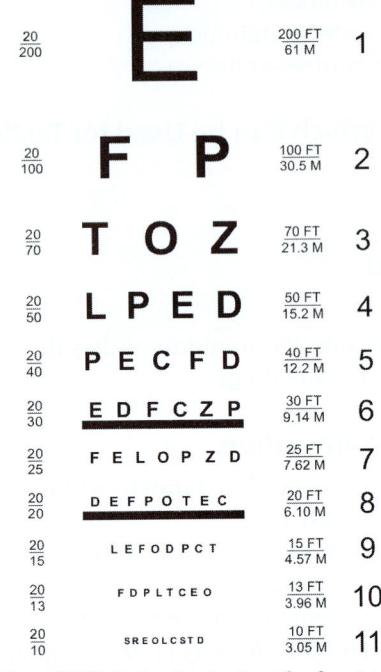

Fig. 6D(iii).2: Snellen's chart for far vision.

0.37 M	I walked up the cheapness I bade him give me three sort. he gave me three puffy rolls. penny worth of any sort. he gave me three puffy rolls. I was sort. he gave me three puffy any worth of any sort. he gave me three puffy . passing by the house. He rolls. I but I took it, and walked off with a rod under each arm with a rod under each arm up Market Street as far as Fourth e a most awkward appearance.Street, passing by the house	J2
0.50 M	the difference of money and the greater cheapness I bade him give me three penny worth of any sort. he gave me three puffy rolls. I was surprised at the quantity but I took it, and walked off with a rod under each arm. Thus I walked up Market Street as far as Fourth Street, passing by the house	J3
0.62 M	of Mr. Read, my future wife's father. She, standing at the door, saw me and thought I made a most awkward appearance, as I certainly did. Then I turned and went down Chesnut street and a part of Walnut Street. Being filled with one of my rolls. I gave the other two to a women	J4
0.75 M	and her child. But this time the street hand many clean and well dressed people in it, all walking the same way. I joined them and was led into the great meeting house of the Quakers'. I sat down among them and after looking around a while and hearing nohting said.	J5
1.00 M	I fell fast asleep. this was the first house I was in, or slept in, in Philadelphia. Looking in the faces of people, I met a young man whose countenance I liked, and asked	J7
1.25 M	if he would tell me where a stranger could get lodging. "Here", and he, "is one place that entertains strangers."	J8

Fig. 6D(iii).3: Jaeger's chart for near vision.

Visual Field Testing

- In formal Visual field testing, central field tested by tangent screen, peripheral field by perimetry.
- Objects are better visible when moving.

Confrontation Method

Prerequisites: Close cooperation, good fixation and adequate illumination.
Testing distance: 1 m or one full hands distance [**Figs. 6D(iii).4A to C**]

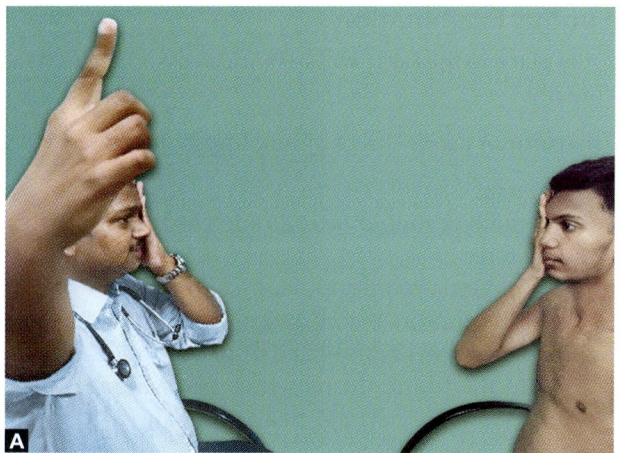
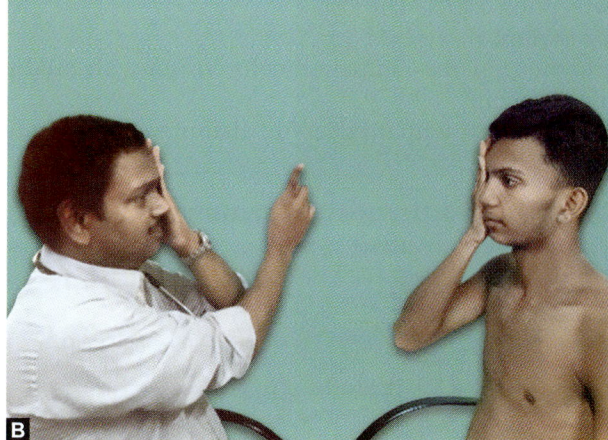
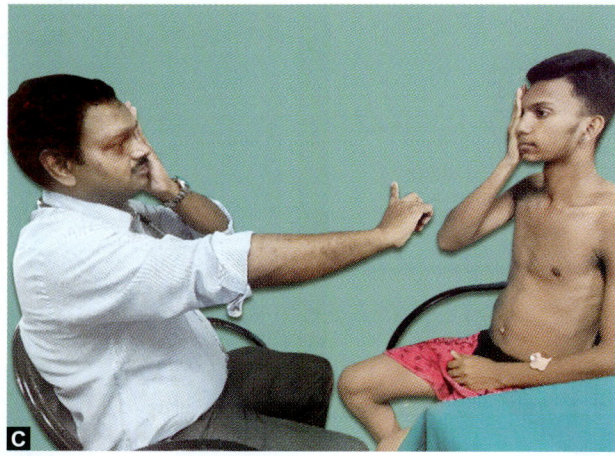

Figs. 6D(iii).4A to C: Method of examination (confrontation method).

Instructions:
- Subject and examiner should be sitting at the same height with each one looking into each other's eye separated by distance of 1 m.
- For checking the visual field of right eye of the subject, he is instructed to close his left eye with his left hand while the examiner closes his right eye with right hand. Now, the examiner brings in the flickering index finger of left hand from extremes of all four directions/quadrants diagonally toward the center of the visual field.
- The subject is instructed to give the signal at the first instance of perceiving the flickering finger movement.
- Normal extent of visual field of individual eye:
  - Vertically up 60°
  - Vertically down 75°
  - Medially 60°
  - Laterally 100°
- Normal extent of visual field in binocular vision:
  - Horizontally = 200°
  - Vertically = 140°

Shortcomings of Confrontation Method
1. Field and defects [Figs. 6D(iii).5 and 6D(iii).6]:

Visual field defect	
Site of lesion	Types of defect
1. **Optic nerve**	Total loss of vision in left eye
2. **Optic chiasma**	Bitemporal hemianopia

Contd...

Contd...

3.	**Optic tract**	Right homonymous hemianopia
4.	**Geniculocalcarine tract**	▪ Upper right quadrantanopia ▪ Lower right quadrantanopia
5.	**Occipital pole**	Right homonymous hemianopia with macular sparing

Notes:
- Visual field defect produced by papilledema—enlarged blind spot
- Visual field can be grossly checked by doing Menace reflex.
- Binasal hemianopsia can be caused by congenital hydrocephalus, atherosclerosis of the internal carotid artery, ischemic optic neuropathy, optic nerve drusen, glaucoma, retinitis pigmentosa, and keratoconus.
- Macular sparing is due to: dual representation of macula in each occipital pole, dual blood supply by ACA and MCA, dual cortical representation both at occipital pole and calcarine fissure.

Color Vision (Red/Green/Blue)

Chart used: Ishihara chart [Figs. 6D(iii).7 and 6D(iii).8]
Crude estimate: Colors in a fabric.
Achromatopsia: Color blindness (loss of color vision may precede other visual deficits).

Congenital anomalies:
- **Red and green** = chromosome X (mnemonic: remember Red, Green and Symbol X all are traffic symbols)
- **Blue** = chromosome 7 (mnemonic: remember sky is **blue** which has rainbow containing 7 colors).

Acquired defects: Occur in macular and optic nerve diseases, and due to certain **drugs (e.g., ethambutol, chloroquine, digitalis, and sildenafil).**

Red perception is first to be lost.

Interpretation:
- Optic neuropathy—impaired color vision with mildly reduced acuity.
- Maculopathy—impaired color vision with severely reduced acuity.

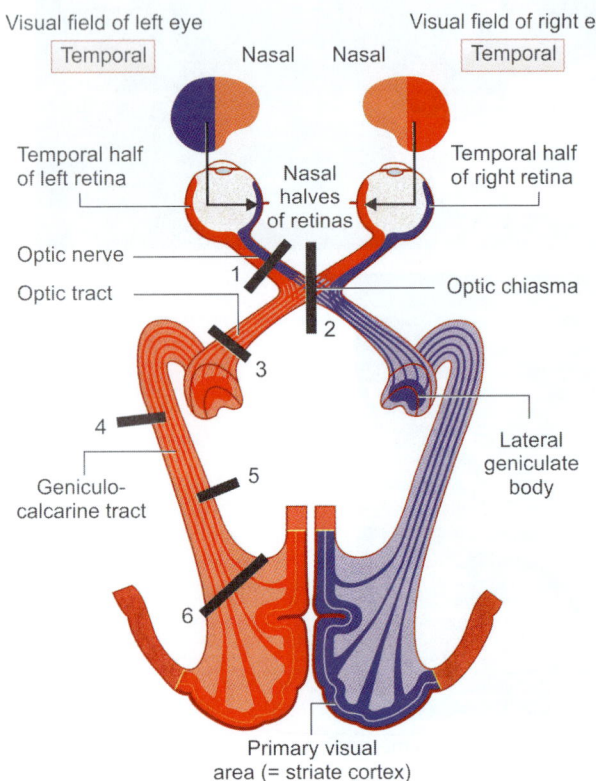

Fig. 6D(iii).5: Sites of lesions causing visual field defects.

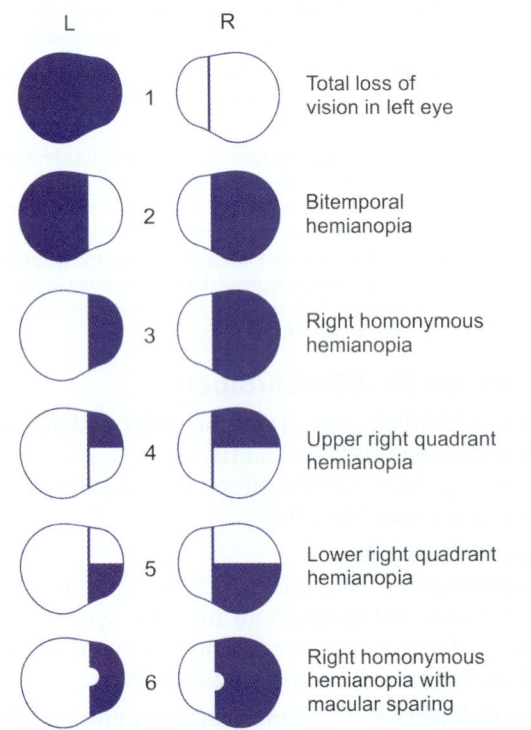

Fig. 6D(iii).6: Visual field defects.

Fundus Examination

Only place in the body where blood vessels can be visualized directly.

Instrument used: Direct ophthalmoscope.

How to use:
- The subject should be examined in sitting or lying down position.
- Examination room should be semidark.
- Routine fundus examination in neurologic patients is done through an undilated pupil.
- Avoid mydriatic drops when assessment of pupillary function is critical (e.g., head trauma).

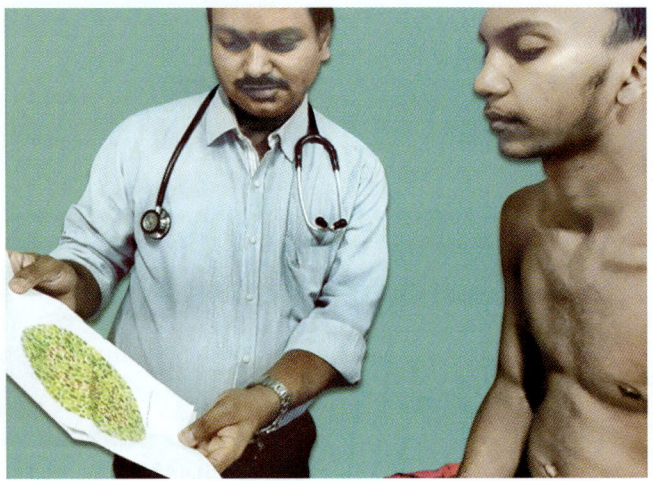

Fig. 6D(iii).7: Method of examining color vision.

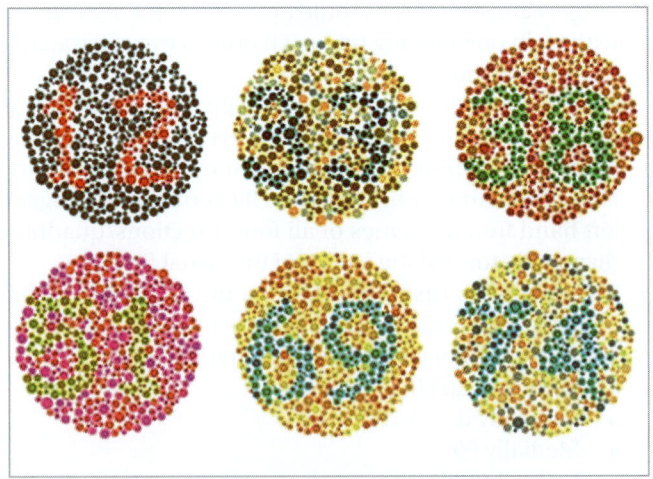

Fig. 6D(iii).8: Ishihara chart for color vision.

- Keep the eye as still as possible.
- Hold ophthalmoscope in same hand as the eye you are looking at, and looking through (e.g., hold ophthalmoscope in the left hand for examining patients left eye, through your left eye) **[Figs. 6D(iii).9 and 6D(iii).10]**.
- Hold head steady with thumb above eyebrow, or hold shoulder.

Nervous System

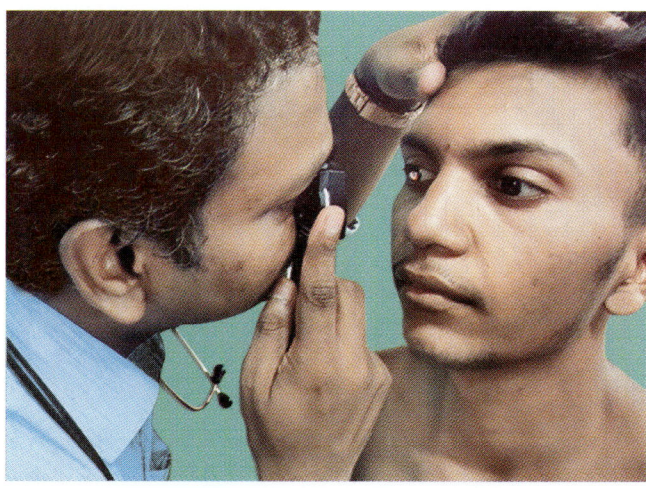

Fig. 6D(iii).9: Fundus examination of right eye.

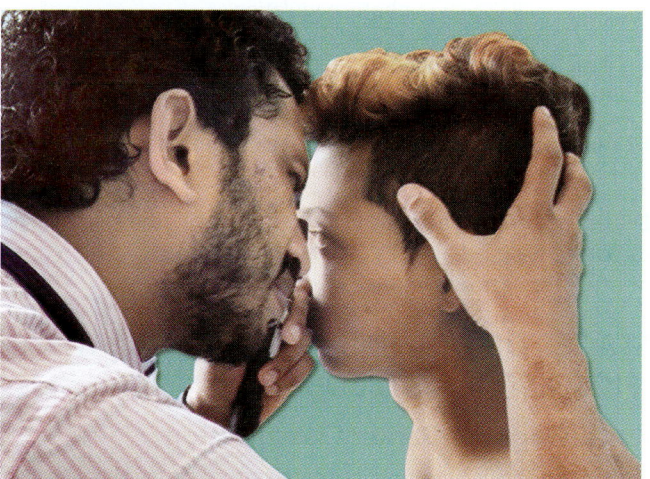

Fig. 6D(iii).10: Fundus examination of left eye.

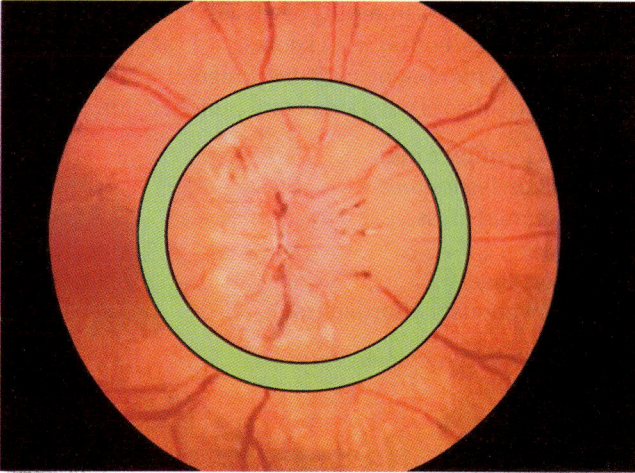

Fig. 6D(iii).11: Papilledema.

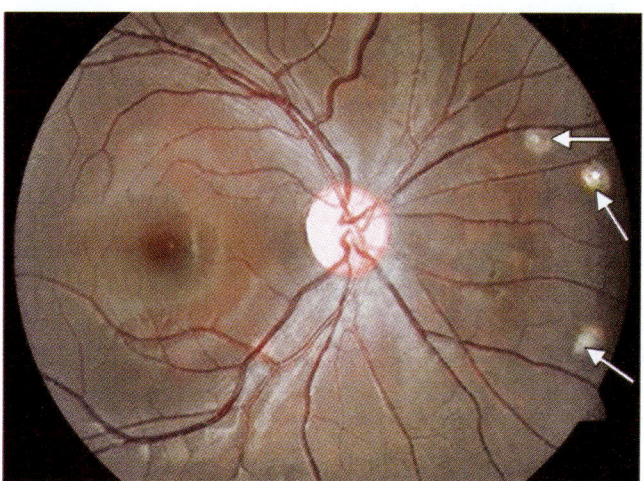

Fig. 6D(iii).12: Choroid tubercles in tuberculosis.

- At about 30 cm distance with light on eye, locate red reflex (seen as an orange glow in the pupil).
- Follow red reflex into the eye as this will get you directly into the optic disc.
- If you cannot find the disc, trace any blood vessels back to it.
- Examine vessels in all four quadrants of eye (upper and lower, nasal and temporal quadrants).
- Identify macula—slightly darker pigmented area, two optic disc widths lateral away from the optic disc.
- Look for optic atrophy and papilledema.

Also watch for feature of retinopathy like hemorrhages, exudates, cotton wool spots, and arteriolar changes.

Fundoscopic Finding

Papilledema is a disease entity which refers to the swelling of the optic disc as a result of impaired axoplasmic flow secondary to elevated intracranial pressure (ICP) [Fig. 6D(iii).11]. Choroid tubercle of tuberculosis is shown in **Figure 6D(iii).12.**

Stages of papilledema:

Grade	Description
1	Disruption of the normal radial arrangement of nerve fiber bundles with a blurring of the nasal border of the optic disc and normal temporal margin
2	Nasal and temporal (circumferential) blurring of the optic disc with more pronounced changes from grade 1
3	The elevated and blurred disc margin borders obscure one or more major retinal vessel segments
4	More pronounced changes than from grade 3 and with total obscuration of a segment of the central retinal artery or vein
5	More pronounced changes than from grade 4 and with total obscuration of all disc vessels

- Early—loss of previously observed spontaneous venous pulsations best seen at site where large vessels dive into hyperemic disc.

- Fully developed—humping of vessels, obliteration of disc, hemorrhages, cotton wool spots.
- Chronic—champagne cork disc bulge.
- Atrophic—disc is pale, small and punched out.

Causes of papilledema:
Space-occupying lesions:
- Intracranial mass
- Abscess
- Hemorrhage
- Arteriovenous malformation

Focal or diffuse cerebral edema:
- Trauma
- Toxic
- Anoxia

Blockage of CSF flow: Noncommunicating hydrocephalus

Reduction in CSF reabsorption:
- Meningitis
- Elevated cerebral venous sinus pressure
- Elevated CSF protein—Guillain-Barré syndrome

Pseudopapilledema: Disc color normal with SVP intact.
Causes: Myelinated nerve fibres, optic nerve drusens, primitive hyaloid remnants.

Pseudotumor cerebri
Systemic causes:
- Hypercarbia
- Hypertension
- Hypercalcemia
- Hypoparathyroidism.

STAGES OF DIABETIC RETINOPATHY

Nonproliferative Diabetic Retinopathy
1. **Mild NPDR:** Microaneurysms only
2. **Moderate NPDR:**
   - Atleast one hemorrhage or micro aneurysm and/or at least one of the following
   - Retinal hemorrhages, hard exduates, cotton wool spots, venous beading.
3. **Severe NPDR:**
   The 4-2-1 rule:
   - Severe retinal hemorrhages in all 4 quadrants
   - Significant venous beading in ³2 quadrants
   - Moderate IRMA in ³1 quadrants.
4. **Proliferative Diabetic Retinopathy [Fig. 6D(iii).13]**
   Mild-moderate:
   - New vessels on the disc (NVD) <1/3 disc area
   - New vessels elsewhere (NVE) <1/2 disc area.

High-risk:
- NVD >1/3 disc area
- Any NVD with vitreous or preretinal hemorrhage
- NVE >1/2 disc area with vitreous or preretinal hemorrhage.

Advanced diabetic eye disease:
- Preretinal (retrohyaloid) and/or intragel hemorrhage
- Tractional retinal detachment

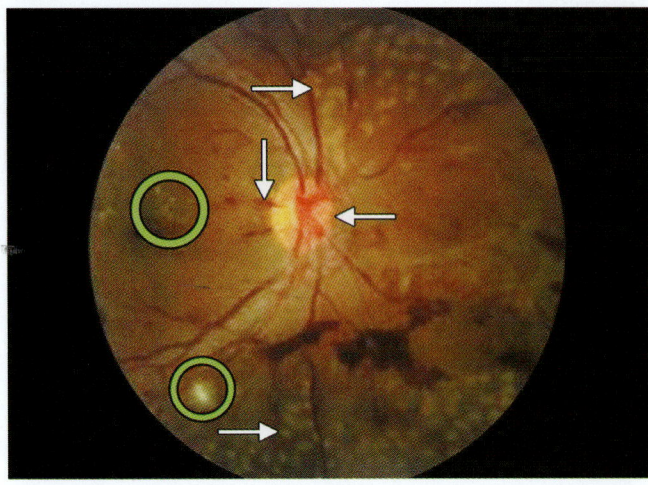

Fig. 6D(iii).13: Proliferative diabetic retinopathy with panretinal photocoagulation.

- Tractional retinoschisis
- Rubeosis iridis (iris neovascularization).

Diabetic maculopathy: Refers to presence of any retinopathy at the macula.

Diabetic papillopathy: It is a form of optic neuropathy seen in young type I diabetics. It is unrelated to glycemic control or any other known feature of diabetes.

STAGES OF HYPERTENSIVE RETINOPATHY [FIGS. 6D(iii).14 TO 6D(iii).17]

Keith-Wagener-Barker Classification
- Group 1: Slight constriction of retinal arterioles
- Group 2: Group 1 + focal narrowing of retinal arterioles + AV nicking
- Group 3: Group 2 + flame-shaped hemorrhages + cotton-wool spots + hard exudates and copper wiring
- Group 4: Group 3 + optic disc swelling and silver wiring.

CAUSES OF OPTIC ATROPHY
1. Inflammation
2. Ischemia

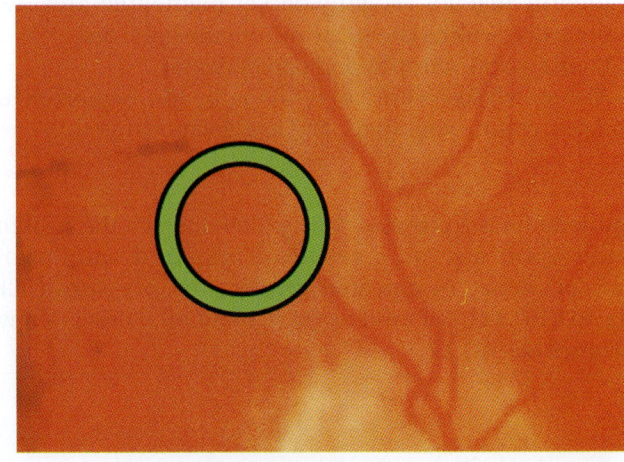

Fig. 6D(iii).14: Focal arteriolar narrowing.

Nervous System

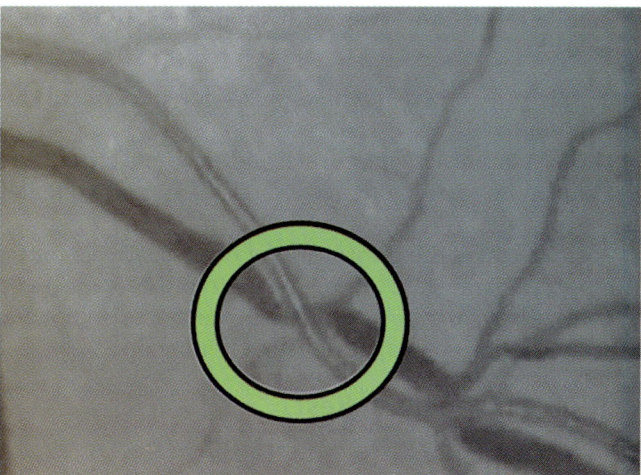

Fig. 6D(iii).15: AV nipping.

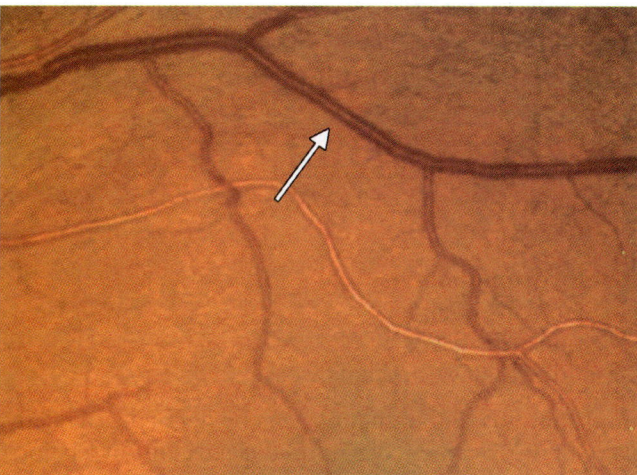

Fig. 6D(iii).16: Copper wiring.

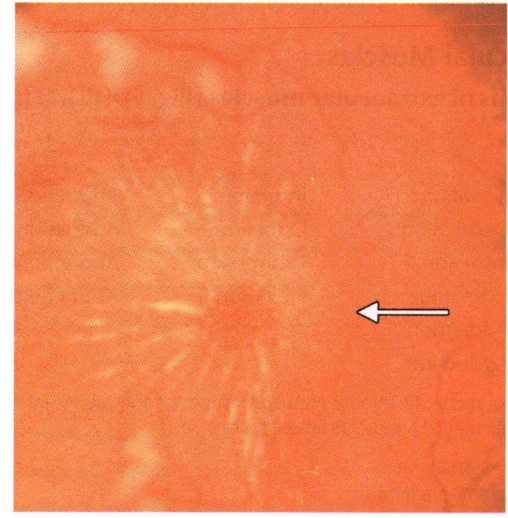

Fig. 6D(iii).17: Cotton wool spots and exudates forming macular star.

3. Compression, including raised ICP
4. Nutritional deficiencies/effect of toxins
5. Trauma

6. Hereditary conditions and childhood optic atrophy
7. Glaucoma.

CRANIAL NERVES III, IV AND VI—OCULOMOTOR, TROCHLEAR AND ABDUCENS

Anatomy:

Nuclei	Location	Additional points
III	Upper midbrain	▪ Four paired nuclei (SR, IR, MR, and IO muscles) ▪ One unpaired nuclei (LPS muscles of both sides)
IV	Midbrain	At level of inferior colliculus (SO muscle)
VI	Mid to lower pons	LR muscle

(SR: superior rectus; IR: inferior rectus; SO: superior oblique; IO: inferior oblique; MR: medial rectus; LR: lateral rectus; LPS: levator palpabrae superioris)

Examined under following headings:
1. Eyelids
2. Eyeballs at rest
3. Extraocular muscles
4. Pupils
5. Nystagmus.

Eyelids

Ptosis: The narrowing of the palpebral fissures due to inability to open an upper eyelid is called ptosis **(Figs. 6D(iii).18 and 6D(iii).19)**.

Ptosis can be due to	
↓	↓
Paralysis of levator palpebrae superioris (LPS)	*Paralysis of tarsal muscle*
LPS supplied by III cranial nerve	Tarsal muscle supplied by sympathetic system
LPS is paralyzed and the patient cannot voluntarily rise the eyelid, he compensates by contracting frontalis muscle and thus there is wrinkling of forehead seen in long-standing cases	Here since the III nerve is intact and LPS is not paralyzed, ptosis disappears on voluntary contraction of LPS

Cause of ptosis:

1. Congenital ptosis: Usually has lid lag in downgaze, differentiating from acquired	
2. Acquired ptosis	
Neurogenic	▪ Horner's syndrome ▪ III nerve palsy
Neuromuscular disorder	▪ Myasthenia gravis (fatigable ptosis) ▪ Poisoning (snake bite/botulism)
Myogenic	▪ Mitochondrial myopathy ▪ Oculopharyngeal muscle dystrophy ▪ Myotonic dystrophy
Mechanical ptosis	Due to eyelid edema or tumors

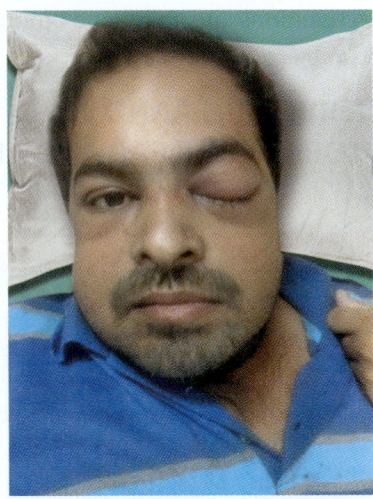

Fig. 6D(iii).18: Neurogenic ptosis.

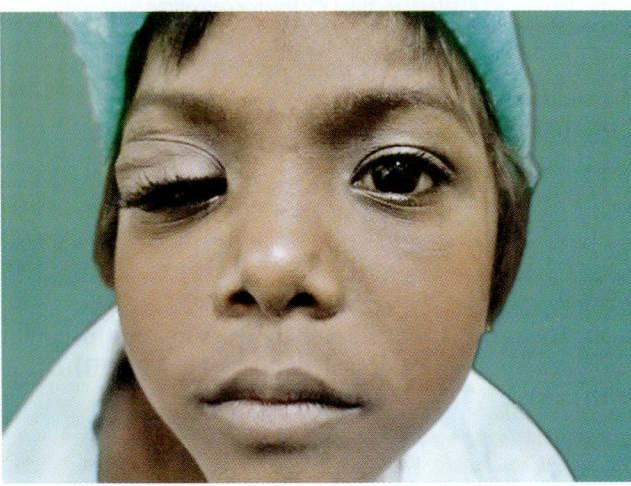

Fig. 6D(iii).19: Mechanical ptosis secondary to edema.

Unilateral and bilateral ptosis:

Unilateral ptosis	Bilateral ptosis
▪ Third cranial nerve lesion ▪ Lesion of cervical sympathetic pathway (Horner's syndrome) ▪ Lesions of the upper eyelid	▪ Myopathies ▪ Myasthenia gravis ▪ Bilateral Horner's syndrome ▪ Snake bite ▪ Botulism

Ptosis and pupil size:

	Ptosis with
Small pupil	Horner's syndrome
Large pupil	IIIrd nerve palsy (compressive lesions)
Normal pupillary size	Infarction of IIIrd nerve, myasthenia gravis, myopathies or Guillain–Barré syndrome

Pseudo ptosis—seen in strabismus, lid disorders, blepharospasm.

Lid retraction:
- Lid is buried under the brow
- Sclera clearly visible above iris
- Example—hyperthyroidism, large doses of anticholinesterases
- Collier's sign: Seen in Parinaud's syndrome. Produces retraction nystagmus.

Pseudo retraction—seen with strabismus, i/l proptosis, c/l ptosis.

Reversible ptosis: Myasthenia gravis—**ice pack test [Figs. 6D(iii).20A to C]**
- The ice pack test is cheap, safe, and very quick to perform as it can be carried out at the bedside in approximately 3–5 minutes
- Positive test is the improvement of ptosis by >2 mm or more. This transient improvement in ptosis is due to the **cold** decreasing the acetylcholinesterase breakdown of acetylcholine at the neuromuscular junction.

Position of Eyeballs at Rest

Exophthalmos:
- Proptosis of eye
- Most commonly seen in hyperthyroidism.

Unilateral exophthalmos:
- Carotid-cavernous fistula (pulsatile exophthalmos)
- Thyroid disorder—hyperthyroidism
- Orbital mass lesion
- Cavernous sinus thrombosis
- Sphenoid wing meningioma
- Meningocele
- Mucormycosis.

Bilateral exophthalmos:
- Thyroid disorder
- Craniosynostosis
- Hand-Schuller-Christian disease

Enophthalmos: Enophthalmos can be defined as a relative, posterior displacement of a normal-sized globe in relation to the bony orbital margin. Causes are trauma, microphthalmia, postradiation, Horner's syndrome (apparent enophthalmos), Marfan syndrome, Duane's syndrome, or phthisis bulbi.

Extraocular Muscles

Functions of extraocular muscles [Fig. 6D(iii).21]:

	Primary function	Secondary function	Tertiary function
SR	Elevation	Intorsion	Adduction
IR	Depression	Extorsion	Adduction
SO	Intorsion	Depression	Abduction
IO	Extorsion	Elevation	Abduction
MR	Adduction		
LR	Abduction		

(SR: superior rectus; IR: inferior rectus; SO: superior oblique; IO: inferior oblique; MR: medial rectus; LR: lateral rectus)

Mnemonic: **SinRad**
- All **S**uperiors are **IN**tortors
- All **R**ecti are **AD**ductors except lateral rectus
- Function of **R**ecti is **R**egular (superior rectus is for elevation)
- Function of **O**blique is **O**pposite (superior oblique is for depression)
- In adducted eye—elevation is by inferior oblique and depression is by superior oblique
- In abducted eye—elevation is by superior rectus and depression is by inferior rectus.

Note: Position of testing the muscle and actual action of the muscle usually is opposite with respect to horizontal gaze.

Nervous System

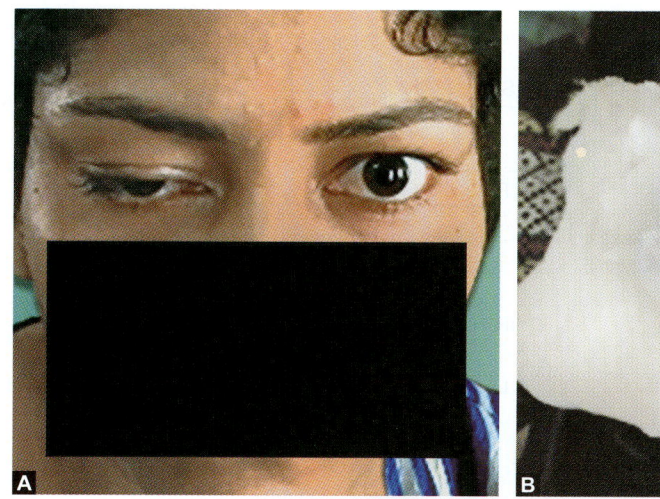
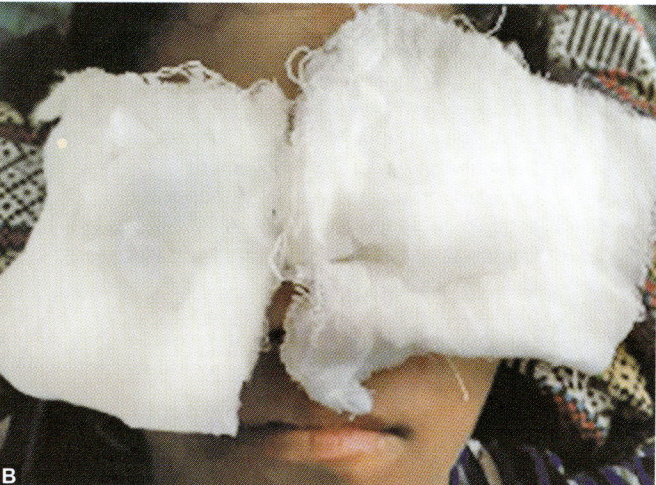
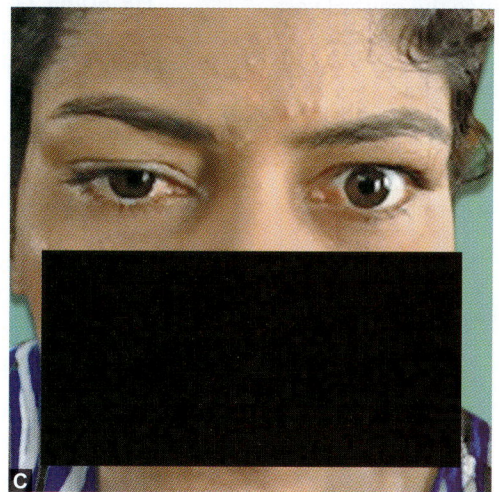

Figs. 6D(iii).20A to C: Reversible ptosis (ice pack test).

Muscle tested	Clinical testing	Movement
SR		Look laterally and upward
IR		Look laterally and downward
LR		Look laterally
MR		Look medially
IO		Look medially and upward
SO		Look medially and downward

Fig. 6D(iii).21: Extraocular movements.
(SR: superior rectus; IR: inferior rectus; SO: superior oblique; IO: inferior oblique; MR: medial rectus; LR: lateral rectus)

Ocular Movements

Uniocular—ductions

Binocular conjugate—versions

Binocular dysconjugate—vergences

Center for conjugate eye movements: Frontal eye field area number 8.

Saccades:
- Conjugate rapid eye movements
- Frontal lobe (premotor area number 6) controls saccadic movements.

Pursuits:
- Slow and smooth movement of eye following a moving target
- Occipital lobe is connected to the PPRF which is responsible for the horizontal pursuit movements.

Reflexes:
- Dolls eye reflex (oculocephalic reflex)
- Caloric stimulation test (vestibuloocular reflex).

Uniocular Movements

Nerve involved and features:

Nerve involved	Clinical features
III cranial nerve	- Down and out eye - Divergent squint - Ptosis - Dilatation of pupil
IV cranial nerve	- Defective downward eye movement - Outward rotation of eyeball by unopposed action of inferior rectus - Compensated by head tilt to opposite side
VI cranial nerve	- Defective lateral gaze - Medial squint - Patient may have diplopia on lateral gaze - Compensated by head turn to same side

In the oculomotor nerve [Fig. 6D(iii).22], the pupillary fibers are peripherally located. In compressive lesions from outside (tumor and hematoma), pupils are involved early. In ischemic lesions, pupils are spared since the central vasa nervosum is affected early.

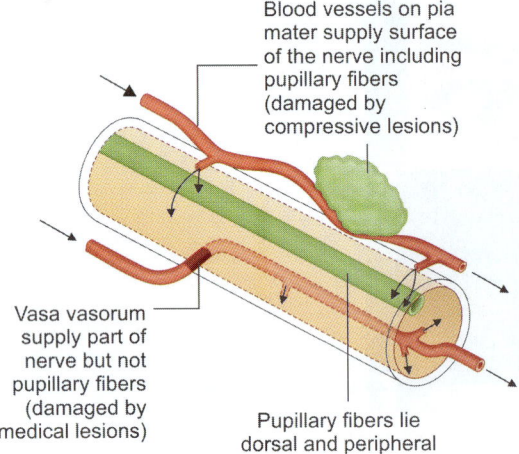

Fig. 6D(iii).22: Oculomotor nerve.

OCULAR MOVEMENT TESTING

Ask the patient to follow the examiner's finger or a red topped hat pin which is kept 60 cm away from the patient's face in all directions [Figs. 6D(iii).23 and 6D(iii).24]. A linear target should be held perpendicular to direction of gaze (vertical for testing horizontal gaze and horizontal for testing vertical gaze).

Etiology of III, IV, and VI nerve palsies		
	Medical palsy	*Surgical palsy*
III nerve ophthal-moplegia	Pupil sparing	Pupil involving
	Due to vascular causes where in the central part of nerve is involved (as visualized from the cut section)	Due to compression from the outside on the peripheral part of nerve (as visualized from the cut section)
	- Diabetes - Vasculitis - Myasthenia gravis - Myopathy	- Posterior communicating aneurysm - Tumors of base of skull
IV nerve palsy	Nuclear lesion	
VI nerve palsy	- Pontine lesions - False localizing sign wherein raised ICT is the cause for palsy	

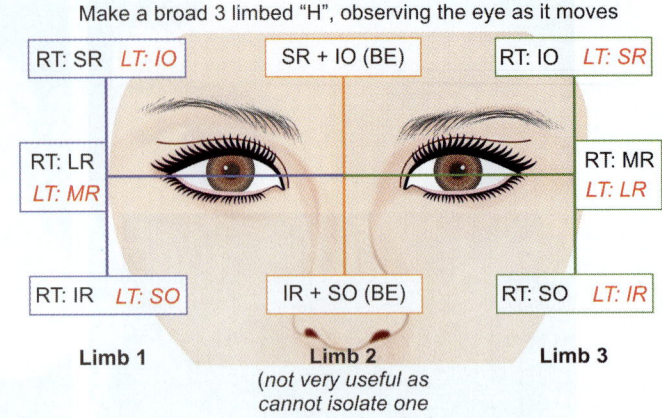

Fig. 6D(iii).23: Ocular movements testing method.
(RT: right; SR: superior rectus; IO: inferior oblique; LT: left; LR: lateral rectus; MR: medial rectus; IR: inferior rectus; SO: superior oblique; IO: inferior oblique)

DIPLOPIA

Diplopia means double vision. Most common subjective complaint elicited by lesions in the oculomotor system. Occurs more frequently with lesions of the extraocular muscles or oculomotor nerves than with supranuclear lesions which result in gaze palsies.

Monocular Diplopia

- The first point to clarify is whether diplopia persists in either eye after covering the fellow eye. If it does, the diagnosis is monocular diplopia.
- The cause is usually intrinsic to the eye. For example, corneal aberrations, uncorrected refractive error, cataract, foveal traction or foreign body in the aqueous or vitreous may give rise to monocular diplopia.

Binocular Diplopia

Diplopia improved by covering one eye is binocular diplopia and is caused by disruption of ocular alignment. Occurs only if both eyes are open.

Binocular diplopia occurs from a wide range or processes: For example, infectious, neoplastic, metabolic, degenerative, inflammatory, and vascular.

Assessment of Diplopia

- Cover one of the patient's eye with a transparent red shield. Move a point of light in the direction of action of each muscle.
- Ask the patient if he sees one object or two.
- If double, do the images lie side by side or one above the other?
  - Side by side—medial rectus (MR)/lateral rectus (LR)
  - One above the other—superior rectus (SR)/inferior rectus (IR) and superior oblique (SO)/inferior oblique (IO)

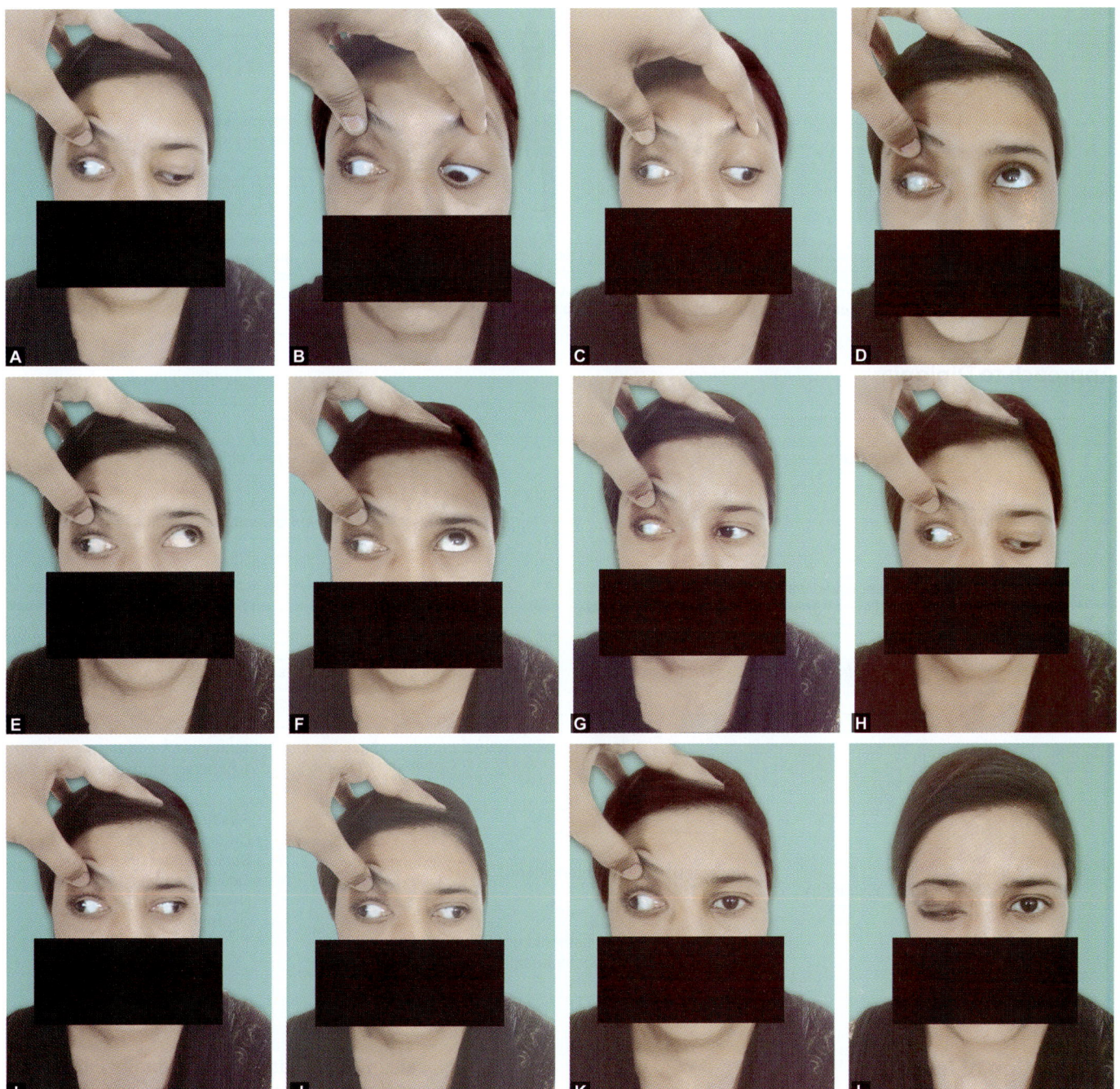

Figs. 6D(iii).24A to L: Ocular movements testing in a patient with right complete ophthalmoplegia.

- Which is the red image?
- In which position the images are the farthest.

Points to note:
- In diplopia two images, one real and one false are formed. The real image is closer to the eye and distinct; the false image is farther away from eye and indistinct.
- Separation of images is maximum in the direction of action of weak muscle.

Intermittent versus Constant Diplopia

- Diplopia that is intermittent tends to either be situation dependent (i.e., only noticeable with certain tasks or in specific environments) or worsen with fatigue.
- The former may suggest a tendency toward ocular misalignment or exacerbating elements that are amenable to modification and therefore may eliminate the symptoms.
- Diplopia that worsens with fatigue immediately raises suspicion for myasthenia gravis (MG).

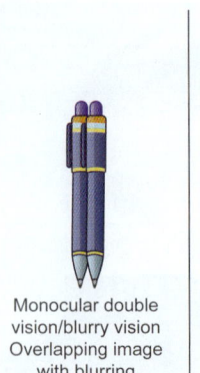 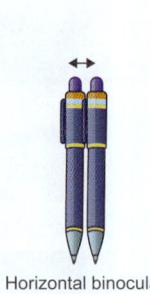 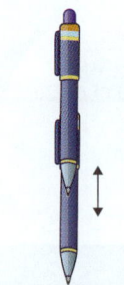 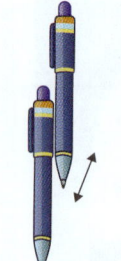 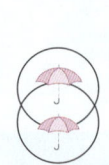 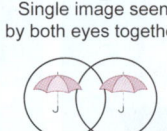 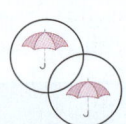

Monocular double vision/blurry vision Overlapping image with blurring | Horizontal binocular double vision Two identical images next to each other | Vertical binocular double vision Two identical images on top of each other | Oblique binocular double vision Two identical images at an angle to each other | Up-and-down double vision (vertical diplopia) | Side-by-side double vision (horizontal diplopia) | Combined side-by-side and up-and-down double vision (oblique diplopia) | Single image seen by both eyes together

Approach to Diplopia

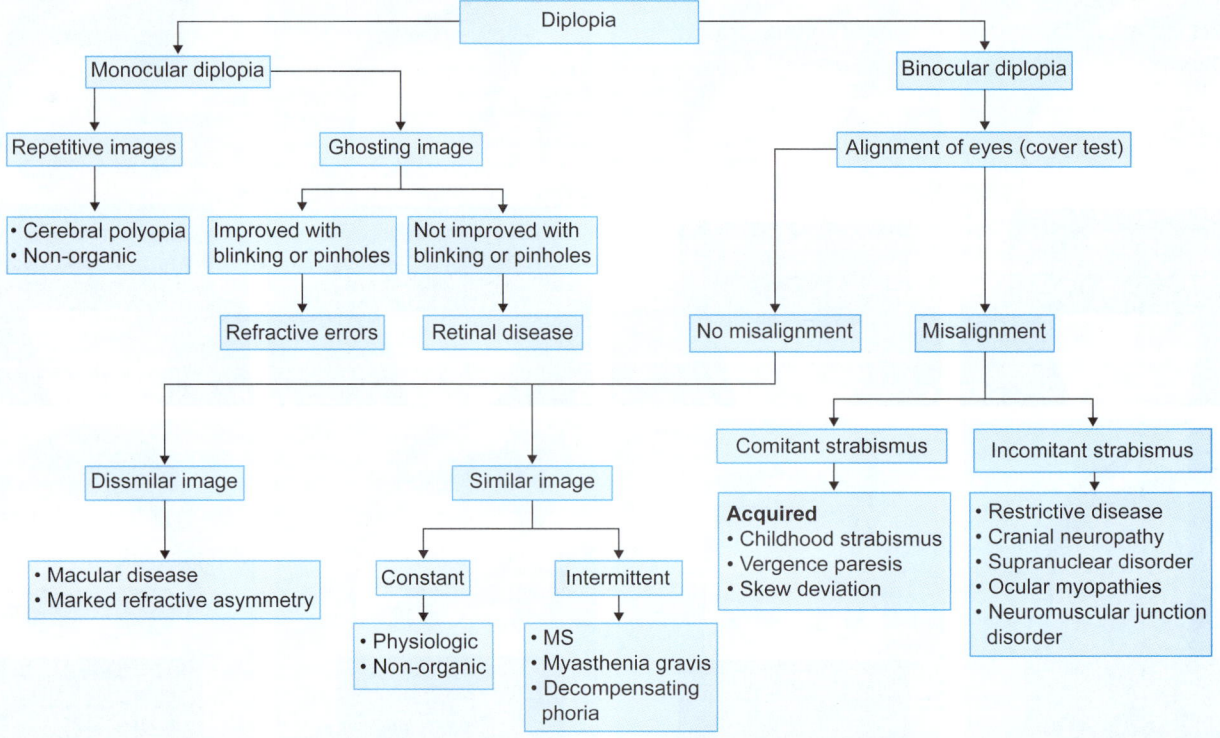

Orientation of Images

- Binocular diplopia that is horizontal in orientation suggests involvement of the medial or lateral rectus muscle.
- Diplopia that is vertical and torsional (with the lower image tilted) suggests involvement of the superior oblique muscle (particularly if associated with a compensatory head tilt to the side opposite the weak muscle).
- Pure vertical diplopia is more likely to reflect brainstem or cerebellar pathology (manifesting as an acquired vertical misalignment of the eyes, referred to as skew deviation).
- Diplopia that is oblique/diagonal, reflecting dysfunction of both vertical and horizontal muscles, suggests dysfunction of the oculomotor nerve (involving some combination of the inferior rectus, superior rectus and inferior oblique muscles).
- Further localizing information can be obtained by asking the patient whether the diplopia is worse in a specific direction of gaze (e.g., diplopia that is most pronounced on gaze to the left is supportive of dysfunction of the left lateral rectus muscle/cranial nerve VI).

Examination of Diplopia

- The red glass test can be helpful in examining patients with diplopia.
- A transparent piece of red glass or plastic is held over one eye, usually the right, and a small white light is held directly in front of the patient.
- The image seen by the right eye is therefore red, and the image seen by the left eye is white.
- The patient is then asked to follow the light as it is moved to nine different positions of gaze, and to report the locations of the white and red images.

- Normally the white and red images are fused in all positions of gaze.

Cover-Uncover Test

- Ask the patient to fix at an object (both near and distant, i.e., 30 cm and 6 m)
- While he fixates on the object, cover the right eye, and observe the left eye
- If the left eye moves to the target, it suggests that the left eye was not fixating. Note the angle of deviation of the left eye
- As the patient fixates with his left eye, uncover the right eye and cover the left eye. Note the angle of deviation
- Whichever angle of deviation is greater is the secondary deviation, while the lesser angle indicates the primary deviation (Hering's law)
- The eye with the primary deviation is the non-fixating (paretic) eye.

Muscle	Movement affected	Squint	Diplopia	
LR	Abduction	Convergent	Uncrossed	Maximum on looking laterally
MR	Adduction	Divergent	Crossed	Maximum on looking medially
SO	Downward movement in adduction	Convergent—in elevation and extorsion	Uncrossed	Maximum on looking down and medially
IO	Upward movement in adduction	Convergent—in depression and intorsion	Uncrossed	Maximum on looking up and medially
SR	Upward movement in abduction	Divergent—in depression and extorsion	Crossed	Maximum on looking up and laterally
IR	Downward movement in abduction	Divergent—in elevation and intorsion	Crossed	Maximum on looking down and laterally

(LR: lateral rectus; MR: medial rectus; SO: superior oblique; IO: inferior oblique; SR: superior rectus; IR: inferior rectus)

STRABISMUS/SQUINT

- Loss of parallelism of eyeball resulting in abnormal position of eyes.
- Primary deviation—deviation in the paralyzed eye
- Secondary deviation—deviation in the normal eye.

Types of Squint

Paralytic	Nonparalytic/Concomitant
Secondary deviation > primary deviation	Secondary deviation = primary deviation
Acquired	- Usually congenital - Starts in childhood
Diplopia present	No diplopia
Ocular movements affected	Ocular movements are full in all directions

Pupils

Miotic: <2 mm
Dilated: >6 mm
Inter pupil difference of 2 mm is significant

Miosis and mydriasis:

Large pupils	Small pupils
Unilateral: - Physiological - Pharmacological - Oculomotor nerve palsy - Adie's pupil - Uncal herniation - Traumatic sphincter paralysis - Iris ischemia - Ocular siderosis	**Unilateral:** - Physiological - Horner's syndrome - Anterior uveitis - Long standing Adie's pupil - Pharmacological
Bilateral: - Pharmacological - Parinaud's dorsal midbrain syndrome - Benign periodic mydriasis - Brainstem death	**Bilateral:** - Physiological senile miosis - Pharmacological - Argyll Robertson pupil - Lepromatous miosis - Congenital microcoria - Myotonic dystrophy

Cranial nerve palsy of CN 3, 4 and 6 is shown in Figure 6D(iii).25.

Light reflex:
- Mediated by retinal photoreceptors.
    - Subserved by four neurons [Fig. 6D(iii).26]
        1. First (sensory)—connects each retina with both pretectal nuclei, nasal fibers decussate, and temporal fibers uncrossed
        2. Second (internuncial)—connects each pretectal nucleus to both Edinger-Westphal nuclei— indirect reflex
        3. Third (preganglionic motor)—connects Edinger-Westphal nucleus to ciliary ganglion.
            ○ Parasympathetic fibers pass through III nerve inferior division and reach the ciliary ganglion via the nerve to the inferior oblique muscle.
        4. Fourth (postganglionic motor) leaves the ciliary ganglion and passes in the short ciliary nerves to innervate the sphincter pupillae.
- Tested in each eye individually
- Patient fixing at a distance
- Light shown to the eye obliquely.
- Cover uncover technique—uses ambient light

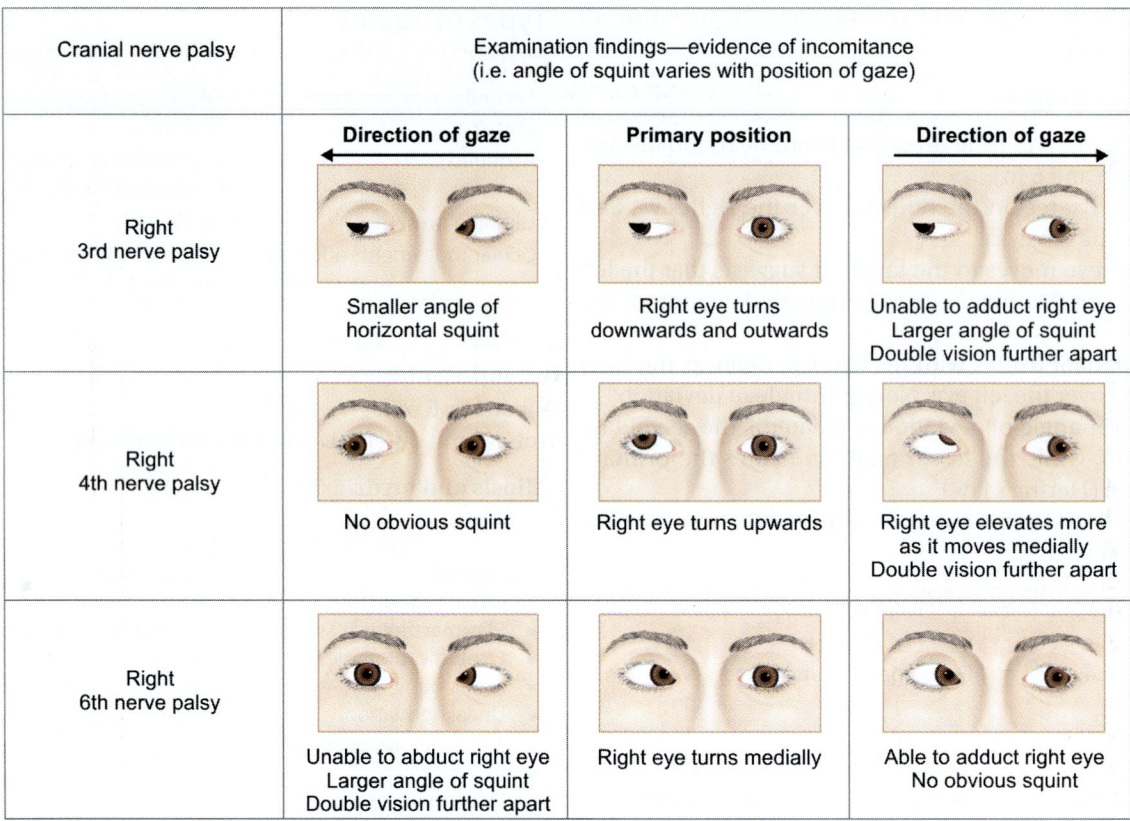

Fig. 6D(iii).25: Cranial nerve 3, 4, and 6 palsy.

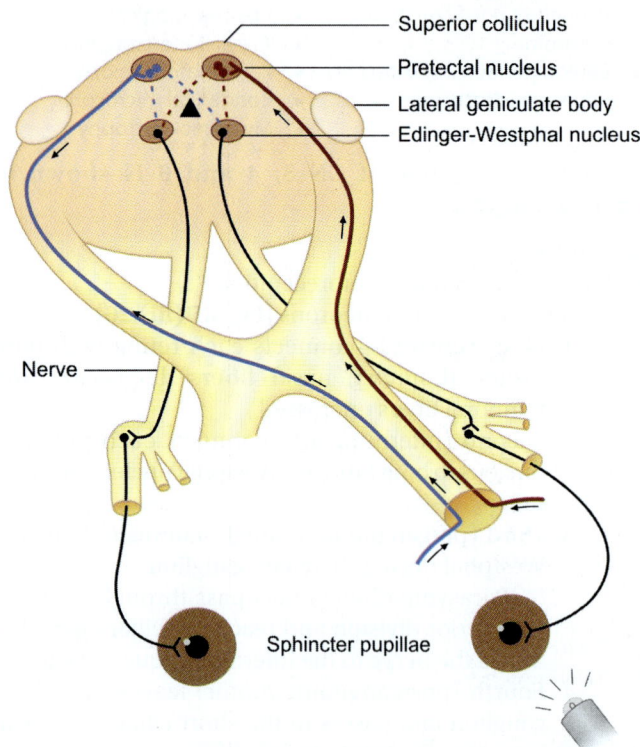

Fig. 6D(iii).26: Light reflex pathway.

- Normal response: Brisk constriction—slight dilatation back to an intermediate state.
- Can be recorded: Prompt, sluggish, and absent—graded 0–4+

The accommodation reflex:
- Relax accommodation by gazing at a distant object.
- Shifting gaze to some near object.
- The primary stimulus for accommodation is blurring.
- Response: Accommodation (thickening of the lens), convergence, and miosis. Pathway similar to light reflex till **[Fig. 6D(iii).27]**
- Fibers of Edinger–Westphal nucleus when entering the eye will cause constriction of the pupil and stimulation of ciliary muscle, so the parasympathetic causes the two changes (constriction of the pupil and contraction of ciliary muscle that increases the thickness of the lens thus increasing its power).
- The third change is convergence (adduction of both eyes by stimulating medial rectus on both sides); this is achieved by the vergence center that affects the oculomotor nucleus in the midbrain on this side and the other. Fibers coming from the oculomotor nucleus will enter and stimulate the medial rectus on both sides, when both eyes are adducted, the image will be on the same area (focus) of the retina.

PUPILLARY ABNORMALITIES

Argyll Robertson Pupil

- Small irregular pupil having light near dissociation **[Fig. 6D(iii).28]**
  Characteristic feature:
  - In dim light, both pupils are small and may be irregular.

Nervous System

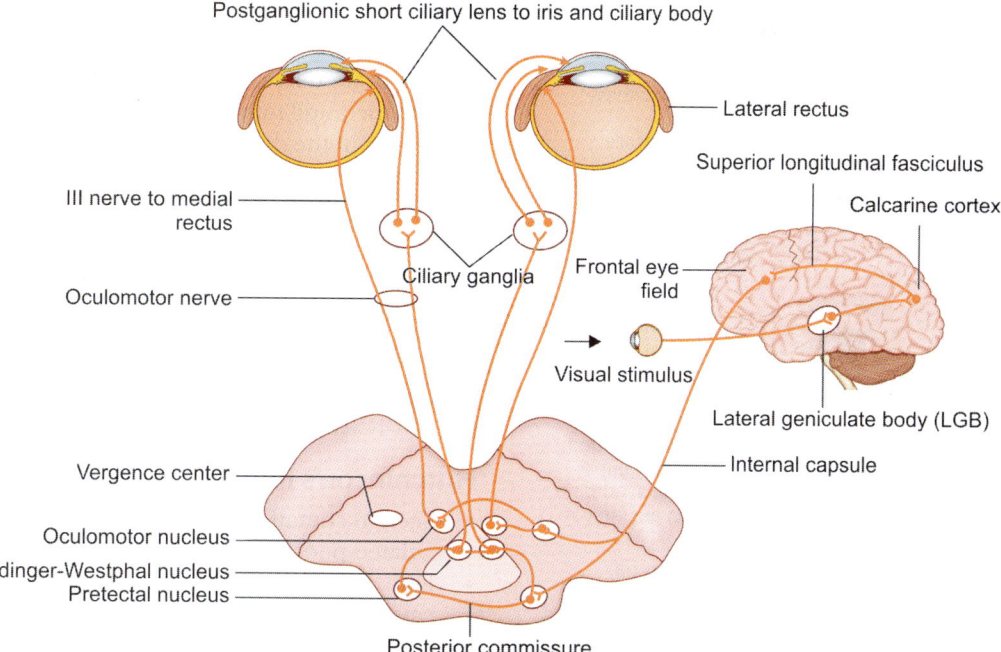

Fig. 6D(iii).27: Accommodation of reflex pathway.

- In bright light, neither pupil constricts.
- On accommodation both pupils constrict (light near dissociation).

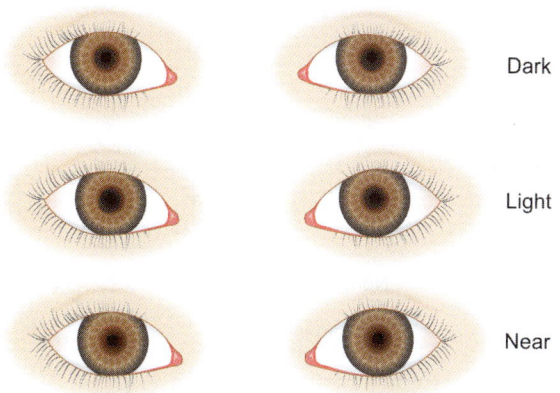

Fig. 6D(iii).28: Argyll Robertson pupil.

- After instillation of pilocarpine 0.1% into both eyes, neither pupil constricts.
- Described for neurosyphilis.
- Lesion in periaqueductal region, pretectal, and rostral midbrain.

Other causes: Diabetes mellitus, chronic alcoholism, multiple sclerosis, and sarcoidosis.

Reverse Argyll Robertson Pupil

In this accommodation, reflex on the pupil is absent.
Cause: Diphtheria and tumors at corpora quadrigemina.

Wernicke's Hemianopic Pupil

- It indicates lesion of the optic tract.
- In this condition, light reflex (ipsilateral direct and contralateral consensual) is absent when light is thrown on the temporal half of the retina of the affected side and nasal half of the opposite side; while it is present when the light is thrown on the nasal half of the affected side and temporal half of the opposite side.

The Adie's Tonic Pupil

In this condition, reaction to light is absent and to near reflex is very slow and tonic.
- The affected pupil is larger (anisocoria).
- Its exact cause is not known.
- It is usually unilateral, associated with absent knee jerk and occurs more often in young women.
- Adie's pupil constricts with weak pilocarpine (0.125%) drops, while normal pupil does not.
- In long-standing cases, the pupil may become small ("little old Adie").
- In some cases, are diminished deep tendon reflexes (Holmes-Adie syndrome).

Afferent Pupillary Defect or Marcus Gunn Pupil

- The status of the light reflex must be judged by comparing the two eyes [Fig. 6D(iii).29]

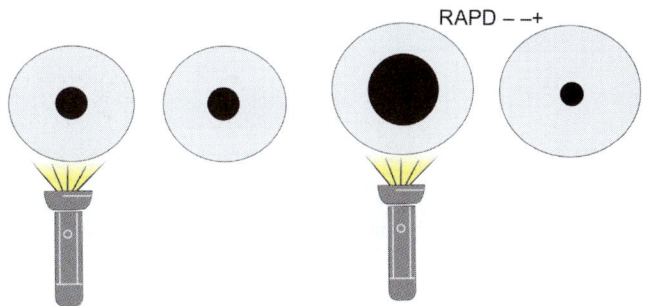

Fig. 6D(iii).29: Relative afferent pupillary defect (RAPD)/Marcus Gunn pupil.

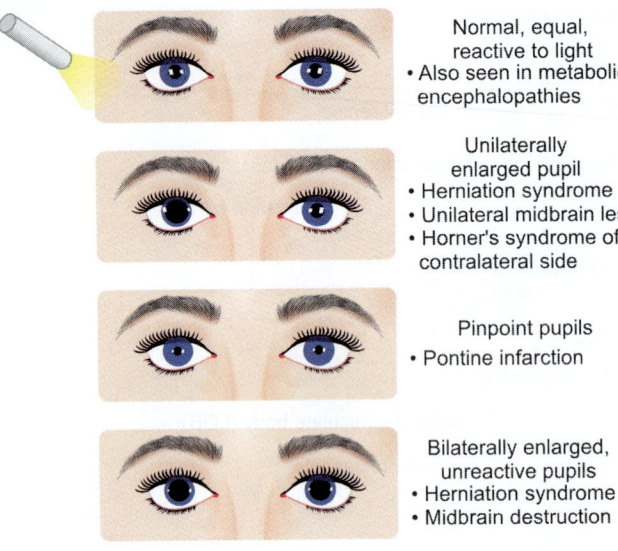

- Normal, equal, reactive to light
  - Also seen in metabolic encephalopathies
- Unilaterally enlarged pupil
  - Herniation syndrome
  - Unilateral midbrain lesion
  - Horner's syndrome of the contralateral side
- Pinpoint pupils
  - Pontine infarction
- Bilaterally enlarged, unreactive pupils
  - Herniation syndrome
  - Midbrain destruction

Fig. 6D(iii).30: Pupillary abnormalities in coma.

- Indicator of optic nerve function
- Swinging flashlight test: Light is held about 1 inch from the eye and just below the visual axis; the light is rapidly alternated.
  - The examiner attends only to the stimulated eye.
  - Comparing the amplitude and velocity of the initial constriction in the two eyes.
- The reaction is relatively weaker when the bad eye is illuminated.
- The brain detects a relative diminution in light intensity and the pupil may dilate a bit in response.
- Bring out the dynamic anisocoria.
- The weaker direct response or the paradoxical dilation of the light-stimulated pupil is termed as an afferent pupillary defect (APD).
- Trace APD: Pupil that has an initial constriction, but then it escapes to a larger intermediate position than in the other eye.
- 1 to 2+ APD: No change in pupil size initially, then dilation.
- 3 to 4+ APD: Immediate dilation of the affected pupil.

Hutchinson's Pupil

- Seen in comatose patients
- Dilated poorly reactive pupil
- Due to expanding intracranial supratentorial mass causing uncal herniation and III nerve compression.

Hippus

- Irregular rhythmic visible pupillary oscillations 2 mm/more in amplitude irregular dilating and constricting movements are observed
- Also called as pupillary athetosis.

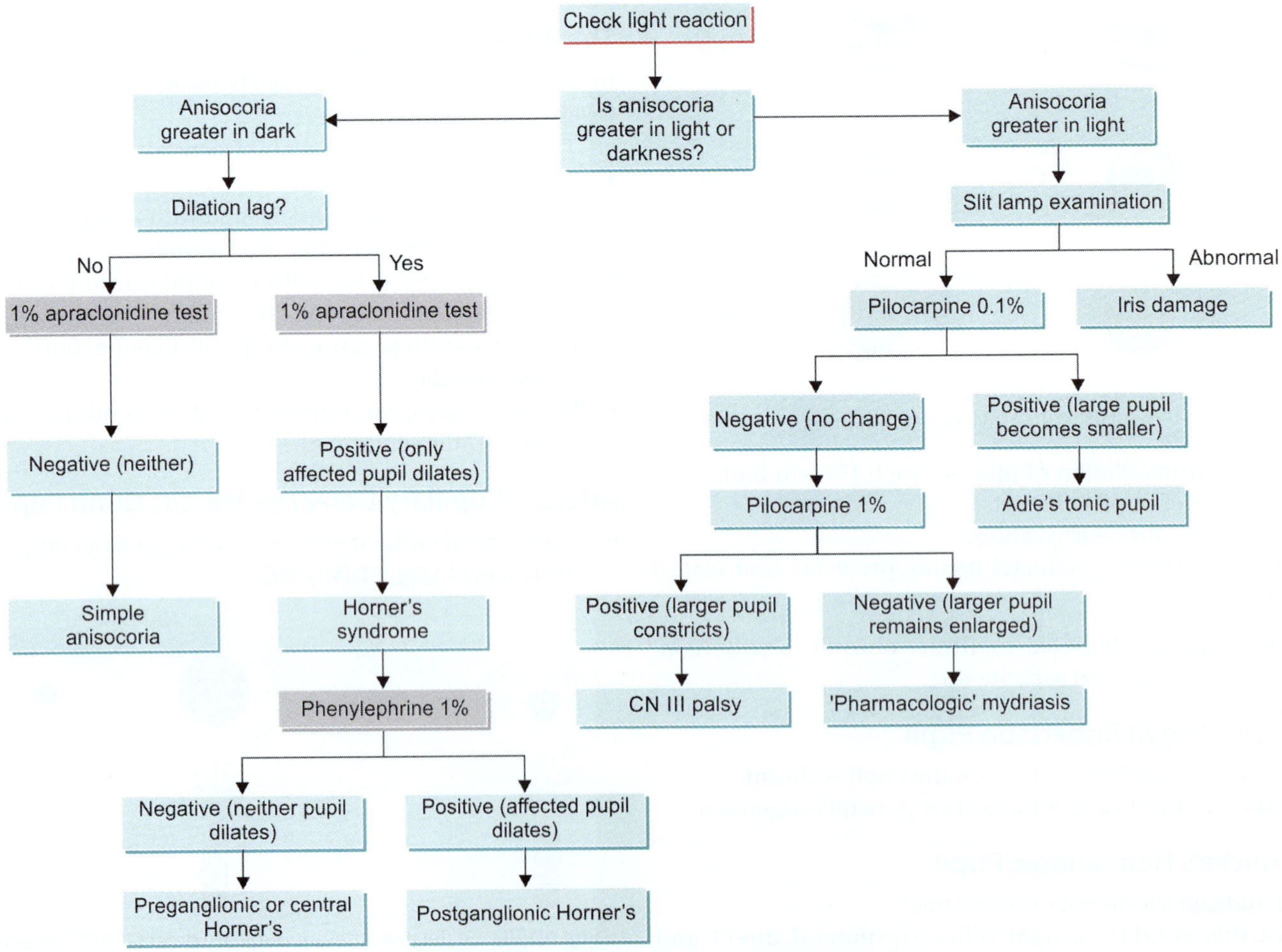

Fig. 6D(iii).31: Approach to pupillary abnormalities.

Unilateral (dilated)			Reaction to light (direct)	Associated signs
Third nerve palsy			None	Ptosis (partial or complete), external ophthalmoplegia
Holmes-Adie syndrome			Slow	Better response to accommodation, lower limb areflexia
Marcus Gunn pupil			Slow and incomplete	Normal consensual response, optic atrophy, central scotoma, impaired color vision
Local lesion of the iris			Variable depending on extent of local damage	Irregular pupil
Unilateral (constricted)				
Horner's syndrome			Reduced dilatation to shade	Ptosis (partial), ipsilateral facial anhidrosis, "enophthalmos"
Bilateral (dilated)				
Midbrain lesion			None	Mid-position pupils; impaired vertical gaze
Iatrogenic/atropine, tricyclic antidepressants			None or reduced	
Bilateral (constricted)				
Senile			None or reduced	
Iatrogenic, pilocarpine drops			None or reduced	
Pontine lesion			None	Pin-point pupils, coma, Cheyne-Stokes respiration
Argyll-Robertson			None	Irregular pupils, normal accommodation

Fig. 6D(iii).32: Summary of pupillary abnormalities.

- It is related to abnormal activity of the autonomic nervous system.
- **Cause:** Aconite poisoning, encephalopathies

Tectal Pupils

Large pupils with light near dissociation: Seen in lesions affecting the upper midbrain.

Pupillary abnormalities in Coma, Approach to Patient with Pupillary abnormalities and Summary of Pupillary Abnormalities is shown in **Figures. 6D(iii).30 to 6D(iii).32**.

Horner's Syndrome: Oculosympathetic Palsy

- **P**tosis: Denervation of Müller's muscles
- **M**iosis: Denervation of dilators
- **E**nophthalmos: Narrowing of palpebral fissure
- **A**nhidrosis: Sympathetic denervation
- **L**oss of ciliospinal reflex. Mnemonic—**P**rotein **MEAL** [Fig. 6D(iii).33].

Usually unilateral: The smooth muscle fibers of the lower eyelid retractors also lose their sympathetic supply in patients with Horner's syndrome and, thus, the lower eyelid appears slightly elevated. This appearance has been termed "**upside-down ptosis**" or "**reverse ptosis**".

- Hypochromic heterochromia (iris of different color—Horner is lighter) may be seen if congenital or long-standing. Sympathetic innervation is thought to be required for the formation of melanin by stromal melanocytes.
- Reduced ipsilateral sweating if the lesion is below the superior cervical ganglion, because the sudomotor fibers supplying the skin of the face run along the external carotid artery.

- Horner's syndrome is usually characterized by "**partial ptosis**" and "**apparent enophthalmos**".

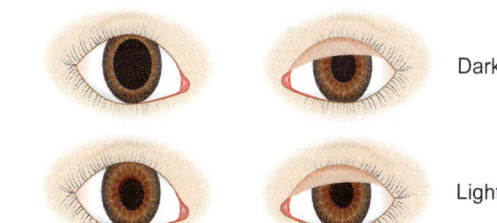

Dark

Light

Fig. 6D(iii).33: Horner's syndrome.

Causes of Horner's Syndrome [Figs. 6D(iii).34]

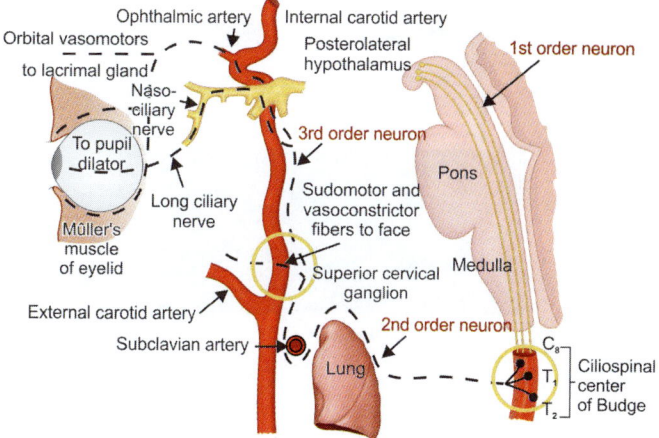

Fig. 6D(iii).34: Diagrammatic representation of sites of involvement of Horner's syndrome.

Unilateral [Figs. 6D(iii).35 and 6D(iii).36]	Bilateral
Central (1st order neurons): Brainstem disease (tumor, vascular, and demyelination), syringomyelia, lateral medullary (Wallenberg) syndrome, spinal cord tumor, and base of skull tumors/injury **Preganglionic (2nd order neuron):**<ul><li>Pancoast tumor, carotid and aortic aneurysm and dissection, neck lesions (glands, trauma, and postsurgical)</li><li>Birth trauma with lower brachial plexus injury and cervical rib</li></ul>**Postganglionic (3rd order neuron):** Cluster headaches (migrainous neuralgia), internal carotid artery dissection, nasopharyngeal tumor, otitis media, cavernous sinus mass, Raeder syndrome (paratrigeminal syndrome), and carotid cavernous fistula	Diabetic autonomic neuropathy, amyloidosis, pure autonomic failure, Anderson–Fabry disease, familial dysautonomia, and paraneoplastic syndrome

- **1st neuron:** Associated symptoms of brainstem involvement, such as dizziness, vertigo, transient ischemic attacks suggestive of hemianopia with/without long tract signs
  - Hydroxyamphetamine—dilates both pupils
  - Phenylephrine—dilates both pupils
  - Cocaine—Horner's pupil dilates more poorly than normal pupil
- **2nd neuron:** Chest mass with arm pain, phrenic nerve paralysis, supraclavicular nodes, neck mass, thyroid enlargement, neck surgery, neck injury, cervical osteoarthritis with bone spurs
  - Hydroxyamphetamine—dilates both pupils
  - Phenylephrine—dilates both pupils
  - Cocaine—Horner's pupil dilates more poorly than normal pupil
- **3rd neuron:** History of vascular headache (migraine, Raeder's, cluster), carotid artery disease with ipsilateral visual loss and contralateral motor and sensory signs. Sweating present if above bifurcation of carotid artery and absent if below bifurcation
  - Hydroxyamphetamine—Horner's pupil dilates less or not at all
  - Phenylephrine—Horner's pupil dilates more
  - Cocaine—Horner's pupil dilates more poorly or not at all

Fig. 6D(iii).35: Differentiating features of 1st order, 2nd order, and 3rd order Horner's syndrome.

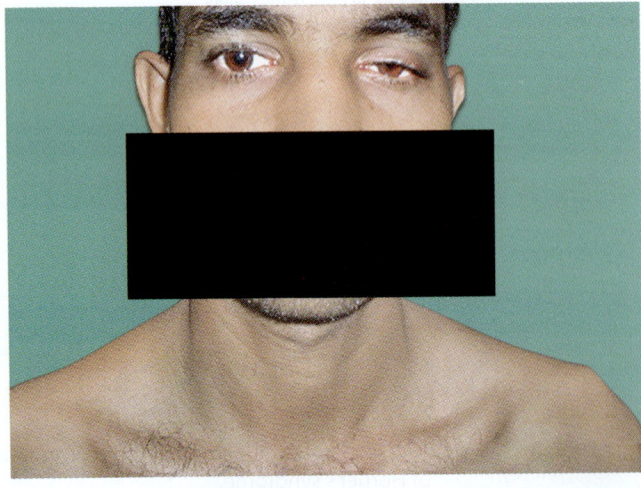

Fig. 6D(iii).36: Horner's syndrome.

OPHTHALMOPLEGIA

Definitions

- **Supranuclear ophthalmoplegia:** Also called as gaze palsies. It is due to involvement of corticonuclear fibers of the III, IV, and VI cranial nerves.
- **Internuclear ophthalmoplegia:** It is due to involvement of medial longitudinal fascicle (MLF) and paramedian pontine reticular formation (PPRF) which connect the III nerve to the contralateral VI nerve.
- **Nuclear/Infranuclear ophthalmoplegia:** Involvement of individual cranial nerves (CN III, IV, and VI).
- **Internal ophthalmoplegia:** Paralysis of constrictor pupillae and ciliary muscle.
- **External ophthalmoplegia:** Paralysis of extraocular muscles.
- **Total ophthalmoplegia:** Combination of external and internal ophthalmoplegia.

Gaze Palsies/Supranuclear Ophthalmoplegia

Vertical Gaze Palsies

Upward gaze palsy:
- Lesions at the superior colliculus—Parinaud's syndrome
- Progressive supranuclear palsy [Fig. 6D(iii).37].

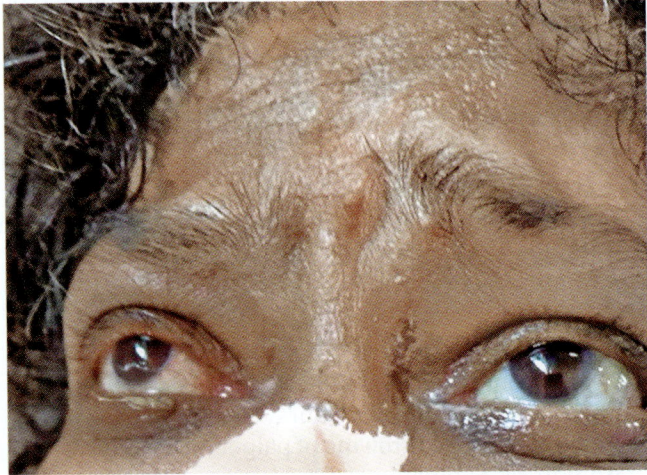

Fig. 6D(iii).37: Reptilian stare in progressive supranuclear palsy.

- Parkinson's disease
- Wernicke's encephalopathy
- Thalamic hemorrhage (Sunset sign).

Downward gaze palsy:
- Huntington's chorea
- Niemann–Pick disease
- Olivopontocerebellar ataxia
- Progressive supranuclear palsy
- Parkinson's disease.

Combined upward and downward gaze palsy:
- Bilateral frontal lobe lesions
- Progressive supranuclear palsy
- Parkinson's disease.

Nervous System

Horizontal Gaze Palsies

- Frontal eye field (Area number 8)
- Destructive lesion—gaze deviation towards diseased side both eyes will turn toward the side of lesion (Vulpian sign)
- Irritative lesion—gaze deviation towards normal side
- Pontine lateral gaze center
- Destructive lesion— gaze deviation towards normal side

Internuclear Ophthalmoplegia

- Caused by a lesion of the medial longitudinal fascicle (MLF), which carries signals from the abducens nucleus to the contralateral medial rectus oculomotor subnucleus [Fig. 6D(iii).38].
- The abducens nerve and MLF coordinate conjugate horizontal eye movements with co-contraction of ipsilateral lateral rectus and contralateral medial rectus muscles.
- Classic signs of unilateral internuclear ophthalmoplegia include impaired adduction of the ipsilesional eye and abducting nystagmus of the contralateral eye.
- Despite ipsilateral adduction weakness with direct motility testing, adduction is often intact with convergence because convergence signals to the medial rectus nucleus are distinct from the MLF.
- Multiple sclerosis and microvascular brainstem ischemia are the most common causes.
- Less common causes for an INO include traumatic, neoplastic, inflammatory (e.g., sarcoid, Behcet's disease, lupus), or infectious [e,g., cryptococcosis, *Borrelia burgdorferi* (Lyme disease)] etiologies.
- INO is rare in children but may result from neoplasms (e.g., medulloblastomas or pontine gliomas).

Note: Normality of lid and pupil distinguishes an INO from third nerve palsy.

Superior INO (Lhermitte's syndrome)	Lesions in the brainstem
Inferior INO (Lutz syndrome)	Lesions in the pontine lateral gaze center → to the abducens nucleus
Pseudo-INO	- Myasthenia gravis - Wernicke's encephalopathy - Thyroid eye disease
WEBINO syndrome (wall-eyed bilateral INO)	Bilateral MLF and bilateral medial rectus nucleus
WEMINO syndrome (wall-eyed monocular INO)	Unilateral MLF and unilateral medial rectus nucleus
One and a half syndrome	Involvement of pontine PPRF and adjacent MLF
Eight and a half syndrome	One and a half syndrome + 7th nerve palsy

(INO: internuclear ophthalmoplegia; MLF: medial longitudinal fasciculus; PPRF: paramedian pontine reticular formation; WEBINO: wall-eyed bilateral internuclear ophthalmoplegia; WEMINO: wall-eyed monocular internuclear ophthalmoplegia)

Etiology of Nuclear or Infranuclear Palsy

Site	Oculomotor nerve palsy	Trochlear nerve palsy	Abducens nerve palsy
Brainstem	- Weber's syndrome - Nothnagel syndrome - Benedict's syndrome - Claude's syndrome	Midbrain syndromes	- Millard–Gubler syndrome - Raymond-Céstan syndrome - Foville's syndrome - Möbius syndrome
Subarachnoid space	+	+	–
Petrous apex—Dorello's canal	–	–	+ (Gradenigo's syndrome)
Cavernous sinus	+	+	+
Superior orbital fissure	+	+	+
Orbit	+/–	+	–

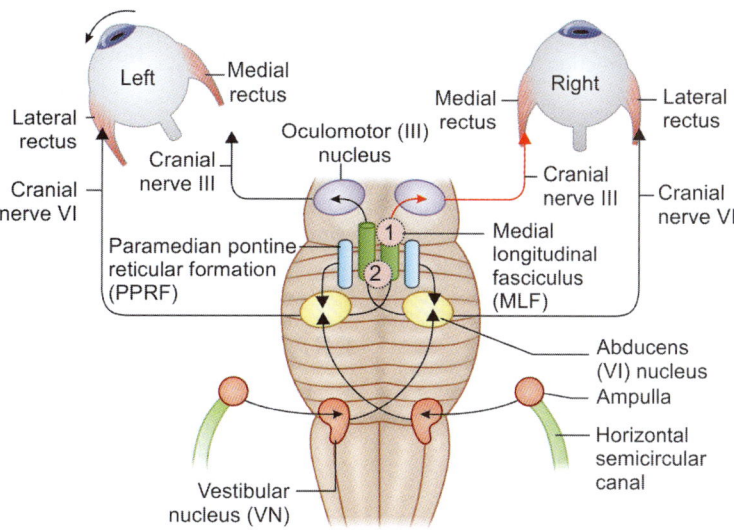

Fig. 6D(iii).38: Internuclear ophthalmoplegia.

Painful Ophthalmoplegia

- Cavernous sinus thrombosis
- Superior orbital fissure syndrome—Tolosa-Hunt syndrome
- Ophthalmoplegic migraine
- Pituitary apoplexy
- Orbital cellulitis
- Orbital tumors.

	Supranuclear ophthalmoplegia	Nuclear/infranuclear ophthalmoplegia
Movements affected	Gaze	Individual muscle movements
Diplopia and squint	Absent	Present
Pupils	Normal	May or may not be involved
Vestibulo-ocular reflex (cold caloric)	+	–

NYSTAGMUS

Definition: Nystagmus is involuntary, conjugate, repetitive, and rhythmic movements of eyeball.

Method of examination: Eyes should be deviated in all four directions for at least 5 seconds and deviation should not be of extremes.

Grading/degrees of nystagmus	
I	Nystagmus only on deviation of eyes
II	Nystagmus on looking forward
III	Direction of nystagmus opposite to the fast beating component

Types of Nystagmus

Physiological nystagmus—end point, OKN, induced vestibular.

Pendular nystagmus	Jerk nystagmus			Nystagmus of dissociated rhythm
In this type amplitude of nystagmus is equal in either directions	In this type of nystagmus, there is slow component followed by fast (jerk) component due to cortical correction			Usually gaze evoked nystagmus
	Horizontal	*Vertical*	*Rotatory*	
These are predominantly seen in congenital conditions especially due to visual defects from earlier years	- Labyrinthine disorders - Cerebellar disorders - Uppermost cervical lesion	- Never labyrinthine - Cerebellar disorders - Brainstem lesions - Drugs like benzodiazepines and barbiturate	- Labyrinthine disorders - Brainstem lesions	MLF lesions Multiple sclerosis

Other Common Types of Nystagmus

	Description	Condition seen
Seesaw nystagmus	Upward deflection of one eyeball with downward deflection on the contralateral eyeball	Suprasellar region anterior to III ventricle/craniopharyngioma
Up beat nystagmus	Fast movement upward	Lesions in the vermis of the cerebellum
Down beat nystagmus	Fast component is down	Foramen magnum lesions
Optokinetic nystagmus	Railway track nystagmus	**Physiological**, changes occur in deep parietal lobe lesions
Convergence retraction nystagmus	Convergent motions with globe retractions into orbit	Lesion at superior colliculus—Parinaud's syndrome

Non-nystagmus Oscillations of Eyeball

Ocular flutter	Periodic horizontal saccades	Cerebellar and PPRF lesions
Opsoclonus	Irregular oscillations with different amplitude and directions	- Toxins - Encephalitis
Ocular bobbing	Rapid downstroke followed by slow uprise of eyeball	Pontine destruction
Ocular dipping	Slow downstroke followed by rapid uprise of the eyeball	Toxic encephalopathy

(PPRF: paramedian pontine reticular formation)

	Central nystagmus	Peripheral nystagmus
Fast component	Fast component is toward same side of pathology	Fast component is to the opposite of the pathology
Duration of episode	Long lasting	Acute and transient
Vertigo	Less prominent	Usually associated
Suppression on fixation using Fresnel lens	Not suppressed	Suppressed
Pursuits and saccades	Usually present	Absent
Other clinical finding	CNS involvement is seen	Hardness of hearing and tinnitus is seen

(CNS: central nervous system)

CRANIAL NERVE V—TRIGEMINAL NERVE

- Largest among cranial nerves
- Most complex of the cranial nerves. We shall discuss trigeminal nerve under:
  1. Sensory component and motor components
  2. Reflexes
  3. Disorders of trigeminal nerve dysfunction

Sensory and Motor Component

Component	Sensory part	Motor part
Size	Larger	Smaller
Nuclei	Three nuclei	One nuclei
Distribution	• Face (except angle of mandible) • Teeth • Oral cavity • Nasal cavity • Scalp to vertex • Intracranial dura • Cerebral vasculature • Proprioception to muscles of mastication	Muscles of mastication

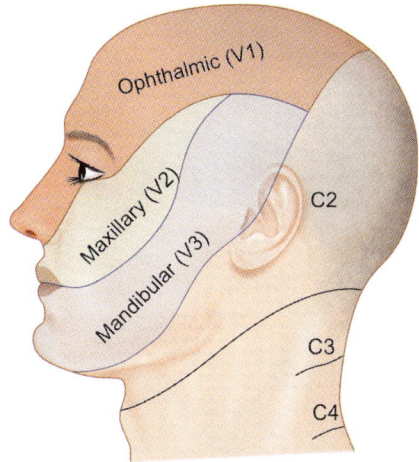

Fig. 6D(iii).39: Image showing sensory distribution of three divisions of trigeminal nerve.

Distribution [Fig. 6D(iii).39]: The distribution of CN V3 does not extend to the jaw line; there is a large "notch" at the angle of the jaw innervated by the greater auricular nerve (C2-3).

Nuclei and functions:

Nuclei	Location	Function
Motor nuclei	Pons	• **M**uscles of mastication • **M**ylohyoid • **A**nterior belly of digastric • **T**ensor veli palatini • **T**ensor tympani
Principle sensory nucleus	Pons	• Pressure • Touch • Vibration
Mesencephalic nuclei	Extends to midbrain	Proprioception of muscles of mastication, extraocular muscle (EOM), facial expression
Spinal nucleus	Extends to spinal nucleus (C3, 4) via medulla—quintothalamic tract	• Pain • Temperature

Notes:
- All the sensory supply relay via trigeminal ganglion which is also called as Gasserian ganglion or semilunar ganglion.
- It is largest ganglion located at Meckel's cave, lateral to ICA and posterior to cavernous sinus.
- It is analogous to dorsal root ganglion.

Testing of sensory component:
- Test the sensation of the face for touch, pain, and temperature in each of the divisions.
- Sensation should be compared in each trigeminal division, and the perioral region compared to the posterior face to exclude an onion skin pattern **[Figs. 6D(iii).40 to 6D(iii).43]**
- Pain or temperature should be compared with touch to exclude dissociated sensory loss (a common finding in lateral medullary syndrome).

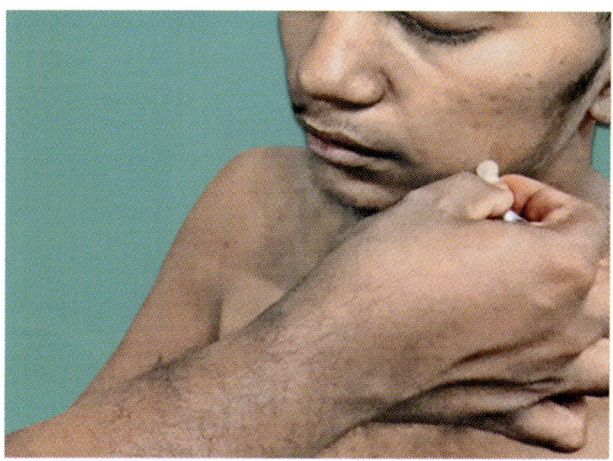

Fig. 6D(iii).40: Examination of sensory component of trigeminal nerve.

- On the trunk, organic sensory loss typically stops short of midline because of the overlap from the opposite side, and crossing of the midline suggests nonorganic nature of the symptoms. However, this finding is not reliable on the face because there is less midline overlap, so organic facial sensory loss may extend to the midline.

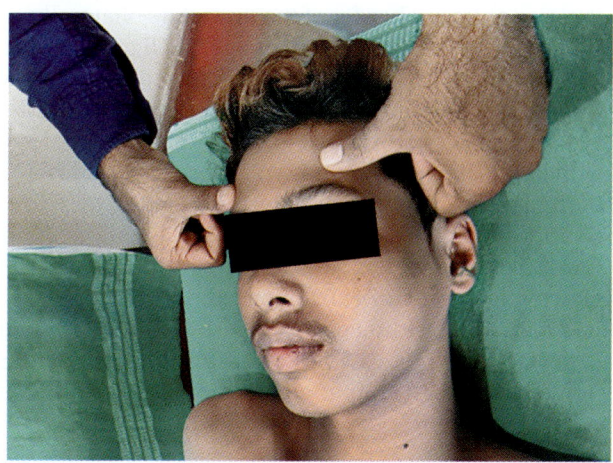

Fig. 6D(iii).41: Examination of ophthalmic division of trigeminal nerve.

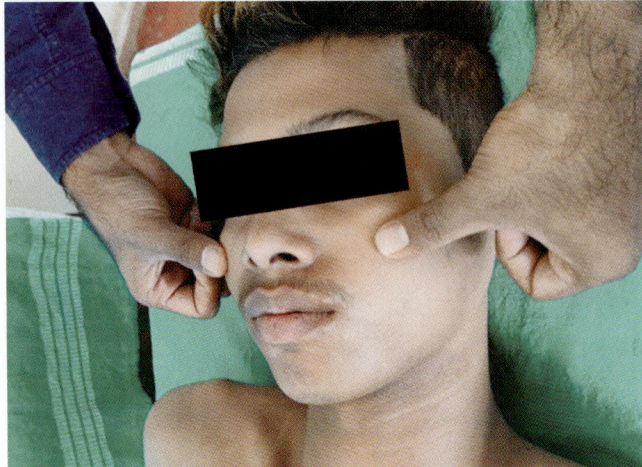

Fig. 6D(iii).42: Examination of maxillary division of trigeminal nerve.

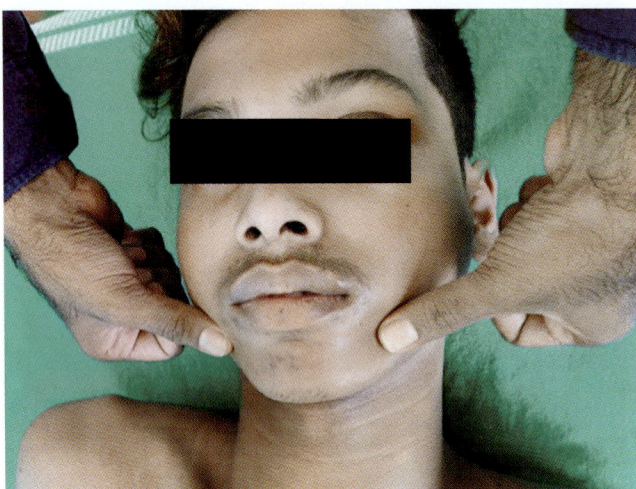

Fig. 6D(iii).43: Examination of mandibular division of trigeminal nerve.

Unilateral weakness of CN V innervated muscles	Bilateral weakness of the muscles of mastication with inability to close the mouth (dangling jaw)
Suggests: - The brainstem - Gasserian ganglion pathology - The motor root of CN V at the base of the skull	**Suggests:** - Motor neuron disease - Neuromuscular transmission disorder - Myopathy

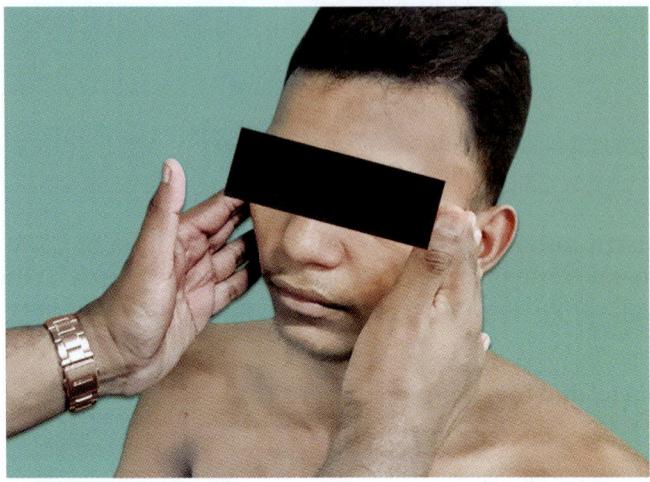

Fig. 6D(iii).44: Examination of motor component of trigeminal nerve (masseter muscle).

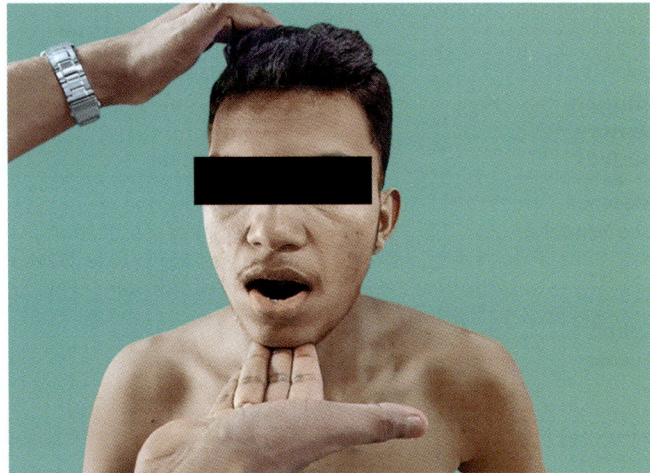

Fig. 6D(iii).45: Examination of motor component of trigeminal nerve (pterygoid muscle).

Testing of motor component [Figs. 6D(iii).44 and 6D(iii).45]:
- Motor component can be gauged by palpating these muscles as the patient clinches the jaw. An effective technique is to place the examining fingers along the anterior or lateral border of the masseters bilaterally.
- When the jaw is clenched, the fingers will move forward (when fingers placed anteriorly) or sideward (when fingers placed laterally); this movement should be symmetric on the two sides.
- Unilateral trigeminal motor weakness causes deviation of the jaw toward the weak side on opening, due to the unopposed action of the contralateral lateral pterygoid. Careful observation of jaw opening is often the earliest clue to the presence of an abnormality.
- It is occasionally difficult to be certain whether the jaw is deviating or not. Note the relationship of the midline notch between the upper and lower incisor teeth; it is a reliable indicator.

Rule of 17 (10 + 7 and 12 + 5)
- **10 + 7** → In facial nerve weakness and vagus nerve involvement, the deviation will be toward the normal side - The levator anguli oris (in CN 7) and palatopharyngeus (in CN 10) are 'pulling' muscles. Hence, the normal side 'pulls' the angle of mouth/uvula toward the normal side - **12 + 5** → In trigeminal nerve and hypoglossal nerve weakness, the deviation will be toward the affected side - The lateral pterygoid (CN 5) and the genioglossus (CN 12) are 'pushing' muscles. Hence, the normal side 'pushes' the angle of jaw/tongue toward the affected side

Reflexes

Reflexes associated with V nerve:
1. Jaw jerk [Fig. 6D(iii).46]
2. Sternutatory reflex
3. Corneal reflex
4. Conjunctival reflex

Jaw Jerk or Masseter or Mandibular Reflex

Theory: Sensory fibers → mesencephalic nucleus → reflex center in pons → motor nucleus → motor fibers. Afferent and efferent both are by trigeminal nerve.

Normal	Minimal or absent response
Limb hyperreflexia due to cervical spinal lesion	Normal jaw reflex
Generalized hyperreflexia	Exaggerated jaw reflex

Note: Exaggerated reflex is due to lesion in the bilateral corticobulbar tracts above motor nucleus, e.g., pseudobulbar palsy or amyotrophic lateral sclerosis.

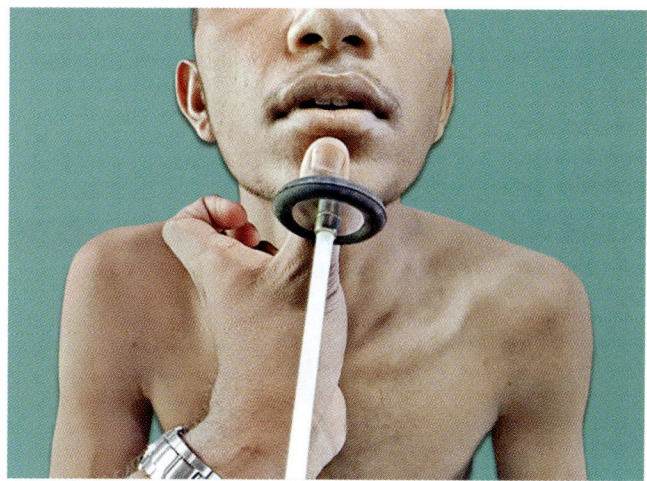

Fig. 6D(iii).47: Examination of jaw jerk.

Sternutatory/Nasal/Sneeze Reflex

Primary clinical use is to cross check the corneal reflex.

Method: Stimulation of nasal mucous membrane with cotton, a spear of tissue or similar object → wrinkling of nose, eye closure, and often a forceful exhalation resembling a feeble sneeze.

Theory: The ophthalmic division of trigeminal innervates the nasal septum and anterior nasal passages.

Afferent limb	Center	Efferent limb
V1	Brainstem and upper spinal cord	V VII IX X

Corneal Reflex

- Elicited by lightly touching the cornea with wisp of cotton or tissue [Fig. 6D(iii).48].
- Stimulus is ideally delivered to upper cornea because the lower cornea may be innervated by CN V2 in some individuals.
- Stimulus should be ideally brought in from the side so that patient cannot see it.
- Stimulus must be delivered to cornea but not sclera.

Afferent limb	Efferent limb
V1	VII

Conjunctival Reflex

- Same as corneal reflex [Fig. 6D(iii).48]
- However, the sensitivity of corneal reflex is more.

Trigeminal lesion (complete)		
	Direct reflex	Consensual (indirect) reflex
Stimulus to involved eye	Absent	Absent
Stimulus to opposite eye	Present	Present

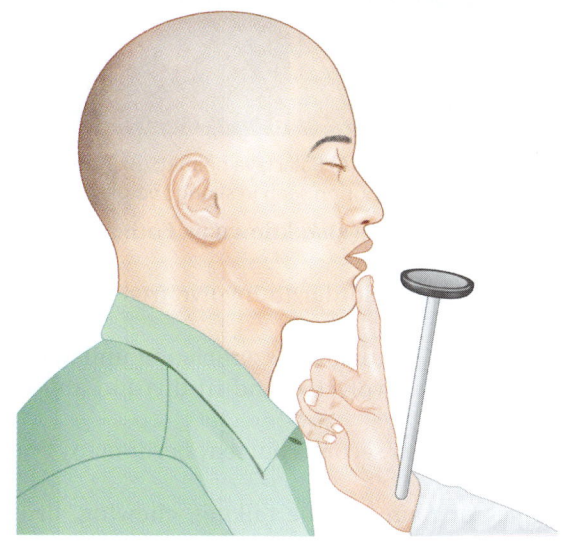

Fig. 6D(iii).46: Illustration showing examination of jaw jerk.

Testing [Fig. 6D(iii).47]:
- Examiner places the index finger or thumb over the middle of patient's chin, holding the mouth open about midway with jaw relaxed and then taps the finger with reflex hammer.
- The response is upward jerk of mandible.

Other methods:
- For bilateral response:
  - Tapping chin directly
  - Placing the tongue blade over the tongue or lower incisor and tapping the protruding end.
- For unilateral response:
  - Tapping the angle of the jaw
  - Placing the tongue blade over the lower molar teeth of one side and tapping the protruding end.

Facial nerve lesion (complete)		
	Direct reflex	Consensual (indirect) reflex
Stimulus to involved eye	Absent	Present
Stimulus to opposite side	Present	Absent

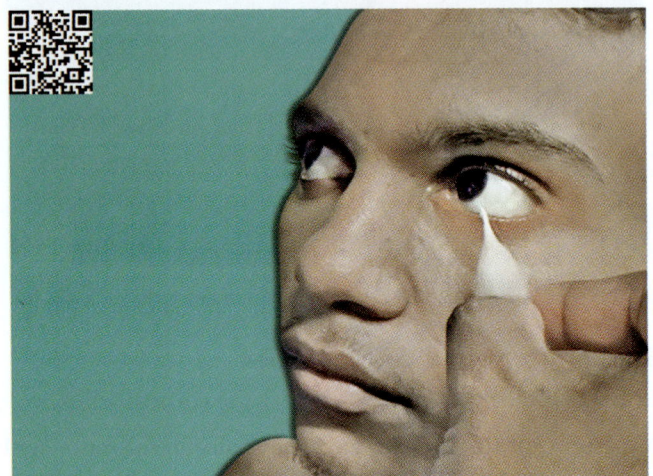

Fig. 6D(iii).48: Demonstration of corneal/conjunctival reflex.

Disorders of V Nerve Dysfunction

1. Motor Dysfunction

- Unilateral UMN lesion—generally no weakness observed.
- Bilateral UMN lesion—pseudobulbar palsy—marked weakness seen with exaggerated jaw jerk.
- Myasthenia gravis—masticatory fatigue (not to be confused with claudication pain of giant cell arteritis)
- ALS: Jaw drop with—dysphagia and difficulty in swallowing their own saliva.
- Involuntary movements include—dystonia (extrapyramidal symptoms of antipsychotic drugs), Meige syndrome (oromandibular dystonia with blepharospasm), and trismus.

Causes of trigeminal nerve involvement
▪ Supranuclear—bilateral (pseudobulbar) palsy
▪ Nuclear—syringobulbia
▪ Nerve root—cerebellopontine angle tumor
▪ Gasserian ganglion—Gradenigo syndrome, otitis media, meningitis, and aneurysms of internal carotid artery
▪ Cavernous sinus—thrombosis/tumor
▪ Superior orbital fissure—Tolosa–Hunt
▪ Individual branches involvement

Sensory Dysfunction

Site of lesion	Disease	Manifestation
Parietal lobe or sensory radiation (supranuclear lesion)	Stroke/tumors	May raise the sensory threshold of contralateral face
Thalamic lesion	Stroke/tumors	Facial hypoesthesia with hyperpathia or allodynia

Contd...

Contd...

Principal sensory nucleus: Pressure Touch Vibration	Stroke/tumors	Diminished tactile sensation of skin and mucous membrane of that side
Spinal nucleus	Lateral medullary or pontine lesion/tumors	Pain and temperature loss
Intramedullary lesion Extramedullary lesion	Syringomyelia/syringobulbia/tumors [Figs. 6D(iii).49A and B]	Dissociative loss of sensation Diminution or loss of all exteroceptive sensations.

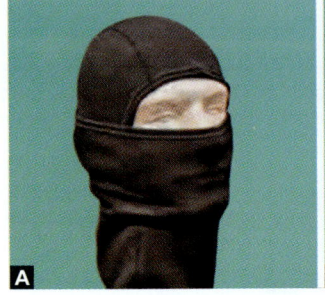 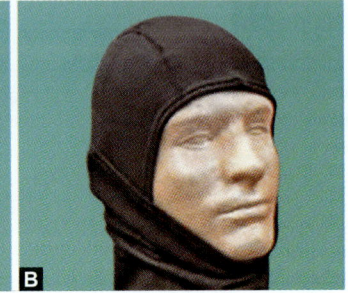

Figs. 6D(iii).49A and B: (A) Balaclava helmet; (B) Dejerine onion skin distribution seen in syringobulbia.

Trigeminal neuralgia (also known as Fothergill's disease tic douloureux)

- Most common disorder to involve trigeminal sensory function.
- Paroxysms of fleeting but excruciation unilateral facial pain—usually involves II and III division and rarely I division.
- Pain lasts for few seconds but may occur many times per day.
- Trigger for pain may be talking, chewing, brushing, exposure to cold or by wind on face.
- Most common cause for compression of sensory root by ecstatic arterial loop of the basilar artery (AICA or superior cerebellar artery)
- Other causes include MS, tumors of CP angle—bilateral is suggestive of MS.

2. Postherpetic Neuralgia

Acute herpes zoster is extremely painful.

- Usually in CN V1—pain in vesicles in forehead, eyelid, and cornea but may affect other division also.
- Persistent neuralgic pain syndrome after 3 months of acute eruption is appropriately labeled as postherpetic neuralgia. It is a dysesthetic with burning component, constant but with superimposed paroxysm of lancinating pain that may be provoked by touching certain spots in affected area.

3. Facial Numbness

- *Numb chin syndrome:* In distribution of mental nerve—due to metastatic process in mental foramen.
- *Numb cheek syndrome:* Involvement of infraorbital nerve.

4. Other Trigeminal Nerve Disorders

Marcus-Gunn phenomenon or jaw winking phenomenon	Seen in congenital ptosis: Opening the mouth, chewing or lateral jaw movements cause an exaggerated reflex elevation of the ptotic lid due to proprioceptive impulses form the pterygoid muscles being misdirected to the oculomotor nucleus
Reversed Gunn phenomenon or inverse jaw winking or Marin-Amat sign	Synkinesis due to aberrant regeneration of facial nerve where there is involuntary closure of one eye on mouth opening
Frey syndrome	Flushing, warmness, and excessive perspiration over the cheek and pinna on one side following ingestion of spicy food— due to misdirection of secretory fibers to parotid gland to the sweat glands and vasodilator ending in the auriculotemporal nerve distribution—usually follows trauma or infection of parotid gland or local nerve injury
Sturge–Weber or Weber–Dimitri disease	Congenital nevi or angiomas over the side of face in the trigeminal distribution with associated ipsilateral leptomeningeal angiomas and intracortical calcification with attendant neurologic complications
Raeder's paratrigeminal syndrome	▪ Unilateral oculosympathetic paresis (differential diagnosis with Horner) ▪ pain in the distribution of the ophthalmic branch of the trigeminal nerve (V1)
Gradenigo's syndrome	▪ Damage to V1 division of trigeminal nerve ▪ Ipsilateral 6th nerve palsy
Cavernous sinus syndrome	3, 4, 6 nerves with V1 and V2 (less often)
Superior orbital fissure syndrome	Never involving V2, other than that similar to cavernous sinus syndrome. Exophthalmos and blindness can be present
V1: Bilateral corneal anesthesia	Diabetic neuropathy
V2: Numb cheek syndrome	▪ Infraorbital nerve ▪ Distribution: Squamous cell carcinoma, skin and LASIK
V2: Trumpet player's neuropathy	Anterior superior alveolar nerve
V3: Tongue numbness	▪ Lingual nerve in temporal ▪ Arteritis
V3: Numb chin syndrome/ Roger's sign	Mental neuropathy: Cancer of breast and lung, giant cell arteritis, Burkitt lymphoma, and sickle cell disease

FACIAL NERVE

Motor (70%)	Sensory	Parasympathetic
▪ Muscles of facial expression ▪ Scalp ▪ Ear ▪ Buccinators ▪ Platysma ▪ Stapedius ▪ Stylohyoid ▪ Posterior belly of digastrics	**Taste:** Anterior 2/3 **Exteroceptive:** ▪ Eardrum ▪ EAC **Proprioception:** From the muscles supplied by it **GVS:** ▪ Salivary glands ▪ Mucosa of nose and pharynx	▪ Submandibular ▪ Sublingual ▪ Lacrimal ▪ Mucous membrane of oral and nasal mucosa

(EAC: external auditory canal)
Notes:
- There is anatomical segregation of motor component from sensory and autonomic fibers.
- Sensory root (nervus intermedius of Wrisberg)—contains both sensory and autonomic fibers.

Examination of Motor Function

Inspection:
- Facial asymmetry, nasolabial fold with forehead wrinkles, and movements during spontaneous facial expression
- Tone of the muscles of facial expression
- Atrophy and fasciculations
- Abnormal muscle contractions and involuntary movements
- Spontaneous blinking for frequency and symmetry

Testing the temporal branches of the facial nerve:
Patient is asked to frown and wrinkle his or her forehead

Testing the zygomatic branches of the facial nerve:
Patient is asked to close their eyes tightly

Testing the buccal branches of the facial nerve:
- Puff up cheeks (buccinator)
- Tap with finger over each cheek to detect ease of air expulsion on the affected side

Testing the mandibular branches of the facial nerve:
- Smile and show teeth (orbicularis oris)

Testing the cervical branches of the facial nerve:
Ask the patient to clench his/her teeth and simultaneously depress the angles of mouth

Muscle tested	Instruction	Response in palsy
Frontal belly of Occipitofrontalis [Fig. 6D(iii).50]	Ask the patient to wrinkle his/her Forehead	Asymmetry as he/she cannot wrinkle his forehead on the side of palsy in lower motor neuron (LMN) Palsy
Orbicularis oculi [Fig. 6D(iii).51]	Ask the patient to close his/her eyes forcibly while you try to open the eyelids with your Fingers	In LMN palsy, eyelids do not close completely. Instead the eyeball rolls up. This is known as Bell's phenomenon. In healthy individuals, eyelids cannot be opened with mild force against patient's resistance

Contd...

Contd...

Levator anguli oris, zygomatic major and minor, depressor anguli oris, buccinator, and risorius [Fig. 6D(iii).52]	Ask the patient to show his/her teeth or smile	Angle of mouth deviates toward normal side
Orbicularis oris and buccinators [Fig. 6D(iii).53]	Ask the patient to blowout cheeks with mouth closed, i.e., puff the cheeks and assess power by your attempt to deflate the cheek. Ask the patient to whistle	Patient cannot blowout his cheek as air escapes from affected side
Platysma [Fig. 6D(iii).54]	Ask the patient to clench his/her teeth and simultaneously depress the angles of mouth	Folds of platysma is seen in the neck as flat

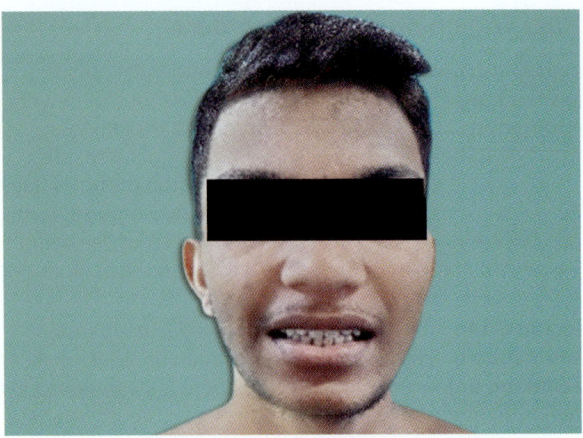

Fig. 6D(iii).52: Examination of levator anguli oris.

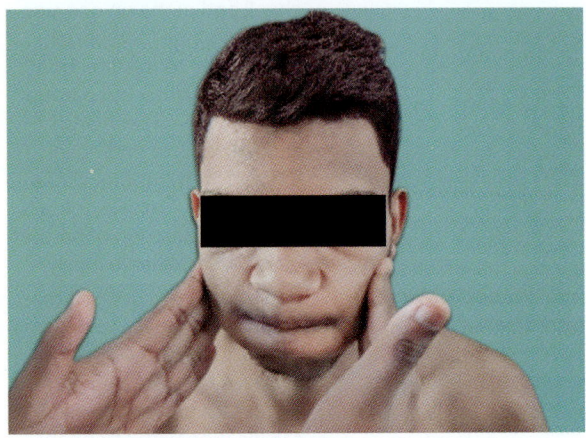

Fig. 6D(iii).53: Examination of buccinator.

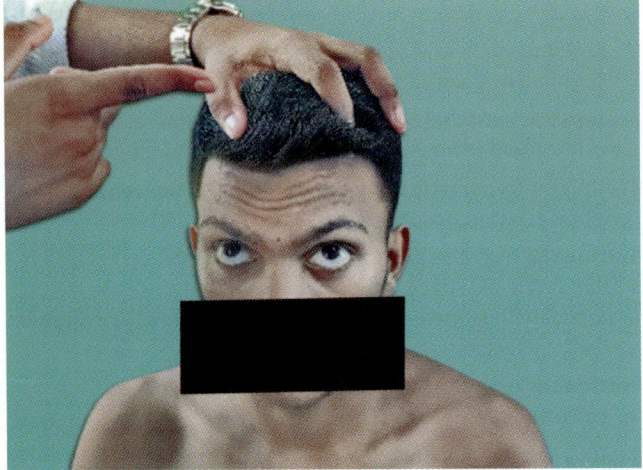

Fig. 6D(iii).50: Examination of frontal belly of occipitofrontalis.

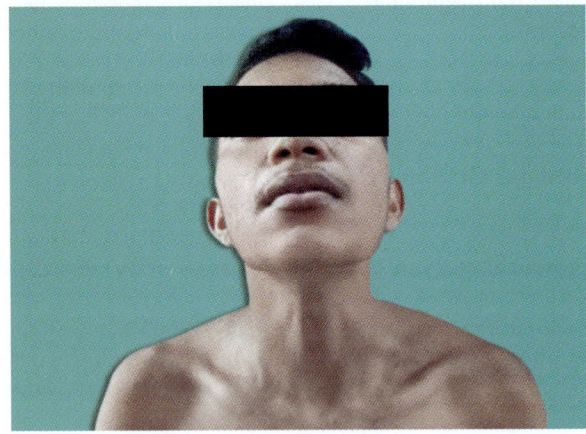

Fig. 6D(iii).54: Examination of platysma.

Examination of Sensory System

Anterior two-thirds of tongue [Fig. 6D(iii).55]
- Tongue protruded
- Hold with soft gauze
- With applicator's tip apply over the dorsum of the tongue
- Rinse after each test with water
- Sensations from the tip to deep—follow sweet → salt → sour → bitter (last)
- Fifth modality—umami appreciated with compounds of some amino acids

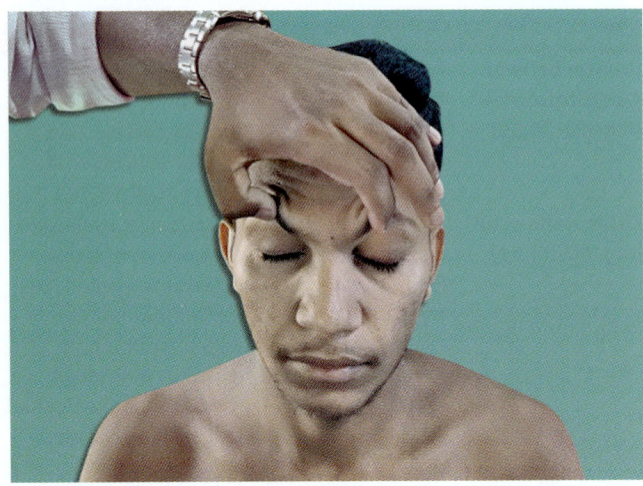

Fig. 6D(iii).51: Examination of orbicularis oculi.

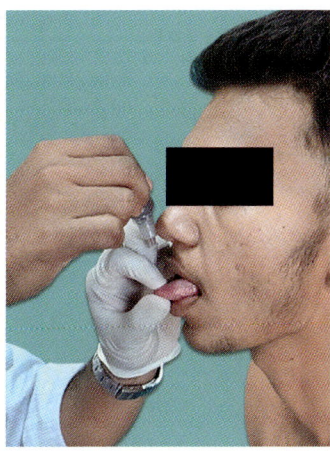

Fig. 6D(iii).55: Examination of taste sensation.

- Normally taste is appreciated within 10 seconds
- Artificial sweeteners make better test substances than ordinary sugar.
- Patient will be unable to speak so use some signaling system.

Ageusia	Complete inability to perceive taste
Hypogeusia	Blunted or delayed taste
Parageusia	Perversions of taste
Impaired taste	Lesion is proximal to junction with chorda tympani
Not affected	Lesion is at or distal to stylomastoid foramen

Secretory Function

1. Lacrimation: Schirmer's test → 10 mm is normal
2. Nasolacrimal test: By diluted solution of ammonium and formaldehyde—trigeminal nerve → greater superficial petrosal nerve.

Reflexes
Orbicularis oculi reflex

- Percussion causes reflex contraction of the eye muscle. The reflex is known as the supraorbital, glabellar, or nasopalpebral reflex, depending upon the site of the stimulus. Both eyes usually close, with the contralateral response being weaker. The trigeminal nerve is the afferent side and the facial nerve the efferent side of the reflex. Light and sound can also produce the reflex, with the optic and acoustic nerves providing the afferent side.
- The response is weak or abolished in nuclear and peripheral lesions, and present or exaggerated in supranuclear lesions. It is exaggerated in Parkinsonism and cannot be voluntarily inhibited

Palpebral oculogyric reflex

- The eyeballs deviate upward when the eyes are closed, both when awake and asleep. The afferent arc is proprioceptive impulses carried through the facial nerve to the medial longitudinal fasciculus. The oculomotor nerve to the superior rectus muscles forms the efferent side
- In peripheral and nuclear lesions, an exaggeration of this reflex is known as **Bell's phenomenon**

Orbicularis oris reflex

- Percussion on the side of the nose or the upper lip causes ipsilateral elevation of the angle of the mouth and upper lip. The reflex arc is composed of the fifth and seventh nerves. *Synonyms:* Nasomental, buccal, oral, or perioral reflex

Contd...

Contd...

- This reflex disappears after about the first year of life, recurring with supranuclear facial nerve lesions and with extrapyramidal diseases, such as Parkinsonism

Snout reflex

- Tapping the upper lip lightly with a reflex hammer, tongue blade, or finger causes bilateral contraction of the muscles around the mouth and base of the nose. The mouth resembles a snout
- This is an exaggeration of the orbicularis oris reflex. It is present with bilateral supranuclear lesions and in diffuse cerebral diseases, such as various causes of dementia

Sucking reflex

- Sucking movements of lips, tongue, and mouth are brought about by lightly touching or tapping on the lips. At times, merely bringing an object near the lips produces the reflex
- Occurs in patients with diffuse cerebral lesions. The snout reflex occurs in similar circumstances

Palmomental reflex

- A stimulus of the thenar area of the hand causes a reflex contraction ipsilaterally of the orbicularis oris and mentalis muscles
- A number of normal individuals have this reflex, and also patients with diffuse cerebral disease. It is significant when other similar reflexes are also present

Corneal reflex

Stimulation of the cornea with a wisp of cotton produces reflex closure of both ipsilateral (strongest) and contralateral eyelids. The fifth nerve carries the afferent impulses, and the facial nerve the efferent impulses

Stapedius reflex

- Both stapedius muscles contract reflexively in response to the loudness of a sound presented to either ear
- Also known as the acoustic reflex, it is best measured with an electroacoustic immittance audiometer that can test the reflex ipsilaterally and contralaterally

Testing for Emotional Function

The examiner should provoke a spontaneous smile by asking funny questions and telling hilarious stories during conversation to assess the emotional component of facial paresis. Emotional component is preserved in UMN facial palsy.

Site of cranial nerve 7 (CN VII) lesion and associated manifestation:

Lesion location	Manifestations
Above the facial nucleus (supranuclear lesion)	Contralateral paralysis of lower facial muscles with relative preservation of upper muscles. Lesion located cortex, internal capsule or midbrain
Pons (nuclear or fascicular lesion)	Ventral pontine lesion (of Millard–Gubler): Ipsilateral facial monoplegia, lateral rectus palsy (VI), and contralateral hemiplegia (corticospinal fibers). Pontine tegmentum lesion (of Foville): Ipsilateral facial monoplegia; contralateral hemiplegia (corticospinal fibers); paralysis of conjugate gaze to side of lesion (pontine paramedian reticular formation)

Contd...

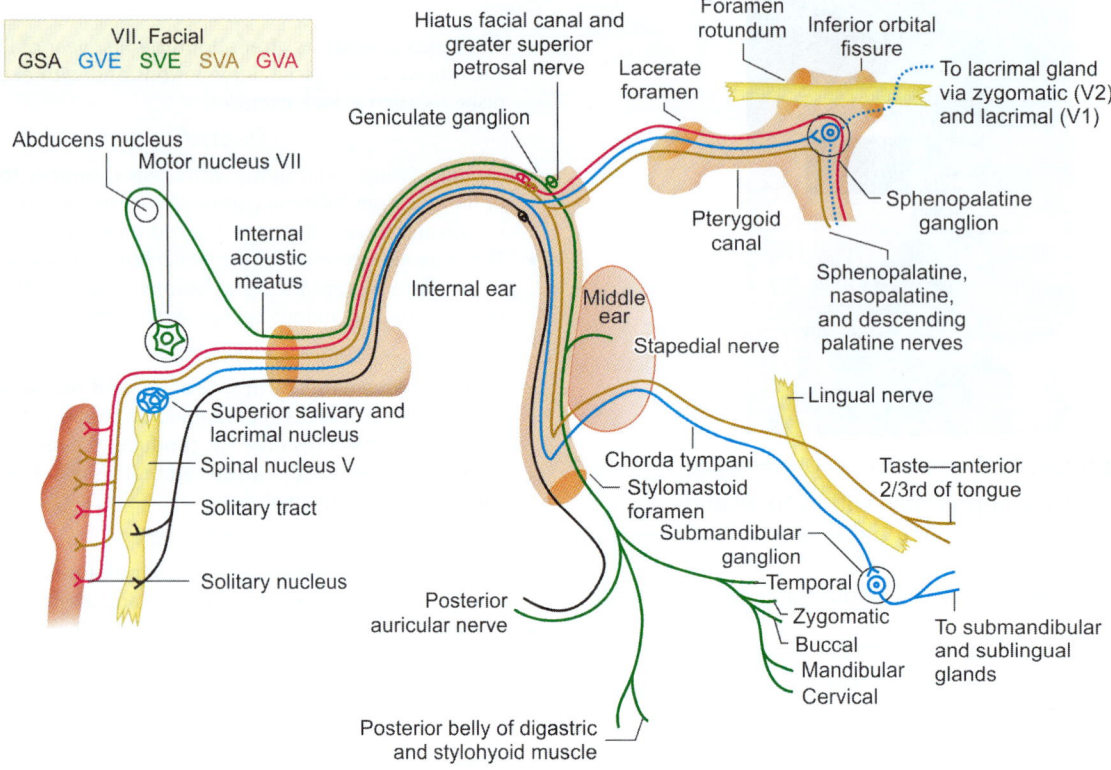

Fig. 6D(iii).56: Facial nerve pathway.

Contd...	
Cerebellopontine angle (peripheral nerve lesion)	Ipsilateral facial monoplegia, loss of taste to anterior two-thirds of tongue, impairment of salivary and tear secretion, hyperacusis (if VIII is not affected). Additional cranial nerves may be involved: deafness, tinnitus, and vertigo (VIII): sensory loss over face and absence of corneal reflex (V); ipsilateral ataxia (cerebellar peduncle)
Facial canal between internal auditory meatus and geniculate ganglion (peripheral nerve type lesion here and subsequently)	Same as above except cranial nerves other than VII are not involved
Facial canal between geniculate ganglion and nerve to stapedius muscle	Facial monoplegia; impaired salivary secretion; loss of taste; and hyperacusis
Facial canal between nerve to stapedius and leaving of chorda tympani	Facial monoplegia; impaired salivary secretion; and loss of taste
After branching of chorda tympani	Facial paralysis, distribution related to site of lesion (partial involvement)

FACIAL NERVE PALSY

Facial nerve pathway and innervation is shown in **Figures 6D(iii).56 and 6D(iii).57**.

Peripheral Facial Palsy

There is flaccid weakness of all the muscles of facial expression on the involved side, both upper and lower face, and the paralysis is usually complete.

Signs in LMN Facial Palsy

Bell's phenomenon	Attempting to close involved eye causes a reflex upturning of the eyeball
Levator sign of Dutemps and Céstan	Patient look down, then close the eyes slowly; because the function of levator palpebrae superioris is no longer counteracted by orbicularis oculi, upper lid on the paralyzed side moves upward slightly [**Figs. 6D(iii).58 and 6D(iii).59**]
Negro's sign	Eyeball on the paralyzed side deviates outward and elevates more than the normal one when the patient raises her eyes
Bergara–Wartenberg sign	Loss of the fine vibrations palpable with the thumbs or fingertips resting lightly on the lids as the patient tries to close the eyes as tightly as possible
Platysma sign of Babinski	Asymmetric contraction of the platysma, less on the involved side, when the mouth is opened

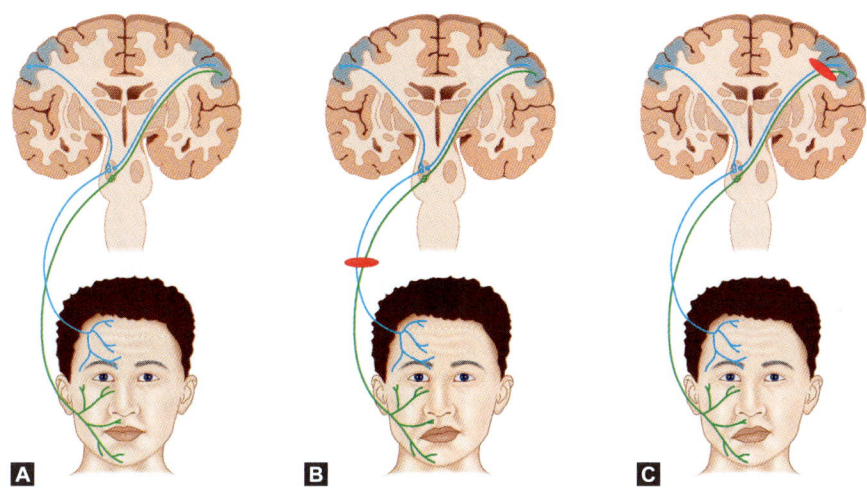

Figs. 6D(iii).57A to C: Innervation by facial nerve.

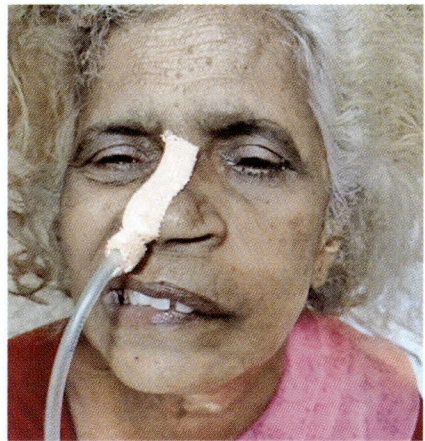

Fig. 6D(iii).58: Image showing deviation of angle of mouth.

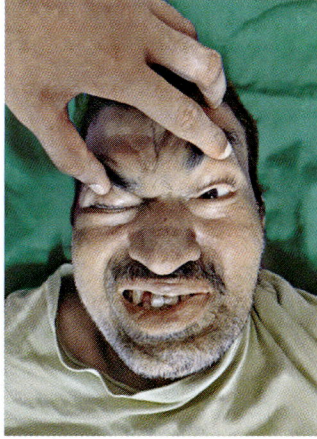

Fig. 6D(iii).59: Weakness of orbicularis oculi.

House–Brackmann grading system of LMN facial palsy	
Grade I	Normal
Grade II	Mild dysfunction, slight weakness on close inspection, and normal symmetry at rest
Grade III	Moderate dysfunction, obvious but not disfiguring difference between sides, eye can be completely closed with effort
Grade IV	Moderately severe, normal tone at rest, obvious weakness or asymmetry with movement, incomplete closure of eye
Grade V	Severe dysfunction, only barely perceptible motion, and asymmetry at rest
Grade VI	No movement

Causes of LMN Facial Palsy

Congenital:
- Möbius syndrome
- Goldenhar syndrome
- Melkersson–Rosenthal syndrome
- **Birth related:** Forceps delivery
- **Idiopathic:** Bell's palsy

Infection:
- Viral infection, i.e., varicella zoster (Ramsay Hunt), herpes zoster, herpes simplex, and HIV
- Otitis media
- Cholesteatoma
- Necrotizing otitis externa
- Skull base osteomyelitis
- Lyme disease
- Leprosy.

Trauma:
- Temporal bone fracture
- Gunshot or penetrating injury
- Laceration.

Neoplastic:
- Schwannoma
- Meningioma
- Hemangioma
- Parotid malignancy.

Iatrogenic: Brain, middle ear, mastoid, parotid or facial surgery.

Neurological:
- Lacunar or brainstem infarct
- Guillain–Barré syndrome
- Myasthenia gravis
- Multiple sclerosis.

Metabolic:
- Diabetes mellitus
- Hypertension

- Pregnancy
- Vitamin A deficiency.

Central Facial Nerve Palsy (UMN Facial Nerve Palsy)

Facial weakness of central origin/UMN facial palsy-rarely complete	
■ Weakness of the lower face, with relative sparing of upper face ■ Upper face is not necessarily completely spared, but it is always involved to a lesser degree than the lower face	
Volitional or voluntary	*Emotional or mimetic*
Lesion of the cortical center in the lower third of the precentral gyrus that controls facial movements, or the corticobulbar tract	Thalamic or striatocapsular lesions, usually infarction
Weakness more marked on voluntary contraction, when patient is asked to smile or bare her teeth	Facial asymmetry more apparent with spontaneous expression, as when laughing

Differences between UMN and LMN type of facial nerve palsy:

	UMN type	LMN type
Facial motor function	Wrinkling of forehead preserved (frontalis unaffected)	Total face is involved
Bell's phenomenon [Figs. 6D(iii).60A to C]	Absent	Present
Facial muscles	Not atrophied	Fasciculations, atrophied
Taste sensation	Preserved	May be lost
Corneal reflex	Preserved	Lost
Hemiplegia	Contralateral	Ipsilateral
Babinski reflex	Present	Absent

(UMN: upper motor neuron; LMN: lower motor neuron)

Emotional Facial Paresis (EFP)/Mimic Paralysis

- This is characterized by the weakness of emotionally evoked facial movements.
- The corticopontine fibers that control spontaneous smiling arise from the medial surface of the prefrontal cortex and descend through the anterior limb of the internal capsule, thalamus, and brainstem, independently from those that control voluntary movement.
- The clinical picture consists of a supranuclear hemifacial paresis exclusively in spontaneous smiling (inverse automatic-voluntary dissociation). This is a sign of anterolateral thalamic infarction, secondarily to tuberothalamic artery ischemia.

Bilateral VII Nerve Palsy

Bilateral UMN palsy	Bilateral LMN palsy
■ Emotional fibers—spared ■ Emotional incontinence—present ■ Associated with bilateral long tract signs ■ Jaw jerk—exaggerated ■ Corneal reflex—present ■ Taste sensation—spared ■ Gag reflex—exaggerated	■ Bell's phenomenon present ■ Emotional fibers—affected ■ Long tract signs—absent ■ Jaw jerk—normal ■ Corneal reflex—absent ■ Taste sensation—absent

(UMN: upper motor neuron; LMN: lower motor neuron)

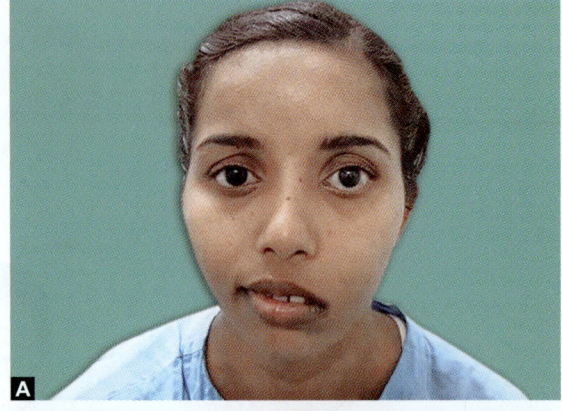
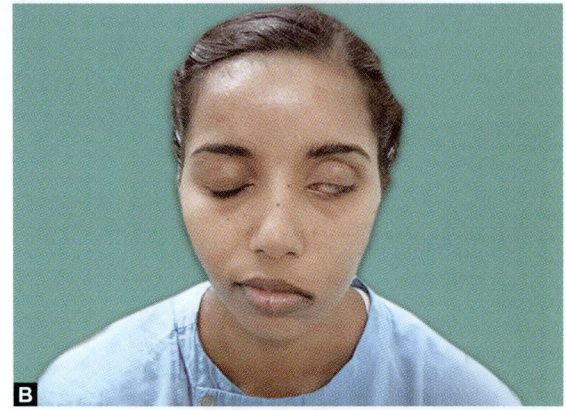
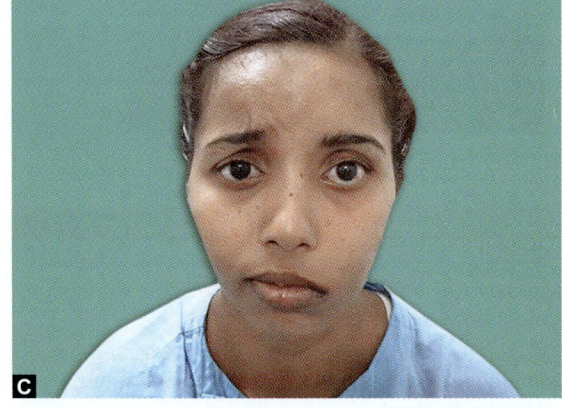

Figs. 6D(iii).60A to C: Bell's phenomenon.

Causes of bilateral facial nerve palsy:
- Diabetes
- Bilateral Bell's palsy
- Borreliosis
- *Mycoplasma pneumoniae* infection
- Guillain-Barré syndrome* and Miller–Fisher syndrome
- Sarcoidosis
- Möbius syndrome
- HIV
- Syphilis
- Basal skull fractures
- Pontine gliomas
- Leprosy
- Mononucleosis
- Brainstem encephalitis
- Hansen's disease
- Cryptococcal meningitis
- Pontine tegmental hemorrhage

*Most common cause

Syndromes of Facial Palsy

Syndromes with facial nerve palsy
- Foville's syndrome
- Millard–Gubler syndrome
- Möbius syndrome
- Ramsay Hunt syndrome
- Melkersson–Rosenthal syndrome [triad of recurrent infranuclear facial paralysis, orofacial edema (predominantly of the lips), and lingua plicata]
- Guillain–Barré syndrome
- Progressive hemifacial atrophy (Parry–Romberg syndrome)
- Meige syndrome (blepharospasm oromandibular dystonia, orofacial cervical dystonia, and Brueghel's syndrome)
- Uveoparotid fever (Heerfordt's disease)
- Goldenhar syndrome
- Crocodile tear syndrome
- Frey's syndrome

CRANIAL NERVE VIII—VESTIBULOCOCHLEAR NERVE

Contains two components	
Vestibular component	Cochlear component
↓	↓
Responsible for equilibrium	Responsible for hearing
Pathway	
For linear accelerations Macula utricle saccule **For angular acceleration** Ampulla	Organ of Corti ↓ Cochlear nuclei ↓ Lateral lemnisci ↓ Inferior colliculus ↓ Medial geniculate body ↓ Brodmann areas 41 and 42 (transverse temporal gyrus of Heschl)
↓ Vestibular ganglia ↓ Vestibular nerve	

Examination	
Vestibular component	Cochlear component
Rotational test	Rubbing fingers
Calorie test [Fig. 6D(iii).61]	Rinne's test and Weber's test
Electronystagmography	Audiometric tests: - Pure tone audiometry - Tone decay - Bekesy audiometry

- Whispered voice is a good recommended hearing screening test.
- Due to bilaterality of central pathways, unilateral central lesions do not cause any detectable deficit.

Testing for vertigo and nystagmus
In sitting position, turn the head to one side by 45°
↓
Make the patient to lie down abruptly with the head hanging down from the edge of cot

Contd...

Contd...

↓

This position is maintained for at least a minute

↓

Watch for nystagmus

↓

Fast component is toward the lower ear suggests following possibilities

↓

Benign paroxysmal positional vertigo	Central cause
Starts after short latency (3–10 sec), patient will have nystagmus associated with vertigo	Immediate nystagmus
Rapid adaptation	No adaptation

Testing the vestibular component of VIII nerve
Rotational test
Patient is seated in a chair that can be rotated with his head well supported and fixed in head rest
↓
To test   Horizontal canal—head in flexed at 30°   Vertical canal—head is flexed at 120°
↓
Chair is rotated 10 times in 20 seconds
↓
Normally when the rotation to the right has stopped, there is nystagmus with its slow phase to the right and vice versa
Calorie test
The patient is placed supine with the head tilted up by 30°. In this way, the horizontal semicircular canal is oriented in a vertical plane
↓
2–10 mL usually but, 30–50 mL in comatose of water (or air at controlled temperature) is irrigated through the external auditory meatus over period of 40 seconds, first using 30°C and later using 44°C
↓
Patient fixes his eyes on the given point immediately above his head
↓
After ceasing the irrigation, the time in seconds is measured during which nystagmus on the forward gaze persist
↓
Now the test is repeated on the other ear. Latency and duration of nystagmus is compared on both sides.
↓
Normal response is cold water produces fast component toward the opposite side and warm water produces a fast component toward the same side (mnemonic—**COWS**)

Contd...

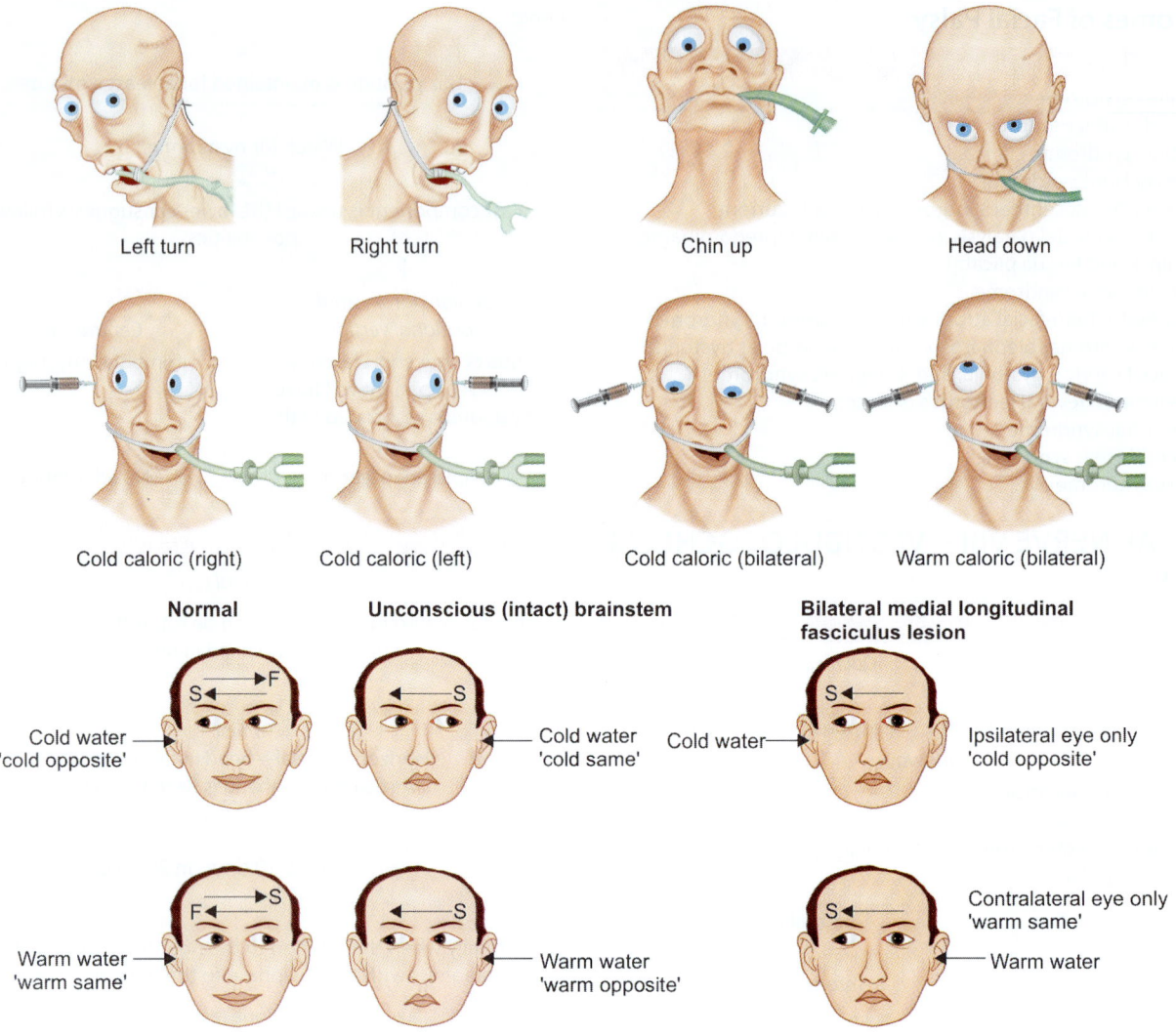

Fig. 6D(iii).61: Illustration demonstrating calorie test.

Interpretation	
No response (canal paresis)	▪ Meniere's disease ▪ Acoustic nerve tumor ▪ Vestibular neuronitis ▪ Lesions of vestibular nuclei
Directional preponderance	▪ Lesions of peripheral or central vestibular apparatus ▪ Cerebellum ▪ Corticofugal fibers deep in the temporal ▪ Lobe
Combination of above two	Vestibular nerve or labyrinth lesions

Testing the Cochlear Component of VIII Nerve

Rinne's and Weber's Test [Figs. 6D(iii).62 to 6D(iii).65]

- Done with 256/512 Hz tuning fork
- The prongs should be put equidistant on either ears while examining
- Examination should be done in quite room

Rinne's test	Weber test
By two methods: 1. An activated fork may be placed first on the mastoid process, then immediately beside the ear and patient asked which is louder 2. Traditional method where—place the tuning fork on the mastoid and when no longer heard there move it beside the ear, where it should still be Audible	A vibrating tuning fork is placed in the midline on the vertex of the skull. Normally the sound is heard equally in both ears
Interpretation	
In conductive hearing loss	
BC > AC (Rinne negative)	Lateralized to abnormal side
In sensorineural hearing loss	
AC > BC (Rinne positive)	Lateralized to normal side

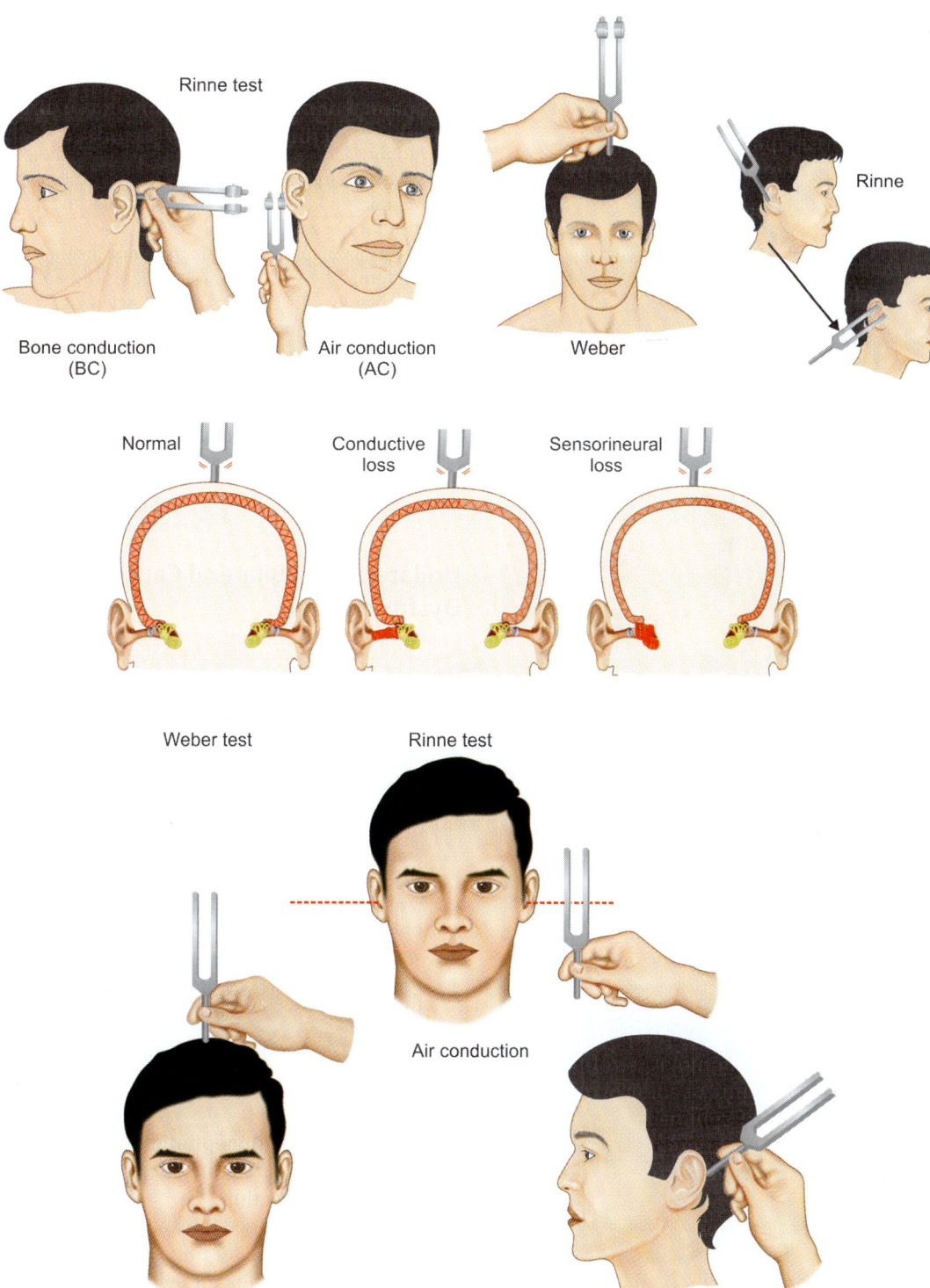

Fig. 6D(iii).62: Illustration showing demonstration of Rinne's test and Weber's test.

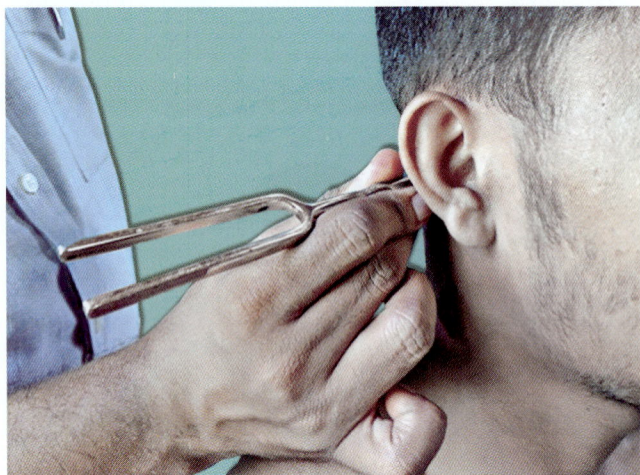

Fig. 6D(iii).63: Rinne's test: Placement of tuning fork on the mastoid process.

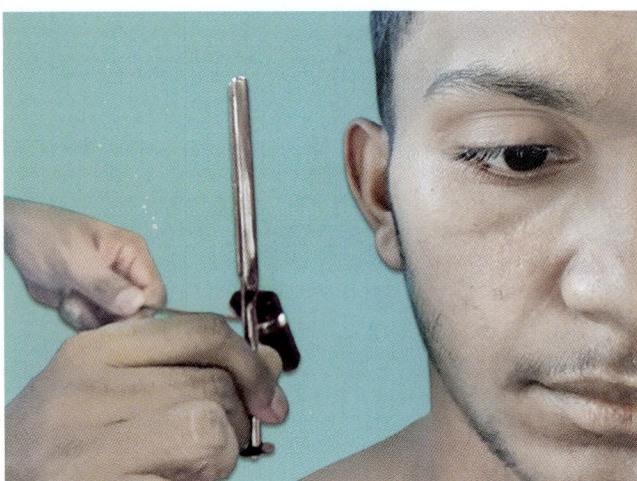

Fig. 6D(iii).64: Rinne's test: Placement of tuning fork beside the ear parallel to tympanic membrane.

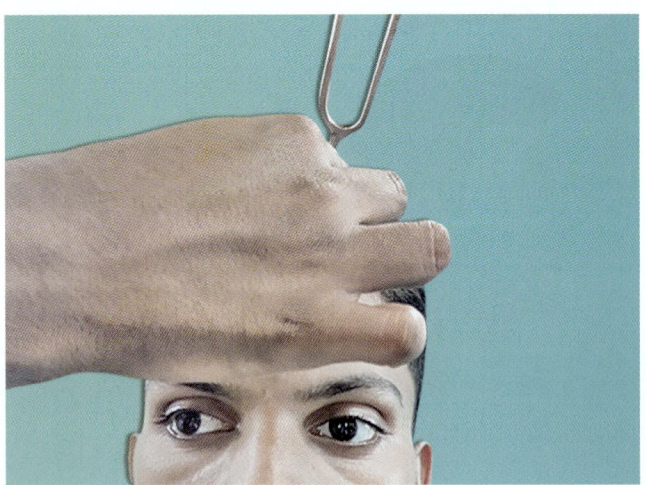

Fig. 6D(iii).65: Weber's test: Placement of tuning fork in midline on the vertex.

Causes of VIII Nerve Dysfunction Based on Site of Involvement

Vestibular component	Cochlear component
At level of labyrinth: - Meniere's disease - Motion sickness - Drug toxicity - Migraine **Vestibular nerve:** - Vestibular neuronitis **Brainstem:** - Vascular insufficiency - Cerebellar tumors - IV ventricle tumors - Acute demyelinating diseases **Temporal lobe:** As epileptic manifestation	**Conduction defects:** - External meatus obstruction - Middle ear pathology - Eustachian tube block - Intracranial infection - Middle ear infection **Cochlear pathology:** - Meniere's disease - Osteosclerosis - Internal auditory meatus occlusion **Nerve trunk:** - Old age - Meningitis - Cerebellopontine angle tumors **Brainstem:** - Vascular pathology - Demyelination disease **Cerebrum:** Temporal disease

Unilateral and Bilateral Causes of VIII Nerve Dysfunction

Vestibular component		Cochlear component	
Unilateral	*Bilateral*	*Unilateral*	*Bilateral*
- Tumor (cerebellopontine angle and acoustic neuroma) - Fracture of the petrous temporal bone - Vascular disease of the internal auditory artery - Vestibular neuritis	- Demyelinating illness, e.g., multiple sclerosis - Migraine	- Tumor (cerebellopontine angle and acoustic neuroma) - Fracture of the petrous temporal bone - Vascular disease of the internal auditory artery	- Industrial deafness - Presbycusis - Drug toxicity (gentamicin, salicylate, etc.) - Meniere's disease - Brainstem lesion (e.g., stroke)

The "doll's eye" oculocephalic reflex:
- Turning the head in one direction causes the eyes to turn in opposite direction.
- Tests the vestibulocochlear nerve, the brainstem nuclei of the vestibulocochlear nerve, the fibers to the cerebellum, the fibers from the cerebellum, the medial longitudinal fasciculus (MLF), and the 3rd and 6th cranial nerves.
- The cause of the unconsciousness in a patient with a negative oculocephalic reflex is some sort of destructive brainstem pathology or brain death. Conversely, an intact oculocephalic reflex suggests that the coma is of a nonstructural cause, because much of the brainstem must be intact.

CRANIAL NERVE IX AND X: GLOSSOPHARYNGEAL AND VAGUS

The two nerves:
- Have motor and autonomic branches with nuclei of origin in the medulla.
- Both conduct general somatic afferent (GSA) as well as general visceral afferent (GVA) fibers to related or identical fiber tracts and nuclei in the brainstem.
- Both have a parasympathetic, or general visceral efferent, and a branchiomotor, or special visceral efferent (SVE), component
- Both leave the skull together
- Remain close in their course through the neck
- Both supply some of the same structures.
- They are often involved in the same disease processes
- Involvement of one may be difficult to differentiate from involvement of the other.

For these reasons, the two nerves are discussed together.

Muscles innervated by cranial nerve IX and X:

IX nerve	
Muscular branch	Stylopharyngeus
X nerve	
Pharyngeal branch [Figs. 6D(iii).66A and B]	▪ Musculus uvulae (azygos uvulae) ▪ Levator veli palatini ▪ Palatopharyngeus ▪ Salpingopharyngeus ▪ Palatoglossus ▪ Superior, middle, and inferior constrictors of the pharynx
Superior laryngeal nerve	Cricothyroid
Recurrent laryngeal nerve	▪ Posterior cricoarytenoids ▪ Lateral cricoarytenoids ▪ Thyroarytenoids (vocalis) ▪ Arytenoid

GLOSSOPHARYNGEAL NERVE IX

Functions:

Glossopharyngeal nerve: Sensory supply to posterior one-third of tongue, taste sensation, and pharyngeal mucosa.

Testing of IX Nerve

Cranial nerve IX is difficult to examine because most or all of its functions are shared by other nerves and because many of the structures it supplies are inaccessible.

Gag Reflex [Fig. 6D(iii).67]

- The gag reflex is protective; it is designed to prevent noxious substances or foreign objects from going beyond the oral cavity.
- **Components of gag reflex:** There are three motor components: Elevation of the soft palate to seal off the nasopharynx, closure of the glottis to protect the airway, and constriction of the pharynx to prevent entry of the substance.

- **Pathway:** The afferent limb of the reflex is mediated by CN IX and the efferent limb through CNs IX and X. The reflex center is in the medulla.

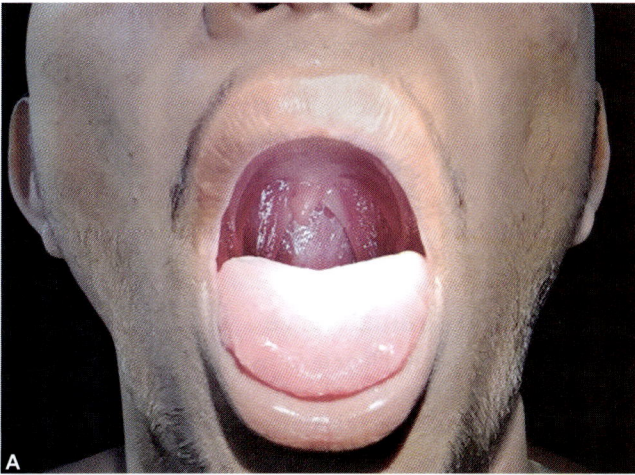
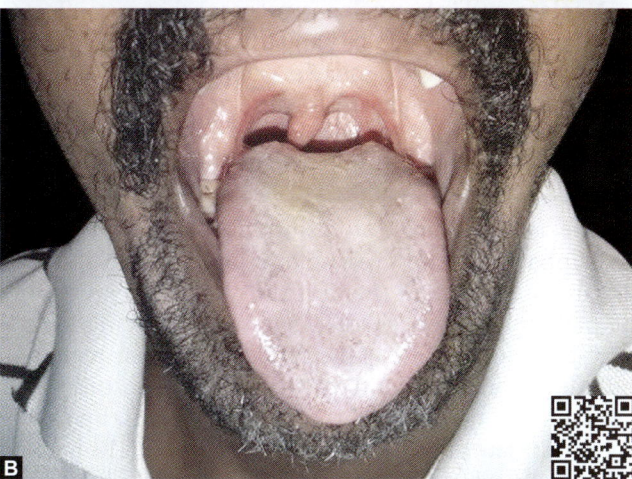

Figs. 6D(iii).66A and B: (A) Examination of deviation of uvula; (B) Deviation of uvula to right side.

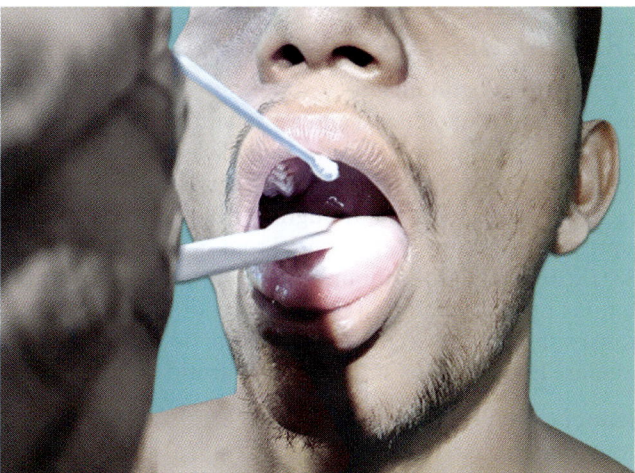

Fig. 6D(iii).67: Examination of gag reflex.

- **Testing of gag reflex:** The reflex is elicited by touching the lateral oropharynx in the region of the anterior faucial pillar with a tongue blade, applicator stick, or similar object (pharyngeal reflex), or by touching one side of

the soft palate or uvula (palatal reflex). The reflex also occurs with touching the base of the tongue or posterior pharyngeal wall.
- **Clinical implication:** May be bilaterally absent in some normal individuals.
Unilateral absence signifies a lower motor neuron lesion. Like most bulbar muscles, the pharynx receives bilateral supranuclear innervation, and a unilateral cerebral lesion does not cause detectable weakness. A hyperactive gag reflex may occur with bilateral cerebral lesions, as in pseudobulbar palsy and amyotrophic lateral sclerosis (ALS).

Disorders of IX Cranial Nerve

- **Unilateral supranuclear lesions** cause no deficit because of the bilateral corticobulbar innervation.
- **Bilateral supranuclear lesions** may cause pseudobulbar palsy.
- **Nuclear and infranuclear processes** that may affect CN IX include intramedullary and extramedullary neoplasms and other mass lesions (e.g., glomus jugulare tumor), trauma (e.g., basilar skull fracture or surgical dissection), motor neuron disease, syringobulbia, retropharyngeal abscess, demyelinating disease, birth injury, and brainstem ischemia.

The most important lesion of the ninth nerve is glossopharyngeal (or vago-glossopharyngeal) neuralgia or "tic douloureux of the ninth nerve". In this condition, the patient experiences attacks of severe lancinating pain originating in one side of the throat or tonsillar region and radiating along the course of the eustachian tube to the tympanic membrane, external auditory canal, behind the angle of the jaw, and adjacent portion of the ear. The pain may be brought on by talking, eating, swallowing, or coughing. It can lead to syncope, convulsions, and rarely to cardiac arrest because of stimulation of the carotid sinus reflex.

CRANIAL NERVE X—VAGUS

The vagus (in Latin means "wandering," because of its wide distribution) is the longest and most widely distributed.

The vagus emerges from the medulla as a series of rootlets just below those of the glossopharyngeal.

CN X leaves the skull through the jugular foramen in the same neural sheath as the cranial root of CN XI and behind CN IX. In the jugular foramen, the nerve lies close to the jugular bulb, a dilatation of the internal jugular vein that houses the glomus jugulare (tympanic body). The glomus jugulare has functions similar to the carotid body.

Branches of cranial nerves: There are 10 major terminal branches that arise at different levels: (a) meningeal, (b) auricular, (c) pharyngeal, (d) carotid, (e) superior laryngeal, (f) recurrent laryngeal, (g) cardiac, (h) esophageal, (i) pulmonary, and (j) gastrointestinal.

Motor: The vagus, with a contribution from the bulbar portion of CN XI, supplies all the striated muscles of the soft palate, pharynx, and larynx except for the stylopharyngeus (CN IX) and tensor veli palatini (CN V).

Parasympathetic: The vagus is the longest parasympathetic nerve in the body and a vagal discharge causes bradycardia, hypotension, bronchoconstriction, bronchorrhea, increased peristalsis, increased gastric secretion, and inhibition of adrenal function. The vagal centers in the medulla that control these functions are themselves under the control of higher centers in the cortex and hypothalamus. Inhibition of vagal function produces the opposite effects.

Sensory: Both vagal ganglia are sensory. The superior ganglion primarily conveys somatic sensation, and most of its communication is with the auricular nerve. The inferior ganglion relays general visceral sensation and taste.

Normal functions mediated by CNs IX and X include swallowing, phonation, and airway protection and modulation.

Examination

Motor function: The character of the voice and the ability to swallow provide information about the branchiomotor functions of the vagus.

Clinical implications:
A unilateral vagal lesion causes weakness of the soft palate, pharynx, and larynx. Acute lesions may produce difficulty swallowing both liquids and solids and hoarseness or a nasal quality to the voice. Sensory change is anesthesia of the larynx due to involvement of the superior laryngeal nerve. The gag reflex is absent on the involved side. Autonomic reflexes (vomiting, coughing, and sneezing) are not usually affected.

Bilateral complete vagal paralysis is incompatible with life. It causes complete paralysis of the palate, pharynx, and larynx, with marked dysphagia and dysarthria; tachycardia; slow, irregular, and respiration; vomiting; and gastrointestinal atonia.

Disorders of Cranial Nerve X

Unilateral supranuclear lesions generally cause no dysfunction because of bilateral innervation.

Bilateral supranuclear lesions, as from pseudobulbar palsy, cause dysphagia and dysarthria.

Extrapyramidal disorders may produce difficulty with swallowing and talking. Patients with Parkinson's disease typically have a hypokinetic dysarthria. Laryngeal spasm with stridor may occur in Parkinson's disease.

Nuclear lesions bulbar ALS, syringomyelia, and some neoplasms, may cause fasciculations in the palatal, pharyngeal, and laryngeal muscles.

Infranuclear: Extramedullary and intracranial involvement can occur in processes involving the meninges, extramedullary tumors, aneurysms, trauma, sarcoidosis, and skull fractures.

Lesions at the jugular foramen or in the retroparotid space usually involve some combination of IX, X, XI, XII, and the cervical sympathetics.

Palatal myoclonus: Seen in lesions at Mollaret triangle.
Jacobson's neuralgia: Involvement of tympanic branch of CN IX.

Recurrent laryngeal nerve palsy:
Causes:
- Unilateral:
  - Mitral stenosis
  - Bronchogenic carcinoma
  - Aortic aneurysm
  - Hodgkin's disease
- Bilateral:
  - Guillain-Barré syndrome
  - Thyroidectomy
  - Lymphomas.

CRANIAL NERVE XI—SPINAL ACCESSORY

The spinal accessory (SA) nerve, cranial nerve XI (CN XI), is actually two nerves that run together in a common bundle for a short distance [Fig. 6D(iii).68].

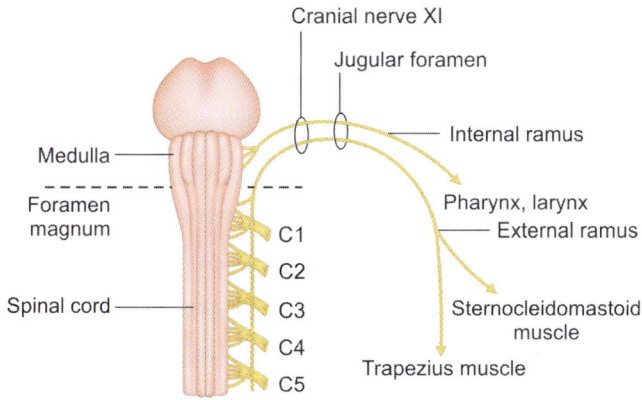

Fig. 6D(iii).68: Anatomy of spinal accessory nerve

Cranial part (ramus internus): The smaller cranial portion is a special visceral efferent (SVE) accessory to the vagus. It emerges from the medulla laterally as four or five rootlets caudal to the vagal filaments. The cranial root runs to the jugular foramen and unites with the spinal portion, traveling with it for only a few millimeters to form the main trunk of CN XI.

The cranial root communicates with the jugular ganglion of the vagus, and then exits through the jugular foramen separately from the spinal portion. It is distributed principally with the recurrent laryngeal nerve to sixth branchial arch muscles in the larynx.

Spinal part (ramus externus): The major part of CN XI is the spinal portion. Its function is to innervate the sternocleidomastoid (SCM) and trapezius muscles. The fibers of the spinal root arise from SVE motor cells in the SA nuclei in the ventral horn from C2 to C5, or even C6. These unite into a single trunk, which ascends between the denticulate ligaments and the posterior roots. The nerve enters the skull through the foramen magnum, ascends the clivus for a short distance, and then curves laterally. The spinal root joins the cranial root for a short distance, probably receiving one or two filaments from it. It exits through the jugular foramen in company with CNs IX and X.

C1-2 supplies sternocleidomastoid.
C3-4 supplies trapezius.

Testing the Spinal Accessory Nerve

Cranial Part

The functions of the cranial portion of CN XI cannot be distinguished from those of CN X, and examination is limited to evaluation of the functions of the spinal portion.

Spinal Part

Testing SCM [Figs. 6D(iii).69 and 6D(iii).70]:

Testing one muscle at a time: To assess SCM power, have the patient turn the head fully to one side and hold it there, then try to turn the head back to midline, avoiding any tilting or leaning motion. The muscle usually stands out well, and its contraction can be seen and felt. Significant weakness of rotation can be detected if the patient tries to counteract firm resistance.

Testing two muscle at a time: The two SCM muscles can be examined simultaneously by having the patient flex his neck while the examiner exerts pressure on the forehead or by having the patient turn the head from side to side. Flexion of the head against resistance may cause deviation of the head toward the paralyzed side.

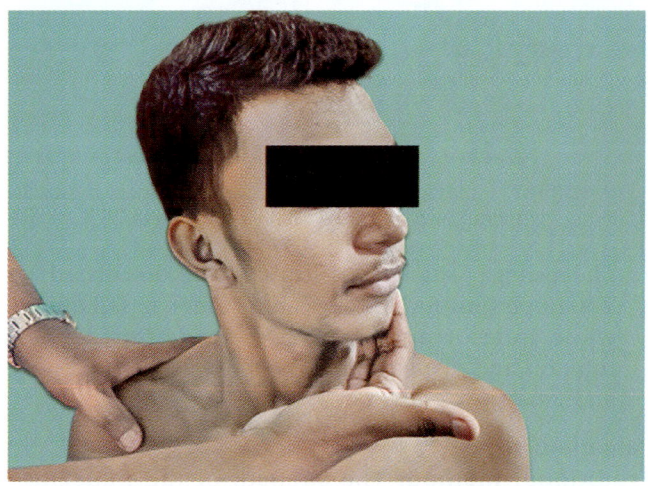

Fig. 6D(iii).69: Examination of sternocleidomastoid muscle (testing one muscle at a time).

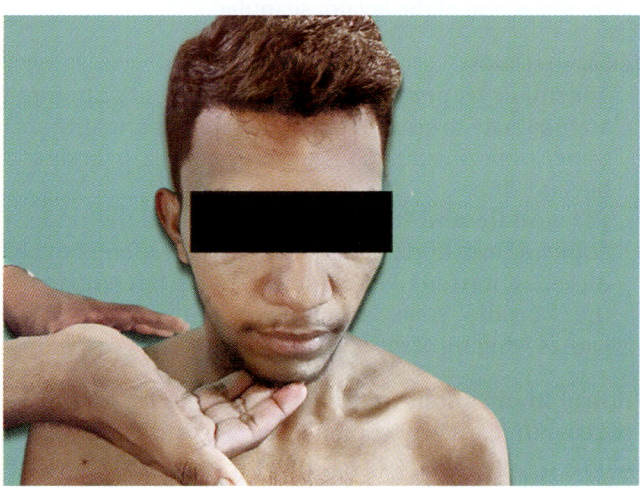

Fig. 6D(iii).70: Examination of sternocleidomastoid (testing both muscles at a time).

Interpretation: With unilateral paralysis, the involved muscle is flat and does not contract or become tense when attempting to turn the head contralaterally or to flex the neck against resistance. Weakness of both SCMs causes difficulty in anteroflexion of the neck, and the head may assume an extended position.

Testing trapezius muscle [Fig. 6D(iii).71]:
Inspection: With trapezius atrophy, inspection findings include:
- Depression or drooping of the shoulder contour
- Flattening of the trapezius ridge
- Sagging of the shoulder

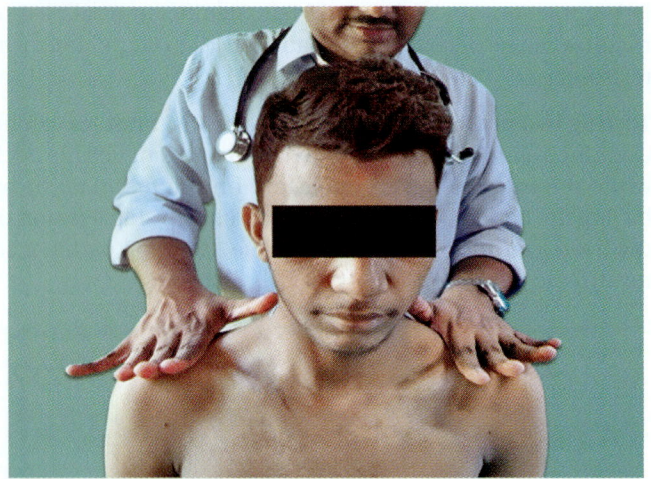

Fig. 6D(iii).71: Traditional method of assessing trapezius muscle (shrugging shoulders against resistance).

- The resting position of the scapula shifts downward
- The upper portion of the scapula tends to fall laterally while inferior angle moves inward (this scapular rotation and displacement are more obvious with arm abduction).

Palpation:
Traditional method: The strength of the trapezius is traditionally tested by having the patient shrug the shoulders against resistance. However, much of shoulder shrugging is due to the action of the levator scapulae.

Newer methods:
- **For upper trapezius:** Resisting the patient's attempt to approximate the occiput to the acromion. Impairment of upper trapezius function causes weakness of abduction beyond 90°.
- **For middle and lower trapezius:** Place the patient's abducted arm horizontally, palm up, and attempt to push the elbow forward. Muscle power should be compared on the two sides. Weakness of the middle trapezius muscle causes winging of the scapula.

Clinical implication: Weakness of the muscles supplied by CN XI may be caused by supranuclear, nuclear, or infranuclear lesions.
- **Supranuclear involvement:** Irritative supranuclear lesions may cause head turning away from the discharging hemisphere. This turning of the head (or head and eyes) may occur as part of a controversive, ipsiversive, or Jacksonian seizure and is often the first manifestation of the seizure. Extrapyramidal lesions may also involve the SCM and trapezius muscles, causing rigidity, akinesia, or hyperkinesis.
- **Nuclear involvement** of the SA nerve may occur in motor neuron disease, syringobulbia, and syringomyelia. In nuclear lesions, the weakness is frequently accompanied by atrophy and fasciculations.
- **Infranuclear or peripheral lesions**—either extramedullary but within the skull, in the jugular foramen, or in the neck—are the most common causes of impairment of function of the SA nerve. Tumors in the foramen magnum, lesions of the cerebellopontine angle, basal skull fractures, and meningitis.

"Dropped Head Syndrome"/Floppy Head Syndrome/Broken Neck Sign

This syndrome, characterized by weakness of the extensor muscles of neck with or without involvement of neck flexors, can be caused by:
- Myasthenia gravis
- Inflammatory myopathy—polymyositis
- Hypothyroid myopathy
- Guillain–Barré syndrome
- Amyotrophic lateral sclerosis (ALS)/bulbar polio
- Facio-scapulo-humeral dystrophy
- Neurotoxic snake bite/organophosphorus compound poisoning.

CRANIAL NERVE XII—HYPOGLOSSAL NERVE

Function: CN XII supplies the intrinsic muscles, and all of the extrinsic muscles of the tongue except the palatoglossus.

Anatomy [Fig. 6D(iii).72]: Nucleus located in medial medulla. Distribution of fibers from rostral to caudal, the innervation is intrinsic tongue muscles, then genioglossus, hyoglossus, and styloglossus.

Examination

The clinical examination of hypoglossal nerve function consists of evaluating the strength, bulk, and dexterity of the tongue—looking especially for weakness, atrophy, abnormal movements (particularly fasciculations), and impairment of rapid movements.

Inspection:
- **Tongue deviation:** To look for tongue deviation by asking the patient to protrude the tongue and also to move the tongue to either sides.
- **Fasciculations:** Ask the patient to open the mouth and with the tongue inside the mouth look for the fasciculations.
- Tremors usually disappear when tongue lies at rest in the mouth, helps to differentiate from fasciculations.

Nervous System

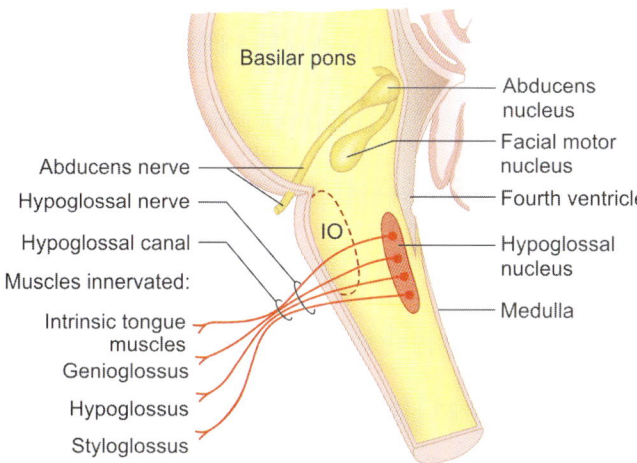

Fig. 6D(iii).72: Location of hypoglossal nerve.

Palpation:
- Hold the tongue with gauze and palpate the tongue with gloved finger to examine the consistency of the tongue [Fig. 6D(iii).73].
- To examine the power of the tongue patient is instructed to push the tongue against the cheek while giving the counter resistance from outside [Fig. 6D(iii).74].

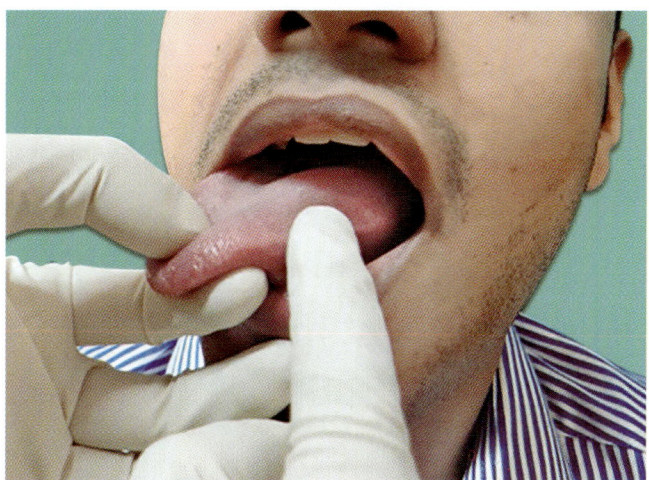

Fig. 6D(iii).73: Palpation of tongue.

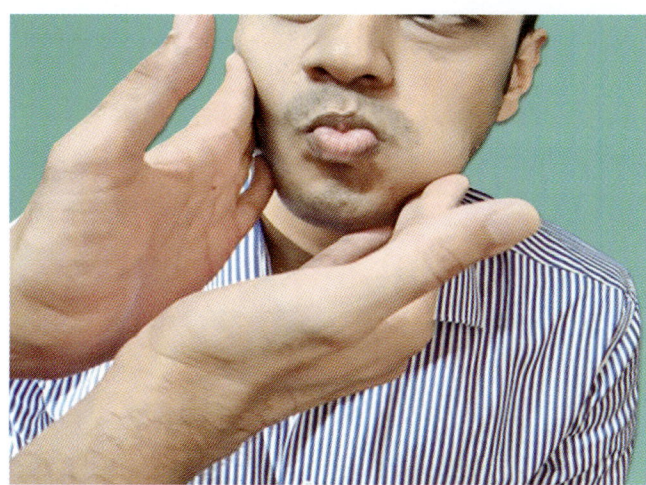

Fig. 6D(iii).74: Examining the motor power of tongue.

Interpretation

On inspection:
- **Tongue deviation [Fig. 6D(iii).75]:** When unilateral weakness is present, the tongue deviates toward the weak side on protrusion because of the action of the normal genioglossus. And also there is impairment of the ability to deviate the protruded tongue toward the opposite side.
- Fasciculations: Presence of fasciculations suggests LMN paralysis of the 12th cranial nerve.

On palpation:
- **Small and stiff tongue:** Suggestive of UMN type of 12th nerve palsy.
- **Flabby tongue with fasciculations:** Suggestive of LMN type of 12th nerve palsy.

Other clinical aspects: The neck-tongue syndrome, consisting of pain in the neck and numbness or tingling in the ipsilateral half of the tongue on sharp rotation of the head, has been attributed to damage to lingual afferent fibers traveling in the hypoglossal nerve to the C2 spinal roots through the atlantoaxial space.

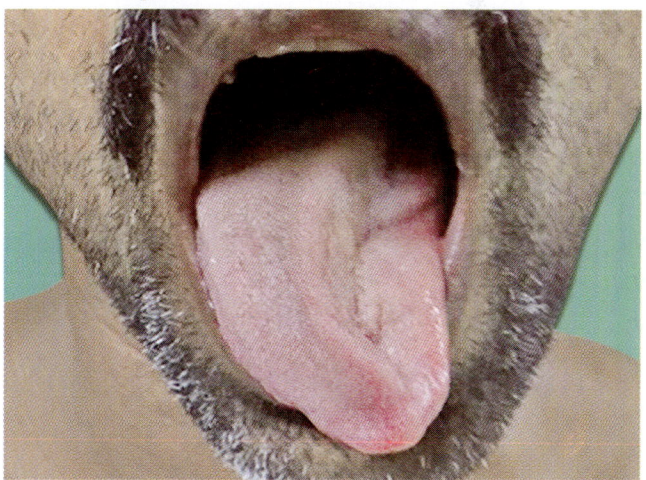

Fig. 6D(iii).75: Tongue deviation to the left suggestive of weakness of left hypoglossal muscle.

Bulbar palsy	Pseudobulbar palsy
Etiology:	**Etiology:**
<ul><li>Motor neuron disease</li><li>Syringobulbia</li><li>Guillain-Barré syndrome</li><li>Poliomyelitis</li><li>Subacute meningitis (carcinoma and lymphoma)</li><li>Neurosyphilis</li><li>Brainstem CVA</li><li>Bilateral damage or injury of the nerve nuclei of cranial nerves IX, X, XI, and XII</li><li>Lower motor neuron palsy of the respective muscles</li><li>Gag reflex—absent</li><li>Tongue—wasted, fasciculations</li></ul>	The most common cause is bilateral CVAs affecting the internal capsule Other causes include:<ul><li>Multiple sclerosis</li><li>Motor neuron disease</li><li>High brainstem tumors</li><li>Head injury</li><li>Bilateral damage or injury of corticobulbar tracts to nerve nuclei of cranial nerves V, VII, X, XI, and XII</li><li>Upper motor neuron palsy of the respective muscles</li><li>Gag reflex—increased or normal</li><li>Tongue—spastic</li></ul>

Contd...

Contd...

"Wasted, wrinkled, thrown into folds, and increasingly motionless" - Palatal movement—absent - Jaw jerk—absent or normal - Speech—nasal "Indistinct (flaccid dysarthria), lacks modulation, and has a nasal twang"	"It cannot be protruded, lies on the floor of the mouth and is small and tight" - Palatal movement— absent - Jaw jerk—increased - Speech—spastic: "A monotonous, slurred, high-pitched, 'Donald Duck', dysarthria" that "sounds as if the patient is trying to squeeze out words from tight lips". "Hot potato voice"

Contd...

- Emotions – normal - Other—signs of the underlying cause, e.g., limb fasciculations	- Emotions—labile - Other—bilateral upper motor neuron (long tract) limb signs. Bilateral extensor plantar and bilateral exaggerated reflexes

Contd...

MULTIPLE CRANIAL NERVE PALSIES

Cranial nerve	Cavernous sinus thrombosis	Superior orbital fissure syndrome	Orbital apex syndrome	Jacod (retro-sphenoid space) syndrome	Petrous apex Gradenigo syndrome	Tolosa-Hunt, lateral cavernous sinus syndrome	CP angle tumor	Vernet jugular foramen syndrome	Villaret, post-retroparotid syndrome	Collet-Sicard syndrome
II			√	√						
III	√	√	√	√		√				
IV	√	√	√	√		√				
V1	√	√	√	√	√	√	√			
V2	√+/−		√	√	√	√+/−				
V3				√	√					
VI	√	√	√	√	√	√	√			
VII							√			
VIII							√			
IX								√	√	√
X								√	√	√
XI								√	√	√
XII									√	√
Horner	√								√	

NOTES

D(iv). MOTOR SYSTEM EXAMINATION

Motor system examination includes examination of:
1. Attitude of the limbs
2. Bulk/nutrition
3. Assessment of tone
4. Examination of power
5. Reflexes
6. Coordination
7. Gait

Reflexes, coordination, and gait have been discussed separately in the successive sections.

ATTITUDE

Attitude is the position of the limbs which it adopts when the patient is in resting position.

In a patient with hemiplegia	
Upper limb	*Lower limb*
▪ Adduction at shoulder ▪ Flexion at elbow ▪ Semipronated ▪ Thumb tucked into the palm	▪ Extended at hip and knee ▪ Externally rotated at hip ▪ Foot inverted ▪ Plantar flexed

Few common attitudes

Paraplegia	Bilateral lower limbs are: ▪ Extended at hip and knee ▪ Externally rotated at hip ▪ Foot inverted ▪ Plantar flexed
Erb's palsy	On the affected side: ▪ Arm: Adducted and internally rotated ▪ Forearm: Extended and pronated ▪ Wrist: Flexed ▪ "Waiter's tip deformity"

MUSCLE BULK/NUTRITION

- Muscle bulk is assessed by inspection as well as measurements at corresponding sites in the extremities.
- Symmetry is important with consideration given to handedness and overall body habitus.
- Wasting is considered if there is >1 cm reduction on the dominant extremity and >2 cm in the nondominant extremity. In some areas, just inspection is adequate (thenar eminence, hypothenar eminence, shoulder) whereas in other areas (thighs, legs, arms and forearms) measurement is required.
- Measurements of the circumferences of the limb are done at corresponding areas at fixed distances from bony landmarks, which are part of that limb. **Example:** 10 cm below the olecranon **[Fig. 6D(iv).1]**, 10 cm above the medial humeral epicondyle **[Fig. 6D(iv).2]**, 18 cm above the patella, and 10 cm below the tibial tuberosity.

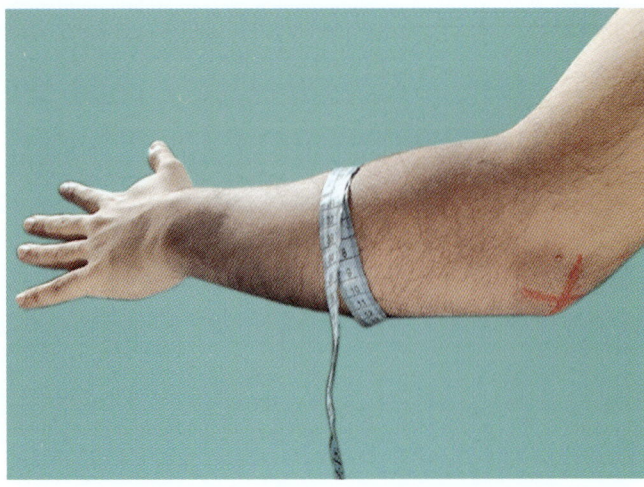

Fig. 6D(iv).1: Measurement of bulk in the forearm.

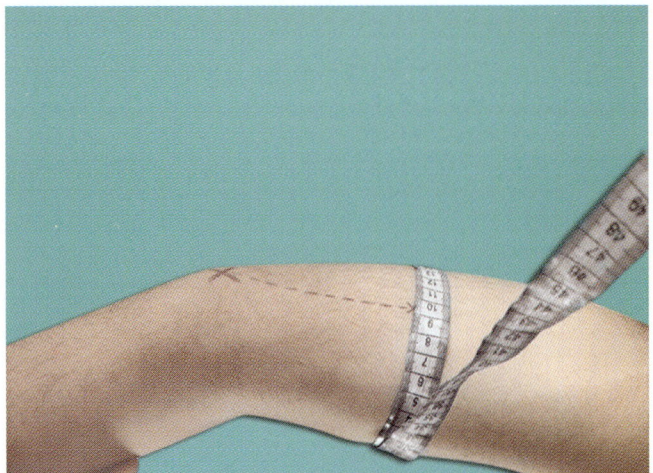

Fig. 6D(iv).2: Measurement of bulk in the arm.

Causes for Muscle Hypertrophy (Usually in the Calf) [Fig. 6D(iv).3]

True hypertrophy	Pseudohypertrophy (due to increased fat in muscle)
Exercise	▪ Duchene's muscular dystrophy ▪ Becker's muscular dystrophy ▪ Myotonia congenita—Thomson's disease ▪ Kugelberg Welander spinal muscular atrophy ▪ Hypothyroidism (infantile Hercules/Kocher–Debré–Semelaigne syndrome) ▪ Storage disorders

Localized muscle swelling—muscle hemorrhage, myositis ossificans, abscess, tumor, muscle rupture or cysts (cysticercosis).

Nervous System

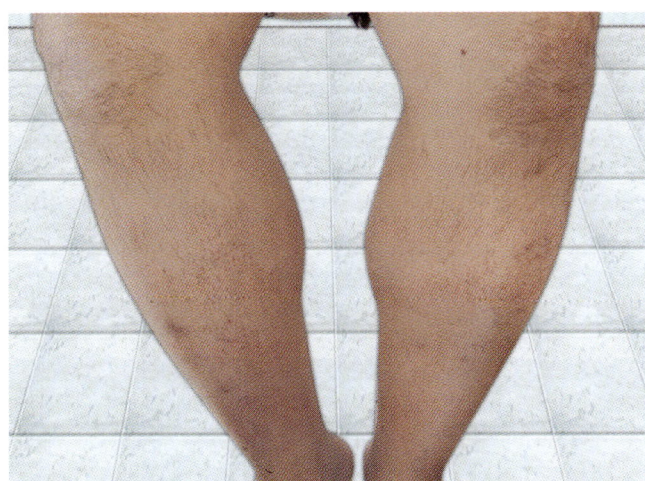

Fig. 6D(iv).3: Pseudohypertrophy of calf muscle.

Causes of Muscle Wasting

Generalized wasting	Proximal wasting	Distal wasting
- Malignancy - Cachexia - Tuberculosis - Thyrotoxicosis - Addison's disease - HIV/AIDS	- Motor neuron disease: Juvenile SMA (Kugelberg Welander) - Muscular dystrophy: FSHD [Fig. 6D(iv).4], limb girdle dystrophy - Inflammatory myopathies - Brachial plexopathy - Axillary neuropathy	- Anterior horn cell disease—polio, motor neuron disease - Syringomyelia, intramedullary tumors - Peripheral neuropathies—leprosy, carpal tunnel syndrome - Myotonic dystrophy - Plexopathies—lower brachial plexus - Arthritis—rheumatoid - Disuse atrophy

Causes of hand muscle wasting [Fig. 6D(iv).5]:

Anterior horn cell disease	- Motor neuron disease - Syringomyelia - Polio - Spinal muscular atrophy
Nerve root	- T1 compression by disc lesion - Pachymeningitis - Cervical spondylosis - Syphilitic amyotrophy - C8–T1 tumors
Brachial plexus	- Pancoast tumor - Thoracic outlet obstruction, cervical rib - Trauma, Klumpke's paralysis - Other—infiltration, irradiation
Lesions of peripheral nerve (ulnar or median)	- Trauma - Acute compression (coma, anesthesia, deep sleep) - Chronic compression (entrapment) - Acute ischemia (collagen vascular disease, diabetes)
Muscle disease	- Myotonic dystrophy - Distal myopathy—Welander, Udd, Miyoshi, Nonaka, Markesbery
Others	- Rheumatoid arthritis - Disuse atrophy - Rarely—parietal lobe lesions

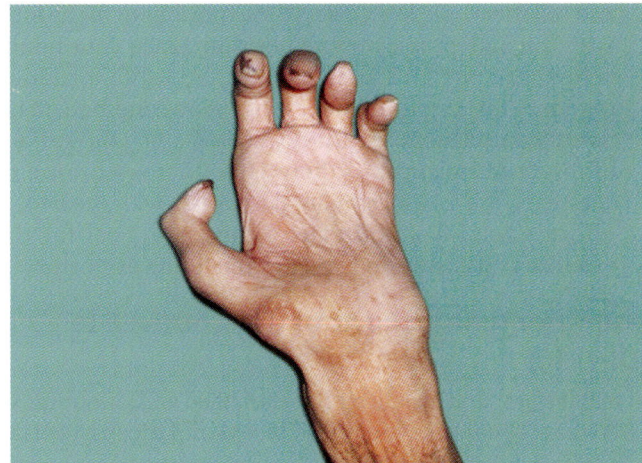

Fig. 6D(iv).5: Small muscle wasting of the hand.

The Split Hand Sign

- It is highly specific for amyotrophic lateral sclerosis (ALS).
- Amyotrophic lateral sclerosis (ALS) is a pure motor neurodegenerative disease where there is asymmetric involvement of the upper and lower motor neurons. In the intrinsic muscles of the hands, there is preferential wasting of the abductor pollicis brevis (APB) and first dorsal interosseous muscle (FDI) (thenar muscles) as compared to the abductor digiti minimi (ADM) (hypothenar muscle)
- The clinical deficit is loss of the pincer grasp.
- APB, FDI, and ADM are innervated by spinal motor neurons of the same segments (C8 and T1), and FDI and ADM have the same ulnar nerve supply. It is not known why APB and FDI are preferentially affected compared with ADM in those with ALS.

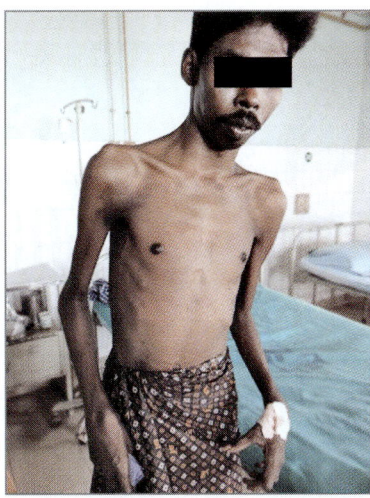

Fig. 6D(iv).4: Proximal muscle wasting seen in facioscapulohumeral dystrophy (FSHD).

- This is in contrast to a C8-T1 root lesion, which will cause wasting of both thenar and hypothenar muscle as both median and ulnar nerves receive C8-T1 innervation.

Other dissociated patterns of muscle atrophy in ALS:
- The split-hand plus (preferential dysfunction of thenar muscles compared with flexor pollicis longus)
- Split-elbow (preferential weakness of biceps brachii compared with triceps muscle)
- Split-leg signs (preferential dysfunction of ankle plantar flexor compared with the dorsiflexor muscles)

MUSCLE TONE

Definition

Tone is defined as partial state of contraction of the muscle at rest which is demonstrated by resistance offered by the muscle to passive movement across the joint.

Tone is examined in the upper limb (wrist and elbow joint) and the lower limb (knee and ankle joint).

Testing for Tone in the Legs [Figs. 6D(iv).6 and 6D(iv).7]

- With the patient relaxed, place your hands on the thigh and roll the whole leg. Observe the movement of the foot.
- With the patient in a supine position, place your hands behind the patient's knee, and lift the leg in a sudden motion. Observe if the heel drags along the bed. With normal muscle tone, the heel will drag along the surface of the bed. However, if there is an increased tone or spasticity, the foot may not make contact with the bed.
- Alternatively, flex and extend the knee. Feel for the extensors during flexion and flexors during extension.

Testing for Tone in the Arms [Figs. 6D(iv).8 to 6D(iv).10]

- Lift the arm and let it drop. See the speed and smoothness.
- At the elbow, check for tone in biceps and triceps. Feel the biceps while extending the arm and feel the triceps while flexing the arm.

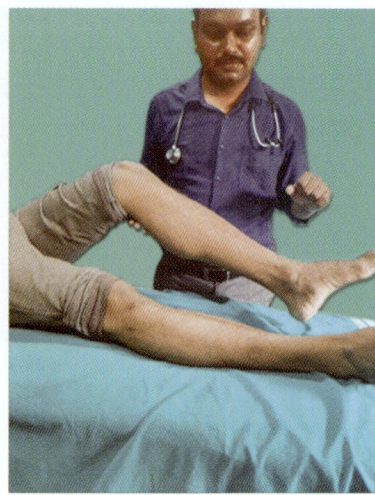

Fig. 6D(iv).7: Assessment of tone in the lower limbs.

- At the wrist, take the hand as if to shake it. First pronate and supinate the forearm. Then roll the hand around at the wrist. This demonstrates cogwheel rigidity [**Fig. 6D(iv).11**].

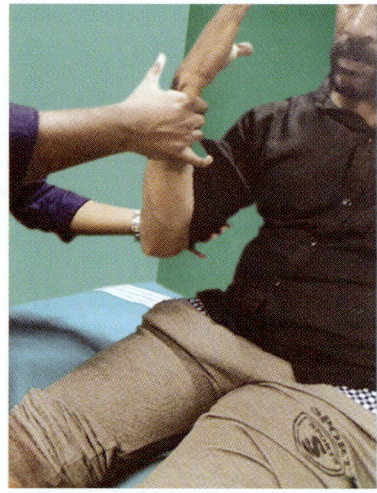

Fig. 6D(iv).8: Examining tone of triceps.

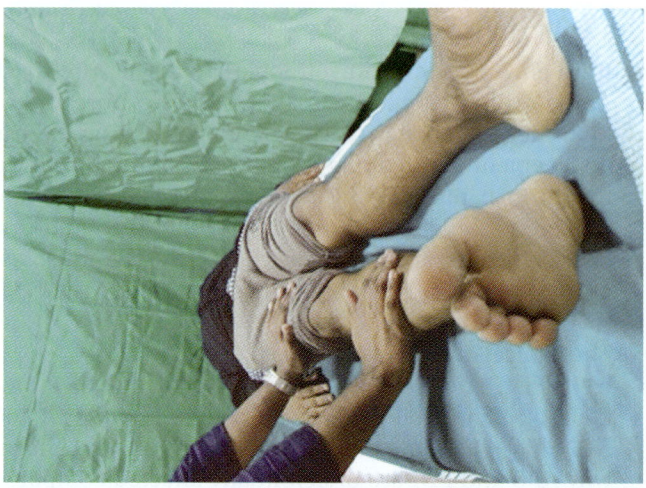

Fig. 6D(iv).6: Assessment of tone in the lower limbs.

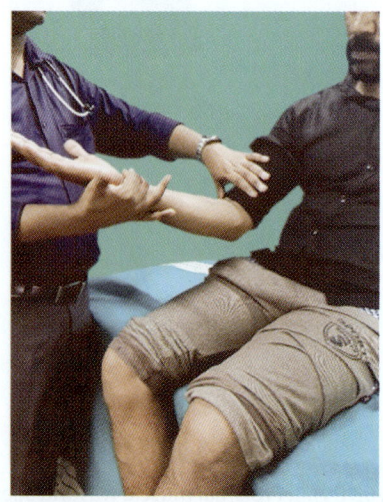

Fig. 6D(iv).9: Examining the tone of biceps.

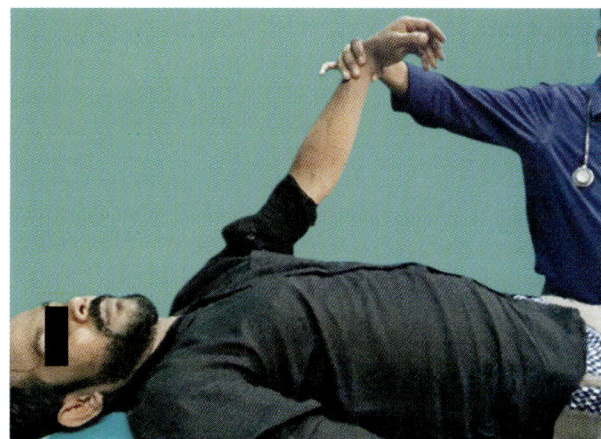

Fig. 6D(iv).10: Examining the tone in the upper limb.

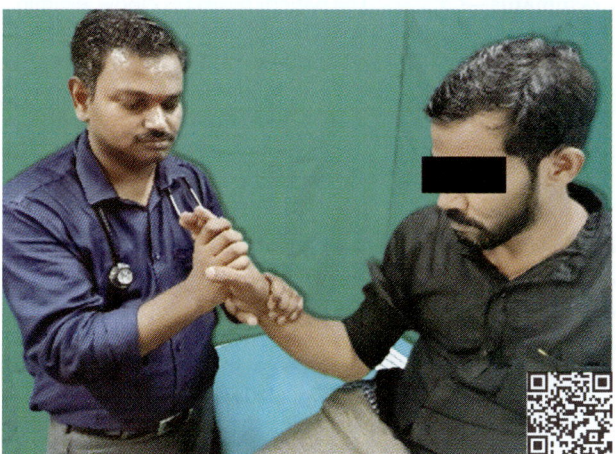

Fig. 6D(iv).11: Examining for cogwheeling/rigidity.

Abnormalities of Tone

Spasticity: JW Lance defined spasticity as "a motor disorder characterized by a velocity dependent increase in tonic stretch reflexes (muscle tone) with exaggerated tendon jerks, resulting from hyperexcitability of the stretch reflex, as one component of the upper motor neuron syndrome".
Rigidity, in contrast to spasticity, does not depend on the velocity of movement. It equally affects flexors and extensors and gives rise to uniform resistance to passive stretching in all directions known as 'lead pipe' phenomenon.
Hypotonia—decreased tone.

Causes:
- Lower motor neuron (LMN) disease
- Cerebellar disease
- Hypothyroidism
- Upper motor neuron (UMN) disease in a state of neuronal shock
- Chorea
- Hypermagnesemia
- Down syndrome
- Anesthesia and muscle relaxants.

Hypertonia—increased tone. Two principal types:
1. Spasticity
2. Rigidity

	Spasticity	Rigidity
Synonym	Clasp-knife	Lead-pipe/Cogwheel
Diseases	Pyramidal	Extrapyramidal
Pathophysiology	Increased gamma activity	Increased gamma and alpha activity
Description	■ Tone increased in the initial part of movement followed by sudden release—clasp-knife effect* ■ Supination-pronation of the forearm will reveal the so-called supinator catch	■ Increased tone present continuously throughout the complete range of movement—lead-pipe ■ With associated tremors—cogwheel**
Muscles involved	Anti-gravity muscles (flexors in the UL and extensors in the LL)	Both groups of muscles
Velocity	Velocity dependent (more with fast movements)	Velocity independent
Associated features	Hyperreflexia, extensor plantar	Tremors, bradykinesia

*__Clasp knife phenomenon:__ The muscles at rest do not have excessive tone but a brisk stretch will produce a catch at about mid-length of the muscle followed by a sudden release of the catch and relaxation of the muscle. The giving away or the release portion of the clasp-knife phenomenon is due to the increased firing of the inhibitory Golgi tendon organs. To elicit this phenomenon, the clinician extends the patient's knee using a constant velocity, but as the patient's knee nears full extension, the muscle tone of the quadriceps muscles increases dramatically and completes the movement, just as the blade of a pocketknife opens under the influence of its spring.
**__Cogwheel rigidity:__ Lead pipe rigidity superimposed with tremors (Negro sign).

Causes of hypertonia:
- UMN disease—pyramidal and extrapyramidal
- Tetanus
- Tetany
- Strychnine poisoning
- Tonic phase of seizure
- Catatonia (seen in schizophrenia where there is increased tone for all movements)

Paratonia—altered tone seen in psychiatric diseases and frontal lobe dysfunction which is characterized by inability to relax the muscle during muscle tone assessment. Can be of two types:
1. Oppositional paratonia **(Gegenhalten)**—where the subjects involuntarily resist passive movements
2. Facilitatory paratonia **(Mitgehen)**—where the subject involuntarily assists passive movement.

Paratonia is present in bilateral frontal lobe dysfunction and diffuse cerebellar disorders.

Myotonia—Slow relaxation of muscle after voluntary contraction or contraction provoked by muscle percussion. Examples: Myotonic dystrophy, congenital myotonia, hypothyroidism, neuromyotonia congenita, Issac syndrome **[Fig. 6D(iv).12]**.

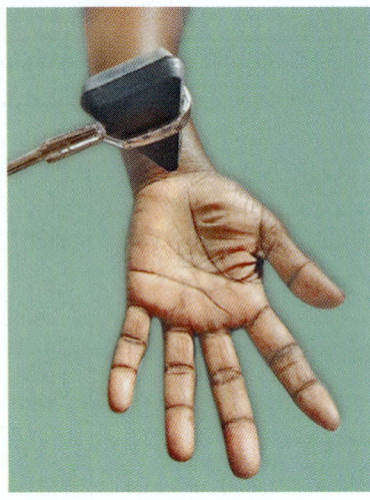

Fig. 6D(iv).12: Demonstration of myotonia.

Myoedema:
Stationary muscle mounding after muscle percussion without electrical muscle activity is called myoedema. Myoedema is due to prolonged muscle contraction caused by delayed calcium reuptake by sarcoplasmic reticulum, following local calcium ion release brought out by percussion or pressure.

Can be seen in hypothyroidism, chronic debilitating diseases, severe cachexia as in TB.

MOTOR POWER

Prerequisites
- Explain the test and the movements you are planning to do clearly to the patient before performing the test.
- Position the patient according to the muscle which is being tested.

State of Muscle during Examination
- Fully contracted muscle
    - Muscle is at maximum advantage (small muscle)
- Fully relaxed muscle
    - Muscle at maximum disadvantage (may detect mild degrees of weakness)
- Mid-contracted muscle
    - Most feasible method
    - Used for most large muscles

Qualitative Assessment of Weakness (MRC Grading)

Grade	Description
Grade 0	no contraction
Grade 1	Flicker or trace of contraction
Grade 2	active movement, with gravity eliminated
Grade 3	active movement against gravity
Grade 4	active movement against gravity and resistance
Grade 5	normal power

Grades 4-, 4, and 4+ may be used to indicate movement against slight, moderate, and strong resistance, respectively.

Muscle of neck	
Flexion of neck (sternocleidomastoid/platysma)	The patient attempts to flex his neck against resistance while supporting the chest [Fig. 6D(iv).13]
Extensor of neck	The patient attempts to extend their neck against resistance; contraction of the trapezius and other extensor muscles can be seen and felt, and strength of movement can be judged [Fig. 6D(iv).14]
Upper limb	
Supraspinatus—C5	Patient initiates abduction of arm from side against resistance [Fig. 6D(iv).15]
Deltoid—C5	Patient holds his hand at 60° against resistance [Fig. 6D(iv).16]
Infraspinatus—C5	The patient flexes his elbow, examiner holds the elbow to his side, and then attempts external rotation of the forearm against resistance [Fig. 6D(iv).17]
Rhomboids—C5	With hands on hip ask the patient to force the elbow backward [Fig. 6D(iv).18]
Serratus anterior—C5, 6, 7	The patient pushes his arms forward against firm resistance [Fig. 6D(iv).19]
Pectoralis major—C6, 7, 8	• Placing hand on hip and pressing inward, sternocostal part of muscle can be seen and felt to contract [Fig. 6D(iv).20] • Raising the arm forward above 90° and attempting to adduct clavicular portion can be felt
Latissimus dorsi—C7	• While palpating muscles ask the patient to cough • Resist the patients attempt to adduct the arm when abducted to above 90° [Fig. 6D(iv).21]
Biceps—C5	Ask the patient to flex at the forearm with hand in supine position, against resistance [Fig. 6D(iv).22]
Brachioradialis—C5, 6	The patient is asked to flex the elbow with the forearm midway between pronation and supination [Fig. 6D(iv).23]
Triceps—C7	The patient attempts to extend elbow against resistance [Fig. 6D(iv).24]
Extensor carpi radialis longus—C6, 7	The patient makes a fist and extends the wrist towards the radial side [Fig. 6D(iv).25]
Extensor carpi ulnaris—C7	The patient makes a fist and extends the wrist towards the ulnar side [Fig. 6D(iv).26]
Extensor digitorium—C7	The examiner attempts to flex the patient's extended fingers at the metacarpophalangeal joints [Figs. 6D(iv).27A and B]
Flexor carpi radialis—C6, 7	The examiner attempts to flex the wrist toward the radial side [Fig. 6D(iv).28]

Contd...

Contd...

Flexor carpi ulnaris—C8	Best seen while testing the abductor digiti minimi when it fixes its point of origin [**Figs. 6D(iv).29A and B**]
Abductor pollicis longus—C8	Patient maintains their thumb in the abduction against the examiner's resistance [**Fig. 6D(iv).30**]
Extensor pollicis brevis—C8	The patient attempts to extend the thumb while the examiner attempts to flex it at the **metacarpophalangeal joint** [**Fig. 6D(iv).31**]
Extensor pollicis longus—C8	The patient attempts to extend the thumb while the examiner attempts to flex it at the **interphalangeal joint**
Opponens pollicis—T1	The patient attempts to touch the little finger with the thumb [**Fig. 6D(iv).32**]
Abductor pollicis brevis—T1	Place an object between the thumb and base of forefinger to prevent full adduction Patient attempts to raise the edge of the thumb vertically against the resistance [**Fig. 6D(iv).33**]
Flexor pollicis longus— C8	Tested by attempting to extend the distal phalanx of the thumb against resistance, while holding the proximal phalanx [**Fig. 6D(iv).34**]
Adductor pollicis—T1	The patient attempts to hold a piece of paper between the thumb and the palmar aspect of forefinger and examiner tries to pull the paper [**Fig. 6D(iv).35**]
Lumbricals—C8, T1	The patient tries to flex the extended fingers at the metacarpophalangeal joints [**Fig. 6D(iv).36**]
Dorsal interossei	The patient attempts to keep the fingers abducted against resistance [**Fig. 6D(iv).37**]
First dorsal interossei and palmar interossei	Place the hand flat on table and the patient tries to abduct and adduct the forefinger against the resistance [**Figs. 6D(iv).38 and 6D(iv).39**]
Flexor digitorum sublimis—C8	The patient flexes the fingers at the proximal interphalangeal joint against resistance from the examiner's fingers placed on the middle phalanx [**Fig. 6D(iv).40**]
Flexor digitorum profundus—C8	The patient keeps his hand on a flat surface. The examiner holds the middle phalanx down; the patient flexes the distal phalanx against resistance [**Fig. 6D(iv).41**]
Flexor digiti minimi—T1	The back of hand is placed on the table and the little finger abducted against resistance (often the only sign of an ulnar lesion) [**Fig. 6D(iv).42**]
Trunk muscles	
Abdominal muscles	The recumbent patient attempts to raise his head against resistance [**Fig. 6D(iv).43**]

Contd...

Contd...

Extensors of spine	The patient, lying prone, attempts to raise the head and upper part of the chest [**Fig. 6D(iv).44**]
Lower limb	
Iliopsoas—L1, 2, 3	The patient lies supine and attempts to flex the thigh against resistance [**Fig. 6D(iv).45**]
Adductor femoris—L5, S1 (adductor magnus, longus and brevis)	The patient attempts to adduct the leg against resistance [**Fig. 6D(iv).46**]
Gluteus medius and minimus—L2, 3	Patient in prone, flexes the knee, and then forces the foot outward against resistance [**Fig. 6D(iv).47**]
Gluteus maximus—L5, S1	Patient in prone raises the thigh against resistance with the knee flexed to minimize the contribution from the hamstrings [**Fig. 6D(iv).48**]
Hamstrings—L4, 5, S1, 2 (biceps, semi-membranosus, and semitendinosus)	Patient in prone and attempts to flex the knee against resistance [**Fig. 6D(iv).49**]
Quadriceps femoris—L3, 4	Patient is supine and extends the knee against resistance [**Fig. 6D(iv).50**]
Tibialis anterior—L4, 5	The patient dorsiflexes the foot against the resistance of examiner [**Fig. 6D(iv).51**]
Tibialis posterior— L4	The patient plantar flexes the foot slightly and then tries to invert it against resistance [**Fig. 6D(iv).52**]
Peronei—L5, S1	The patient everts the foot against resistance [**Fig. 6D(iv).53**]
Extensor digitorum longus—L5	Patient asked to dorsiflex the foot against resistance [**Fig. 6D(iv).54**]
Flexor digitorum longus—S1, 2	Patient asked to flex the terminal phalanges against resistance [**Fig. 6D(iv).55**]
Extensor hallucis longus—L5, S1	Patient asked to dorsiflex the great toe against resistance [**Fig. 6D(iv).56**]
Extensor digitorum brevis—S1	The patient dorsiflexes the toes against resistance [**Fig. 6D(iv).57**]

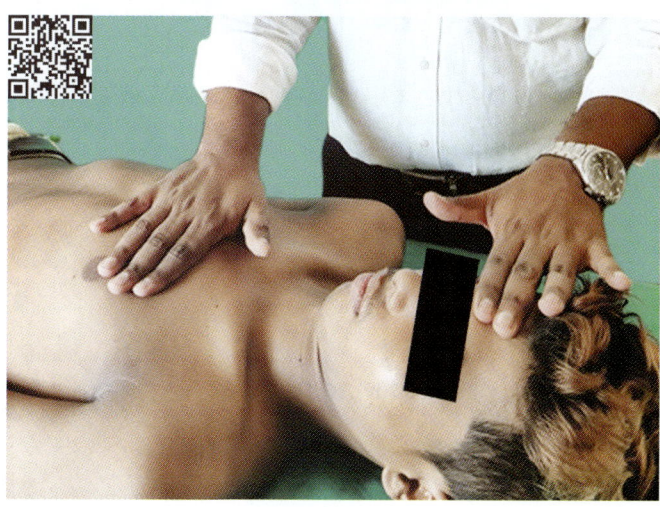

Fig. 6D(iv).13: Flexion of neck (sternocleidomastoid/platysma).

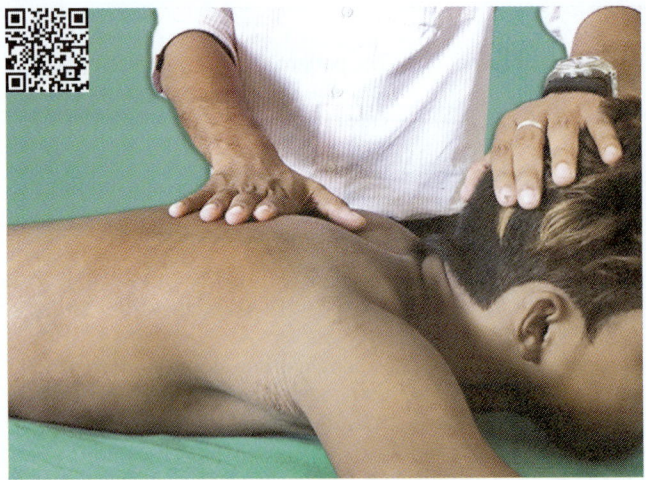

Fig. 6D(iv).14: Extensor of neck.

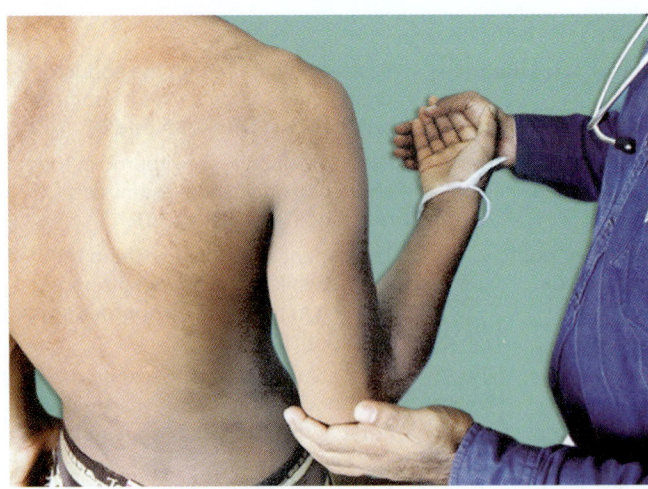

Fig. 6D(iv).17: Infraspinatus—C5.

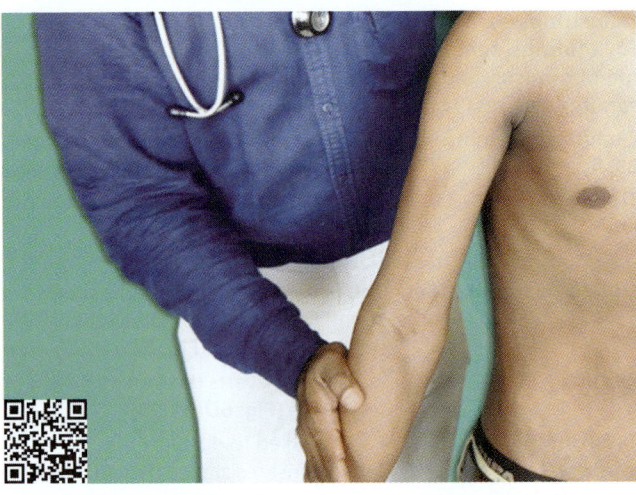

Fig. 6D(iv).15: Supraspinatus—C5. Patient initiates abduction of arm from side against resistance.

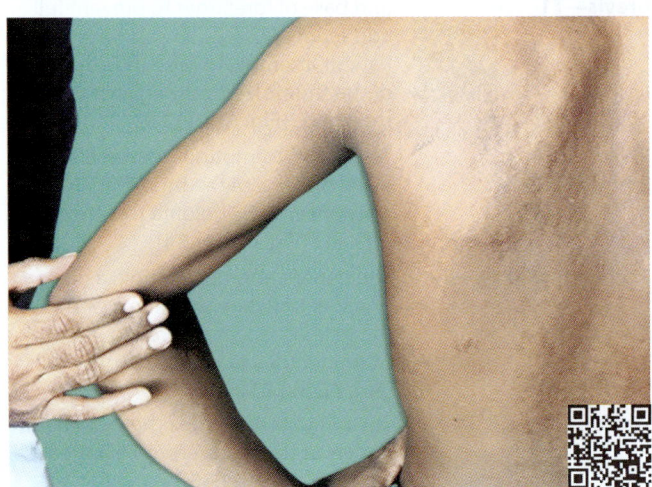

Fig. 6D(iv).18: Rhomboids—C5.

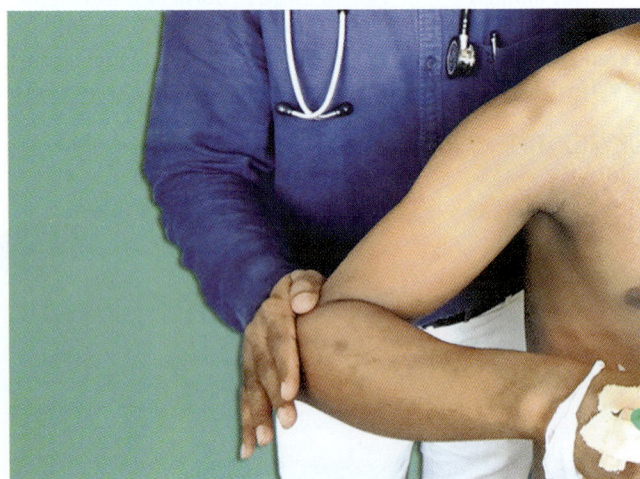

Fig. 6D(iv).16: Deltoid C5.

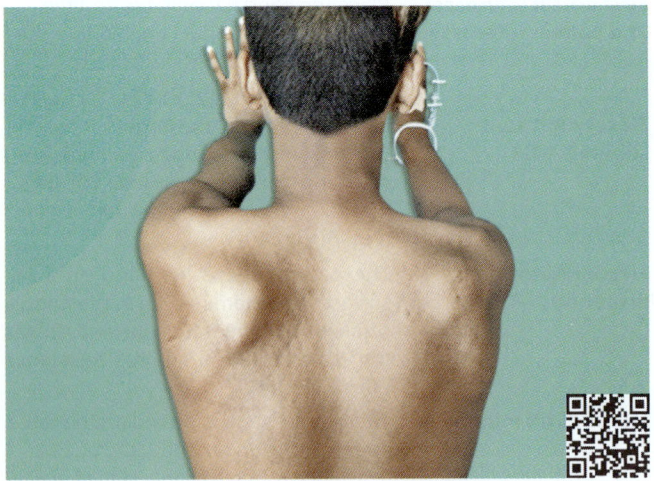

Fig. 6D(iv).19: Serratus anterior—C5, 6, 7.

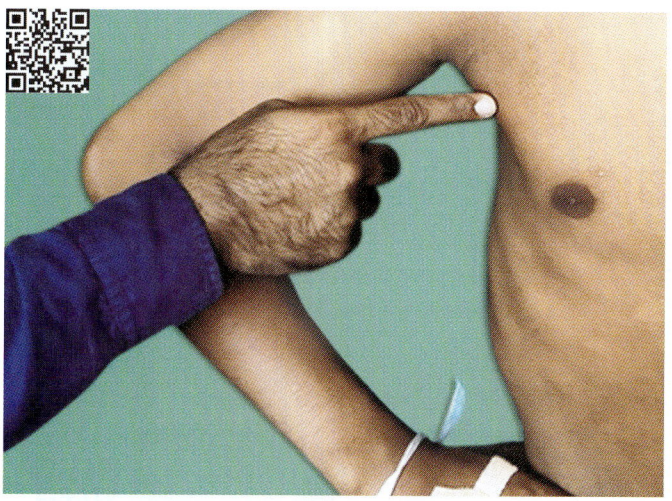

Fig. 6D(iv).20: Pectoralis major—C6, 7, 8.

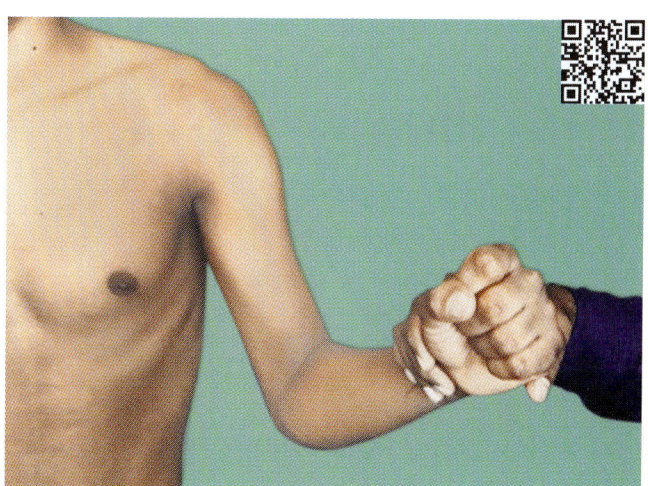

Fig. 6D(iv).23: Brachioradialis—C5, 6.

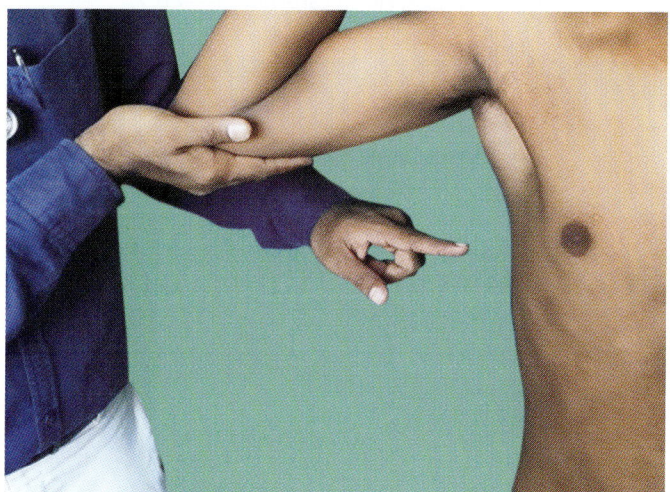

Fig. 6D(iv).21: Latissimus dorsi—C7.

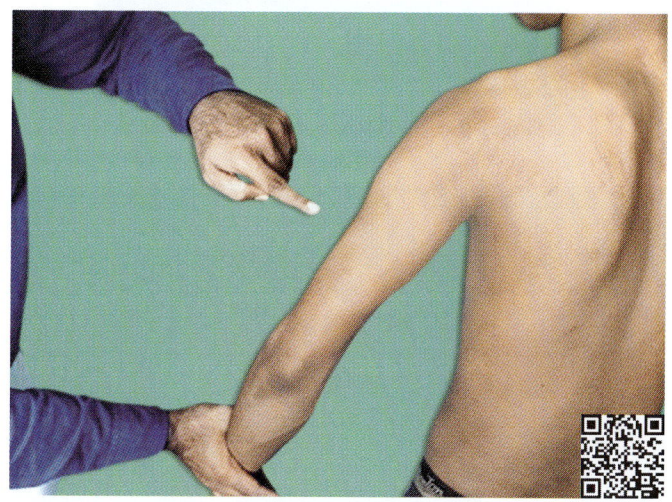

Fig. 6D(iv).24: Triceps—C7.

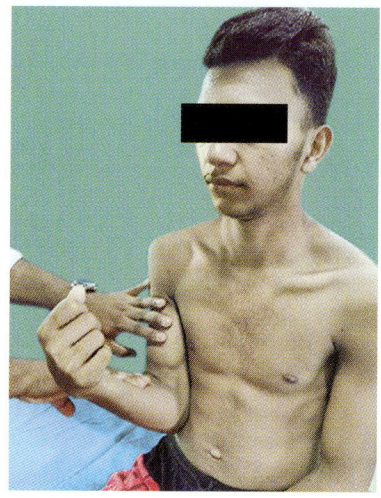

Fig. 6D(iv).22: Biceps—C5.

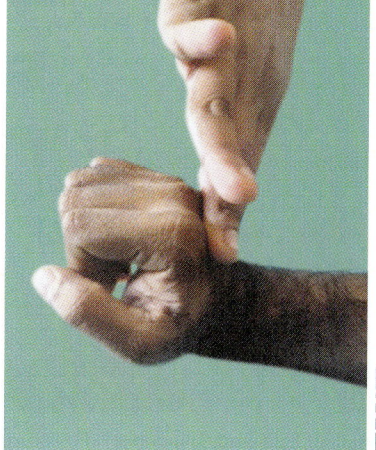

Fig. 6D(iv).25: Extensor carpi radialis longus—C6, 7.

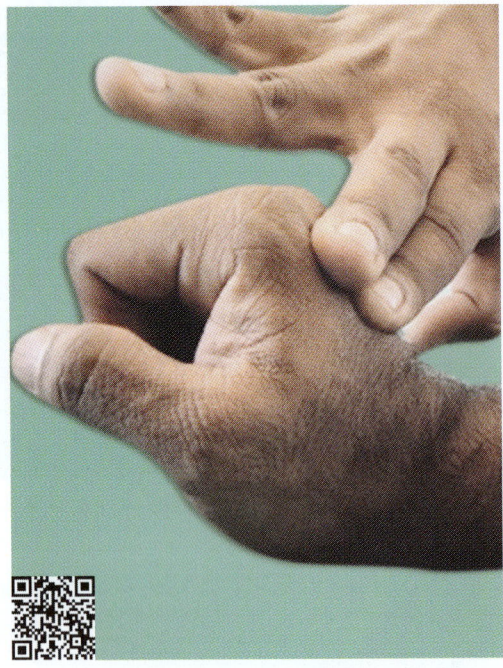

Fig. 6D(iv).26: Extensor carpi ulnaris—C7.

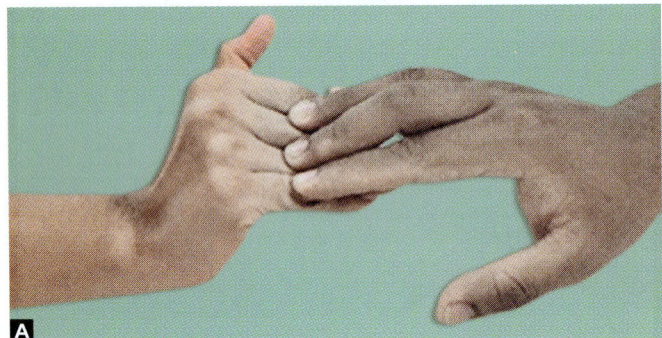

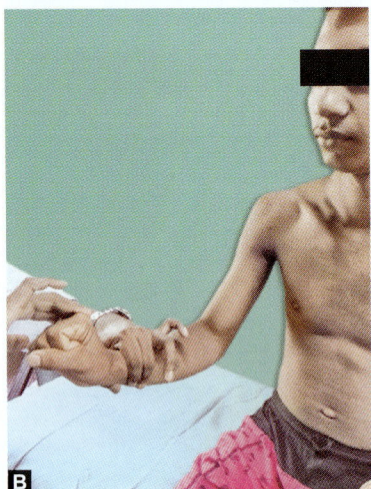

Figs. 6D(iv).27A and B: Extensor digitorum—C7.

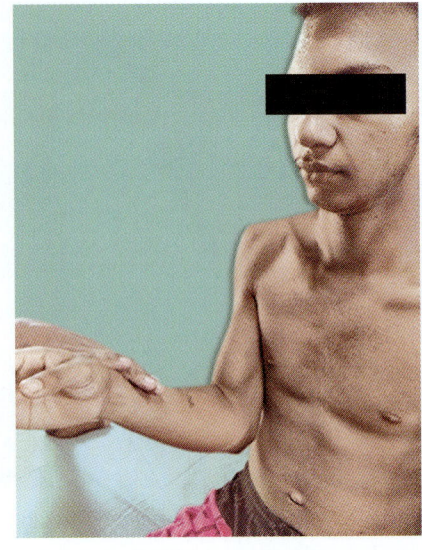

Fig. 6D(iv).28: Flexor carpi radialis—C6, 7.

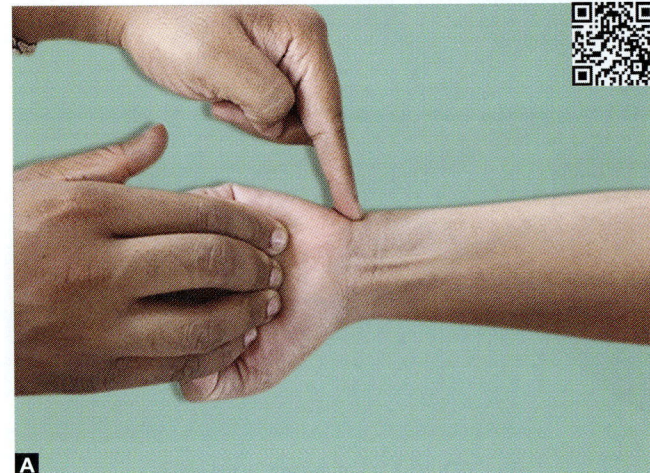

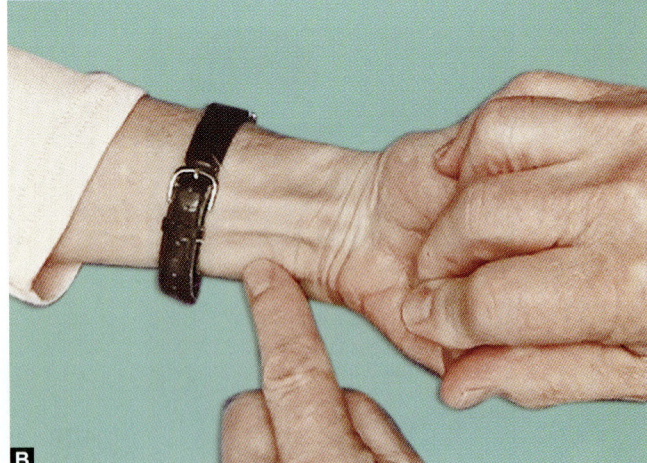

Figs. 6D(iv).29A and B: Flexor carpi ulnaris—C8.

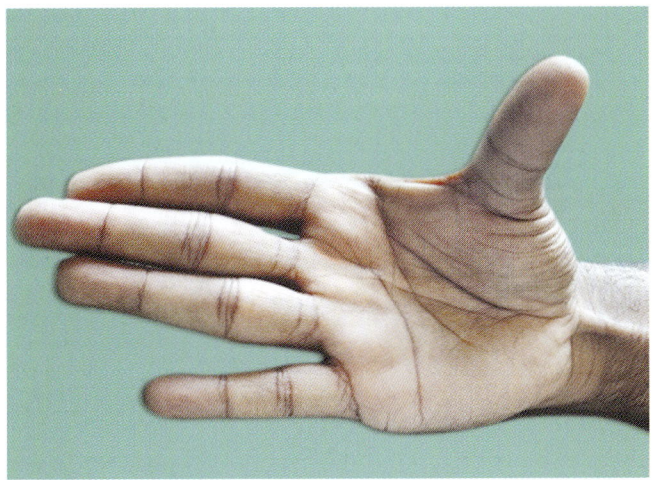

Fig. 6D(iv).30: Thumb abduction.

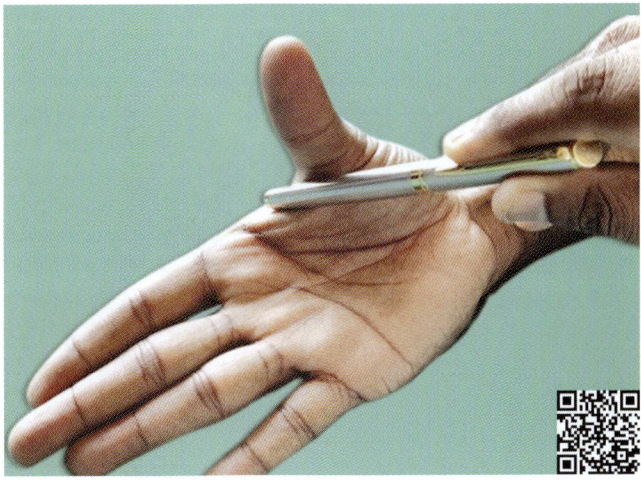

Fig. 6D(iv).33: Abductor pollicis brevis—T1.

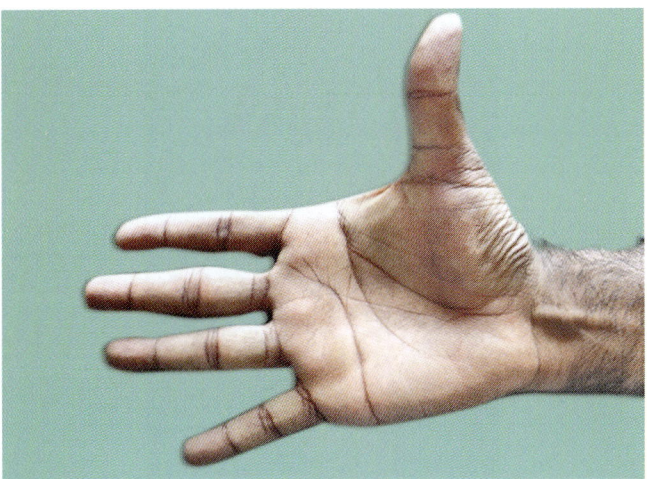

Fig. 6D(iv).31: Thumb extension.

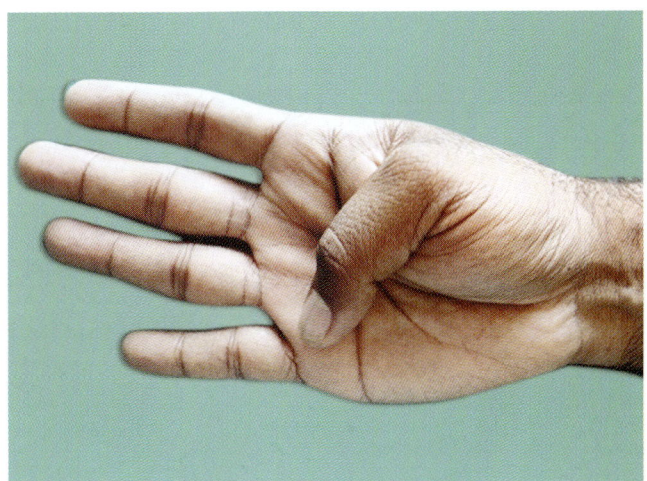

Fig. 6D(iv).34: Thumb flexion.

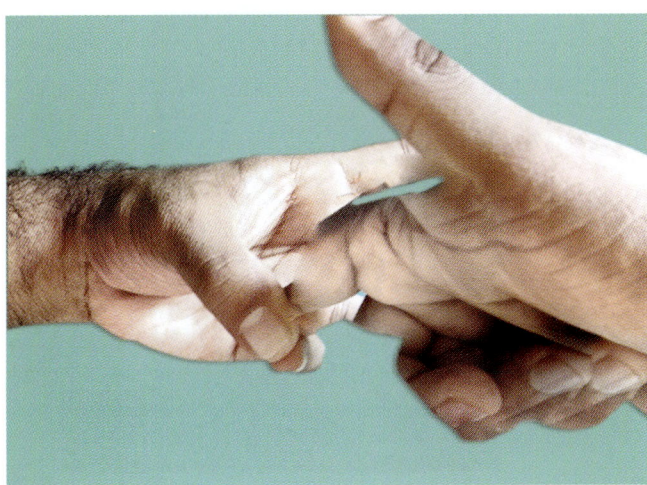

Fig. 6D(iv).32: Opponens pollicis—T1.

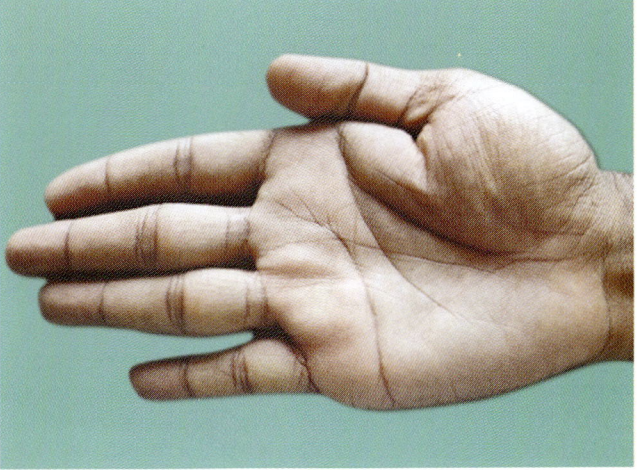

Fig. 6D(iv).35: Thumb adduction.

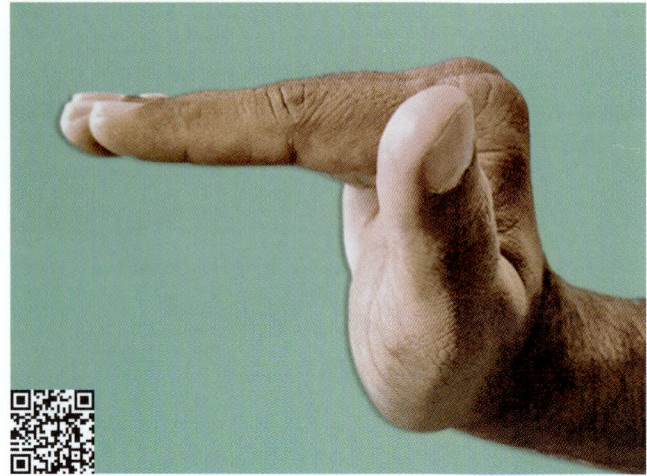

Fig. 6D(iv).36: Lumbricals—C8, T1.

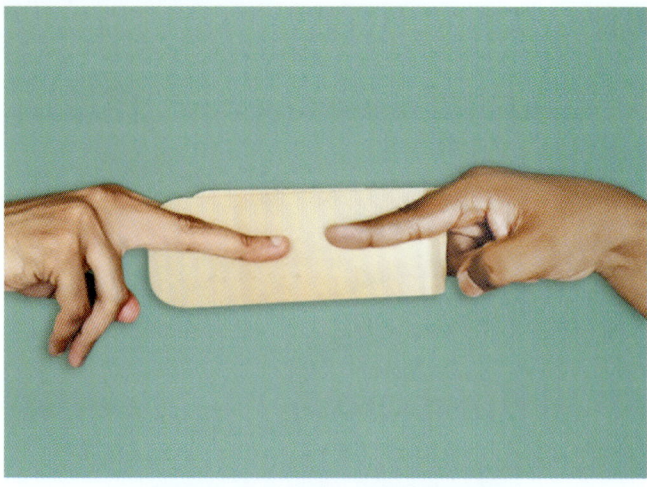

Fig. 6D(iv).39: Card test for palmar interossei.

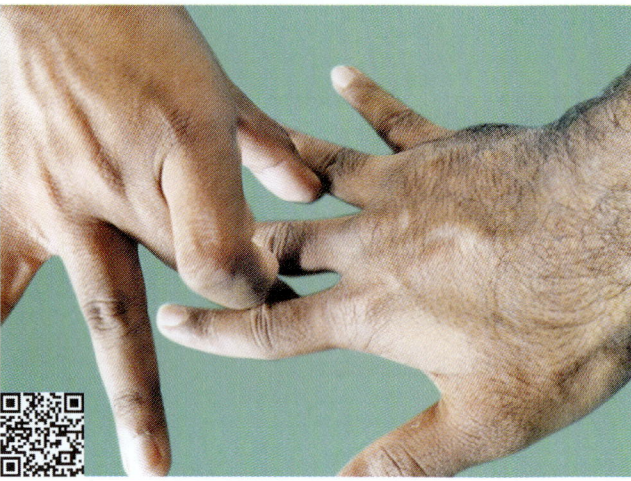

Fig. 6D(iv).37: Dorsal interossei.

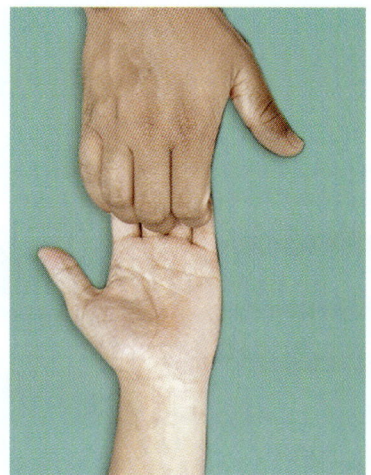

Fig. 6D(iv).40: Flexor digitorum sublimis.

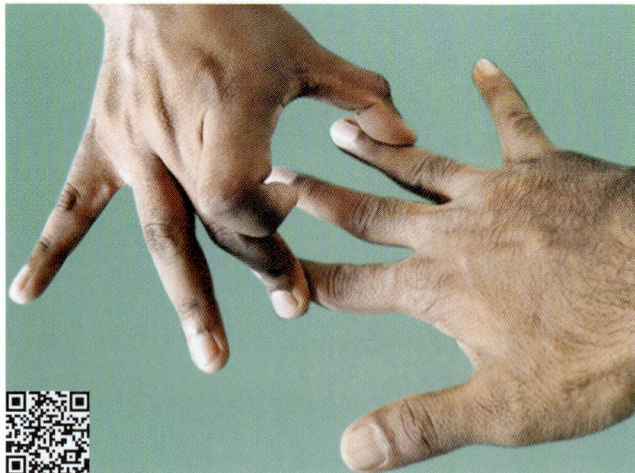

Fig. 6D(iv).38: Palmar interossei.

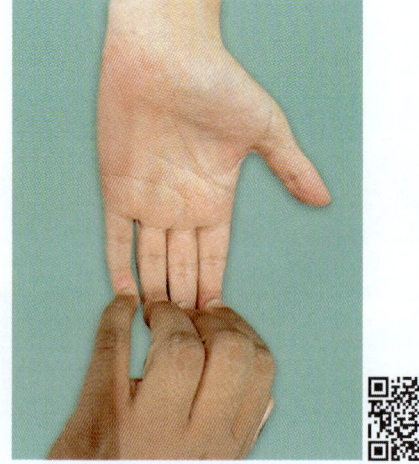

Fig. 6D(iv).41: Flexor digitorum profundus.

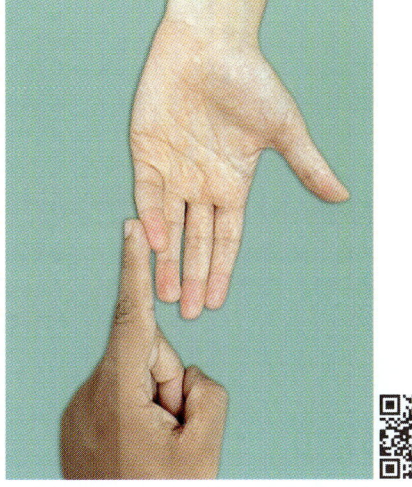

Fig. 6D(iv).42: Abductor digiti minimi.

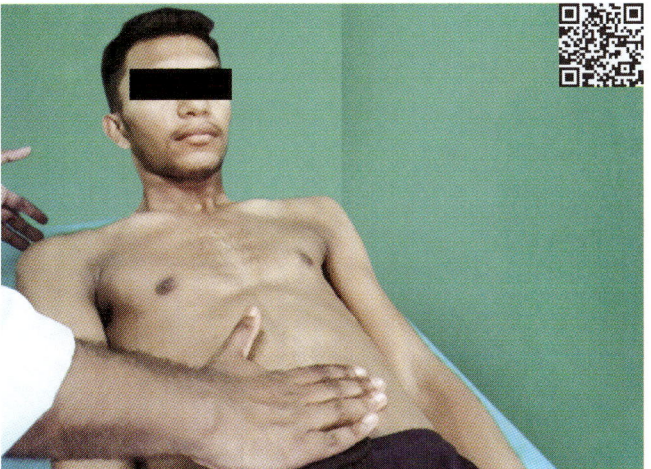

Fig. 6D(iv).43: Abdominal muscles—T5-L1.

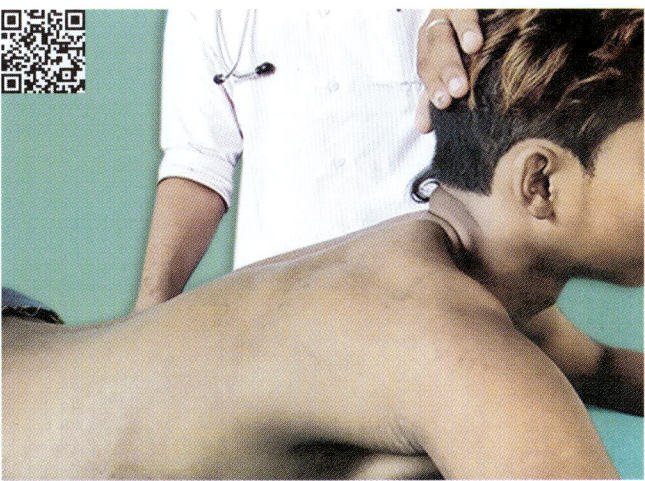

Fig. 6D(iv).44: Extensors of spine.

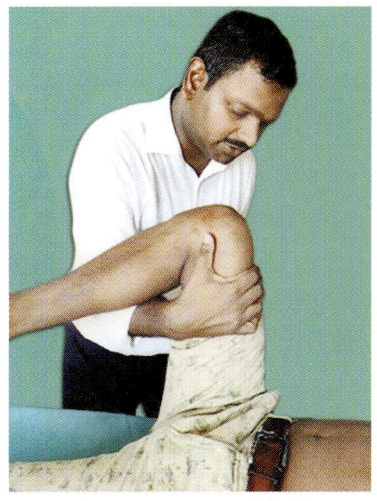

Fig. 6D(iv).45: Iliopsoas—L1, 2, and 3.

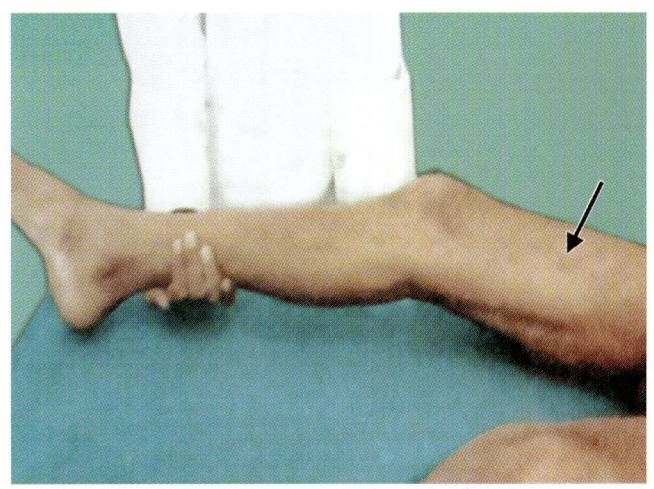

Fig. 6D(iv).46: Adductor femoris—L5, S1.

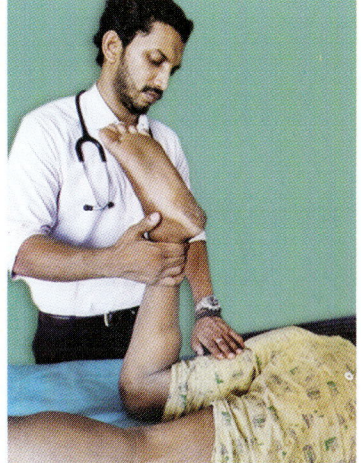

Fig. 6D(iv).47: Gluteus medius and minimus—L2, 3.

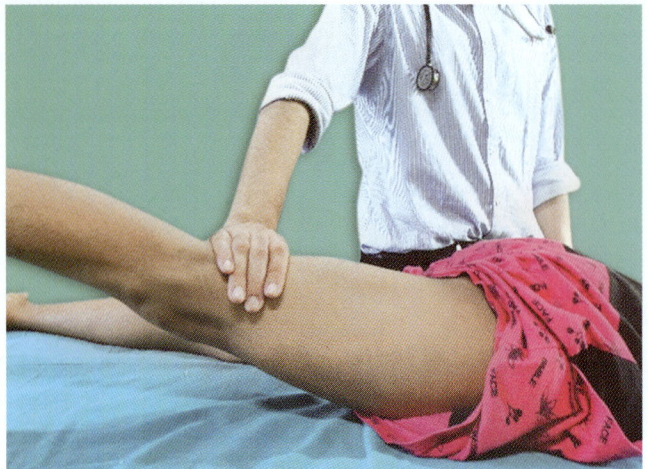

Fig. 6D(iv).48: Gluteus maximus—L5, S1.

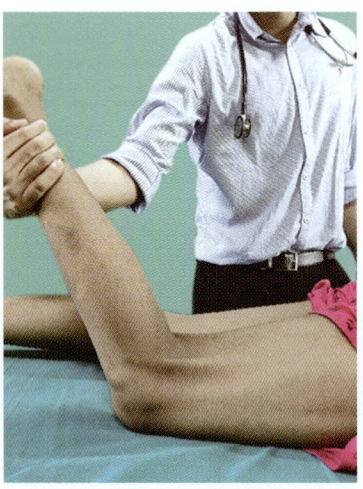

Fig. 6D(iv).49: Hamstrings—L4, 5, S1, 2 (biceps, semimembranosus, and semitendinosus).

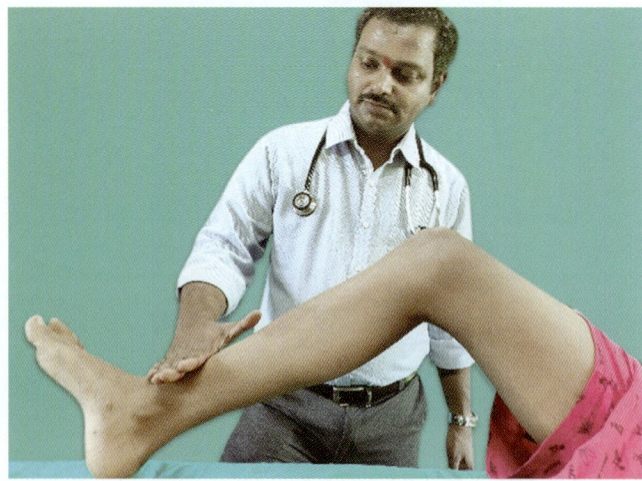

Fig. 6D(iv).50: Quadriceps femoris—L3, 4.

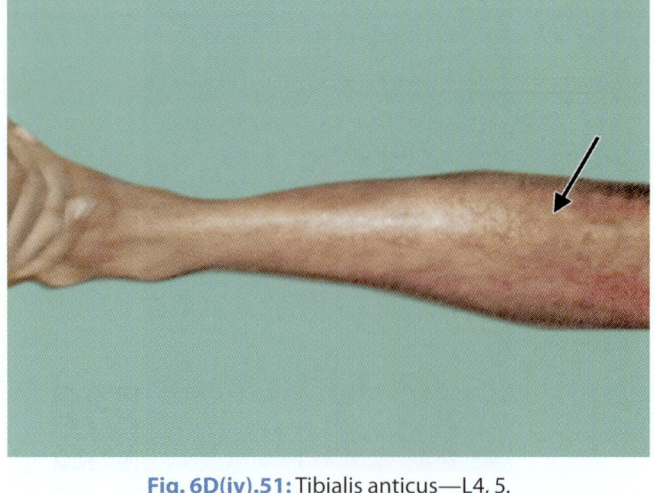

Fig. 6D(iv).51: Tibialis anticus—L4, 5.

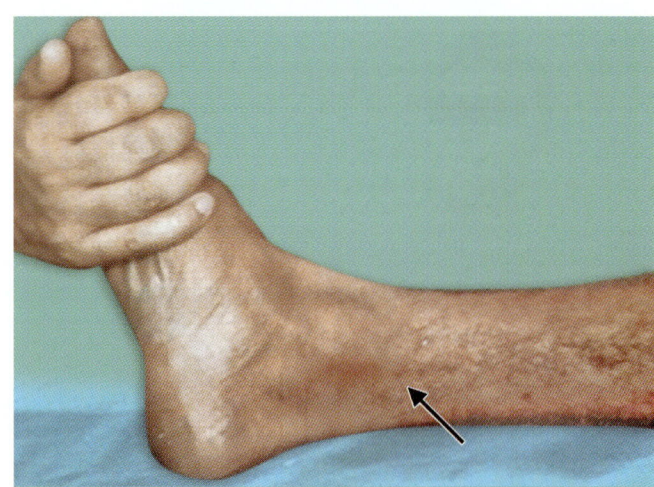

Fig. 6D(iv).52: Tibialis posticus—L4.

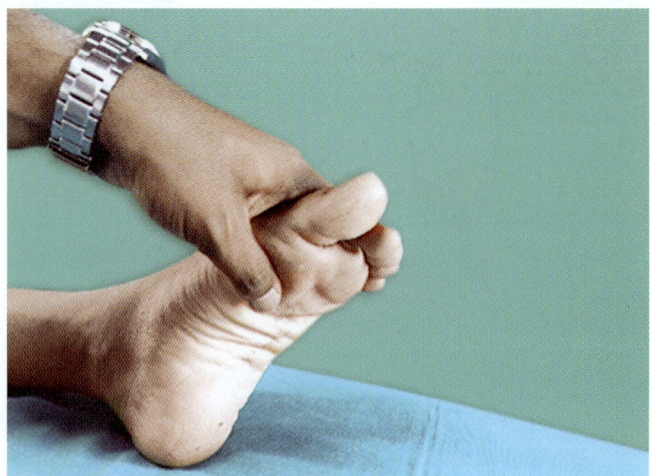

Fig. 6D(iv).53: Peronei—L5, S1.

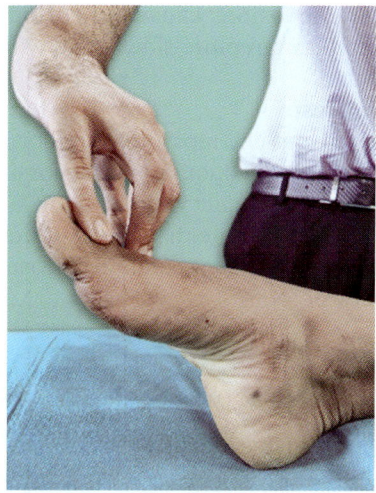

Fig. 6D(iv).54: Extensor digitorum longus—L5.

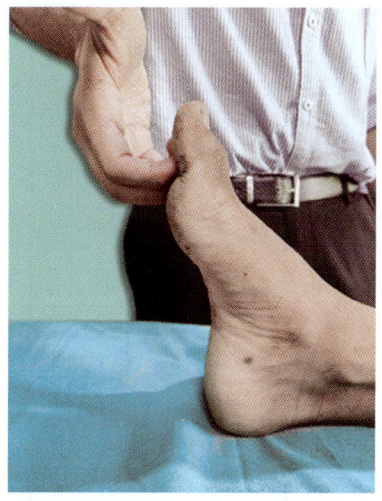

Fig. 6D(iv).55: Flexor digitorum longus—S1, 2.

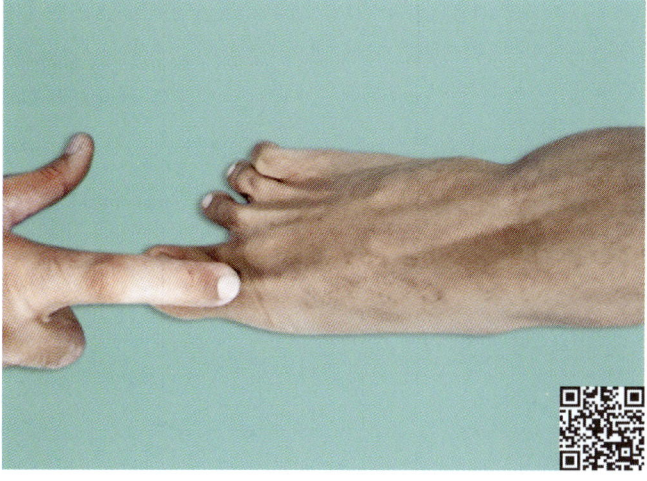

Fig. 6D(iv).56: Extensor hallucis longus—L5, S1.

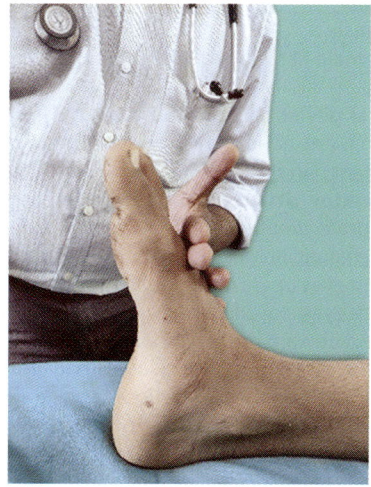

Fig. 6D(iv).57: Extensor digitorum brevis—S1.

EXAMINATION FOR SUBTLE HEMIPARESIS [FIG. 6D(iv).58]

1. **Pronator drift (Barre's sign):**
   - The patient stretches out both arms directly in front of him or her with palms upright (i.e., forearms supinated) and closes his or her eyes.
   - This position is held for 20–30 seconds.

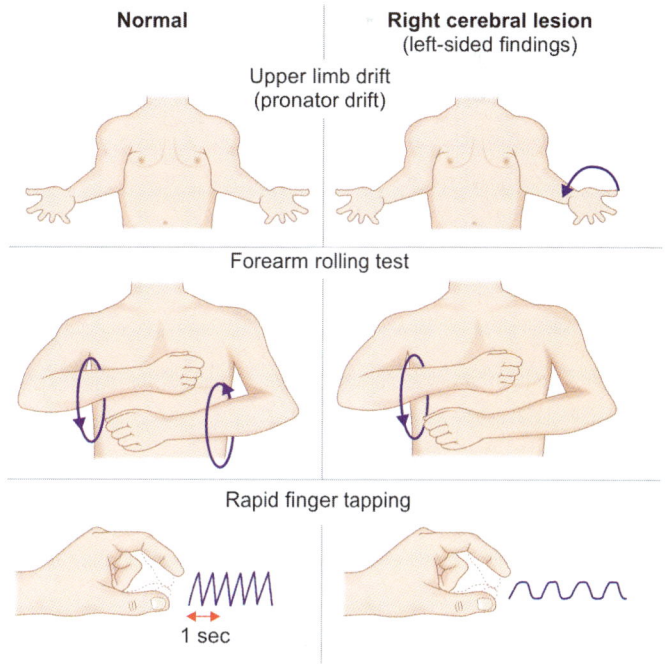

Fig. 6D(iv).58: Examination for subtle hemiparesis.

Normal response:
- Palm will remain flat, elbows straight and the limbs horizontal OR
- Symmetrical deviation from this position (i.e., on both the sides—dominant hand may pronate slightly more than the non-dominant hand)

Positive pronator drift: Components of pronator drift as mentioned above are seen in the weaker side (asymmetric response) which indicates a lesion in contralateral cortex
- Positive with eyes open: Motor deficit
- Positive with eyes closed: Sensory deficit (posterior column)
- Outward and upward drift: Cerebellar drift
- "Updrift" (involved arm rising overhead without patient awareness): Parietal lobe lesions (loss of position sense)
- Drift without pronation: Functional upper limb paresis (conversion disorder)

2. **Forearm rolling test [Fig. 6D(iv).59]:**
   - The patient bends each elbow and places both forearms parallel to each other.
   - He or she then rotates the forearms about each other, first in one direction and then the other.
   - In the abnormal response, the forearm contralateral to the lesion appears fixed while the other arm rotates around it.

3. **Rapid finger tapping test:**
   - The patient rapidly taps the thumb and index finger repeatedly at a speed of about two taps per second.
   - Hemispheric lesions cause the contralateral finger and thumb to tap more slowly and with diminished amplitude.

4. **Foot tapping test:**
   - The seated patient taps one forefoot at a time for 10 seconds on the floor, as fast as possible, while the heel maintains contact with the floor.
   - A discrepancy of more than five taps between the left and right foot indicates cerebral disease contralateral to the slower foot.

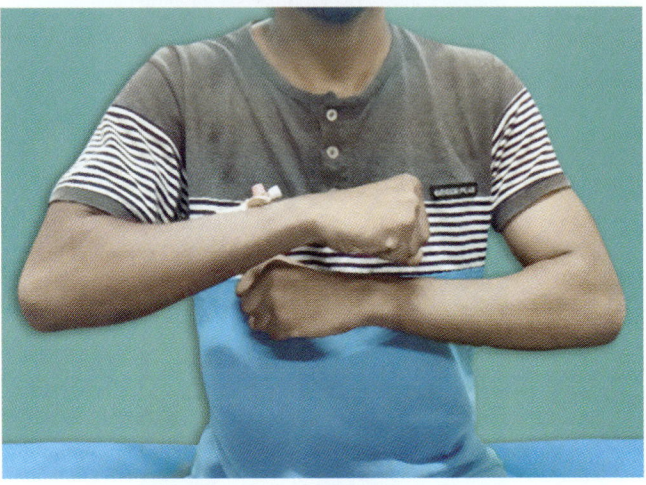

Fig. 6D(iv).59: Forearm rolling test.

D(v). REFLEXES

DEFINITION

A reflex is an involuntary response to a sensory stimulus.

MECHANISM OF REFLEX GENERATION [FIG. 6D(v).1]

Afferent impulses arising in a sensory organ produce a response in the effector organ. The response can be sensory, motor or autonomic.

It has two components:

Segmental component	Suprasegmental component
It consists of a local reflex center in the spinal cord or brainstem and its afferent and efferent connections	It is made up of descending central pathways that control, modulate, and regulate the segmental activity
	Diseases may increase the activity of some reflexes, decrease activity of others, and causes reflexes to appear that are not normally seen

TYPES OF REFLEXES

1. Deep tendon reflexes (monosynaptic reflex)
2. Superficial reflex (polysynaptic reflex)
3. Plantar reflex
4. Latent reflex
5. Primitive reflexes
6. Inverted and perverted reflexes.

GRADING OF REFLEXES (FOR DTRs) NINDS SCALE

Absent reflex (even after reinforcement)	Grade 0
Present but diminished	Grade 1+
Normal	Grade 2+
Increased but not necessarily to pathologic degree	Grade 3+
Markedly hyperactive, pathologic, often with extra beats or accompanying sustained clonus	Grade 4+

REINFORCEMENT MECHANISM AND METHODS

Mechanism

Normally, when a muscle spindle is stimulated two kinds of responses are seen via the following nerves:

Alpha motor neuron	Gamma motor neuron*	Inhibitory neuron
Causes: Contraction of **E**xtrafusal fibers of muscle	**Causes:** Contraction of **I**ntrafusal fibers of muscle	**Causes:** Inhibition of reciprocal muscle contraction

*Normally gamma motor neurons are under the inhibitory control of upper motor neurons and reinforcement maneuvers remove the inhibitory effect on gamma motor neurons [**Fig. 6D(v).1**].

Note: Mnemonic—**A**nti**E**pileptics cause **G**astro**I**ntestinal disturbance. (**A:** Alpha neuron, **E:** Extrafusal fibers), (**G:** Gamma neuron, **I:** Intrafusal fibers).

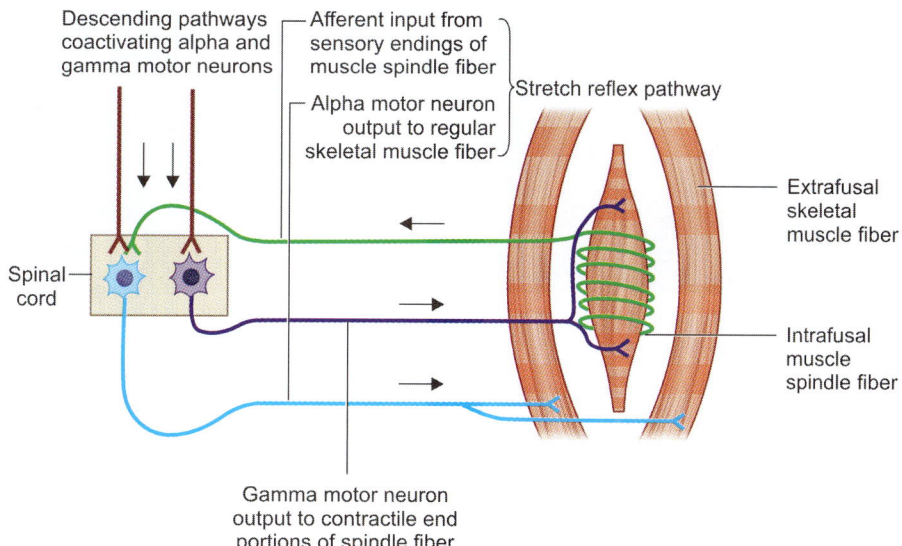

Fig. 6D(v).1: Schematic representation of innervation of muscle fiber and pathways.

Reinforcement Maneuvers for Deep Tendon Reflexes (DTRs)

Distraction	Talk to the patient and cause diversion of thought process
Clenching the teeth or clenching the fist of the other arm [Fig. 6D(v).2]	Traditionally done for upper limb
Jendrassik maneuver (interlocking the flexed fingers of the two hands and pull one against each other) [Fig. 6D(v).3]	Preferably done for lower limb

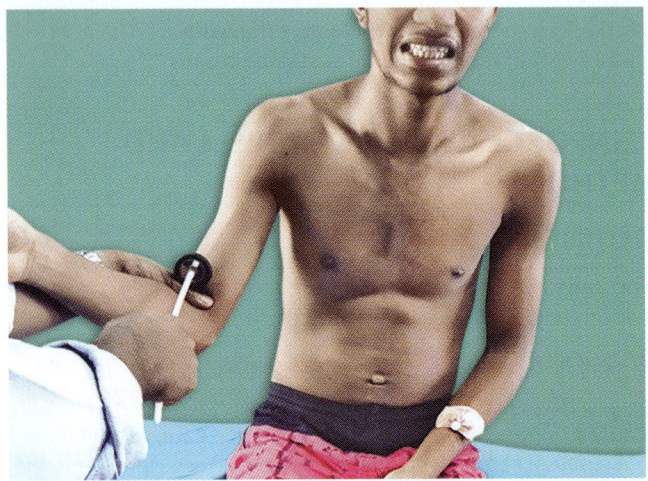

Fig. 6D(v).2: Clenching the teeth for reinforcement of upper limb reflexes.

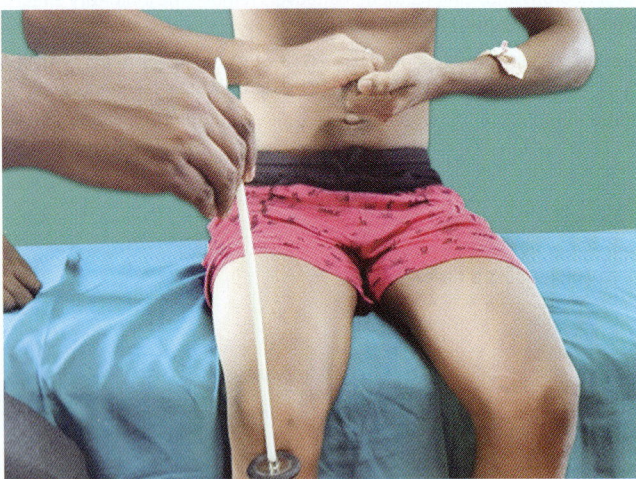

Fig. 6D(v).3: Jendrassik maneuver for reinforcement of lower limb reflexes.

DEEP TENDON REFLEXES

These are monosynaptic reflexes.
Prerequisite for examination:
- Good knee hammer (preferably Queen Square reflex hammer)
- Expose adequately the muscle to be tested
- Make sure patient is not anxious
- The muscle should be placed in optimum position, slightly on stretch, but with plenty of room for contraction.

The most commonly used specialized reflex hammers are grouped into three types by the shape of the head: triangular/tomahawk shaped (Taylor), T-shaped (Tromner, Buck), or circular (Queen Square, Babinski)

Tromner neurological reflex hammer

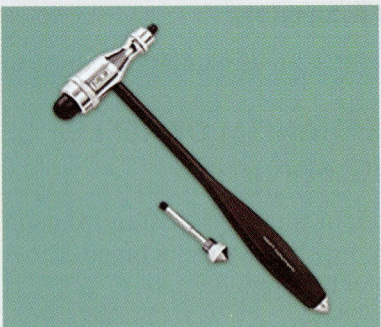

Taylor hammer

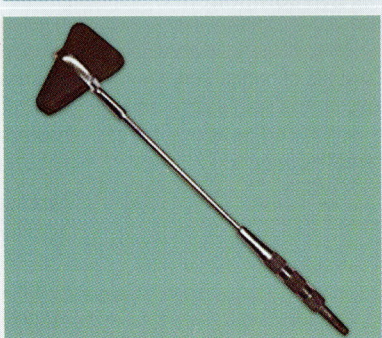

Babinski neurological reflex hammer

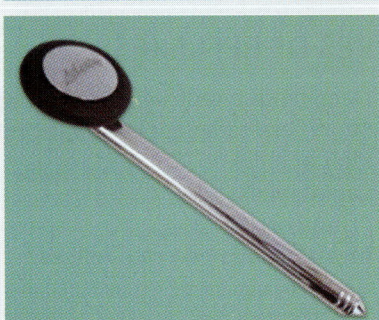

Queen square neurological reflex hammer

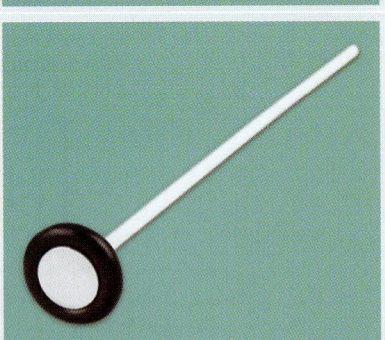

Buck neurological reflex hammer

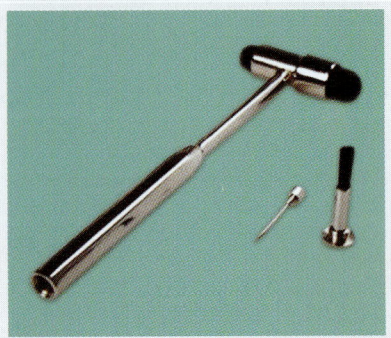

Nervous System

Reflex	Root value
Biceps	C5C6 (musculocutaneous nerve)
Supinator (brachioradialis)	C5C6 (radial nerve)
Triceps	C7C8 (radial nerve)
Knee	L3L4 (femoral nerve)
Ankle	S1S2 (medial popliteal nerve)
Mnemonic—S1,2 : L3,4 : C5,6 : C7,8 (in sequence from below)	
Few others	
Pectoral	C5-T1 (medial and lateral pectoral nerves)
Finger flexion	C6-T1 (median nerve)

Reflex	Method of elicitation	Normal response
Biceps [Figs. 6D(v).4A to C]	Press the forefinger gently on the biceps tendon in the antecubital fossa and then strike the finger with the hammer	Flexion of the elbow with visible contraction of the biceps muscle
Supinator [Figs. 6D(v).5A to C]	Strike the lower end of the radius about 5 cm above the wrist and watch for the movement of forearm and fingers	Contraction of brachioradialis and flexion of elbow
Triceps [Figs. 6D(v).6A to D]	By holding the patient's hand draw the arm across the trunk and allow it to lie loosely in the new position. Then strike the triceps tendon 5 cm above the elbow	Extension of elbow with visible contraction of triceps muscle
Knee [Figs. 6D(v).7A to C]	For right-handed examiner, the left arm is under both the knees in order to flex them together and tap the patellar tendon lightly on each side and compare the movements of lower leg and of quadriceps muscle	Extension of the knee and visible contraction of the quadriceps (in case of lower leg amputation keep finger just above the patella with legs extended and strike it in peripheral direction and look for upward pull of patella)
Ankle [Figs. 6D(v).8A to E]	Patient's leg should be externally rotated and slightly flexed at the knee. Examiner uses the left hand to dorsiflex the foot. For the left leg move to the other side of the bed. The Achilles tendon is then struck	Plantar flexion of foot and contraction of gastrocnemius
Pectoral [Fig. 6D(v).9]	With patients arm in the mid position between adduction and abduction hook your index finger on the tendon of the pectoralis major muscle in the anterior fold of axilla and strike with hammer	Adduction of the arm and visible contraction of the pectoralis major

Contd...

Finger flexion test [Fig. 6D(v).10]	Allow the patient's hand to rest palm upwards, the fingers slightly flexed. The examiner interlocks his fingers with patient's fingers and strikes them with the hammer	Slight flexion of all the fingers and of the interphalangeal joint of the thumb

The adductor reflex of the thigh is elicited by tapping either the medial epicondyle of the femur or the medial condyle of the tibia, located on the inner side of the thigh, causing the adductor muscles to contract and thigh moving towards the midline. The root value of this reflex is L2-L4. The Hannington-Kiff sign is a clinical sign in which there is an absent adductor reflex in the thigh in the presence of a positive patellar reflex. It occurs in patients with an obturator hernia, due to compression of the obturator nerve.

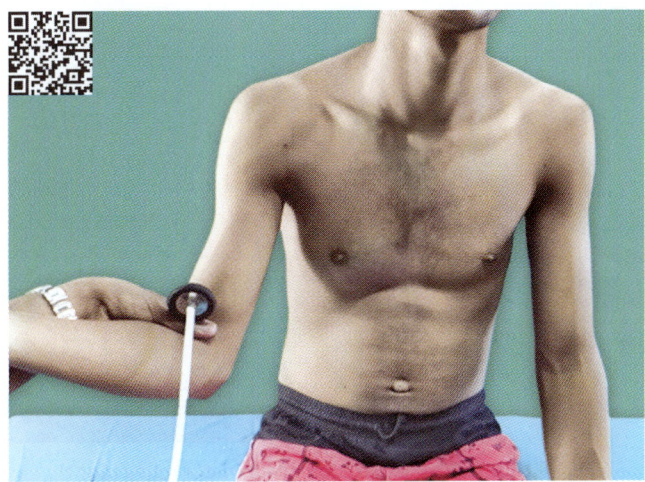

Fig. 6D(v).4A: Demonstration of biceps reflex (right hand).

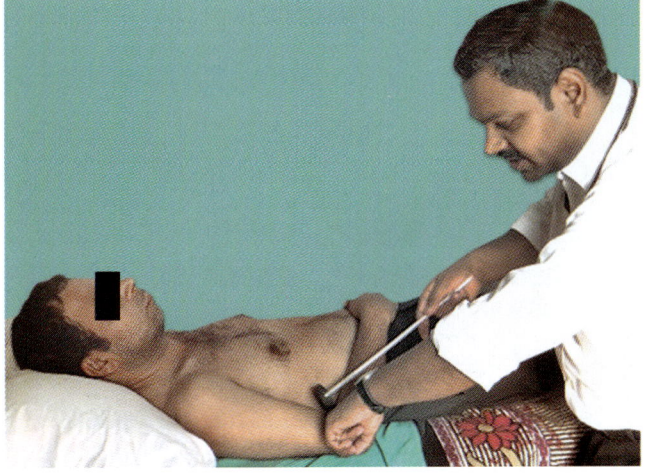

Fig. 6D(v).4B: Demonstration of biceps reflex supine position (right side).

Contd...

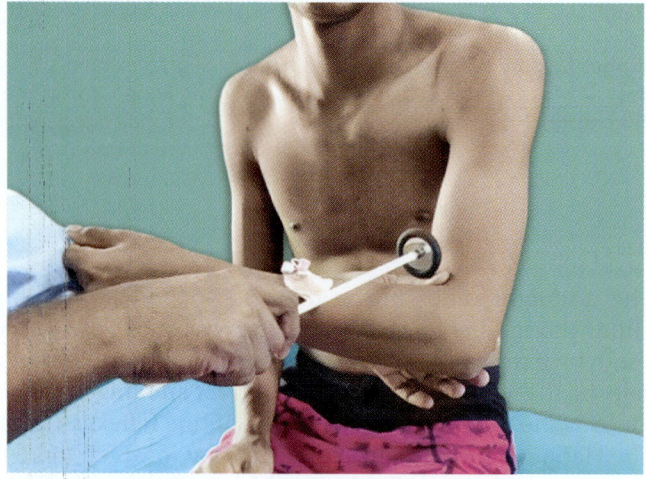

Fig. 6D(v).4C: Demonstration of biceps reflex (left side).

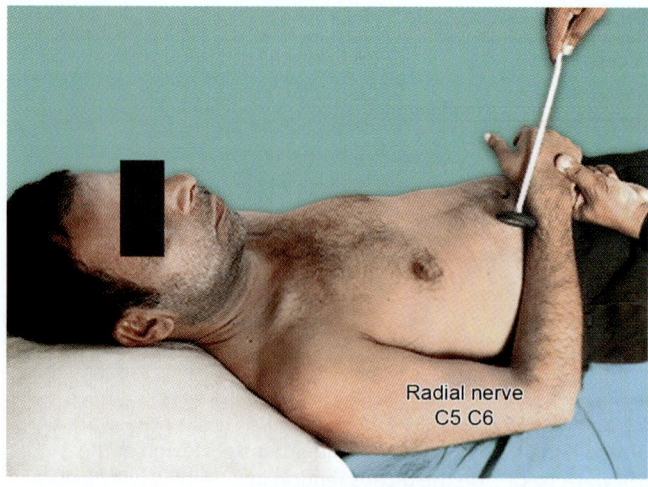

Fig. 6D(v).5C: Demonstration of supinator reflex in supine position.

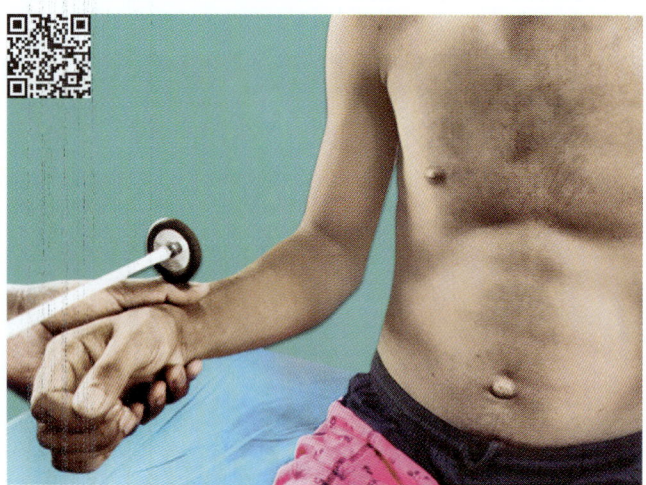

Fig. 6D(v).5A: Demonstration of supinator reflex (right).

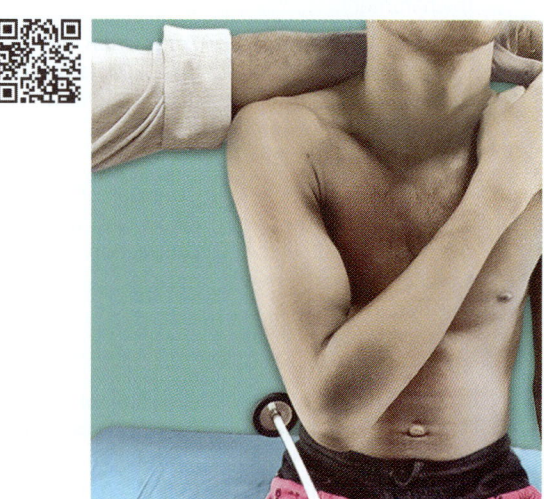

Fig. 6D(v).6A: Demonstration of triceps reflex (right side).

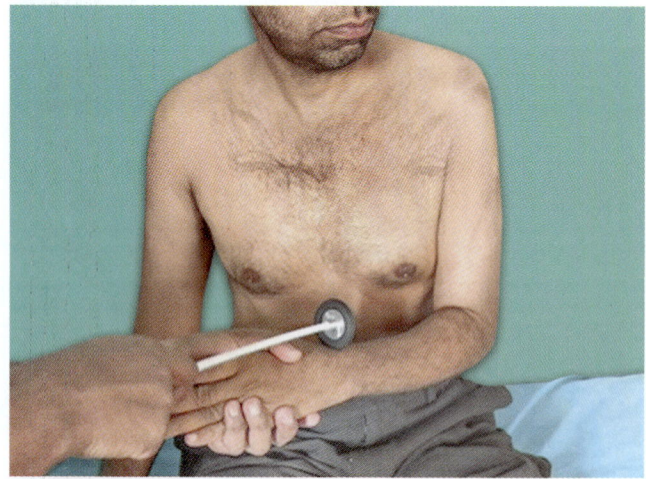

Fig. 6D(v).5B: Demonstration of supinator reflex (left).

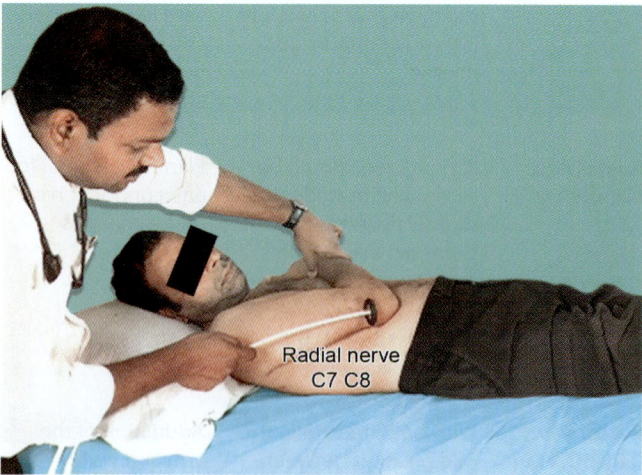

Fig. 6D(v).6B: Demonstration of triceps reflex (right side) in supine position.

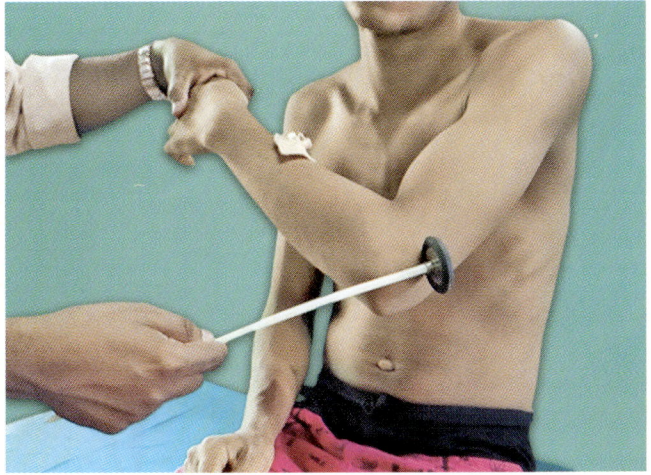

Fig. 6D(v).6C: Demonstration of triceps reflex (left side).

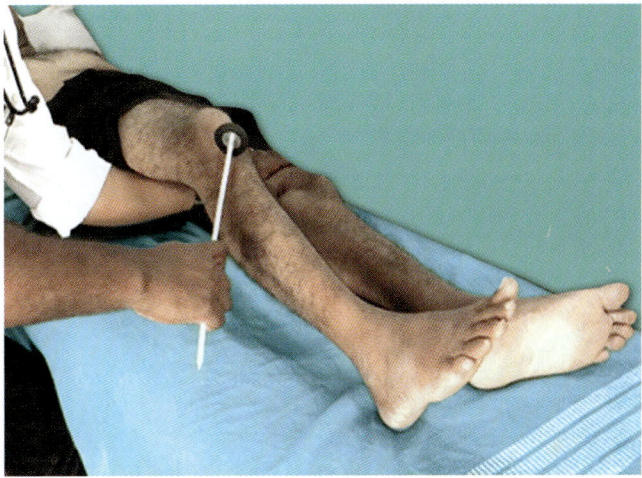

Fig. 6D(v).7B: Demonstration of right knee jerk in supine position.

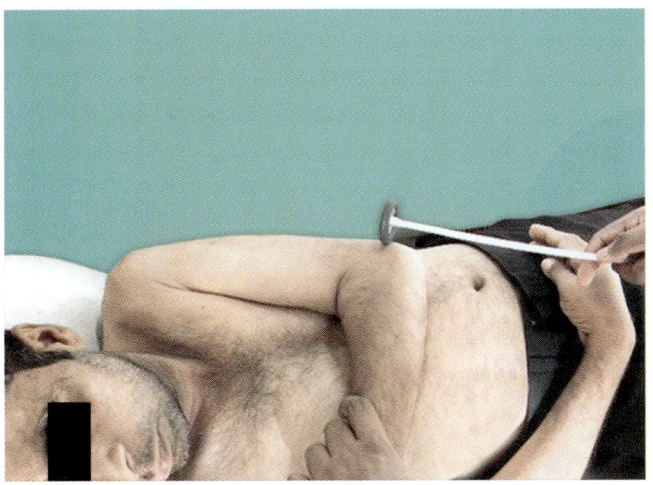

Fig. 6D(v).6D: Demonstration of triceps reflex (left side) in supine position.

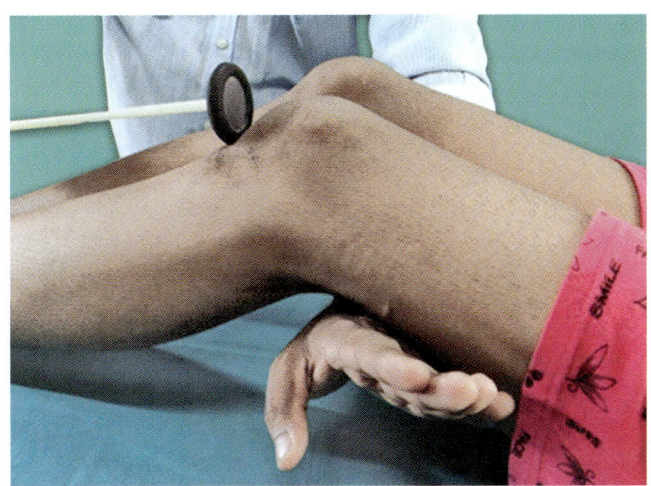

Fig. 6D(v).7C: Demonstration of knee jerk (for comparing both sides).

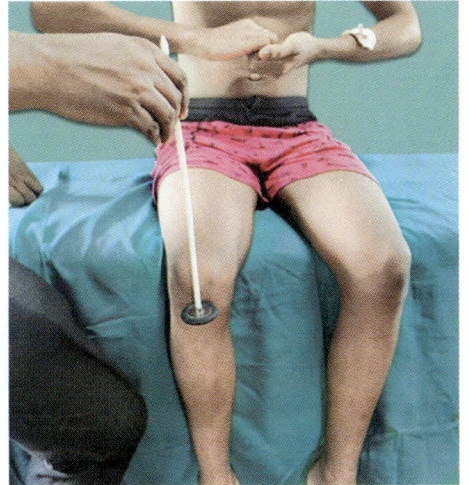

Fig. 6D(v).7A: Demonstration of knee jerk sitting position (for pendular movement).

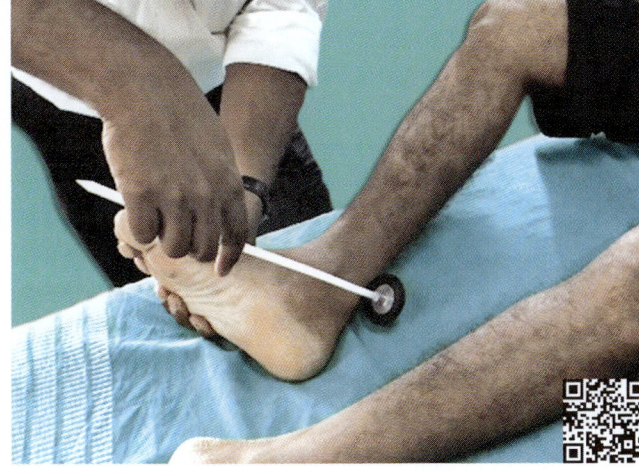

Fig. 6D(v).8A: Demonstration of ankle reflex of right leg.

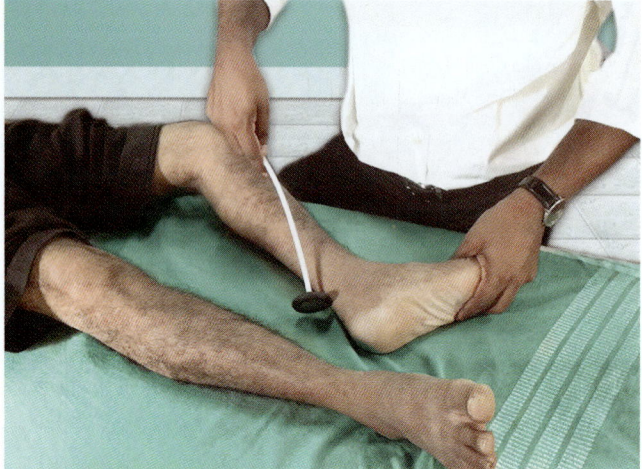

Fig. 6D(v).8B: Demonstration of ankle reflex of left leg.

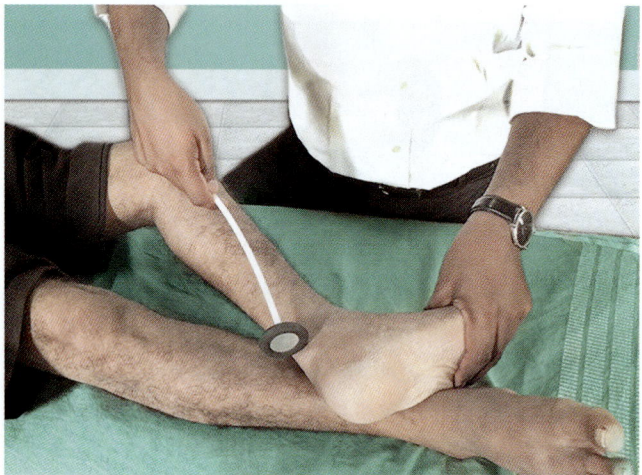

Fig. 6D(v).8C: Demonstration of ankle reflex of left leg.

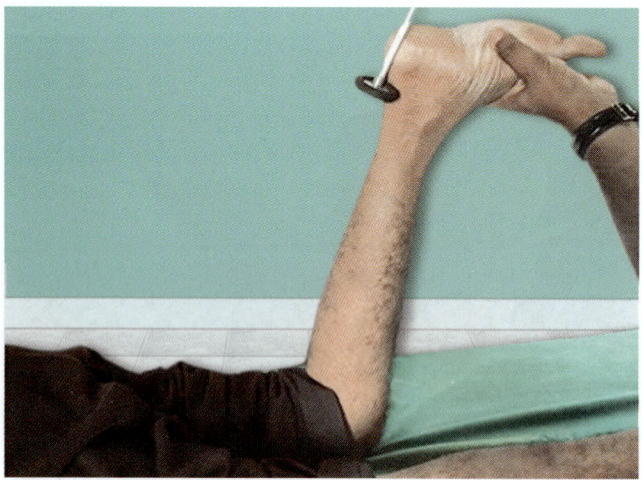

Fig. 6D(v).8D: Demonstration of ankle reflex in prone position.

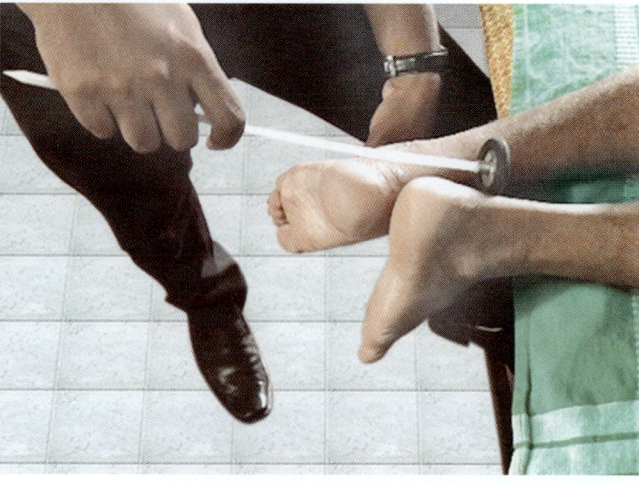

Fig. 6D(v).8E: Demonstration of ankle reflex with foot dangling over the edge of table.

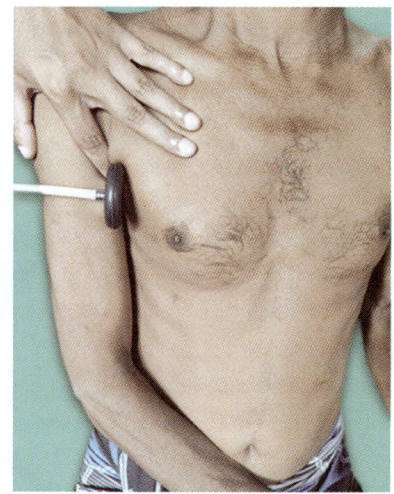

Fig. 6D(v).9: Demonstration of pectoral reflex.

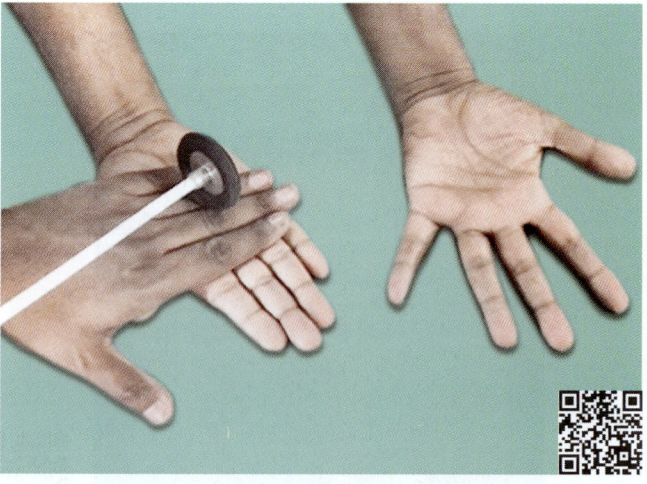

Fig. 6D(v).10: Demonstration of finger flexion reflex.

Clonus

Clonus is a series of rhythmic involuntary muscular contractions induced by the sudden passive stretching of a muscle or tendon.

Clonus	Demonstration
Ankle clonus [Figs. 6D(v).11A and B]	Examiner supports the leg, preferably with one hand under the knee, grasps the foot from below with the other hand, and quickly dorsiflexes the foot while maintaining slight pressure on the sole at the end of the dorsiflexion • The leg and foot should be well relaxed, the knee and ankle in moderate flexion, and the foot slightly everted • Right ankle clonus is examined by standing on the right side of the patient and left ankle clonus by standing on the left side • Unsustained clonus fades away after a few beats; sustained clonus persists as long as the examiner continues to hold slight dorsiflexion pressure on the foot
Patellar clonus [Figs. 6D(v).12A and B]	Examiner grasps the patella between index finger and thumb and executes a sudden, sharp, downward thrust, holding downward pressure at the end of the movement
Wrist clonus	Sudden passive extension of the wrist produces wrist clonus

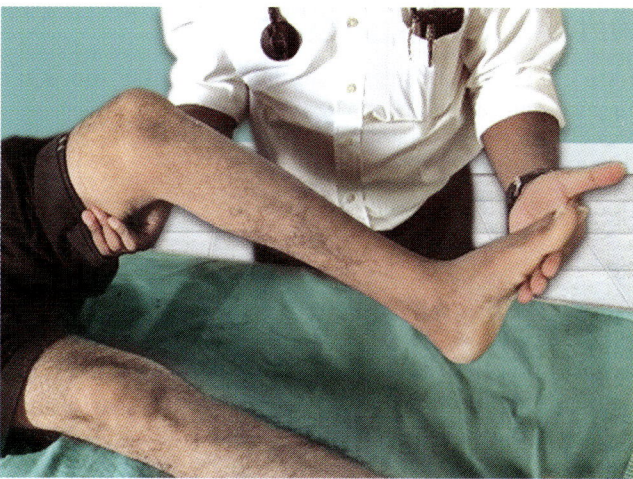

Fig. 6D(v).11B: Demonstration of left ankle clonus.

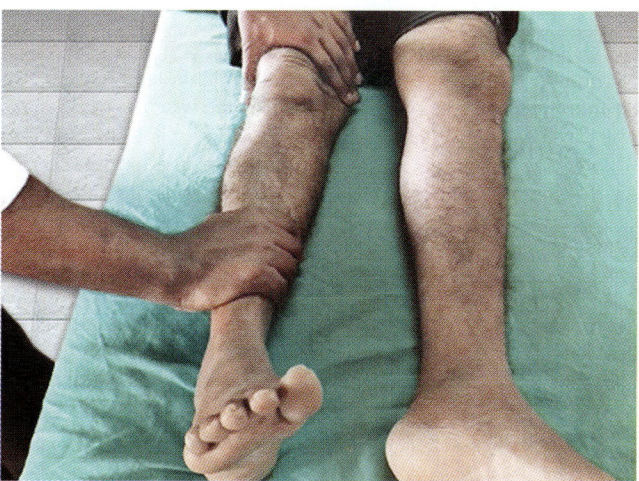

Fig. 6D(v).12A: Demonstration of right patellar clonus.

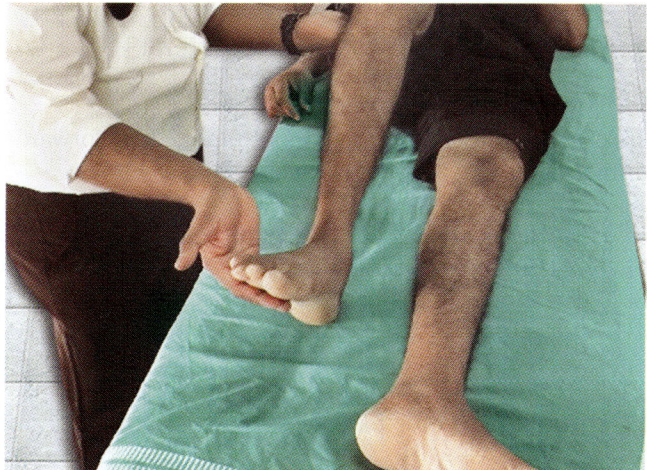

Fig. 6D(v).11A: Demonstration of right ankle clonus.

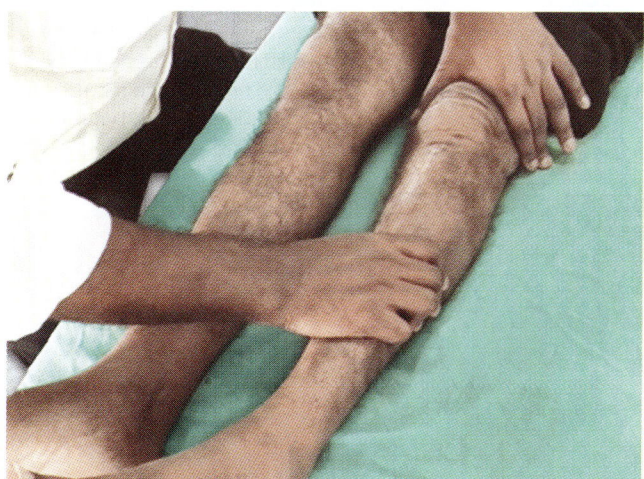

Fig. 6D(v).12B: Demonstration of left patellar clonus.

SUPERFICIAL REFLEXES

These are the responses to stimulation of either the skin or mucous membrane.

Clinical Significance

Superficial reflexes are abolished by pyramidal tract lesions.

Superficial reflex	Deep tendon reflex
Polysynaptic reflexes	Monosynaptic reflexes
Respond slowly	Faster response
Latency is longer	Latency is slower
Fatigue easily	Fatigue slowly
Not as consistently present as deep tendon reflexes	Consistently present
Abolished by pyramidal tract lesions	Exaggerated by pyramidal tract lesions

Superficial reflex	Elicitation
Corneal (cranial nerve V and VII)	Lightly touching the upper cornea with wisp of cotton or tissue, brought in from the side so the patient cannot see
Abdominal [Fig. 6D(v).13] ■ Epigastric (T6-T9) ■ Mid abdominal (T9-T11) ■ Hypogastric (T11-L1)	Stimulus is delivered by stroking the abdominal wall (preferably towards the umbilicus) and watch for contractions
Cremasteric [Fig. 6D(v).14] (L1, L2)	Stroking the skin in upper inner aspect of thigh and watch for the upward movement of testes in scrotum
Anal reflex (S2, S3)	Contraction of external sphincter in response to stroking the skin or mucous membrane in the perianal region
Bulbocavernosus reflex (S2, S3) [Fig. 6D(v).15]	Contraction of anal sphincter which is best appreciated by a gloved finger in the rectum on stimulation of glans penis or clitoris

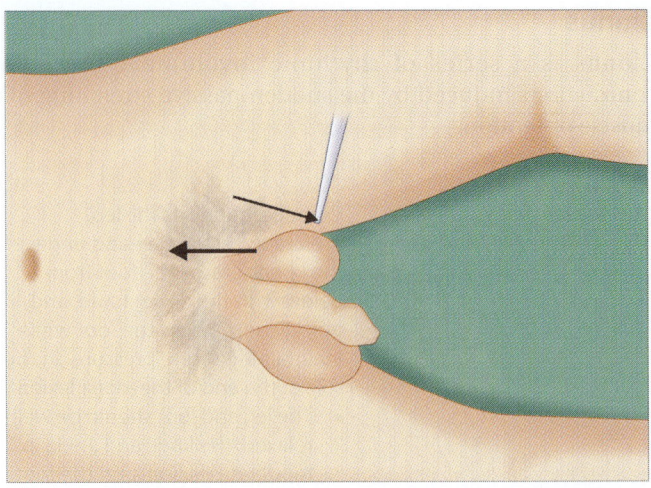

Fig. 6D(v).14: Direction of stimulus and movement of testes in cremasteric reflex.

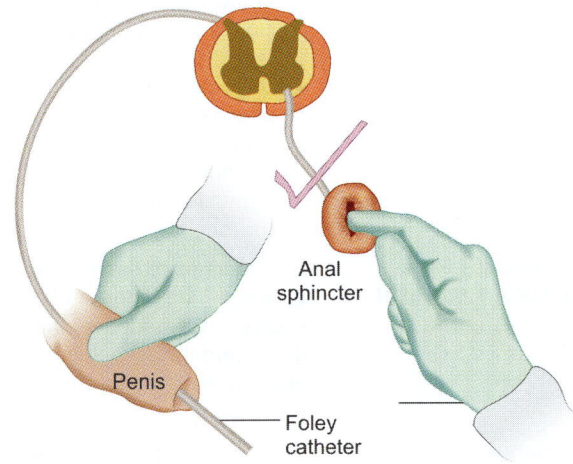

Fig. 6D(v).15: Pictorial representation of bulbocavernosus reflex.

PLANTAR REFLEX AND VARIATIONS

Plantar Reflex

Stroking the plantar surface of foot from the heel forward is normally followed by plantar flexion of foot and toes.

Babinski Sign

It is the pathologic variation of plantar reflex (i.e., extensor plantar response). It is part of primitive flexion reflex. In higher vertebrates, the flexion response includes flexion at hip, flexion at knee, and dorsiflexion of ankle (all of which help in removing the threatened part form danger). Normally, the descending motor pathway suppresses the primitive flexion response.

Positioning of patient [Fig. 6D(v).16]	■ Best position is supine ■ Knee must be extended ■ Heels should rest on the bed
Prerequisites	Rule out ankylosis of great toe

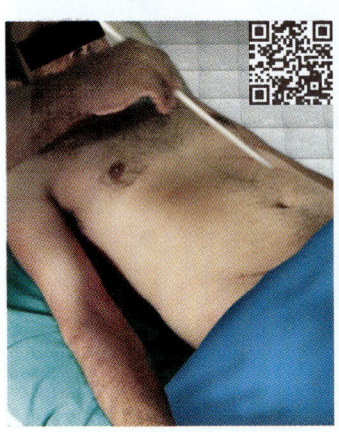
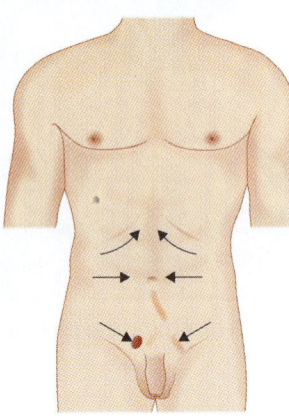

Fig. 6D(v).13: Demonstration of abdominal reflex.

Contd...

Contd...

Stimulating agent	- Applicator stick - Blunt key - Hand of reflex hammer - Broken tongue blade - Thumb nail
Strength of stimulus	Variable strength with strong stimulus for thick soles and minimal stimulation when response is strongly extensor
Site of stimulus	- Reflexogenic area of S1 - Stimulus should begin near the heel on the lateral aspect of sole and carried up to metatarsophalangeal joint of little toe and then carried medially falling short of 1st metatarsophalangeal joint **[Fig. 6D(v).17]**
Normal response	Flexion of the great toe and other toes
Abnormal response (Babinski sign)	- Dorsiflexion of great toe and small toes - Fanning of toes - Dorsiflexion of ankle - Flexion of knee joint - Flexion at hip joint - Contraction of tensor fascia lata
Reinforcement of plantar reflex	By asking patient to rotate the head to opposite side

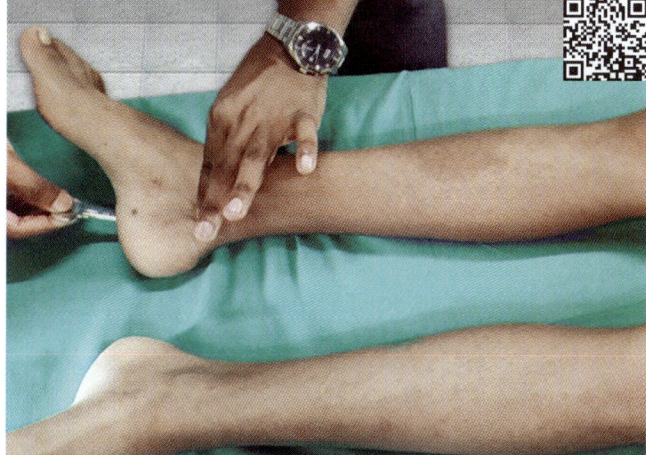

Fig. 6D(v).16: Position of leg for demonstration of plantar reflex.

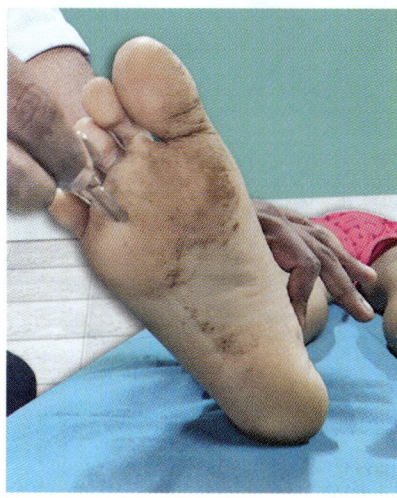

Fig. 6D(v).17: Direction of stimuli for demonstrating the plantar reflex.

Variants of Plantar Response

Equivocal response	- Rapid extension followed by flexion - Only great toe extension - Extension of great toe with flexion of fingers - No response to the plantar stimulus - Flexion at hip and knee, but no movement of toes
Minimal plantar response	- No toe movement - Contraction of tensor fascia lata with mild internal rotation and abduction of hip
Pseudo Babinski	- Voluntary extension of great toe due to hyperesthesia or strong painful stimulus - Dystonic posturing of great toe

Other methods of obtaining plantar reflex work by increasing the reflexogenic zone

Method	Elicitation
Chaddock [Fig. 6D(v).18]	- Elicited by stimulating the lateral aspect of the foot, not the sole, beginning about under the lateral malleolus near the junction of the dorsal and plantar skin, drawing the stimulus from the heel forward to the small toe - The Chaddock is the only alternative toe sign that is truly useful - It may be more sensitive than the Babinski but is less specific - It produces less withdrawal than plantar stimulation
Reverse Chaddock	The stimulus moves from the small toe toward the heel
Oppenheim [Fig. 6D(v).19]	- Dragging the knuckles heavily down the anteromedial surface of the tibia from the infrapatellar region to the ankle. - The response is slow and often occurs toward the end of stimulation
Schaeffer's sign [Fig. 6D(v).20]	Deep pressure on Achilles tendon
Gordon's sign [Fig. 6D(v).21]	Squeezing of calf muscles
Bing's sign [Fig. 6D(v).22]	Pricking dorsum of foot with a pin
Moniz' sign [Fig. 6D(v).23]	Forceful passive plantar flexion at ankle
Throckmorton's sign	Percussing over dorsal aspect of metatarsophalangeal joint of great toe just medial to EHL tendon
Stransky	Small toe forcibly abducted, then released
Szapiro	Pressure against dorsum of second through fifth toes, causing firm passive plantar flexion while stimulating plantar surface of foot
Strümpell's phenomenon	Forceful pressure over anterior tibial region
Cornell response	Scratching dorsum of foot along inner side of EHL tendon

Combining two methods may elicit minimal reflexes **[Fig. 6D(v).24]**

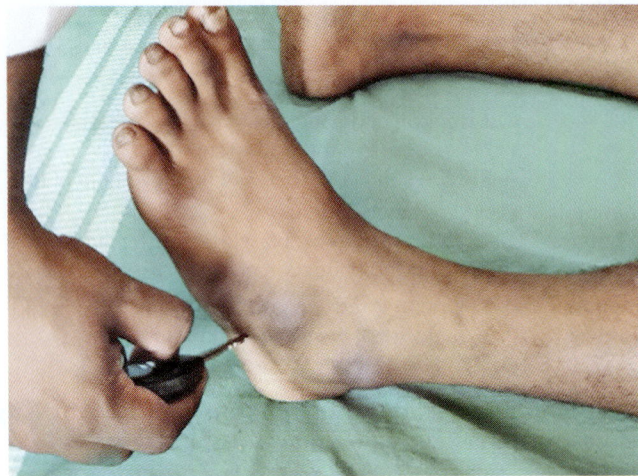

Fig. 6D(v).18: Chaddock's sign.

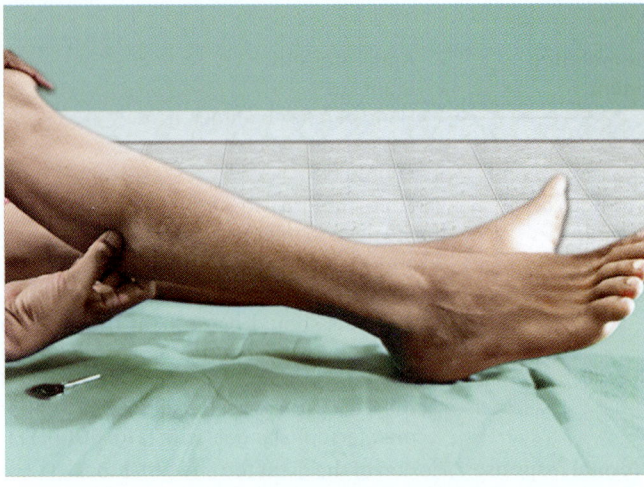

Fig. 6D(v).21: Gordon's technique.

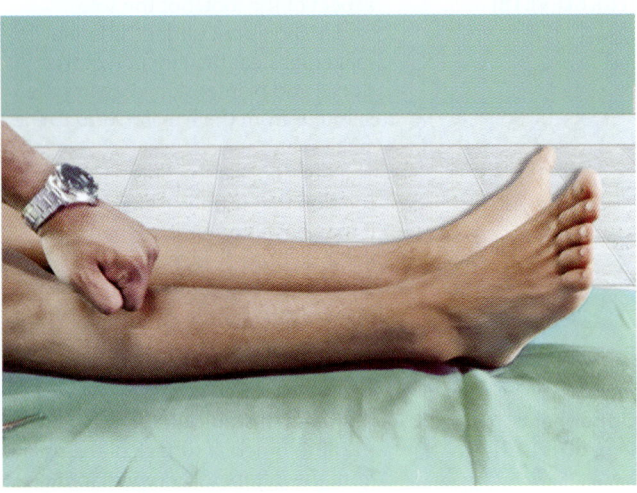

Fig. 6D(v).19: Openheim's technique.

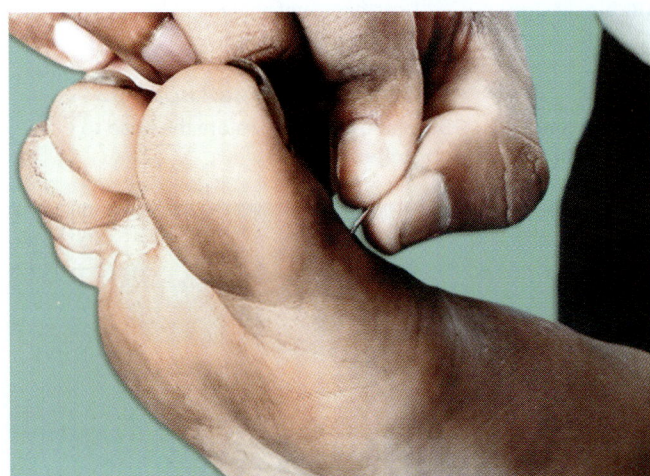

Fig. 6D(v).22: Bing's sign.

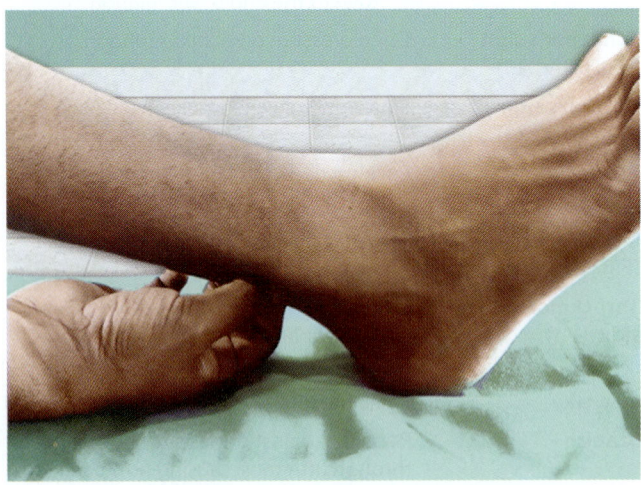

Fig. 6D(v).20: Schaeffer's technique.

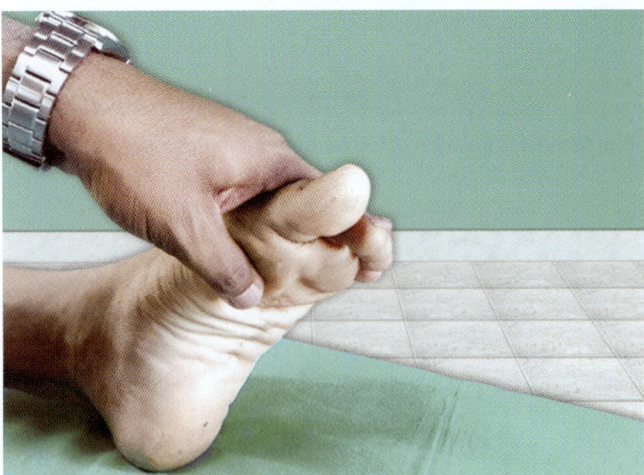

Fig. 6D(v).23: Moniz's sign.

Nervous System

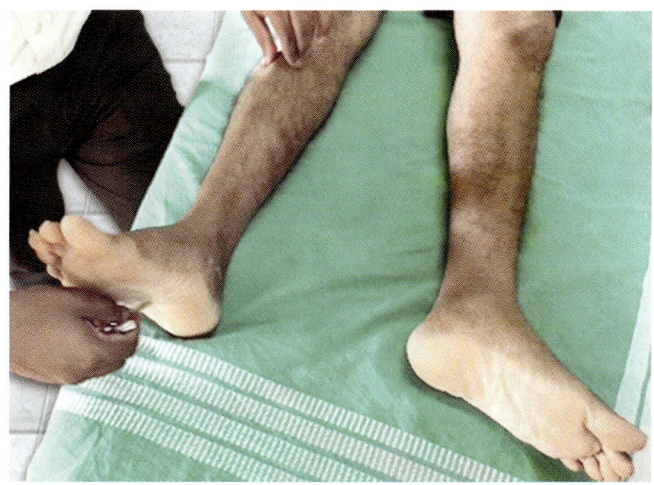

Fig. 6D(v).24: Eliciting plantar by simultaneous stimulus from Openheim's and plantar strike.

LATENT REFLEXES OF UPPER LIMB

Reflex	Elicitation
Wartenberg's reflex [Fig. 6D(v).25]	Patient's fingers are interlocked with examiner's fingers and pulled apart. Normally thumb extends. However, in pyramidal lesions thumb is adducted and flexed. This sign is equivalent of Babinski of lower limb
Hoffman's reflex [Fig. 6D(v).26]	Flexion of the interphalangeal joint of middle finger of patient produces flexion response in other fingers along with adduction of thumb
Tromner's reflex [Fig. 6D(v).27]	Examiner holds the patient's partially extended middle finger, letting the hand dangle, then, with the other hand, thumps or flicks the finger pad. The response is the same as that in the Hoffmann test

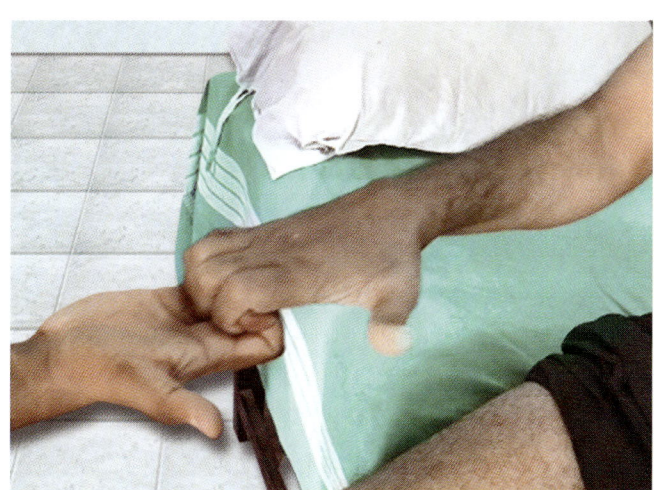

Fig. 6D(v).25: Wartenberg's sign.

Fig. 6D(v).26: Hoffman's reflex.

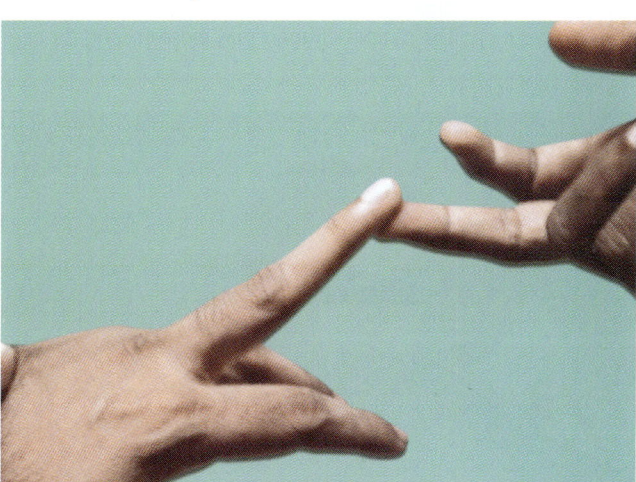

Fig. 6D(v).27: Tromner's reflex.

PRIMITIVE REFLEXES

Reflex	Elicitation
Glabellar tap (Myerson's sign) [Fig. 6D(v).28]	Repetitive tapping of the forehead between the eyebrows causing blinking, which usually stops within few taps. However, if blinking persists, it suggests positive frontal release sign. *Note:* To avoid visual stimulus bring the hand from above and behind
Palmomental reflex of Marinesco–Radovici [Fig. 6D(v).29]	■ Stroke the thenar eminence in a proximal to distal direction using a sharp object such as the pointed end of a reflex hammer, key, paper clip, or fingernail and watch for twitch of chin muscle ■ This reflex does not have any localizing value, and is commonly seen in elderly patients with degenerative disease of the cortex

Contd...

Contd...

Sucking reflex [Fig. 6D(v).30]	Sucking reflexes may be seen in response to tactile stimulation in the oral region, or in response to the insertion of an object (for example, a spatula) into the mouth
Rooting reflex [Fig. 6D(v).31]	Rooting responses are seen when the mouth turns towards an object gently stroking the cheek (tactile rooting), or towards an object (for example, tendon hammer) brought into the patient's field of view (visual rooting)
Pout and snout reflex [Fig. 6D(v).32]	The snout reflex is present when the lips pucker in response to gentle pressure over the nasal philtrum
Grasp reflex [Fig. 6D(v).33]	If the examiner's fingers are placed in the patient's hand, especially between the thumb and forefinger, or if the palmar skin is stimulated gently, there is slow flexion of the digits. The patient's fingers may close around the examiner's fingers

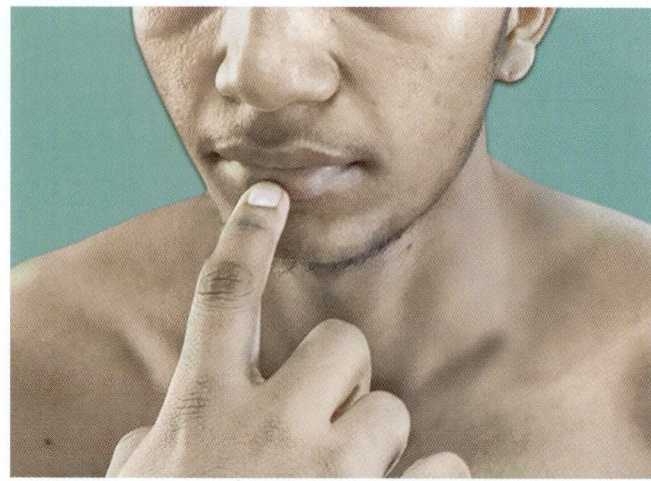

Fig. 6D(v).30: Sucking reflex.

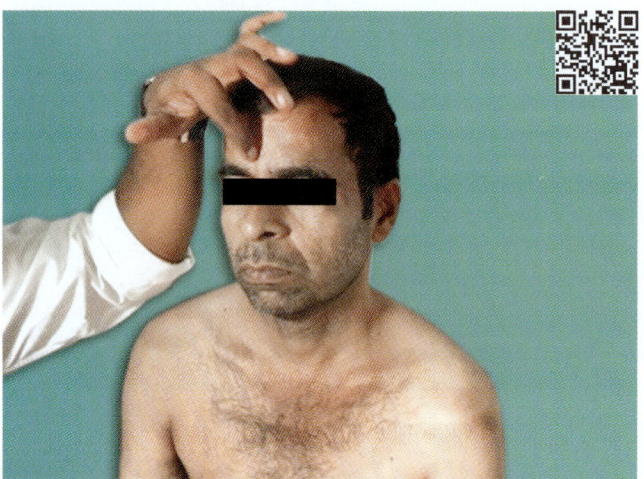

Fig. 6D(v).28: Glabellar tap.

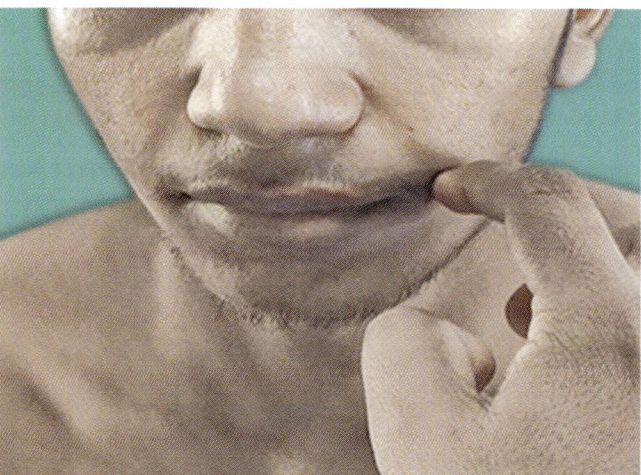

Fig. 6D(v).31: Rooting reflex.

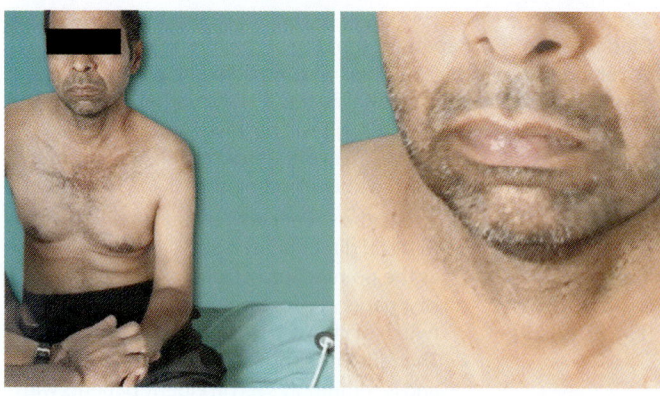

Fig. 6D(v).29: Palmomental reflex.

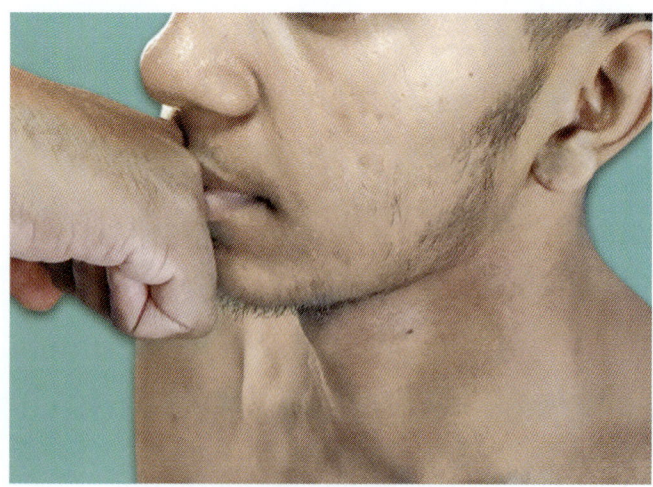

Fig. 6D(v).32: Pout reflex.

Nervous System

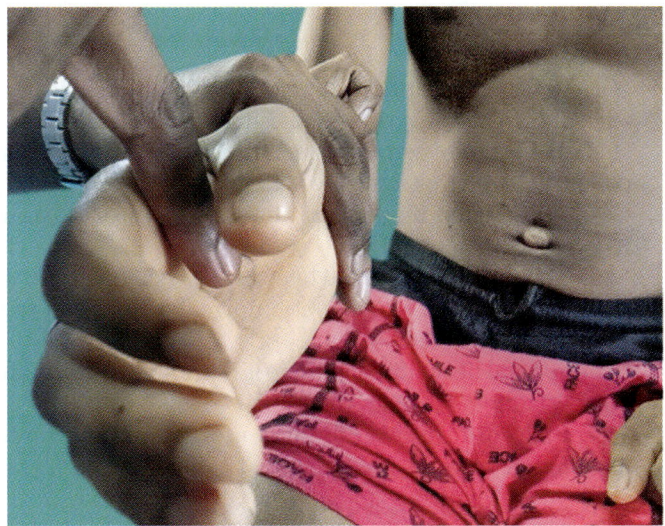

Fig. 6D(v).33: Grasp reflex.

INVERTED AND PERVERTED REFLEXES

Reflex	Description and example

Inverted reflex	Contractions opposite to that of expected
	For example:
	An inverted brachioradialis reflex
	• When the supinator reflex elicits finger flexion and not elbow flexion
	• Is associated with an absent biceps jerk and an exaggerated triceps jerk
	• Is indicative of a spinal cord lesion at C5 or C6, e.g., due to trauma, syringomyelia, or disc prolapse
	Inversion of biceps reflex
	• On eliciting bicep reflex the following are noticed:
	  • There is no flexion at the elbow
	  • But instead there is extension at the elbow due contraction of the triceps muscle
	• Presence of this reflex indicates that the lesion is at the level of C5 segment
	Inversion of triceps reflex
	With disc protrusions at C6/7 there is a "paradoxical triceps reflex" with forearm muscles acting to flex the elbow against no triceps resistance
	Inversion of knee reflex
	• On eliciting the knee jerk
	• There is no extension of the knee joint
	• But instead there is flexion of the knee due to contraction of the hamstring muscles
	• Presence of this indicates that the lesion is at the level of L3, L4

Perverted reflex	It is false inverted reflex where there is an alteration in the response rather than true inversion For example: When supinator jerk is elicited there is a perverted response of finger flexion. (*Note:* In the presence of brachioradialis reflex this phenomenon is called as spread of reflex, while in the absent of brachioradialis reflex this is considered as pseudo inverted reflex or perverted reflex)

Other causes of altered reflexes

Woltman's sign of myxedema, is the delayed relaxation phase of the muscle stretch reflex. In hypothermia or β-blockade, the relaxation phase of the ankle jerk may be prolonged.

Chorea: "Hungup" knee jerk is a specific but rarely appreciated clinical sign of Huntington disease (HD) and Sydenham chorea. During an elicited knee jerk, the extended lower leg may not relax immediately but may remain elevated for several seconds due to sustained contraction of the quadriceps femoris.

Very brisk reflexes—even with a few beats of clonus can be seen in anxious individuals, as well as in hyperthyroidism and in tetany.

Electrolyte disturbances
Absent reflexes is seen with hypermagnesemia.
In the **Holmes-Adie syndrome,** absent deep tendon reflexes are seen.

SIGNS TO IDENTIFY HYSTERICAL WEAKNESS

Hoover's Sign

Weakness on one side of the body may be masked by increased strength when trying to move the other leg. A subject with hemiparesis of organic cause while asked to flex the hip of normal leg against resistance will not exert pressure on the hand of examiner placed under the heel on the affected side while in hysterical weakness heightened pressure will be felt on the examiner's hand.

Barré's Sign (Manoeuvre de la jambe)

The affected leg may not fall or drop when the patient lies on their stomach with knees bent.

Abductor Sign

The examiner tells the patient to abduct each leg, and opposes this movement with his hands placed on the lateral surfaces of the patient's legs. The leg contralateral to the abducted one shows opposite actions for organic paresis and non-organic paresis: for example, when the paretic leg is abducted, the sound leg stayed fixed in organic paresis, but moves in the hyperadducting direction in non-organic paresis.

Give-way Weakness/Collapsing Weakness

In cases of hysterical weakness, the examined limb can exhibit abrupt fluctuations in force when resistance is applied. In contrast, Organic weakness will demonstrate sustained resistance without abrupt changes in force.

The Elbow Flex-ex Sign

The examiner holds both forearms near the wrists while asking the patient to flex or extend the normal arm at the elbow and simultaneously feeling for flexion or extension of the contralateral (paretic) arm. In patients with organic paresis, there is not a significant detectable force of contralateral opposition of the paretic limb. Patients with non-organic arm weakness havedetectable strength of contralateral opposition in the paretic arm when the normal arm was tested.

Others tests include—abductor sign, abduction finger sign, spinal injuries center test, drift without pronation sign.

D(vi). SENSORY SYSTEM EXAMINATION

Sensations can be grossly divided into primary and secondary modalities

Primary modalities	Secondary modalities (cortical sensation)
Touch	Tactile localization
Pressure	Two-point discrimination
Pain	Sensory inattention
Temperature	Stereognosis
Joint position sense	Graphesthesia
Vibration	These require secondary association area in parietal lobe

Note: When primary sensation are normal but secondary modalities are lost it implies a parietal lobe lesion.

Sherrington classification of sensory system	
Exteroceptive system	Information about the external environment, including somatosensory functions and special senses
Proprioceptive system	Senses the orientation of the limbs and body in space
Interoceptive system	Information about internal functions, blood pressure, or the concentration of chemical constituents in bodily fluids

PRIMARY MODALITIES

Examination of Exteroceptive System (Spinothalamic Tract)

Pain

- Ask the patient to close his eyes.
- Sharp end of pin is applied mildly sufficient to produce pain but not to penetrate the skin **[Fig. 6D(vi).1]**.
- Compare adjacent normal area and corresponding area on the opposite side (commonly used technique is to ask patient to compare one side with other in monitory terms like percentages)
- A useful trick is to hold the pin or shaft of the applicator stick lightly between thumb and fingertip and allow the shaft to slide between fingertip and thumb. This ensures consistent stimulus intensity.
- Commonly used objects are the safety pin or broken wooden applicator stick.
- Avoid too sharp objects and hypodermic needles.
- Indicates whether sensation is normal, decreased (or absent) or increased.
- In peripheral nerve disease, there is more anesthesia than analgesia.
- In spinal cord disease, there is more analgesia than anesthesia.

Temperature [Fig. 6D(vi).2]

- With the patient's eyes closed, apply the warm and cold test tubes randomly over the skin in dermatomal pattern.
- Instruct the patient to say what he feels–hot/cold/no response.
- Cold = 5–10°C (41–50°F) (crushed ice can be used).
- Warmth = 40–45°C (104–113°F) (warm water can be used).
- Temperature much lower or higher than these elicit pains rather than temperature sensations.
- In lesions of leprosy, temperature may be lost prior to pain. (Note = In majority of cases heat and cold sensations are equally affected)

Tactile Sensation

- Light touch can be tested with a:
  - Wisp of cotton **[Fig. 6D(vi).3]**
  - Feather
  - Soft brush **[Fig. 6D(vi).4]**
  - Light touch of the fingertip
- For diabetic neuropathies
  - Von Grey's hairs
  - Semmes-Weinstein monofilament

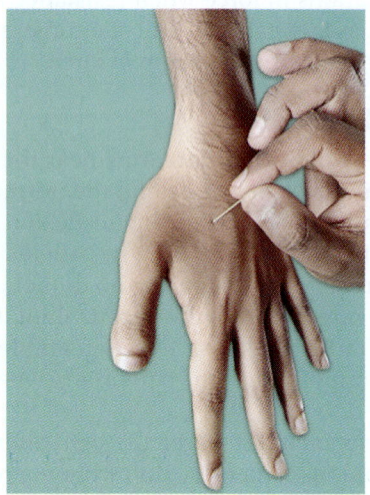

Fig. 6D(vi).1: Examination of pin prick sensation.

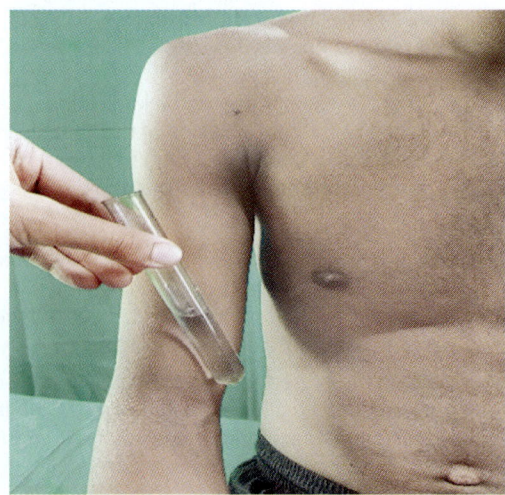

Fig. 6D(vi).2: Examination of temperature.

- With patient's eyes closed, gently touch the skin (preferably nonhairy region) without exerting pressure.
- Ask the patient whether he can feel the touch.
- Tactile response can be graded as per international spinal injury standards as:
  - 0 = absent
  - 1 = altered response (impaired/increased)
  - 2 = normal/intact response

- Noninvasive methods = quantifying Meissner's corpuscles and dermal papillae by reflectance confluence microscopy.

Examination of Proprioceptive System

Proprioception (Proprioception refers to either the sense of position of a body part or motion of a body part) Also called as kinesthesia Primary receptors = muscle spindles	
Conscious component	*Unconscious component*
Travels with the fibers subserving fine, discriminative touch. These include: - Motion - Position - Vibration - Pressure	Via spinocerebellar tract

Examination of different components of proprioception:

Joint Motion and Position

- Usually tested together
- In the lower extremity **[Figs. 6D(vi).5A and B]**:
- Tested at the metatarsophalangeal joint of the great toe
- In the upper extremity **[Figs. 6D(vi).6A to C]**:
  At one of the distal interphalangeal joints. If these distal joints are normal, there is no need to test more proximally.

Joint Motion

- Testing is done with the patient's eyes closed.
- It is extremely helpful to instruct the patient, eyes open, about the responses expected before beginning the test.

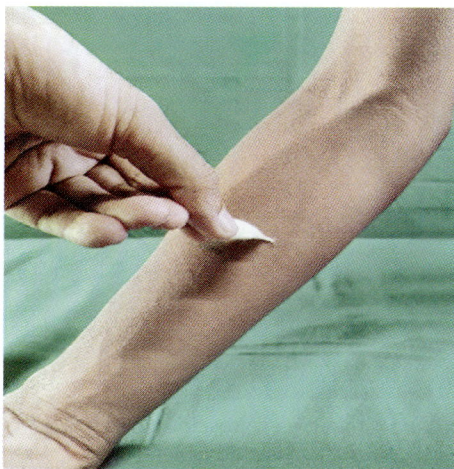

Fig. 6D(vi).3: Examination of tactile sensation with wisp of cotton.

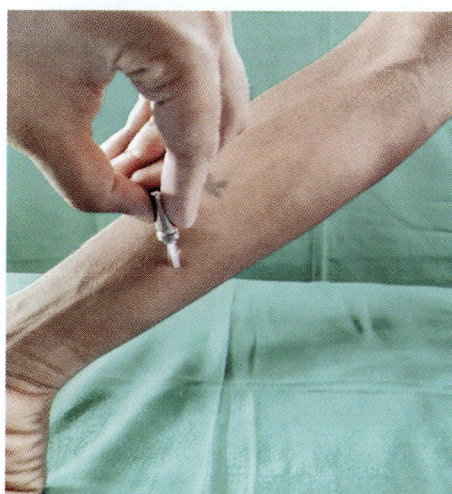

Fig. 6D(vi).4: Examination of tactile sensation with soft brush.

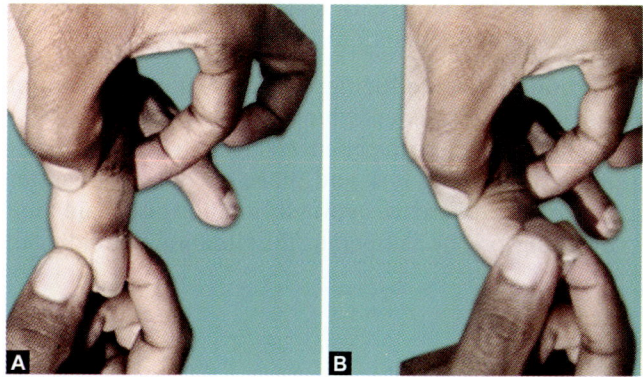

Figs. 6D(vi).5A and B: Examination of joint sense in the lower limb.

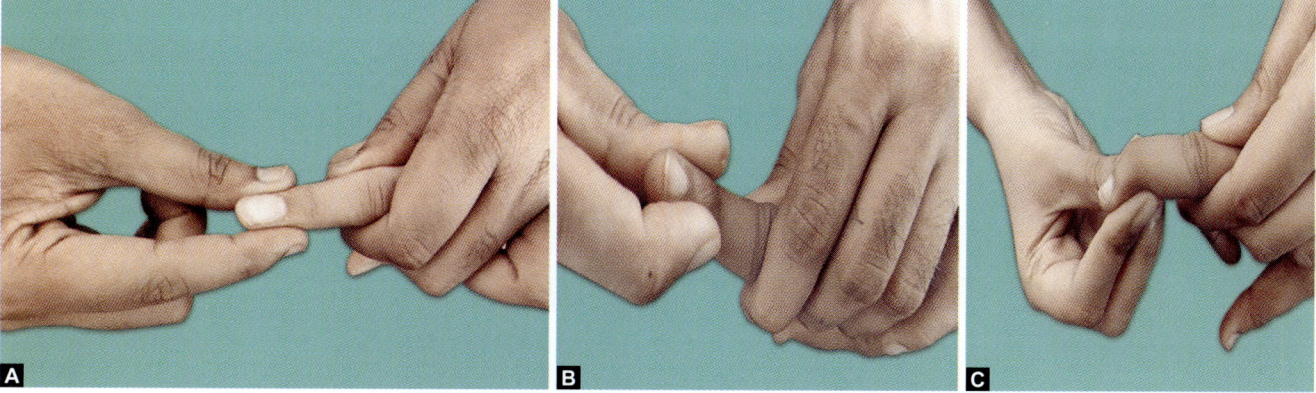

Figs. 6D(vi).6A to C: Examination of joint sense in upper limb.

- Show the patient up or down movements and instruct him to reply "up" or "down".
- The examiner should hold the patient's completely relaxed digit on the sides, away from the neighboring digits, parallel to the plane of movement, exerting as little pressure as possible to eliminate clues from variations in pressure.
- The part is then passively moved up or down, and the patient is instructed to indicate the direction of movement from the last position.
- Healthy young individuals can detect great toe movements of about 1 mm, or 2° to 3°; and in the fingers virtually invisible movements, 1° or less, at the distal interphalangeal joints are accurately detected.

Position Sense
- Tested by placing the fingers of one of the patient's hands in a certain position (like "OK" sign) **[Fig. 6D(vi).7]** while his eyes are closed, and then asking him to imitate it with the other hand OR do passive movement in one hand and ask the patient to do in similar way in other hand **[Fig. 6D(vi).8]**.
- This is sometimes referred to as **parietal copy**. Both parietal lobes (and their connections) must be intact: one side to register the position and the other side to copy it.
- Loss of position sense may cause involuntary movements called pseudoathetosis.

Vibration (Pallesthesia) [Figs. 6D(vi).9A to C]
Preferentially using a tuning fork of 128 Hz due to slow decay (256 Hz is used to detect early changes in cases like subacute combined cord degeneration).

The graduated Rydel-Seiffer tuning fork provides more quantitative assessment of vibration.
- Explain procedure to patient clearly.
- Strike the tuning fork and place on the forehead and explain the difference between vibration and plain touch of tuning fork, by dampening the vibration by holding the prongs.
- Keep the vibrating tuning fork, starting from the distal most bony prominence and proceed proximally.
- Ask the patient to say when he ceases to feel the vibration.
- Loss of vibration sense due to peripheral neuropathy is distal loss and normal proximal but if it is due to posterior column disease there is uniform loss of vibration.

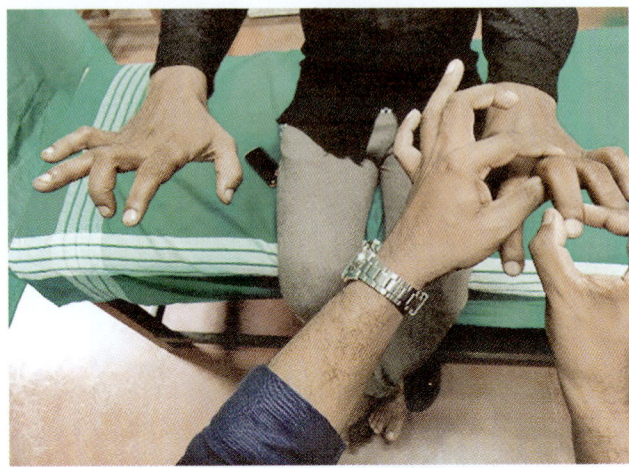
Fig. 6D(vi).8: Examination of position sense by asking to copy passive movement.

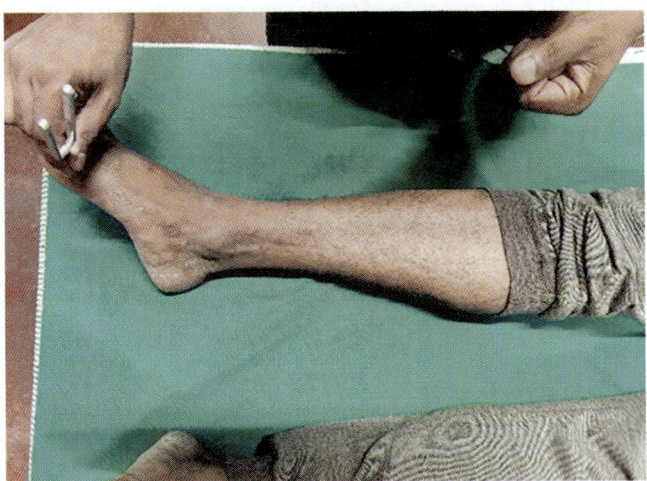
Fig. 6D(vi).9A: Demonstration of vibration over proximal great toe.

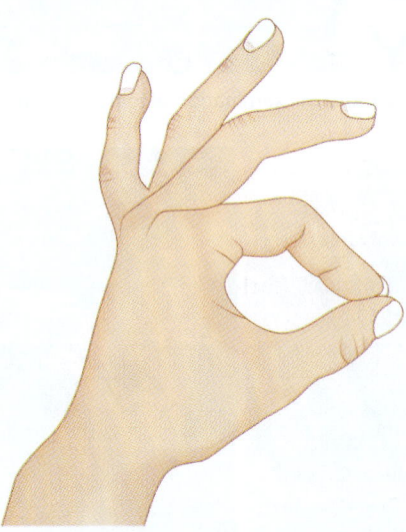
Fig. 6D(vi).7: Examination of position sense (OK sign).

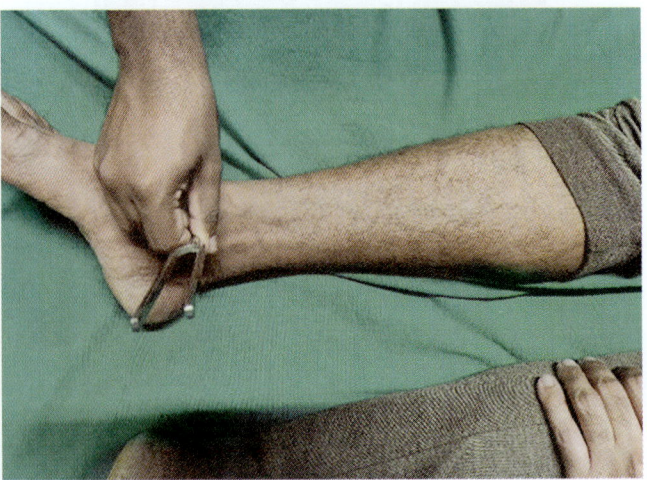
Fig. 6D(vi).9B: Demonstration of vibration over medial malleolus.

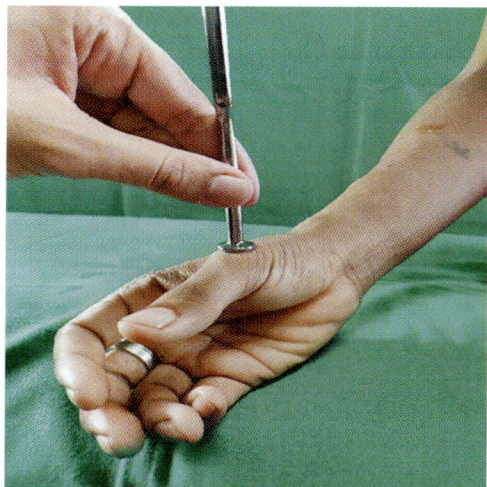

Fig. 6D(vi).9C: Demonstration of vibration over the proximal 1st metacarpophalangeal joint.

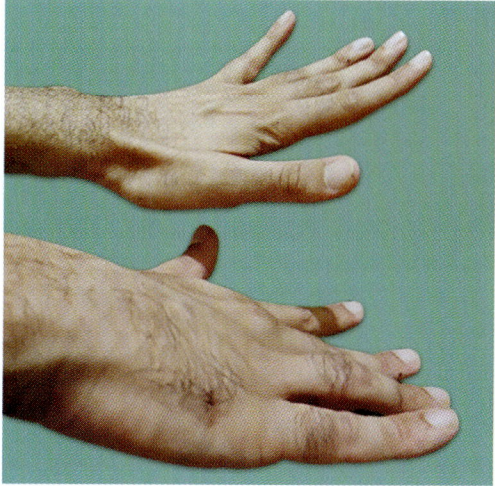

Fig. 6D(vi).11: Demonstration of pseudoathetosis in upper limb.

Timed vibration test:
- It is the most sensitive and simple method to quantify defects in vibration.
- Note the time duration of perception of vibration after the tuning fork is set into vibration.
- Normally:
  - ≥10 seconds in lower limb
  - ≥20 seconds in upper limb

Romberg's Sign [Figs. 6D(vi).10A and B]
- It is a sign of posterior column dysfunction.
- Ask the patient to stand upright with feet/heels close together, arms by the side and eyes open.
- Any significant swaying is noted.
- Now, ask the patient to close the eyes while taking adequate measures to make sure patient does not fall and hurt himself.
- The Romberg sign is said to be positive in a patient who can stand with his feet placed together and eyes open but paradoxically sways or falls while closing his eyes, thereby eliminating his visual cues.

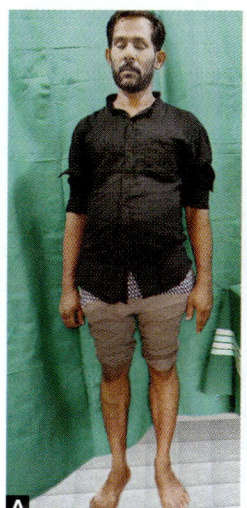 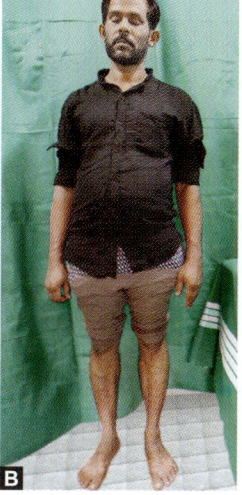

Figs. 6D(vi).10A and B: Demonstration of Romberg's sign.

- In cerebellar disease, the patient is often unsteady with the eyes open as well.
- In vestibular diseases, the patient significantly tends to fall to the side of the affected labyrinth during the test.
- "Sharpened Romberg test"—narrowing the patient's base of support with feet in a heel-to-toe tandem position or
- Conducting the test in foam rubber to nullify the proprioceptive inputs from the foot.

Pseudoathetosis [Fig. 6D(vi).11]:
- It is an upper limb equivalent of examination of posterior column dysfunction.
- Ask the patient to hold the upper limb in extended position and close the eyes.
- Watch for slow writhing movements of fingers (piano-playing movement) which disappear on opening the eyes.

Pressure pain:
- Tested by squeezing the Achilles tendon or calf muscle.
- Abadie's sign is loss of deep pain (seen with diseases affecting the posterior column like neurosyphilis–tabes dorsalis).
- Pitres sign—the loss of sensation in the scrotum and testicles, a symptom of tabes dorsalis.

SECONDARY MODALITIES

Cortical Sensations

Cortical sensations cannot reliably be tested unless primary sensation is intact bilaterally.

Two-point discrimination [Fig. 6D(vi).12]: Ability to recognize simultaneous stimulation by two blunt points. Measured by the distance between the points required for recognition. Two-point discrimination is assessed in two forms: static and moving. Static two-point discrimination is tested by applying the instrument to the skin and maintaining contact for several seconds. Moving two-point discrimination, typically performed on the fingertip, involves drawing the instrument from the distal interphalangeal joint crease toward the fingertip over a span of several seconds.

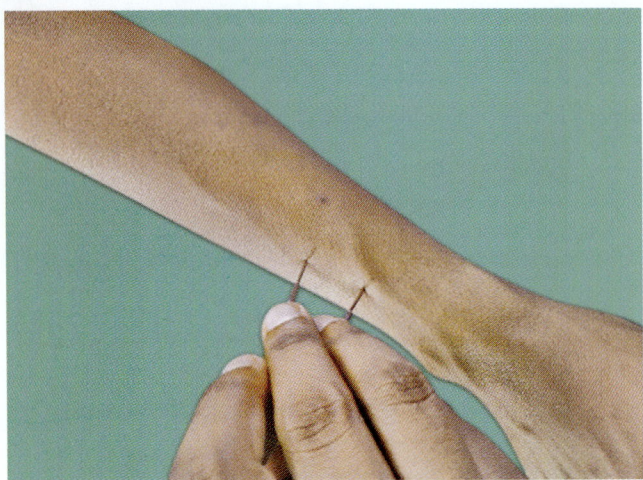

Fig. 6D(vi).12: Demonstration of two-point discrimination.

Tactile extinction (double simultaneous stimulation) [Figs. 6D(vi).15A and B]:

- Ability to perceive a sensory stimulus when corresponding areas on the opposite side of the body are stimulated simultaneously. Loss of this ability is termed sensory extinction (perceptual rivalry/sensory suppression).
- The site of lesion is contralateral parietal lobe.

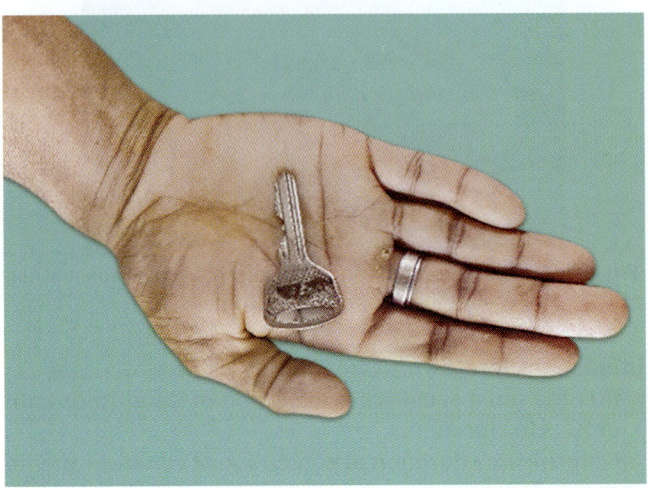

Fig. 6D(vi).14A: Demonstration of stereognosis with key.

This examination may also assist in identifying a sensory level on the trunk in patients with suspected myelopathy. The normal distances at which two points can be discriminated on various body parts:
- Tongue tip: 1 mm
- Fingertip: 2–4 mm
- Dorsum of fingers: 4–6 mm
- Palm: 8–12 mm
- Dorsum of hand: 20–30 mm
- Skin over the back : 30–40 mm

Tactile localization (topognosis):
Ability to localize stimuli to parts of the body. Topagnosia is the absence of this ability.

Graphesthesia [Fig. 6D(vi).13]:
Ask the patient to close their eyes and identify letters or numbers that are being traced onto their palm or the tip of their finger. Loss of this ability is known as agraphesthesia.

Stereognosis [Figs. 6D(vi).14A and B]:
Ask the patient to close their eyes and identify various objects by touch using one hand at a time.

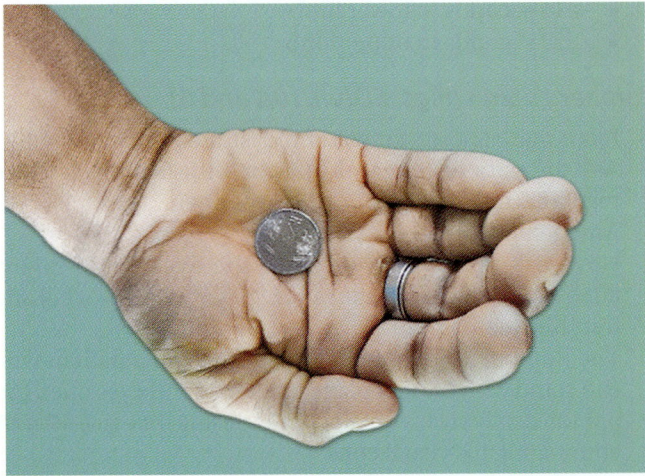

Fig. 6D(vi).14B: Demonstration of stereognosis with coin.

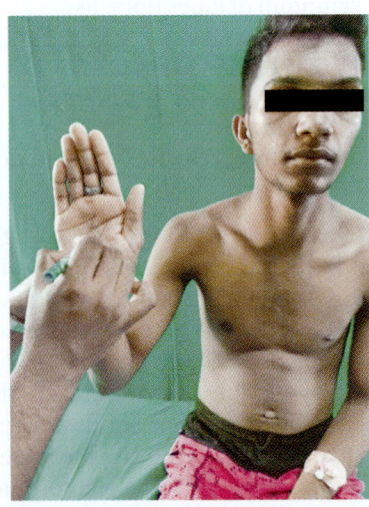

Fig. 6D(vi).13: Demonstration of graphesthesia.

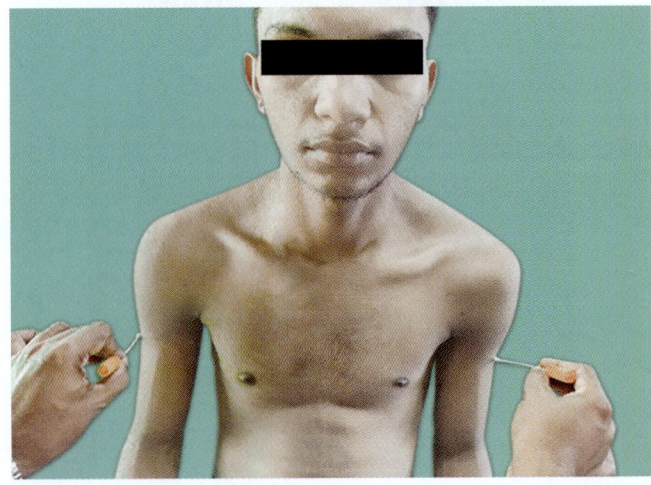

Fig. 6D(vi).15A: Demonstration of tactile extinction in upper limb.

Nervous System

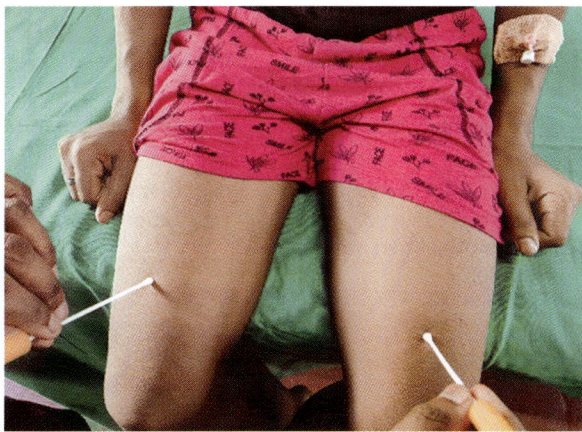

Fig. 6D(vi).15B: Demonstration of tactile extinction in lower limb.

HOMUNCULUS, SENSORY PATHWAY, DERMATOMES AND CLINICAL PATTERNS OF SENSORY LOSS (FIGS. 6D(vi).16 AND 6D(vi).17)

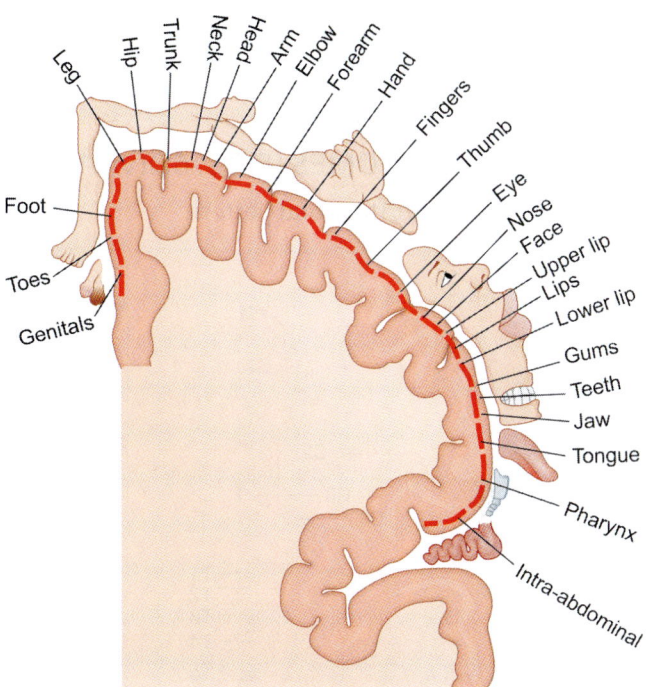

Fig. 6D(vi).16: Sensory homunculus.

Disorders of touch	
Anesthesia	Absence of touch appreciation absence of all sensations
Hypoesthesia	Decrease in touch appreciation
Hyperesthesia	Exaggeration of touch sensation, which is often unpleasant
Paresthesia	Abnormal sensations perceived without specific stimulation. They can include a wide variety of abnormal sensations except pain; episodic or constant
Hyperpathia	Exaggerated reaction to any stimuli (touch/pressure/pain)
Disorders of pain	
Analgesia	Absence of pain appreciation
Hypoalgesia	Decrease in pain appreciation
Hyperalgesia	Exaggeration of pain appreciation, which is often unpleasant
Allodynia	Perception of nonpainful stimulus as painful
Causalgia	Persistent pain, allodynia or hyperalgesia along with abnormal pseudomotor activity (edema and blood flow changes). It is also called as reflex sympathetic dystrophy
Phantom limb pain	Individuals who have had a limb amputated may experience pain or tingling sensations that feel as if they were coming from the amputated limb, just as if that limb were still present
Central or thalamic pain	Spontaneous, inexplicable, agonizing pain and other unusual sensations in the anesthetic parts
Disorders of temperature	
Thermanalgesia	Absence of temperature appreciation
Thermhypoesthesia	Decrease of temperature appreciation
Thermhyperesthesia	Exaggeration of temperature sensation, which is often unpleasant
Disorders of posterior column sensations	
Arthranesthesia	Absence of joint position sense (**Arthresthesia**—perception of joint position sense)
Apallesthesia/pallanesthesia	Absence of vibration sense

Barognosis (recognition of weight)
- The ability to recognize different weights.
- A set of discrimination weights consisting of small objects of the same size and shape but of graduated weights are used.

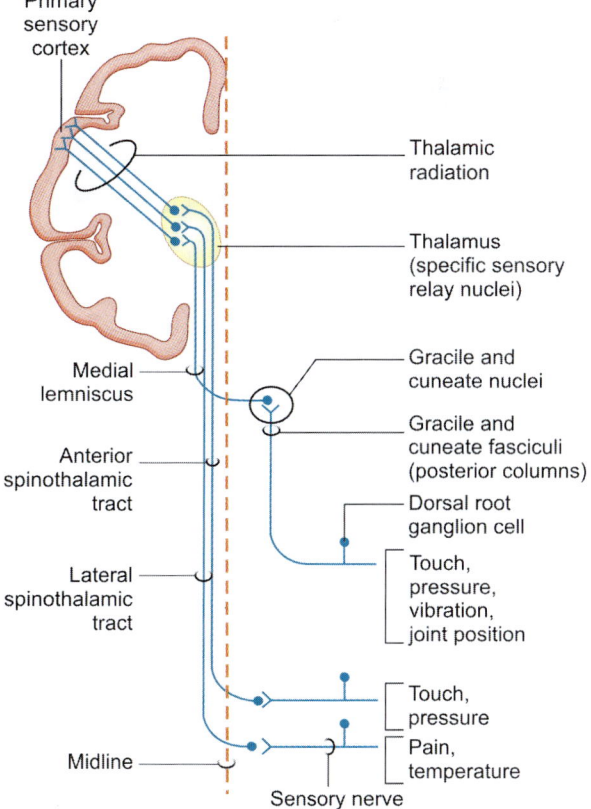

Fig. 6D(vi).17: Sensory pathway.

Sensation	Receptor	Pathway	Decussation
Pain and thermal sense from the body	A δ and C fiber endings	Spinothalamic tract of anterolateral system (ALS)	Anterior white commissure
Nondiscriminative (crude) touch and superficial pressure from the body	Free nerve endings, Merkel's disks, peritrichial nerve endings	Spinothalamic tract of ALS	Anterior white commissure
Two-point discriminative (fine) touch, vibratory sense, proprioceptive sense from muscles and joints of body	Meissner's corpuscles, Pacinian corpuscles, muscle stretch receptors, Golgi tendon organs	First-order fibers: Fasciculi gracilis and cuneatus Second-order fibers: Medial lemniscus	Medial lemniscal decussation

SENSORY DERMATOMES [FIGS. 6D(vi).18 AND 6D(vi).19]

Keegan and garret dermatomal pattern

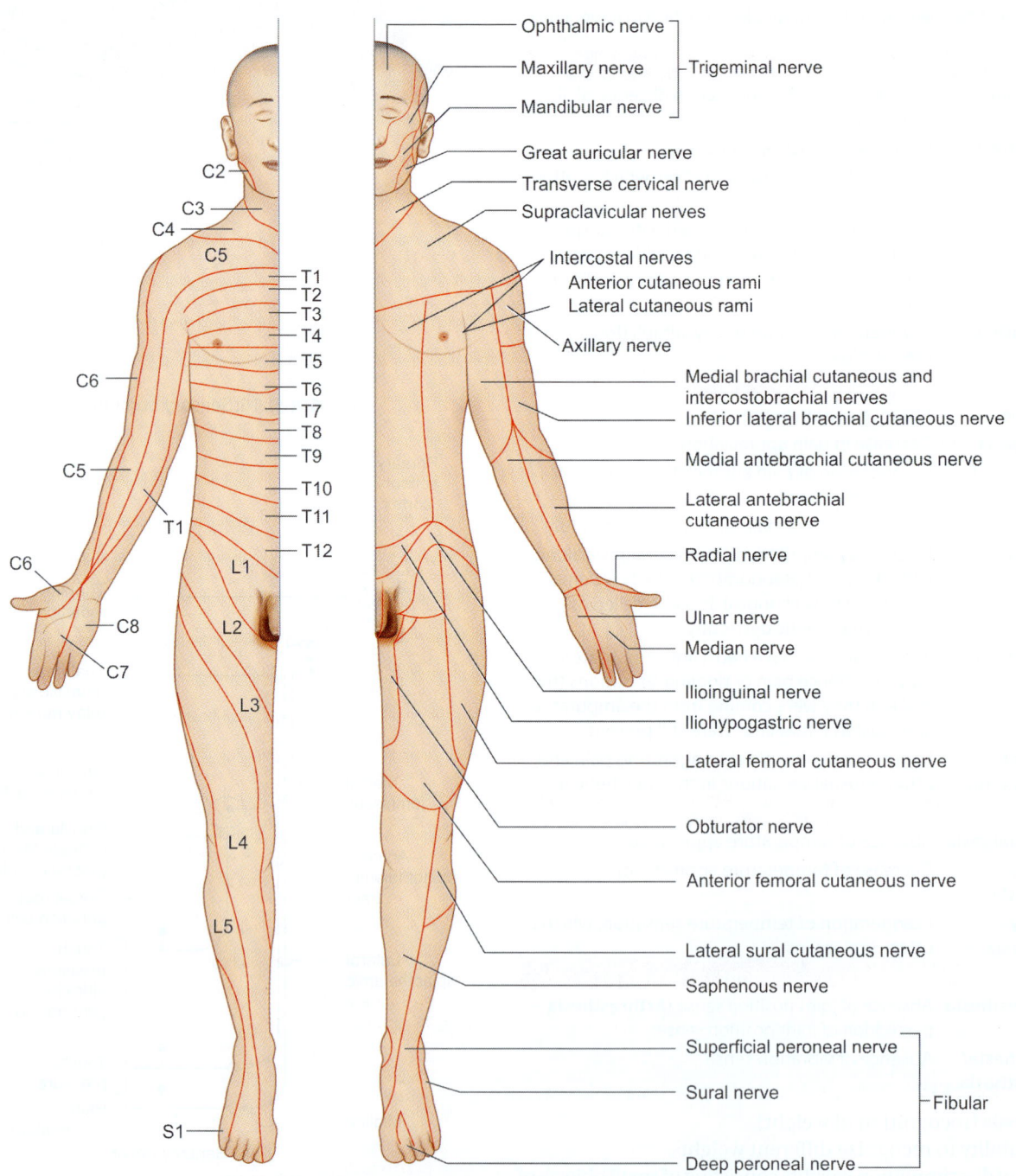

Fig. 6D(vi).18: Anterior view of skin segment innervation.

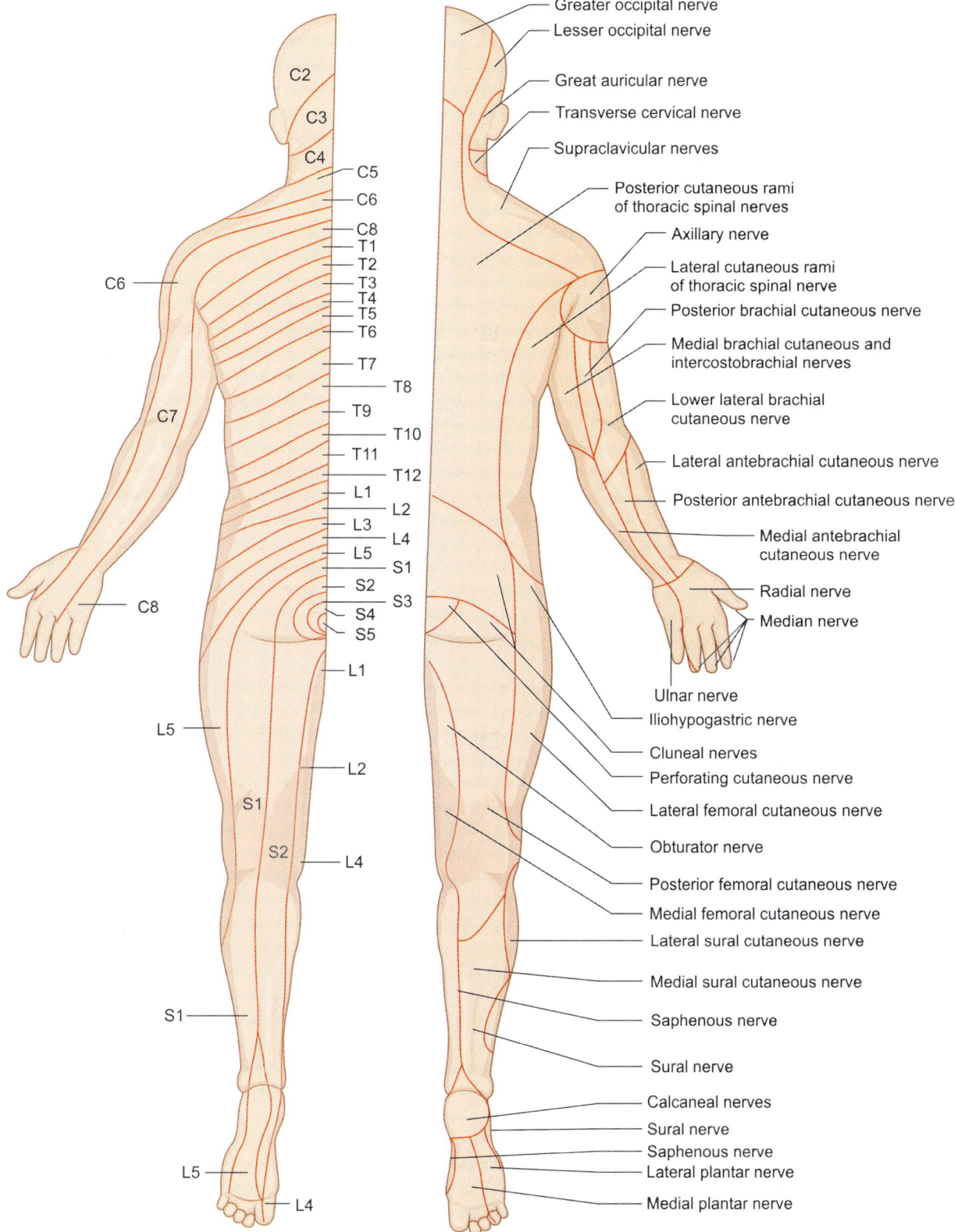

Fig. 6D(vi).19: Posterior view of skin segment innervation.

NONORGANIC SENSORY LOSS [FIGS. 6D(vi).20A TO H]

Features of Functional Sensory Loss
- **Nonanatomical distribution:** Sensory deficits do not follow known dermatomal or peripheral nerve patterns.
- **Inconsistencies over time:** Symptoms may vary upon repeated examinations, lacking a consistent neurological pattern.

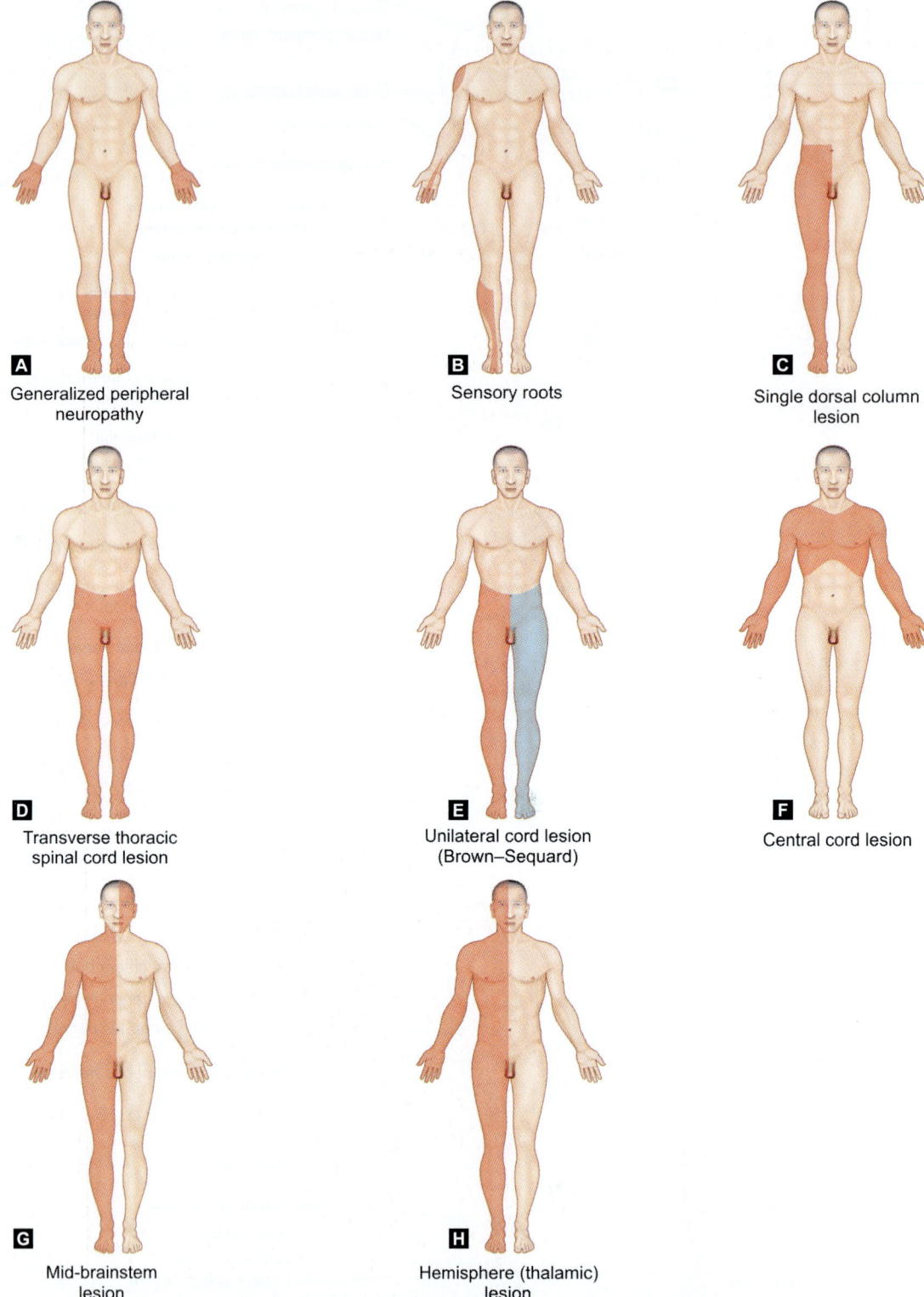

Figs. 6D(vi).20A to H: Clinical patterns of sensory dysfunction.

- **Positive signs.**
- **Yes-no test:** Assesses the patient's ability to perceive and respond to sensory stimuli.
- **Bowlus-Currier test:** Evaluates sensory perception by testing the patient's response to stimuli in a forced-choice format.

D(vii). CEREBELLUM AND COORDINATION

SIGNS OF CEREBELLAR DISORDERS

Deficit	Manifestation
Ataxia	Reeling, wide-based gait
Decomposition of movement	Inability to sequence fine, coordinate acts correctly. *This is usually tested while performing the finger-nose test, which requires a fine coordination between shoulder, elbow, and wrist joint. Patients with a cerebellar lesion will find it difficult to perform such movements*
Dysarthria	Inability to articulate words correctly, usually manifesting as slurring and/or inappropriate phrasing
Dysdiadochokinesia	Inability to perform rapid, alternating movements
Dysmetria	Inability to control or limit the range of movement
Hypotonia	Decrease in muscle tone
Nystagmus	Involuntary rapid oscillation of eyeballs in a horizontal, vertical or rotationary fashion with the fast component of nystagmus maximal towards the side of the cerebellar lesion
Scanning/staccato speech	Slow explosive enunciation with a tendency to hesitate at the beginning of each word or each syllable. *Asking the patient to pronounce a word with multiple syllables, such as Mississippi or Venkataramana will elicit distinct pauses before each syllable*
Tremor	Rhythmic, alternating, oscillatory movements which affect a limb as it approaches a target (intention tremor) or of proximal musculature when attempting to bear weight (postural tremor)

Scan QR code for Wide-based gait

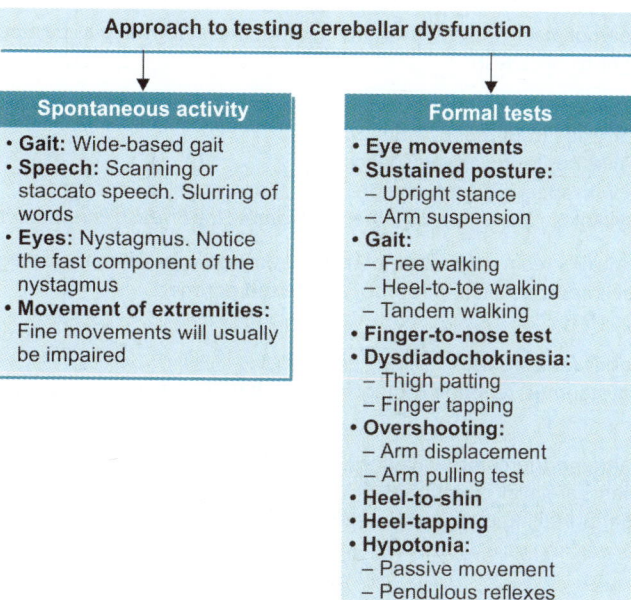

Hypotonia
- Usually accompanies acute hemispheric lesions.
- Interestingly, it is seen less often in chronic lesions.
- Ipsilateral to the side of a cerebellar lesion.
- More noticeable in upper limbs and proximal muscles.
- Pendular knee jerk: Leg keeps swinging after knee jerk more than 4 times (4 or less is considered normal). It occurs due to hypotonia and lack of normal checking of reflex response.

Ataxia
- Defective timing of sequential contraction of agonist/antagonist muscles.
- Results in a disturbance in smooth performance of voluntary acts (errors in rate, range, force, duration).
- May affect limbs, trunk, gait (depends on the part of cerebellum involved).

Asynergia
Lack of synergy of various muscles while performing complex movements (movements are broken up into isolated, successive parts. This is known as decomposition of movement).

Contd...

Contd...

Dysmetria or abnormal excursions in movement
- **Finger-to-nose test**
  - With eyes open, the patient is asked to partially extend elbow and rapidly bring tip of index finger in a wide arc to tip of his nose.
  - In cerebellar disease, the action may manifest an intention tremor.
  - With eyes closed, sense of position in the shoulder and elbow is tested.
- **Heel-to-shin test**
  - Patient is asked to place one heel on opposite knee and slide the heel down the shin of tibia with foot dorsiflexed.
  - Movement should be performed accurately.
  - In cerebellar disease, the arc of the movement is jerky/wavering.
  - The slide down the shin may manifest an action tremor.

Dysdiadochokinesia or impaired performance of rapidly alternating movement
Normal coordination includes ability to arrest one motor impulse and substitute the opposite. There are several simple clinical methods to test this:
- Alternating movements (pronate and supinate forearm and hand quickly): In cerebellar disease, the movements tend to overshoot or are inadequate resulting in irregular or inaccurate movements.
- Rapidly tap fingers on the table
- Open and close fists
- Stewart–Holmes rebound sign

Have the patient pull on your hand and when they do, slip your hand out of their grasp. Normally the antagonist's muscles will contract and stop their arm from moving in the desired direction. A positive sign is seen in a spastic limb where the exaggerated "rebound" occurs with movement in the opposite direction. However, in cerebellar disease, this response is completely absent causing the limb to continue moving in the desired direction. (Be careful that you protect the patient from the unrestricted movement causing them to strike themselves).

Past pointing
Overshoot is also commonly seen as part of ataxic movements and is sometimes referred to as past pointing, when the patient overshoots while reaching target (finger-to-nose test)

Cerebellar dysarthria
- Abnormalities in articulation and prosody (together or independent).
- Scanning, slurring, staccato, explosive, hesitant, garbled speech.
- Hemisphere lesions are associated with speech disorders more often than vermal lesions.
- Causes enunciation of individual syllables: *"the British Parliament" becomes "the Brit-tish Par-la-ment."*

Intention tremor—occurs during goal-directed movements. Intention tremor results when the antagonist activation that normally stops a goal-directed movement as the goal is approached is inappropriately sized or timed.

Oculomotor dysfunction
- Nystagmus frequently seen in cerebellar disorders.
- Gaze-evoked nystagmus, upbeat nystagmus, rebound nystagmus, optokinetic nystagmus may all be seen in midline cerebellar lesions.

Gait
- In cerebellar disease, the gait is staggering/lurching/wavering.
- Lesion in mid-cerebellum: Movements are in all directions.
- Lesion in lateral cerebellum: Staggering/falling is toward the side of the lesion.
- Somewhat steadied by standing or walking on a wide base.

Position of feet
Ataxia from cerebellar disease is less when the patient stands on a broad base (feet widely apart).

Eyes open or closed
Cerebellar ataxia is not improved by visual orientation; ataxia from posterior column disease (disordered proprioception) is worsened with the eyes closed.

Direction of falling
Disease of lateral lobe of cerebellum causes falling to ipsilateral side.
Lesions of midline/vermis cause indiscriminate falling depending on initial stance of the patient.

Titubation
Consists of a rhythmic body or head tremor. There is a rotatory, rocking or bobbing movement. *Clinically, this does not have significant value in localizing the lesion with respect to the part of the cerebellum involved.*

HEEL KNEE TEST [FIGS. 6D(vii). 1A TO D]

The patient is asked to touch the heel of one foot to the opposite knee and then to drag their heel in a straight line all the way down the front of their shin and back up again. In order to eliminate the effect of gravity in moving the heel down the shin, this test should always be done in the supine position.

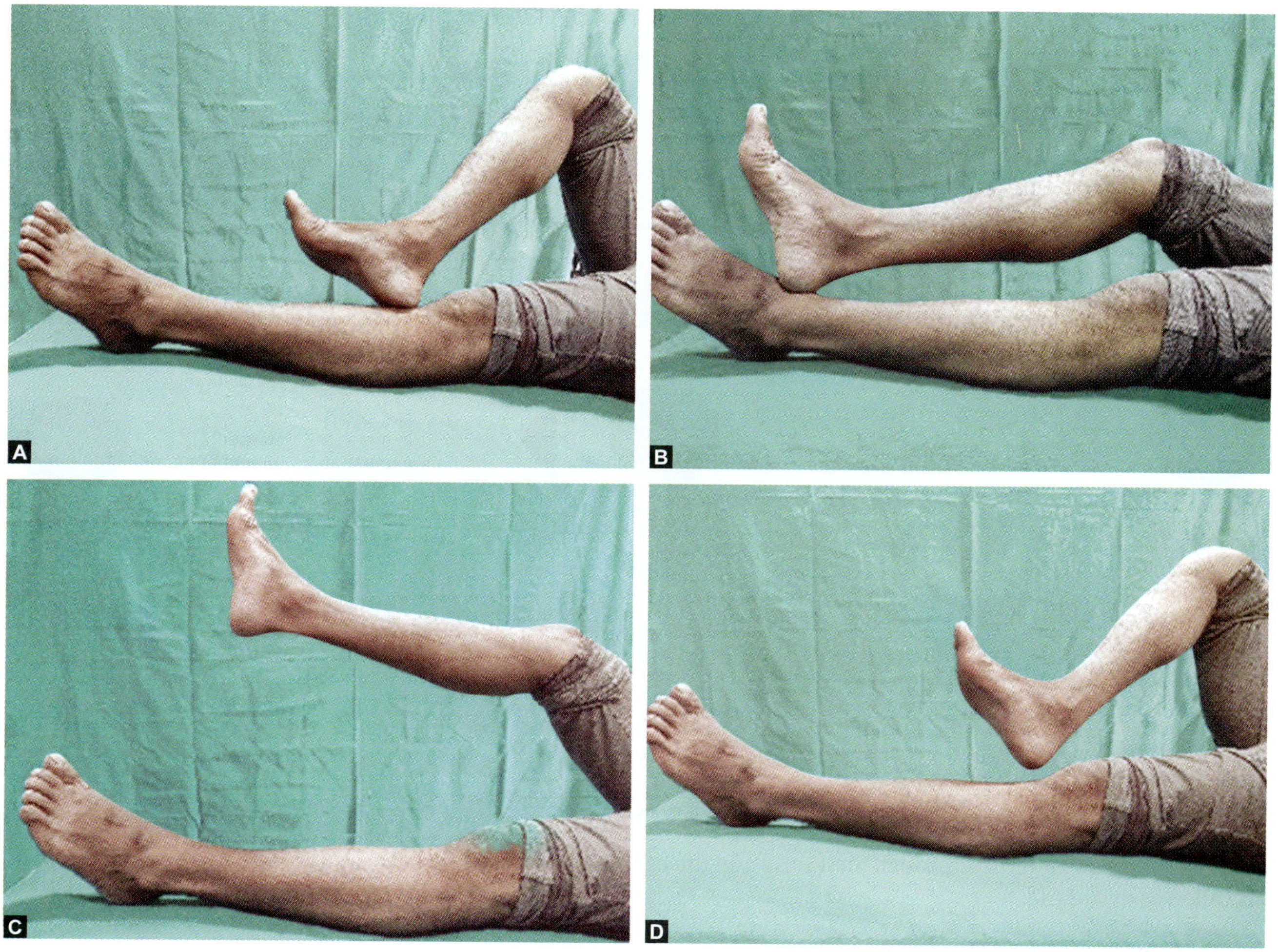

Figs. 6D(vii).1A to D: Demonstration of heel knee test.

TOE FINGER TEST [FIGS. 6D(vii).2A AND B]

Patient lies in bed and is asked to touch his great toe to the examiners fingers or any object held above the bed within his reach.

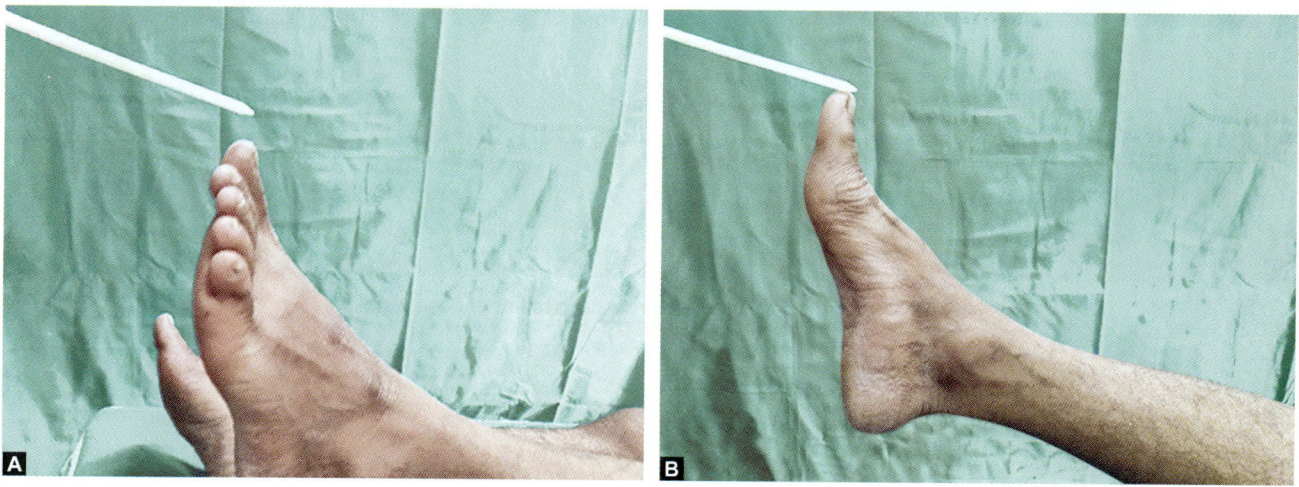

Figs. 6D(vii).2A and B: Demonstration of toe finger test.

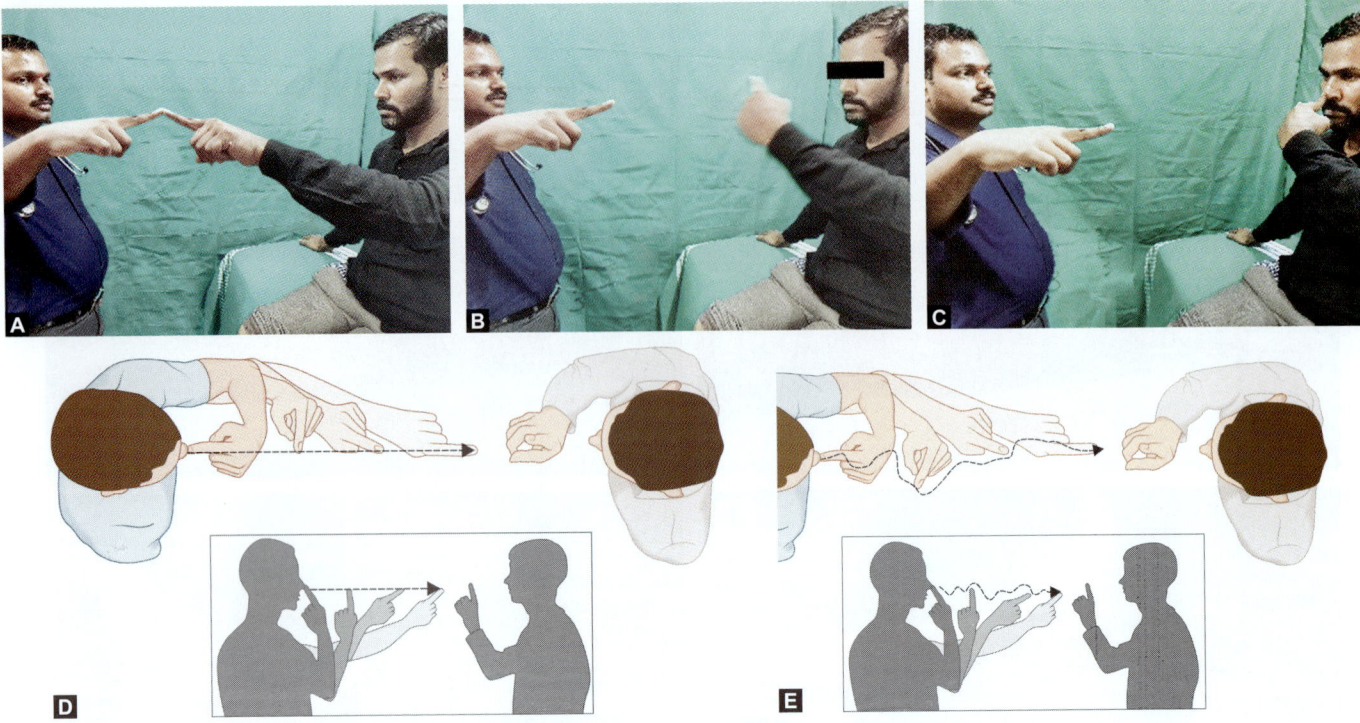

Figs. 6D(vii).3A to E: Showing demonstration of nose finger nose test.

NOSE-FINGER-NOSE TEST [FIGS. 6D(VII).3A TO E]

The patient is asked to alternately touch their nose and the examiner's finger as quickly as possible. Abnormality of this is called as dysmetria.

Finger Nose Test [Figs. 6D(vii).4A and B]

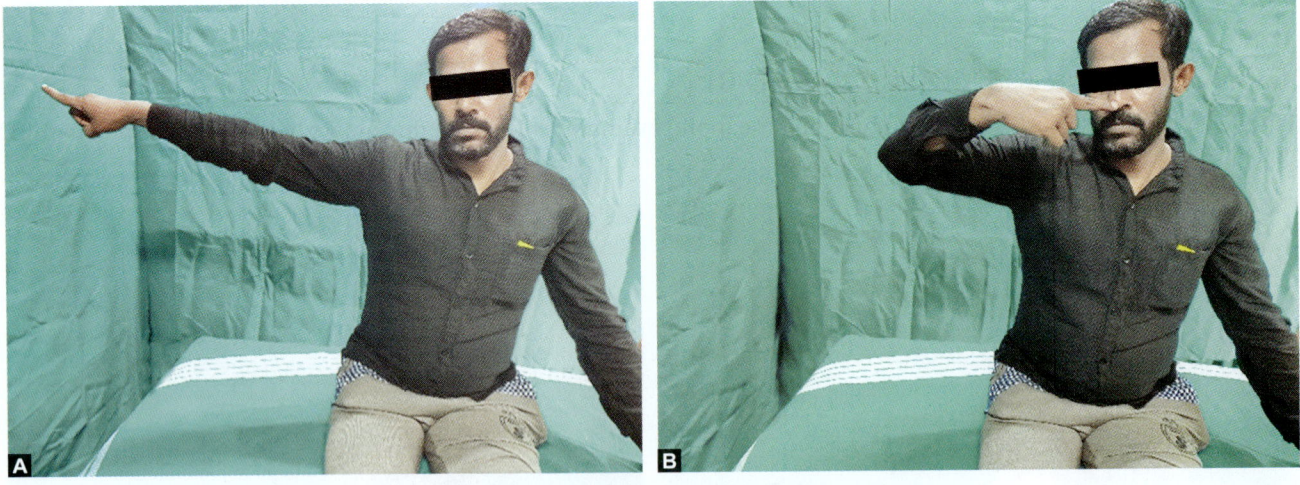

Figs. 6D(vii).4A and B: Demonstration of finger nose test.

Rebound Phenomenon [Fig. 6D(vii).5]

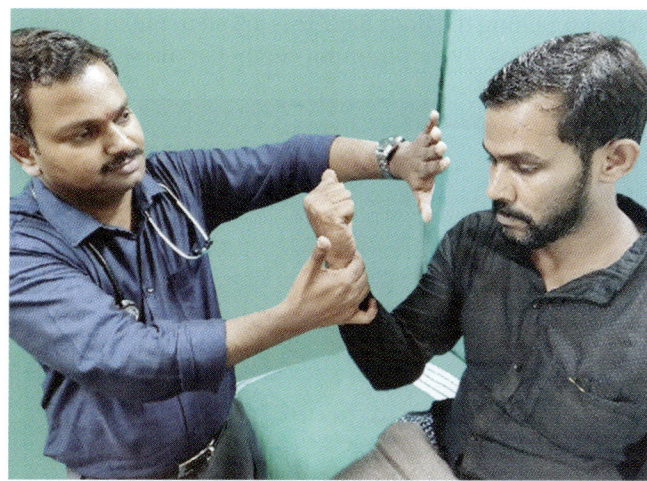

Fig. 6D(vii).5: Demonstration of rebound phenomenon.

DYSDIADOCHOKINESIA [FIGS. 6D(vii).6A TO D]

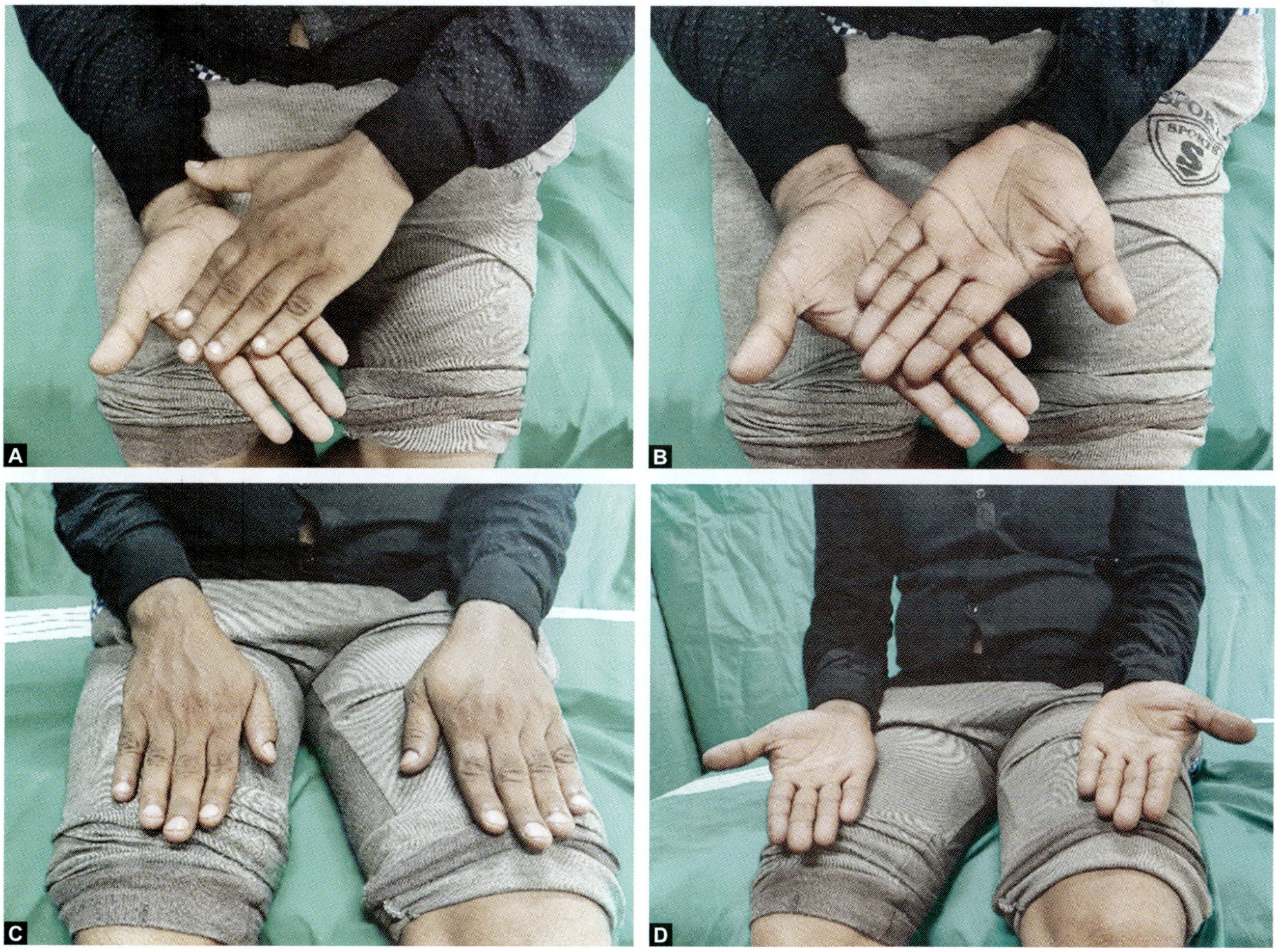

Figs. 6D(vii).6A to D: Demonstration of dysdiadochokinesia.

FOOT TAPPING/FOOT PAT TEST [FIGS. 6D(vii).7A TO C]

Patient is made to sit on chair with feet touching the floor flat. He is asked to pat the floor with his forefoot. The rate, rhythm and speed of patting is compared on both sides. Even minimum cerebellar disease can be picked up by this test.

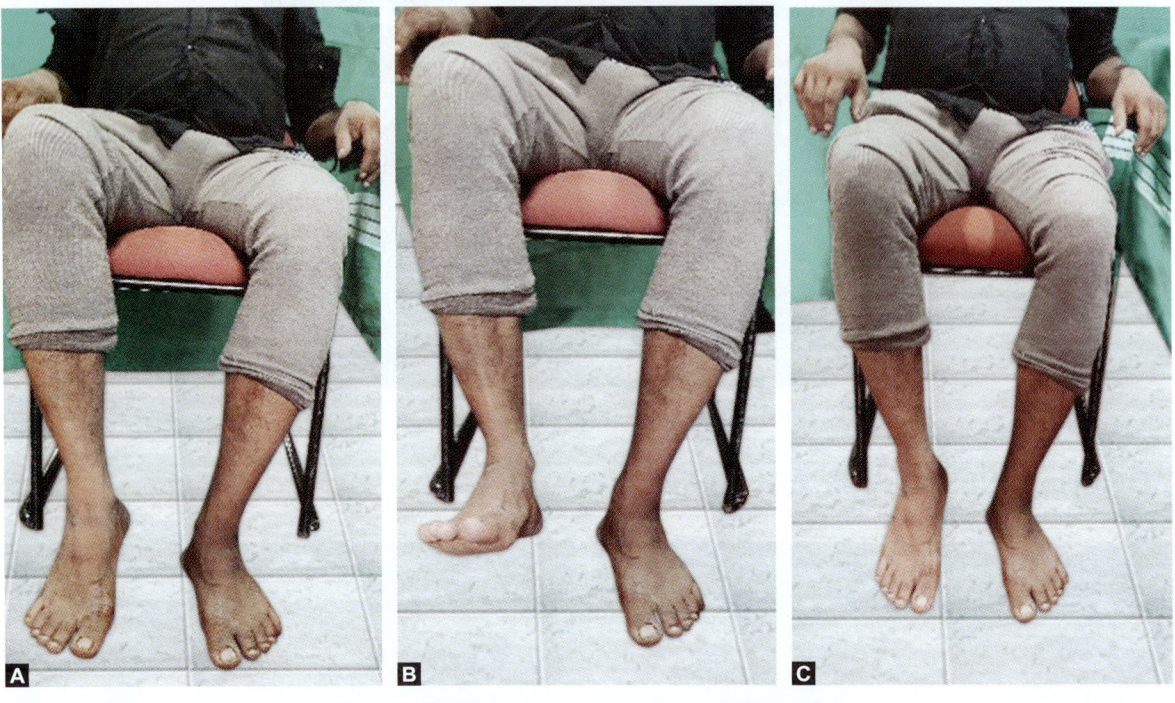

Figs. 6D(vii).7A to C: Demonstration of foot tapping.

STRAIGHT LINE WALKING [FIGS. 6D(vii).8A AND B]

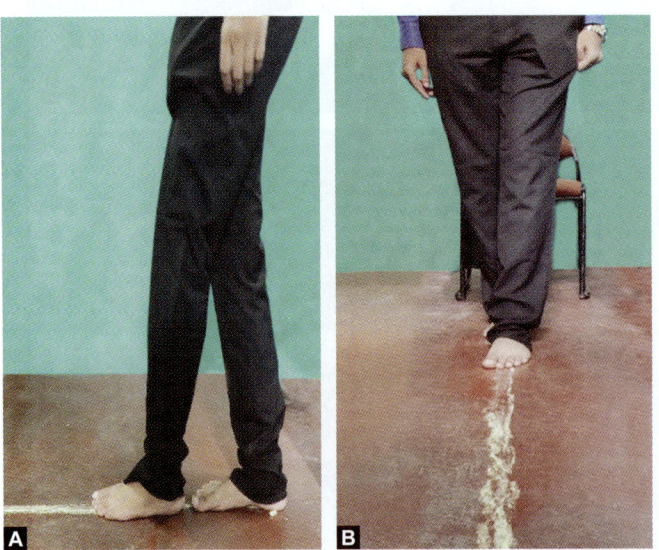

Figs. 6D(vii).8A and B: Straight line walking.

TANDEM WALKING [FIGS. 6D(vii).9A AND B]

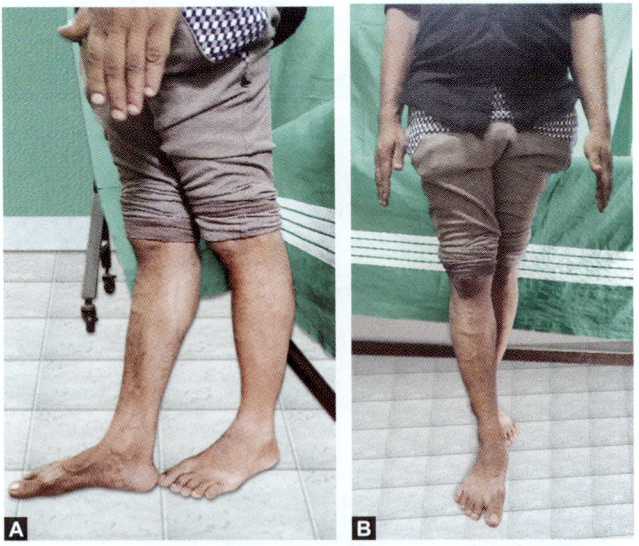

Figs. 6D(vii).9A and B: Demonstration of tandem walking.

APPROACH TO ATAXIA

- Ataxia, defined as impaired coordination of voluntary muscle movement affecting the rate, range, direction and force of movements.
- It is a physical finding, not a disease.
- Types of ataxia:
  1. Cerebellar
  2. Sensory
  3. Vestibular
  4. Optic
  5. Frontal

Type of ataxia	Cerebellar	Sensory	Frontal
Stance and support	Wide based	Narrow based; looking down	Wide based
Velocity	Variable	Slow	Very slow
Stride	Irregular, lurching	Regular with path deviation	Short, shuffling
Romberg	+/−	Unsteady; patient falls	+/−
Heel-shin	Abnormal	+/−	Normal
Initiation	Normal	Normal	Hesitant
Postural instability	+	+++	+++++
Falls	Late event	Frequent	Frequent
Turns	Unsteady	+/−	Multistepped; hesitant

Sensory ataxia is due to a severe sensory neuropathy, ganglionopathy or lesions of the posterior column of the spinal cord, e.g., Sjogren's syndrome, cisplatin, chronic inflammatory demyelinating polyradiculoneuropathy (CIDP), paraneoplastic disorders, subacute combined degeneration (SACD), tabes dorsalis, Miller–Fisher syndrome, celiac disease.

- Ataxia more at night or while walking through narrow passages (coffee plantations).
- A history of falling into the sink or imbalance when splashing water on the face (wash-basin sign), passing a towel over the face or pulling a shirt over the head should also be sought.
- Pseudoathetosis/sensory wandering—"piano-playing" movements—when the patient has his arms outstretched and eyes closed, the affected arm will wander from its original position.
- Vibration and position sense are usually lost together.
- Positive Romberg's test is a hallmark of sensory ataxia.

Vestibular ataxia is due to lesion of vestibular pathways resulting in impairment and imbalance of vestibular inputs, e.g., vestibular neuronitis, and streptomycin toxicity.
- Vertigo and associated tinnitus and hearing loss.
- Direction of the nystagmus is away from the lesion.

Optic ataxia was first described in a man with lesions of the posterior parietal lobe on both sides of the brain, later known as **Balint syndrome**.
- Among the symptoms that characterize the syndrome are a restriction of visual attention to single objects and a paucity of spontaneous eye movements.
- Patients have difficulty in completing visually guided reaching tasks in the absence of other sensory cues.

Frontal lobe ataxia (Brun's ataxia) is due to involvement of subcortical small vessels, Binswanger's disease, multi-infarct state or normal pressure hydrocephalus (NPH).
- The gait may appear to be a combination of awkward, magnetic (stuck to the floor), cautious, slow, and shuffling. This is also known as a frontal gait disorder, referring to the frontal lobe conditions which often cause **gait apraxia.**

CEREBELLAR ATAXIA

Zone [Fig. 6D(vii).10]	Corresponding anatomical site	Function	Loss of function
Midline zone	Anterior and posterior parts of the vermis, fastigial nucleus	Posture, locomotion, position of head relative to trunk, control of extra ocular movements	Disorders of stance/gait, truncal postural disturbances, rotated postures of the head, disturbances of eye movements
Intermediate zone	Paravermal region of cerebellum and interposed nuclei *(emboliform, globose)*	Control of velocity, force and pattern of muscle activity	—
Lateral zone	Cerebellar hemisphere and dentate nucleus	Planning of fine and skilled movement *(in connection with neurons in the Rolandic region of the cerebral cortex)*	Hypotonia, dysarthria, dysmetria, dysdiadochokinesia, excessive rebound, impaired check, kinetic and static tremors, past pointing

CAUSES OF CEREBELLAR ATAXIA

Symmetrical Cerebellar Ataxias

Acute	Subacute	Chronic
- Drugs: Phenytoin, phenobarbitone, lithium, chemotherapeutic agents - Alcohol - Infectious: Acute viral cerebellitis, post-infectious - Toxins: Toluene, glue, gasoline, methyl mercury	- Alcohol, or nutritional (B_1, B_{12}) - Paraneoplastic - Antigliadin or anti-GAD antibody - Prion diseases	- MSA-C - Hypothyroidism - Phenytoin toxicity

(GAD: glutamic acid decarboxylase; MSA-C: multiple system atrophy with cerebellar ataxia)

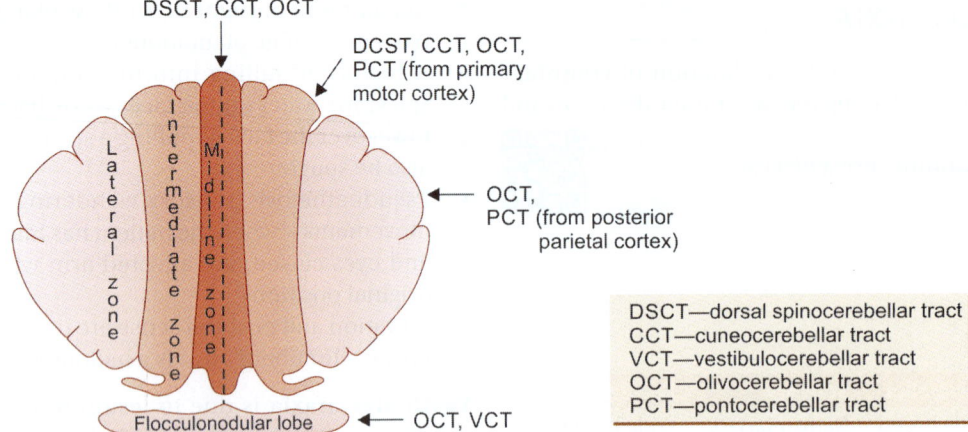

Fig. 6D(vii).10: Anatomical and functional areas of cerebellum.

Asymmetrical Cerebellar Ataxias

Acute	Subacute	Chronic
Vascular: Cerebellar infarction or hemorrhage, subdural hematoma ■ Infectious: Abscess	■ Neoplastic: Glioma, metastases, lymphoma ■ Demyelination: MS ■ HIV related: Progressive multifocal leukoencephalopathy	■ Congenital lesions: Arnold–Chiari malformation, Dandy–Walker syndrome

Treatable Causes of Ataxia

- Hypothyroidism
- Ataxia with vitamin E deficiency (AVED)
- Vitamin B_{12} deficiency
- Wilson's disease
- Ataxia with antigliadin antibodies and gluten sensitive enteropathy
- Ataxia due to malabsorption syndromes
- Lyme's disease
- Mitochondrial encephalomyopathies, aminoacidopathies, leukodystrophies and urea cycle abnormalities
- Wernicke's encephalopathy

Cerebellar Syndromes

Rostral vermis syndrome (anterior lobe) *For example, alcoholics*	■ Wide-based stance and gait. ■ Ataxia of gait; proportionally less ataxia is seen on performing heel-shin test while the patient is lying down. ■ Normal or slightly impaired arm coordination. ■ Infrequent hypotonia, nystagmus and/or dysarthria.
Caudal vermis syndrome (flocculonodular, posterior lobe) *For example, tumors (medulloblastoma)*	■ Axial disequilibrium; staggering gait. ■ Little or no limb ataxia. ■ Spontaneous nystagmus might be seen. Rotated postures of head.
Hemispheric syndrome (posterior lobe, anterior variants also possible) *For example, infarcts, neoplasms, abscesses*	■ Incoordination of ipsilateral limb movements. ■ More noticeable with fine motor skills. ■ Incoordination affects most noticeably muscles involved in speech and finger movements.

Contd...

Contd...

Pancerebellar syndrome *For example, infectious/parainfectious processes, hypoglycemia, paraneoplastic disorders, toxic-metabolic disorders*	■ Combination of all the other syndromes. ■ Bilateral signs of cerebellar dysfunction involving trunk, limbs, cranial musculature.

LOCALIZATION OF CEREBELLAR LESIONS

Signs and symptoms	Most probable region of involvement
Higher cognitive changes	Lateral hemispheres
Action tremor	Dentate and interposed nuclei OR cerebellar outflow to ventral thalamus
Palatal tremor	Dentate nucleus, Guillain Mollaret triangle
Titubation	Any zone; especially anterior vermis and associated deep nuclei
Dysarthria	Posterior left hemisphere and vermis
Gait ataxia	Anterior vermis
Limb ataxia	Lateral hemispheres
Saccadic dysmetria	Dorsal vermis
Square wave jerks	Cerebellar outflow
Gaze-evoked nystagmus	Flocculus and paraflocculus

Mnemonics for cerebellar signs:

Danish pen	Vanishd
Dysdiadochokinesia	**V**ertigo
Ataxic gait	**A**taxia
Nystagmus	**N**ystagmus
Intention tremor	**I**ntentional tremor
Scanning/**S**taccato speech	**S**canning speech
Hypotonia/**H**eel-shin test	**H**ypotonia
Pendular knee jerk	**D**ysdiadochokinesia

D(viii). GAIT

NORMAL GAIT CYCLE [FIGS. 6D(viii).1A TO G]

The gait cycle is the time interval or sequence of motions occurring between two consecutive initial contacts of the same foot, i.e., cycle of stance and swing by one foot.

Observation to be noted while the patient walks:
1. Posture of the body while walking
2. The regularity of the movement
3. The position and movement of the arms
4. The relative ease and smoothness of the movement of the legs
5. The distance between the feet both in forward and lateral directions
6. The ability to maintain a straight course
7. The ease of turning
8. Stopping
9. Position of feet and posture just before initiation of gait.

ABNORMALITIES OF GAIT

Neurogenic gait disorders should be differentiated from those due to skeletal abnormalities (characterized by pain producing an antalgic gait, or limp).

Gait abnormalities incompatible with any anatomical or physiological deficit may be due to functional disorders.

Pyramidal (Circumduction/Hemiplegic) Gait [Fig. 6D(viii).2]

- Lesions of the upper motor neuron lesions produce characteristic extension of the affected leg. There is tendency for the toes to strike the ground on walking and outward throwing/swing of lower limbs. This movement occurring at the hip joint is called circumduction. There is leaning towards the opposite normal side. The arm of the affected side is adducted at the shoulder and flexed at the elbow, wrist, and fingers.

- In hemiplegia/hemiparesis, there is a clear asymmetry between affected and normal sides on walking, but in paraparesis both lower legs swing slowly from the hips in extension and are stiffly dragged over the ground (walking in mud).

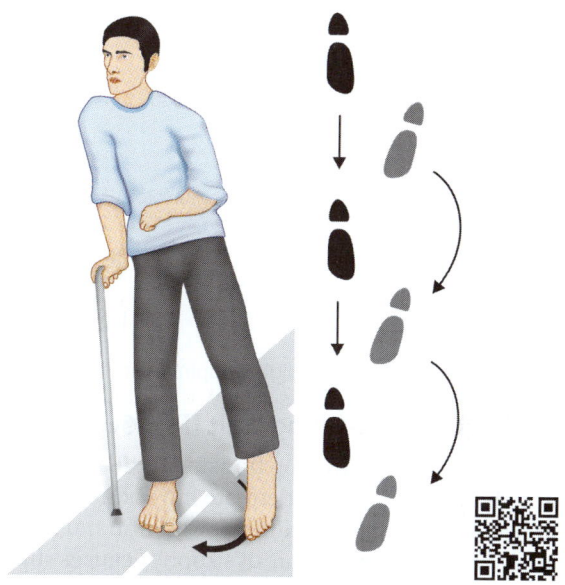

Fig. 6D(viii).2: Circumduction gait.

Foot Drop (High Stepping/Slapping Gait) [Fig. 6D(viii).3]

In normal walking, the heel is the first part of the foot to hit the ground. A lower motor neuron lesion affecting the leg will cause weakness of ankle dorsiflexion, resulting in a less controlled descent of the foot, which makes slapping noise as it hits the ground. In severe cases, the foot will have to be lifted higher at the knee to allow room for the inadequately dorsiflexed foot to swing through, resulting in a high-stepping gait. Cause, e.g., common peroneal nerve palsy.

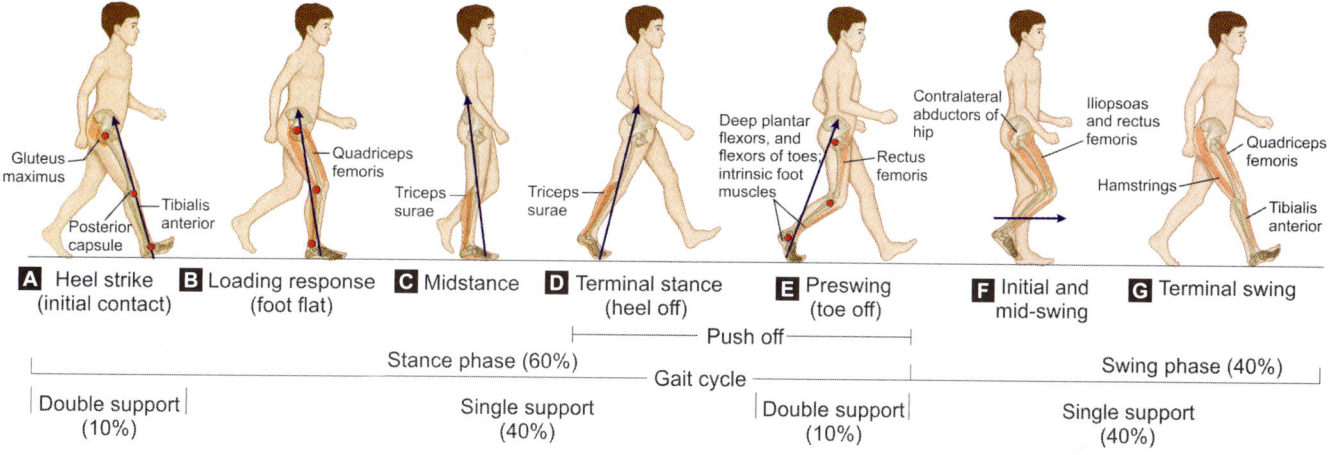

Figs. 6D(viii).1A to G: Normal gait cycle.

Ataxic Gait (Cerebellar Ataxia: Broad-based Gait) [Fig. 6D(viii).5]

- In this type of gait, the patient, unstable, tremulous and reels in any direction (including backwards) and walks on a broad base. Ataxia describes this incoordination. The patient finds difficulty in executing tandem walking.
- **Causes:** Lesions of the cerebellum, vestibular apparatus or peripheral nerves. When walking, the patient tends to veer to the side of the affected cerebellar lobe. When the disease involves cerebellar vermis, the trunk becomes unsteady without limb ataxia, with a tendency to fall backwards or sideways and is termed truncal ataxia.

In a typical walking pattern, the distance between the feet during the double support phase (when both feet are on the ground) is relatively narrow, usually around 2–4 inches. In contrast, individuals with a broad-based gait exhibit a wider stance, with their feet placed further apart. This wider stance is an attempt to increase stability and compensate for impaired balance and coordination.

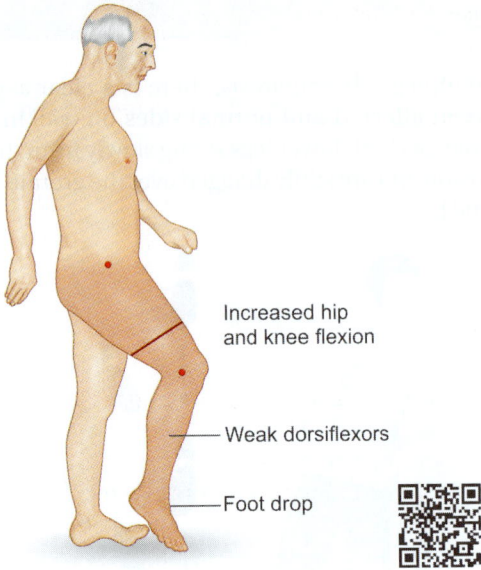

Fig. 6D(viii).3: High stepping gait.

Myopathic Gait/Waddling Gait [Fig. 6D(viii).4]

- During walking, alternating transfer of the body's weight through each leg, needs adequate hip abduction.
- **Causes:** Weakness of proximal lower limb muscles (e.g., polymyositis and muscular dystrophy) causes difficulty rising from sitting. The hips are not properly fixed by these muscles and trunk movements are exaggerated, and walking becomes a waddle or rolling. The pelvis is poorly supported by each leg. This may be seen with bilateral congenital dislocation of hip (**Trendelenburg gait**). The patient walks on a broad base with exaggerated lumbar lordosis.

Gluteus Medius Gait or Abductor Lurch

Lurch of body towards affected side in every stance phase (abductor lurch). Seen with congenital coxa vara, gluteus medius paralysis, polio, and Perthes disease.

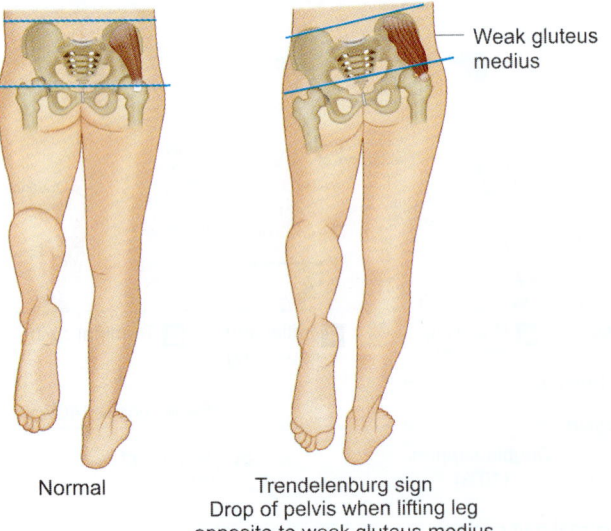

Fig. 6D(viii).4: Waddling gait.

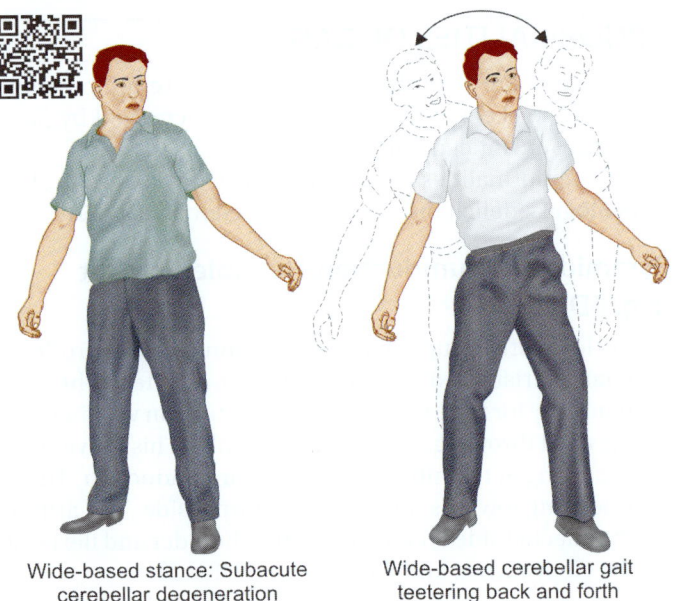

Fig. 6D(viii).5: Cerebellar/ataxic gait.

Apraxic Gait

- In an apraxic gait, the acquired walking skills become disorganized. On examination of the legs, the power, cerebellar function, and proprioception are normal. Leg movement is normal when sitting or lying and the patient can carry out complex motor tasks (e.g., bicycling motion). But patient cannot initiate and organize the motor act of walking. The feet appear stuck to the floor and the patient cannot walk.
- **Causes:** Diffuse bilateral hemisphere disease or diffuse frontal lobe disease (e.g., tumor, hydrocephalus, and infarction).

Marche à petits pas

- It is characterized by small, slow steps, and marked instability. In contrast to the festination found in Parkinson's disease, it lacks increasing pace and freezing.

- **Cause:** Small-vessel cerebrovascular disease and accompanying bilateral upper motor neuron signs.

Extrapyramidal/Shuffling/Festinant Gait [Fig. 6D(viii).6]

- It is characterized by stooped posture and gait difficulties with problems initiating walking and controlling the pace of the gait. Patients make a series of small, flat-footed shuffles, and become stuck while trying to start walking or when walking through doorways (freezing). The center of gravity will be moved forwards to aid propulsion and difficulty in stopping. It is characterized by muscular rigidity throughout extensors and flexors. Power is preserved, pace is shortened and slows to a shuffle, and its base remains narrow. There is a stoop and diminished arm swinging and gait becomes festinant (hurried) with short rapid steps. Patient will be having difficulty in turning quickly and initiating movement. Retropulsion, i.e., small backward steps are taken involuntarily when a patient halts.
- **Cause:** Parkinsonism.
  [**Kinesia paradoxa**—presented in Parkinson's disease patients, who generally cannot move but under certain circumstances of need exhibit a sudden, brief period of mobility (walking or even running)]

Scissoring Gait [Figs. 6D(viii).7A and B]

Seen classically with cerebral palsy due to bilateral spasticity.

Sensory Ataxia: Stamping Gait [Fig. 6D(viii).8]

- It is characterized by broad based, high stepping, stamping gait, and ataxia due to loss of proprioception (position sense). This type of ataxia becomes more prominent by removal of sensory input (e.g., walks with eyes closed) and becomes worse in the dark. Romberg's test is positive.
- **Cause:** Peripheral sensory (large fiber) lesions (e.g., polyneuropathy), posterior column lesion (vitamin B_{12} deficiency or tabes dorsalis).

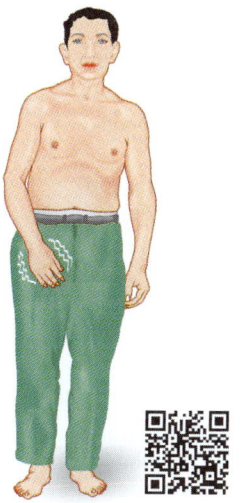
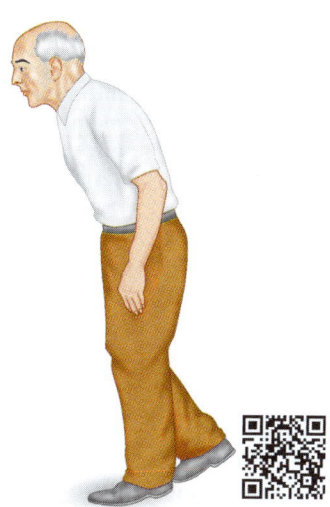
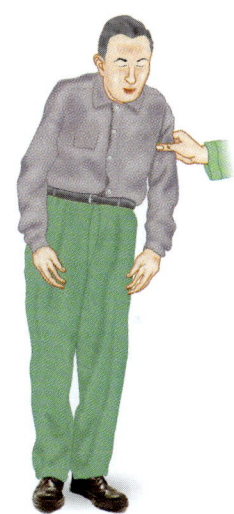

Stage 1: Unilateral involvement; early masking of facial expresion; affected arm is semiflexed position with tremor

Stage 2: Bilateral involvement with early postural changes; slow, shuffling gait with decreased excursion of legs

Stage 3: Pronounced gait disturbances and moderate generalized disability; postural instability with tendency to fall

Fig. 6D(viii).6: Stages of Parkinson's gait.

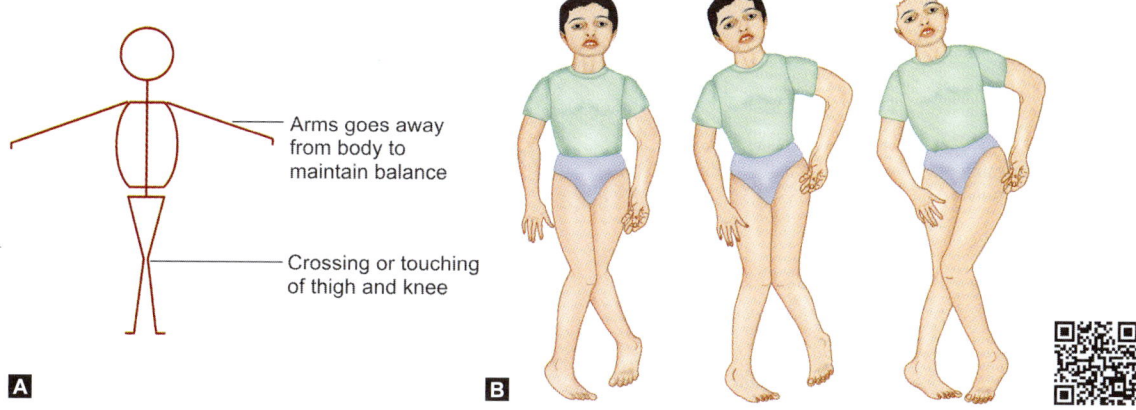

Figs. 6D(viii).7A and B: Scissoring gait.

Nervous System

Toe-walking or Equinus Gait
Heel strike is avoided. It is seen in patients with heel pain, clubfoot, congenital short Achilles tendon, and cerebral palsy.

Quadriceps Weakness Gait
Inability to maintain knee extension at heel-strike and patient may push on thigh to extend the knee and lock. It is seen in quadriceps paralysis.

Astasia-Abasia
It is a psychogenic pattern of walking in which the patient seems to alternate between a broad base for stability and a narrow, tightrope-like stance, with contortions of the trunk, and limbs that give the appearance of an imminent fall.

Alderman's Gait
Patient walks with chest and head thrown backwards with protuberant abdomen and legs thrown wide apart. It is seen in tuberculosis of lower thoracic and upper lumbar vertebra.

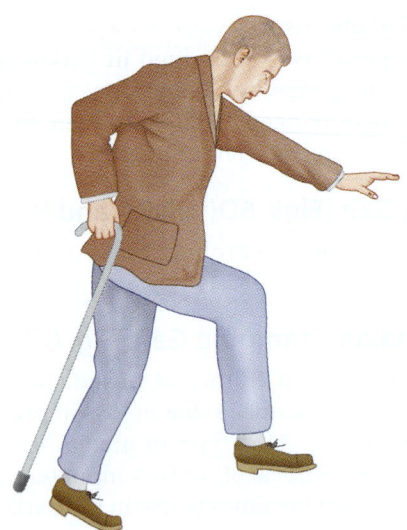

Fig. 6D(viii).8: Sensory ataxia.

Choreiform Gait (Hyperkinetic Gait)
- The patient will display irregular, jerky, and involuntary movements in all extremities. Walking may accentuate their baseline movement disorder.
- **Cause:** Sydenham's chorea, Huntington's disease, and other forms of chorea, athetosis or dystonia.

Antalgic or Painful Gait
Decreased duration of stance phase as the painful limb is unable to bear full weight. It is seen in any painful lesion of the lower extremity, i.e., foot, knee, and hip.

Coxalgic Gait [Figs. 6D(viii).9A and B]
In patients with hip pain, the upper trunk is typically shifted towards the affected side during the stance phase on the affected leg. This is an unconscious adaptive maneuver which reduces the force exerted on the affected hip during the stance phase.

GAIT ABNORMALITIES ANALYSIS

Gait initiation, maintenance, and termination	Difficulty starting	PD, atypical parkinsonism
	Freezing of gait	PD, atypical parkinsonism
	Inability to stop (festination)	PD, atypical parkinsonism
Stance width	Narrowed base of support	PD, spastic paraparesis
	Widened base of support	Cerebellar ataxia, sensory ataxia, vestibular ataxia
	Scissoring of the legs	Spastic paraparesis
	Unable to walk in a straight line, sideways deviation (veering) of gait	Unilateral vestibular ataxia, unilateral cerebellar ataxia
Step length, height, and cadence	Reduced step height	PD, parkinsonism; foot drop
	Small steps	PD, atypical parkinsonism, normal pressure hydrocephalus
	Irregular step size	Cerebellar ataxia, vestibular ataxia, chorea
	Reduced stance phase on the affected side (limping)	Pain (antalgic gait)
Arm swing	Unilaterally reduced	Hemiparesis, dystonia, PD
	Bilaterally reduced	PD, parkinsonism, dystonia
	Excessive	Chorea, levodopa-induced dyskinesias, NPH
	Tremor appearing in hand during walking	PD, parkinsonism

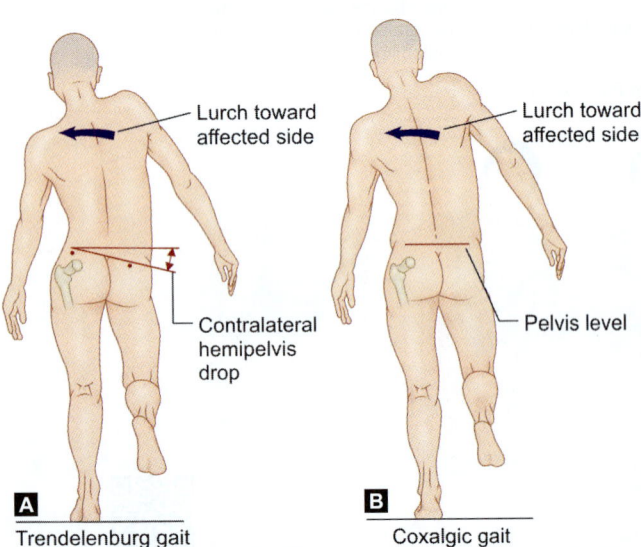

A Trendelenburg gait — Lurch toward affected side, Contralateral hemipelvis drop
B Coxalgic gait — Lurch toward affected side, Pelvis level

Figs. 6D(viii).9A and B: Trendelenburg gait versus coxalgic gait.

Contd...

Contd...

Movement fluidity	Dropped foot, lifting the leg higher than normal (steppage gait)	Neuropathy of common fibular nerve or sciatic nerve, L5 radiculopathy, Charcot–Marie–Tooth disease
	Knees giving way (buckling of the knees)	Quadriceps weakness (for example, limb-girdle myopathy, IBM)
	Locking of the knees	Cerebellar ataxia
	Pelvis drop at side of the swing leg, resulting in alternating lateral trunk movements (waddling gait and bilateral Trendelenburg gait)	Bilateral proximal muscle weakness in the leg and hip girdle
	Bizarre gait pattern	Chorea
Gait speed	Slow	PD
	Fast	Vestibular disease, Alzheimer's disease

(PD: Parkinson's disease; NPH: normal pressure hydrocephalus; IBM: inclusion body myositis)

BEDSIDE TESTS TO DIAGNOSE PES CAVUS AND PES PLANUS

Wet Test [Fig. 6D(viii).10]

There are three basic foot types, each based on the height of the arches. The quickest and easiest way to determine your foot type is by taking the "wet test," below. (1) Pour a thin layer of water into a shallow pan. (2) Wet the sole of your foot. (3) Step onto a shopping bag or a blank piece of heavy paper. (4) Step off and look down. Observe the shape of your foot.

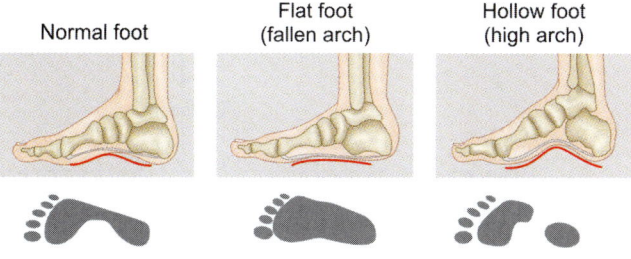

Fig. 6D(viii).10: Wet test and appearance.

D(ix). APPROACH TO INVOLUNTARY MOVEMENTS

MOVEMENT DISORDERS

Dyskinesia is abnormal uncontrolled movement and is a common symptom of many movement disorders [Flowcharts 6D(ix).1 and 6D(ix).2].

Movement disorders disrupt motor function by:
1. Abnormal, involuntary, unwanted movements (hyperkinetic movement disorders).
2. Curtailing (restricting) the amount of normal free flowing, fluid movement (hypokinetic movement disorders).

Flowchart 6D(ix).1: Categorization of movement disorders.

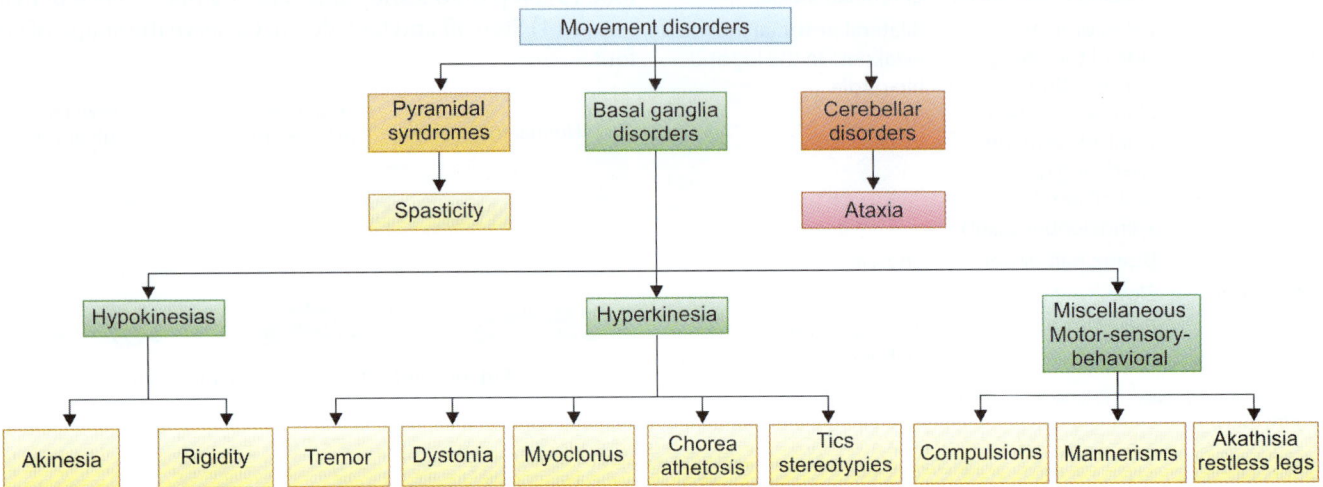

Flowchart 6D(ix).2: Systematic approach to movement disorders.

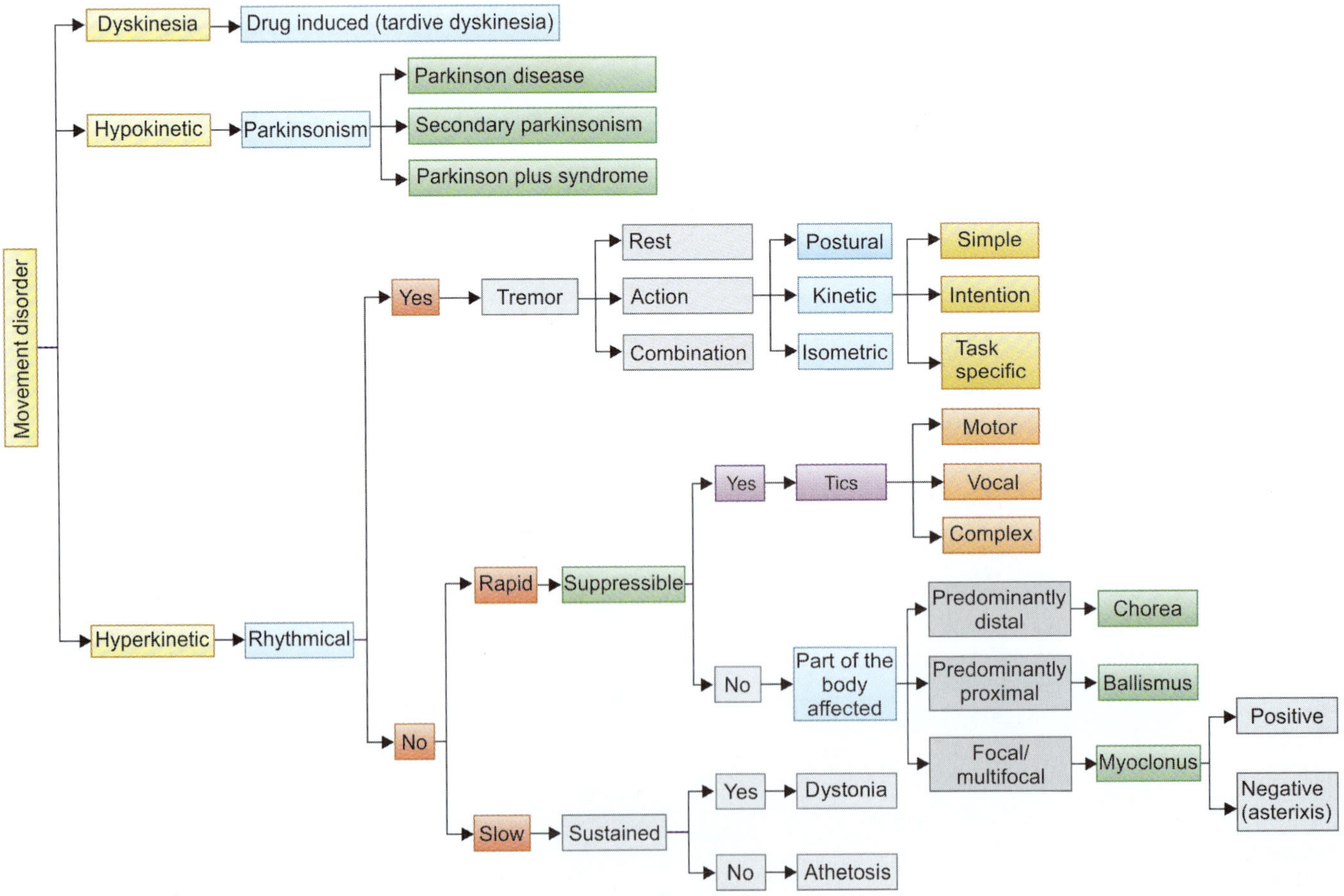

Site of Lesion

1. Parkinsonism → Contralateral substantia nigra
2. Unilateral hemiballismus → contralateral subthalamic nucleus
3. Chronic chorea → Caudate nucleus/putamen
4. Athetosis, dystonia → Contralateral putamen or thalamus
5. Myoclonus → Cerebellar cortex/thalamus
6. Rhythmic palatal/facial myoclonus → Central tegmental tract, inferior olivary nucleus, olivodentate fibers.

TREMOR

Series of involuntary, relatively rhythmic, purposeless, oscillatory movements due to intermittent muscle contractions:

- Simple tremor involves only a single muscle group
- Compound tremor involves several muscle groups
  - Several elements in combination
  - Resulting in a series of complex movements
- May be unilateral or bilateral
- Most commonly involves distal parts of the extremities—fingers or hands
- May also affect the arms, feet, legs, tongue, eyelids, jaw, and head
- May occasionally involve the entire body
  - Rate may be slow, medium, or fast
    - Slow: Oscillations of 3–5 Hz
    - Rapid: Oscillations of 10–20 Hz
  - Amplitude may be fine, coarse, or medium
  - The relationship to rest or activity is the basis for classification into two primary tremor types:
    1. Resting
    2. Action

Resting (static)
- Tremors are present mainly during relaxation (e.g., with the hands in the lap)
- Attenuate when the part is used
- Rest tremor is seen primarily in PD and other Parkinsonian syndromes

Action tremors

Postural tremors become evident when the limbs are: Maintained in an antigravity position (e.g., arms outstretched) *Types of postural tremor:* <ul><li>Enhanced physiological tremor (EPT)</li><li>Essential tremor (ET)</li></ul>	**Kinetic tremor:** Appears when making a voluntary movement. May occur at the beginning, during or at the end of the movement. For example, intention (terminal) tremor seen primarily in cerebellar disease	**Task specific tremor:** Occurs when performing highly skilled, goal-oriented tasks. For example, while writing or speaking

CHOREA

- Characterized by involuntary, irregular, purposeless, random, nonrhythmic hyperkinesias.
- Movements are spontaneous, abrupt, brief, rapid, jerky, and unsustained.
- Movements are actually random and aimless:
  - Rather than disrupting a voluntary task, it appears as if fragments of movements intrude; in some cases, there is loss of motor tone, known as "**motor impersistence**", which appears due to lapses in the ability to perform desired action.
- When asked to hold the hands outstretched, there may be constant random movements of individual fingers (**piano-playing** movements).
- If the patient holds the examiner's finger in her fist, there are constant twitches of individual fingers (**milkmaid grip**):
  - "**Jack in the box**" **tongue**/harlequin's tongue: Patient is unable to maintain tongue in protruded state and the tongue moves in and out.
- Blink rate is increased.

Causes

- Hereditary: Huntington's disease, benign chorea
- Drugs: Antiparkinsonian drugs, oral contraceptives
- Toxin: Alcohol, carbon monoxide poisoning
- Infections: Sydenham's chorea, encephalitis
- Metabolic: Hyperthyroidism, hypocalcemia
- Immunological: SLE, polyarteritis nodosa
- Vascular – chorea in primary polycythemia
- Pregnancy (chorea gravidarum)

ATHETOSIS

- Involuntary, irregular, coarse, somewhat rhythmic, and writhing or squirming in character (twisting).
- Hyperkinesias are slower, more sustained, and larger in amplitude than those in chorea.
- May involve the extremities, face, neck, and trunk.
- In the extremities, they affect mainly the distal portions, the fingers, hands, and toes:
  - Affected limbs are in constant motion (athetosis means "without fixed position")
  - Choreoathetosis refers to movements that lie between chorea and athetosis in rate and rhythmicity and may represent a transitional form.

Causes

- Cerebral palsy
- Congenital due to perinatal injury to the basal ganglia

HEMIBALLISMUS

Dramatic neurologic syndrome of wild, flinging (forceful), incessant (uninterrupted or continuous) movements that occur on one side of the body.

Due to infarction or hemorrhage in the region of the contralateral subthalamic nucleus.

- More rapid and forceful
- Involve the proximal portions of the extremities
- When fully developed, there are continuous, violent, swinging, flinging, rolling, throwing, flailing (thrashing) movements of the involved extremities.

- They are usually unilateral and involve one entire half of the body.
- Rarely, they are bilateral (biballismus or paraballismus) or involve a single extremity (monoballismus).

MYOCLONUS

Single or repetitive, abrupt, brief, rapid, lightning-like, jerky, arrhythmic, asynergic, involuntary contractions, involving portions of muscles, entire muscles, or groups of muscles.
- Seen principally in the muscles of the extremities and trunk, but the involvement is often multifocal, diffuse, or widespread.
- May involve the facial muscles, jaws, tongue, pharynx, and larynx.
- Myoclonus may appear symmetrically on both sides. Such synchrony may be an attribute unique to myoclonus.

Myoclonus has been classified in numerous ways including the following:
i. Positive versus negative
ii. Epileptic versus nonepileptic
iii. Stimulus sensitive (reflex) versus spontaneous
iv. Rhythmic versus arrhythmic
v. Anatomically (peripheral, spinal, segmental, brainstem, or cortical)
vi. By etiology (physiologic, essential, epileptic, and symptomatic)

- Encephalitis
- Juvenile myoclonic epilepsy (JME, Janz syndrome)
- Drug overdose
- Hypnic jerks (appear during the process of falling asleep)
- Hiccup
- Creutzfeldt–Jakob disease
- Subacute sclerosing panencephalitis (SSPE)
- Anoxic encephalopathy (Lance-Adams syndrome)

TIC

A "tic" is an involuntary movement or vocalization that is usually sudden onset, brief, repetitive, stereotyped but nonrhythmical in character, can be suppressed.

Types

Motor tics are associated with movements. Categorized as simple or complex.
Simple motor tics involve only a few muscles usually restricted to a specific body part.
- Examples of simple motor tics include eye blinking, shoulder shrugging, facial grimacing, neck stretching, mouth movements, jaw clenching, and spitting.

Vocal/phonic tics are associated with sound.
Simple vocal tics consist of sounds that do not form words, such as, throat clearing, grunting, coughing, and sniffing.
   Common complex vocal tics include repeating words or phrases out of context.
- Coprolalia: Use of socially unacceptable words, frequently obscene.
- Palilalia: Repeating one's own sounds or words.
- Echolalia: Repeating the last-heard sound, word, or phrase.

Gilles de la Tourette syndrome—associated with chronic motor and phonic tics.

DYSTONIA

- Refers to a syndrome of involuntary sustained or spasmodic muscle contractions involving cocontraction of the agonist and the antagonist.
- The movements are usually slow and sustained, and they often occur in a repetitive and patterned manner.
- They can be unpredictable and fluctuate.

Partial or focal	Generalized
- Spasmodic torticollis - Blepharospasm - Oromandibular dystonia - Writers cramp - Hemiplegic dystonia after stroke	- Dystonia musculorum deformans (idiopathic torsion dystonia) - Dopamine responsive dystonia: In childhood and generally involves the legs only - Drug-induced dystonia (metoclopramide, phenothiazine, haloperidol, chlorpromazine) - Symptomatic dystonia (after encephalitis, Wilsons disease)

Blepharospasm and Oromandibular Dystonia

Involuntary prolonged tight eye closure (blepharospasm) is associated with dystonia of mouth, tongue or jaw muscles (jaw clenching and tongue protrusion).

Writer's Cramp = Mogigraphia = Scrivener's Palsy

Symptoms usually appear when a person is trying to do a task that requires fine motor movements such as writing or playing a musical instrument.

MYOKYMIA

Myokymia, a form of involuntary muscular movement, usually can be visualized on the skin as vermicular or continuous rippling movements. This is common in outer aspect of thigh or upper arm.

AKATHISIA

Akathisia is a movement disorder characterized by a feeling of inner restlessness and a compelling need to be in constant motion, as well as by actions such as:
- Rocking while standing or sitting
- Lifting the feet as if marching on the spot
- Crossing and uncrossing the legs while sitting

RESTLESS LEGS SYNDROME/ "EKBOM'S SYNDROME"

- Spontaneous, continuous leg movements associated with paresthesia.
- These sensations occur only at the rest and relieved by movement.
- Causes: Familial, lumbar root disease, polyneuropathy, renal failure, and iron deficiency.

SYNKINESIS/MIRROR MOVEMENTS

Mirror movements are characterized by involuntary movements on one side of the body mirroring voluntary movements of the other side.

FASCICULATIONS

Fasciculations are visible, fine and fast, sometimes vermicular contractions of fine muscle fibers that occur spontaneously and intermittently but usually do not generate sufficient force to move a limb. Described as verminosis, because they look like *worms* moving below the dermis.

Involuntary contraction of the muscle fibers innervated by a motor unit.

Causes of Fasciculations

Fasciculations in healthy subjects	Coffee; exhaustive physical activity/fatigue; stress; **Benign fasciculations**
Fasciculations associated with movement disorders	Spinocerebellar degeneration-type 3; spinocerebellar degeneration-type 36; Parkinsonism (multiple system atrophy, ALS-plus syndromes)
Motor neuron diseases	**Amyotrophic lateral sclerosis;** progressive spinal muscular atrophies; benign monomelic amyotrophy; postpolio syndrome; Kennedy disease
Systemic diseases	**Hyperthyroidism;** hypophosphatemia; calcium disorders secondary to hyperparathyroidism; paraneoplastic myopathy
Drugs and/or intoxications by heavy metals pollutants	**Organophosphorus poisoning;** neostigmine; corticosteroids; succinylcholine; elemental mercury intoxication; atropine; lithium; nortriptyline; flunarizine; isoniazid

D(x). MENINGEAL SIGNS, SKULL, AND SPINE

SIGNS OF MENINGEAL IRRITATION

Nuchal Rigidity/Meningeal Stiffness

Meningeal tightness is a contracture of the paravertebral muscles, a defense against the secondary pain stemming from inflammation of the meninges.

Painful and permanent, it sometimes presents with the subject lying down, curled up with his or her back to the light, head back, and extremities half-bent. All attempts to flex the head provoke insurmountable and painful resistance. There is extreme neck stiffness; rotational and side-to-side movements are possible but aggravate the headache [**Fig. 6D(x).1**].

In **Kernig's sign**, patient is kept in supine position, hip and knee are flexed to a right angle, and then knee is slowly extended by the examiner. The appearance of resistance or pain during extension of the patient's knees beyond 135° constitutes a positive Kernig's sign [**Figs. 6D(x).2 and 6D(x).3**].

Brudzinski's Sign

Josef Brudzinski described four maneuvers for the clinical diagnosis of meningitis: The cheek sign, symphyseal sign, Brudzinski's leg sign/reflex, and Brudzinski's neck sign.

1.	**The cheek sign**	A positive cheek sign is elicited by applying pressure on both cheeks inferior to the zygomatic arch that leads to spontaneous flexion of the forearm and arm
2.	**Symphyseal sign** [Fig. 6D(x).4]	A positive symphyseal sign occurs when pressure applied to the pubic symphysis elicits a reflex hip and knee flexion and abduction of the leg

Contd...

Contd...

3.	**Brudzinski's leg sign/reflex** [Fig. 6D(x).5]	Brudzinski's contralateral reflex sign consists of reflex flexion of a lower extremity after passive flexion of the opposite extremity
4.	**Brudzinski's neck sign** [Figs. 6D(x).6 and 6D(x).7]	Brudzinski's neck sign is performed with the patient in the supine position. The examiner keeps one hand behind the patient's head and the other on chest in order to prevent the patient from rising. Reflex flexion of the patient's hips and knees after passive flexion of the neck constitutes a positive Brudzinski's sign

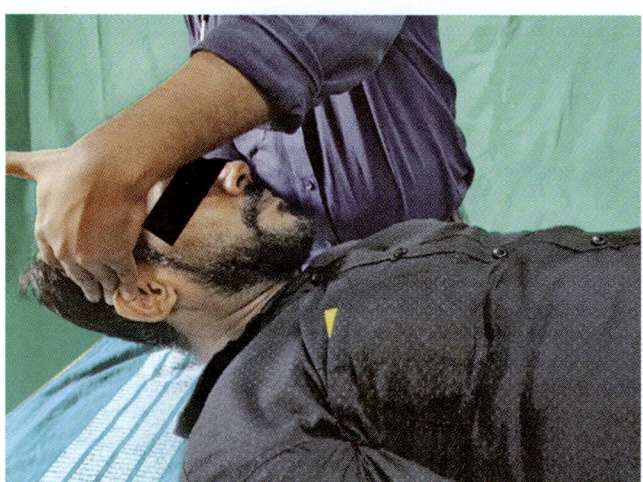

Fig. 6D(x).1: Examination of neck stiffness.

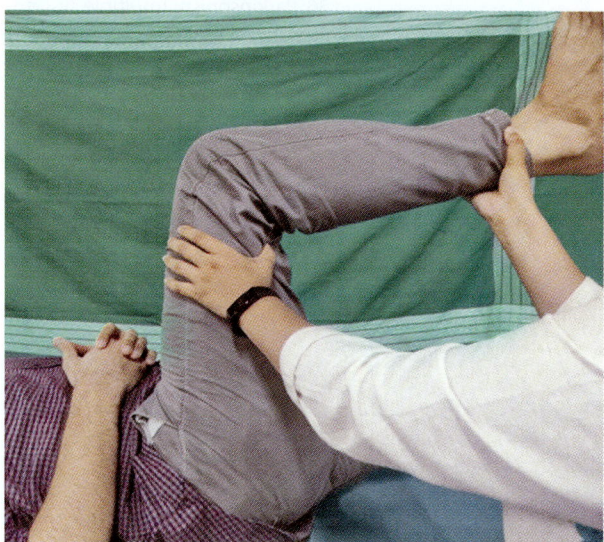

Fig. 6D(x).2: Demonstration of Kernig's sign.

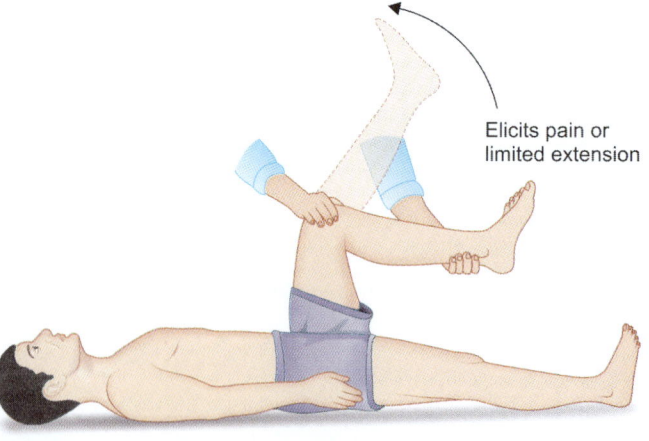

Fig. 6D(x).3: Illustration of Kernig's sign.

the arms brought back in a plane posterior to the pelvis to support the thorax.

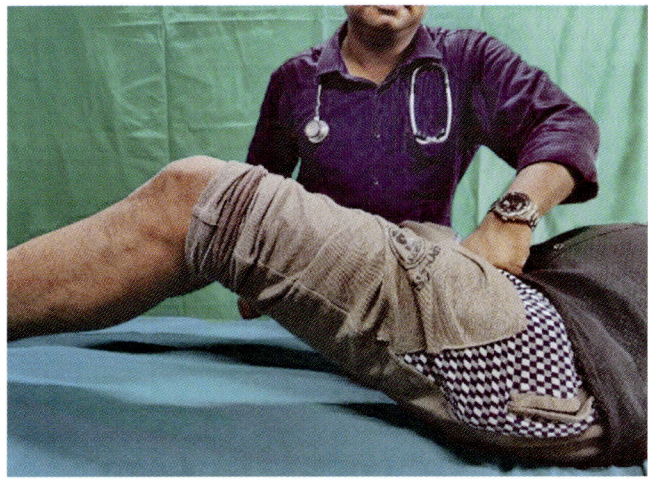

Fig. 6D(x).4: Symphyseal sign.

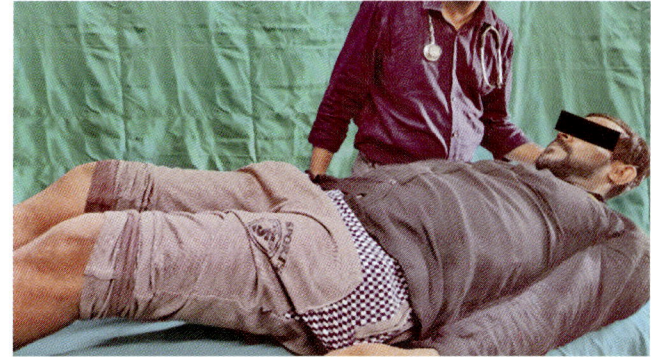

Fig. 6D(x).7: Brudzinski's neck sign.

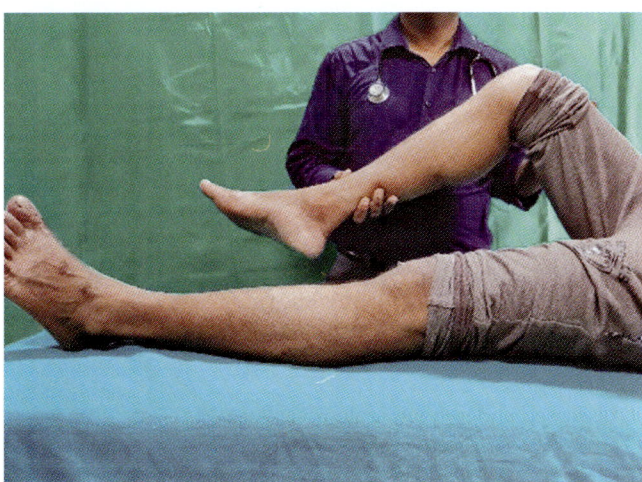

Fig. 6D(x).5: Brudzinski's leg sign/reflex.

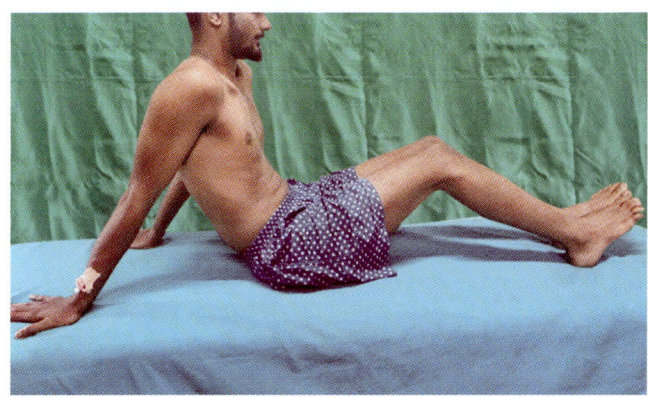

Fig. 6D(x).8: Tripod sign (Amoss's sign).

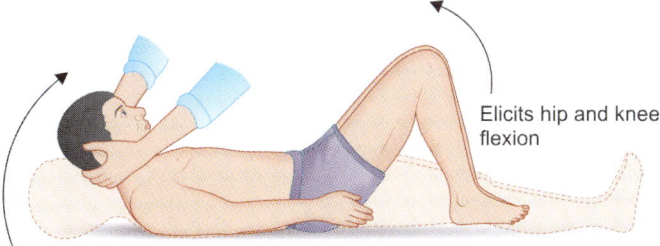

- Passive flexion of neck

Fig. 6D(x).6: Illustration of Brudzinski's sign.

Tripod sign, also known as the "Amoss's sign", is a useful sign of meningeal irritation.

The patient is asked to sit up in bed. This action requires active movement involving flexion of the neck. Although a normal patient sits up without supporting himself, a patient with meningeal irritation tries to sit up by supporting himself with his hands placed far behind him in the bed (like a tripod), in order to take the weight off the spine and prevent its flexion **[Fig. 6D(x).8]**. Severe meningeal irritation may result in the patient assuming the tripod position with the knees and hips flexed, the back arched lordotically, the neck extended, and

MENINGISM

Meningism, also called meningismus or pseudomeningitis, is a set of symptoms similar to those of meningitis but not caused by meningitis. Whereas meningitis is inflammation of the meninges (membranes that cover the central nervous system), meningism is caused by nonmeningitic irritation of the meninges usually associated with acute febrile illness, especially in children and adolescents.

Causes

Meningism:
- Meningitis
- Subarachnoid hemorrhage.

Other conditions that mimic meningism (also resist cervical rotation):
- Cervical spondylosis
- After cervical fusion
- Parkinson's disease
- Raised intracranial pressure, especially if there is impending tonsillar herniation
- Acute dystonic reaction
- Tetanus
- Strychnine poisoning

Intermittent neck stiffness is characteristic of Arnold–Chiari malformation.

EXAMINATION OF SKULL

- Size of skull—microcephaly, macrocephaly
- Shape/deformities
- Tenderness—fracture/metastasis
- Crackpot sound on percussion—hydrocephalus
- Bruits on auscultation—arteriovenous malformation (AVM), hemangioma

EXAMINATION OF SPINE

- Inspection—deformities, curvature—kyphosis, scoliosis, lordosis, dimple, tuft of hair, Pott's spine, and meningioma
- Palpation—tenderness, paraspinal spasm, and deformities
- Movements [Figs. 6D(x).9A and B].

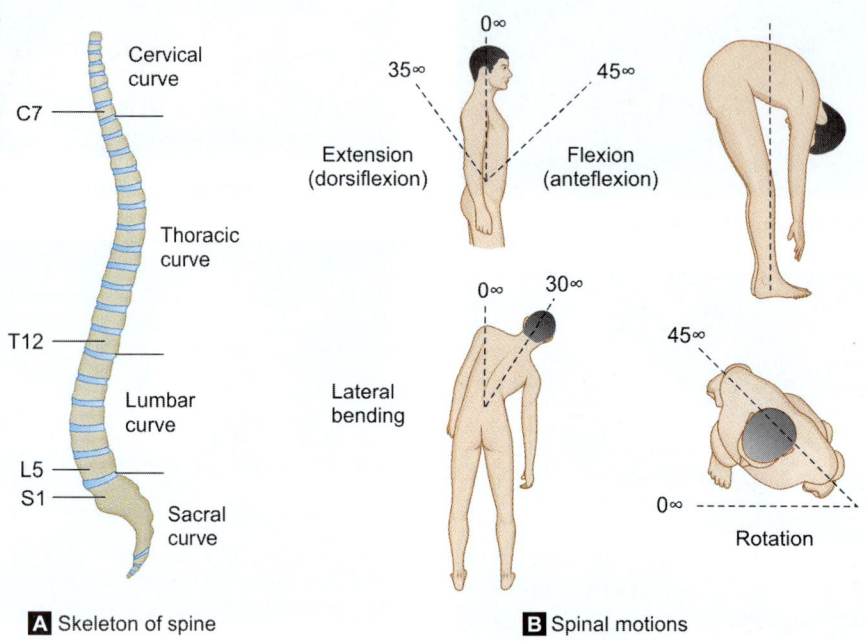

Figs. 6D(x).9A and B: Movements of spine (details discussed under rheumatology section).

AUTONOMIC NERVOUS SYSTEM TESTING

Common autonomic symptoms	Signs
▪ Orthostatic intolerance ▪ Dizziness ▪ Lightheadedness ▪ Fatigue ▪ "Coat hanger" headache ▪ Nausea ▪ Palpitations ▪ Near syncope and syncope **Genitourinary** ▪ Bladder urgency or frequency ▪ Incontinence ▪ Nocturia ▪ Erectile dysfunction ▪ Ejaculatory disturbances **Gastrointestinal** ▪ Diarrhea ▪ Constipation ▪ Fecal incontinence ▪ Postprandial fullness, cramping, or bloating **Sudomotor** ▪ Hyperhidrosis ▪ Hypohidrosis and anhidrosis	▪ Pupils—mid-dilated sluggish reacting pupil ▪ Pedal edema ▪ Resting tachycardia ▪ Postural hypotension ▪ Palpable urinary bladder ▪ Sweating abnormalities

Contd...

Contd...

Tests	
Cardiovagal innervation (parasympathetic innervation) - Heart rate (HR) response to deep breathing - Valsalva ratio, and - HR response to standing (30:15 ratio)	**"Spoon test":** A kitchen soup spoon, with its curved surface resting on the skin, was held between the thumb and forefinger, and was drawn slowly on the skin, using sufficient energy to overcome its weight without lifting it from the skin. When "sympathectomized" skin was crossed, the pull was smooth and unopposed; but where sweat gland innervation and sympathetic function was intact, the skin was moist, and the flow of the spoon was interrupted, and became sticky requiring readjustment of the strength of pull
Adrenergic - Beat-to-beat blood pressure (BP) responses to the Valsalva maneuver, sustained handgrip/diastolic hand grip test** and - BP and HR responses to tilt-up or active standing	**"Sustained handgrip test (SHT)":** This parameter indicates cardiac sympathetic response and DBP response to the sustained handgrip test—taken as the difference between the DBP just before release of handgrip and the mean of three resting DBP readings. The change in mean DBP in response to sustained handgrip test was interpreted as: - ≥16 mm Hg was taken as normal - 11–15 mm Hg as borderline - ≤10 mm Hg as abnormal
Sudomotor: - Quantitative sudomotor axon reflex test (QSART) - Thermoregulatory sweat test (TST) - Sympathetic skin response (SSR), and - Silastic sweat imprint - Quantitative direct and indirect test of sudomotor function (QIRT) - Sensitive sweat test (SST) - Sudoscan	

Head-Up Tilt-Table Testing

The patient lies supine on the tilt table. Beat-to-beat and oscillometric BP instruments are attached to each arm. ECG monitoring should take place throughout the test. Once the patient is comfortable, with feet resting on the footboard, a baseline BP is recorded for at least 3 minutes. The patient is then slowly tilted upright to an angle of 60–80°.

During testing, the patient is asked to report any symptoms. Both BP and HR are recorded throughout tilt-table testing, after which the patient is returned to a horizontal supine position.

Three well-described patterns of neurally-mediated syncope can occur during head-up tilt-table testing:
1. Vasodepression resulting in hypotension without bradycardia.
2. Cardioinhibition with a marked bradycardia (fewer than 40 beats/min) with or without significant hypotension.
3. Mixed, with both bradycardia and hypotension.

Valsalva Ratio

The Valsalva maneuver consists of respiratory strain which increases intrathoracic and intra-abdominal pressures and alters hemodynamic and cardiac functions.
- The patient is supine or with head slightly elevated to about 30°.
- The patient generates the increase in intrathoracic and intra-abdominal pressure of 40 mm Hg for 10–20 s by exhaling through a special mouthpiece (e.g., a 5 or 10 mL syringe, the plunger rod of which has been removed and which is fitted with a small hole and connected to a blood pressure measuring device.
- Following cessation of the Valsalva strain, the patient relaxes and breathes at a normal comfortable rate.
- The ECG is monitored during the strain and 30–45 seconds following its release.
- The maximal heart rate of phase II actually occurs about 1 second following cessation of the strain.
- The minimal heart rate occurs about 15–20 seconds after releasing the strain.

Lesion	Phase I	Phase II (early)	Phase II (late)	Phase III	Phase IV
None	Stress dependent increase in blood pressure	Arterial pressure drop	Increase in arterial blood pressure	Short-term drop in blood pressure	Excessive rise in blood pressure
Parasympathetic	Normal	Reduced blood pressure	Normal	Normal	Normal
Sympathetic, slight	Normal	Slight increase in blood pressure drop	Reduced to missing blood pressure increase	Normal	Slight reduction of the increase in blood pressure
Sympathetic, moderate	Normal	Significant increase in blood pressure drop	Missing blood pressure increase	Normal	Significant reduction in blood pressure increase
Sympathetic, severe	Normal	Severe drop in blood pressure	Missing blood pressure increase	Normal	Missing blood pressure increase

Physiological and pathological changes in arterial blood pressure during the various phases of the Valsalva maneuver.

Pressor Functional Tests

The isometric hand grip test evaluates changes in heart rate and blood pressure over a 3 min compression of a hand dynamometer or a partially inflated blood pressure cuff to approximately one-third of the maximum fist closure force. In the cold pressor test, the stimulus lies in the 2 min immersion of one hand in ice water. In the mental arithmetic test, the patient must solve a complex sequential arithmetic problem during a 2 min interval.

All pressor tests lead to an increase in blood pressure and heart rate. In the isometric hand grip test and cold pressor test, peripheral receptors are activated in addition to an important cerebral activation. The effect of other stimuli, such as the mental arithmetic test, depends primarily on cerebral activation.

DISEASES ASSOCIATED WITH AUTONOMIC DYSFUNCTION [TABLE 6D(x).1]

Table 6D(x).1: Diseases commonly associated with autonomic dysfunction.

- **Preganglionic autonomic failure:**
  - Multiple system atrophy
  - Parkinson's disease with autonomic failure
- **Ganglionic and postganglionic disorders**
  - Pure autonomic failure
- **Peripheral neuropathies and neuronopathies with autonomic dysfunction**
  - *Acute and subacute (preganglionic and postganglionic):*
    - Acute pandysautonomia
    - Guillain–Barré syndrome
    - Paraneoplastic pandysautonomia
    - Others (porphyria, toxins, drugs)
  - *Chronic small fiber (postganglionic) neuropathies:*
    - Diabetes
    - Amyloidosis
    - Hereditary (familial dysautonomia, Fabry's disease)
  - *Subacute or chronic sensory and autonomic ganglionopathies:*
    - Paraneoplastic
    - Sjogren's syndrome
  - *Other peripheral neuropathies:*
    - Infections (human immunodeficiency virus)
    - Connective tissue disease (systemic lupus erythematosus)
  - Metabolic-nutritional (alcohol, uremia, vitamin B_{12} deficiency)

CHAPTER 7

Rheumatology

A. CASE SHEET FORMAT

HISTORY TAKING

Name:
Age:
Sex:
Residence:
Occupation:

Chief Complaints

1. _____ × days
2. _____ × days
3. _____ × days

History of Presenting Illness

Joint pain:
- Duration:
- Onset:
- No. of joints involved:
- Symmetry:
- Progression:
- Variation:
- Aggravating factors:
- Relieving factors:

Morning stiffness:
- Duration of stiffness:
- Onset:
- Progression:
- Variation:
- Aggravating:
- Relieving factors:

Deformities:
- Duration:
- Onset:

Ulcers:
- Duration:
- Onset:
- Progression:

Fever:
- Episodic or continuous
- Grade
- Chill and rigors
- Aggravating factors
- Relieving factors
- Variation
  - Diurnal variation

History of:
- Petechiae
- Purpura
- Other bleeding manifestations
- Breathing difficulty
- Dyspnea on exertion
- Numbness and tingling of legs
- Skin lesions
- Endocrine abnormalities

Past history:
- Asthma
- Chronic obstructive airway disease
- Tuberculosis
- History of contact with tuberculosis
- Diabetes mellitus (DM)
- Hypertension (HTN)
- Ischemic heart disease (IHD)
- Seizure disorder

Family history:
(Draw pedigree chart representing three generations)

Personal history:
- Bowel habits
- Bladder habits
- Appetite
- Loss of weight
- Occupational exposure
- Sleep
- Dietary habits and taboo
- Food allergies

- Smoking (in smoking Index or Pack years)
- Alcohol history (_____grams of alcohol/day or_____ units of alcohol/week)

Menstrual and obstetric history:
- G_P_L_A_
- Age of menarche
- Menopause at
- Flow—amenorrhea/oligomenorrhea/menorrhagia

Summarize:

Differential diagnosis:
1.
2.
3.

EXAMINATION

Rheumatological examination includes a thorough general examination and systemic examination along with examination of locomotor system.

General Examination

Patient
- Conscious
- Oriented
- Cooperative
- Obeying commands

Body Mass Index (BMI)
- Weight (in kg)/height^2 (in meters)
- Grading according to WHO for Southeast Asian countries

Vitals
- **Pulse**
  - Rate
  - Rhythm
  - Volume
  - Character
  - Vessel wall thickening
  - Radio-radial delay and radio-femoral delay
  - Peripheral pulses
- **Blood pressure**
  - Right arm
  - Left arm
  - Both lower limbs
- **Respiration**
  - Rate
  - Abdominothoracic (male) or thoracoabdominal (female)
  - Usage of accessory muscles
- **Jugular venous pulse**
  - Waveform
- **Jugular venous pressure**
  - _____cm of blood above sternal angle (+ 5 cm water)
- **Temperature**_____degree of Celsius or Fahrenheit measured at_____site.

Physical Examination
- Pallor
- Icterus
- Cyanosis
- Clubbing
- Lymphadenopathy [systemic lupus erythematosus (SLE) and Still's disease]
- Edema

Other Head to Toe
- Skin
- Nails
- Oral cavity
- Mucous membrane
- Eyes

Locomotor System Examination

Rapid screening of the locomotor system can be done by **GALS screen** (**G**ait-**A**rms-**L**egs-**S**pine) with the patient undressed, observe the patient from front, back, and sides. Observe his gait, check his arms (inspect and palpate), check his legs (inspect and palpate), and check his spine (inspect and palpate).

Examination of the Individual Joints

[Regional Examination of Musculoskeletal System (REMS)]

We have 14 joint areas in the body on either side namely:
1. Proximal and distal interphalangeal joints
2. Metacarpophalangeal joints
3. Carpometacarpal joints of thumb
4. Wrist joint
5. Elbow joint
6. Shoulder joint
7. Acromioclavicular joint
8. Sternoclavicular joint
9. Temporomandibular joint
10. Hip joint
11. Knee joint
12. Ankle joint
13. Subtalar joint
14. Small joints of foot including midtarsal, metatarsophalangeal, and interphalangeal joints

Each of the joints is examined under the following headings:

Inspection: Look for swelling, skin, and deformity

Palpation
- Look for tenderness and warmth
- Palpate for synovial thickening
- Look for **crepitus** (crepitus can also be auscultated) (Fine crepitus—synovitis or bursitis; coarse crepitus—cartilage or bone damage)

- Look for range of movement of joint (both active and passive movements)

Example: *At knee joint there is swelling on inspection and on palpation synovial thickening present, warmth and tenderness present, crepitus felt. The range of movement is painful and restricted in both active and passive movement at the joint.* Also examine the **tendons, bursae, ligaments, synovium, and muscles** around the joint.

Examination of Spine

Look for the curvature of the spine. Normally there is cervical lordosis, thoracic kyphosis, lumbar lordosis, and sacral kyphosis. List if any deformities present.

Movements of the spine	
Cervical spine	- Rotation - Flexion - Extension - Lateral bending
Thoracolumbar spine	- Flexion - Extension - Lateral bending - Rotation - Schober's test - Straight leg raising test
Sacroiliac joint	- Direct pressure - Patrick's test - Gaenslen's test

B. DIAGNOSIS FORMAT

Based on chronicity
Acute/chronic

Based on symmetry
Symmetrical/nonsymmetrical

Based on inflammation
Inflammatory/non-inflammatory

Based on number of joints involved
Mono/oligo/polyarthritis

Associated features
- With/without deformities
- With/without axial spine involvement
- With systemic manifestations in the form (pleural effusion, anemia, uveitis, etc.)

Disease severity
- DAS28
- Simplified and clinical disease activity indices (SDAI and CDAI)
- Rheumatoid arthritis severity scale (RASS)

EXAMPLES

Example 1

Chronic symmetrical inflammatory polyarthritis with swan neck deformity of fingers, with no axial spine involvement, with systemic features in the form of anemia and interstitial lung disease—I would like to consider diagnosis of **rheumatoid arthritis.**

CDAI score 7

Example 2

Chronic recurrent inflammatory monoarthritis involving right first MTP joint with deformities, without axial spine involvement or systemic manifestations—I would like to consider diagnosis of **gout.**

NOTES

C. DISCUSSION ON SYMPTOMATOLOGY AND EXAMINATION

DISCUSSED IN THE FOLLOWING HEADINGS

1. Symptomatology
2. Examination of skin, hands, and eyes
3. Examination pattern of musculoskeletal system
4. Examination of upper limbs
5. Examination of lower limbs
6. Examination of spine
7. Examination of other joints
8. Examination of other systems in rheumatological disorders
9. Discussion on common rheumatological diseases
10. Scoring systems

1. SYMPTOMATOLOGY

Arthralgia (subjective): Only pain around the joint

Arthritis (objective): Pain + other signs of inflammation (redness/swelling/increased temperature/loss of function)

Synovitis: Inflammation of synovial membrane

Tenosynovitis: Inflammation of the tendon sheath

Enthesitis: Inflammation of site of attachment of ligament, tendon or capsule to the periosteum or bone

Myositis: Inflammation of muscle

Arthritis—presentation	
Duration	• Acute (presenting within hours to days) Chronic (persisting for weeks or longer)
Number of joints involved	• Monoarticular (only 1 joint) • Oligoarticular/pauciarticular (2–4 joints) • Polyarticular (5 joints or more)
If more than one joint is involved	• Symmetric (or) asymmetric • Additive (or) migratory
Type	Inflammatory or noninflammatory (see below)
Deformities	Present (or) absent Deformities are usually seen in: • Rheumatoid arthritis • Psoriatic arthritis • Osteoarthritis • Reiter's disease • Chronic gout
Precipitating factors like	• Sexually transmitted disease (STD) • Infection • Trauma • Alcohol • Diarrhea
Associated features	Constitutional symptoms: • Fever, fatigue, and weight loss • Extra-articular manifestations and systemic manifestations • Comorbid conditions

Note: Treatment history should be taken in detail.

Inflammatory versus Noninflammatory Disease

Features	Inflammatory (rheumatoid arthritis)	Noninflammatory (osteoarthritis)
Age of onset	Usually 20–40 years but may begin at any age	Most commonly over 50 years of age
Speed of onset	Rapid over weeks to months	Slow; over years
Systemic symptoms	Fatigue, low-grade fever, anorexia. Extra-articular manifestations: Rheumatoid nodules, Sjogren's syndrome, Felty syndrome	No systemic symptoms
Joint affection	Symmetrical	Asymmetrical
Joint symptoms	Painful, swollen, stiff joints, and muscle aches	Joints painful without-swelling
Joints involved	Primarily affects small joints [metacarpophalangeal (MCP) and proximal interphalangeal (PIP)] with sparing of DIP	Affects large weight bearing joints (hip, knee or the spine). Affects proximal interphalangeal (PIP) and distal interphalangeal (DIP) joints
Stiffness	Morning stiffness for >1 hour. Stiffness occurs after periods of rest/inactivity (the so-called "gel phenomenon")	Morning stiffness for <30 minutes. Stiffness is generally mild and occurs after periods of activity
Relation of movement with pain	Movement or mild to moderate activity decreases pain	Movement increases the pain (worsens with activity) and improves with rest
Examination of joint	Swollen, red, warm, tender, and painful	Swollen, cool, and hard on palpation. When severely inflamed (as in acute gout or septic arthritis), can have erythema of the overlying skin
Radiological findings	Bony erosions, soft-tissue swelling, angular deformities, periarticular osteopenia	Loss of joint space and damage to articular cartilage, osteophytes
Rheumatoid factor (RF) and antinuclear antibody (ANA)	Positive	Negative

Contd...

Contd...

Erythrocyte sedimentation rate (ESR) and C-reactive protein	Both are often raised	Usually normal but transient elevation of ESR may occur due to synovitis
White blood cell (WBC) count in the synovial fluid	WBC count is >2,000/mm³ in septic arthritis and not in rheumatoid arthritis	WBC count is <2,000/mm³

Causes of Arthritis

Acute monoarthritis	
Inflammatory	Crystal disease (e.g., gout), infectious disease, spondyloarthropathy, rheumatoid arthritis
Mechanical	Trauma, avascular necrosis

Acute polyarthritis	
Infectious	Bacterial, human immunodeficiency virus (HIV)
Noninfectious	Rheumatoid arthritis, spondyloarthropathy, other connective tissue diseases, crystal (gout), sarcoidosis, malignancy, leukemia, sickle cell anemia

Chronic monoarthritis	
Inflammatory	Crystal disease, infectious disease (e.g., tuberculosis, fungal), spondyloarthropathy, rheumatoid arthritis
Noninflammatory	Osteoarthritis, avascular necrosis, neuropathic arthropathy, villonodular synovitis

Chronic polyarthritis	
Inflammatory	Rheumatoid arthritis, spondyloarthropathy, other connective tissue diseases
Mechanical	Osteoarthritis
Crystal	Gout
Metabolic	Infiltrative, metabolic, hypothyroidism

Approach to Musculoskeletal Complaint

	Musculoskeletal Complaint				
	Distribution				
	Polyarthritis (≤4 Joints)		Monoarthritis/oligoarthritis (1–3 joints)		Non-articular
	Acute	Chronic	Acute	Chronic	
Non-inflammatory	• Hemoglobinopathies • Amyloid arthropathies	• Osteoarthritis	• Meniscal tear • Ostearthritis flare • Reflax sympathetic dystrophy	• Osteoarthritis • Osteonecrosis • Neuropathic arthritis • Hemochromatosis • Pigmented villonodular synovitis	• Trauma • Fracture • Fibromyalgia • Reflex sympathetic dystrophy
Inflammatory	• Viral arthritis • Serum sicknenss • Drug-induced arthritis • Early onset CTC • Rheumatic fever • Palindromic rheumatism • Remitting seronegative symmetrical synovitis with pitting edema (RS3PE)	• Rheumatoid arthritis • Undifferentiated polyarthritis • Inflammatory osteoarthritis • Mixed connective tissue disease (MCTD) • Lupus, scleroderma • Polyarticular JIA • Adult syphilis disease	• Infectious arthritis • Gout • Pseudogout • Reactive arthritis • Chlamydial arthritis	• Psoriatic arthritis • Spondylo-arthropathies • Pauciarticular JIA • Indolent infectious arthritis	• Bursitis • Tendinitis • Polymyalgia rheumatica

2. EXAMINATION OF SKIN, HANDS, AND EYES

Skin changes in rheumatology	
Erythema	Septic arthritis crystal arthropathy
Palpable purpura (Fig. 7C.1)	Vasculitis
Ulcers over skin (Fig. 7C.2)	Vasculitis
Rash	Systemic lupus erythematosus (SLE) [malar or discoid rash (Fig. 7C.3)] Vasculitis Drugs Stills disease
Violaceous scaly lesions	Psoriasis

Contd...

Keratoderma blennorrhagica Circinate balanitis	Reiter's disease
Mucosal ulcers (Fig. 7C.4)	Behcet's disease SLE
Dryness of skin	Sjogren's disease
Thickened hard skin (Figs. 7C.5A to C)	Systemic sclerosis Scleroderma
Pyoderma gangrenosum	Inflammatory bowel disease
Palmar erythema	Rheumatoid arthritis
Photosensitivity	Development of rash on exposure to sunlight of less than 30 minutes (SLE)

Contd...

Rheumatology

Contd...

Digital gangrene	Raynaud's and medium vessel vasculitis
Alopecia	SLE Scleroderma
Heliotrope rash and Gottron's papules	Dermatomyositis
Salt and pepper appearance	Scleroderma (most prominently on the upper back and chest)
Livedo reticularis (Fig. 7C.6)	SLE Antiphospholipid antibody (APLA) syndrome Sneddon's syndrome, polyarteritis nodosa
Raynaud's	Systemic sclerosis, vasculitis Mixed connective tissue disorder
Sclerodactyly	Progressive systemic sclerosis

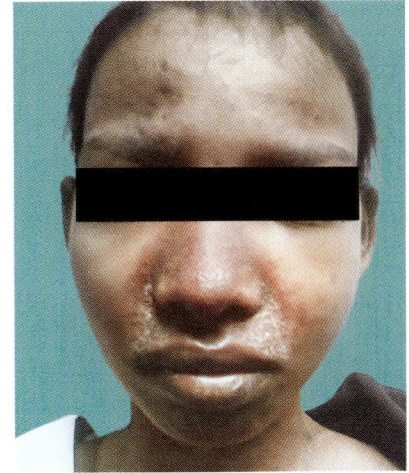

Fig. 7C.3: Systemic lupus erythematosus with malar rash and alopecia.

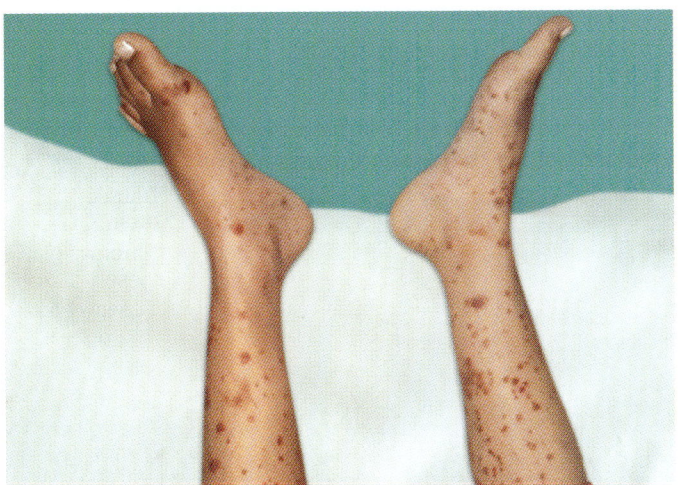

Fig. 7C.1: Palpable purpura over lower legs in Henoch–Schönlein purpura.

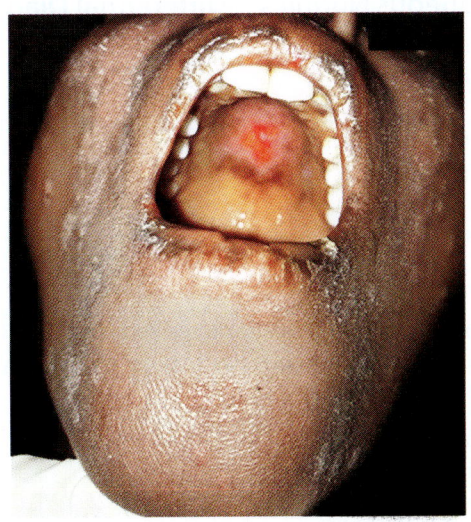

Fig. 7C.4: Mucosal ulcers in SLE.

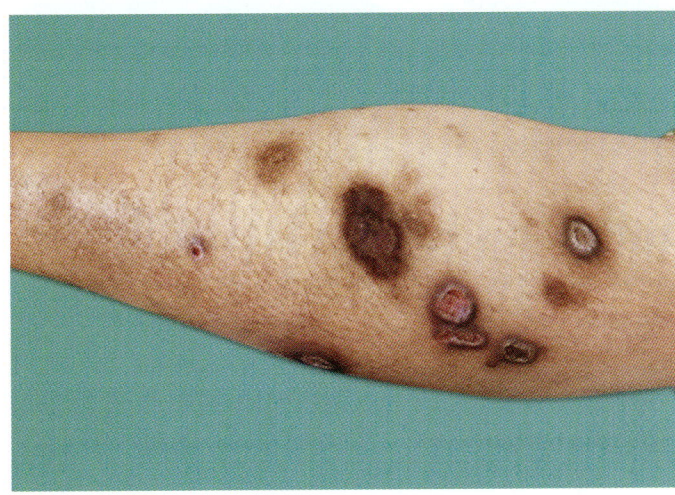

Fig. 7C.2: Ulcers on the leg in medium vessel vasculitis.

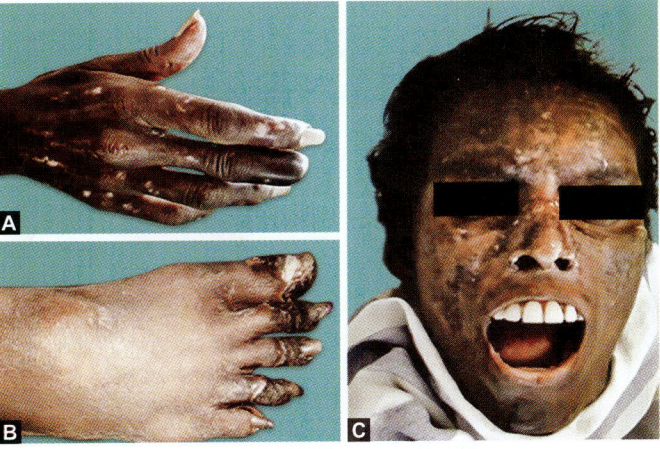

Figs. 7C.5A to C: Systemic sclerosis: (A and B) Shiny and thickened skin of hands and feet; (C) Mask-like face with decreased oral aperture.

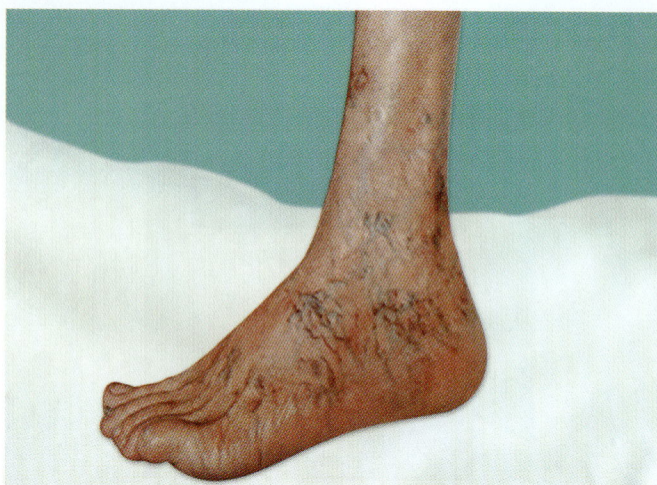

Fig. 7C.6: Livedo reticularis—mottled reticulated vascular pattern that appears as a lace-like purplish discoloration of the skin. It is due to swelling of the venules caused by obstruction of capillaries.

Subcutaneous Nodules—Differential Diagnosis

- Rheumatoid arthritis
- Rheumatic fever
- Gout
- Erythema nodosum*
- Sarcoidosis
- SLE
- Hyperlipidemia.

*Erythema Nodosum (Fig. 7C.7)

It is a type of panniculitis characterized by painful reddish nodules in the subcutaneous tissue most commonly seen on the shin.

Common causes include:
- Tuberculosis
- Leprosy
- Sulfonamides and other drugs
- Streptococcal infection
- Sarcoidosis
- Inflammatory bowel disease.

Nail Changes

Clubbing	▪ Fibrosing alveolitis ▪ Hypertrophic Osteoarthropathy
Pitting and onycholysis (Fig. 7C.8)	Psoriasis*
Splinter hemorrhages	Vasculitis

*Nail Changes in Psoriasis

Involvement is common and may be observed up to 50% of patients with psoriasis. These include:
a. "Thimble pitting" of the nail plate;
b. Distal separation of the nail plate from the nail bed (onycholysis);
c. Yellow-brown discoloration underneath the nail plate ("oil drop" sign);
d. Subungual hyperkeratosis; and
e. Thickening of the nail (onychodystrophy).

For diagnosis of nail involvement: >6 nails should be involved with each nail should have >20 pits.

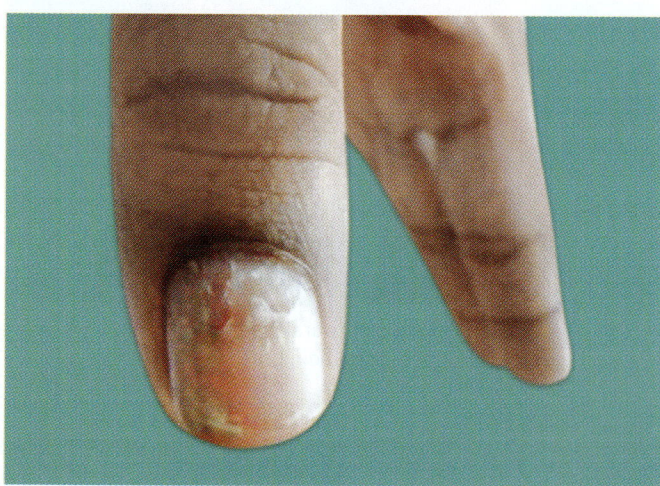

Fig. 7C.8: Nail changes in psoriasis.

Eye Changes

Dryness of eyes	Sjogren's syndrome
Episcleritis/scleritis (Fig. 7C.9)	Rheumatoid arthritis
Iritis/iridocyclitis	Ankylosing spondylitis
Conjunctivitis	Reiter's disease
Tenosynovitis of superior oblique	Rheumatoid arthritis (Brown's syndrome)
Scleromalacia perforans	Rheumatoid arthritis

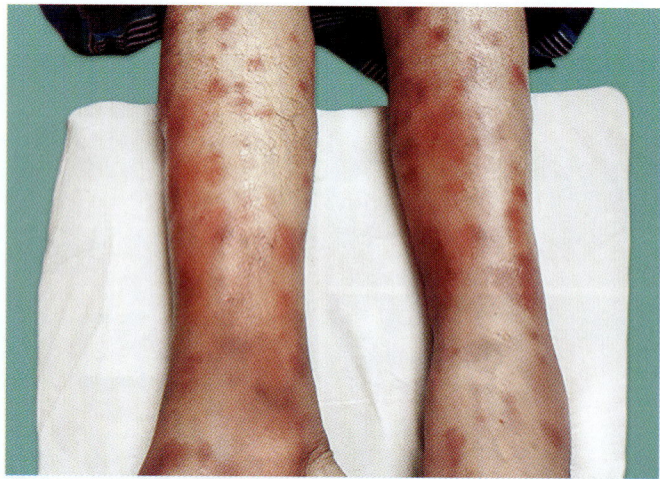

Fig. 7C.7: Erythema nodosum.

Rheumatology

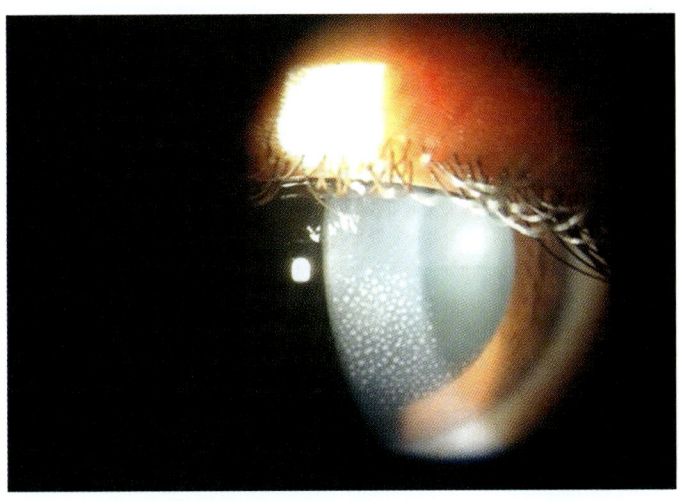

Fig. 7C.9: Slit-lamp examination showing keratitis.

3. EXAMINATION PATTERN OF MUSCULOSKELETAL SYSTEM

Gait, arms, legs, spine (GALS) screening

Gait	Observe the gait
Arms	- Examine the range of movement of joints - Joint deformities - Synovial thickening
Legs	- Examine the range of movement of joints - Joint deformities - Synovial thickening - Special tests
Spine	- Look for spine deformity - Special test

Regional examination of musculoskeletal system (REMS) examination (look, feel, move)	
Look for	- Swellings - Redness - Rashes - Scars - Muscle wasting
Feel for	- Temperature - Swelling - Tenderness
Move	- Full range of movement—active and passive (refer the table and figure) **(Figs. 7C.10A to H)** - Restriction—mild/moderate/severe
Function	- Functional assessment of joint
All the joints have to be examined in the above headings.	

Range of movement of joints (Figs. 7C.10A to H):

	Flexion	Extension	Abduction	Adduction	Rotation
Wrist	70°	70°	30°	30°	
MCP	45°	90°			
PIP	120°				
DIP	90°	10°			
Elbow	160°	5°			
Shoulder	160°	60°	175°	50°	70°
Hip	110°	30°	30°	30°	45°
Knee	130°				
Ankle	40° (dorsiflexion)	50° (plantar flexion)			

Others:
Subtalar joint—has 5° of inversion and eversion.
Midtarsal joint—has 30° of inversion and eversion.

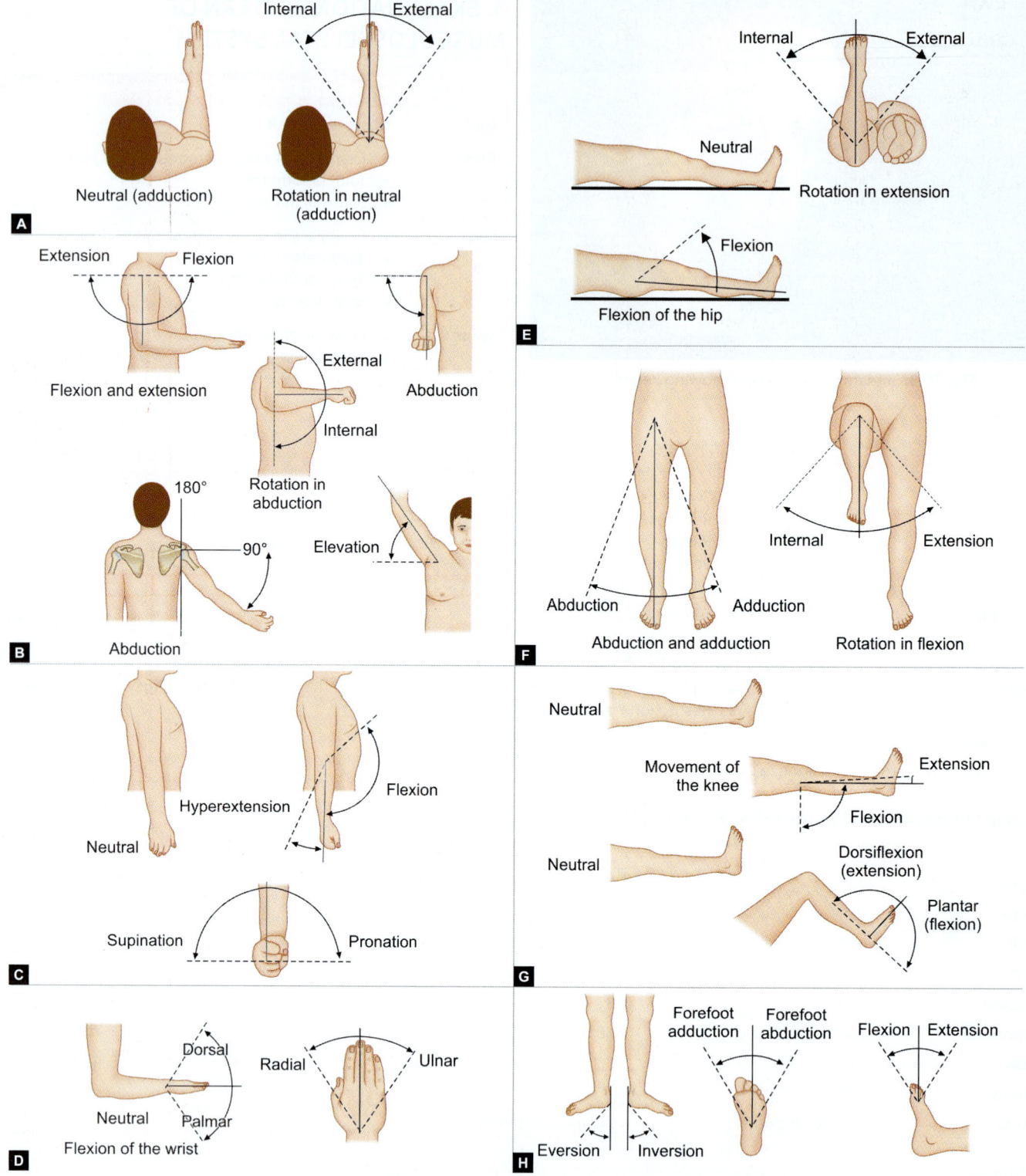

Figs. 7C.10A to H: Demonstration of range of movement of joints.

4. EXAMINATION OF UPPER LIMBS

Examination of Shoulder

Examination of glenohumeral joint (Fig. 7C.11):
- Examine for tenderness and swelling along the joint line as shown in **Figure 7C.11**.

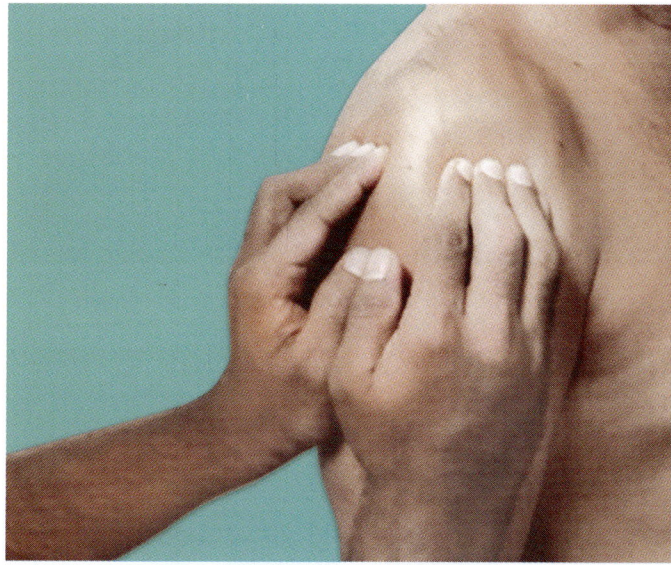

Fig. 7C.11: Image showing examination of tenderness and swelling along the joint line of shoulder joint.

Impingement test (Fig. 7C.12):

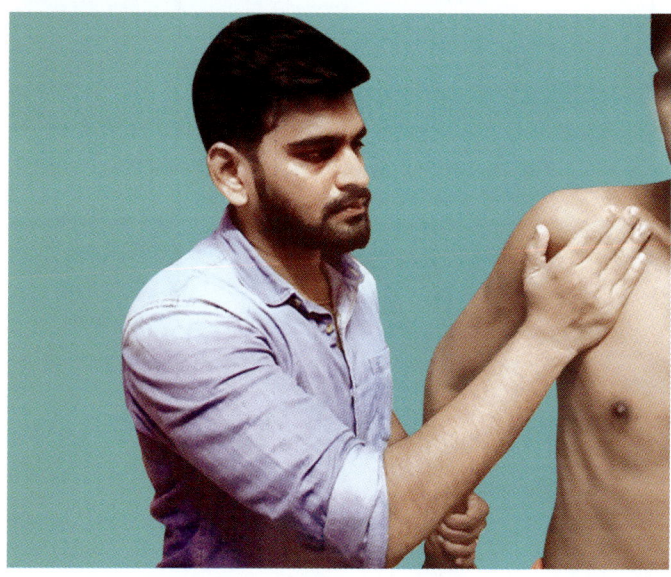

Fig. 7C.12: Demonstration of impingement test.

Apprehension test (Fig. 7C.13):
- Flex the patients elbow to 90°
- Abduct the patients shoulder to 90°
- Now attempt external rotation of the shoulder
- Apprehension to the test is considered positive suggesting glenohumeral instability with possibility of labral tear.

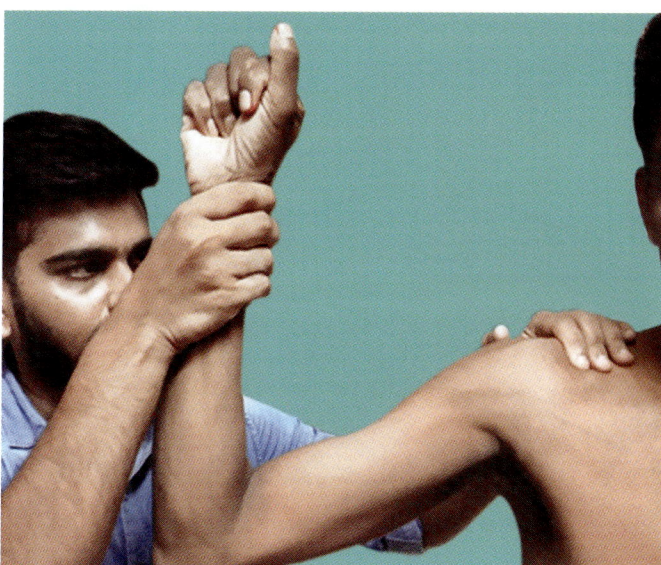

Fig. 7C.13: Demonstration of apprehension test.

Examination of Elbow (Fig. 7C.14)
- Palpate the joint for tenderness and synovial thickening along the joint line as shown in **Figure 7C.14**.

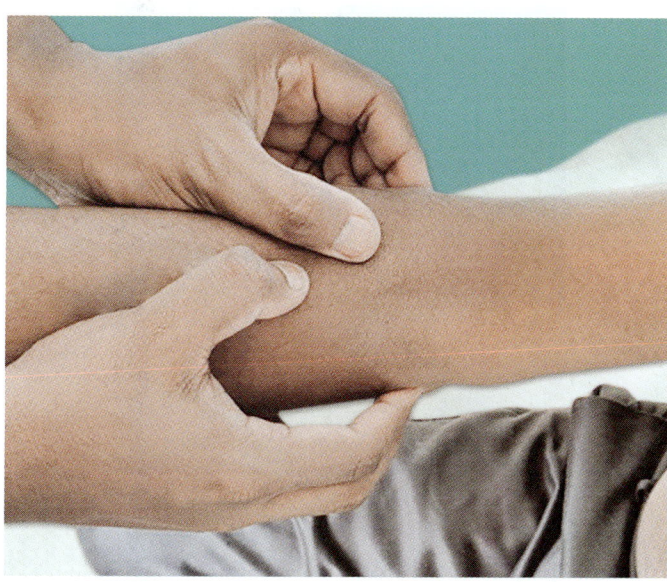

Fig. 7C.14: Palpation of elbow.

Examination of Wrist Joint

(Two-thumb technique) (Fig. 7C.15):
- The examiner's thumb should follow the third metacarpal bone on the dorsal aspect of the hand until a dimple is reached at the capitate level.
- Continuous pressure is exerted by the thumb.
- The other thumb is used to intermittently apply pressure approximately half an inch away on the wrist joint in order to identify swelling and/or tenderness.

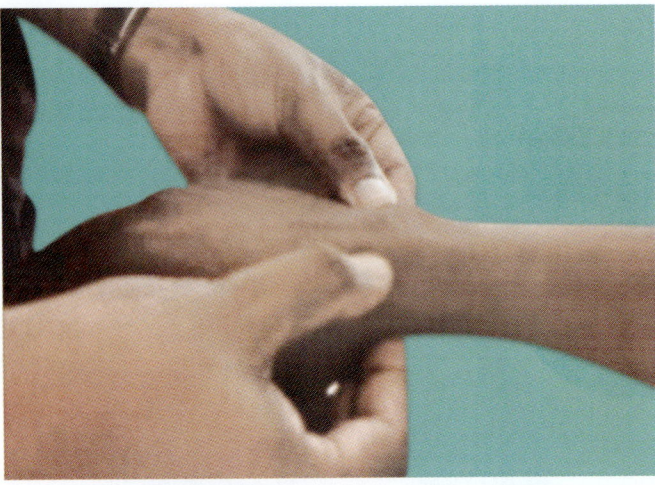

Fig. 7C.15: Examination of wrist joint.

Prayer sign (Fig. 7C.16):
- The patient is asked to dorsiflex both the wrist and hold the palms together actively as in praying
- Pain or inability to perform this activity would suggest joint involvement or carpal tunnel syndrome
- Also seen with diabetic cheiroarthropathy.

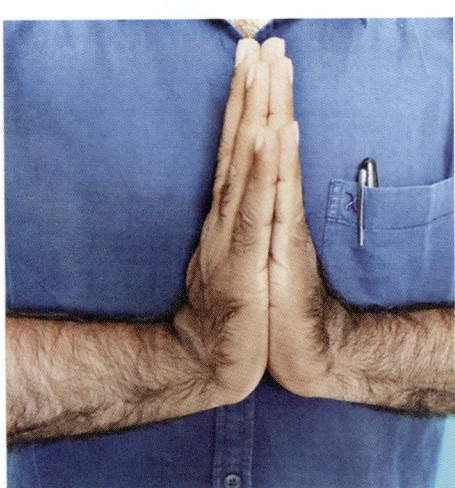

Fig. 7C.16: Demonstration of prayer sign.

Metacarpophalangeal Joint Assessment (Figs. 7C.17A to C)

- **Scissor technique:** A scissor-like shape is made with the fingers. The patient's hand is held from the sides at the MCP level **(Fig. 7C.17A)**.
- The MCPs are flexed to 90°. The thumbs are used to palpate the joint—one to apply pressure to the joint, the other to assess for effusion, swelling, and/or tenderness **(Fig. 7C.17B)**.
- **Squeeze test:** Squeeze the metacarpophalangeal joints as shown in **Figure 7C.17C** and watch for tenderness.

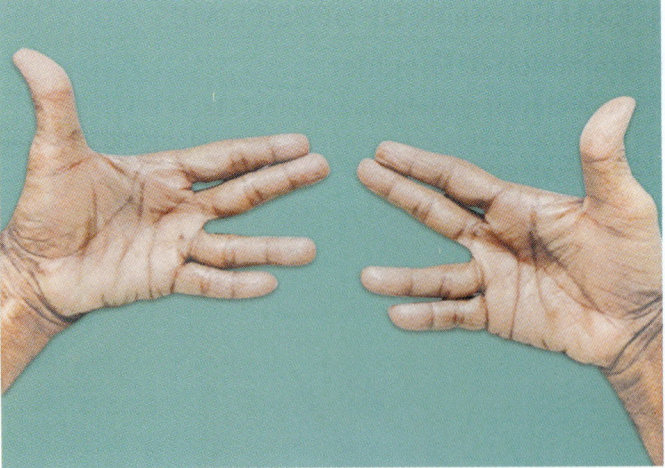

Fig. 7C.17A: Scissor-like shape is made with the fingers.

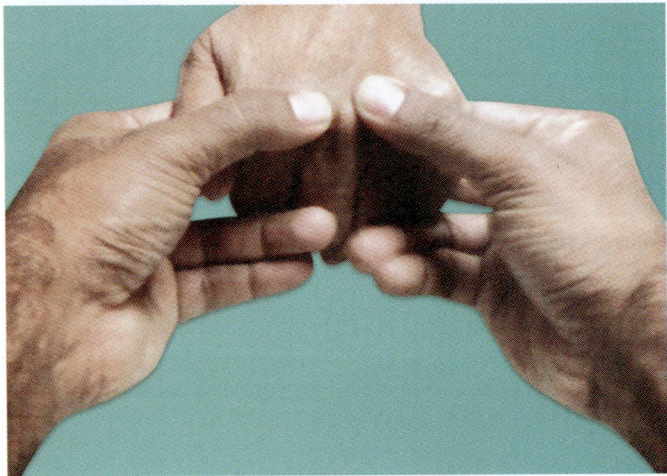

Fig. 7C.17B: Applying pressure on the MCP.

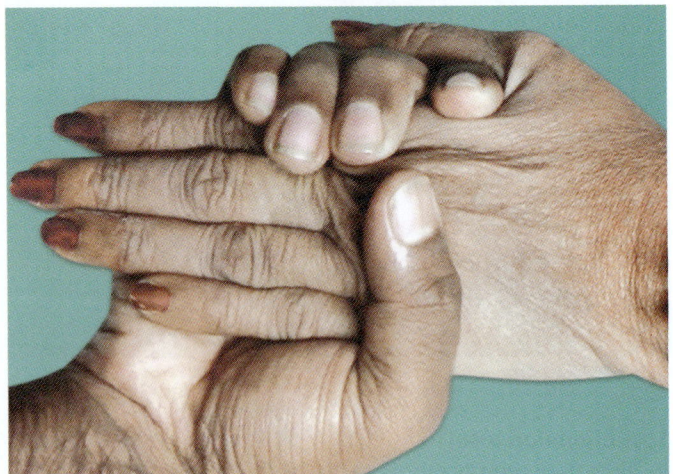

Fig. 7C.17C: Squeeze test of hand for assessment of metacarpophalangeal joint.

Interphalangeal Joint Assessment (Fig. 7C.18)

Four-finger technique:
Each interphalangeal joint is held by the thumb and index finger of one hand of the examiner. Pressure is applied until the distal finger becomes whitened due to low blood supply. The thumb and index finger of the examiner's other hand are used palpate the joint to identify effusion, swelling, and/or tenderness.

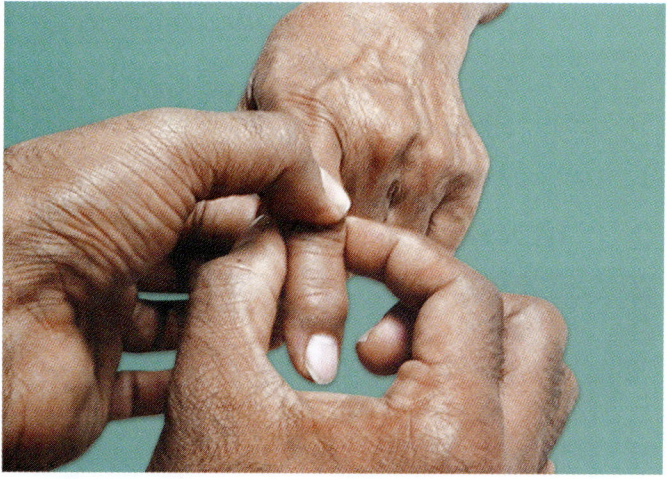

Fig. 7C.18: Examination of interphalangeal joints (four finger technique).

Deformities of hand	
Spindling of the fingers	It is the earliest finding characterized by swelling of the proximal, but not the distal interphalangeal joints.
Swan-neck deformity (Figs. 7C.19 and 7C.20)	It is due to hyperextension of the proximal interphalangeal joints (PIP) with flexion of the distal interphalangeal joints (DIP). At DIP joint, there is elongation or rupture of attachment of the extensor tendon to the base of the distal phalanx; this results in mallet deformity of distal joint and in addition, an extensor tendon imbalance, leading to hyperextension deformity at PIP joint.
Boutonniere' or "button-hole" deformity (Figs. 7C.19 and 7C.21)	This deformity is due to flexion of the PIP joints and extension of the DIP joints. Disruption of the central slip of the extensor tendon and the triangular ligament allows each of the conjoint lateral bands of the digit to slide volarly resulting in a pathologic flexion force and an extension lag; all tendons traversing the PIP joint in this setting elicit flexion of the joint.
Ulnar deviation (Fig. 7C.22)	It results from subluxation of the metacarpophalangeal (MCP) joints, with subluxation of the proximal phalanx to the volar side of the hand.

Contd...

Contd...

Hitchhiker's thumb (Fig. 7C.23)	A condition where the thumb can bend backwards to an angle of almost 45°. Thumb flexes at the metacarpophalangeal joint and hyperextends at the interphalangeal joint.
"Z" deformity (Fig. 7C.24)	It is due to radial deviation of the wrist, ulnar deviation of the digits with palmar subluxation of the first MCP joint with hyperextension of the first interphalangeal (IP) joint.
Carpal tunnel syndrome	Due to synovial proliferation in and around the wrists producing compression of the median nerve.
Bow string sign	Prominence of the tendons in the extensor compartment of the hand.
Heberden's nodes (Fig. 7C.25)	DIP swelling in osteoarthritis.
Bouchard's node (Fig. 7C.25)	PIP swelling in osteoarthritis.
Sausage digits (Fig. 7C.26)	Dactylitis involving both PIP and DIP as seen in psoriatic arthritis.
Pencil in cup deformity	Psoriatic arthritis.
Arthritis mutilans	Psoriatic arthritis.

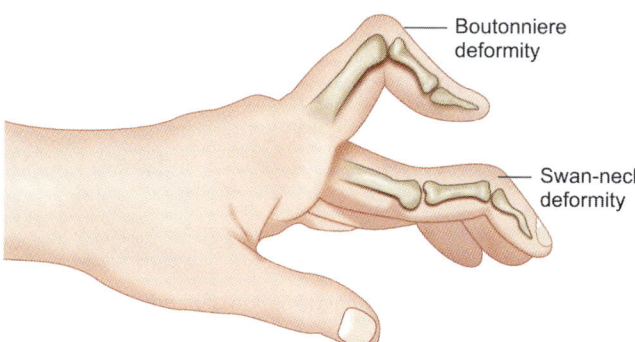

Fig. 7C.19: Boutonniere and swan-neck deformity.

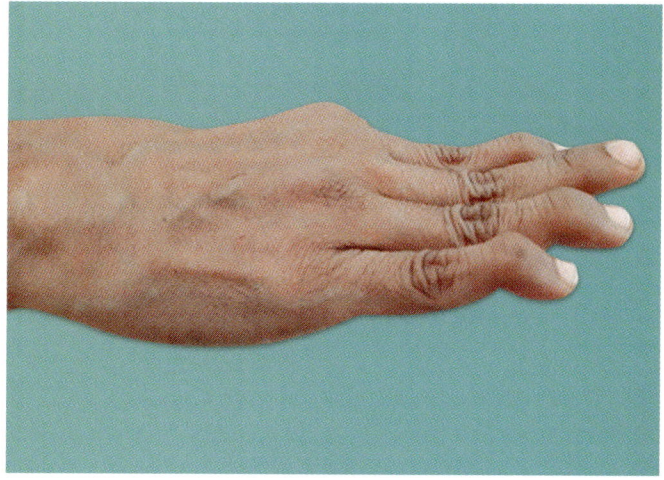

Fig. 7C.20: Swan-neck deformity.

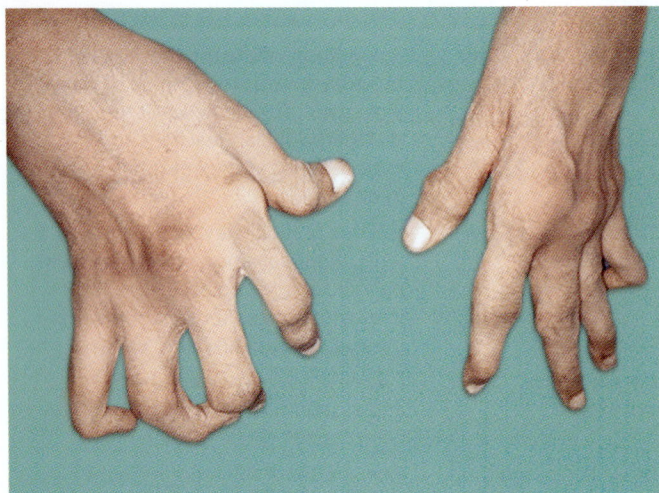

Fig. 7C.21: Boutonniere deformity.

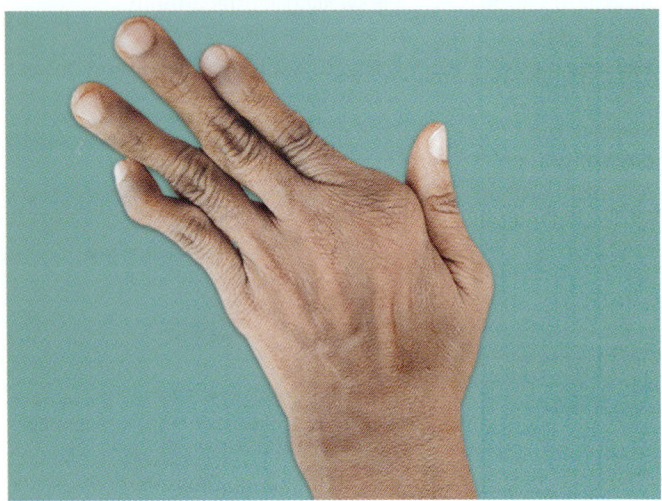

Fig. 7C.22: Ulnar deviation of hand.

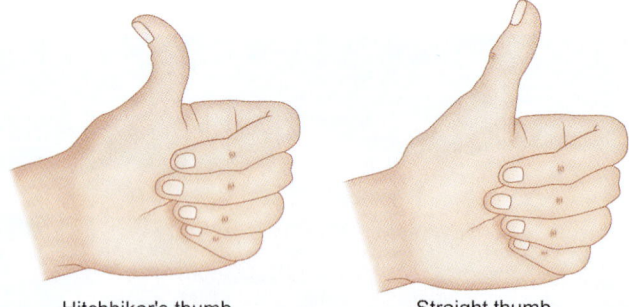

Fig. 7C.23: Hitchhiker's thumb.

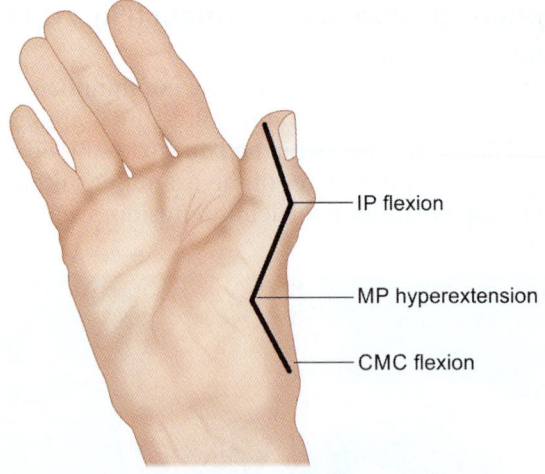

Fig. 7C.24: Z-shaped deformity of thumb in RA.

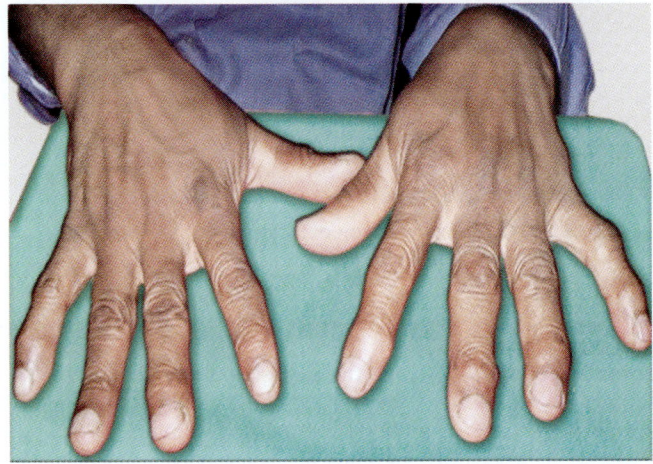

Fig. 7C.25: Osteoarthritis showing Heberden's nodes (on DIP) and Bouchard's nodes (on PIP).

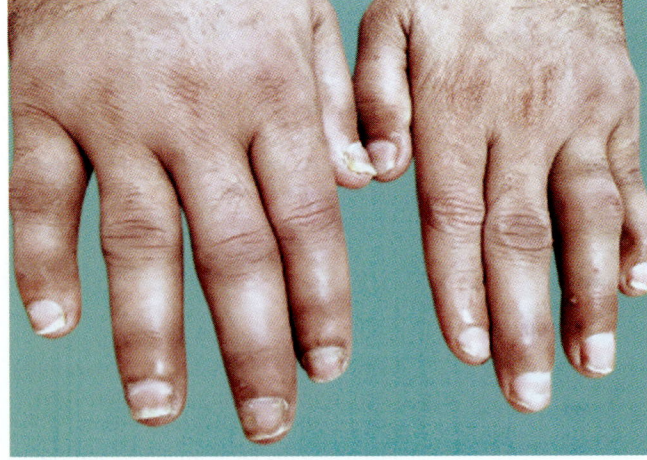

Fig. 7C.26: Sausage digits in psoriatic arthritis and psoriatic nails.

Rheumatology

5. EXAMINATION OF LOWER LIMB

Examination Hip Joint

Trendelenburg Test (Fig. 7C.27)
- Assesses the proximal hip muscles strength.
- This involves patient alternately standing on each leg alone.
- In a negative test, the pelvis remains level.
- In an abnormal test, the pelvis will dip to the contralateral side suggesting gluteus medius weakness.
- This test is abnormal, if the hip is involved either due to arthritis or avascular necrosis. Also proximal muscle weakness can be secondary to drugs used like steroids.

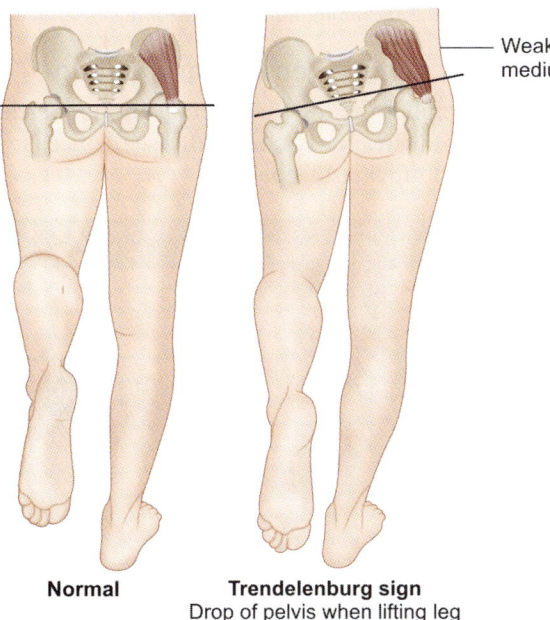

Fig. 7C.27: Trendelenburg sign.

Thomas Test (Fig. 7C.28)
- To look for fixed flexion deformity of hip.
- Keep one hand under the patient's back to ensure that there is no lumbar lordosis.
- Fully flex one hip.
- If the opposite leg lifts off the couch, there is a fixed flexion deformity (normally as the pelvis tilts, the hip would extend allowing the leg to remain on the couch).

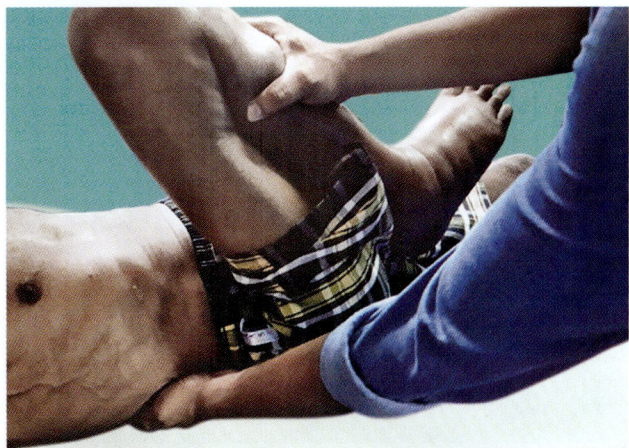

Fig. 7C.28: Demonstration of Thomas test.

Examination of Knee Joint
- Palpation of knee joint to look for tenderness and synovial thickening (**Fig. 7C.29**).

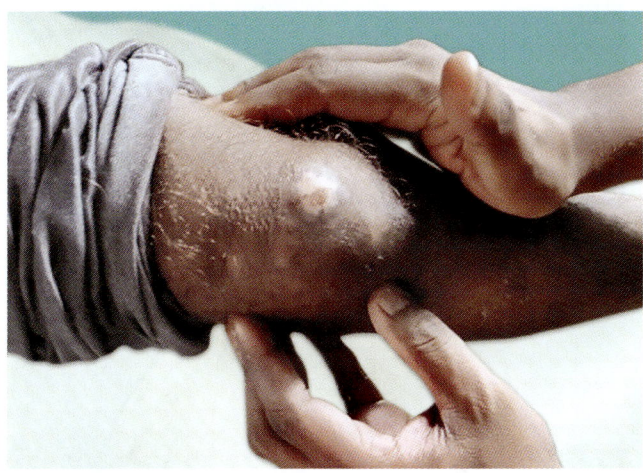

Fig. 7C.29: Demonstration of palpation of knee joint.

Patellar Tap Test
- Used to detect effusion in the knee joint.
- Slide your hand down the patient's thigh compressing the suprapatellar pouch (**Fig. 7C.30**).
- This forces all the fluid to collect behind the patella.
- With two fingers of the other hand push the patella down gently (**Fig. 7C.31**).
- In a positive test, the patella will bounce back with the tap.

Bulge Sign/Cross Fluctuation Sign (Figs. 7C.32A and B)
- Stroke the medial side of the knee upwards towards the suprapatellar pouch.
- This empties the medial compartment of the fluid.
- Now stroke the lateral side downwards.
- The medial side will now refill and bulge indicating joint effusion.

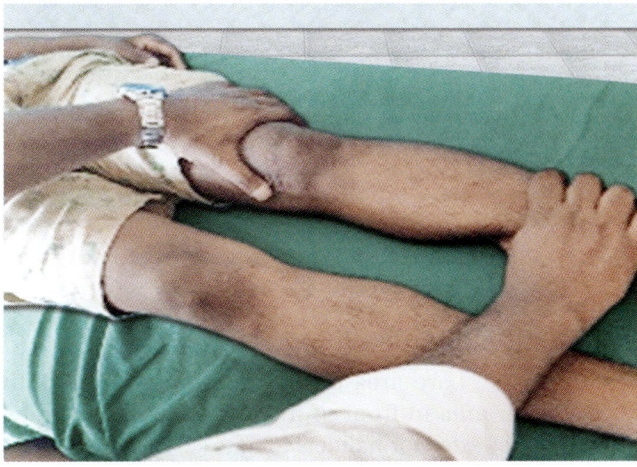

Fig. 7C.30: Slide your hand down the patient's thigh compressing the suprapatellar pouch.

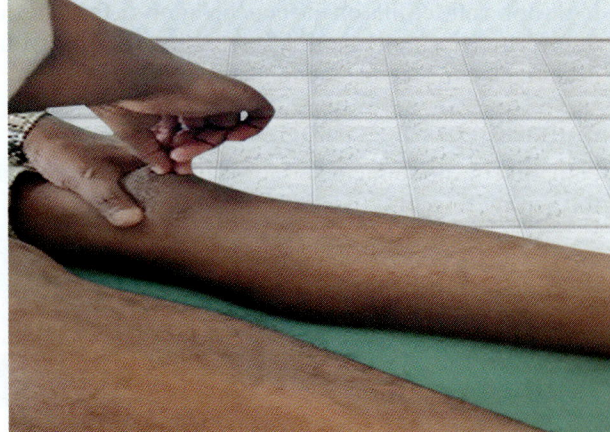

Fig. 7C.31: With two fingers of the other hand push the patella down gently.

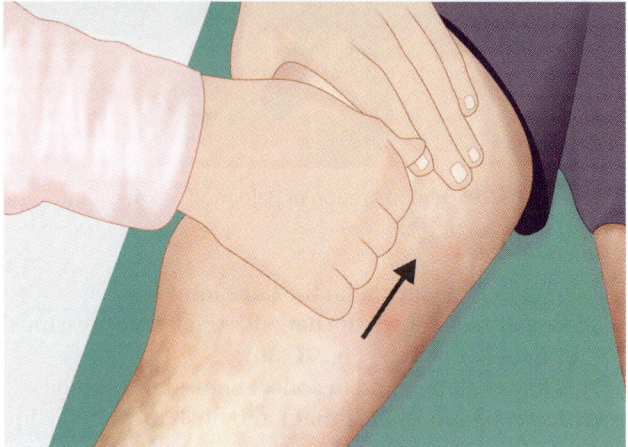

Fig. 7C.32A: The cross fluctuation sign (bulge sign): Stroke the medial side of the knee upwards towards the suprapatellar pouch.

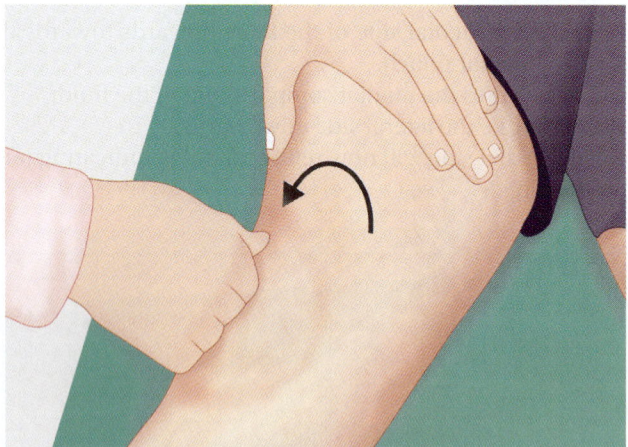

Fig. 7C.32B: The cross fluctuation sign (bulge sign): Stroke the lateral side downwards.

Examination of Ankle Joint

- Palpate the bare area of the ankle [bare area is the triangular area in front of the ankle, between the two tendons of extensor hallucis longus (EHL) and extensor digitorum longus (EDL)] for tenderness and synovial thickening **(Fig. 7C.33)**.

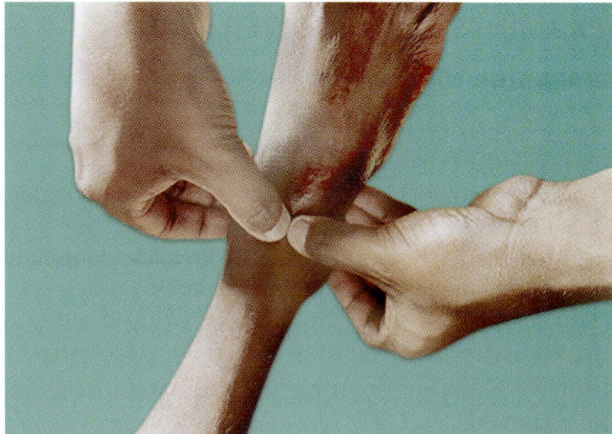

Fig. 7C.33: Examination of ankle joint.

Examination of Achilles Tendon for Swelling

- Palpate the Achilles tendon for swelling and tenderness **(Fig. 7C.34)**. Enthesitis is classically seen in case of seronegative spondyloarthropathies.

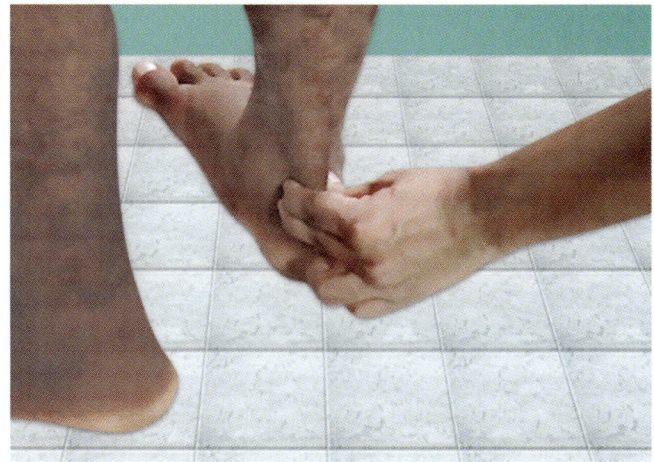

Fig. 7C.34: Examination of swelling over Achilles tendon.

Examination of Metatarsophalangeal Joints

- Squeezing the metatarsophalangeal joints to look for pain **(Fig. 7C.35)**

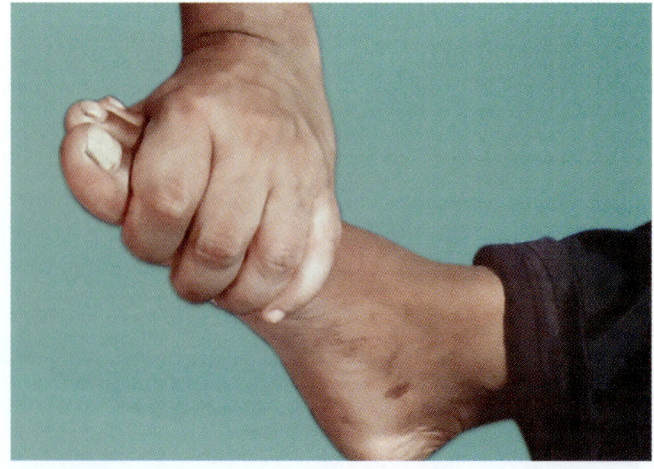

Fig. 7C.35: Examination of metatarsophalangeal joints.

Rheumatology

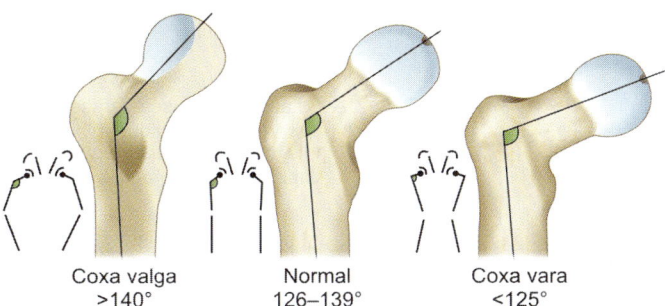

Fig. 7C.36: Hip joint deformities.

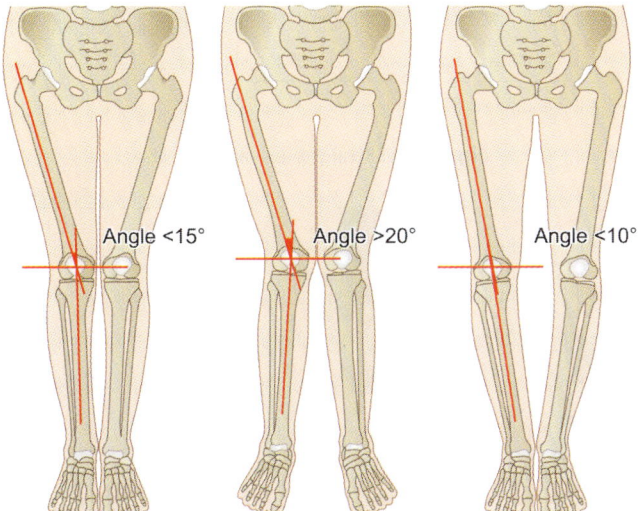

Figs. 7C.37A to C: Knee joint deformities: (A) Normal; (B) Genu valgus (knock knees); (C) Genu varus (bow legs).

Deformities of leg:

Hip joint (Fig. 7C.36)	Coxa vara/valgum
Knee joint (Figs. 7C.37A to C)	Genu varum (bow legs)/Genu valgum (knock knee)
Foot (Fig. 7C.38)	Hallux varus/hallux valgus/hammer toes
Metatarsophalangeal (Fig. 7C.39)	Gout/podagra

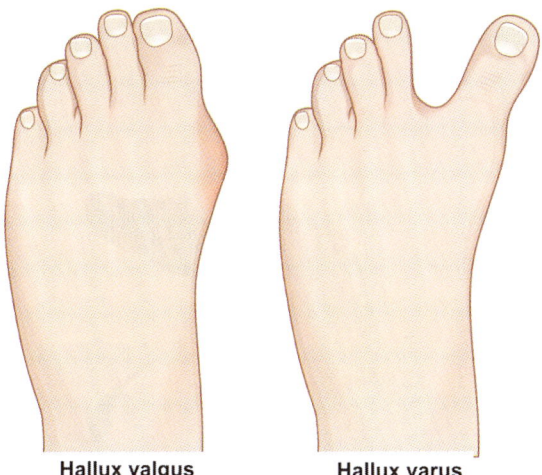

Fig. 7C.38: Hallux valgus and hallux varus deformity.

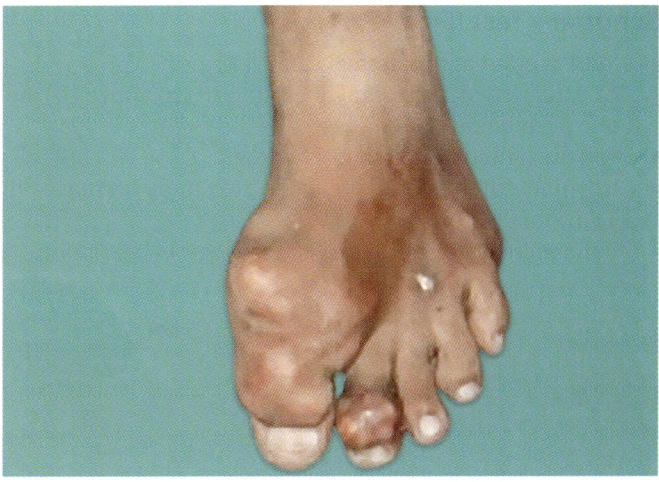

Fig. 7C.39: Acute gouty arthritis involving the first metatarsophalangeal (MTP) joint (termed podagra).

6. EXAMINATION OF SPINE

Occiput to Wall Distance/Flesche Test (Fig. 7C.40)

- Ask the patient to stand erect against a wall, with heels and buttocks placed against a wall.
- Now, ask the patient to extend the neck maximally.
- The distance between the occiput and the wall is measured in degree of flexion deformity of cervical spine.
- Normally the occiput to wall distance is zero.
- It is increased in cervical flexion deformity as in ankylosing spondylitis.

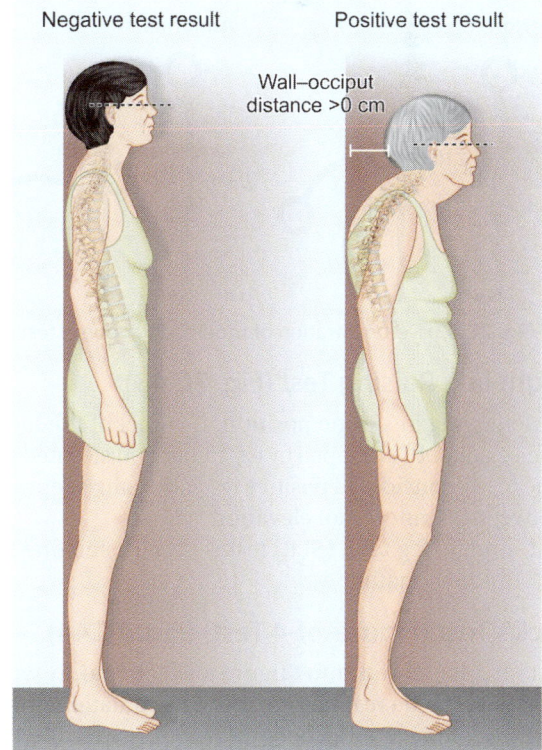

Fig. 7C.40: Demonstration of Flesche test.

Schober's Test (Fig. 7C.41)

- Mark a point approximately at L5 (A)
- Now mark two horizontal lines, one 10 cm above (B) and one 5 cm below L5 (C)
- Ask the patient to touch his/her toes
- Normally the distance between two lines increases by 5 cm (total >20 cm)
- If the increase is less than 5 cm, it suggests restriction.

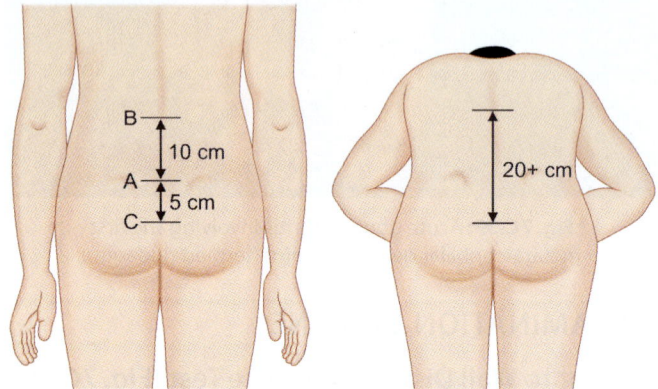

Fig. 7C.41: Demonstration of Schober's test.

Modified Schober's Test (Fig. 7C.42)

- Mark a line connecting two posterior superior iliac spine.
- Draw a parallel line 10 cm above this line.
- Now ask the patient to bend and touch his toes as much as possible.
- The distance between the two lines must be >15 cm. If it is less than 15 cm, it indicates restricted movement of the lumbar spine as seen **in ankylosing spondylosis.**

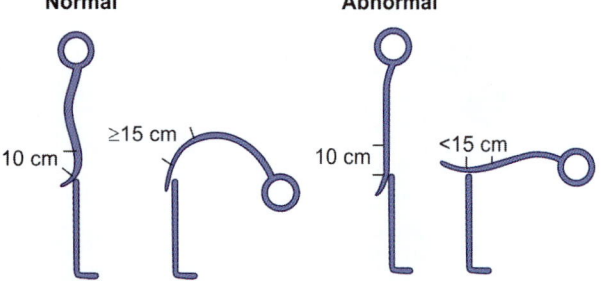

Fig. 7C.42: Demonstration of modified Schober's test.

Straight Leg Raising Test (Fig. 7C.43)

- Patient lying in supine position, the heel of the leg (with knee extended) is cupped by examiner and elevated slowly.
- The test is considered positive if sciatic pain is reproduced between 35° and 70° of elevation.
- The straight leg raise (SLR) test is best for eliciting L4, L5, or S1 radiculopathy.

Patrick's Test (Figure-of-4 Test) (Fig. 7C.44)

- One leg is guided into "figure-of-4" position with the ipsilateral ankle resting across the contralateral thigh.
- The ipsilateral knee is then pressed downwards with one hand while providing counter pressure with the other hand on the contralateral anterior superior iliac spine.
- Pain indicates **sacroiliac joint involvement.**

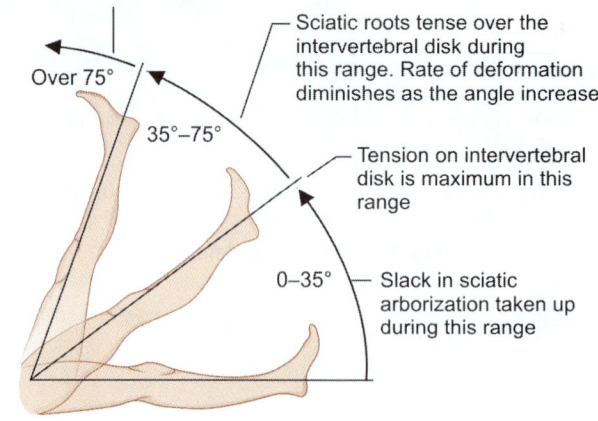

Fig. 7C.43: Straight leg raising test.

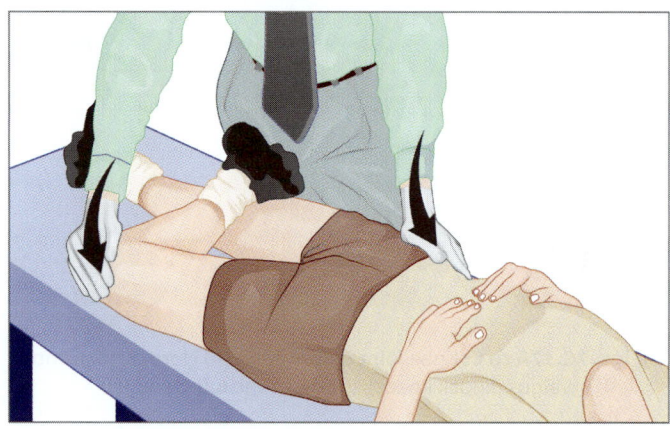

Fig. 7C.44: Demonstration of Patrick's test (figure-of-4).

Gaenslen Maneuver (Fig. 7C.45)

- Ask the patient to lie down on supine.
- One hip if flexed maximally and the other hip is extended by allowing the leg to dangle off the side of the examining table as shown in **Figure 7C.45**.
- Pain **indicates sacroiliac joint involvement.**

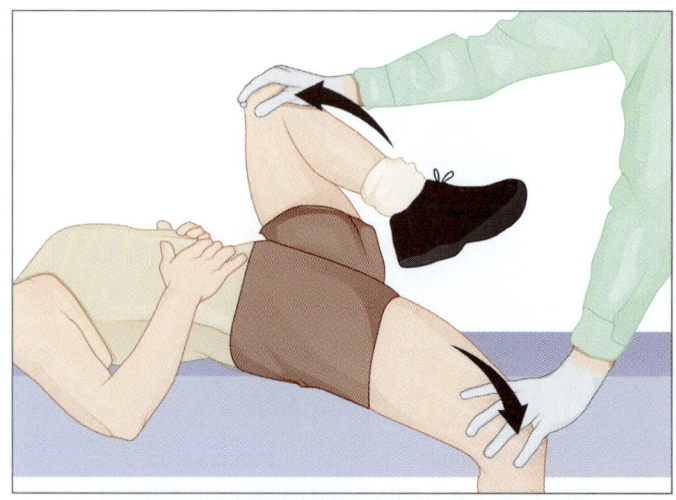

Fig. 7C.45: Demonstration of Gaenslen test.

Deformities of spine (Fig. 7C.46)	
Lordosis	Anterior curvature
Kyphosis	Posterior curvature
Scoliosis	Lateral curvature
Knuckle deformity or step deformity	Prominence of one spinous process
Gibbus deformity (e.g., Pott's spine/metastasis)	Prominence of two spinous processes

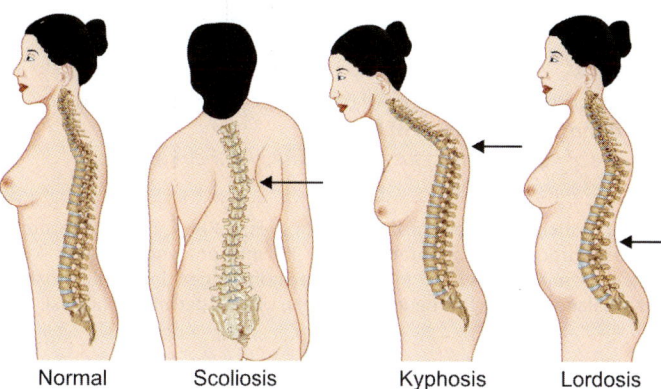

Fig. 7C.46: Various spine deformities.

7. EXAMINATION OF OTHER JOINTS

Temporomandibular Joints (Fig. 7C.47)

- Palpate the temporomandibular joint by asking the patient to open the mouth.
- Observe for tenderness, synovial thickening, and crepitus.

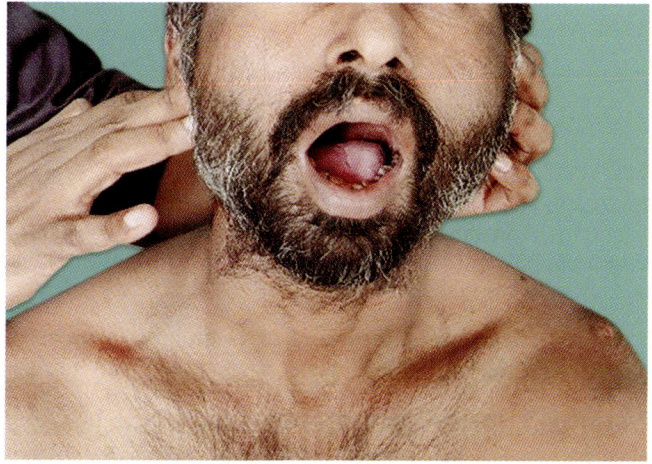

Fig. 7C.47: Examination of temporomandibular joint (TMJ).

Examination of Sternoclavicular Joint (Fig. 7C.48)

- Palpate the sternoclavicular joint.
- Look for tenderness and synovial thickening.

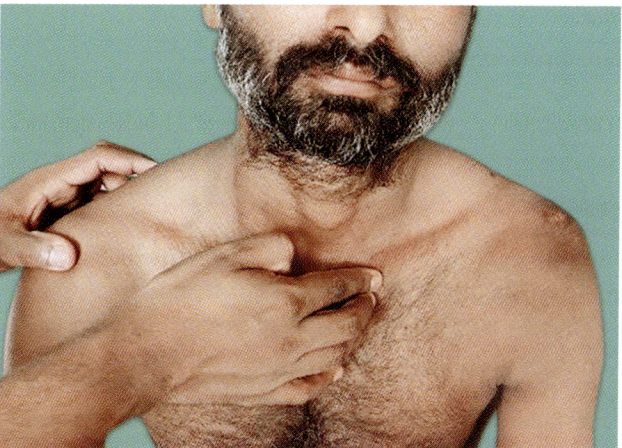

Fig. 7C.48: Examination of sternoclavicular joint.

8. EXAMINATION OF OTHER SYSTEMS IN RHEUMATOLOGICAL DISORDERS

Cardiovascular system	
Pericarditis	RA SLE
Endocarditis	SLE
Aortitis and aortic regurgitation	- RA - Psoriasis - Ankylosing spondylitis - Reiter's
Conduction defects	SLE
Nervous system	
Myelopathy	- RA—atlantoaxial dislocation Vasculitis
Neuropathy (entrapment/mononeuritis multiplex)	- RA SLE - Vasculitis (especially PAN)
Stroke	- RA SLE APLA - Vasculitis
Myopathy	- Polymyositis - Dermatomyositis
Respiratory system	
Upper respiratory tract	Wegener's granulomatosis
Pleural effusion	- RA - SLE
Fibrosis	- RA - SLE - Systemic sclerosis
Lung nodules	RA (Caplan's syndrome)
Alveolar hemorrhage	- Microscopic polyangiitis - Goodpasture's syndrome - Wegener's granulomatosis
Asthma	Churg–Strauss syndrome
Decreased chest expansion	Ankylosing spondylosis
Gastrointestinal system	
Oral ulcers	- SLE - Behcet's disease
IBD	Seronegative spondyloarthropathies

Contd...

Contd...

Hepatosplenomegaly	- SLE RA - Stills disease
GI bleeding	- Henoch-Schönlein purpura Other vasculitis - Analgesic use
Genitourinary system	
Urethritis	- Reactive arthritis

Glomerulonephritis	- SLE
	- Microscopic polyangiitis
	  Goodpasture's syndrome
	  Wegener's granulomatosis

Renal failure	- Analgesics use, vasculitis
Endocrinology	
Diabetes	- Steroid induced
Thyroid disease	- Associated autoimmune conditions
Blood	
- Anemia - Thrombocytopenia Pancytopenia	- SLE - RA (Felty's syndrome)

9. DISCUSSION ON COMMON RHEUMATOLOGICAL DISEASES

Rheumatoid Arthritis

American College of Rheumatology (ACR) criteria for rheumatoid arthritis
Morning stiffness Arthritis of 3 joint areas Arthritis of the hands Symmetric arthritis Rheumatoid nodules Serum rheumatoid factor positive Radiographic changes These criteria *must be* present for more than 6 weeks. Presence of *four or more criteria* favors definite diagnosis of RA.
European League against Rheumatism (EULAR) Classification criteria for rheumatoid arthritis: 2010
A. Joint involvement **(Fig. 7C.49)**

1 large joint (shoulder, elbow, hip, knee, ankle)	0
2–10 large joints	1
1–3 small joints (MCP, PIP, thumb IP, MTP, wrists) + involvement of large joints	2
4–10 small joints + involvement of large joints	3
>10 joints (at least 1 small joint)	5

Contd...

Contd...

B. Serology (at least one test result is needed for classification)	
Negative RF and negative ACPA	0
Low-positive RF or low-positive ACPA (≤3 times ULN)	2
High-positive RF or high-positive ACPA (≥3 times ULN)	3
C. Acute-phase reactants (at least one test result is needed for classification)	
Normal CRP and normal ESR	0
Abnormal CRP or abnormal ESR	1
D. Duration of symptoms	
<6 weeks	0
≥6 weeks	1
Above criteria yields a score of 0–10. A score of **≥6 required for definitive diagnosis of RA.** *A score of <6/10 are not classifiable as RA, but their status to be reassessed over time.*	

(ACPA: anticitrullinated protein antibodies; CRP: C-reactive protein; ESR: erythrocyte sedimentation rate; IP: interphalangeal joint; MCP: metacarpophalangeal joint; MTP: metatarsophalangeal joint; PIP: proximal interphalangeal joint; RF: rheumatoid factor; ULN: upper limit of normal)

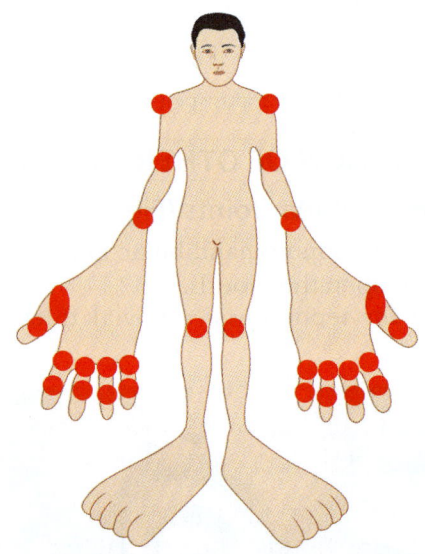

Fig. 7C.49: The 28 joints to be examined in rheumatoid arthritis include the 5 proximal interphalangeal joints of the 2 hands, the 5 metacarpophalangeal joints of the 2 hands, the 2 wrists, the 2 elbows, the 2 shoulders, and the 2 knees.

Extra-articular manifestations of rheumatoid arthritis are shown in **Figure 7C.50**.

Systemic Lupus Erythematosus (Fig. 7C.51)

2019 European League Against Rheumatism (EULAR)/ American College of Rheumatology (ACR) classification criteria for systemic lupus erythematosus

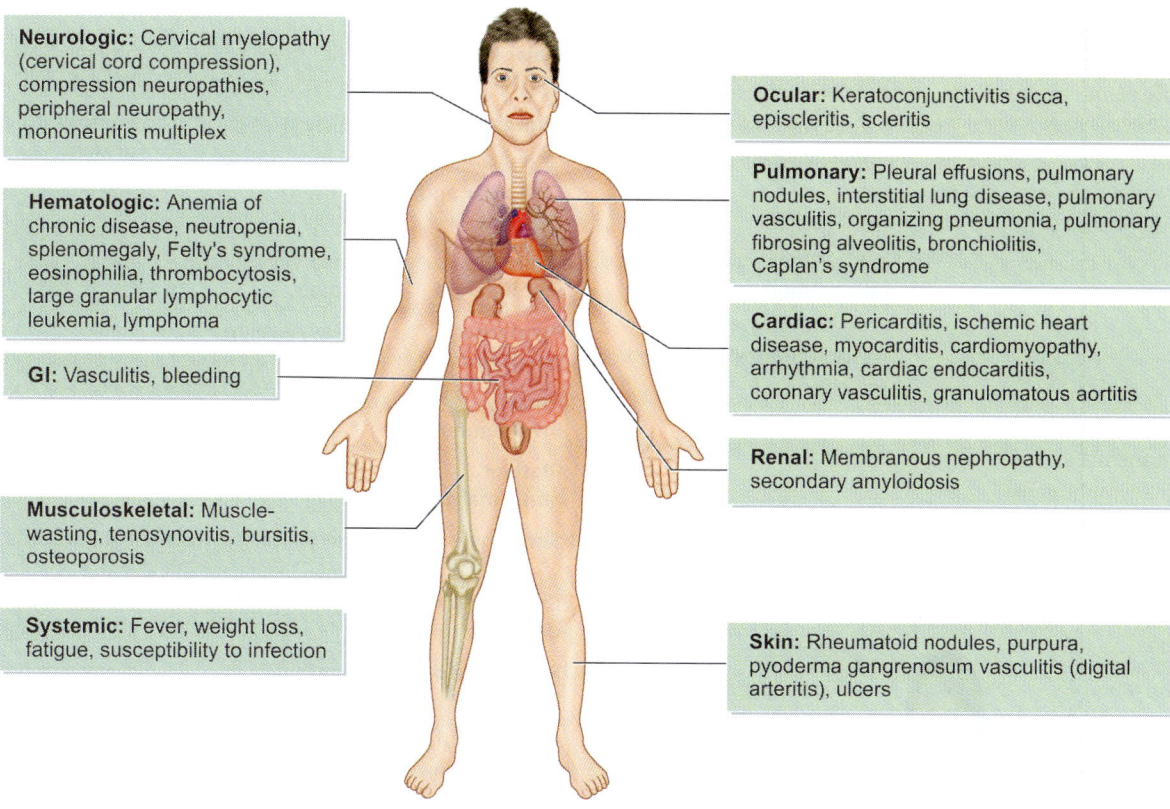

Fig. 7C.50: Extra-articular manifestations of rheumatoid arthritis.

ENTRY CRITERION
Antinuclear antibodies (ANA) at a titer of ≥1:80 on HEp-2 cells or an equivalent positive test (ever)

↓

If absent, do not classify as SLE
If present, apply additive criteria

↓

Additive criteria
Do not count a criterion if there is a more likely explanation than SLE.
Occurrence of a criterion on at least one occasion is sufficient.
SLE classification requires at least one clinical criterion and ≥10 points.
Criteria need not occur simultaneously.
Within each domain, only the highest weighted criterion is counted toward the total score§.

Clinical domains and criteria	Weight	Immunology domains and criteria	Weight
Constitutional Fever	2	**Antiphospholipid antibodies** Anticardiolipin antibodies or Anti-β2GP1 antibodies or Lupus anticoagulant	2
Hematologic Leukopenia Thrombocytopenia Autoimmune hemolysis	3 4 4	**Complement proteins** Low C3 or low C4 Low C3 and low C4	3 4
Neuropsychiatric Delirium Psychosis Seizure	2 3 5	**SLE-specific antibodies** Anti-dsDNA antibody* or Anti-Smith antibody	6
Mucocutaneous Non-scarring alopecia Oral ulcers Subacute cutaneous or discoid lupus Acute cutaneous lupus	2 2 4 6		
Serosal Pleural or pericardial effusion Acute pericarditis	5 6	*Note:* § = additional criteria within the same domain will not be counted *= in an assay with 90% specificity against relevant disease controls Anti-β2GPI = anti–β2-glycoprotein I anti-dsDNA = anti-double-stranded DNA.	
Musculoskeletal Joint involvement **Renal** Proteinuria >0.5 g/24 h Renal biopsy Class II or V lupus nephritis Renal biopsy Class III or IV lupus nephritis	6 4 8 10	**2019 Classification Criteria for Systemic Lupus Erythematosus (SLE)**	

Total score:
↓
Classify as systemic lupus erythematosus with a score of 10 or more if entry criterion fulfilled.

Contd...

Systemic Lupus International Collaborating Clinics (SLICC) Classification 2012 criteria	
Biopsy proven lupus nephritis and ANA/anti-DNA (or) at least four criteria (one needs to be immunological)	
Clinical	Immunological
Acute cutaneous LE	ANA
Chronic cutaneous LE	Anti-dsDNA
Oral ulcer	Anti-Sm
Alopecia	aPL antibodies
Synovitis	Low complement
Serositis	Direct Coombs' test Positive
Renal	
Neurologic	
Hemolytic anemia	
Leukopenia/lymphopenia	
Thrombocytopenia	

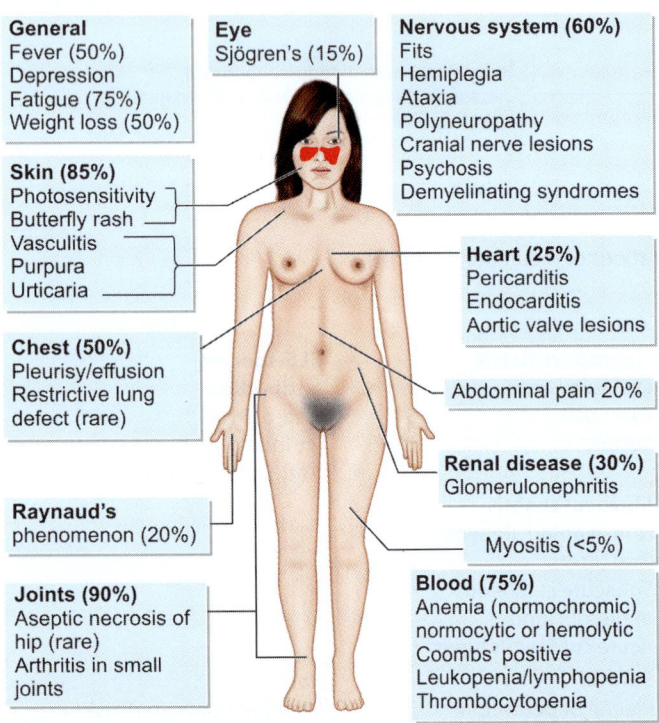

Fig. 7C.51: Clinical features of systemic lupus erythematosus (SLE).

Differences between rheumatoid arthritis and SLE		
Features	Rheumatoid arthritis	Systemic lupus erythematosus
Smoking	Predisposing factor	No relation
Female: Male	3:1	9:1
Type of arthritis	Erosive	Nonerosive
Deformities	Common	Rare, Jaccoud's arthropathy (10%)
Systemic involvement	Relatively less	Marked
Nodules	Rheumatoid nodules	Absent

Contd...

Malar (skin) rash	Nil	Striking feature: Malar rash, discoid rash
Photosensitivity	Absent	Photosensitivity present
Oral ulcer and alopecia	Absent	Present
Spine involvement	Involves cervical spine	Rare
Pyoderma gangrenosum	May develop	Rare
Renal involvement	Uncommon	Common and severe
Platelet abnormality	Thrombocythemia	Thrombocytopenia
Serology	RA factor and ACPA	ANA and anti-dsDNA
Criteria for diagnosis	ACR/EULAR	SLICC/ACR
Response to DMARDs	Present	Less response

(ACPA: anticyclic citrullinated peptide antibodies; ACR: American College of Rheumatology; ANA: antinuclear antibodies; DMARD: disease-modifying antirheumatic drugs; dsDNA: double-stranded deoxyribonucleic acid; EULAR: European League against Rheumatism; RA: rheumatoid arthritis; SLICC: Systemic Lupus International Collaborating Clinics)

Osteoarthritis (Fig. 7C.52)

Osteoarthritis (OA) is a **noninflammatory, slowly progressive joint disease**, mainly **involving the cartilage**. It shows **progressive destruction of articular cartilage** of weight-bearing joints of **genetically susceptible older persons**. It leads to narrowing of joint space, subchondral bone thickening and finally **painful and nonfunctioning joints**.

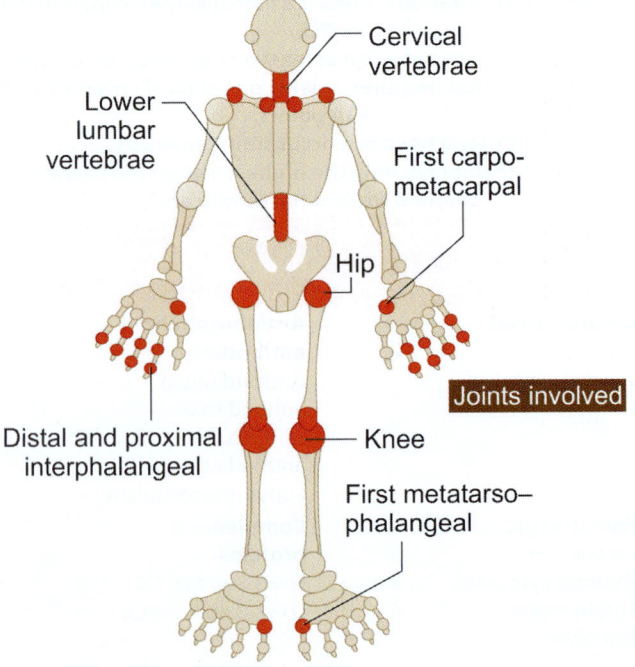

Fig. 7C.52: Pattern of joint involvement in osteoarthritis.

Ankylosing Spondylitis

Diagnostic Criteria

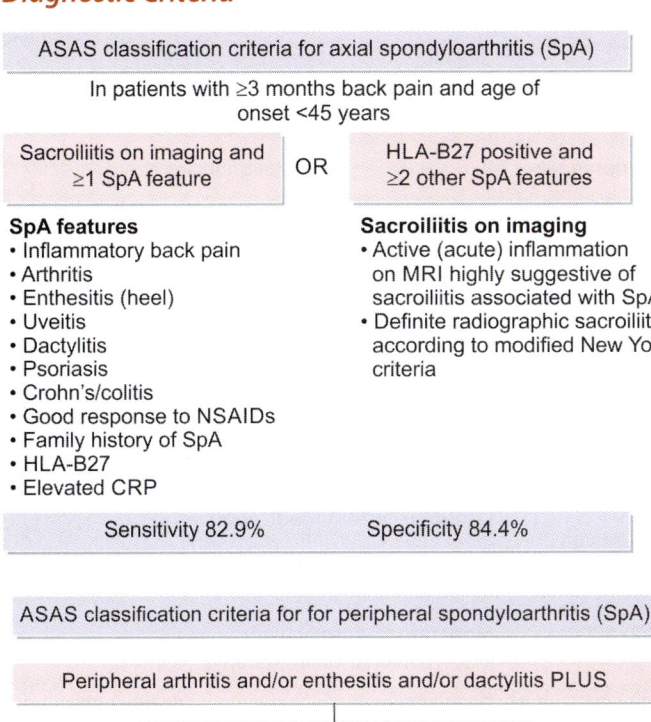

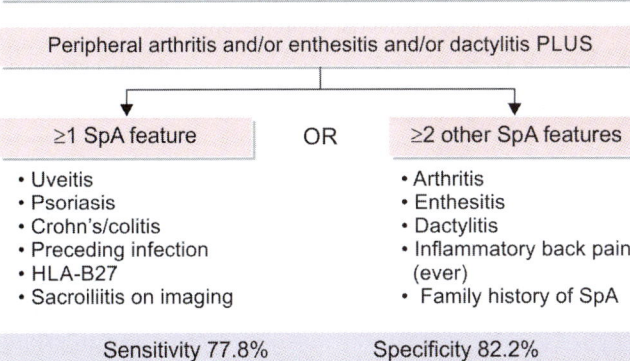

Fibromyalgia

Fibromyalgia syndrome (FMS) is characterized by chronic widespread pain, and is defined as pain for more than 3 months both above and below the waist.

Diagnostic Criteria for FMS

- At least 3 months of widespread pain that is bilateral, above and below the waist.
- It includes axial skeletal pain and pain to palpation at a minimum of 11 of 18 predefined tender points **(Fig. 7C.53)**.
- The diagnosis of other diseases does not exclude the diagnosis of FMS.

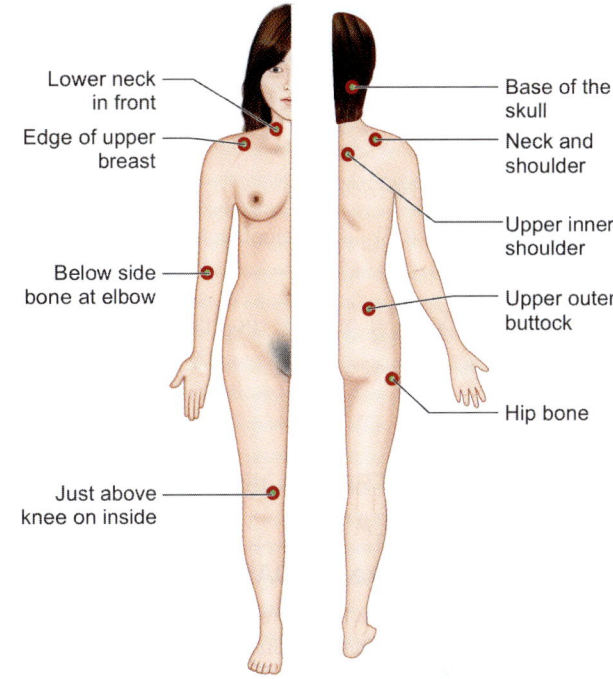

Fig. 7C.53: Trigger points in fibromyalgia.

Psoriatic Arthritis

It is called **ClAS**sification for **P**soriatic **AR**thritis (the CASPAR criteria)

Classification of Psoriatic-Arthritis: CASPAR Criteria

To meet the CASPAR criteria for PsA, a patient must have inflammatory articular disease (joint, spine or entheseal) and score ≥3 points based on these categories.	
	Points
1. **Evidence of psoriasis** Current psoriasis Personal history of psoriasis Family history of psoriasis	2 or 1 or 1
2. **Psoriatic nail dystrophy** Pitting, onycholysis, hyperkeratosis	1
3. **Negative test result for rheumatoid factor**	1
4. **Dactylitis** Current swelling of an entire digit History of dactylitis	1 or 1
5. **Radiologic evidence of juxta-articular new bone formation** Ill-defined ossification near joint margins on plain X-rays of hand and foot	1

Source: Taylor W, et al. CASPAR, ClASsification criteria for Psoriatic ARthritis Arthritis Rheum. 2006;54:2665-73.

Adult Onset Still's Disease

Yamaguchi's Criteria		
Five or more criteria are required. Two or more criteria must be major.		
Major criteria	Minor criteria	Exclusion criteria
Fever >39°C lasting 7 days or longer	Sore throat	Infections
Arthralgias or arthritis for 14 days or longer	Hepatomegaly or splenomegaly	Malignancies
Typical rash	Lymphadenopathy	Other rheumatic disease
WBC count >10,000/μL with >80% neutrophils	Abnormal aminotransferases	
	Negative rheumatoid factor and anti-nuclear antibody	

10. SCORING SYSTEMS FOR SEVERITY OF DISEASE

Disease Activity Score 28 (DAS28)

DAS28 is a common measurement of disease activity in RA and provides score that tells you how well controlled your RA is and whether treatment is working.

Twenty-eight joints (20 hand joints, 2 shoulder joints, 2 elbow joints, 2 wrist joints, and 2 knee joints) are examined throughout your body. Each joint is squeezed and the number of tender and swollen joints is calculated.

DAS28	Implication
Less than 2.6	Disease remission Usually no action necessary Continue current medication
2.6–3.2	Low disease activity May merit change in therapy for some patients
3.2–5.1	Moderate disease activity May merit change in therapy
More than 5.1	Severe disease activity require change in therapy Consider biologic treatment

Clinical Disease Activity Index (CDAI) (Fig. 7C.54)

Clinical Disease Activity Index (CDAI)

Joint	Left		Right	
	Tender	Swollen	Tender	Swollen
Shoulder				
Elbow				
Wrist				
MCP 1				
MCP 2				
MCP 3				
MCP 4				
MCP 5				
PIP 1				
PIP 2				
PIP 3				
PIP 4				
PIP 5				
Knee				
Total	Tender:		Swollen:	

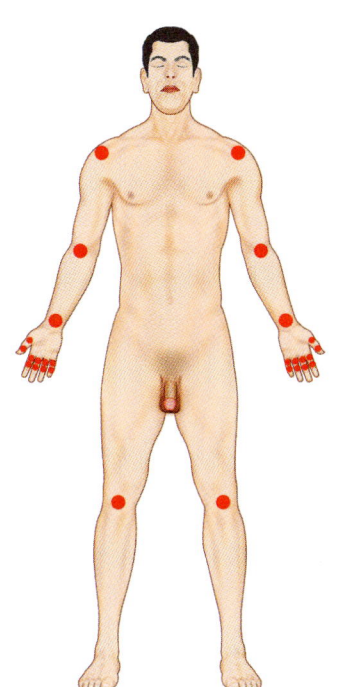

Patient global assessment of disease activity

Considering all the ways your arthritis affects you, rate how well you are doing on the following scale:

Very Well 0 0.5 1.0 1.5 2.0 2.5 3.0 3.5 4.0 4.5 5.0 5.5 6.0 6.5 7.0 7.5 8.0 8.5 9.0 9.5 10 Very Poor

Your name_____ Date of birth_____ Today's date_____

Provider global assessment of disease activity

Very Well 0 0.5 1.0 1.5 2.0 2.5 3.0 3.5 4.0 4.5 5.0 5.5 6.0 6.5 7.0 7.5 8.0 8.5 9.0 9.5 10 Very Poor

How to score the CDAI

Variable	Range	Value
Tender joint score	(0–2.8)	
Swollen joint score	(0–2.8)	
Patient global score	(0–10)	
Provider global score	(0–10)	
Add the above values to calculate the CDAI score	(0–76)	

CDAI Score Interpretation	
0.0–2.8	Remission
2.9–10.0	Low activity
10.1–22.0	Moderate activity
22.1–76.0	High activity

Fig. 7C.54: Clinical disease activity index.

NOTES

CHAPTER 8

Comprehensive Geriatric Assessment

Sheetal Raj M

CASE SHEET FORMAT

HISTORY TAKING

Name:

Hospital number:

Age:

Sex:

Date of examination:

Address/contact:

Name/relationship of contact person:

Contact address/number:

Problem list	Duration

Past Medical History:

Medical condition	Duration
Vision impaired	
Hearing impaired	
Cancer	
OA	
Thyroid	

Family History:

Hypertension	
Diabetes	
Heart disease	
Dementia	
Cancer	

Social Assessment:

Married:	Yes	No
Spouse living:	Yes	No
Living with:		
No. of children		
How often do you see them?		
Who assists you?		
Is it sufficient?	Yes	No
Native language		
Type of house	Independent	Apartment
Stairs	Present	Absent

Personal History:

Do you exercise daily?	Yes	No
If yes, minutes/day?		
What type?		
Weight loss/gain (3 kg)	Yes	No
Smoker	Yes	No
Duration		
Alcohol	Yes	No
Duration		

Level of independence (tick one of them)	Independent
	Dependent
	Needs assistance

Caregiver fatigue	Yes	No

10-minute comprehensive screening			
Memory	3 objects named	Yes	No
Depression	Are you often sad/depressed?	Yes	No
Falls	Fallen more than twice in last 1 year	Yes	No
	Able to walk around chair?	Yes	No

Urinary incontinence	Lost urine/got wet in past 1 year?	Yes		No
Memory recall	One object	Two objects	Three objects	None
Imagine this is a clock and add numbers to make it look like a clock. Draw the clock hand to show ten minutes past eleven	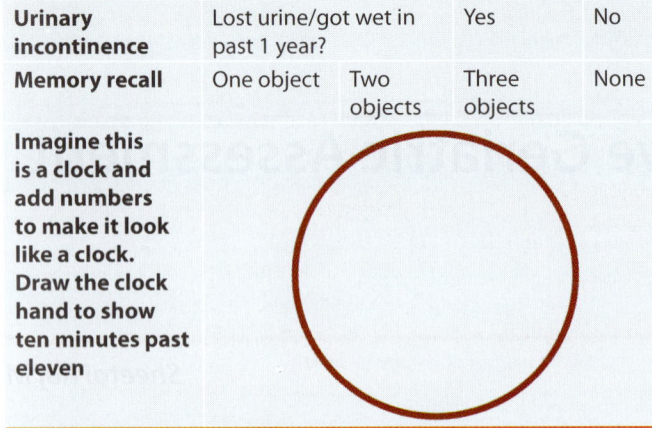			

Vision	Difficulty in reading	Right eye	Left eye
Hearing		Right ear	Left ear
6, 1, 9 test—stand behind the patient and say 6, 1 and 9 in normal tone and in whisper	Normally	Yes/no	Yes/No
	Softly	Yes/No	Yes/No
Constipation		Yes	No
Insomnia		Yes	No

Physical Functional Capacity:

Are you able to _____?

Run/walk fast to catch a bus	Yes	No
Do heavy work at home	Yes	No
Go shopping for groceries/clothes	Yes	No
Get to places out of walking distance? (drive/take a bus)	Yes	No
Bath using shower/bucket	Yes	No
Put on clothes/footwear	Yes	No

Basic Activities of Daily Living:

Bath	Yes	No	Transfer	Yes	No
Dress	Yes	No	Continence	Yes	No
Toilet	Yes	No	Feeding	Yes	No

Montreal cognitive assessment score	
Geriatric depression score	

Physical Examination:

Height (m)	
Weight (kg)	
Body mass index (BMI) (W/H^2)	
Pulse	
Blood pressure (BP) (sitting/supine)	
BP (standing 1 minute/3 minutes)	

Contd...

Contd...

Anemia	Yes/No
Skin	Normal/abnormal
Teeth	Normal/abnormal
Any other GPE abnormality	

Systemic Examination:

	Normal/abnormal	Describe	
Joints			
Cervical spine			
Thoracic spine			
Lumbar spine			
RS			
CVS			
P/A			
Neurological examination		**R**	**L**
Muscle strength	Upper limb		
	Shoulder		
	Elbow		
	Wrist		
	Small muscles of hand		
	Lower limb		
	Hip		
	Knee		
	Ankle		
Tone (describe)	Rigidity/hypotonia/spasticity		
Balance	Normal/abnormal	▪ Sensory ▪ Cerebellar ▪ Vestibular	
Gait			
Timed up and go test (seconds)			

Current Treatment Details:
Write down name of drug, dose and dosing frequency of all the medications the patient is currently consuming, including over the counter medications and those from alternative systems of medicine

....

Polypharmacy: Yes/No

Investigations:

Investigations	Date	Values
Complete blood picture		
Creatinine		
Electrolytes, blood sugar		
PSA (for males)		
Urine routine		
Ultrasonography (USG) abdomen and pelvis		

DIAGNOSIS FORMAT

Comprehensive Geriatric Assessment Report:

Acute illness	
Comorbidity	
Geriatric giants	
Other age-related problems	
Social problems	
Economic problems	
Prescription modification	

Examples:

Acute illness	Memory issues, abnormal behavior, temper tantrums, knee pain, backache, repetition

Contd...

Contd...

Comorbidity	Diabetes, hypertension, dyslipidemia
Geriatric giants	- Fall risk, fear of fall - Moderate impairment of cognition
Other age-related problems	- Cataract - Bilateral hearing loss (sensorineural, age-related)
Social problems	- Living alone - Feels lonely - Has nobody for emergency help
Economic problems	None. Earning a pension
Prescription modification	Avoid benzodiazepines (Lorazepam as it increases fall risk)

DISCUSSION

Comprehensive Geriatric Assessment (CGA)

Comprehensive geriatric assessment (CGA) **(Fig. 8.1)** is a multidimensional, multidisciplinary diagnostic, and therapeutic process conducted to determine the medical, mental, and functional problems of older people with frailty so that a coordinated and integrated plan for treatment and follow-up can be developed.

Factors which make assessment/treatment of elderly different are as follows:
- Individuals become more dissimilar as they grow
- Abrupt decline in any system is always due to disease and not due to normal aging
- Multiple pathology
- Missing symptoms (e.g., angina in an elderly patient with osteoarthritis—may not manifest)
- Masking symptoms (e.g., history of fall and fracture neck of femur in an elderly female-masked a coexistent hemiparesis due to an internal capsule infarct).

When an older person is identified as being at risk of frailty, whether in an acute hospital, day hospital, community or residential care, they should be considered for a CGA. CGA should be initiated as soon as possible after admission to hospital by a skilled, senior member of the multidisciplinary team, and used to identify reversible medical problems, target rehabilitation goals, and plan all the components of discharge and post-discharge support needs.

The CGA multidisciplinary team may include:
- Physician, e.g., geriatrician, or general practitioner (GP)
- Nurse
- Medical social worker
- Physiotherapist
- Occupational therapist
- Speech and language therapist
- Dietitian
- Clinical pharmacist
- Podiatrist.

Benefits of Comprehensive Geriatric Assessment
- Improves diagnostic accuracy
- Decreases long-term home placement
- Minimizes the impact of "geriatric syndromes" such as cognitive impairment, urinary incontinence and falls.
- Optimizes medical and rehabilitation treatment
- Enhances health and functional outcomes
- Informs the development of individualized care plans
- Assists in avoiding the potential complications of hospitalization
- Facilitates effective discharge planning.

The **four main dimensions** covered in a CGA should include physical, functional, psychological, and social assessment as follows:

Four main dimensions	
Physical assessment	*Functional assessment*
- Presenting complaint (problem list) - Past medical history - Screening for geriatric syndromes - Assessment of senses (hearing, vision) - Medication reconciliation and review - Nutritional status - Alcohol/smoking - Immunization status - Advanced directives	- Activities of daily living/instrumental activities of daily living - Balance assessment - Mobility/gait assessment
Psychological assessment	*Social assessment*
- Cognition and mood - Spiritual assessment	- Living arrangements - Social support - Career stress - Financial circumstances - Living environment

Identifying Elderly Patients who would Benefit from Such an Assessment

Strongly consider doing a CGA if three or more of the Red Flags are present
- >75 years - Needs help with activities of daily living/instrumental activities for daily living (ADLs/IADLs) by caregiver - Lives alone - Falls - Delirium/confusion - Incontinence - >2 admissions to acute care hospital/year - "Failure to thrive"

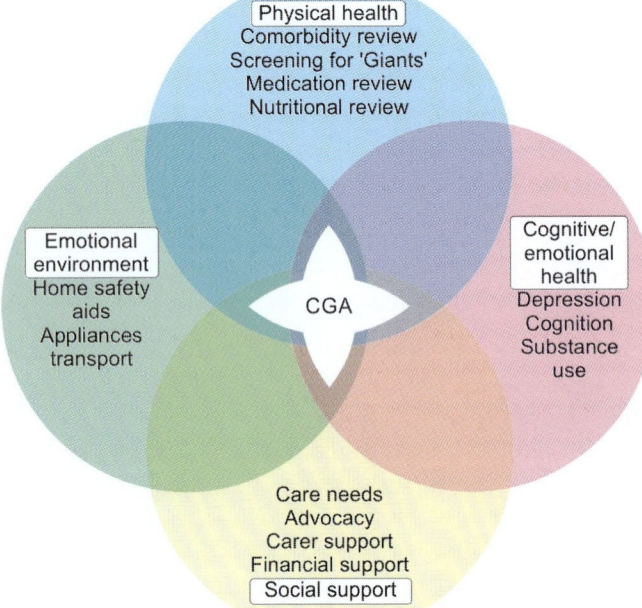

Fig. 8.1: Components of comprehensive geriatric assessment (CGA).

Basic Activities of Daily Living

Basic activities of daily livings (BADLs) are fundamental activities, such as personal cares which are basic to independent living. Loss of basic ADLs places a heavy burden on the caregivers and is a marker of complete dependence.

For assessing autonomy in daily activities:
- Toileting, self-hygiene, bathing, grooming, dressing, feeding, and ambulation (stairs too).
- For each of the questions, inquire whether the person can perform it independently, whether he/she needs assistance or he/she is completely caregiver-dependent.

Instrumental Activities of Daily Living

Instrumental activities of daily living (IADLs) are complex tasks which enable an older adult to live independently and safely. They are not necessary for fundamental existence in the way that basic ADLs are necessary, but are an indicator of functional independence and are culturally dependent. Assessment of IADLs is useful during baseline and follow-up assessments among older adults. Loss of IADLs may be the first indication of deterioration in an older adult.

Examples for IADLs: Complex tasks and roles you do at home such as shopping, meal planning and preparation, housekeeping, laundry, transit, financial management, using a telephone, medication management, and driving.

Geriatric Giants (Fig. 8.2)

The term geriatric giant was coined by Sir Bernard Isaacs. He identified a set of medical problems or syndromes which were common in older adults and which crossed several organ systems and were difficult to manage. These geriatric giant are chronic disabilities which impact multiple domains such as physical, psychological, and social domains. Although geriatric giants are commonly misperceived to be an unavoidable part of old age, they can often be improved if they are identified and managed.

FRAILTY SYNDROME

Frailty is defined as the loss of an individual's ability to withstand minor stresses because of decreased functional reserve of several organ systems.

Some of the scales used in diagnosing frailty are Linda Fried, Johns Hopkins Frailty criteria and the Rockwood Clinical Frailty Scale.

Five key elements form the core of the frailty cycle (phenotypic definition)
Frailty is defined as the presence of three or more of following conditions
1. Unexplained weight loss (>5% over a year)
2. Poor endurance and energy (self-reported)
3. Poor strength (in lowest 20th percentile)
4. Slow walking speed (poor "Get up and Go" test)
5. Low physical activity (lowest 20th percentile)

Assessment of Functioning

Functional assessment can decline in older adults following acute illnesses, advancing age, sudden changes in psychosocial environment, worsening of chronic illnesses, etc.

WHO defines intrinsic capacity as the combination of the individual's physical and mental, including psychological capacities. Functional ability is the combination and interaction of intrinsic capacity with the environment that a person inhabits.

[Integrated care for older people (ICOPE): Guidance for person-centered assessment and pathways in primary care. Geneva: World Health Organization; 2019 (WHO/FWC/ALC/19.1). License: CC BY-NC-SA 3.0 IGO]

The following are some of the measures of physical function in older adults:

Objective measures of physical function	
Timed up and go (TUG) test (Fig. 8.3)	>30 seconds: Fall risk
6-meter walk	<5.8 seconds
Gait speed	>6.0 seconds
6-minute walk	<300 m: Mortality <400 m: Functional impairment
Activities of daily living (Barthel's index)	
Lawton's instrumental activities of daily living	

DEMENTIA

Causes of dementia are given in **Box 8.1.**

Mini-Mental State Examination

- For screening of cognitive impairments
- Time required: 15 minutes
- Mini-mental state examination test a broad range of cognitive functions including orientation, recall, attention, calculation, language manipulation, and constructional praxis.

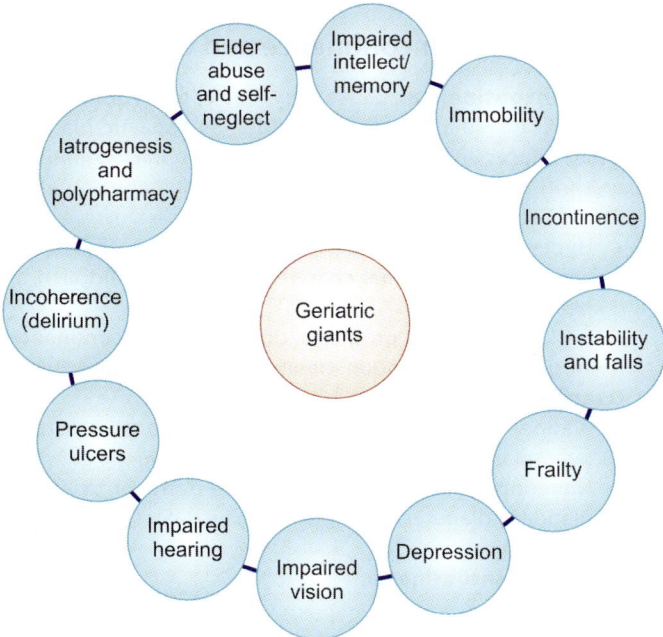

Fig. 8.2: Modern geriatric giants.

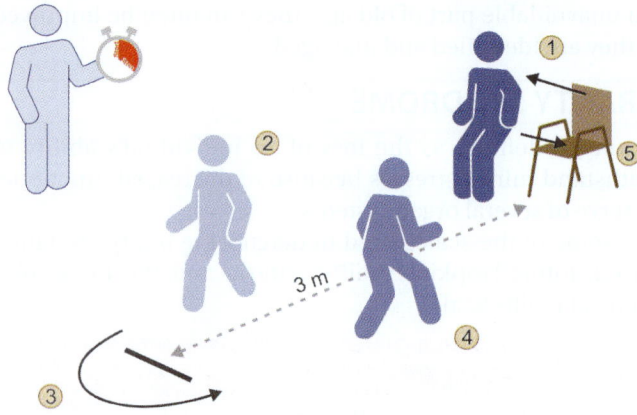

Fig. 8.3: Timed up-and-go (TUG) test.

Principle of the timed up-and-go (TUG) test: (1) on command, the subject rises from the armchair; (2) the subject walks 3 meters; (3) the subject turns around; (4) the subjects walks back to the chair; (5) the subjects sits back on the chair. Interpreting the results:
- A faster time (less than 10–12 seconds) generally indicates better functional mobility and a lower risk of falls.
- A slower time (>12 seconds) may indicate an increased risk of falls, especially in older adults.

Box 8.1: Causes of dementia.

Degenerative/inherited:
- Alzheimer's disease—60–70%
- Neurodegenerative disorders: Frontotemporal dementia (including Pick's disease)—Lewy body disease, Parkinson's disease, Huntington's disease

Vascular dementia (10–20%): Diffuse small vessel disease

Neoplastic: Primary/secondary deposits

Traumatic: Chronic subdural hematoma, post-head injury

Infections: Creutzfeldt–Jakob disease, human immunodeficiency virus (HIV), syphilis

Toxic/nutritional: Alcohol, thiamine deficiency, vitamin B_{12} deficiency

Prion disease

Modifiable/Reversible Causes of Dementia

		Mnemonic—DEMENTIA
▪ Depression also called 'Pseudodementia' ▪ Electrolyte disorders (hyponatremia, hypercalcemia, etc.) ▪ Hypothyroidism ▪ Late onset psychosis ▪ Medication side effects (e.g., sedatives, anticonvulsants, antihypertensives, anticholinergics, first generation neuroleptics)	▪ Vitamin deficiencies (B_{12}, folate) ▪ Obstructive sleep apnea ▪ Normal pressure hydrocephalus (reverse with shunting) ▪ Brain tumor (post-resection) ▪ Subdural hematoma (SDH)	D = Drugs, delirium E = Emotions (such as depression) and endocrine disorders M = Metabolic disturbances E = Eye and ear impairments N = Nutritional disorders T = Tumors, toxicity, trauma to head I = Infectious disorders

Contd...

▪ Ethanol overuse/misuse	▪ Sub-acute CNS infections (i.e., meningitis, encephalitis, syphilis)	A = Alcohol, arteriosclerosis

For assessing cognitive impairment we use Mini-Mental State Examination (MMSE), Montreal Cognitive Assessment (MoCA), or Mini-Cog™.

Montreal Cognitive Assessment

Montreal Cognitive Assessment (MoCA) is a 30-point test that is sensitive for the detection of mild cognitive impairment, and it includes items that sample a wider range of cognitive domains including memory, language, attention, visuospatial, and executive functions.

Mini-Cog™

The Mini-Cog™ serves as an effective triage tool to identify individuals who need more thorough evaluation. **The Clock drawing test (CDT)** component of the Mini-Cog™ allows clinicians to quickly assess numerous cognitive domains including cognitive function, memory, language comprehension, visual-motor skills, and executive function and provides a visible record of both normal and impaired performance that can be tracked over time.

The Clock Drawing Test

Ask patient to draw the face of a clock. After numbers are on the face, ask patient to draw hands to read 10 minutes after 11:00 (or 20 minutes after 8:00).

INCONTINENCE

Involuntary loss of urine or stool in sufficient amount or frequency to constitute a social and/or health problem.

Types of Urinary Incontinence and Causes

- **Urge incontinence:** Caused by detrusor hyperactivity, detrusor instability, irritable bladder, and spastic bladder. Other Causes: Infection, tumor, stones, atrophic vaginitis or urethritis, stroke, Parkinson's disease, and dementia
- **Stress incontinence:**
  - Hypermotility of bladder neck and urethra; associated with aging, hormonal changes, trauma of childbirth or pelvic surgery
  - Intrinsic sphincter problems; due to pelvic/incontinence surgery, pelvic radiation, trauma, and neurogenic causes
- **Overflow incontinence:**
  - Bladder outlet obstruction; stricture, benign prostatic hyperplasia (BPH), cystocele, fecal impaction
  - Noncontractile bladder (hypoactive detrusor or atonic bladder); diabetes, multiple sclerosis (MS), spinal injury, and medications
- **Functional incontinence**

Contd...

FALLS IN THE ELDERLY (FIG. 8.4)

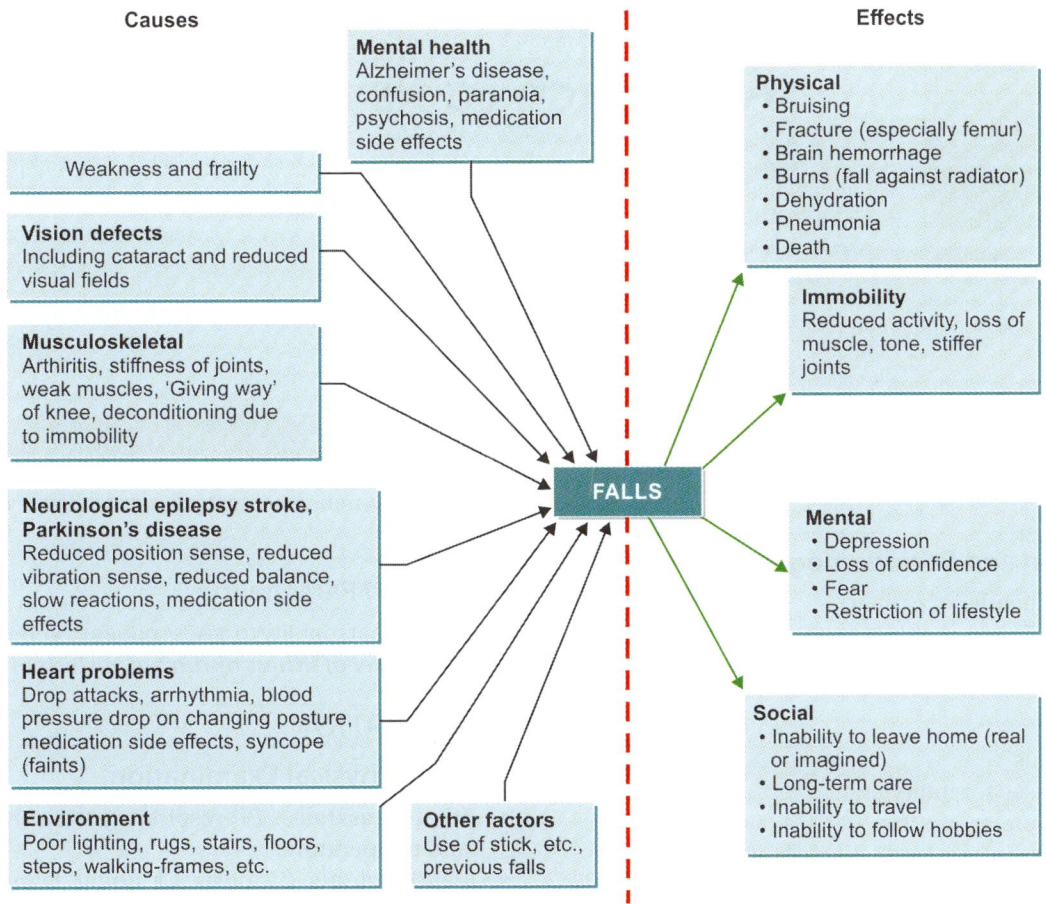

Fig. 8.4: Causes of falls in elderly and their effects.

Balance Test
- Done to assess the risk of falls
- **Side-by-side:** Feet side-by-side, touching
- **Semi-tandem:** Side of the heel of one foot touching the big toe of the other
- **Tandem:** Heel of one foot directly in front of and touching the toes of the other foot.

Note: People unable to hold a position for 10 seconds are not asked to attempt further stands.

Other Geriatric Problems

Failure to Thrive
It is a syndrome of weight loss, decreased appetite, poor nutrition and inactivity, often accompanied by dehydration, depressive symptoms, impaired immune function and low cholesterol

Sarcopenia
- Age-related loss of muscle mass
- Increases the risk for falls, fractures, dependency, use of hospital services, institutionalization, poor quality of life, and mortality

Anorexia of aging
- The multifactorial decrease in appetite and/or food intake that occurs in late life
- Specific geriatric syndrome that can lead to malnutrition if not appropriately diagnosed and treated
- **Multimorbidity:** The coexistence of ≥2 chronic conditions, where one is not necessarily more central than the others
- **Polypharmacy:** Administration of more medications than clinically indicated, representing unnecessary drug use, i.e., ≥5 drugs during a 3-month period

CHAPTER 9: Approach to Psychiatric Illness

Sriraksha Nayak, Vaddi Rohit

CASE SHEET FORMAT

HISTORY

Identification and Sociodemographic Data
- Name, age, gender of patient:
- Name, age, relationship of the informant (caregiver/spouse/parent)
- Education
- Occupation
- Marital status
- Language used for interview
- Use of interpreter: Yes/No
- **Reliability** of informant: Reliable/not reliable
- **Adequacy of history** obtained (from patient and informant) *to make a diagnosis*: Adequate/inadequate.

Presenting Complaints
Presenting complaints to be listed in chronological order of symptom appearance along with duration of each symptom.

History of Present Illness
History of present illness to be obtained *from patient and informant* and *recorded separately*. Describe nature of onset, precipitating incidents if any, course and evolution of symptoms, functional impairment, biological functions and relevant negative history. Also inquire if any **treatment** was sought for the presenting illness.

Past History
Past history of psychiatric and medical/neurological illness in the past.

Family History
Family history to include type of family, family tree, medical/psychiatric disorders in family, etc.

Personal History
Personal history to include significant events during birth and early developmental history, details of education and occupation, menstrual history, sexual history and biological functions.

Premorbid Personality
Premorbid personality to assess patient's general *functioning prior to onset of illness or during periods of remission.*

EXAMINATION

General Physical Examination
- **Vital signs**: Pulse, BP, respiratory rate, oxygen saturation and temperature.
- **P**allor, **I**cterus, **C**yanosis, **C**lubbing, **L**ymphadenopathy, **E**dema
- Built, nourishment and BMI
- **Handedness**
- Conduct a general examination to assess for **stigmata of systemic disease** or any features helping in diagnoses.

Examination of systems (CNS, GI, CVS, RS) to be done as per the format mentioned in respective sections.

Mental Status Examination
- Consciousness and alertness
- General appearance and behavior
- **Rapport** (*therapeutic relationship between patient and caregiver*): Established or not
- Abnormal involuntary movements/hallucinatory behavior/catatonic symptoms
- Speech and language
- Thought
- Mood and affect
- Perception
- Other phenomenon: Compulsion, depersonalization/derealization, made affect/act/impulse, somatic passivity, etc.
- Cognitive functions: Orientation, attention and concentration, memory, general intelligence, abstraction, judgment, insight

- Additional assessment in ***substance use disorders***:
  - *Defense mechanism* used to justify substance taking behavior, e.g., denial, rationalization
  - *Stage of motivation* that the patient is in, i.e., pre-contemplation, contemplation, preparation, action, maintenance, relapse
  - *Locus of control,* i.e., perceived cause/responsibility of substance taking behavior: internal/external

Further Assessments

- **Scales/questionnaires** to assess severity, remission/relapse of symptoms
- **Blood investigations** to obtain baseline values to monitor for drug side effects/toxicity. For example, TC/DC, AST/ALT, serum creatinine, electrolytes, TFT, ECG, serum lithium, etc.
- **Electroencephalogram:** To differentiate pseudoseizure vs true seizure, alcohol withdrawal delirium (fast waves) vs other causes of delirium (slow waves)
- **Neuroimaging:** To look for structural/functional pathology of brain.

Summary/Diagnostic Formulation

Deduce relevant positive and negative findings in history, examination and assessments to provide a gist of significant events/findings that aid in making appropriate diagnosis and in adequate/holistic management of patient.

DIAGNOSIS FORMAT

Axis I:
Clinical syndromes (psychiatric disorder and somatic disease) with:
- Total duration of illness: Since first onset of illness
- Current duration: Since onset of current episode/illness.

Axis II:
Disability in POFS functioning: Ranging from normal (grade 1) to complete loss of function (grade 4).
- **A:** **P**ersonal
- **B:** **O**ccupational
- **C:** **F**amily
- **D:** **S**ocial

Axis III:
Environmental/circumstantial and personal lifestyle **factors contributing to the manifestation of disorder.**

Example 1

Axis I:
Bipolar affective disorder, current episode mania without psychotic symptoms and hypertension
   Total duration of illness 5 years, current episode 1 week.

Axis II:
A3 **B**2 **C**2 **D**2

Axis III:
Family history of other mental and behavioral disorders.

Example 2

Axis I:
Paranoid schizophrenia episodic with stable deficit and diabetes mellitus.
   Total duration of illness 8 years, current duration 1 month.

Axis II:
A3 **B**2 **C**2 **D**4

Axis III:
Problems in relationship with spouse or partner.

DISCUSSION ON HISTORY AND EXAMINATION

SALIENT POINTS IN HISTORY

Identification and Sociodemographic Data

- **Reliability of informant (reliable/not reliable)** assessed based on **5Cs**
  1. **C**redibility
  2. **C**ontact during period of illness
  3. **C**ontinuity in history of illness and significant life events
  4. **C**onstancy of information provided
  5. **C**orroboration, i.e., history obtained is similar even when cross-verified from other informants
- Location of residence: To educate regarding immediate available care in case of emergency/drug side effects/relapse.

History of Present Illness

History of present illness to be obtained *from patient and informant* and *recorded separately*. Describe each symptom with the help of following pointers:

- Nature of **onset,** i.e., time taken from normal/baseline behavior to abnormality may be *abrupt* <2 days, *acute* <2 weeks, sub-acute <month, *gradual* >month
- **Precipitating** incidents: Look for **positive or negative stress, substance use, sleep disturbance**, **non-compliance to medication,** e.g., family function/increased work following promotion leading to sleep disturbance or restarting substance use after loss in business/relationship/reputation thereby alteration in body concentration of medications
- **Course and evolution:**
  - What was the first symptom to appear?
  - When and how did other symptoms start?
  - How were the symptoms when they began, how have they progressed and what is the present status?
- Explore for **additional symptoms** other than the ones mentioned in presenting complaints, that would help in **diagnosing a disorder,** e.g., if presenting complaints are decreased sleep and increased activity, inquire:
  - What does the patient do when awake at night?
  - Does he talk/eat/pray/spend excessively?
  - Does he boast of having special powers?
- How has the illness **affected his living**? For example, discontinued school/work, stopped interacting with family/neighbors, impaired self-care
- **Biological functions:** Sleep, appetite, libido
- Relevant **negative history**: Ask for symptoms that would differentiate current disorder from *other psychiatric/substance-induced disorder* and would exclude other *medical/neurological* disorder (trauma to head/loss of consciousness/abnormal involuntary movement/fever, etc.)
- *Additional points* to be elicited **in case of substance use disorder**:
  - *Evolution* from 1st use to pattern of use during past 1 year
  - *Average quantity of use* in the past month, duration since *last consumption*, symptoms of withdrawal/intoxication
  - Explore for *associated* personality traits/conduct disorder in childhood
  - Physical/psychological/psychiatric/legal/social/occupational *consequences*
  - If patient had been abstinent, explore *reasons for relapse*

Treatment History

- Record any form of treatment sought **during the course of present illness** prior to the current consultation and the corresponding response to treatment.
- Details of medications and their side effects, e.g., antipsychotic induced extrapyramidal symptoms, clozapine-induced excessive salivation/weight gain, carbamazepine/oxcarbazepine-induced rash, lithium/valproate-induced tremors.

Past History

- Symptoms during past episodes, severity, response to treatment, reasons for poor compliance
- History of ECT/suicide attempt/untreated episodes in the past
- Assess patient's **functioning** in the **period intervening between two episodes**: Was there complete return to pre-morbid status? Were there any symptoms that persisted/progressively worsened?
- Look for significant *medical/neurological disorders* like head injury, seizure, diabetes mellitus, thyroid disorders, etc.

Family History

- **Type of family** (nuclear, joint, extended) to assess family support for favorable prognosis
- Family tree up to three generations: Inquire for age, education, occupation, personality traits of each member
- Ask for psychiatric (intellectual disability/suicide/epilepsy/substance abuse/abnormal or odd personalities) and medical disorders (dementia, seizure disorder, movement disorders, hypertension, type II diabetes mellitus)
- Assess **interpersonal relationships** among the family members and general beliefs/practices in the family
- **Marital history:** Assess interpersonal relationships with spouse and children. Look for marital discord due to delusion of infidelity/medication induced sexual dysfunction.

Personal History

- **Birth and early developmental history:** Assess for anoxic injury to brain, delayed milestones, health during childhood

- **Education:**
    - Assess interpersonal relationship with peers and teachers, performance in curricular and extra-curricular activities
    - Look for poor *scholastic performance*/discontinuation of studies which may be indicative of unrecognized neurodevelopmental disorder (e.g., learning/intellectual disability)
    - Look for features of other psychiatric disorders of childhood and adolescence, e.g., ADHD (inability to sit at a place, cannot wait for ones turn), autism (poor interaction with peers), conduct disorder (truancy, disciplinary issues)
- **Occupation:** Assess nature of jobs taken, reasons for change of jobs, coping with stress at work, interpersonal relationships with colleagues. Look for *factors* that could *precipitate relapse* or could *exacerbate existing condition*
    - Frequent change of jobs may be suggestive of patients symptoms interfering with normal functioning, e.g., suspicion in paranoid PD or expansive ideas in mania
    - Night-shift working interferes with normal sleep-wake cycle: Necessitates close watch for early signs of relapse, adjustment of medication doses may be needed to avoid occupational hazards due to drowsiness during working hours
    - Individual working at a bar (has easy access to alcohol) may need greater motivation to remain abstinent.
- **Menstrual history:** Assess regularity and flow, LMP, ability to main adequate personal hygiene, emotional/somatic changes during menses. Ask if any alteration in cycles due to medications, antipsychotic-induced galactorrhea/amenorrhea
- **Sexual history:** Assess sexual knowledge, attitude and practices
- **Biological functions:** Sleep, appetite, libido, bowel and bladder habits, personal care.

Premorbid/Inter-morbid Personality

Premorbid/inter-morbid personality (temperament in <18 years age): To be obtained from *neutral informant* to explore following areas of *functioning prior to onset of illness or during periods of remission*:
- Descriptive approach (as compared to use of labels) to be used to get a complete picture
- Ability to make and sustain interpersonal relationships, ability to function in different societal roles
- Intellectual and leisure time activities of preference/interest
- Predominant mood states and energy levels, ability to understand, express and control emotions, coping with stress, degree of optimism
- Practical attitude towards self/others/relationships/health/life, e.g., what are his strengths and abilities? Is he shy/makes friends easily? Does he always want to be the center of attraction? Is he able to live up to moral, religious, social standards?

SALIENT POINTS IN GENERAL PHYSICAL AND SYSTEMIC EXAMINATION

- **Vital signs:**
    - Pulse: β blockers used in anxiety disorders may cause bradycardia
    - Blood pressure: Hypotension caused by antipsychotics and antidepressants
    - Respiratory rate and oxygen saturation: BZD induced respiratory depression
    - Temperature: NMS, drug overdose/withdrawal, delirium
- *Icterus* may be seen in substance use and pedal *edema* could be drug induced
- **Nourishment** is important while making the choice of drugs and monitoring drug related weight gain
- **Handedness**: Electrode placed on nondominant side in unilateral ECT
- *Features substantiating diagnosis*: Hesitation cuts over forearm in case of deliberate self-harm, needle tracks in IV drug abuse, injuries sustained during altercation, conjunctival injection and alcohol smell in breath/from clothes in alcohol intoxication
- Look for *features of drug toxicity/side effects*: Lithium induced tremors, antipsychotic induced EPS
- **Stigmata of intellectual disability** (head to toe): Mongoloid facies, microcephaly, hypertelorism, low set ears, cleft lip/palate, webbed neck, simian crease, saddle gap, etc.
- **Stigmata of alcoholic liver disease**: Palmar erythema, parotid enlargement, spider nevi, gynecomastia, testicular atrophy

Findings of utmost importance in systemic examination:
- **Central nervous system (CNS):** Focal neurological signs, exaggerated reflexes, meningeal signs, cerebellar dysfunction, frontal release signs, drunken gait, involuntary movements, extrapyramidal signs, fundoscopy, lobe function tests. Positive signs obtained point towards organic brain dysfunction
- **Gastrointestinal (GI) system:** Organomegaly, ascites with everted umbilicus, prominent abdominal veins with reversal of flow in alcoholic liver disease
- **Cardiovascular system (CVS):** Cardiac murmurs point to organic causation of anxiety/panic symptoms
- **Respiratory system (RS):** Infection or its treatment may have caused symptom relapse in compliant patient with no other identifiable cause.

MENTAL STATUS EXAMINATION

Level of Consciousness

- Normal consciousness indicates alert, vigilant, lucid individual
- If the subject is not fully alert, mention amount of *stimulation needed for arousal* and duration of time patient can maintain *attention once aroused*

Approach to Psychiatric Illness

Abnormalities of consciousness	
Quantitative	**Qualitative**
▪ **Clouding:** Impaired attention and concentration	▪ **Delirium:** Altered sensorium
▪ **Drowsy:** Drifts to sleep if not actively stimulated, unable to pay attention when aroused	▪ **Twilight:** Disruption in continuity of consciousness
▪ **Sopor/obtundation:** Persistent vigorous stimulation required to elicit response (groaning or mumbling), confused when aroused	▪ **Oneiroid:** Dream like state
	▪ **Stupor:** Akinesia + mutism in awake, alert patient
▪ **Coma:** Complete unawareness, no response to external stimuli	

General Appearance and Behavior

- **Grooming:** Whether the patient's grooming/personal hygiene appropriate to the situation? For example, overdressing in mania, unkempt in psychosis, depression
- **Posture:** Drooping of shoulders in depression
- **Facial expressions:** Happy, sad, *Otto Verugath sign*; increased forehead marking in depression, worried/excess perspiration/tensed voice in anxiety
- **Eye to eye contact** made/maintained or not
- **Attitude towards examiner,** e.g., cooperative/hostile/evasive/guarded
- **Psychomotor activity** (motor execution of psychic events): Agitated/retardation
- **Abnormal motor behavior:** If present, describe rate or speed, purposiveness, goal-directedness, response to command/environmental stimuli and repetitiveness.

Speech

- Assess *phonation, articulation, comprehension* (give a three stage command, e.g., "place index finger of right hand on your nose and then on your left ear"), *repetition* (repeat "No ifs, ands, or buts"), *reading* (ask patient to read and obey a written command on a piece of paper stating "Close your eyes"), *writing* (ask the patient to write a sentence and assess if it is sensible and has a subject and a verb), *naming* (show a pencil and watch and ask them what is it).
- Assess **volume** (quantity), **tone** (pitch/quality), **reaction time** (gap between end of interviewers' question and patients response it), **coherence** (whether patient's response is understandable?), **relevance** (of patients reply to the question asked)
- Slow and low tone speech in depression, excessive and high tone speech in mania, incoherent speech and neologism in schizophrenia

Thought abnormalities: Assessed from overall response during interview and by the *sample of talk* obtained by seeking patient's response to an open-ended, neutral question (e.g., how is a particular festival celebrated?) in the language that the patient is fluent in. Look for following abnormalities:

- Thought **formation:** Look for incoherence, loosening of association, neologism (distorting existing words/coining new words/giving new meaning to existing words)
- Thought **possession:** Are the thoughts one's own/controlled by an external source?
  - *Thought insertion:* Someone else's thoughts are being put in one's mind
  - *Thought withdrawal:* One's thoughts are being removed from one's mind
  - *Thought broadcast:* Many people are getting to know one's thoughts
- Thought **stream/speed:** Increased (pressured speech, flight of ideas), decreased (inhibition, slowing of thinking)
- Thought **continuity:** Perseveration (repetition beyond the point of relevance), thought block
- Thought **content:** Assess for presence of **delusions, obsessions, ideas** of suicide/hopelessness/worthlessness/helplessness

DELUSION

Delusion is a ***false, unshakable*** belief of ***personal significance***, arising out of an ***internal morbid process***, and is ***out of keeping*** with the one's ***sociocultural background***. Yet, the belief is held with ***strong conviction despite evidence to the contrary***.

Types of Delusion Based on Theme

- *Persecution:* Belief that others are out to harm me
- *Grandeur:* Belief of having special powers or status (suggests mania)
- *Guilt/sin:* Belief of having committed sin, blaming oneself
- *Nihilism,* e.g., conviction that 'My head is missing,' 'I have no body', 'I am dead'.
- *Erotomania,* e.g., belief that a movie star secretly loves them
- *Infidelity:* Belief that partner/spouse is unfaithful
- *Reference,* e.g., belief that the story in a book is referring to them
- *Control/passivity* of motor functions or bodily sensations. For example, belief of one's thoughts/emotions/action/sensations being controlled by aliens
- *Misidentification:* Capgras (persecutor coming in disguise of familiar person), Fregoli (known person who wants to harm taking disguise of stranger), intermetamorphosis, delusion of subjective doubles
- *Somatic:* Body parts being abnormal in size and shape (dysmorphophobia), infestation by worms (parasitosis), foul odor (halitosis, olfactory reference syndrome).

Characteristics of Delusion

- Onset: *Primary/secondary* (to psychopathology, previous experience, cultural belief)
- Duration: *Fleeting* (in delirium)/*persistent* (in delusional disorder)
- *Congruence with mood*: Mood-congruent (grandiose delusion in mania/delusion of guilt in depression) or mood-incongruent (in schizophrenia)
- *Well or ill-systematization:* Ability to describe why does he believes a belief
- *Non-bizarre/bizarre,* i.e., culturally inappropriate and implausible

- *Acting out,* i.e., whether patient responds to the delusions or not
- *Active or encapsulated,* i.e., present but decreased
- *Single/multiple*

OBSESSIONS

Obsessions are **thoughts/ideas/images/impulses/urges** that are own's own but involuntary, unpleasantly recurrent, persistent, perceived as unwanted/senseless, unsuccessfully resisted, cause marked anxiety or distress or interfere with activities/**socio-occupational impairment.**

Themes of Obsession

- *Cleanliness:* Fears of contamination
- *Symmetry and numbers,* e.g., need to read a line for a particular number of times
- *Doubt,* e.g., whether door is locked or not
- *Forbidden or taboo thoughts,* e.g., aggressive, sexual or religious obsessions
- *Harm,* i.e., thoughts of causing harm to oneself/others.

MOOD AND AFFECT

Assess *range* of emotions expressed, *reactivity*/response to stimuli, *intensity* of emotion expressed, *appropriateness* to situation, *congruence* to one's thought, *relatedness* and *stability/lability/incontinence* of affect.

Mood

- Mood refers to **pervasive and sustained emotional state** that colors individual's experiences and his perception of environment, i.e., is *subjective and longitudinal*
- Ask the patient how he has been feeling over the past 2 weeks, e.g., sad/happy/anxious/tensed/worried. Feeling guilty or hopeless (in depression). Inquire for thoughts/plans of self-harm, if any. Feeling excessively worried about many things (in anxiety disorders)

Affect

- Affect refers to pattern of **observable behavior** as an expression of subjective experience of one's emotional state, i.e., *objective and cross-sectional emotional state*
- It is assessed by observing facial expression, posture, gesture, general appearance, tone of voice, etc. For example, elated affect (elevated mood with excess energy) seen in mania or depressed affect, i.e., sad mood with low energy/interest in depression.

Perceptual abnormalities: Assess for presence of illusion or hallucination and their *modality, content, frequency, intensity, clarity, association with other sensory stimuli,* etc.

ILLUSIONS

Illusions are **misperceptions of real external stimuli,** e.g., mistaking a shrub for a person in poor light.

HALLUCINATION

- It is **perception in the absence of corresponding external stimuli** that has characteristics of normal perception (i.e., it is clear, involuntary, considered to be real and occurs in external objective space with the patient being conscious) but lacks publicness (patient experiences it but others around him cannot experience it)
- It can occur in any sensory modality; most common in psychiatric disorders being *auditory* (thought echo, command hallucination, running commentary) and most common in organic psychiatric disorders being *visual* (e.g., seeing 'visions', Lilliputian hallucination).
- *Olfactory* and *gustatory* hallucination are usually seen in temporal lobe epilepsy
- *Tactile hallucination* (e.g., cocaine bugs) can be superficial, kinesthetic or visceral
- *Hypnagogic* (occur while going to sleep) and *hypnopompic* (occur while waking up from sleep) are seen in narcolepsy.
- *Other* types of *hallucination*: Functional (simultaneous normal perception and hallucination, both from same modality), reflex (simultaneous normal perception in one modality and hallucination in other modality), extracampine (hallucination occurring beyond the limits of sensory field).

PSEUDOHALLUCINATION

Phenomenon lying in between true hallucination and mental imagery

- Hare described it as hallucination with insight
- Jasper described it as hallucination occurring in inner subjective space
- Kandinsky described it as mental imagery that is clear.

Factors to differentiate	Normal perception	Hallucination	Mental imagery
Actual source of stimuli	Outer objective space, i.e., external world	Inner subjective space, i.e., one's own mind	Inner subjective space
Perceived source of stimuli	Perceived to be coming from external world	Misperceived to be coming from external world	Perceived to be coming from one's mind

Cognitive Functions

- **Orientation to time, place and person:** Assess awareness to passage of time, knowing whereabouts and recognizing self, significant others, etc.
- **Attention and concentration:** May be assessed by:
  - **Serial subtraction test (100–7)** in which the patient is asked to subtract 7 from 100 and then 7 from the answer and so on
  - Month/day backwards
  - Spelling WORLD backwards as DLROW

- **Memory**
  - Based on length of storage of memory
    - *Registration/immediate*: It is judged by asking the patient to **repeat** simple new information (3 unrelated words like apple, penny, Thursday) **immediately** after hearing it.
    - *Recent*: It is judged by asking the patient to repeat simple new information (as mentioned above) **after an interval of 1–2 minutes** during which time the patient's attention should be diverted elsewhere **or 24-hour recall**
    - *Remote:* It is judged by asking the patient to recall past (>24 hours) events, personal and impersonal
  - Based on type of information
    - *Implicit/procedural* memory: *Does not* require **conscious attention to recall** (e.g., memory for procedures, skills, habits)
    - *Explicit/declarative* memory: *Requires* conscious attention to recall. It can be further classified into **episodic memory** (for specific events and contexts) and **semantic memory** (for vocabulary and concepts).

Mini-mental state examination	
Component assessed	Test/total score
Orientation **Time,** day, date, month, year **Place:** Room/floor/building, city, district, state, country	–/5 –/5
Registration: Examiner presents 3 names of unrelated objects that the patient is asked to repeat immediately, e.g., apple, Sunday, blue	–/3
Attention and calculation: *Serial subtraction* of 7 from the answer starting from 100, to continue up to five steps, e.g., 93, 84, 77, 70, 63 OR Spell world *backwards*, e.g., DLROW	–/5
Recall: Patient is asked to recall the 3 words given during registration assessment	–/3
Language *Naming* any 2 objects, (e.g., book, table) *Repeat the sentence* "No, ifs, ands or buts" *Follow a 3 stage command*, e.g., "Pick the paper from table, crumple it and throw in the dustbin" *Read and obey the command*, e.g., "Close your eyes" *Writing a sentence*	–/2 –/1 –/3 –/1 –/1
Copy an *intersecting pentagon*	–/1
Final score	–/30
Interpretation of MMSE score: ≥24: No cognitive impairment, 18–23: Mild cognitive impairment, ≤17: Severe cognitive impairment	

- **Intellectual ability:** Assess general knowledge, simple calculation, vocabulary and concept complexity (i.e., difference between child and dwarf, sea and river)
- **Abstract ability:**
  - Assessed using *proverb test,* i.e., ability to understand and explain inner meaning of a proverb or by *similarity test,* i.e., ask for similarity between chair and table (furnitures), apple and orange (fruits), etc.
  - Patient with poor abstraction/concretization of thinking, may explain "Barking dogs seldom bite" as "Yes, my dog barks but does not bite" or the similarity between table and chair as "having 4 legs"
- **Judgment**
  - *Test* judgment: Give a test situation and inquiring would the patient respond to it. For example, what would you do if you found an addressed letter on road/house on fire/child in pond?
  - *Personal and social* judgment: Opined from historical data and patient's behavior during interview based on ability to conduct oneself (behave/emote) in appropriate manner.
- **Insight** refers to patients' awareness and understanding of his illness, its cause and the need for treatment. **Lack of insight,** i.e., failure to accept that one is ill and/or in need of treatment is a ***feature of psychotic disorders***.

Grading of insight	
Grade 0	Complete denial of illness
Grade 1	Slight awareness of being sick and needing help but denying it at the same time (ambivalent)
Grade 2	Aware of illness but attributes it to external factors (black magic) or to physical illness
Grade 3	Aware of illness, but attributes it to internal, unknown, mysterious factors
Grade 4	Intellectual insight: Aware of illness being caused due to neurophysiological changes in brain causing disturbances in thought and emotion and that it can be alleviated/controlled by adherence to appropriate treatment strategies. However, unable to utilize this knowledge to positively modify one's behavior
Grade 5	Emotional insight: Complete awareness and understanding of illness along with being able to maintain strict adherence to treatment, abstinence from substance, regular follow-up so as to promote remission

Kirby's method for examination of uncooperative patients
(e.g., in catatonia, stupor)

- **Observe** for spontaneous movements, speech and emotional response
- **Examine** for degree of uncooperativeness of patients like negativism, gegenhalten, rigidity, automatic obedience, mitgehen and mitmachen
- **Record** mutism, echo phenomenon, vital parameters including pulse, BP, temperature and respiratory rate
- Assessment to be recorded under following headings:

  - General reaction and posture
  - Facial movements and expression
  - Reaction to examiners questions and tests
  - Emotional responsiveness
  - Eyes and pupils
  - Muscular reactions
  - Speech
  - Writing
  - Vitals

Note:
Mitmachen—the patient's body can be placed in any posture, despite asking the patient to resist all movements. When released, the patient returns to the resting position (cf. waxy flexibility).
Mitgehen—an extreme form of mitmachen in which the patient will move in any direction with very slight pressure.
Gegenhalten (opposition)—the patient will oppose attempts at passive movement with a force equal to that being applied (cf. mitmachen).

DISCUSSION ON DIAGNOSIS OF PSYCHIATRIC DISORDERS

APPROACH TO DIAGNOSIS IN PSYCHIATRY

- **Symptom**s and their **duration** fulfil requisite **criteria** for diagnosis of a particular psychiatric disorder
- Symptoms must cause significant **socio-occupational**, (i.e., education/work, interpersonal relationships, self-care) **disturbance** as perceived by patient/his family
- Symptoms are **not better explained by** diagnostic criteria of **other psychiatric** disorder
- Symptoms are **not caused by** any **substance use** or any **other medical/surgical condition**.

Major/Common Groups of Psychiatric Disorders

- Psychotic disorders: Schizophrenia, delusional disorder, mood disorders
- Neurotic disorders: Anxiety, panic, phobia, PTSD, dissociation, hypochondriasis
- OCD and related disorders: OCD, trichotillomania, skin picking, hoarding disorder
- Organic mental disorders: Delirium, dementia, amnestic disorder
- Substance use disorders
- Others: Disorders of eating, sleep, sexual, menstrual, puerperal, personality
- Neurodevelopmental disorders: Intellectual disability, autism, ADHD.

Features of differentiation	Psychosis	Neurosis
Insight/reality contact/illness awareness	Absent	Present
Delusions/hallucinations (psychotic symptoms)	Present	Absent
Neurotransmitter involved	Dopamine	Serotonin
Pharmacotherapy of choice	Antipsychotics	SSRI
Interpersonal behavior	Impaired	Preserved
Examples	Schizophrenia	Anxiety, phobia

Psychotic disorders: Relationship of various psychiatric illnesses has been shown in **Figure 9.1**.

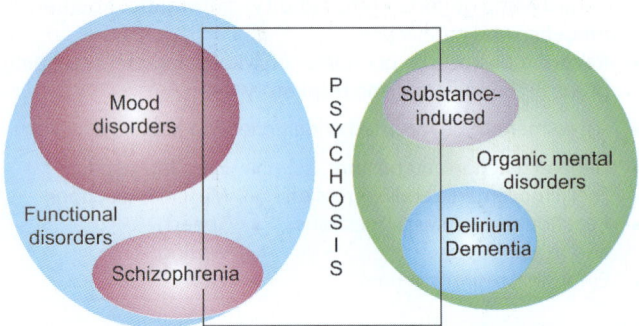

Fig. 9.1: Relationship of various psychiatric illnesses.

Features of differentiation among types of psychosis	Functional psychosis	Organic psychosis
Demonstrable underlying **cause**	Absent	Present (structural defect/physiologic dysfunction of brain)
Predominant type of **hallucination**	Auditory	Visual
Sensorium	Intact	Altered
Onset	Gradual	Acute
Focal neurological deficit	Usually absent	Usually present
Example	Schizophrenia	Delirium

DSM-5 diagnostic criteria for schizophrenia: Symptom and duration criteria

≥**2** of the below symptoms to be present for **at least 6 months** with at least 1 month of active symptoms; **one** symptom **must be** either **a, b, or c**

Positive symptoms
a. **Delusions**
b. **Hallucinations**
c. **Disorganized speech/thought:** Loosening of association, formal thought disorders, neologisms, conceptual disorganization
d. **Disorganized/bizarre behavior:** Aggressive/agitated, odd clothing or appearance, odd social behavior, repetitive stereotyped behavior, catatonia

Negative symptoms
- **Alogia:** 'Lack of words,' including poverty of speech and of speech content in response to a question
- **Affective flattening/blunting:** Lack of expressive gestures
- **Alexithymia:** Inability to describe and express emotions
- **Avolition:** Loss of drive
- **Apathy:** Lack of concern
- **Anhedonia:** Loss of interest in previously pleasurable activities
- **Asociality:** Diminished social engagement, few friends, activities, interests; impaired intimacy
- **Attention impairment**

Differentiating types of **schizophrenia like disorders** based on **duration of symptoms**:
- <1 month: Acute and transient psychotic disorder/brief psychotic disorder
- 1–6 months: Schizophreniform disorder
- >6 months: Schizophrenia

Features of differentiation among types of functional psychosis	Nonaffective psychosis	Affective psychosis
Mood symptoms	Not predominant	Predominant
Includes	- Schizophrenia - Delusional disorder	- Bipolar disorder - Schizoaffective disorder

Approach to Psychiatric Illness

Features of differentiation among types of nonaffective psychosis	Schizophrenia	Delusional disorder
Delusions	Present	Present
Hallucinations	Present	Absent
Behavior	Abnormal	Normal
Socio-occupational functioning	Impaired	Intact

Features of differentiation among types of affective psychosis	Bipolar disorder	Schizophreniform disorder
Episodes	Mania/depression ± psychosis (psychotic symptoms are usually mood congruent)	Mania/depression + psychosis
Intervening period	Normal	Psychotic symptoms always present

Mood Disorders

Figure 9.2 depicts the **spectrum** of mood disorders.

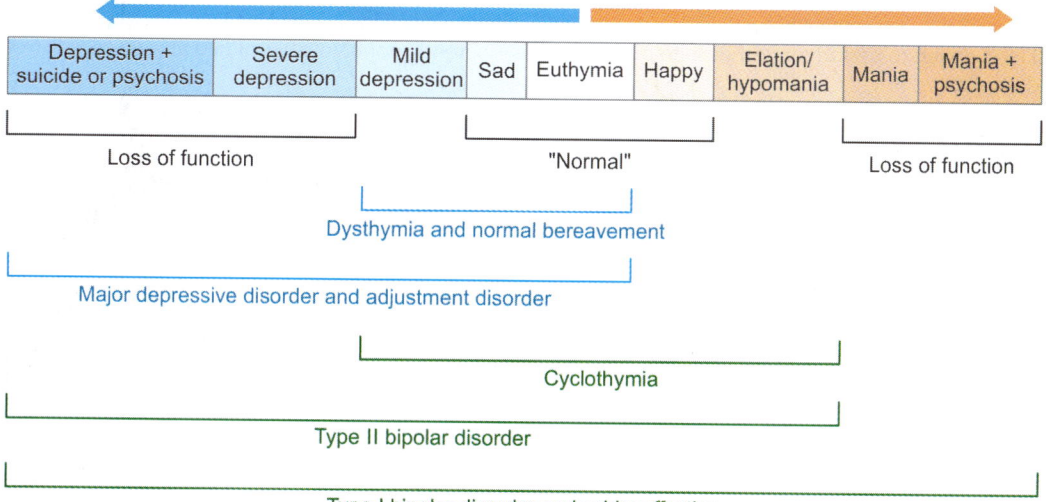

Fig. 9.2: Spectrum of mood disorders.

Classification of mood disorders		
Unipolar	**Bipolar**	**Mood disorders with known etiology**
Major depressive disorder	Bipolar I disorder	Substance-induced mood disorder
Dysthymic disorder	Bipolar II disorder	Mood disorder due to general medical condition
	Cyclothymic disorder	

DSM-5 diagnostic criteria for major depressive episode: Symptom and duration criteria
≥5 of the below symptoms to be present for **at least 2 weeks**; **one** symptom **must be** either **a or b**
a. **Depressed mood**: As reported by patient (feeling sad/empty/hopeless) or observed by others (appears tearful) b. **Loss of interest/pleasure** c. Significant and unintentional **weight loss/gain**, i.e., >5% change in a month **or decrease/increase in appetite** d. **Insomnia or hypersomnia** e. **Psychomotor agitation or retardation** f. Fatigue or **low energy** g. Feelings of **worthlessness** or excessive/inappropriate **guilt** h. Diminished ability to think or **decreased concentration** or indecisiveness i. Recurrent thoughts of death or **suicidal ideation**/plan/attempt

DSM-5 diagnostic criteria for manic episode: Symptom and duration criteria
At least one week of **a + b + c**
a. **Mood disturbance**: Elevated/expansive or irritable mood b. **Increased energy**/goal-directed activity c. **≥3** of the below symptoms (**≥4** if mood is irritable) • **Inflated self-esteem** or grandiosity • **Decreased need for sleep**, rested after only a few hours of sleep • Increased talkativeness, **pressured speech** • **Racing thoughts** and flight of ideas • **Distractibility**: Attention drawn too easily to unimportant/irrelevant external stimuli • Increased activity (goal directed—social/work or school related/sexual) or **psychomotor agitation** (non-goal directed purposeless activity) • Excessive involvement in activities with high potential for painful consequence (**indiscretion** in spending/business investment/travel/sexual engagements)

Features of differentiation among types of *anxiety-predominant neurotic disorders*	Generalized anxiety disorder	Panic disorder	Phobic anxiety disorder
Occurrence	Persistent	Paroxysmal	Situational
Symptoms	Persistent	Episodic	On exposure
Cognitions	Worry	Fear of symptoms	Fear of situation
Behavior	Agitation	Escape	Avoidance

Features of differentiation among neurotic disorders occurring after trauma/stress

Following sudden, life-threatening trauma/stress		After gradual routine life stress
Symptom duration <1 month	Symptom duration >1 month	**Adjustment disorder**
Acute stress reaction	**Post-traumatic stress disorder**	

Diagnostic criteria for obsessive—compulsive disorder

- Presence of **obsession, compulsions or both** for **at least 2 weeks**
- Obsessions: **Thoughts/ideas/images/impulses/urges** that are one's own but involuntary, unpleasantly recurrent, persistent, perceived as unwanted/senseless, unsuccessfully resisted
- Compulsions: Excessive and repetitive **behaviors** (hand washing's, ordering, checking) or **mental acts** (praying, counting, repeating) that the individual feels driven to perform in response to obsession, are inherently nonenjoyable, aimed at reducing distress or preventing some dreaded situation
- Obsessions and compulsions are time-consuming (>1 hour/day) and cause marked anxiety or distress or interfere with activities/**socio-occupational impairment**

Features of differentiation among types of organic mental disorders	Delirium	Dementia	Amnestic disorder
Onset	Acute	Chronic	Chronic
Course	Fluctuating	Progressive	Progressive
Sensorium	Altered	Clear	Clear
Cognitive functions affected	<ul><li>Multiple</li><li>Poor attention and concentration:<ul><li>Recent memory affected</li><li>Remote memory normal</li></ul></li></ul>	<ul><li>Multiple</li><li>Amnesia (remote + recent)</li><li>Apraxia</li><li>Agnosia</li><li>Aphasia</li><li>Loss of executive functions</li></ul>	Only memory affected Recent > remote
Confabulations (filling up gaps in memory)	Absent	Absent	Present
Psychotic symptoms	<ul><li>Present</li><li>Fleeting paranoid delusions</li><li>Transient visual hallucinations</li></ul>	<ul><li>Present</li><li>Fixed paranoid delusions</li><li>Auditory, visual hallucinations</li></ul>	Absent
Cause	Metabolic, infective, endocrine, drug-intoxication/withdrawal	<ul><li>Reversible: Depression, NPH, B_{12} deficiency, hypothyroidism</li><li>Irreversible: Alzheimer's, vascular, Lewy body, frontotemporal</li></ul>	B_{12} deficiency: Korsakoff's amnestic syndrome
Management	Treat the underlying cause	Antidementia drugs	B_{12} supplements

ICD-10 diagnostic criteria for delirium

For a definitive diagnosis, **symptoms** should be present **in each one of the following areas:**
- Impairment of **consciousness and attention**
- Global disturbance of **cognition** (illusions and hallucinations, impaired memory, disorientation)
- **Psychomotor** disturbances (hypo- or hyperactivity)
- Disturbance of the **sleep-wake cycle** (insomnia, reversal of the sleep-wake cycle; daytime drowsiness; nocturnal worsening of symptoms)
- **Emotional** disturbances, e.g., depression, anxiety or fear, irritability, euphoria or wandering perplexity

ICD-10 diagnostic criteria for substance dependence syndrome

For a definite diagnosis of dependence, ≥3 of the **below symptoms** to be **present together** for **at least a month during the previous year:**
- A strong desire or sense of compulsion to take the substance: **Craving**
  Difficulties in controlling substance-taking behavior in terms of its onset, termination, or levels of use: **Loss of control**
- A physiological **withdrawal** state when substance use has ceased or been reduced
- Evidence of **tolerance**, such that increased doses of the psychoactive substance are required in order to achieve effects originally produced by lower doses
- Progressive neglect of alternative interests because of increased amount of time spent to obtain/take/recover from effects of psychoactive substance use: **Salience**
- Persisting with substance use despite clear evidence of overtly harmful consequences, such as harm to the liver through excessive drinking: **Continued use despite harm**

Symptoms of alcohol withdrawal: Based on time elapsed since last alcohol intake

6–8 hours: Tremors (shakes, jitters), autonomic hyperactivity (increased BP, tachycardia, flushing)
8–12 hours: Psychotic and perceptual symptoms (alcoholic paranoia)
12–24 hours: Seizures (rum fits)
Within 72 hours: Delirium tremens—coarse tremors + altered sensorium + visual hallucination

Classification of personality disorders (DSM-5) and their characteristic features

Cluster A Odd, eccentric	Cluster B Dramatic, emotional	Cluster C Anxious, fearful
Schizoid (emotionally detached)	**Borderline** (unstable relationships, mood swings)	**Anxious-avoidant** (sensitive to rejection)
Schizotypal (magical thinking, speech oddities)	**Histrionic** (need to be center of attraction) **Narcissistic** (self-centered)	**Dependent** (need reassurance)
Paranoid (extreme suspiciousness)	**Antisocial** (break rules and laws)	**Anankastic** (perfectionist)

Grading of intellectual disability

Feature	ICD10	ICD11/DSM-5
Severity assessed by	Intelligence quotient	Adaptive functioning
Mild	50–69	2–3 SD below mean
Moderate	35–49	3–4 SD below mean
Severe	20–34	>4 SD below mean
Profound	<20	

ICD-10 diagnostic criteria for mental disorders occurring secondary to brain damage/dysfunction and physical illness

- **Evidence** of cerebral disease/dysfunction or systemic physical disease known to be associated with the mental disorder
- **Temporal relationship** between onset of underlying disease and mental disorder
- **Recovery** from mental disorder following removal/improvement of underlying presumed cause
- **Absence of** evidence to suggest an **alternative cause** of mental disorder (e.g., strong family history or precipitating stress)

Assessment Tools used in Psychiatry

Help to identify the presence, measure of severity, monitoring improvement/worsening from baseline values:
- Psychotic symptoms:
    - Brief psychiatric rating scale (BPRS)
    - Positive and negative symptom scale (PANSS)
    - Bush Francis catatonia rating scale (BFCRS)
- Side effects of antipsychotic drugs
    - Abnormal involuntary movement scale (AIMS)
    - Barnes akathisia rating scale
    - Simpson Angus scale to assess EPS
- Depression
    - Hamilton depression rating scale (HDRS)
    - Becks depression inventory (BDI)
    - Montgomery Asberg depression rating scale (MADRS)
- Suicide
    - Becks hopelessness scale
    - Becks scale for suicidal ideation
    - Columbia suicide severity scale
    - Scale for assessment of lethality of suicidal attempt (SALSA)
- Youngs mania rating scale (YMRS)
- Hamilton anxiety rating scale
- Yale Brown obsessive compulsive scale (Y-BOCS)
- Dementia
    - Mini-mental status examination for screening
    - Clinical dementia rating scale (CDRS)
    - Confusion assessment method (CAM) for delirium
- Alcohol use disorder
    - CAGE questionnaire
    - Alcohol use disorder inventory (AUDIT)
    - Michigan alcoholism screening test (MAST)
    - Severity of alcohol dependence questionnaire (SADQ)
    - Clinical institute withdrawal assessment (CIWA)
    - University of Rhode Island change assessment scale for motivation (URICA)
- Intelligence assessment
    - Weschler's adult intelligence scales (WAIS)
    - Binet-Kamat test
    - Vineland social maturity scale (VSMS)
- Childhood autism rating scale (CARS)
- Conners scale for assessment of ADHD
- Personality
    - 16 personality factor test (16PF)
    - International Personality Disorder Examination (IPDE)
    - Rorschach inkblot technique
    - Thematic apperception test
- Scales to assess general functioning
    - Global Assessment of Functioning (GAF)
    - Clinical Global Impression (CGI)
    - Indian Disability Evaluation and Assessment Scale (IDEAS) for certification of disability due to mental illness (schizophrenia, BPAD, OCD, dementia)

CAGE Questionnaire: Alcohol Abuse Screening Tool

- Have you ever felt that you should **cut** down your drinking?
- Have you ever felt **annoyed** by others criticizing your drinking?
- Have you ever felt **guilty** about your drinking?
- Have you ever had a morning drink (**eye**-opener) after hangover?
- Affirmative response to ≥2 of the following questions (or to the last question alone) indicates a positive screen

CLINICAL INSTITUTE WITHDRAWAL ASSESSMENT FOR ALCOHOL (CIWA-A) SCALE

- Scale includes 10 common signs and symptoms of alcohol withdrawal with the notable exceptions of pulse rate and blood pressure, which must be a part of the assessment of alcohol withdrawal states

Clinical Institute Withdrawal Assessment for Alcohol—revised (CIWA-Ar) Scale

Symptoms	Range of scores
Nausea or vomiting	0 (no nausea, no vomiting) – 7 (constant nausea and/or vomiting)
Tremor	0 (no tremor) – 7 (severe tremors, even with arms not extended)
Paroxysmal sweats	0 (no sweat visible) – 7 (drenching sweats)
Anxiety	0 (no anxiety, at ease) – 7 (acute panic states)
Agitation	0 (normal activity) – 7 (constantly trashes about)
Tactile disturbances	0 (none) – 7 (continuous hallucinations)
Auditory disturbances	0 (not present) – 7 (continuous hallucinations)
Visual disturbances	0 (not present) – 7 (continuous hallucinations)
Headache	0 (not present) – 7 (extremely severe)
Orientation/clouding of sensorium	0 (oriented, can do serial additions) – 4 (disoriented for place and/or person)

- **Score grading:**
  - Less than 8 indicate mild withdrawal,
  - 8–15 indicate moderate withdrawal (marked autonomic arousal)
  - And >15 indicate severe withdrawal and are also predictive of the development of seizures and delirium
- **Score interpretation:**
  - If CIWA-Ar score is <8 pharmacological treatment is not necessary
  - If CIWA-Ar score 8–15 pharmacological treatment may be appropriate to prevent the progression to more severe forms of AWS
  - Pharmacological treatment is strongly indicated in patients with CIWA-Ar score >1

GENERAL OUTLINE OF PLAN OF MANAGEMENT OF PSYCHIATRIC DISORDERS

- **Psychiatric** management:
  - Perform diagnostic evaluation
  - Evaluate safety of patient and others
  - Evaluate and address functional impairment
  - Determine treatment setting: OP/IP
  - Establish and maintain therapeutic alliance
  - Monitor clinical status and safety
  - Psychoeducation of family and patient: Regarding nature, course, prognosis of illness, risk factors for relapse (stress, sleep disturbance, substance use, non-compliance to treatment), recognizing early warning signs of relapse, regular follow-up, relapse prevention strategies, etc.
  - Enhance treatment adherence
  - Address early signs of relapse
- **Pharmacological** management:
  - Antipsychotics
  - Mood stabilizers
  - Antidepressants
  - Benzodiazepines
  - Drugs for substance dependence management
  - Anti-dementia drugs
  - Drugs to manage side effects of psychotropics

Factors guiding *choice of particular drug*

- Efficacy
- Target symptoms
- Tolerability
- Drug-drug interaction
- Drug disease interaction
- Past response
- Patient preference
- Psychiatrist preference
- Financial

- **Psychological** management with suitable psychotherapy
  - Cognitive behavior therapy (CBT) for depression
  - Systematic desensitization for phobia
  - Eye movement desensitization reprocessing (EMDR) for PTSD
  - Aversion therapy for paraphilia
  - Dialectical behavior therapy for borderline personality disorder
  - **FRAMES** principle in **brief intervention** for substance use disorders
    - Give **feedback**
    - Help the patient understand that **responsibility** of behavior change is his own
    - **Advice** on the need for intervention
    - Provide **menu** of options available for de-addiction
    - Express **empathy**
    - Support **self-efficacy**
  - **Motivation enhancement therapy** for substance use disorders (**DARES**)
    - Establish **discrepancy** between patients present and ideal/expected behavior
    - Avoid **arguments**
    - Roll with **resistance** to behavior change
    - Express **empathy**
    - Support **self-efficacy**
- **Physical** methods: ECT, VNS, DBS, rTMS, psychosurgery
  - **Indications for ECT**
    - Severe depression with suicidal ideation
    - Catatonia
    - Resistant cases of schizophrenia, mania
    - Neuroleptic malignant syndrome
  - Left **vagal nerve stimulation** for resistant depression, intractable epilepsy
  - **Direct brain stimulation** for resistant OCD (basal ganglia), Parkinsonism (thalamus)
  - Psychosurgery: **Cingulotomy** for resistant OCD
- **Rehabilitation**: Interventions to reduce disability and facilitate re-integration of individual from treatment setting back into society (taking care of oneself, attending school/work, maintaining good interpersonal relationships)
  - **Vocational**: Identify patients interests/abilities and facilitate him to find a suitable job
  - **Social skills**: Helping patient understand, analyze and respond to social cues
  - **Cognitive**: Reducing neurocognitive deficits

CHAPTER 10

Semilong Cases

SEMILONG/THERAPEUTIC CASES

Therapeutic cases are common cases that will be encountered in outpatient settings. In examination of such cases, candidate is expected to take a brief focused history, do general examination and relevant systemic examination pertaining to the case. Also, the candidate is expected to formulate a management plan for the patient which would include relevant investigations, treatment strategy, and appropriate referral.

Common therapeutic cases kept are diabetes mellitus (DM), chronic kidney disease, thyroid disorders (hypothyroid/hyperthyroid), obesity, hypertension (HTN), fever, chronic obstructive pulmonary disease (COPD), bronchial asthma, anemia, pedal edema, and anasarca.

The format of case taking would include following:
1. History:
    a. Demographic details and presenting complaints
    b. Duration of disease and presence of complications
    c. Treatment details, any surgeries/interventions, and history of hospitalizations
    d. Personal history
    e. Diet history
2. General physical examination:
    a. Vitals
    b. Anthropometry
3. Systemic examination:
    a. Skin
    b. Cardiovascular
    c. Respiratory
    d. Neurological
    e. Gastrointestinal
    f. Musculoskeletal
4. Complete diagnosis
5. Investigations
6. Treatment plan.

A: Diabetes Mellitus	
History	<ul><li>Type of diabetes</li><li>Duration</li><li>Any complications—microvascular/macrovascular</li><li>Other coexistent diseases—hypertension, etc.</li><li>Treatment history</li><li>Diet history</li><li>Family history</li><li>History of hypoglycemia</li></ul>
Vitals	<ul><li>Pulse—peripheral pulses, resting tachycardia, and vessel wall thickening</li><li>Hypertension and postural hypotension</li><li>Raised jugular venous pressure (JVP)</li><li>Pedal edema (renal, cardiac, insulin induced, and autonomic neuropathy)</li></ul>
Anthropometry	Body mass index (BMI), waist circumference, and waist-hip ratio
Skin	<ul><li>Ulcers</li><li>Signs of insulin resistance (acanthosis nigricans, skin tags, and visceral obesity)</li><li>Diabetic dermopathy (shin spots) and blisters</li><li>*Taenia*, intertrigo (**Fig. 10A.1**), balanoposthitis (**Fig. 10A.2**), vulvovaginitis, oral thrush, folliculitis, and carbuncle</li></ul>
Cardiovascular	Orthostatic hypotension, resting tachycardia, evidence of hypertension, and heart failure
Respiratory	Pneumonia and tuberculosis
Neurological	<ul><li>Polyneuropathy and autonomic dysfunction</li><li>Retinopathy (**Figs. 10A.3 and 10A.4**)</li></ul>
Gastrointestinal	Gastroparesis, constipation, and nocturnal diarrhea
Musculoskeletal	Carpal tunnel syndrome, diabetic cheiroarthropathy, Charcot's joint, frozen shoulder, and Dupuytren's contracture

Contd...

Contd...

Others	- Genitourinary—urinary incontinence, recurrent infection, impotence, erectile dysfunction, and retrograde ejaculation - Examination of foot—ulcers, callosities, and vascular and neurological examination
Complete diagnosis	For example, type 2 diabetes mellitus with hypertension and obesity with nonproliferative retinopathy, chronic symmetrical sensorimotor polyneuropathy with autonomic dysfunction
Investigations	Hemoglobin A1c (HbA1c), fasting blood sugar (FBS), postprandial blood sugar (PPBS), serum creatinine, fasting lipid profile, urine routine and microalbuminuria, electrocardiogram (ECG), and thyroid stimulating hormone (TSH)
Treatment plan	- Nutritional and lifestyle modification - Drugs including insulin - Management of complication
Referral	Ophthalmology, nephrology, and neurology

B: Hypertension

History	- Duration - Complications - Treatment details
Vitals	- Signs of atherosclerosis (vessel thickening, bruits, and xanthelasma) - Peripheral pulses and radiofemoral delay—coarctation - Pulse rate and rhythm - Blood pressure (BP) to be checked in all four limbs and postural BP - Edema (cardiac, renal, and drug induced) - Pallor [chronic kidney disease (CKD)]
Anthropometry	BMI and waist-hip ratio
Skin	Hyperpigmentation, striae, signs of CKD, and thyroid disease
Cardiovascular	Signs of left ventricular hypertrophy (LVH) (heaving apex, S4) and heart failure
Respiratory	Obstructive sleep apnea (OSA)
Neurological	- Fundus—hypertensive retinopathy - Evidence of stroke

Contd...

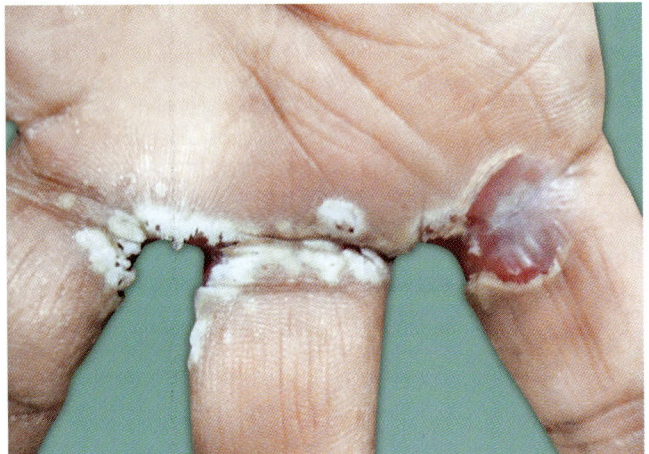

Fig. 10A.1: Intertrigo.

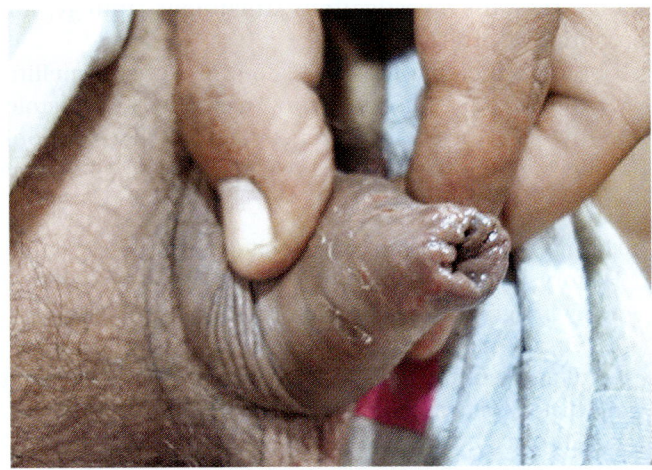

Fig. 10A.2: Balanoposthitis.

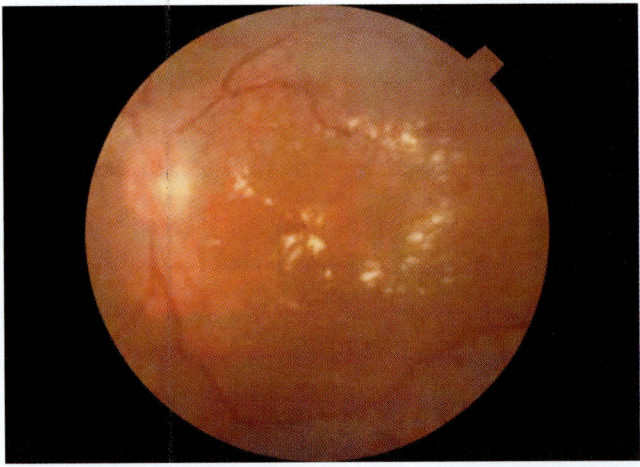

Fig. 10A.3: Nonproliferative diabetic retinopathy.

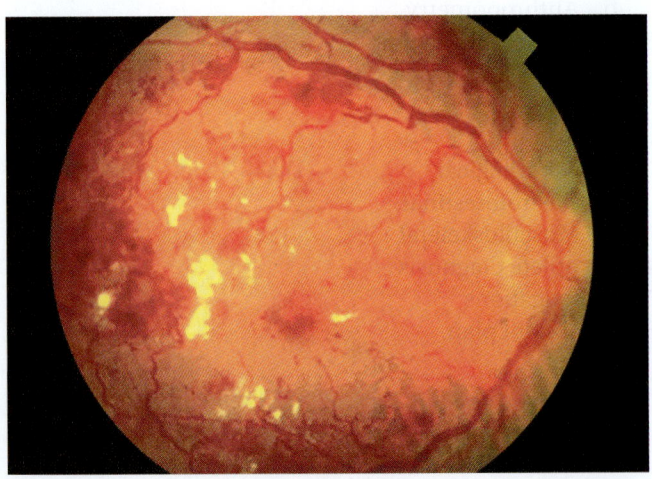

Fig. 10A.4: Proliferative diabetic retinopathy.

Contd...

Renal	Palpable kidney (polycystic kidney) and renal bruit (renal artery stenosis)
Complete diagnosis	Hypertension (primary/secondary) with LVH and retinopathy (Fig. 10B.1)
Investigations	ECG, creatinine, urine routine and protein, echocardiography, FBS, lipid profile, serum uric acid, and evaluation of secondary causes—thyroid, ultrasonography (USG) abdomen
Treatment plan	■ Nutritional and lifestyle modification ■ Drugs ■ Management of complication
Referral	Ophthalmology and nephrology

C: Chronic Kidney Disease (Fig. 10C.1)

History	■ Duration ■ Treatment details and dialysis ■ History for etiology—DM, HTN, drugs, chronic glomerulonephritis, etc. ■ Symptoms of uremia
Vitals	Hypertension, pallor, edema, and raised JVP
Anthropometry	Body mass index (BMI)
Skin	Pruritus/itching, rash, uremic frost, metastatic calcification, arteriovenous (AV) fistula (Fig. 10C.2) and dialysis catheter
Cardiovascular	Atherosclerosis, heart failure, hypertension, and pericarditis
Respiratory	Pulmonary edema, pleural effusion, and interstitial lung disease
Neurological	Peripheral neuropathy, encephalopathy, proximal myopathy, seizures, myoclonic twitching, coma, and restless leg syndrome
Gastrointestinal	Loss of appetite (anorexia), nausea, vomiting, diarrhea, GI bleed
Musculoskeletal	Bone pains
Others	■ Women: Amenorrhea and menorrhagia ■ Males: Erectile dysfunction and oligospermia
Complete diagnosis	For example, chronic kidney disease (stage—) secondary to diabetes, and patient has peripheral neuropathy

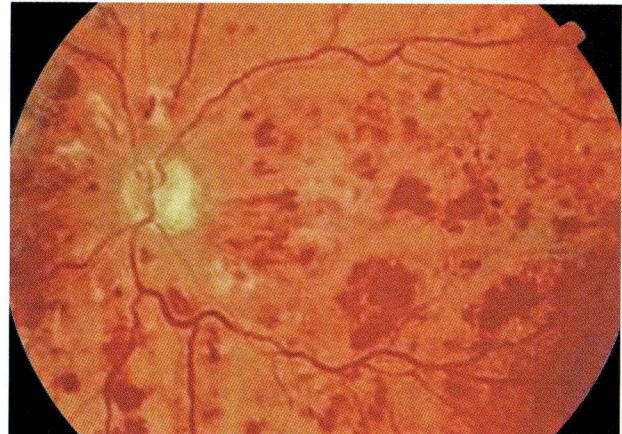

Fig. 10B.1: Fundus image of hypertensive retinopathy.

Contd...

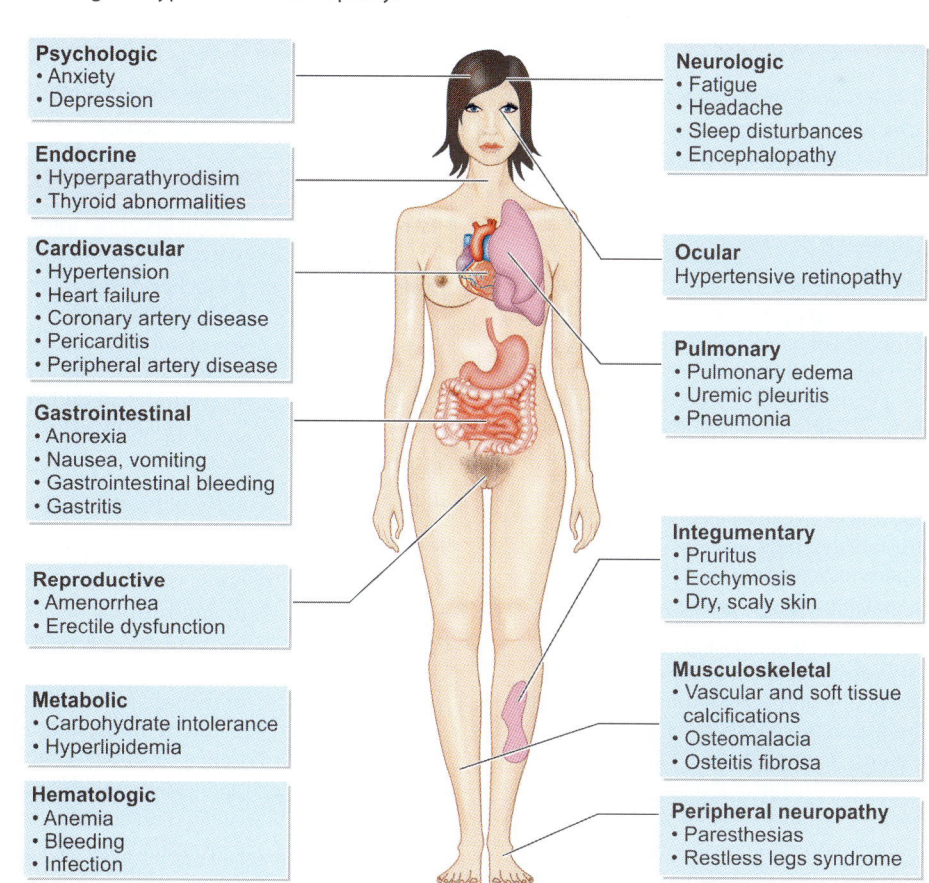

Fig. 10C.1: Various clinical manifestations of chronic kidney disease (CKD).

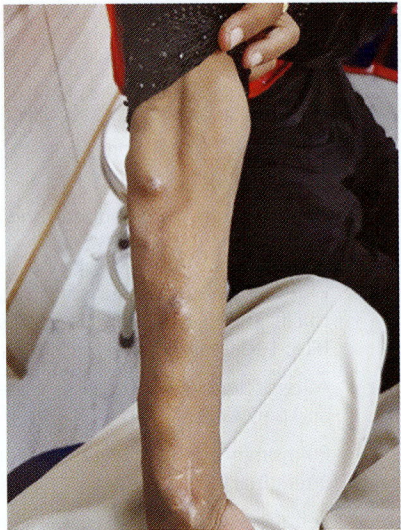

Fig. 10C.2: Arteriovenous fistula (AV) created for dialysis.

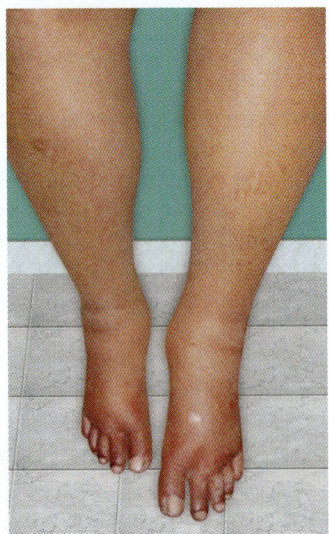

Fig. 10D.1: Nonpitting pedal edema—myxedema.

Contd...

Investigations	Serum creatinine, urea, electrolytes, arterial blood gas (ABG), ECG, ECHO, ultrasound abdomen, urine analysis, and complete blood count (CBC) with peripheral smear
Treatment plan	<ul><li>Nutritional and lifestyle modification drugs medical management</li><li>Hemodialysis</li></ul>
Referral	Nephrology

D: Hypothyroidism

History	<ul><li>Lethargy, somnolence, weight gain, goiter, cold intolerance, and hoarse voice</li><li>Family history</li><li>Drug history</li></ul>
Vitals	<ul><li>Bradycardia, nonpitting edema, diastolic hypertension, and thyromegaly, pallor</li><li>Anemia</li></ul>
Anthropometry	Obesity
Skin	Myxedema **(Fig. 10D.1)** (nonpitting edema of the skin of hands, feet, and eyelids), dry flaky skin and hair, alopecia, vitiligo, purplish lips and malar flush, carotenemia, erythema ab igne, xanthelasmas, and madarosis (thinning of lateral one-third of eyebrows)
Cardiovascular	Angina, bradycardia, hypertension (diastolic), cardiac failure, pericardial effusion, dyslipidemia and hyperhomocysteinemia
Respiratory	Pleural effusion and OSA
Neurological	Aches and pains, muscle stiffness, delayed relaxation of tendon reflexes (Woltman's sign), carpal tunnel syndrome, depression, psychosis, cerebellar ataxia, deafness, myotonia, proximal myopathy, pseudohypertrophy of muscles, and Hashimoto encephalopathy
Gastrointestinal	Reduced appetite, constipation, ileus, ascites, and macroglossia

Contd...

Musculoskeletal	Carpal tunnel syndrome
Others	Menorrhagia, infertility, galactorrhea (hyperprolactinemia), impotence and hyponatremia
Complete diagnosis	Primary hypothyroidism possibly secondary to Hashimoto's disease with bilateral carpal tunnel syndrome and infertility
Investigations	TSH, free thyroxine (FT4), thyroid peroxidase (TPO) antibodies, FBS, lipid profile, CBC with smear, and ECG
Treatment plan	<ul><li>Thyroxine supplementation</li><li>Monitoring with TSH</li></ul>
Referral	Endocrinology

E: Hyperthyroidism

History	Weight loss, heat intolerance, fatigue, gynecomastia, apathy, and thirst
Vitals	<ul><li>Tachycardia, irregularly irregular pulse [atrial fibrillation (AF)], and hypertension</li><li>Anemia</li><li>Thyroid: Diffuse or nodular enlargement, warmth and bruit (due to increased vascularity)</li></ul>
Anthropometry	Low BMI
Skin	Soft, warm, and moist. Increased sweating, pruritus, palmar erythema, spider nevi, onycholysis, pretibial myxedema (Graves'), pigmentation, alopecia, and clubbing (thyroid acropachy)
Cardiovascular	Exertional dyspnea, palpitations, angina, sinus tachycardia, atrial fibrillation, wide pulse pressure, cardiac failure, cardiomyopathy, and "scratchy" midsystolic murmur (Means–Lerman scratch)
Neurological	Nervousness, irritability, psychosis, emotional lability, and fine tremors Inability to concentrate, hyperreflexia, proximal myopathy, bulbar myopathy, ill-sustained clonus

Contd...

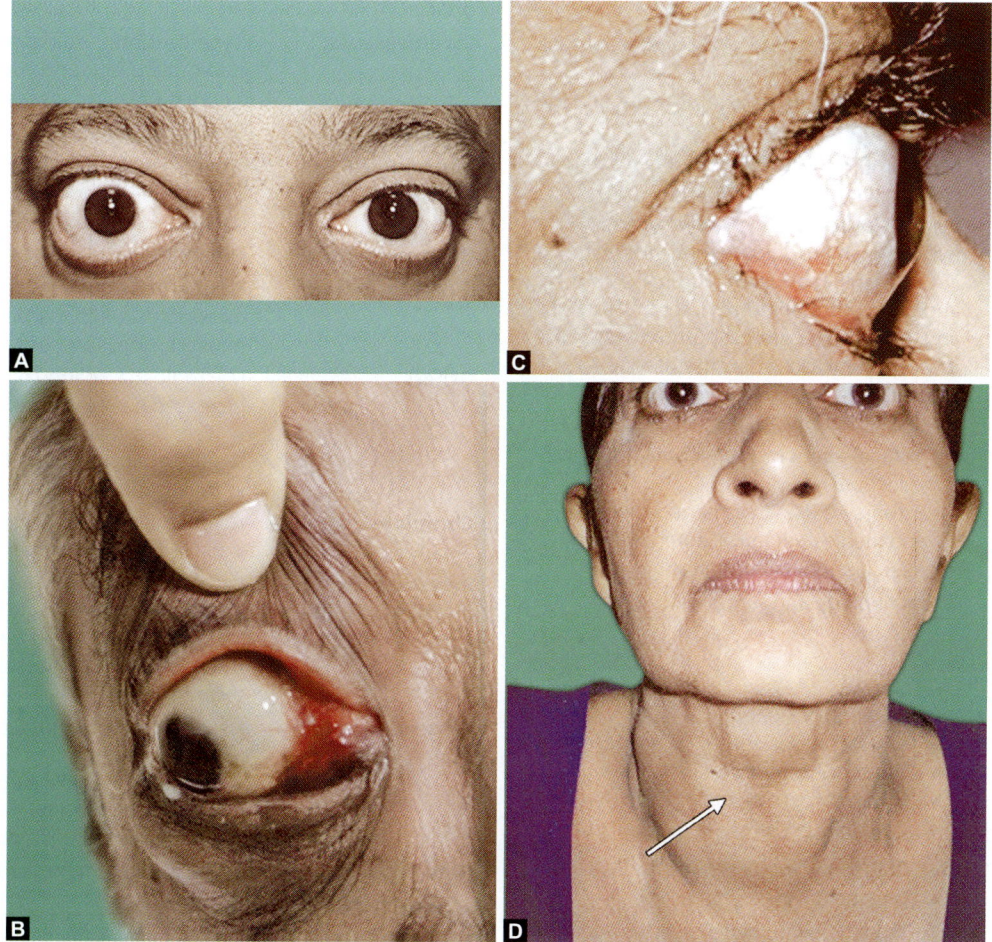

Figs. 10E.1A to D: (A and B) Exophthalmos (front and side view); (C) Infiltration of extraocular muscles in hyperthyroidism; (D) Eye signs and enlarged nodular goiter (arrow).

Contd...

Gastrointestinal	Increased appetite, vomiting, diarrhea, and steatorrhea
Others	- Menstrual disturbances (amenorrhea or oligomenorrhea), repeated abortions, infertility, loss of libido, and impotence - Eye signs **(Figs. 10E.1A to D):** Lid lag, exophthalmos, proptosis, extraocular diplopia, exposure keratitis, and lagophthalmos (classically seen in Graves' disease)
Complete diagnosis	Primary hyperthyroidism due to Graves' disease with thyroid ophthalmopathy and atrial fibrillation
Investigations	TSH, FT4, FT3, TSH receptor antibody, radioactive iodine (RAI) scan, USG neck, ECG, and CBC
Treatment plan	- Antithyroid drugs - Surgery/radioactive iodine ablation - Follow-up
Referral	Endocrinology, nuclear medicine, ophthalmology, and surgery

F: Cushing's Syndrome (Fig. 10F.1)

History	- Onset - Duration - Any complications—cardiovascular system (CVS) and respiratory system (RS) - Other coexistent diseases - Treatment history—chronic steroid use with indication
Vitals	- Hypertension - Pedal edema
Anthropometry	BMI—truncal obesity
Skin (Figs. 10F.2A to D)	- Moon face, buffalo hump, plethora, and purple striae - Easy bruisability, and ecchymosis. Thinning of hair, skin infections, and acne
Cardiovascular	Hypertension, coronary artery disease, and heart failure
Respiratory	Infections—pneumonia and tuberculosis
Neurological	Proximal myopathy, emotional lability, nervousness, irritability, and psychosis
Gastrointestinal	Pain abdomen and peptic ulcer disease
Musculoskeletal	Backache, osteoporosis, and fractures

Contd...

Contd...

Others	- Females: Hirsutism, acne, and menstrual disturbances - Male: Gynecomastia, impotence, and loss of libido
Complete diagnosis	For example, Cushing's syndrome probably due to glucocorticoid therapy
Investigations	Serum electrolytes (hypokalemia and hypochloremia), glucose tolerance test (GTT), CT/MRI abdomen (adrenal lesion) and brain (pituitary tumor), serum cortisol and adrenocorticotropic hormone (ACTH), low dose/high dose dexamethasone suppression test, and 24-hour urinary free cortisol excretion
Treatment plan	- Adrenal adenoma/carcinoma—surgical resection - Ectopic ACTH—treatment of primary and medical/chemical adrenalectomy Management of complications
Referral	Endocrinology and surgery

G: Acromegaly (Figs. 10G.1 to 10G.3)

History	- Onset - Duration - Any complications—CVS and RS - Other coexistent diseases - Husky voice to be noted
Vitals	Hypertension
Anthropometry	- BMI - Gigantism
Skin	- Thick skin with hypertrichosis and exaggerated nasolabial fold - Hyperhidrosis, skin tags, and acanthosis nigricans

Contd...

Contd...

Cardiovascular	Hypertension, cardiomegaly, cardiomyopathy, and congestive cardiac failure (CCF)
Respiratory	OSA
Neurological	Proximal myopathy, bitemporal hemianopia, blindness (optic atrophy), headache, and cranial nerve palsy
Gastrointestinal	Organomegaly
Musculoskeletal	Prognathism, carpal tunnel syndrome, osteoporosis, kyphoscoliosis, dental malocclusion, and frontal bossing
Others	Macroglossia, spade-shaped hand, and increased heel pad thickness - Females: Mild hirsutism, menstrual disturbances, and galactorrhea - Male: Impotence and loss of libido
Complete diagnosis	Acromegaly due to pituitary tumor with impaired glucose tolerance (IGT)
Investigations (Figs.10G.3A to C)	Basal fasting growth hormone (GH) levels, insulin-like growth factor-1 (IGF-1) level, X-ray (skull, hand, and feet), GTT, MRI brain (pituitary tumor), and visual field examination
Treatment plan	- Medical: Octreotide, pegvisomant, and bromocriptine - Trans-sphenoidal surgical removal of pituitary adenoma - Management of complications
Referral	Endocrinology, neurosurgery, and ophthalmology

Fig. 10F.1: Clinical features of Cushing's syndrome.

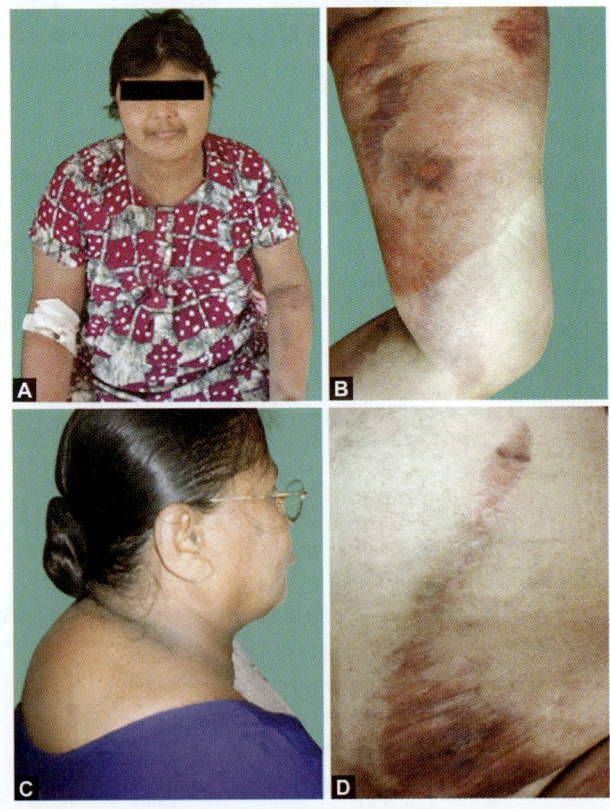

Figs. 10F.2A to D: Features of Cushing's syndrome: (A) Cushing's habitus, obesity and moon facies; (B) Buffalo hump; (C and D) Pigmented striae.

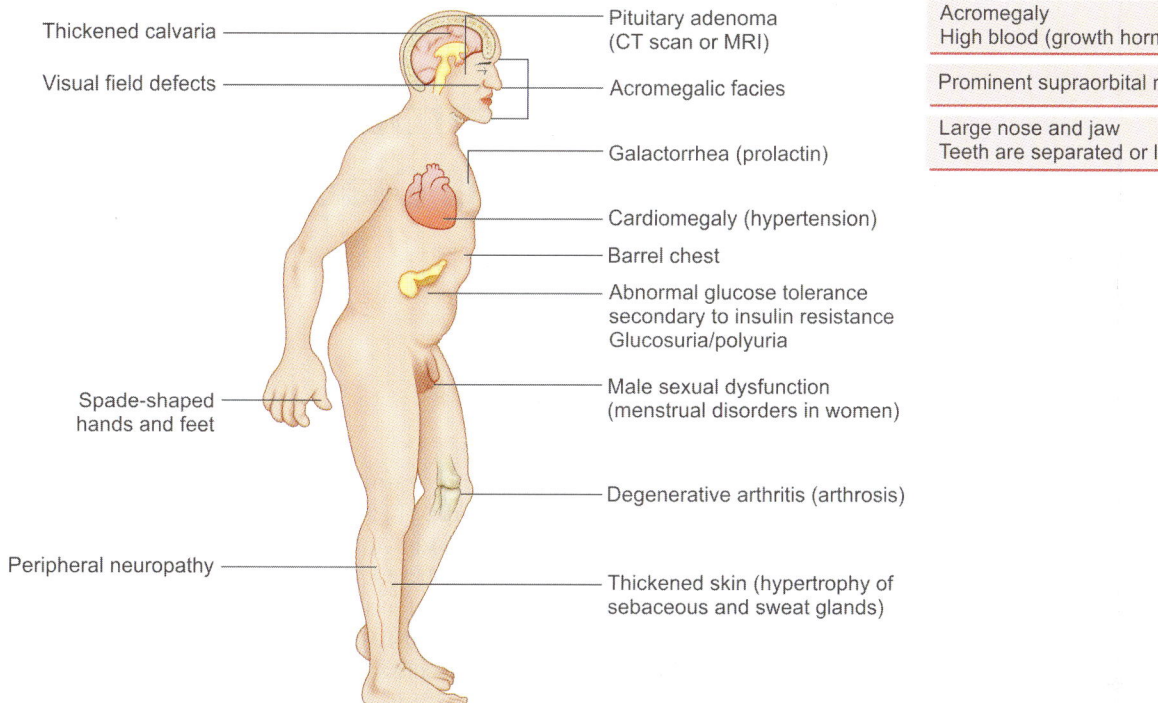

Fig. 10G.1: Summary of various clinical features of acromegaly (diagrammatic).

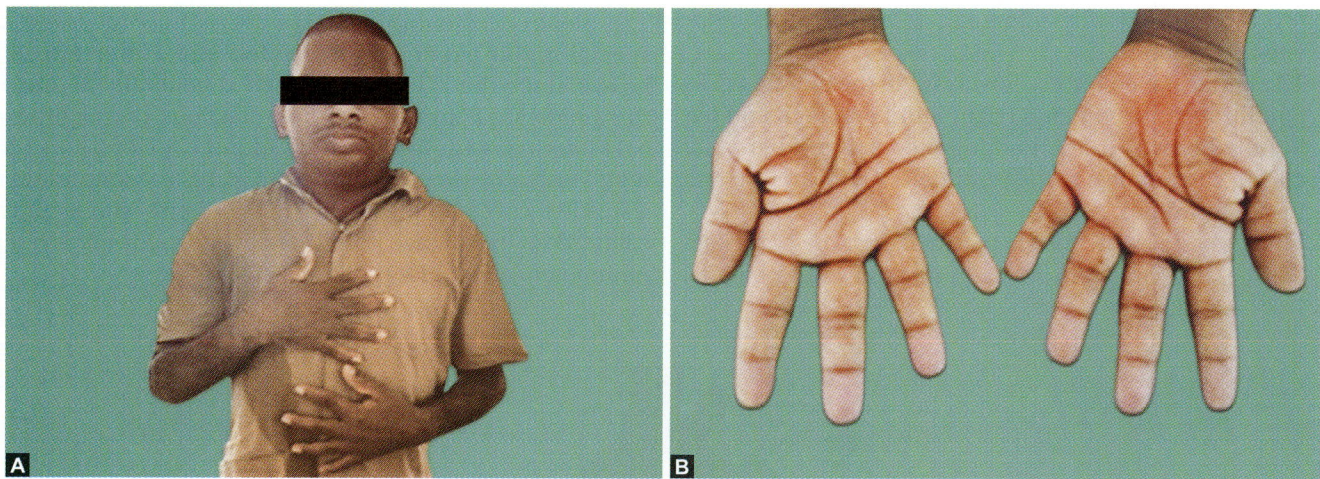

Figs. 10G.2A and B: Acromegalic facies and thick and spade-shaped hands.

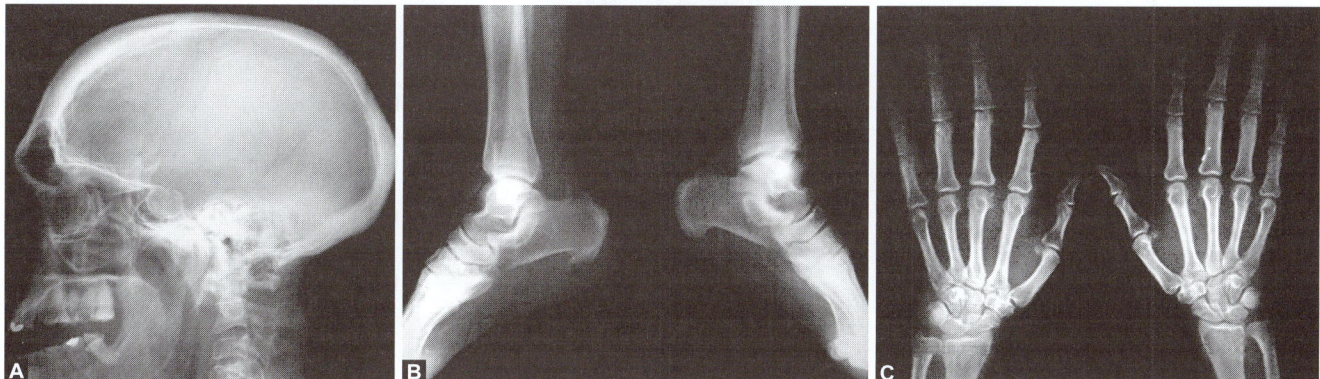

Figs. 10G.3A to C: X-ray findings in acromegaly: (A) Lateral X-ray skull showing sellar enlargement, thickening of the calvarium, enlargement of the frontal and maxillary sinuses, and enlargement of the jaw; (B) X-ray ankle shows increased thickness of the heel pad in acromegaly; (C) X-ray of hand showing increased soft tissue bulk and "arrowhead" tufting of the distal phalanges.

11 CHAPTER

Simplified Approach to ECG (Reading and Diagnosis)

CONDUCTION SYSTEM OF THE HEART (FIG. 11.1)

The rate and rhythm of the heart are controlled by the sinoatrial node (SA node) situated at the junction of superior vena cava and right atrium.

- The impulse from the SA node spreads through the atrial musculature and down to the atrioventricular (AV) node that is situated above the tricuspid valve.
- Passage through the AV node is relatively slow, accounting for the normal physiological delay in ventricular depolarization.
- The impulse then travels downward to the bundle of His and through its branches (right bundle branch and left bundle branch) to the Purkinje network of fibers that convey the impulse to the ventricular endocardium and then epicardium.
- The SA node is the normal pacemaker of the heart as it has the fastest inherent discharge rate. However, potential pacemaking properties also exist in the cells of the AV node, bundle of His, and Purkinje fibers.
- Sinoatrial node—dominant pacemaker with an intrinsic rate of 60–100 beats/minute.
- Atrioventricular node—back-up pacemaker with an intrinsic rate of 40–60 beats/minute.
- Ventricular cells—back-up pacemaker with an intrinsic rate of 20–45 bpm.

ECG WAVEFORMS AND INTERVALS

The electrocardiogram (ECG) ordinarily is recorded on special graph paper that is divided into 1 mm^2 grid-like boxes. Since the ECG paper speed is generally 25 mm/s, the smallest (1 mm) horizontal divisions correspond to 0.04 (40 ms), with heavier lines at intervals of 0.20 s (200 ms). Vertically, the ECG graph measures the amplitude of a specific wave or deflection (1 mV = 10 mm with standard calibration; the voltage criteria for hypertrophy are given in millimeters) **(Fig. 11.2)**.

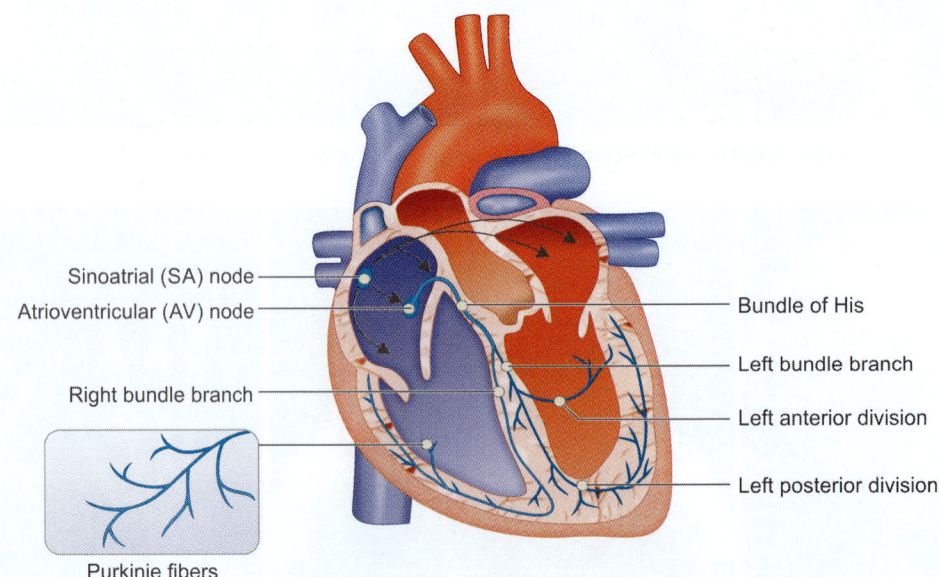

Fig. 11.1: Conduction system of the heart.

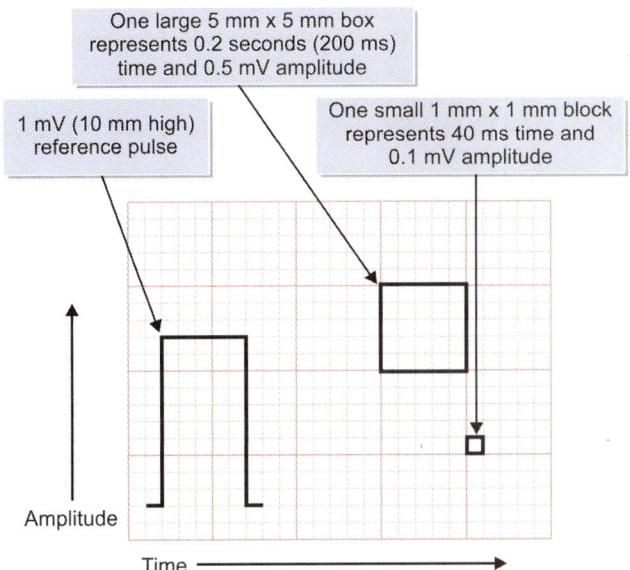

Fig. 11.2: ECG grid and standardization.

The ECG waveforms are labeled alphabetically (Fig. 11.3), beginning with the P wave, which represents atrial depolarization. The QRS complex represents ventricular depolarization, and the ST-T-U complex (ST segment, T wave, and U wave) represents ventricular repolarization. The J point is the junction between the end of the QRS complex and the beginning of the ST segment. *Atrial repolarization is usually too low in amplitude to be detected, but it may become apparent in conditions such as acute pericarditis and atrial infarction.*

There are four major ECG intervals; R-R, PR, QRS, and QT. The heart rate (beats per minute) can be computed readily from the R-R interval [number of small (0.04 s) units into 1,500]. The PR interval measures the time (normally 120–200 ms) between atrial and ventricular depolarization, which includes the physiologic delay imposed by stimulation of cells in the AV junction area. The QRS interval (normally 100–110 ms or less) reflects the duration of ventricular depolarization. The QT interval incudes both ventricular depolarization and repolarization times and varies inversely with the heart rate. A rate-related ("corrected" Bazett's correction) QT interval, QTc, can be calculated as $QT_c = QT/\sqrt{RR}$. The upper normal for QTc is 0.44 s (some references give QTc upper normal limits as 0.43 s in men and 0.45 s in women. Also, a number of different formulas have been proposed, without consensus, for calculating the QTc). The QRS complex is subdivided into specific deflections or waves. If the initial QRS deflection in a particular lead is negative, it is termed the Q wave; the first positive deflection is termed the R wave. A negative deflection after the R wave is termed the S wave. Subsequent positive or negative waves are labeled R' or R prime and S' or S prime, respectively. Lowercase letters (qrs) are used for waves of relatively small amplitude. An entirely negative QRS complex is termed a QS wave.

- U wave: Small, rounded, and upright wave following T wave. Most easily seen with a slow heart rate. Indicates repolarization of Purkinje fibers.

ECG Leads (Figs. 11.4A and B)

The 12 conventional ECG leads record the difference in potential between electrodes placed on the surface of the body. These leads are divided into two groups: six limb (extremity) leads and six chest (precordial) leads. The limb leads record potentials transmitted onto the frontal plane, and the chest leads record potentials transmitted onto the horizontal plane. The spatial orientation and polarity of the six frontal plane leads are represented on the hexaxial diagram. The six chest leads are unipolar recordings obtained by electrodes in the following positions; lead V1, fourth intercostal space, just to the right of the sternum; lead V2, fourth intercostal space, just to the left of the sternum; lead V3, midway between V2 and V4: Lead V4, midclavicular line, fifth intercostal space; and lead V5, anterior axillary line, same level as V4; and lead V6, midaxillary line, same level as V4 and V5.

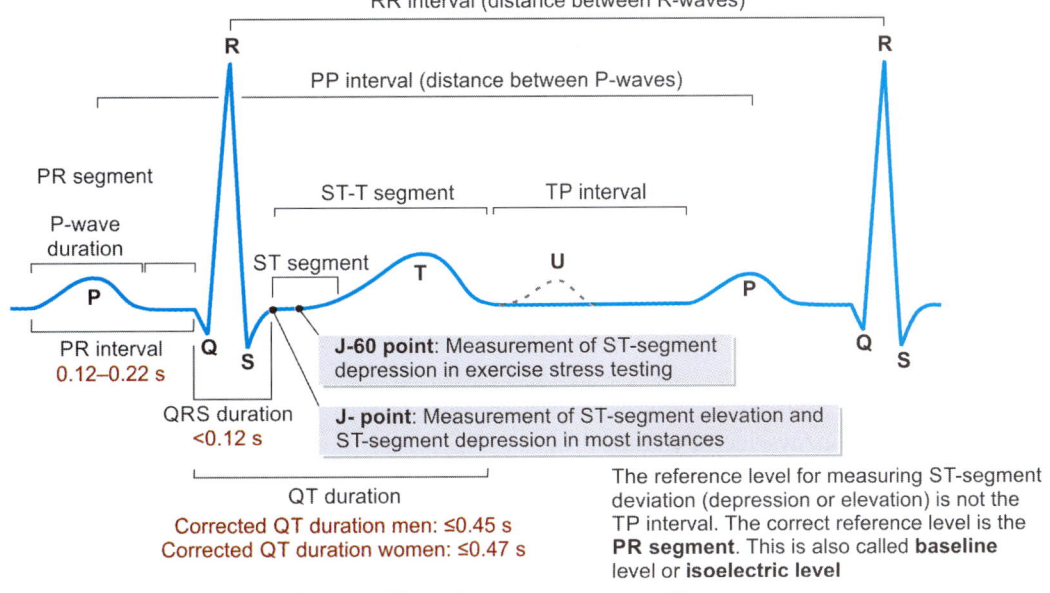

Fig. 11.3: Normal waves, segments and Intervals.

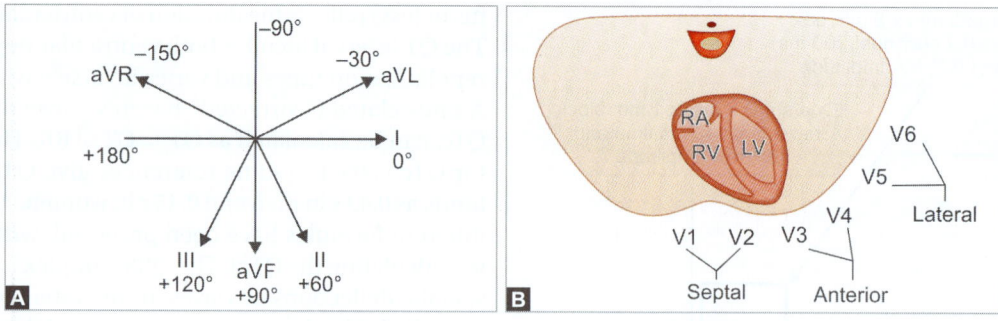

Figs. 11.4A and B: Anatomical relation of leads.

Anatomic Groups of ECG Leads

I Lateral	aVR None	V1 Septal	V4 Anterior
II Inferior	aVL Lateral	V2 Septal	V5 Lateral
III Inferior	aVF Inferior	V3 Anterior	V6 Lateral

Together, the frontal and horizontal plane electrodes provide a three-dimensional representation of cardiac electrical activity. Each lead can be likened to a different video camera angle "looking" at the same events—atrial and ventricular depolarization and repolarization—from different spatial circumstances. For example, right precordial leads V3R, V4R, etc., are useful in detecting evidence of acute right ventricular ischemia. Bedside monitors and ambulatory ECG (Holter) recordings, usually employ only one or two modified leads. The ECG leads are configured so that a positive (upright) deflection is recorded in a lead, if a wave of depolarization spreads toward the positive pole of the lead, and a negative deflection is recorded, if the wave spreads toward the negative pole. If the mean orientation of the depolarization vector is at right angles to a particular lead axis, a biphasic (equally positive and negative) deflection will be recorded.

READING 12-LEAD ECGs

The best way to read 12-lead ECGs is to develop a step-by-step approach (just as we did for analyzing a rhythm strip). In these modules, we present a seven-step approach:
1. Calculate RATE
2. Determine RHYTHM
3. Determine QRS AXIS
4. Check individual WAVES
5. Calculate INTERVALS
6. Assess for CHAMBER ENLARGEMENT
7. Look for evidence of infarction/dyselectrolytemia/drug toxicity.

Step 1: Determining the Heart Rate (Fig. 11.5A)

Rule of 300/1,500

Count the number of "big boxes" between two QRS complexes, and divide this into 300 (smaller boxes with 1,500) for regular rhythms.

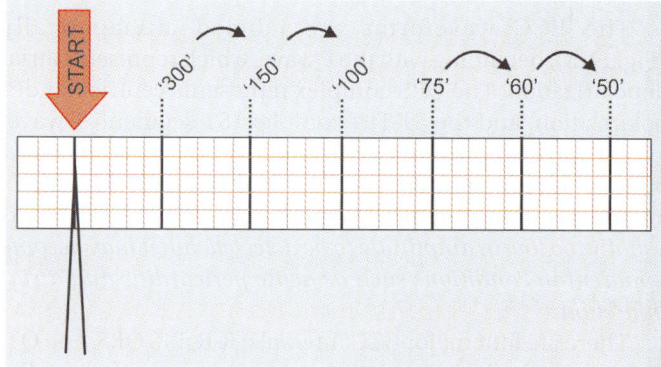

Fig. 11.5A: Calculation of heart rate.

6 Second Rule

- ECGs record 6 seconds of rhythm per page
- Count the number of beats present on the ECG in 6 seconds
- Multiply by 10
- This is useful for irregular rhythms.

Interpretation	bpm	Causes
Normal	60–99	—
Bradycardia	<60	Hypothermia, increased vagal tone (due to vagal stimulation or drugs), athletes (fit people), hypothyroidism, beta blockade, marked intracranial hypertension, obstructive jaundice, uremia, structural SA node disease, or ischemia
Tachycardia	>100	Any cause of adrenergic stimulation (including pain); thyrotoxicosis; hypovolemia; vagolytic drugs (e.g., atropine) anemia, pregnancy; vasodilator drugs, including many hypotensive agents; fever, myocarditis

Step 2: Determine Regularity
- Look at the R-R distances (using a caliper or markings on a pen or paper).
- Regular (are they equidistant apart)? Occasionally irregular? Regularly irregular?
- Irregularly irregular?—atrial fibrillation (AF).

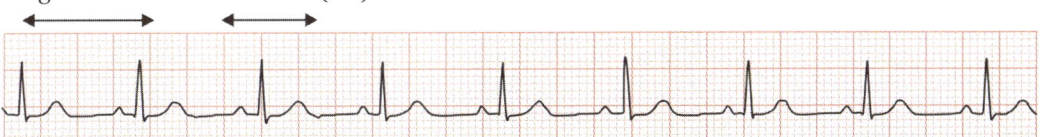

Sinus rhythm
Cardiac impulse originates from the sinus node. Every QRS must be sinus nodal in origin. Every QRS must be preceded by a P wave.

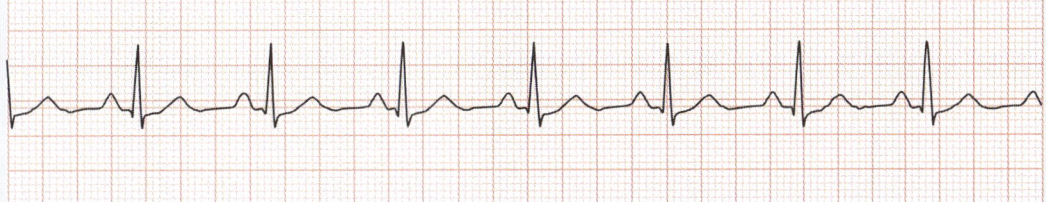

Sinus bradycardia
Rhythm originates in the sinus node. Rate of less than 60 beats per minute.

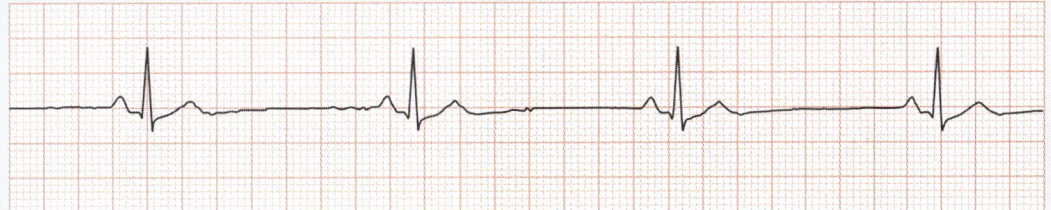

Sinus tachycardia
Rate >100 bpm, otherwise, normal.

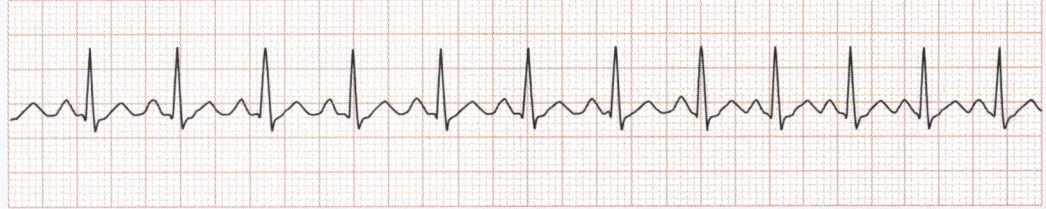

Sinus pause
In disease (e.g., sick sinus syndrome), the SA node can fail in its pacing function. If failure is brief and recovery is prompt, the result is only a missed beat (sinus pause). If recovery is delayed and no other focus assumes pacing function, cardiac arrest follows.

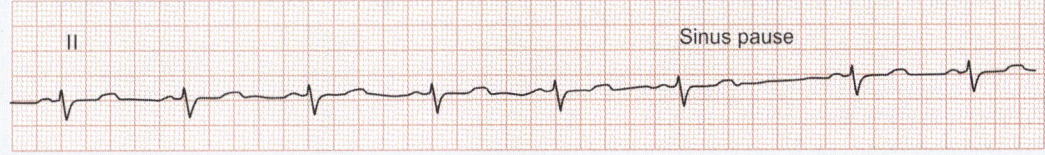

Atrial fibrillation
Atrial rate approximately 400–600; ventricular rate approximately 150 bpm; irregularly irregular, baseline irregularity, no visible p waves, QRS occurs irregularly with its length usually <0.12 s, fibrillary waves.

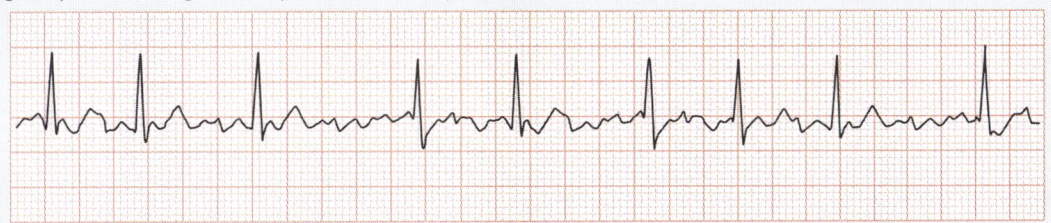

Atrial flutter
Atrial rate =~300 bpm, P waves absent but have flutter waves, ECG baseline adapts "saw-toothed" appearance.

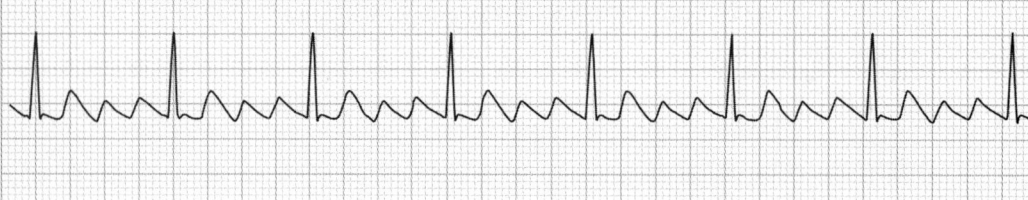

Ventricular fibrillation
Rate cannot be discerned, rhythm unorganized, QRS broad >0.12 s.

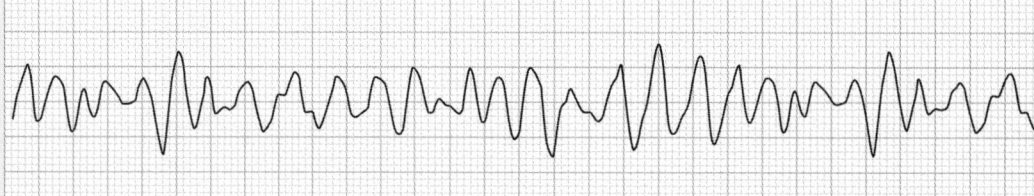

Ventricular tachycardia
Rate = 100–250 bpm, broad QRS, regular.

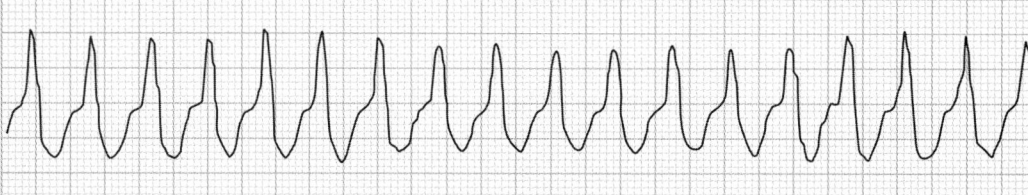

Torsades de pointes
Literally meaning twisting of points is a distinctive form of polymorphic ventricular tachycardia characterized by a gradual change in the amplitude and twisting of the QRS complexes around the isoelectric line.

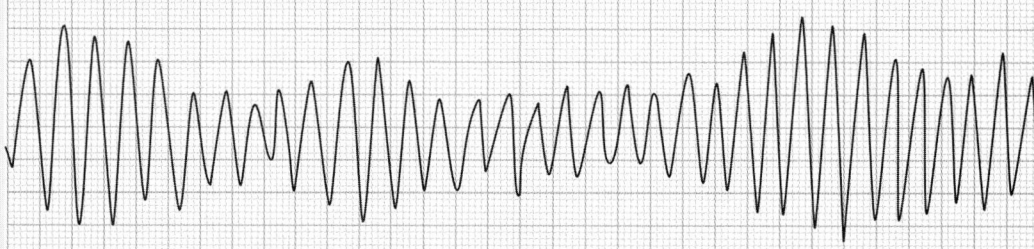

Supraventricular tachycardia
Tachycardic rhythm originating above the ventricular tissue. Atrial and ventricular rate = 150–250 bpm. Regular rhythm, p is usually not discernable.
Note:
Types of SVT:
- Sinoatrial node reentrant tachycardia (SANRT)
- Ectopic (unifocal) atrial tachycardia (EAT)
- Multifocal atrial tachycardia (MAT)
- A-fib or A flutter with rapid ventricular response. Without rapid ventricular response both usually not classified as SVT
- Atrioventricular (AV)-nodal reentrant tachycardia (AVNRT—commonest)
- Permanent (or persistent) junctional reciprocating tachycardia (PJRT)
- Atrioventricular reentrant tachycardia (AVRT)

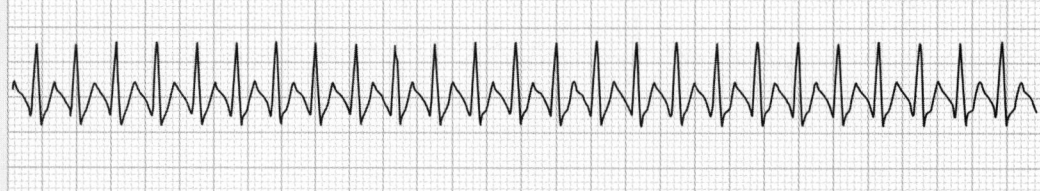

Atrial premature beat (APB)

Arises from an irritable focus in one of the atria. APB produces different looking P wave, because depolarization vector is abnormal. QRS complex has normal duration and same morphology. The premature beat is followed by a pause. This pause is not equal to double the preceding R-R interval (not a full compensatory pause). Atrial premature beats occurring very early in the cycle (e.g., AV node in refractory period) may not conduct to the ventricles. This will produce an abnormal p wave without a QRS complex followed by a pause.

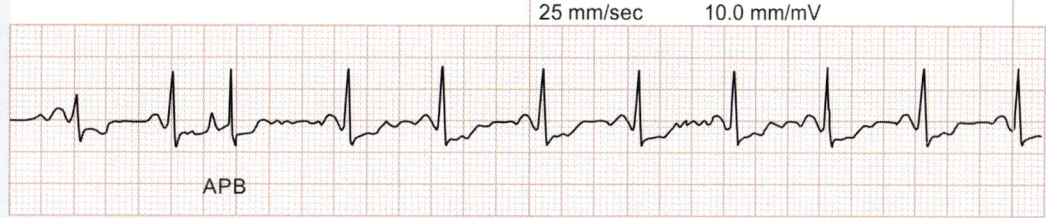

Premature ventricular complexes (PVCs)

Occasionally irregular rhythm, broad QRS arising from ventricles.
No P-wave associated with PVCs. It can be monomorphic/polymorphic.
Followed by a pause, usually equal to twice the preceding R-R interval (full compensatory pause).
PVCs arising from the right ventricle have LBBB morphology and those arising from left ventricle have RBBB morphology.

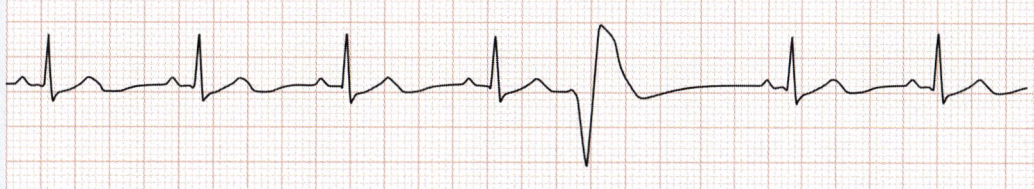

Artificial pacemaker

Sharp, thin spike, before each complex, ventricular paced rhythm shows wide ventricular pacemaker spikes.

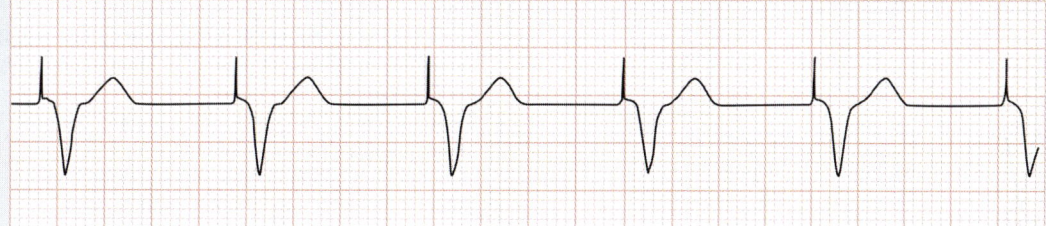

Step 3: Determining the Axis

- Normal QRS axis from −30° to +110°.
- −30° to −90° is referred to as a left axis deviation (LAD).
- +110° to +180° is referred to as a right axis deviation (RAD).
- −180° to −90° is referred as Northwest axis/extreme axis/axis in no man's land as depicted in **Figure 11.5B**.

Axis	LI	LIII or aVF	TIP (Fig. 11.5C)
Normal	Positive	Positive	Both up
Right	Negative	Positive	Meet-**R**EACHING
Left	Positive	Negative	Separate-**L**EAVING
Northwest	Negative	Negative	Both down

- QRS complex in leads I and aVF.
- Determine if they are predominantly positive or negative.
- The combination should place the axis into one of the four quadrants above.

Cardiac axis	Causes
Left axis deviation	▪ Left anterior hemiblock, left ventricular hypertrophy, Wolff-Parkinson-White syndrome (right-sided pathway), inferior myocardial infarction (MI), ostium primum atrial septal defect (ASD), and ventricular tachycardia ▪ Normal variation in pregnancy, obesity; ascites
Right axis deviation	Normal finding in children and tall thin adults, right ventricular hypertrophy (RVH), chronic lung pulmonary disease (COPD), left posterior hemiblock, ostium secundum ASD, Wolff-Parkinson-White syndrome (left sided pathway), and anterolateral MI
Northwest	Dextrocardia, severe emphysema, hyperkalemia, lead transposition, artificial cardiac pacing, and ventricular tachycardia

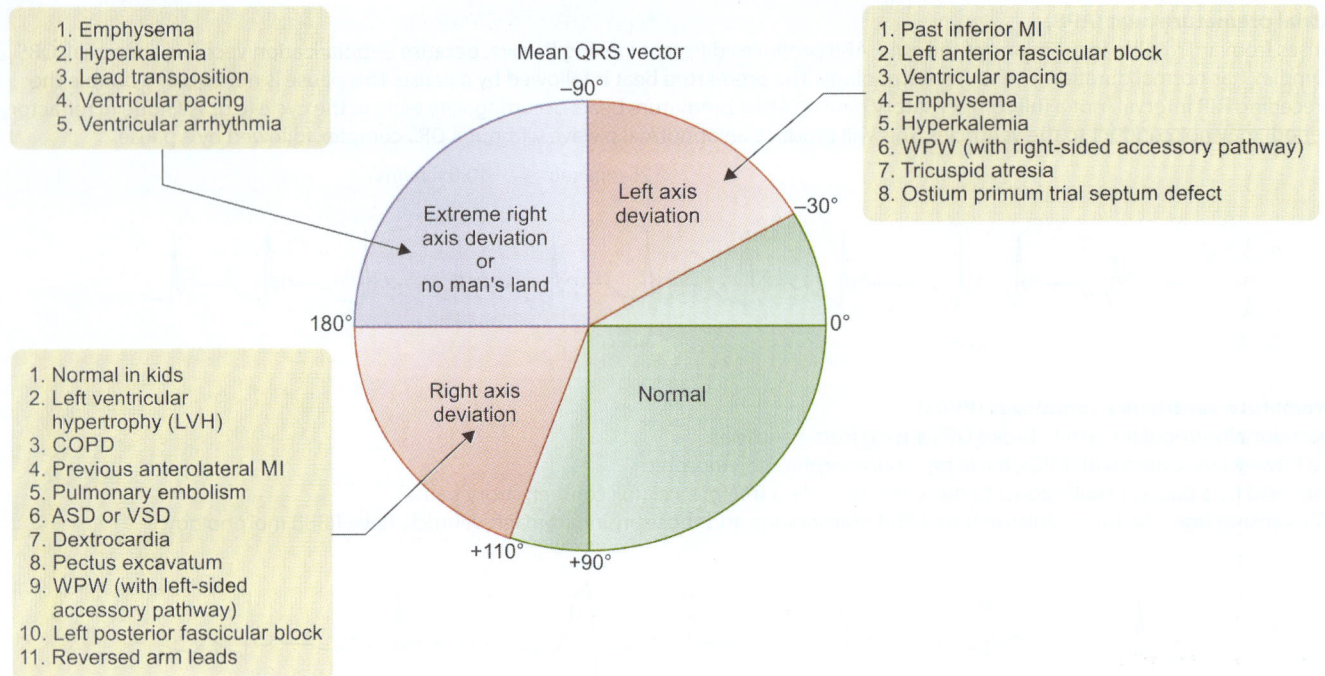

Fig. 11.5B: Pictorial representation of axis deviation with examples.
(COPD: chronic obstructive pulmonary disease; ASD: atrial septal defects; VSD: ventricular septal defects)

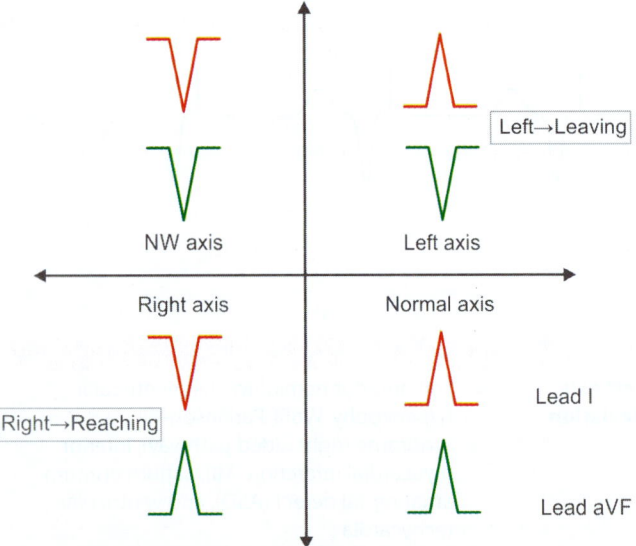

Fig. 11.5C: Axis determination based on direction of lead I and lead aVF.

Step 4: Check Individual Waves

Assess P Waves

- Always positive in lead I and II
- Always negative in lead aVR
- <2.5 small squares in duration
- <2.5 small squares in amplitude
- Commonly biphasic in lead V1
- Best seen in leads II
- Tall (>2.5 mm), pointed P waves **(P pulmonale)**—suggests right atrial enlargement

Contd...

- Seen in chronic obstructive pulmonary disease (COPD), atrial septal defect (ASD), TS, Ebstein anomaly **(Himalayan P waves)**
- Notched/bifid ("M" shaped) P wave **(P "mitrale")** in limb leads—suggests left atrial enlargement
  - Seen in MS, MR, and systemic hypertension
- Absent P waves—atrial fibrillation/flutter
- Inverted P waves in lead II—dextrocardia
- Extremely tall 'Himalayan' P waves—Ebstein anomaly
- **Macruz index** is a proportion between the P wave duration and PQ segment (not interval) duration (P/PQ). Reference range between <1;1,6>, Macruz index >1,6 indicates P mitrale, while <1 indicates P pulmonale
- **Morris index** is the algebraic product of the duration of the terminal P wave force and the amplitude od the force in V1. In LAE it is >40 msec

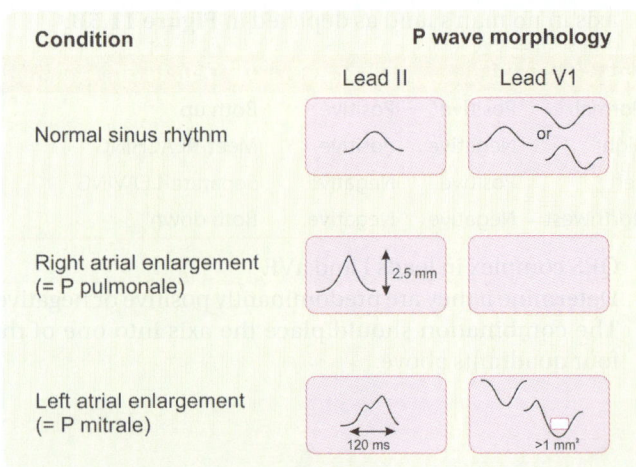

QRS Complex

Normal characteristics:
- Duration: 0.04–0.11 seconds.
  - **Broad/wide QRS** (>0.12 s)
    - Ventricular hypertrophy
    - Intraventricular conduction disturbance
    - Aberrant ventricular conduction
    - Ventricular pre-excitation
    - Ventricular ectopic or escape pacemaker
    - Ventricular pacing by cardiac pacemaker.
- Q <0.04 s, <25% of R wave
- Height of QRS—**Sokolow index** (SV2 + RV5) <35 mm (<45 mm for young)
  - Increased in RV/LV hypertrophy
  - Decreased—**low voltage QRS** (<5 mV in limb leads/<10 mV in chest leads)
    - Obese patient
    - Restrictive cardiomyopathy
    - Pericardial effusion
    - Hypothyroidism
    - Hypothermia
    - Myocarditis.
- Axis of ventricular depolarization −30 to +110° (abnormalities already discussed)
- **Ventricular activation time (vAT)**—time from start of q wave till top of R wave. Normal of LV <0.04 s (V5 and V6 leads), RV <0.03 s (V1 lead).
  - Prolonged in ischemia, bundle branch block
- **Precordial R wave progression**, i.e., R wave amplitude progressively increases from V1 to V6.
  - Absent R wave progression sign of anterior wall MI.

Q Waves
- The normal Q wave in lead I is due to septal depolarization
- It is small in amplitude—less than 25% of the succeeding R wave, or less than 3 mm
- Its duration is <0.04 sec or one small box
- It is seen in L1 and sometimes in V5 and V6
- The pathological Q wave of infarction in the respective leads is due to dead muscle
- It is deep in amplitude—more than 25% of the succeeding R wave, or more than 4 mm. Its duration is >0.04 sec or >1 small box
- Pathological Q waves may be seen in cardiomyopathies—hypertrophic obstructive cardiomyopathy (HOCM), infiltrative myocardial disease
- Absent Q waves in V5–V6 is most commonly due to left bundle branch block (LBBB).

T Wave
- Normally repolarization directs from epicardium to endocardium = T wave is concordant with QRS complex
- Ischemic area: A repolarization is delayed, an action potential is extended
- Vector of repolarization is directed from ischemic area:
  - Subendocardial ischemia—to epicardium—T wave elevation
  - Subepicardial ischemia—to endocardium—T wave inversion
- Asymmetrical T wave inversion—the first half having more gradual slope than the second half
- Symmetrical T wave inversion seen in ischemia
- Amplitude rarely exceeds 10 mm.

Causes of T wave inversions	Tall T waves (more than two-thirds of neighboring QRS)
- CAD/ischemia - Cardiomyopathies—hypertrophic - Myocarditis and pericarditis - Wellens syndrome - Pulmonary embolism - Raised ICT—CNS bleed - Ventricular hypertrophy - Bundle branch block - Pacing - Persistent juvenile T wave pattern	- Hyperkalemia—Steeple T waves - Hyperacute MI - Benign early repolarization (BER)

U Waves
- The U wave is a wave on an electrocardiogram that is not always seen. It is typically small, and, by definition, follows the T wave. U waves are thought to represent repolarization of the papillary muscles or Purkinje fibers.
- Normal U waves are small, round and symmetrical and positive in lead II. It is the same direction as T wave in that lead.
- Prominent U waves are most often seen in hypokalemia, but may be present in hypercalcemia, thyrotoxicosis, or exposure to digitalis, epinephrine, and class 1A and 3 antiarrhythmics, as well as in congenital long QT syndrome, and in the setting of intracranial hemorrhage.
- An inverted U wave may represent myocardial ischemia or left ventricular volume overload.

Other Waves

The Osborn wave (J wave) is a positive deflection at the J point (negative in aVR and V1), characteristically seen in hypothermia (typically temperature <30°C), but also can be seen in raised ICT, hypercalcemia

Delta wave is a slurred upstroke in the QRS complex often associated with a short PR interval which is most commonly seen with pre-excitation syndrome such as Wolff-Parkinson-White syndrome

Epsilon wave is a small positive deflection buried in the end of the QRS complex. It is the characteristic of arrhythmogenic right ventricular dysplasia (ARVD).

Step 5: Calculate Intervals

PR Interval (Figs. 11.6A to C)
Normal: 0.12–0.20 seconds.

Long PR interval may indicate heart block.

First degree heart block

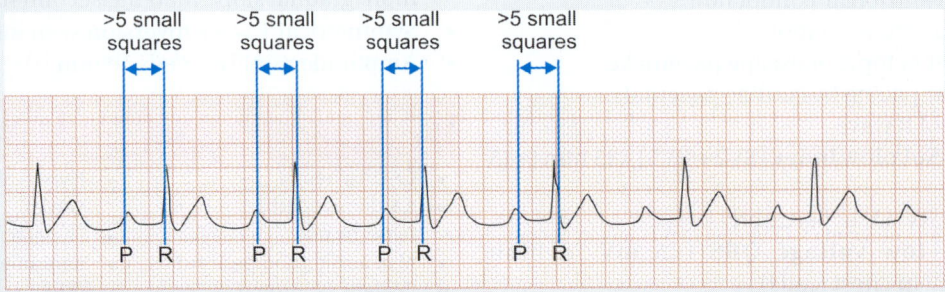

P wave precedes QRS complex but PR intervals prolong (>5 small squares) and remains constant from beat to beat.

Second degree heart block
1. **Mobitz Type I or Wenckebach**
   - Runs in cycle, first PR interval is often normal. With successive beat, PR interval lengthens until there will be a P wave with no following QRS complex.
   - The block is at AV node, often transient, may be asymptomatic.

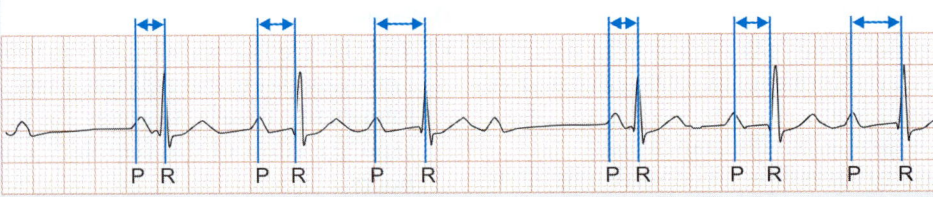

2. **Mobitz Type 2**
   - PR interval is constant, duration is normal/prolonged. Periodically, no conduction between atria and ventricles—producing a p wave with no associated QRS complex (blocked P wave).
   - The block is most often below AV node, at bundle of His or BB.
   - May progress to third degree heart block.

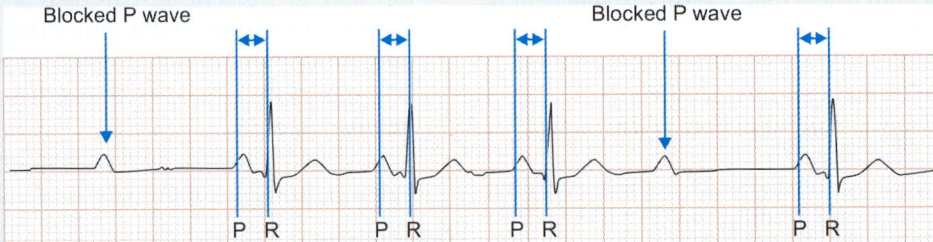

Third degree heart block (complete heart block)
- No relationship between P waves and QRS complexes.
- An accessory pacemaker in the lower chambers will typically activate the ventricles—escape rhythm. Atrial rate = 60–100 bpm. Ventricular rate based on site of escape pacemaker. Atrial and ventricular rhythm, both are regular.

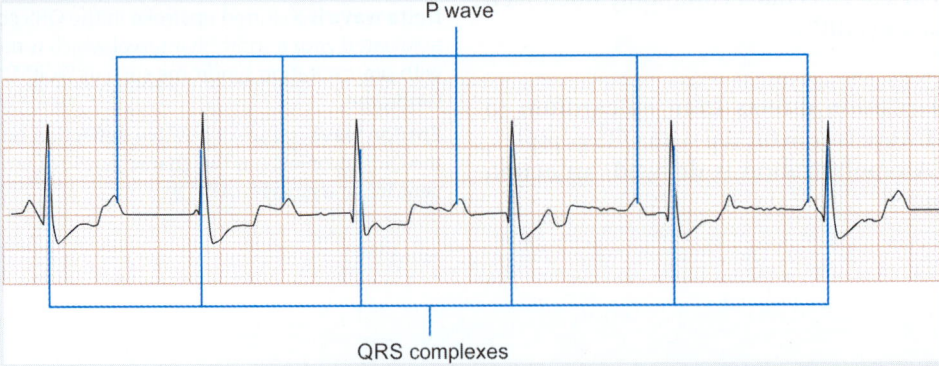

Causes of Conduction Block

- CAD, acute MI, remote MI, pulmonary embolism
- Drugs
- Aortic stenosis
- SABE + abscesses
- Cardiac trauma
- Hyperkalemia
- Lenegre's disease (idiopathic fibrosis of conduction)
- Lev's disease (calcification of the cardiac skeleton)
- Cardiomyopathy—dilated and hypertrophic
- Infiltrative—Chagas disease
- Myxedema, amyloidosis
- Ventricular hypertrophy
- Idiopathic

Short PR Interval

1. Tachycardia
2. Pre-excitation syndromes
   a. Lown–Ganong–Levine syndrome
   b. Wolff-Parkinson-White (WPW) syndrome
   c. Mahaim pathway.

The diagnostic triad of WPW consists of a wide QRS complex associated with a relatively short PR interval and slurring of the initial part of the QRS (delta wave), with the latter effect being due to aberrant activation of ventricular myocardium. The presence of a bypass tract predisposes to re-entrant supraventricular tachyarrhythmias.

QT Interval

It represents the time taken for ventricular depolarization and repolarization.

- The duration of the QT interval is proportionate to the heart rate. The faster the heart beats, the faster the ventricles repolarize so the shorter the QT interval. Therefore, what is a "normal" QT varies with the heart rate.
- QT interval should be 0.35–0.45 s.
- For each heart rate you need to calculate an adjusted QT interval, called the "corrected QT" (QTc): QTc = QT/square root of RR interval—**Bazett's formula**.

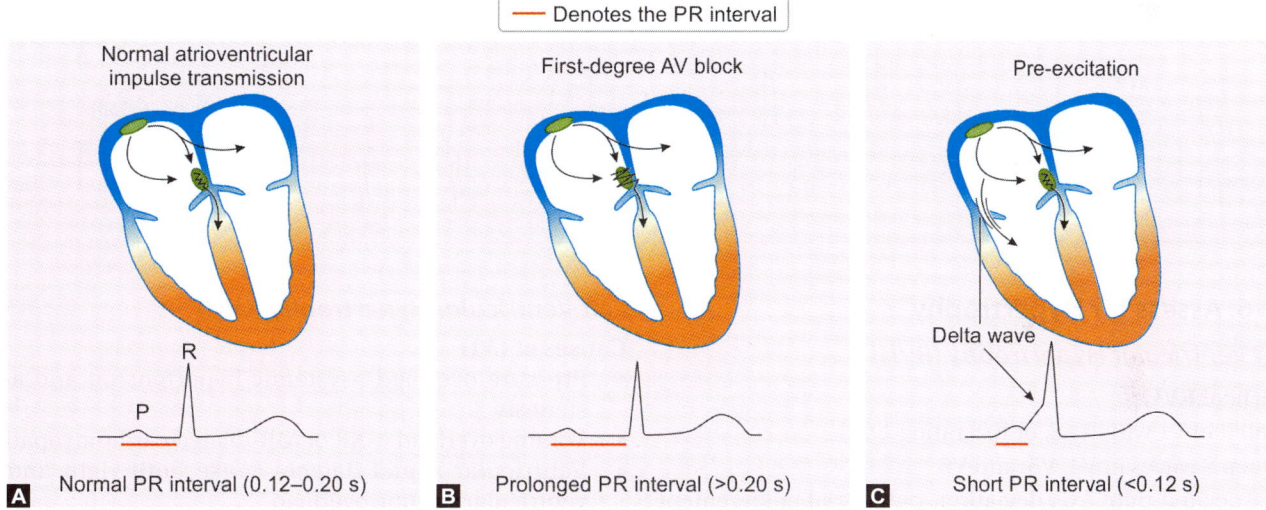

Figs. 11.6A to C: (A) Normal atrioventricular impulse transmissions; (B) First-degree AV block; (C) Pre-excitation.

Prolonged QTc (>440 ms)—a prolonged QT can be very dangerous. It can predispose an individual to a type of ventricular tachycardia—torsades de pointes.
- Hypokalemia
- Hypomagnesemia
- Hypocalcemia
- Hypothermia
- Myocardial ischemia
- Raised intracranial pressure
- Congenital long QT syndrome, e.g., Jervell and Lange–Nielsen syndrome or Romano-Ward syndrome
- Drugs—chlorpromazine, haloperidol, quetiapine, quinidine, procainamide, disopyramide, flecainide, sotalol, amiodarone, amitriptyline, diphenhydramine, astemizole, loratadine, terfenadine, chloroquine, quinine, and macrolides.

Short QTc (<350 ms)
- Hypercalcemia
- Digoxin effect.

Bundle Branch Blocks

Left bundle branch block (LBBB)—*indirect activation causes left ventricle to contract later than the right ventricle*

QS or rS complex in V1—W-shaped RsR' wave in V6—M-shaped

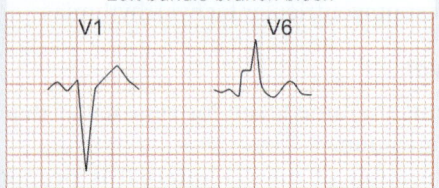

Mnemonic: **WI**LL**IAM**

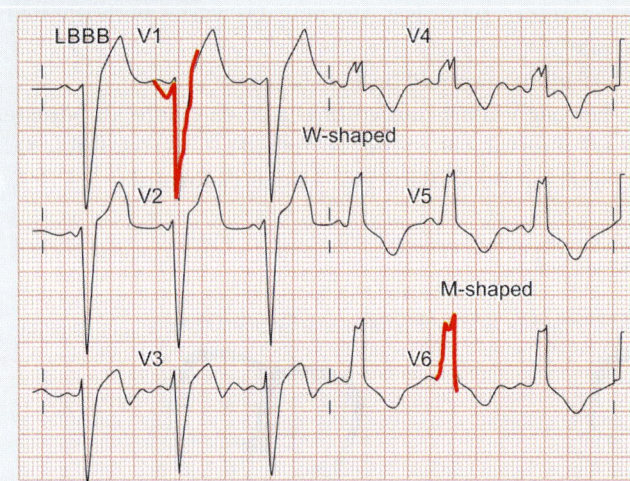

Right bundle branch block (RBBB)—*indirect activation causes right ventricle to contract later than the left ventricle*

Terminal R wave (rSR') in V1—M-shaped slurred S wave in V6—W-shaped

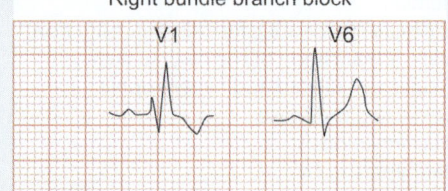

Mnemonic: **MA**RR**OW**

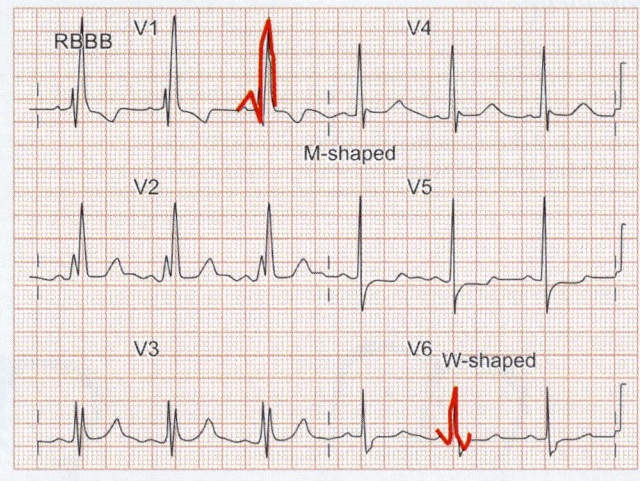

Step 6: Assess for Hypertrophy

Right Ventricular Hypertrophy (RVH)

Criteria of RVH
- Tall R in V1 with R >S, or R/S ratio >1
- Deep S waves in V4, V5, and V6
- Associated right axis deviation, right atrial enlargement (RAE)
- Deep T inversion in V1, V2, and V3.

Cause of RVH
- Long-standing mitral stenosis
- Pulmonary hypertension of any cause
- Ventricular septal defect (VSD) or atrial septal defect (ASD) with initial L to R shunt
- Congenital heart with RV over load
- Tricuspid regurgitation, pulmonary stenosis.

Left Ventricular Hypertrophy (LVH)

Causes of LVH
- Pressure overload—systemic hypertension and aortic stenosis
- Volume overload —AR or MR-dilated cardiomyopathy
- Ventricular septal defect—cause both right and left ventricular volume overload
- Hypertrophic cardiomyopathy.

Criteria of LVH
- High QRS voltages in limb leads:
  - Sokolow and Lyon criteria: S (V1) + R (V5 or V6) >35 mm
  - Cornell criteria: S (V3) + R (aVL) >28 mm (men) or >20 mm (women)
  - Others: R (aVL) >13 mm.
- Deep symmetric T inversion in V4, V5, and V6
- QRS duration >0.09 sec, associated left axis deviation, left atrial enlargement (LAE).

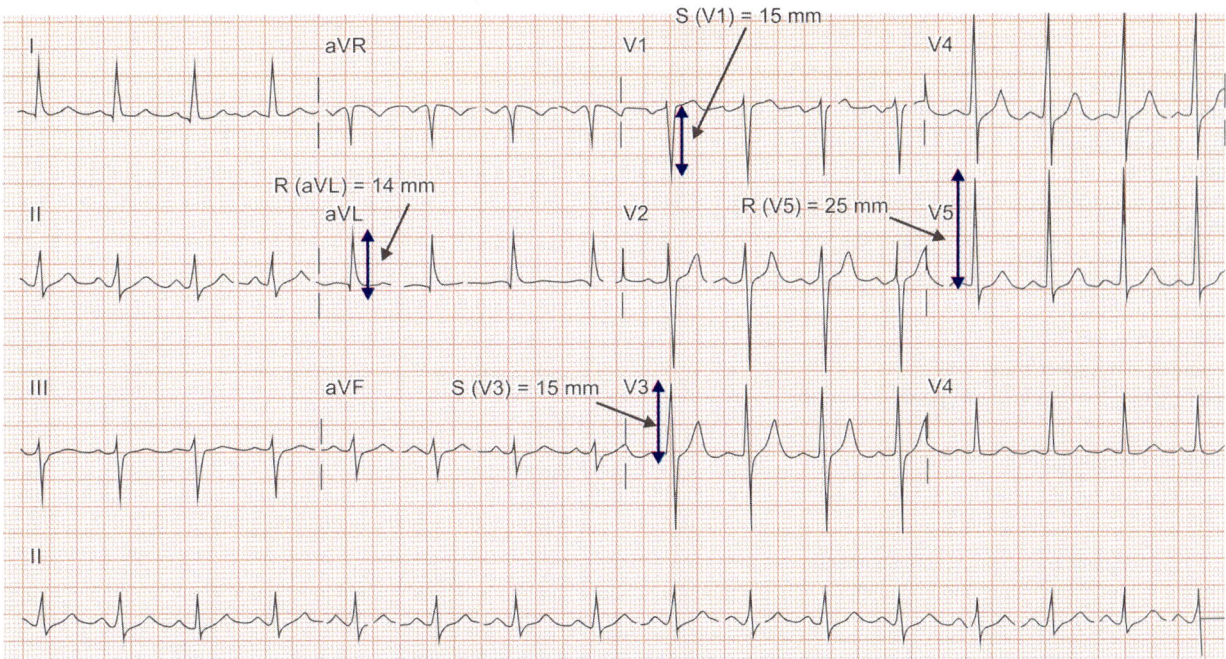

Fig. 11.7: ECG showing voltage criteria for LVH.

Romhilt–Estes Score: Score >5—definite LvH, <3 LvH unlikely

ECG criteria	Points
Voltage criteria (any of) **(Fig. 11.7):** R or S in limb leads ≥20 mm S in V1 or V2 ≥30 mm R in V5 or V6 ≥30 mm	3
ST-T abnormalities: ▪ ST-T vector opposite to QRS without digitalis ▪ ST-T vector opposite to QRS with digitalis	3 1
Negative terminal P mode in V1, 1 mm in depth and 0.04 sec in duration (indicates left atrial enlargement)	3
Left axis deviation (QRS of –30° or more)	2
QRS duration ≥0.09 sec	1
Delayed intrinsicoid deflection in V5 or V6 (>0.05 sec)	1

TYPES OF LVH

Pressure overload	Volume overload
▪ Like in hypertension, ischemic heart disease (IHD) ▪ LV strain pattern—ST depression with T inversion in V5, V6, L1, and aVL leads	▪ Like in mitral or aortic regurgitation ▪ Shows prominent Q waves, positive T waves in V5, V6, L1, and aVL

Biventricular enlargement large diphasic complexes over 50 mm in either leads V2, V3, V4 is usually seen in VSD (**Katz-Wachtel phenomenon**).

Step 7: Look for Evidence of Infarction/ST Segment Abnormalities

ST Segment

- ST segment is isoelectric and at the same level as subsequent PR-interval
- The length between the end of the S wave (end of ventricular depolarization) and the beginning of repolarization
- From J point on the end of QRS complex, to inclination of T wave.

Causes of ST segment elevation

- Ischemia
- Early repolarization
- Acute pericarditis: ST elevation in all leads except aVR
- Pulmonary embolism
- Hypothermia
- Hypertrophic cardiomyopathy
- High potassium
- Cerebrovascular accident
- Acute sympathetic stress
- Brugada syndrome
- Cardiac aneurysm
- Left ventricular hypertrophy
- Idioventricular rhythm including paced rhythm.

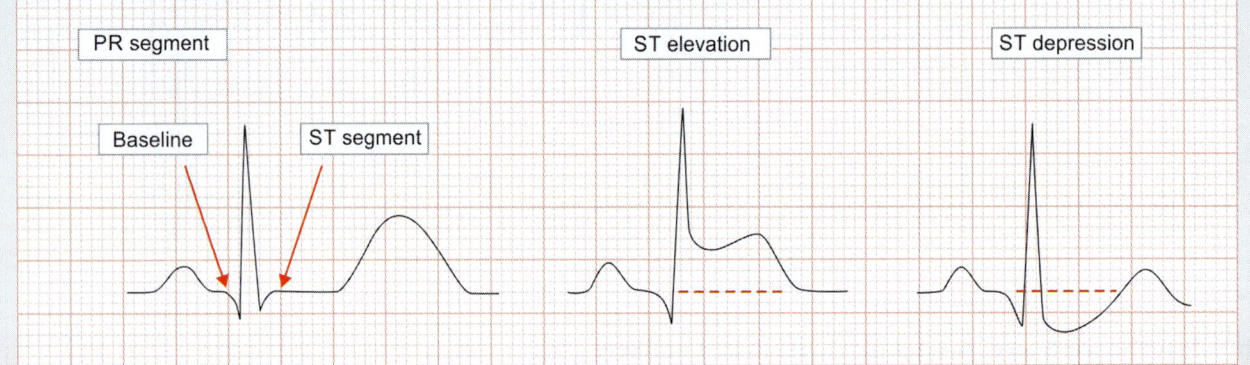

Causes of ST segment depression

- Myocardial ischemia/non-ST-elevation myocardial infarction (NSTEMI)
- Reciprocal change in STEMI
- Posterior MI
- Digoxin effect (reverse tick mark/"sagging" morphology, resembling Salvador Dali's moustache)
- Hypokalemia
- Bundle branch block
- Ventricular hypertrophy
- Ventricular pacing.

ECG CHANGES IN MYOCARDIAL INFARCTION

There are two types of myocardial infarction (MI). ST segment elevation myocardial infarction (STEMI) and non-STEMI (NSTEMI). ST elevation myocardial infarction criteria:
- ST elevation in >2 chest leads >2 mm elevation
- ST elevation in >2 limb leads >1 mm elevation
- Q wave >0.04 s (1 small square).

Location of MI	Lead with ST changes	Affected coronary artery
Anterior	V1, V2, V3, V4	Left anterior descending (LAD) artery
Septal	V1, V2	LAD
Lateral	I, aVL, V5, V6	Left circumflex
Inferior	II, III, aVF	Right coronary artery (RCA)
Right atrium	aVR, V1	RCA
Posterior	Posterior chest leads	RCA
Right ventricle	Right-sided leads	RCA

Simplified Approach to ECG (Reading and Diagnosis)

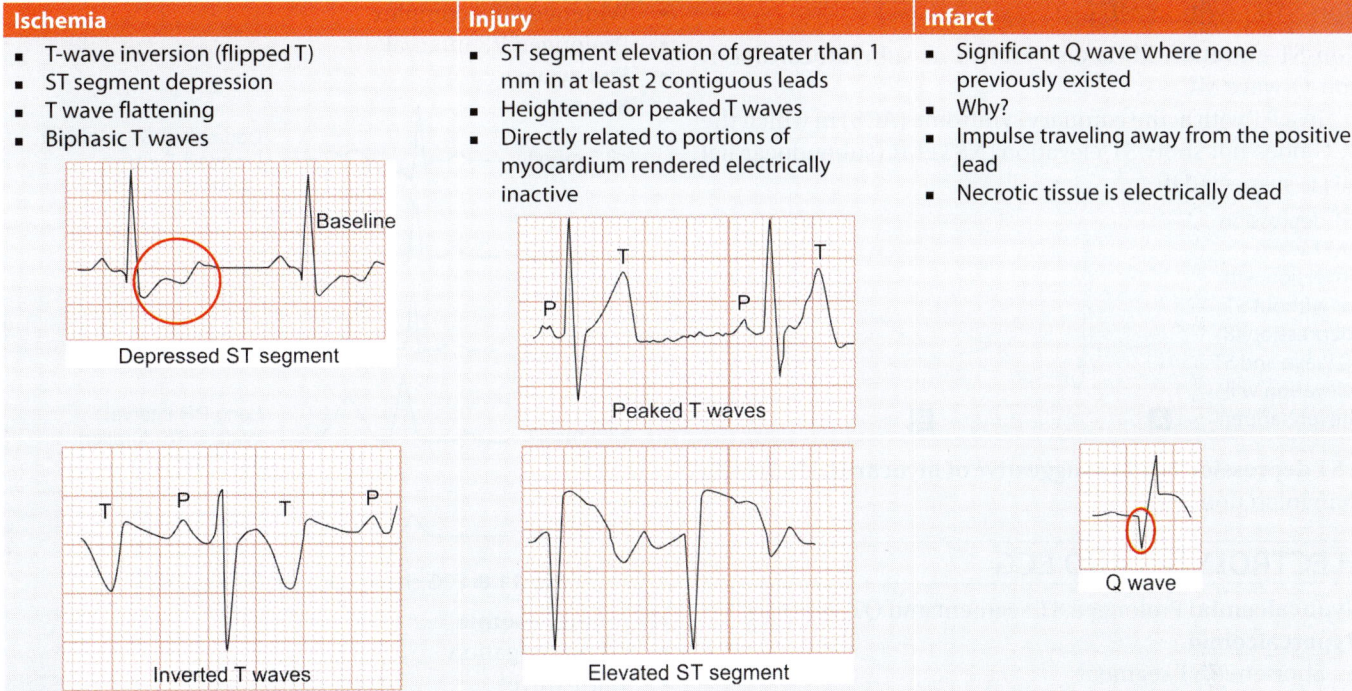

Ischemia	Injury	Infarct
- T-wave inversion (flipped T) - ST segment depression - T wave flattening - Biphasic T waves	- ST segment elevation of greater than 1 mm in at least 2 contiguous leads - Heightened or peaked T waves - Directly related to portions of myocardium rendered electrically inactive	- Significant Q wave where none previously existed - Why? - Impulse traveling away from the positive lead - Necrotic tissue is electrically dead

Sequential ECG changes in STEMI

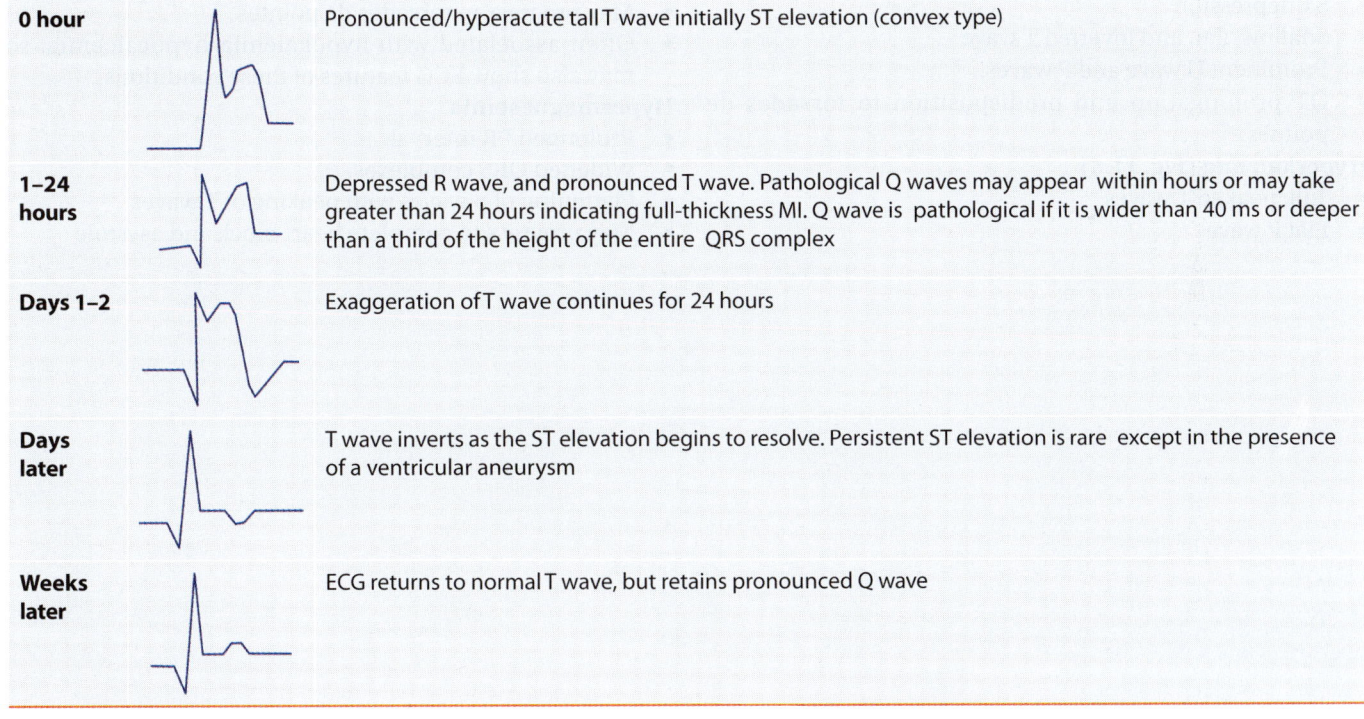

0 hour		Pronounced/hyperacute tall T wave initially ST elevation (convex type)
1–24 hours		Depressed R wave, and pronounced T wave. Pathological Q waves may appear within hours or may take greater than 24 hours indicating full-thickness MI. Q wave is pathological if it is wider than 40 ms or deeper than a third of the height of the entire QRS complex
Days 1–2		Exaggeration of T wave continues for 24 hours
Days later		T wave inverts as the ST elevation begins to resolve. Persistent ST elevation is rare except in the presence of a ventricular aneurysm
Weeks later		ECG returns to normal T wave, but retains pronounced Q wave

Non-ST-Elevation MI

Non-ST-elevation MI is also known as subendocardial or non-Q-wave MI.

In a PT with acute coronary syndrome (ACS) in which the ECG does not show ST elevation, NSTEMI (subendocardial MI) is suspected if:

ST depression (A) T wave inversion with or without ST depression (B) Q wave and ST elevation will never happen

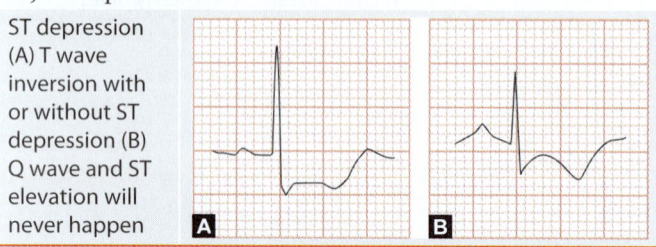

A **ST depression is more suggestive of myocardial ischemia** than infarction.

ELECTROLYTES AND ECG

Hypocalcemia: Prolonged ST segment and QT intervals.

Hypercalcemia
- Shortened ST segment
- Widened T wave and short QT

Hypokalemia (Fig. 11.8)
- ST depression
- Shallow, flat, and inverted T wave
- Prominent U wave and P waves.
- QT prolongation and predisposition to torsades de pointes

Hyperkalemia (Fig. 11.8)
- Tall, peaked T waves
- Flat P waves
- Widened QRS complex
- Prolonged PR interval
- Sine wave.

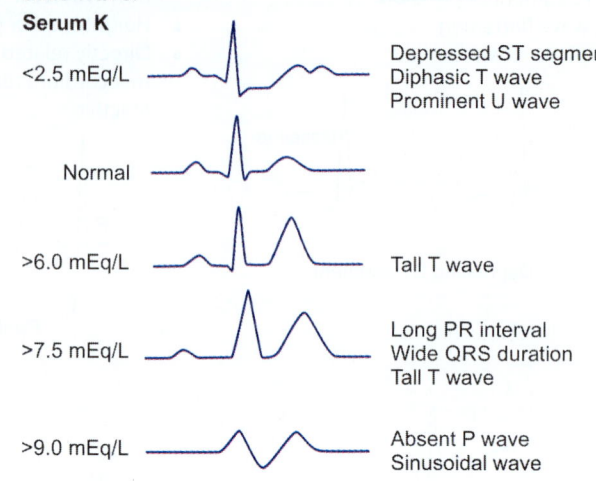

Fig. 11.8: ECG changes in seen with potassium.

Hypomagnesemia
- PR prolongation
- Tall T waves
- Depressed ST segment.
- Prolonged QT interval
- May progress to torsades de pointes
- Often associated with hypokalemia/hypocalcemia, so may also show ECG features of these conditions

Hypermagnesemia
- Prolonged PR interval.
- Widened QRS complexes.
- Flattening of p waves with peaking of T waves
- May progress to complete heart block and asystole

EXAMPLES

Example 1

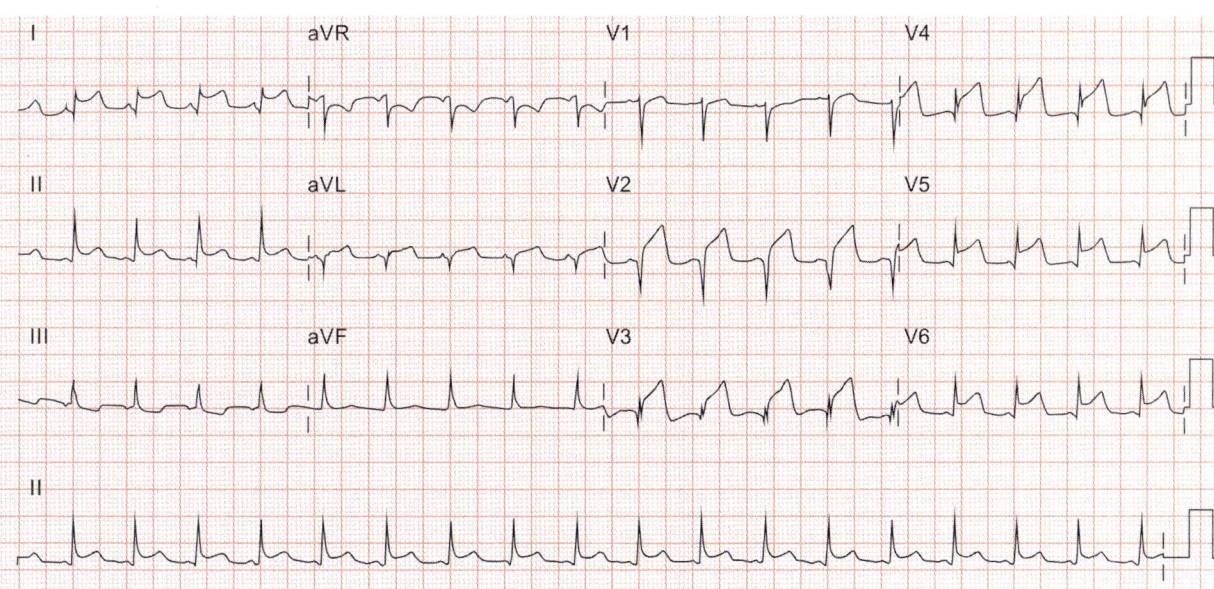

12-lead ECG showing

Rate	110 bpm
Rhythm	Sinus rhythm
Axis	Normal
P wave	Duration 0.08 sec and normal morphology
PR interval/segment	0.12 sec PR segment elevation in aVR
QRS	0.08 sec
ST segment	Elevation in V2–V6, I, aVL depression in aVR
T wave	Normal
QT interval	0.32 sec
Final diagnosis	Acute pericarditis

Example 2

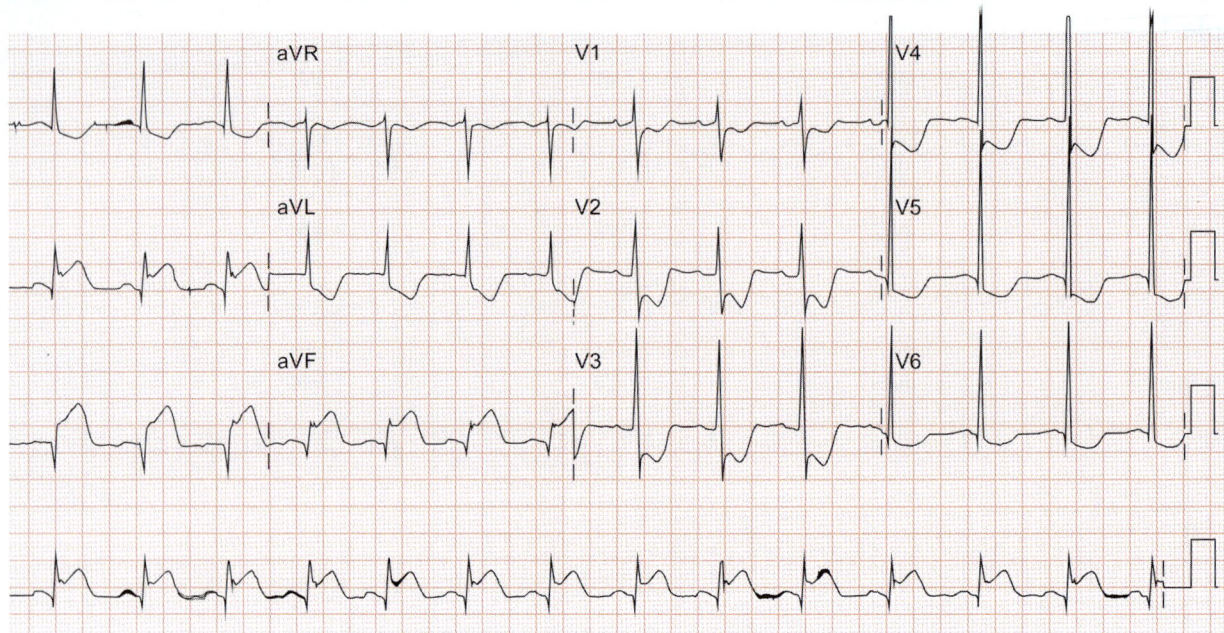

12-lead ECG showing

Rate	85 bpm
Rhythm	Sinus
Axis	Normal
P wave	Duration 0.12 sec and normal morphology
PR interval/segment	0.16 sec
QRS	0.08 sec
ST segment	Elevation in II, III, aVF (elevation in Lead III > II) depression in V1–V6, I, aVL
T wave	Corresponds to ST–T changes
QT interval	0.36 sec
Final diagnosis	Inferior wall MI with signs of RV infarction

Example 3

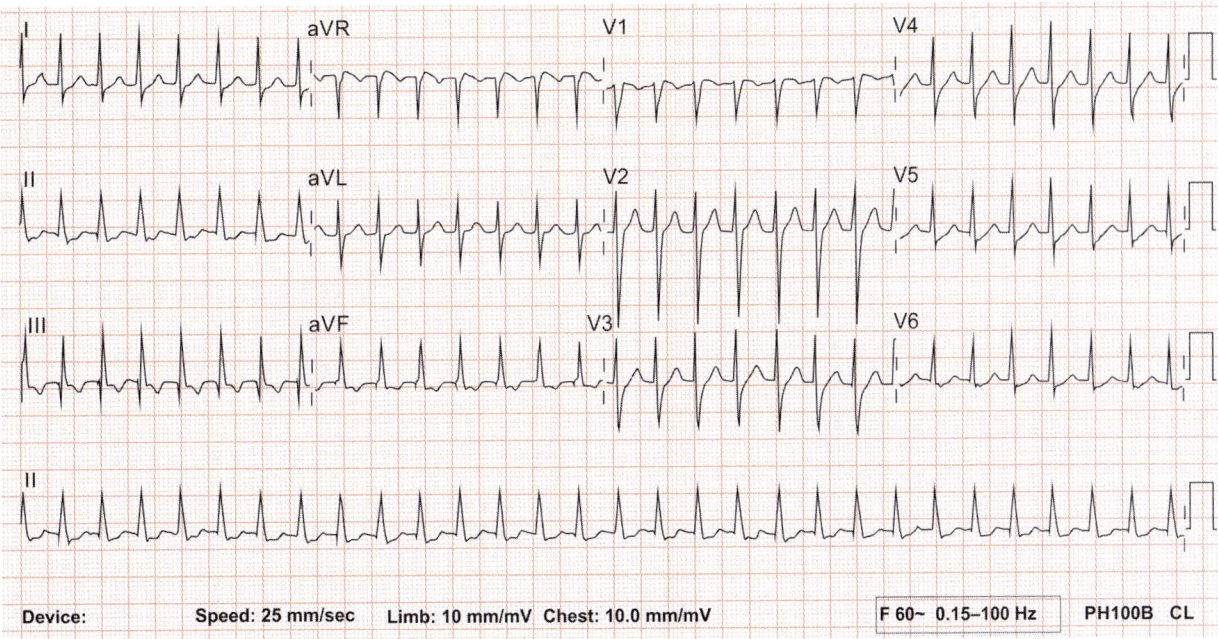

12-lead ECG showing

Rate	200 bpm
Rhythm	Regular
Axis	Normal
P wave	Retrograde
PR interval/segment	—
QRS	0.08 sec (narrow complex)
ST segment	Normal
T wave	Normal
QT interval	0.28 sec
Final diagnosis	Supraventricular tachycardia-atrioventricular nodal reentry tachycardia (SVT-AVNRT)

Example 4

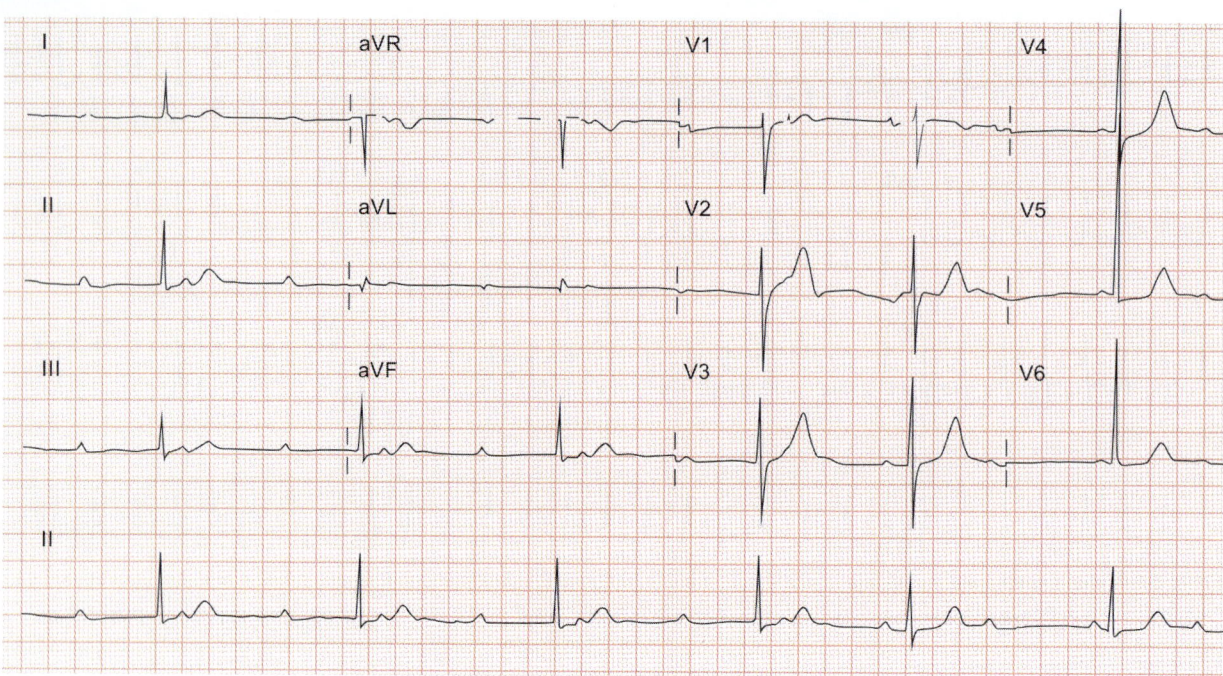

12-lead ECG showing

Rate	Atrial—80 bpm; ventricular—50 bpm
Rhythm	Junctional escape
Axis	Normal
P wave	Present
PR interval/segment	—
QRS	0.08 sec independent of P waves
ST segment	Normal
T wave	Normal
QT interval	0.36 sec
Final diagnosis	Complete heart block

Example 5

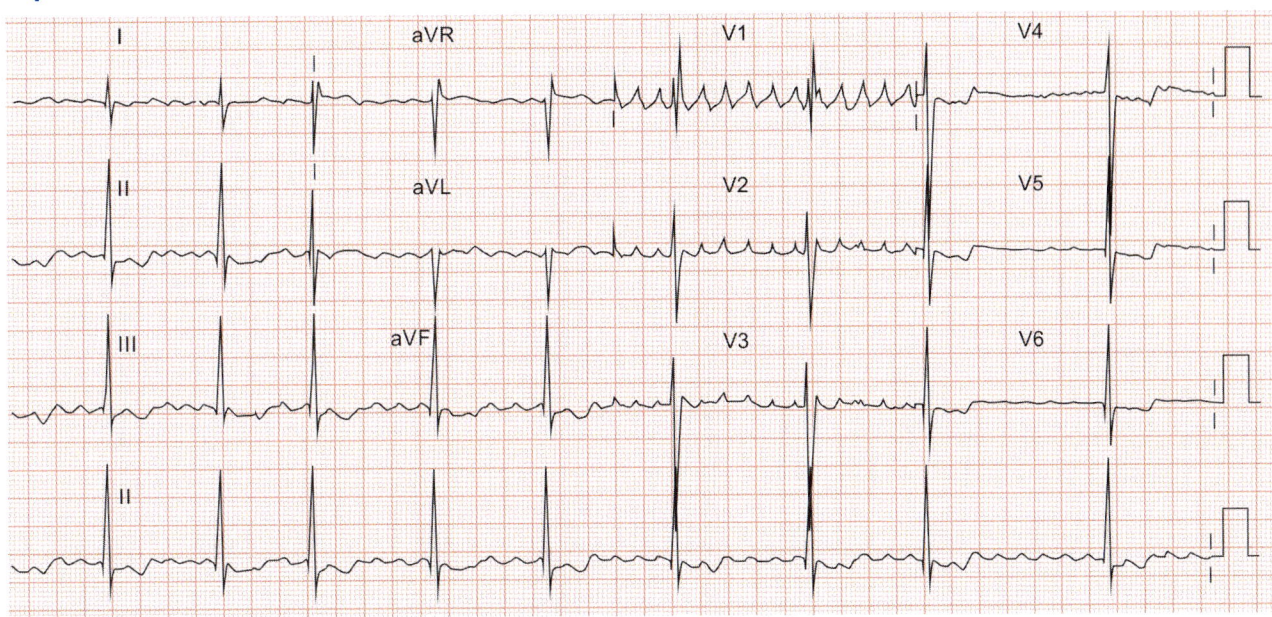

12-lead ECG showing

Rate	70 bpm (6 sec rule)
Rhythm	Irregular
Axis	Normal
P wave	Absent, presence of fibrillary waves
PR interval/segment	—
QRS	0.08 sec varying RR interval
ST segment	Normal
T wave	Normal
QT interval	0.32 sec
Final diagnosis	Atrial fibrillation

Example 6

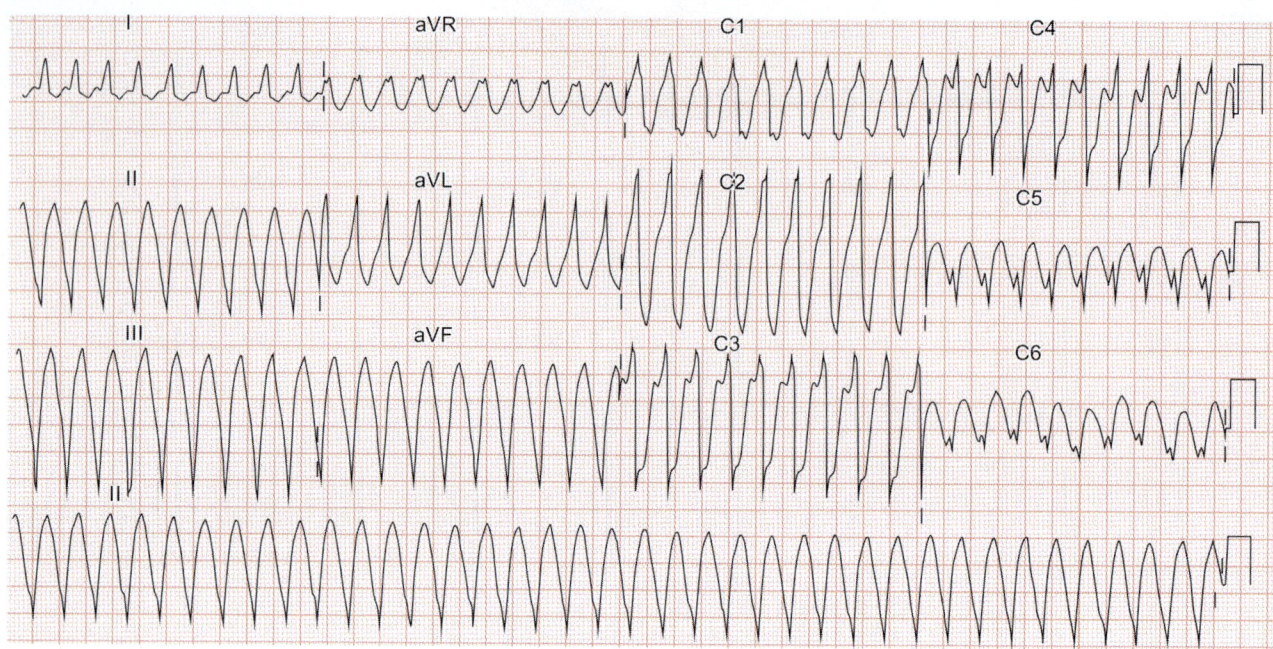

12-lead ECG showing

Rate	250 bpm
Rhythm	Regular
Axis	Left—Northwest
P wave	AV dissociation
PR interval/segment	—
QRS	- 0.28 sec (broad complex) - Positive concordance
ST segment	—
T wave	—
QT interval	—
Final diagnosis	Monomorphic ventricular tachycardia (VT)

Example 7

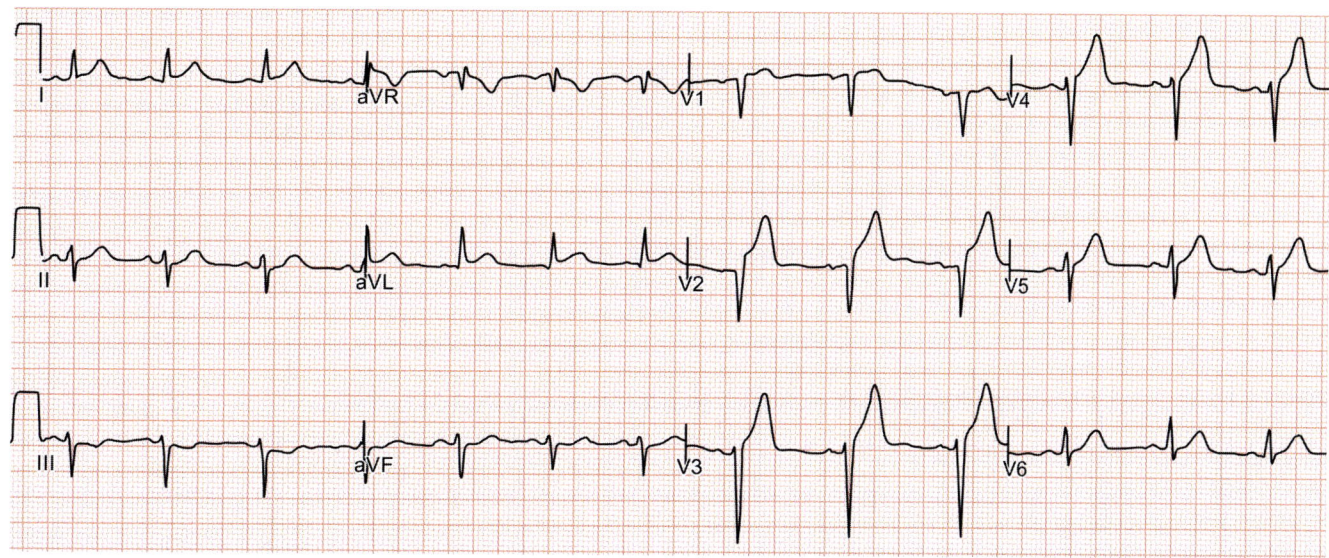

12-lead ECG showing

Rate	71
Rhythm	Regular
Axis	Left
P wave	Normal
PR interval/segment	Normal
QRS	Narrow, QS complexes in septal leads
ST segment	Elevation in I, aVL, V2, depression in III ('South African flag' sign), elevations seen in V1–V4
T wave	Hyperacute T waves seen in V2–V3
QT interval	0.348
Final diagnosis	- High-lateral STEMI - Hyperacute anteroseptal MI

Example 8

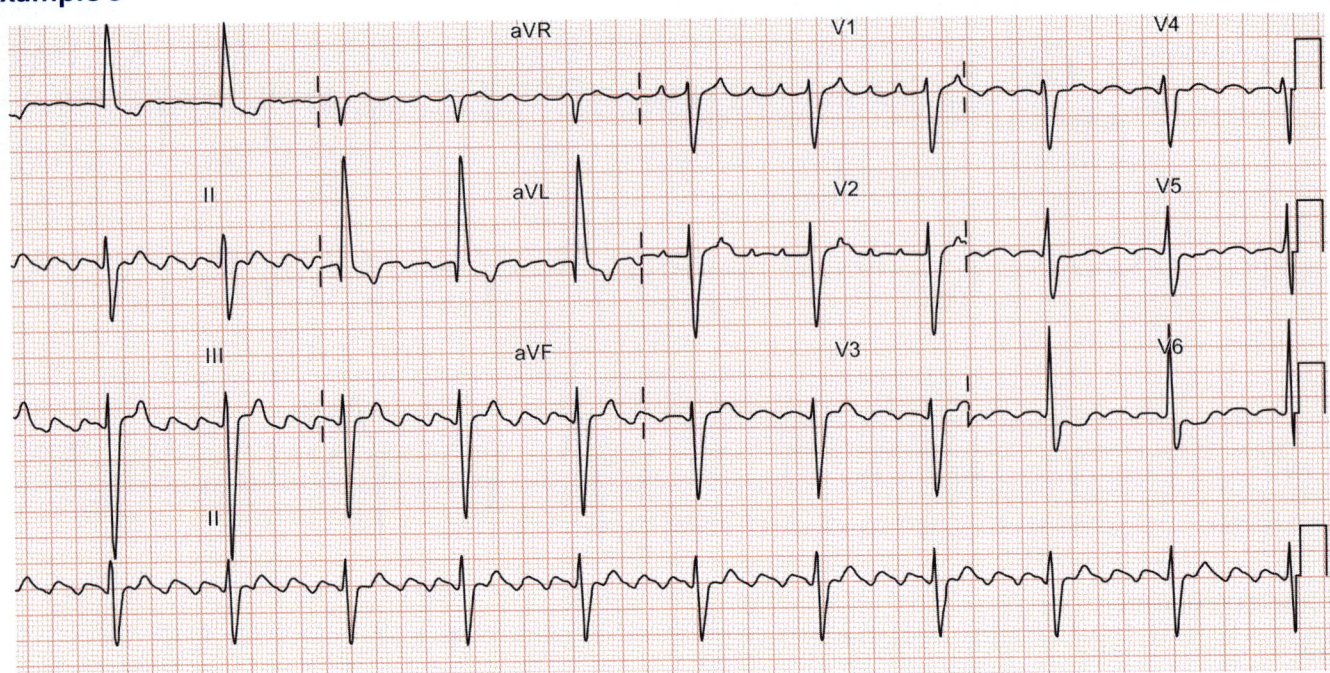

12-lead ECG showing

Rate	Atrial ~250, ventricular ~65
Rhythm	Regular
Axis	Leftward
P wave	"Saw-tooth" pattern
PR interval/segment	No PR interval
QRS	Narrow
ST segment	Cannot be commented
T wave	Superimposed by flutter waves
QT interval	Cannot be commented
Final diagnosis	▪ **Atrial flutter** with fixed AV block (4:1) ▪ LVH (limb lead voltage criteria: R in aVL ≥13 mm, S in III ≥15 mm, R in I+S in III >25 mm)

Example 9

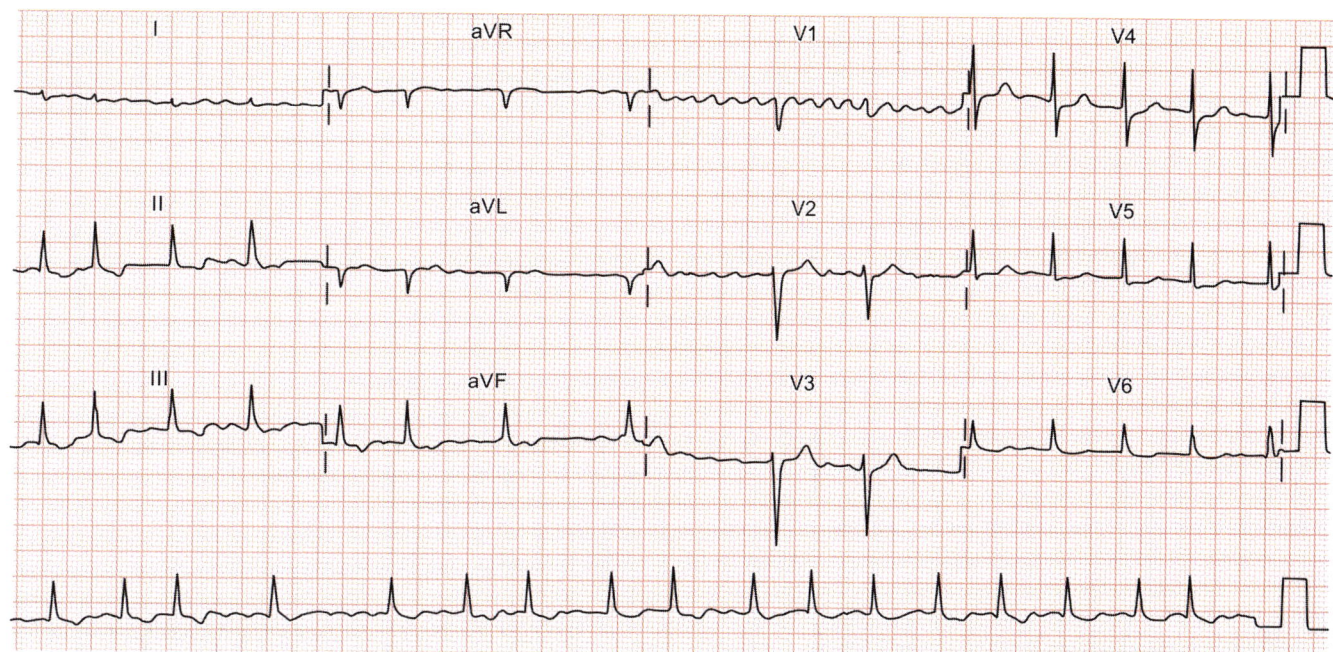

12-lead ECG showing

Rate	102 (number of complexes in 10 sec rhythm strip × 6)
Rhythm	Irregular
Axis	Normal
P wave	Absent, coarse fibrillary waves (V1)
PR interval/segment	Cannot be commented
QRS	Narrow
ST segment	ST segment depression with downward slopping in II, III, aVF
T wave	Normal
QTc interval	0.443
Final diagnosis	- **Atrial fibrillation** with rapid ventricular response - Digoxin effect ("sagging" ST depressions in inferior leads)/MI (reciprocal ST depressions of a high-lateral MI)

Example 10

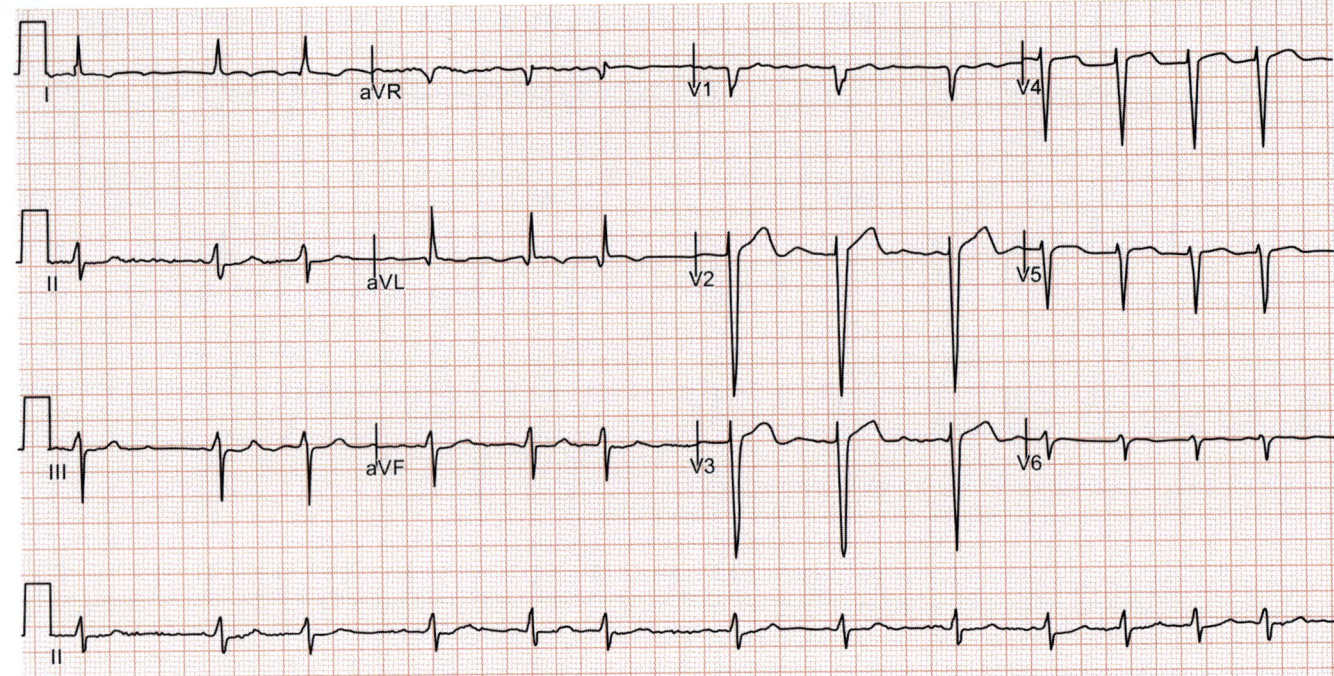

12-lead ECG showing

Rate	78 (number of complexes in 10 sec rhythm strip × 6)
Rhythm	Irregular
Axis	Leftward
P wave	Absent, fine fibrillary waves (V1)
PR interval/segment	Cannot be commented
QRS	Narrow, poor R wave progression
ST segment	Normal
T wave	Flat/inverted in lateral leads
QTc interval	0.410
Final diagnosis	▪ **Atrial fibrillation** ▪ Possible old lateral wall MI

Example 11

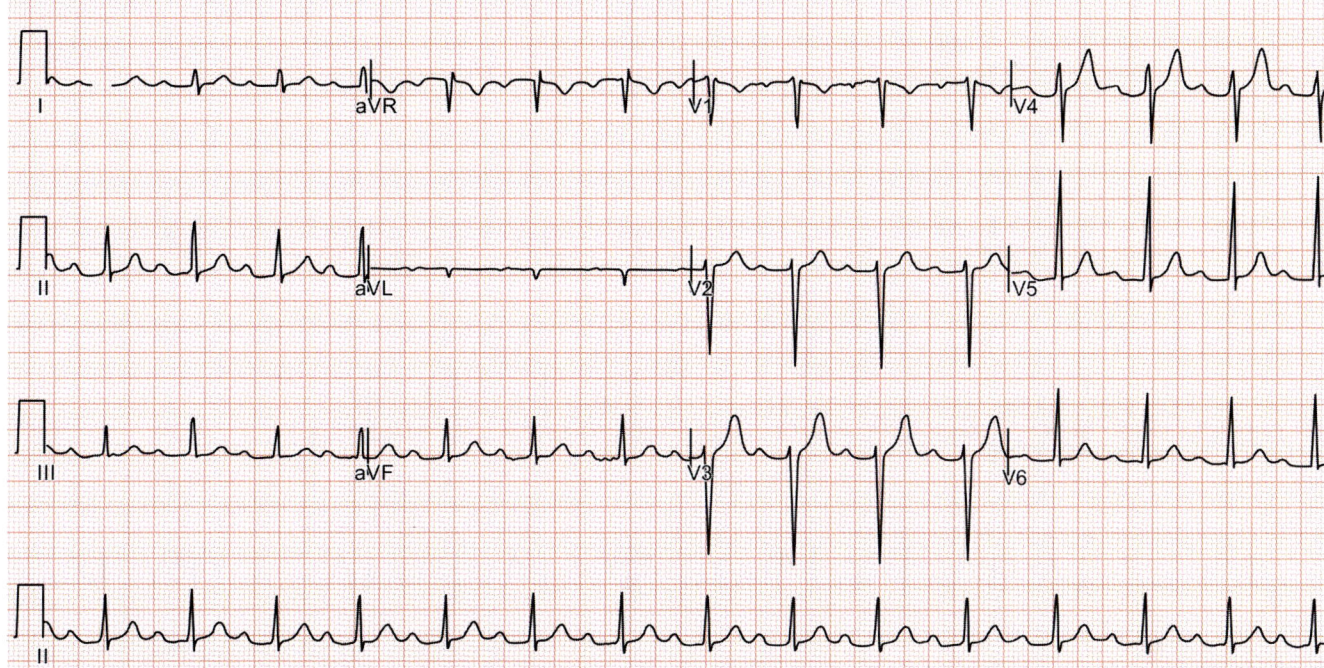

12-lead ECG showing

Rate	88
Rhythm	Regular
Axis	Normal
P wave	Normal
PR interval/segment	0.28, prolonged
QRS	Narrow
ST segment	Normal
T wave	Normal
QTc interval	0.436
Final diagnosis	1st degree AV block

Example 12

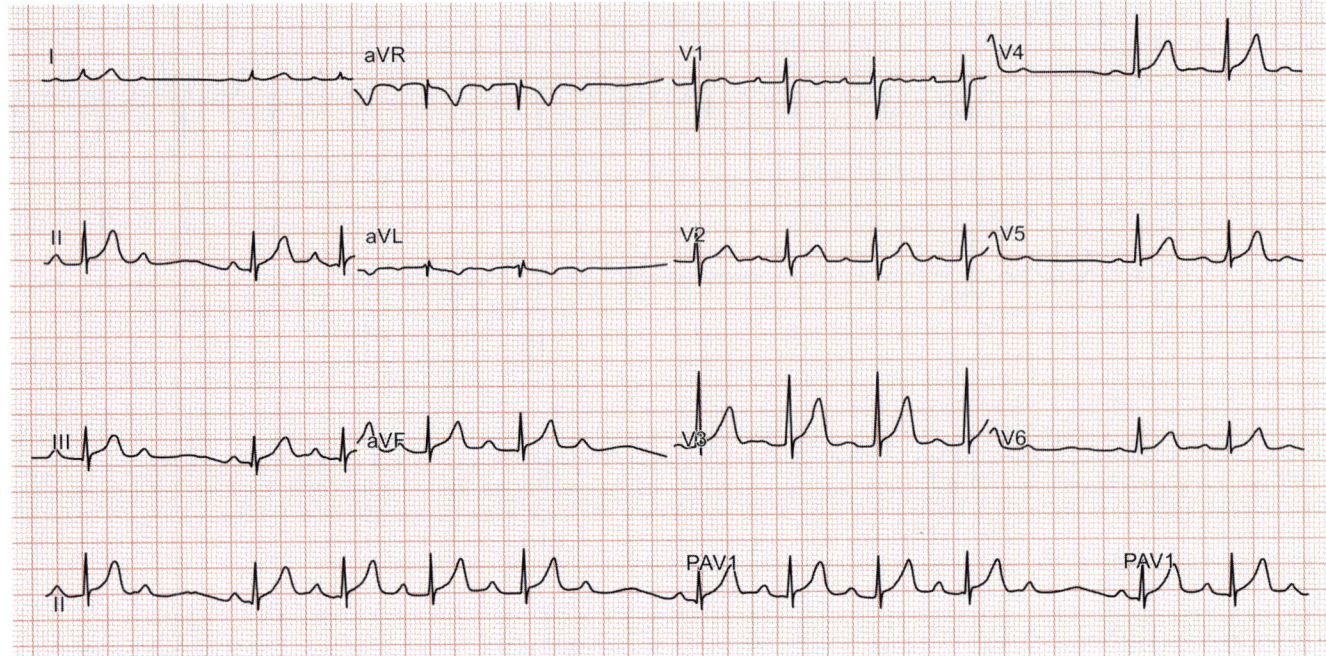

12-lead ECG showing

Rate	88
Rhythm	Regular sinus with dropped beat at regular intervals
Axis	Normal
P wave	Normal
PR interval/segment	Progressive prolongation of PR interval with subsequent non-conducted P wave
QRS	Narrow
ST segment	Normal
T wave	Normal
QTc interval	0.388
Final diagnosis	2nd degree AV block Mobitz type 1 (Wenckebach phenomenon)

Example 13

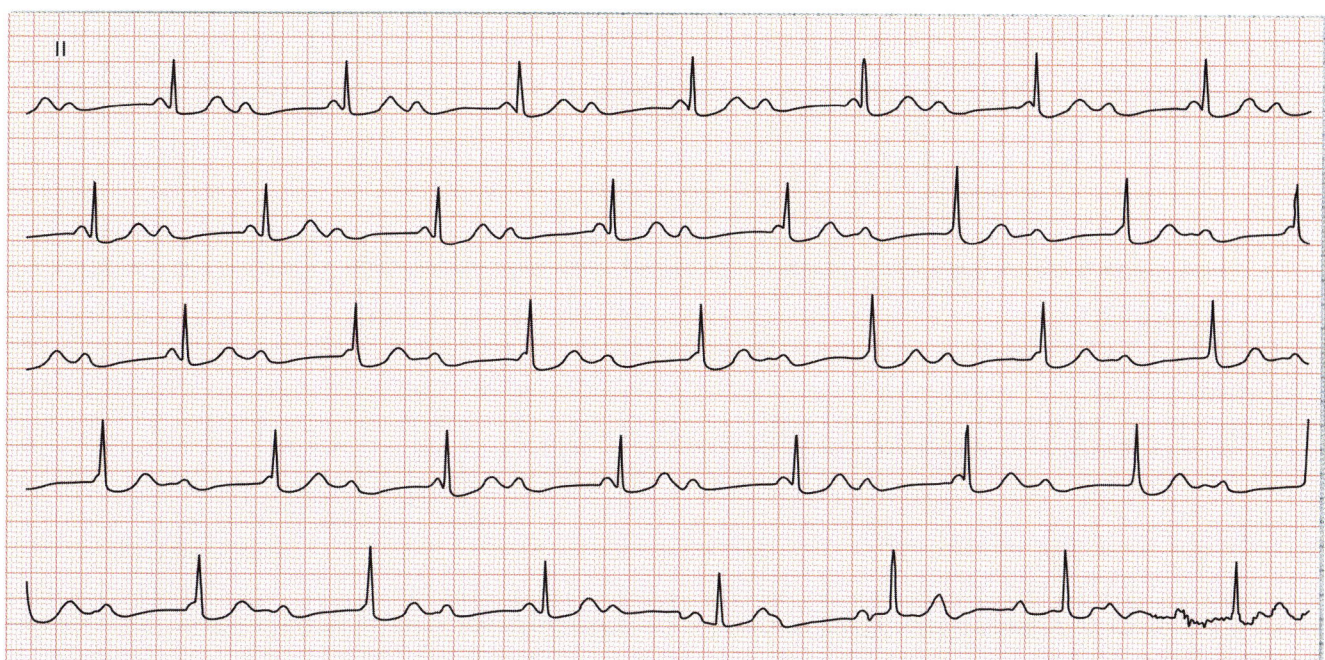

12-lead ECG showing

Rate	Atrial—88, ventricular—42
Rhythm	Regular, junctional escape
Axis	Single lead cannot comment
P wave	Normal
PR interval/segment	Varying, isorhythmic AV dissociation (some P waves appear to conduct, but on closer inspection the PR interval is varying. What appears to be a relationship between the P waves and QRS complexes is purely by chance)
QRS	Narrow
ST segment	Depressions with upsloping (nonspecific)
T wave	Normal
QTc interval	0.418
Final diagnosis	3rd degree (complete) heart block

Example 14

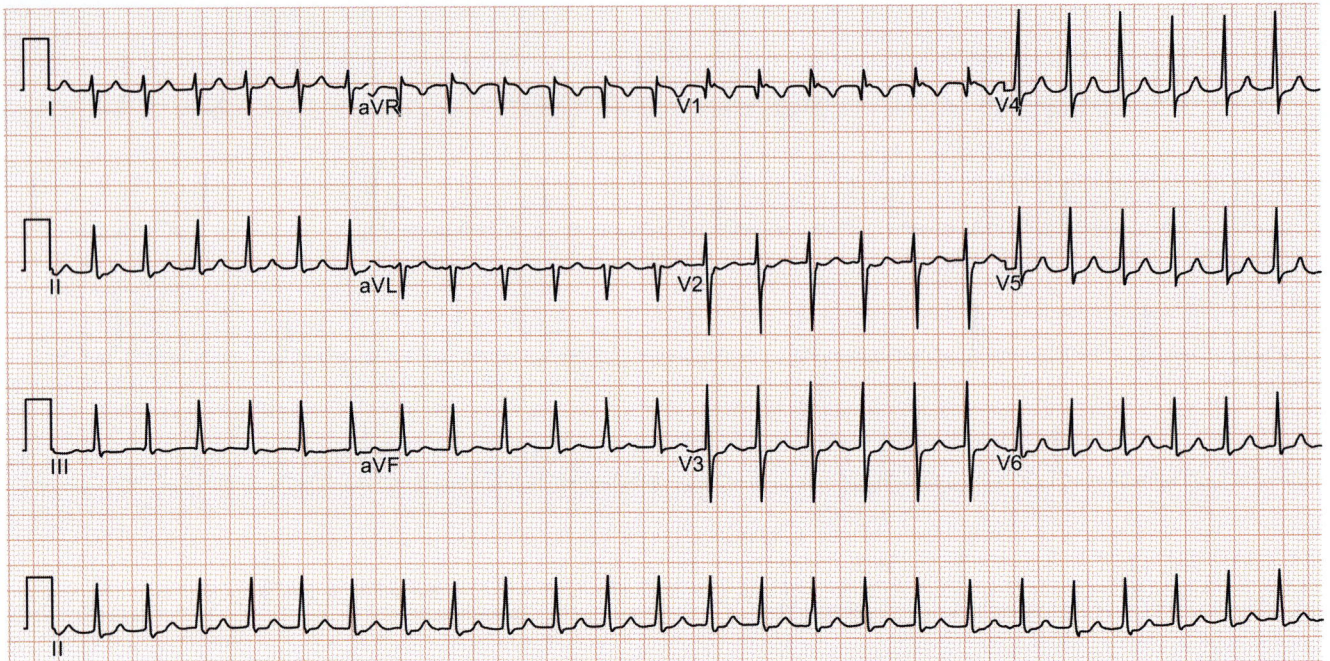

12-lead ECG showing

Rate	150
Rhythm	Regular
Axis	Normal
P wave	Absent (retrograde P waves get buried in the QRS complexes; some retrograde P waves can be seen just before the QRS complexes in leads V1 and V2, termed pseudo R' waves)
PR interval/segment	—
QRS	Narrow
ST segment	Normal
T wave	Normal
QTc interval	379
Final diagnosis	Supraventricular tachycardia (AVNRT slow-fast type)

Example 15

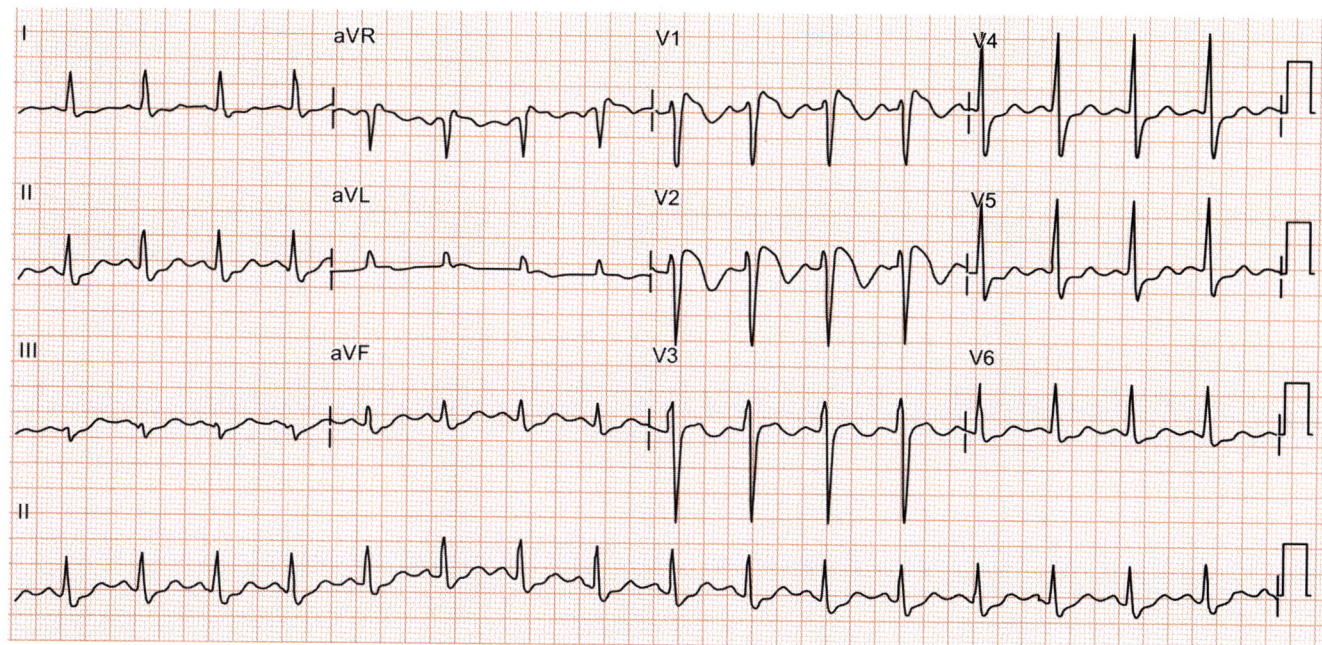

12-lead ECG showing

Rate	100
Rhythm	Regular
Axis	Normal
P wave	Normal
PR interval/segment	Normal
QRS	Narrow, rSR' in V1, V2
ST segment	Coved ST elevation in V1, V2 ST depressions in other leads
T wave	T wave inversions in V1, V2, V3
QTc interval	0.516
Final diagnosis	▪ **Brugada syndrome (type 1)** ▪ Hypokalemia to be considered (generalized ST depressions, QT prolongation, type 1 Brugada like pattern)

Example 16

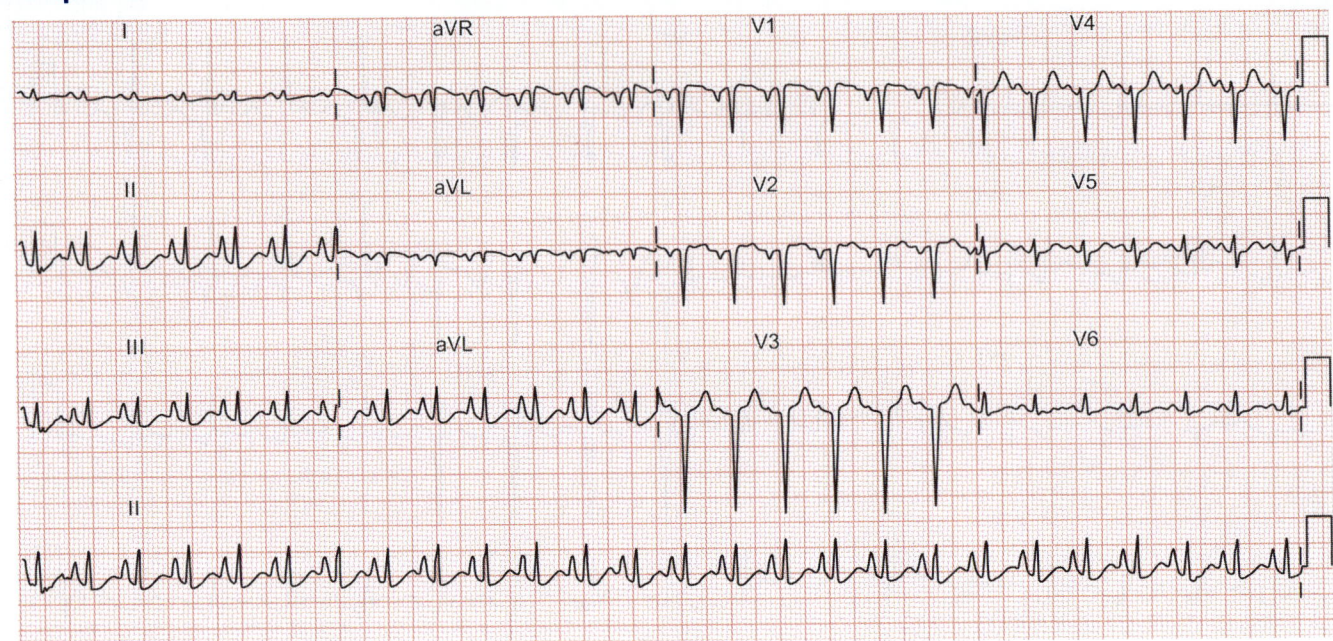

12-lead ECG showing

Rate	150
Rhythm	Regular
Axis	Normal
P wave	Tall (>2.5; P pulmonale)
PR interval/segment	Normal
QRS	Narrow
ST segment	Normal
T wave	Normal
QTc interval	0.443
Final diagnosis	**Right atrial enlargement** [possible etiologies include cor-pulmonale, tricuspid stenosis, pulmonary stenosis, congenital heart diseases—tricuspid atresia, Fallot's tetralogy, Ebstein's anomaly (very tall 'Himalayan' P waves)]

Example 17

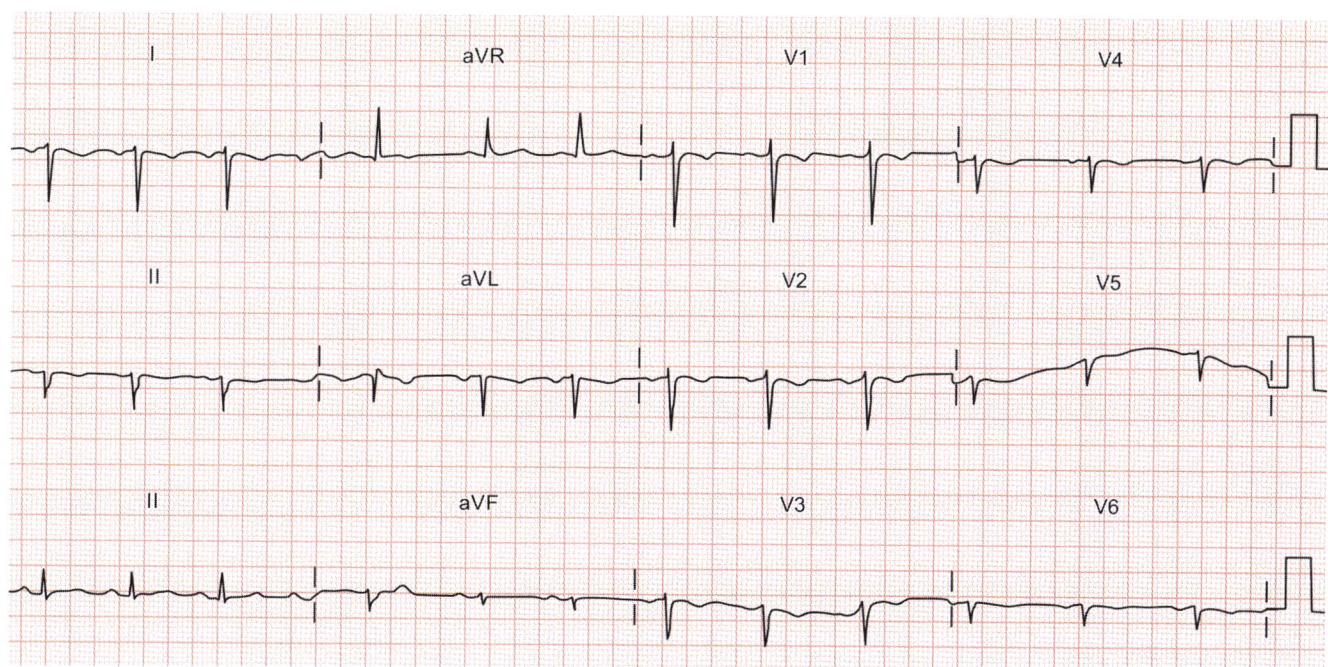

12-lead ECG showing

Rate	75
Rhythm	Regular
Axis	Northwest
P wave	Normal, inverted in most leads
PR interval/segment	Normal
QRS	Narrow, upright in lead aVR, poor R wave progression
ST segment	Normal
T wave	Inverted in most leads
QTc interval	0.358
Final diagnosis	Dextrocardia

Example 18

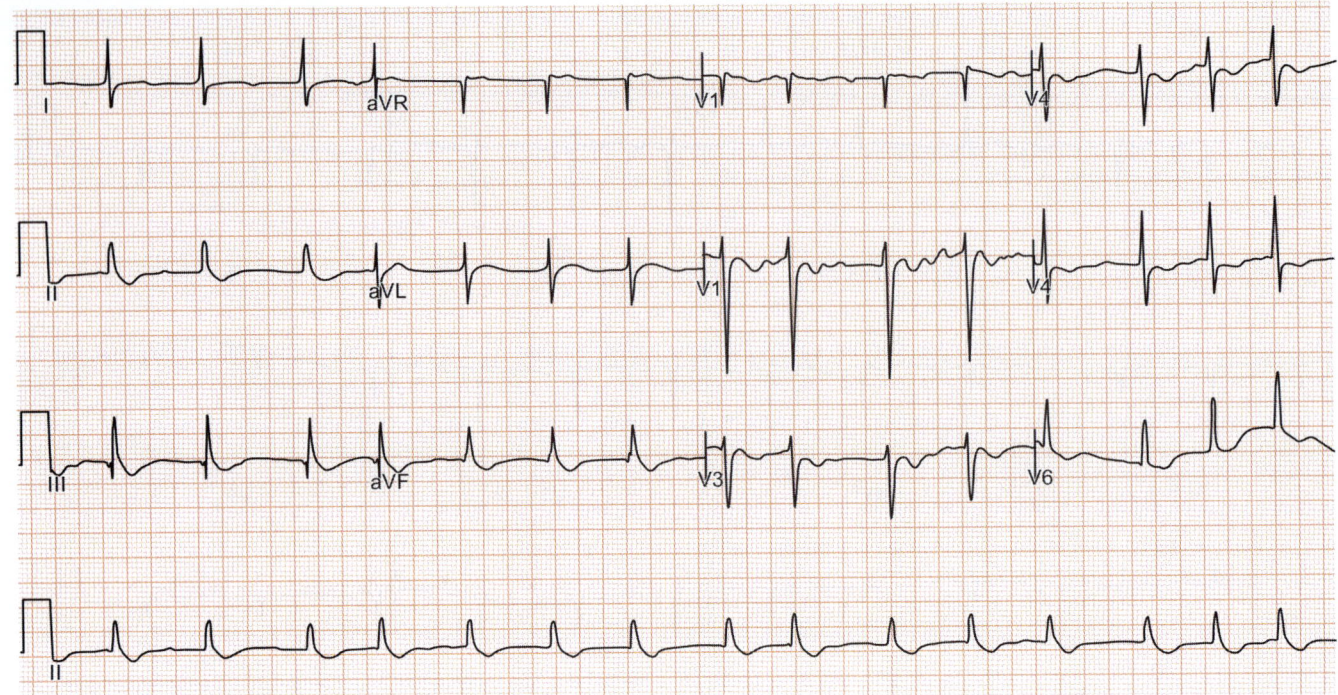

12-lead ECG showing

Rate	~90 (number of complexes in 10 sec rhythm strip × 6)
Rhythm	Irregular
Axis	Normal
P wave	Absent, fibrillary waves seen
PR interval/segment	—
QRS	Narrow
ST segment	Sagging/downsloping ST depressions ('reverse tick' sign or 'Salvador Dali moustache' sign)
T wave	Normal
QTc interval	0.343
Final diagnosis	▪ Digoxin effect ▪ Atrial fibrillation with controlled rate

Example 19

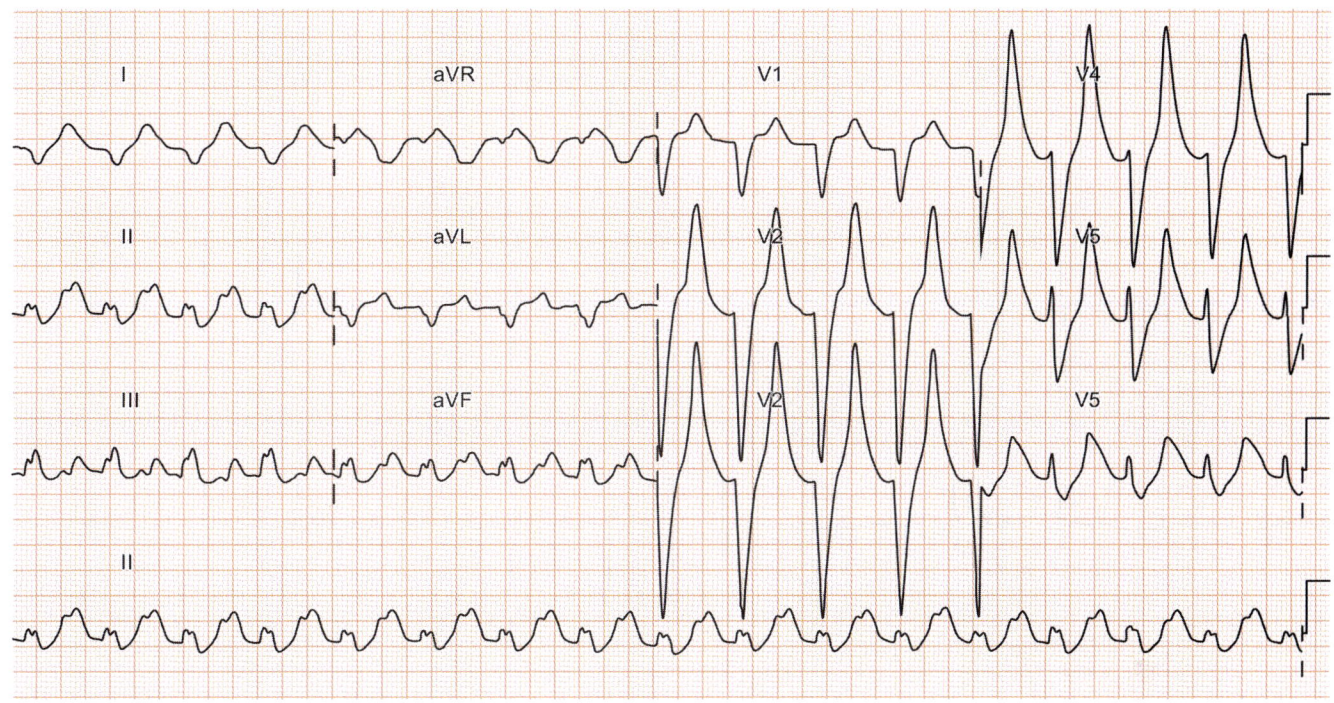

12-lead ECG showing

Rate	~100
Rhythm	Regular
Axis	Right
P wave	Flattened (barely seen)
PR interval/segment	Cannot be commented
QRS	Broad bizarre looking merged
ST segment	Elevations/depressions seen (appropriate discordance)
T wave	Tall peaked (tented)
QT interval	Difficult to comment (almost sine wave like pattern seen)
Final diagnosis	Severe hyperkalemia

Example 20

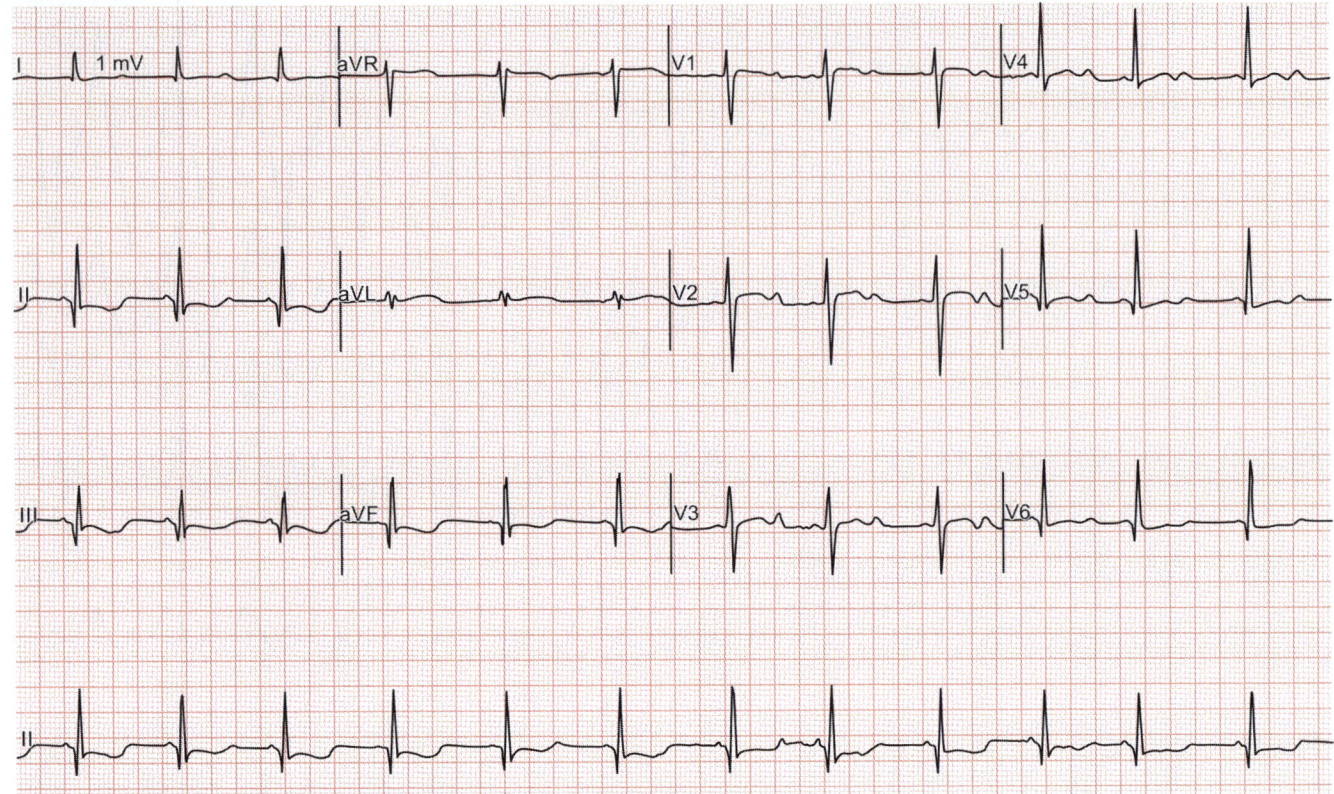

12-lead ECG showing

Rate	68
Rhythm	Regular
Axis	Normal
P wave	Normal
PR interval/segment	Normal
QRS	Narrow, prominent Q waves in inferior leads
ST segment	Depressions in inferior leads
T wave	Flattening
QTc interval	0.511, prominent U waves seen (apparent QT prolongation)
Final diagnosis	- **Severe hypokalemia** - Possible old inferior wall MI

Example 21

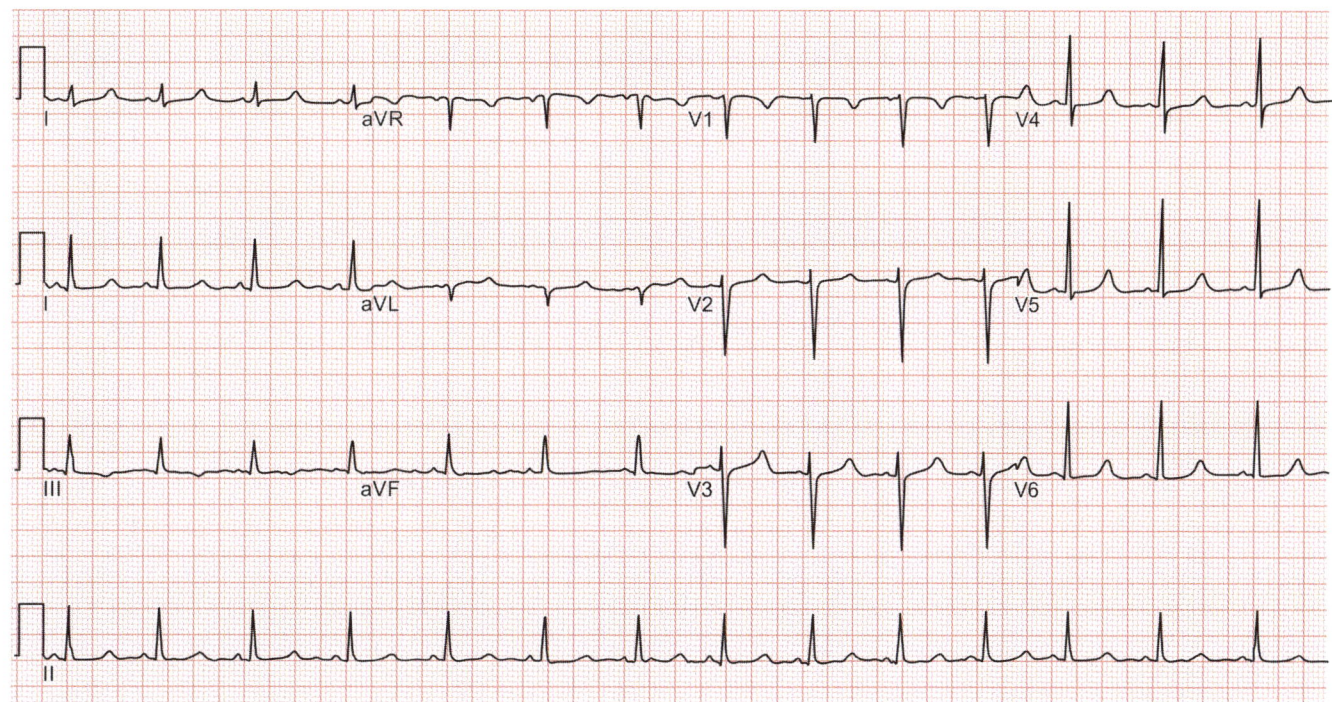

12-lead ECG showing

Rate	83
Rhythm	Regular
Axis	Normal
P wave	Normal
PR interval/segment	Normal
QRS	Narrow
ST segment	Normal
T wave	Normal
QTc interval	0.470
Final diagnosis	Normal ECG

Example 22

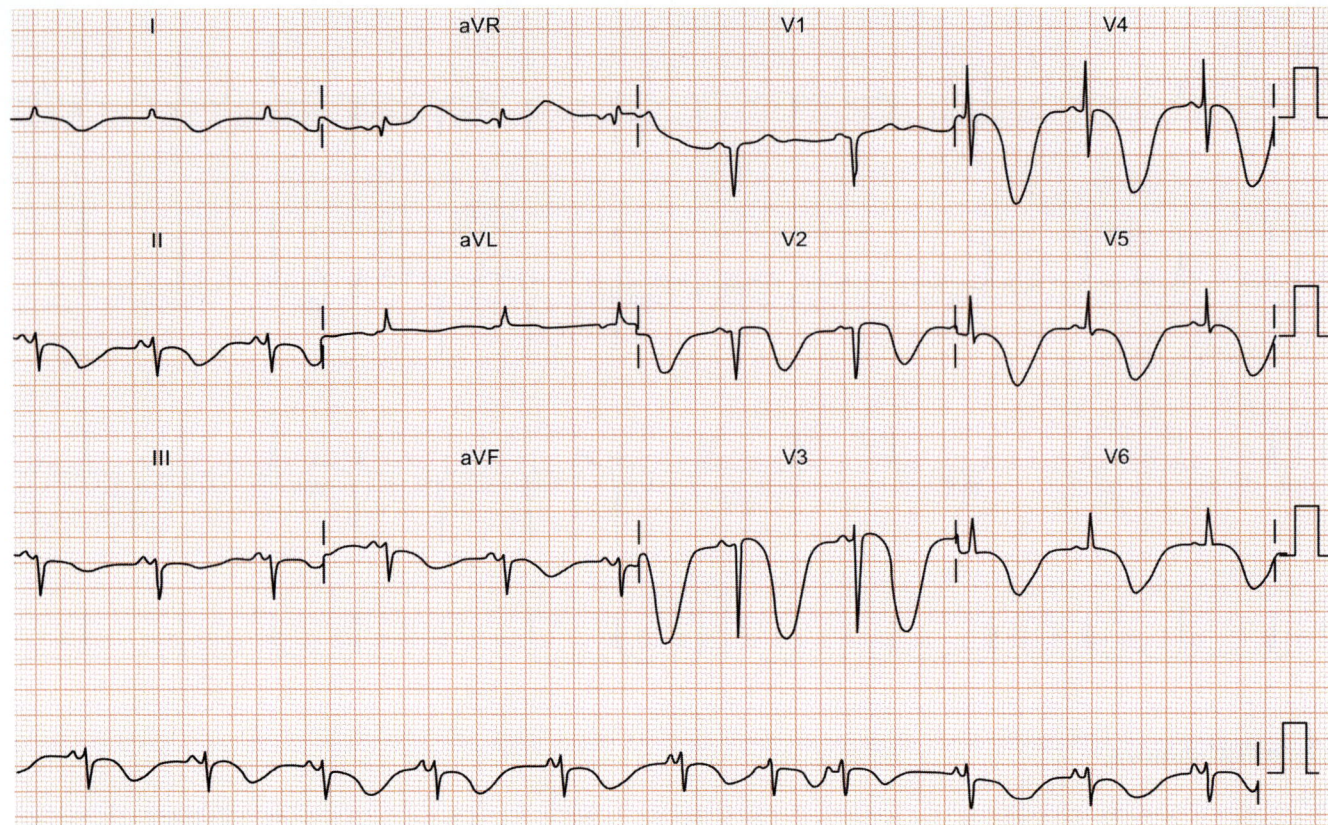

12-lead ECG showing

Rate	63
Rhythm	Regular
Axis	Left
P wave	Normal
PR interval/segment	Normal
QRS	Narrow
ST segment	Normal
T wave	Widespread deep inversions (cerebral T waves)
QTc interval	0.600
Final diagnosis	Features favor raised intracranial tension (if young patient, rule out HOCM)

Example 23

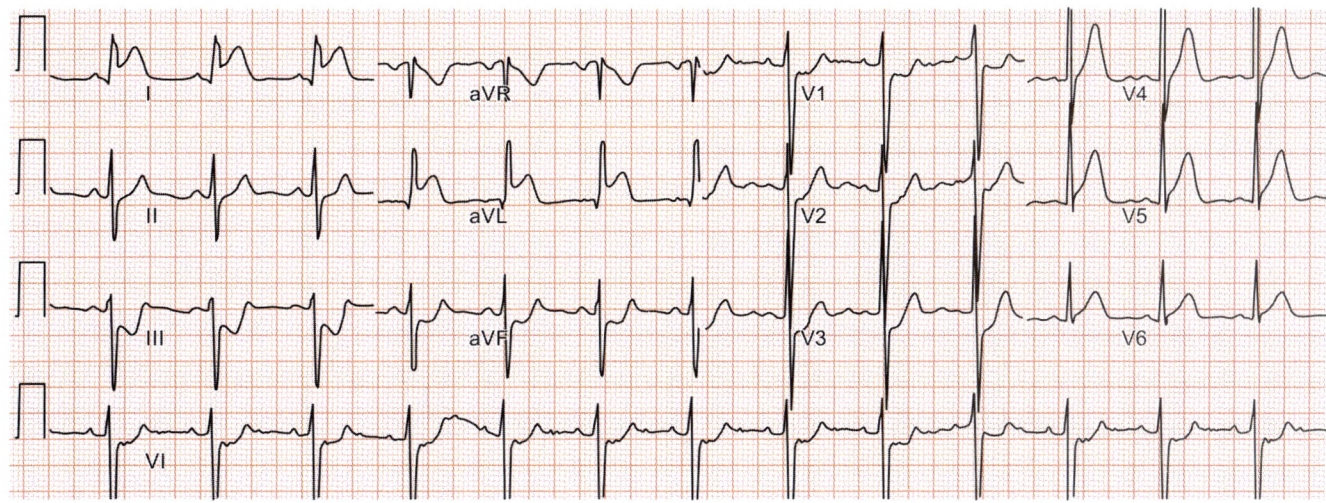

12-lead ECG showing

Rate	88
Rhythm	Regular
Axis	Left
P wave	Normal
PR interval/segment	Normal
QRS	Narrow
ST segment	Elevations in I, aVL; reciprocal depressions in II, III, aVF; depressions in V1–V3 (reciprocal changes or anterior ischemia)
T wave	Normal
QTc interval	0.388
Final diagnosis	Acute **high lateral wall STEMI** with possible anteroseptal ischemia

Example 24

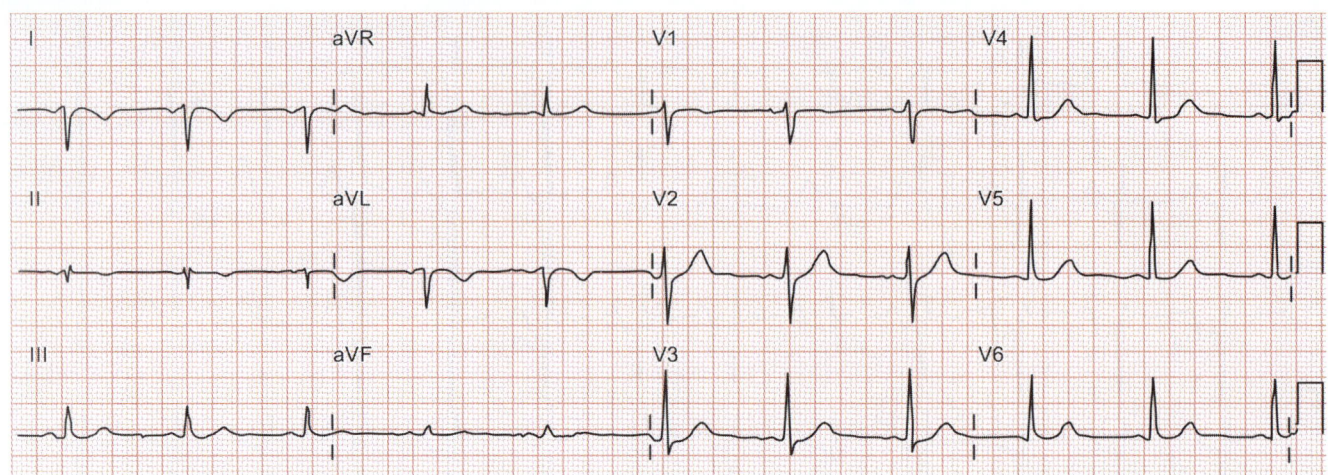

12-lead ECG showing

Rate	63
Rhythm	Regular
Axis	Right
P wave	Normal
PR interval/segment	Normal
QRS	Narrow, normal R wave progression, upright in lead aVR
ST segment	Normal
T wave	Normal
QTc interval	Appears normal (t waves end before mid-point of R-R interval)
Final diagnosis	Incorrect lead (limb lead) placement

Example 25

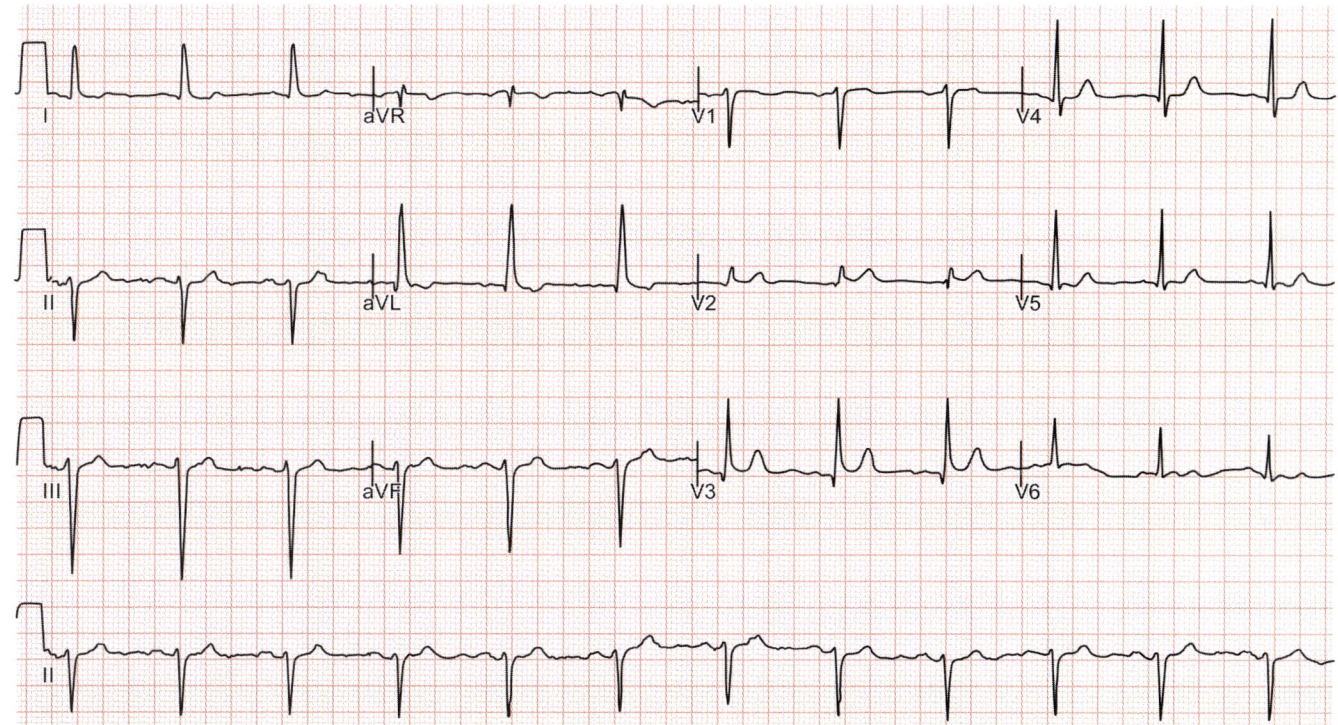

12-lead ECG showing

Rate	75
Rhythm	Regular
Axis	Left
P wave	Normal
PR interval/segment	Normal
QRS	Narrow, q waves in V2–V3
ST segment	Subtle elevations in anteroseptal leads
T wave	Normal
QTc interval	0.402
Final diagnosis	LVH (limb lead voltage criteria: R in aVL ≥13 mm, S in III ≥15 mm, R in I+S in III >25 mm) Possible anteroseptal MI (although changes are not very specific, it should be suspected in the presence of any q waves in anterior/septal leads)

Example 26

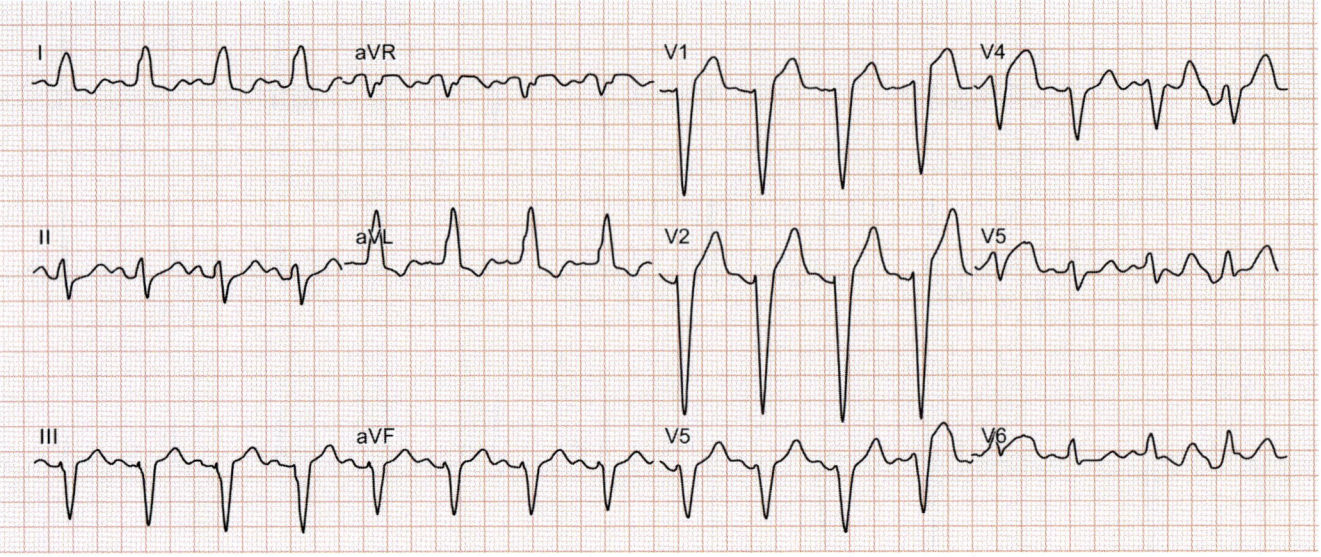

12-lead ECG showing

Rate	100
Rhythm	Regular
Axis	Left
P wave	Normal
PR interval/segment	Normal
QRS	Wide (140 ms), deep S in V1, tall slurred R best seen in I, aVL, absent q in V5–V6
ST segment	Elevations/depressions seen (appropriate discordance)
T wave	Normal
QT interval	0.465
Final diagnosis	LBBB

Contd...
Example 27

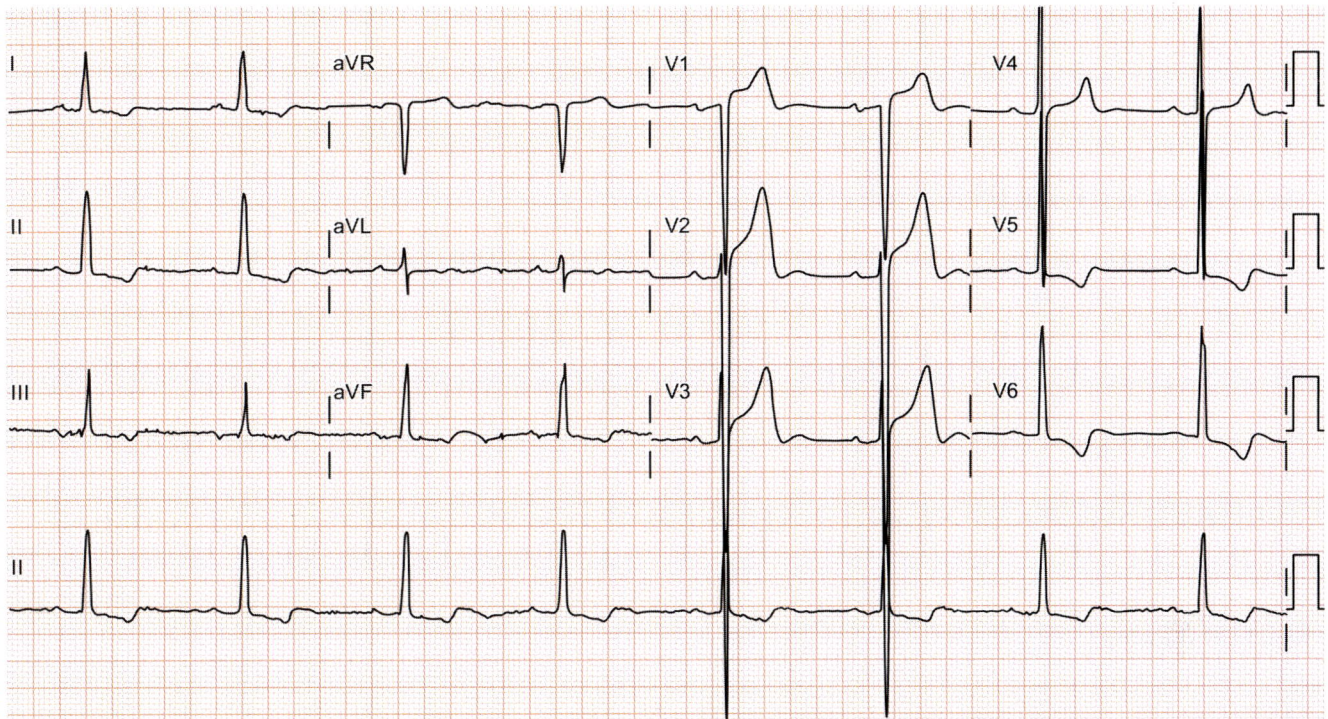

12-lead ECG showing

Rate	50
Rhythm	Regular
Axis	Normal
P wave	Normal
PR interval/segment	Normal
QRS	Narrow
ST segment	Down-sloping depressions in all leads with dominant R wave
T wave	Inversions seen all leads with dominant R wave (strain pattern)
QT interval	0.402
Final diagnosis	▪ Left ventricular hypertrophy with LV strain ▪ Sinus bradycardia

Example 28

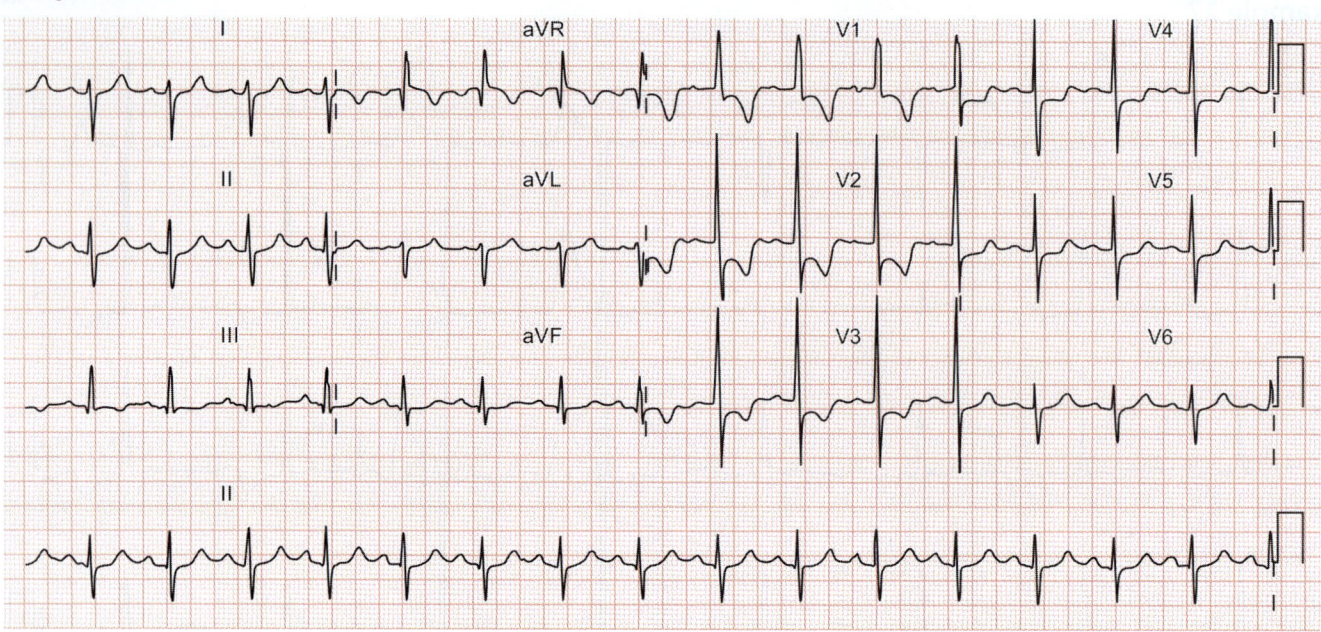

12-lead ECG showing

Rate	94
Rhythm	Regular
Axis	Right
P wave	Normal
PR interval/segment	Normal
QRS	Narrow, tall R in V1 (>7 mm, R/S ratio >1), deep S in V6 (>7 mm, R/S ratio <1)
ST segment	Depressions in V1–V4
T wave	Inversions in V1–V4
QT interval	0.451
Final diagnosis	Right ventricular hypertrophy with RV strain pattern

Example 29

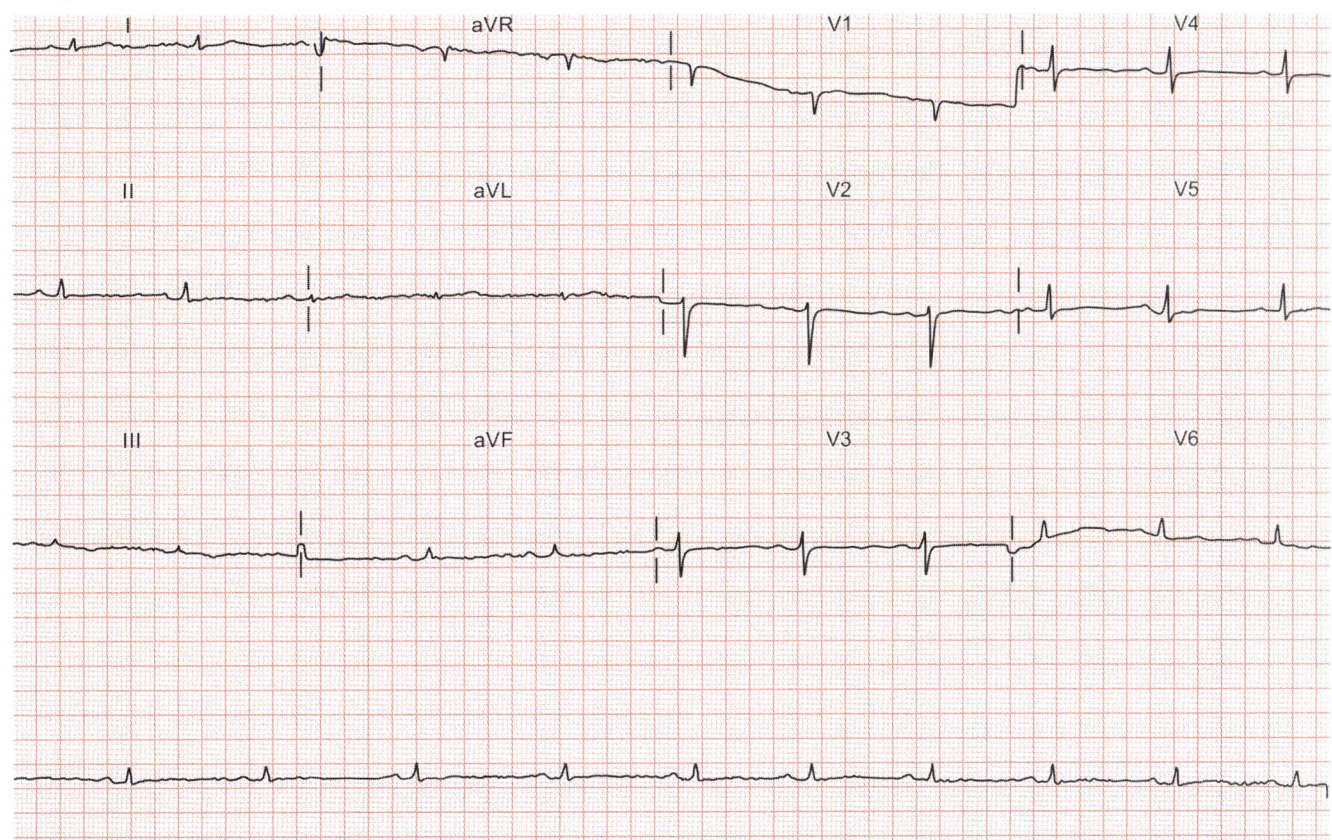

12-lead ECG showing

Rate	68
Rhythm	Regular
Axis	Normal
P wave	Normal
PR interval/segment	Normal
QRS	Narrow, low voltage complexes in all limb leads (<5 mm)
ST segment	Normal
T wave	Generalized flattening
QTc interval	0.383 (T waves are barely visible. T waves in leads I and III used for calculation)
Final diagnosis	▪ **Low QRS voltage** with possible etiology being pericardial effusion, hypothyroidism, hypothermia, emphysema; pneumothorax, amyloidosis, hemochromatosis ▪ Hypokalemia to be ruled out (flat T waves)

Example 30

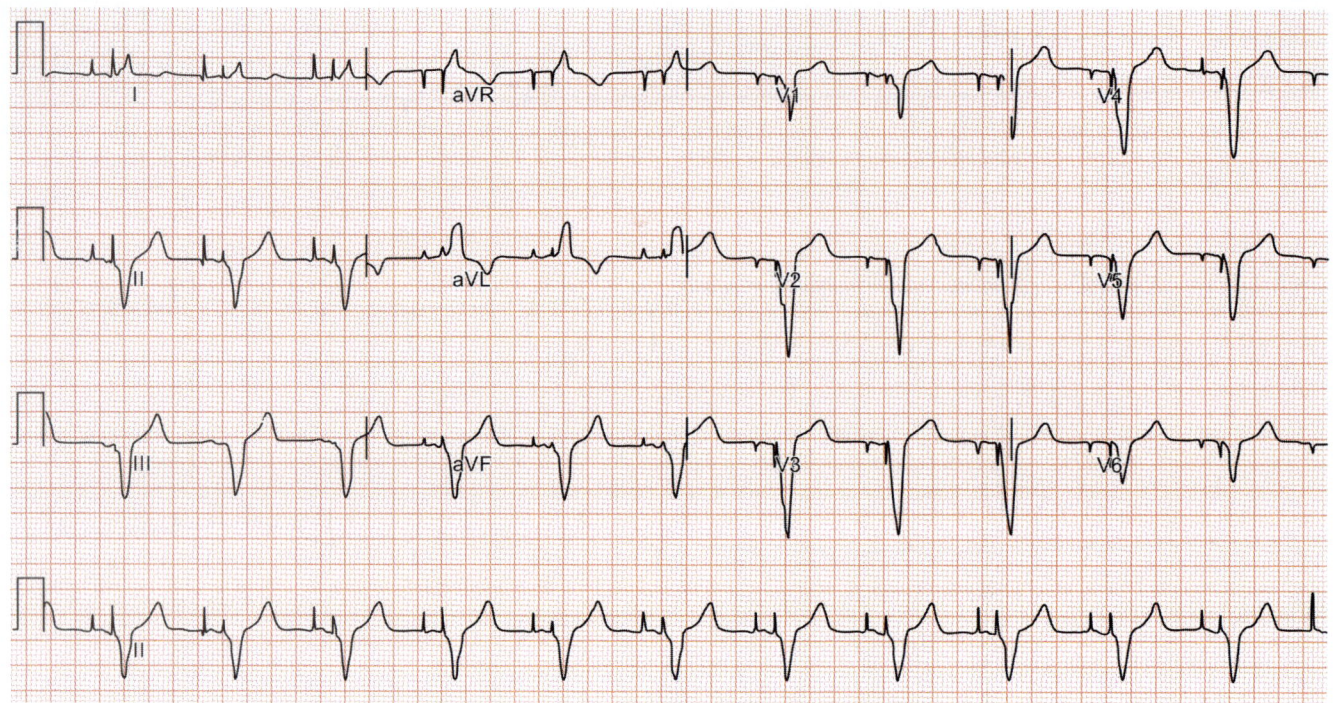

12-lead ECG showing

Rate	71
Rhythm	Regular, pacemaker spikes seen—atrial and ventricular with complete capture
Axis	Left
P wave	Small, normal morphology succeeding each atrial pacemaker spike
PR interval/segment	Normal
QRS	Broad with nonspecific interventricular conduction block morphology (but may be taken as LBBB morphology, note deep slurred S in V1)
ST segment	Normal
T wave	Normal
QT interval	0.479
Final diagnosis	A-V sequential pacing (ventricular pacemaker lead more likely in RV)

Example 31

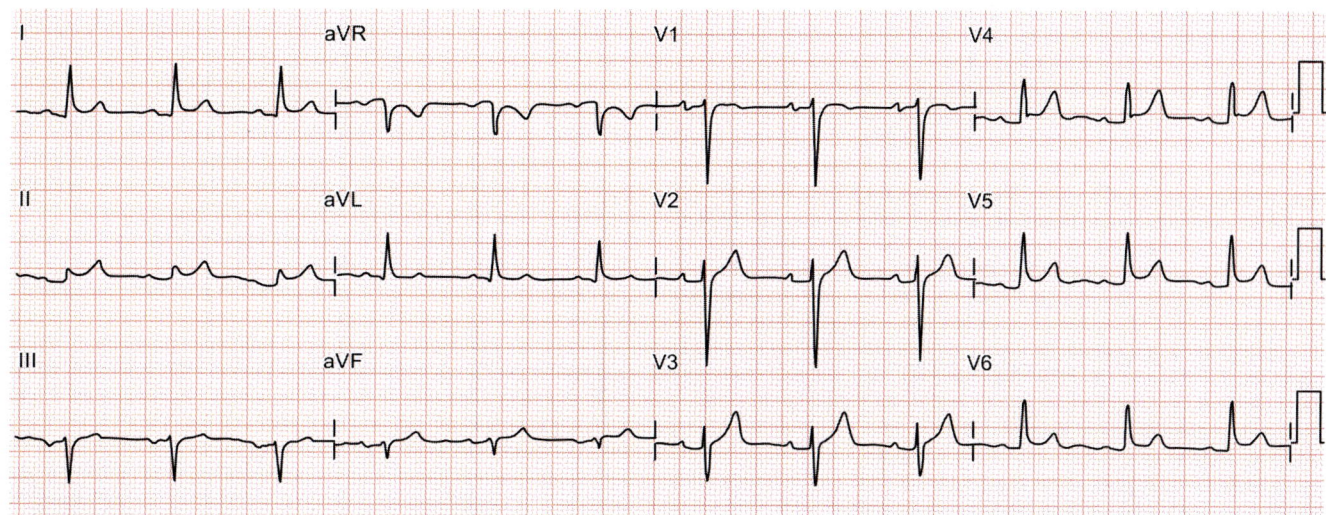

12-lead ECG showing

Rate	75
Rhythm	Regular
Axis	Leftward
P wave	Normal
PR interval/segment	Generalized depressions, except in leads aVR (elevated)
QRS	Narrow
ST segment	Generalized concave elevations, depression in lead aVR
T wave	Normal
QTc interval	0.358
Final diagnosis	Acute pericarditis

Example 32

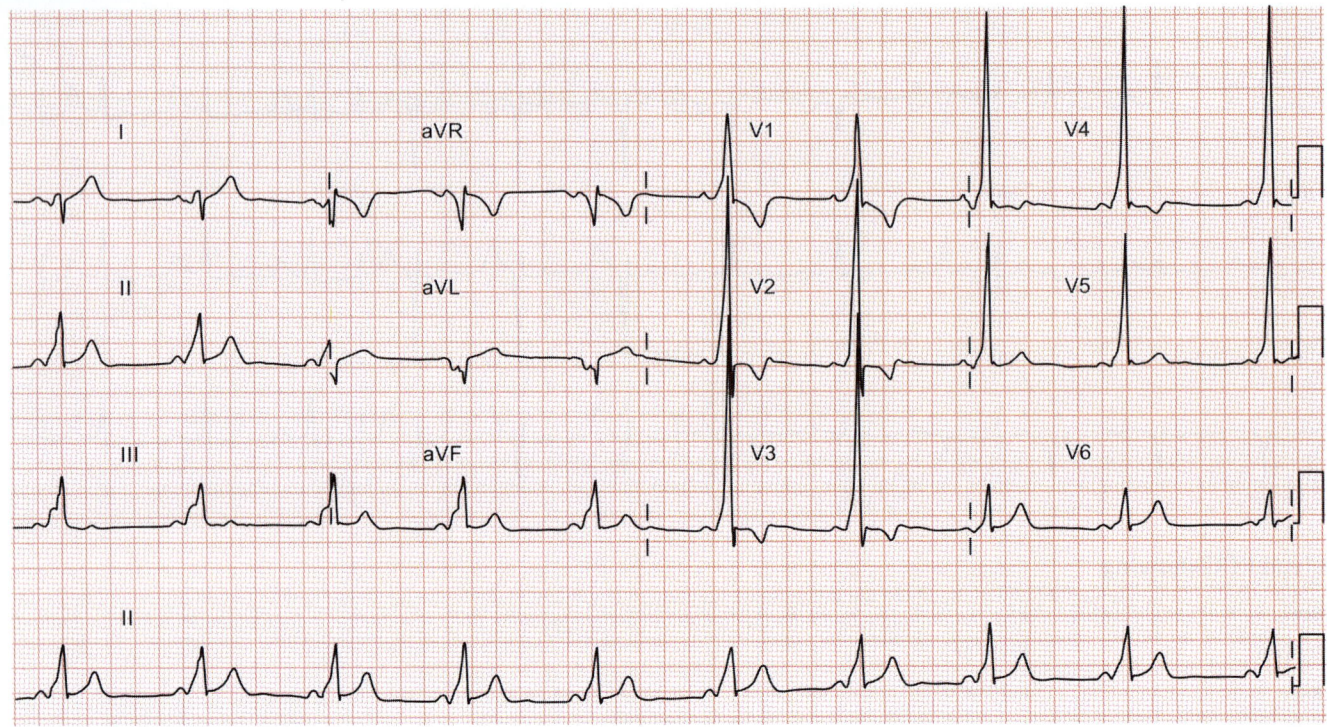

12-lead ECG showing

Rate	60
Rhythm	Regular
Axis	Normal/rightward
P wave	Normal
PR interval/segment	Short (<120 ms)
QRS	Wide (~ 160 ms), slurring of upstroke ('Delta' wave), dominant R wave in V1, apparent Q wave in lead aVL (this is actually a negative delta wave, which simulates a lateral wall MI, hence the name "pseudo-infarction" pattern)
ST segment	Normal
T wave	Inverted in V1–V3 (tall R with T wave inversions in septal leads mimics RVH, but these changes are due to repolarization abnormalities and not RVH)
QTc interval	0.440
Final diagnosis	WPW syndrome (type A)

Example 33

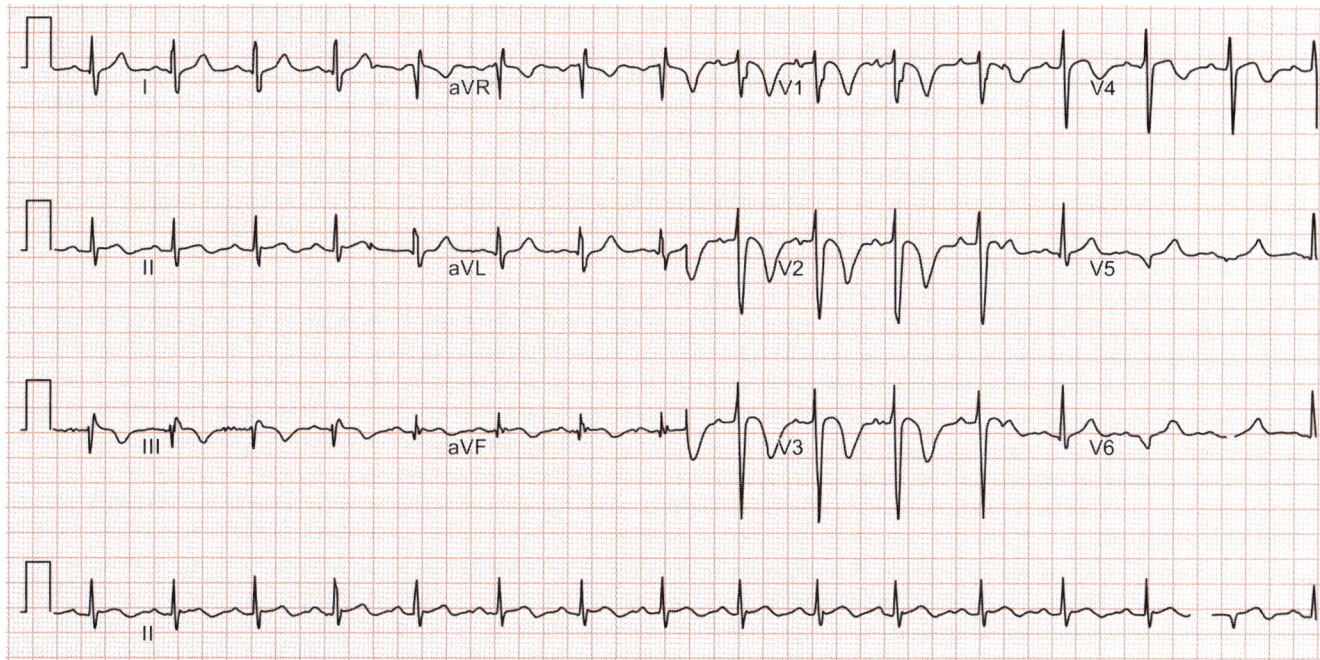

12-lead ECG showing

Rate	94
Rhythm	Regular
Axis	Normal
P wave	Normal
PR interval/segment	Normal
QRS	Narrow, S1Q3T3 pattern (McGinn-White sign)
ST segment	Nonspecific changes in lead III
T wave	Inversions in V1–V3, II, III, aVF (RV strain pattern)
QT interval	0.350
Final diagnosis	Features favor pulmonary embolism (note also the S1Q3T3 pattern)

Example 34

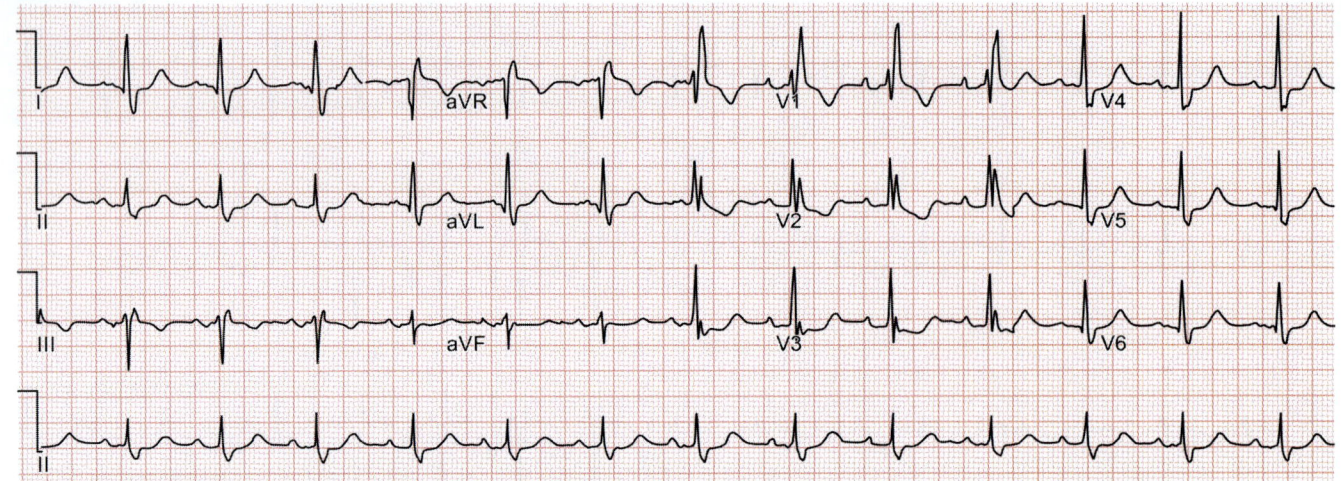

12-lead ECG showing

Rate	79
Rhythm	Regular
Axis	Normal
P wave	Normal
PR interval/segment	Normal
QRS	Wide, rSR' in V1–V2, deep wide slurred S in V5–V6 and I
ST segment	Normal
T wave	Inversions in V1–V2 (appropriate discordance)
QTc interval	0.413
Final diagnosis	Complete RBBB

Example 35

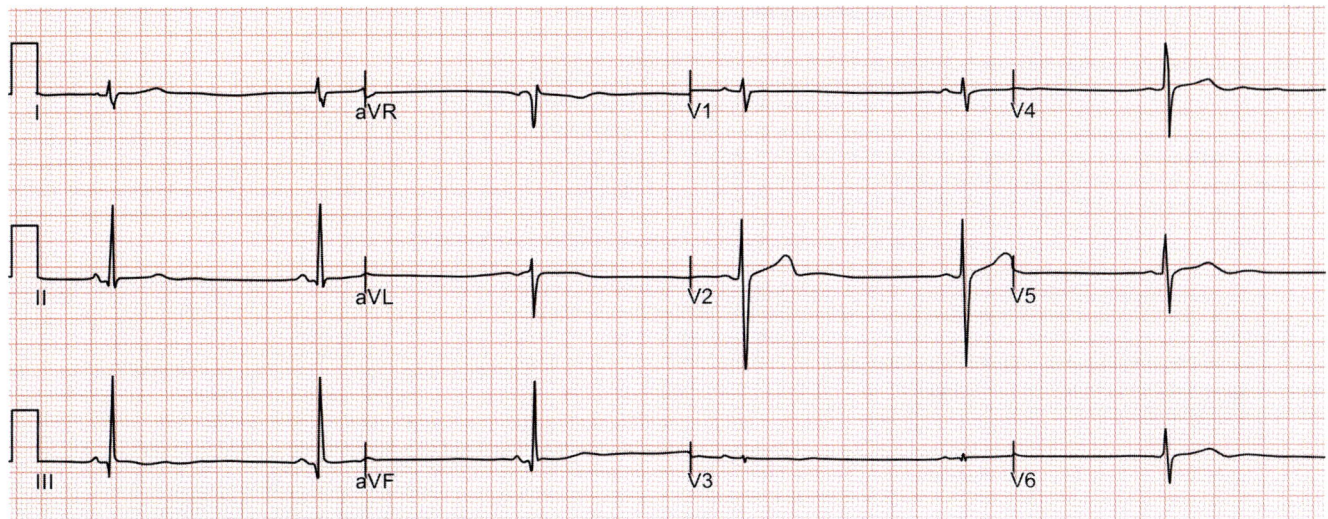

12-lead ECG showing

Rate	~37
Rhythm	Regular
Axis	Normal
P wave	Normal
PR interval/segment	Normal
QRS	Narrow
ST segment	Normal
T wave	Normal
QTc interval	0.346
Final diagnosis	**Sinus bradycardia** Poor R wave progression—possibly normal variant

BASIC INTERPRETATION OF ECG

Looks at the ECG Standardization (10 mm = 1 mV) and speed (25 mm/sec)	
Quickly scans the ECG for obvious abnormalities. Note the overall quality of the tracing (artifact, lead placement issues, etc.).	AVR—always negative Lead I—always positive R wave progression V1 → V6
Rate and rhythm<ul><li>**Heart rate:**<ul><li>Calculates the heart rate</li></ul></li><li>**Rhythm:**<ul><li>Assess for regularity or irregularity.</li><li>Identify the rhythm (e.g., sinus rhythm, atrial fibrillation, etc.).</li></ul></li></ul>	300/LS 1,500/SS For irregular rhythms—6 seconds of rhythm, count the number of beats present on the ECG multiply by 10
<ul><li>**QRS axis:**<ul><li>O Calculate the QRS axis (normal: −30° to +90°).</li></ul></li></ul> Lead I Lead III Q____ Q____ R____ R____ S____ S____ Net QRS I____ Net QRS III____  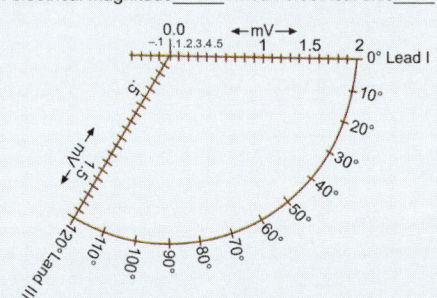	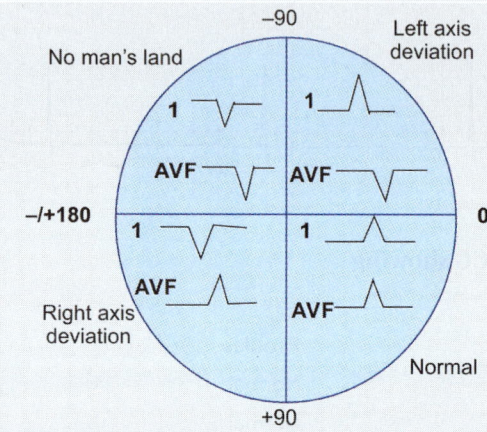
P wave<ul><li>**Presence and morphology:**<ul><li>Check if P waves are present before each QRS complex.</li><li>Evaluate the shape and size of P waves.</li><li>Ensure the P wave is upright in leads I and II.</li></ul></li></ul>	<ul><li>Always positive in lead I and II</li><li>Always negative in lead aVR</li><li><2.5 small squares in duration</li><li><2.5 small squares in amplitude</li><li>Commonly biphasic in lead V1</li><li>Best seen in leads II</li></ul>
PR interval<ul><li>**Duration:**<ul><li>Measure the PR interval (normal: 120–200 ms).</li><li>Check for consistency or variability.</li></ul></li></ul>	**Abnormalities:**<ul><li>Identify any signs of first-degree AV block, second-degree AV block (Mobitz I or II), or third-degree AV block.</li><li>Short PR interval may disease like Wolf-Parkinson-White</li></ul>
QRS complex<ul><li>**Duration:**<ul><li>Measure the width of the QRS complex (normal: ≤120 ms).</li></ul></li><li>**Morphology:**<ul><li>Look for bundle branch blocks (right or left), pathological Q waves, and other abnormalities.</li></ul></li></ul>	RVH: V1 R/S ratio >1 or V6 S/R ratio >1. LVH: S in V1 or V2 + R in V5 or V6 ≥35 mm.
ST segment<ul><li>**Elevation or depression:**<ul><li>Identify any ST segment elevation or depression (e.g., >1 mm in two contiguous leads).</li></ul></li></ul>	<ul><li>**Clinical significance:**<ul><li>Consider the differential diagnosis for ST segment changes (e.g., myocardial infarction, pericarditis, ischemia).</li></ul></li></ul>
T wave<ul><li>**Morphology and symmetry:**<ul><li>Assess T wave height and shape.</li><li>Look for T wave inversions, flattening, or hyperacute T waves.</li></ul></li></ul>	**Tall T waves**<ul><li>Hyperkalemia, hyperacute MI</li></ul>**Deep flipped T waves**<ul><li>CAD/ischemia, HOCM, SAH</li></ul>
QT interval<ul><li>**Duration:**<ul><li>Measure the QT interval and correct it for heart rate (QTc) using Bazett's formula (QTc = QT/√RR)</li></ul></li></ul>	**Prolongation:**<ul><li>Identify QT prolongation (e.g., QTc >450 ms in men, >460 ms in women) and consider hypocalcaemia and congenital long QT syndrome associated with an increased risk of Torsades de pointes</li></ul>

Additional findings:
- **U Waves:**
  - Look for the presence of U waves and assess their significance.
- **Overall ECG pattern:**
  - Evaluate for patterns suggestive of specific conditions.

Prominent U waves are most often seen in hypokalemia:

I Lateral	aVR None	V1 Septal	V4 Anterior
II Inferior	aVL Lateral	V2 Septal	V5 Lateral
III Inferior	aVF Inferior	V3 Anterior	V6 Lateral

Clinical correlation
- **Summary of findings:**
  - Summarize the key findings of the ECG.
- **Potential diagnoses:**
  - Discuss possible clinical diagnoses based on the ECG findings.
- **Next steps:**
  - Suggest appropriate clinical management or further investigations.

CHAPTER 12: A Systematic Approach to Chest X-rays

APPROACH TO CHEST X-RAYS

Reading into the Chest Radiograph

The 11 Step Approach

1. What type of view
2. Exposure/penetration
3. Inspiratory versus expiratory film
4. Rotation
5. Angulation
6. Soft tissues and bony structures
7. Trachea
8. Hilum/mediastinum
9. Diaphragm
10. Lung fields
11. Cardia

Type of View

Chest X-ray
1. PA view
2. AP view
3. Lateral view
   a. **PA view (posteroanterior view) (Fig. 12.1):** The ray of beam is from posteroanteriorly with the film in front of the patient.
   b. **AP view (anteroposterior view) (Fig. 12.2):** The ray of beam is from anteroposteriorly with the film behind the patient.
   c. **Lateral view (Fig. 12.3):** The ray of beam is from one side with the film placed on the opposite side of the patient.

Differences between PA view and AP view of chest X-ray

	PA view (Fig. 12.4)	AP view (Fig. 12.5)
Fundic gas shadow	Usually present	Absent
Clavicles	Seen over the lung fields and more horizontal	Seen above the apex of lung field and more oblique
Scapula	Inner borders are away from the lung fields	Inner borders are seen over the lung fields
Ribs	Posterior ribs are better seen and more oblique	Anterior ribs are better seen
Apparent cardiomegaly	Not seen	Seen
Spine	Better seen	Not seen
The distance between the projector and the patient	6 feet	40 inches

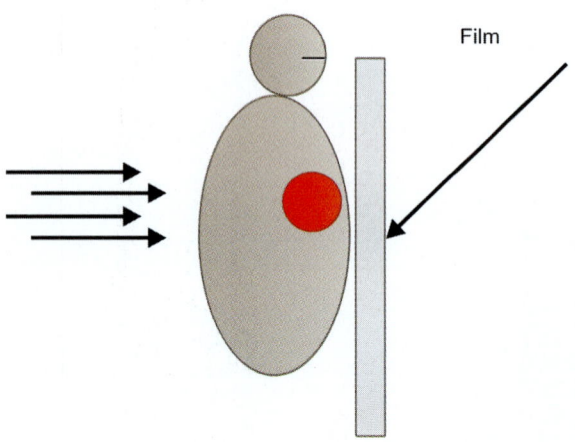

Fig. 12.1: Posteroanterior view.

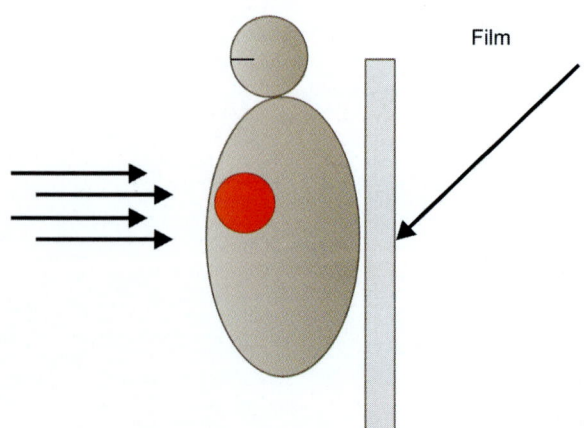

Fig. 12.2: Anteroposterior view.

A Systematic Approach to Chest X-rays

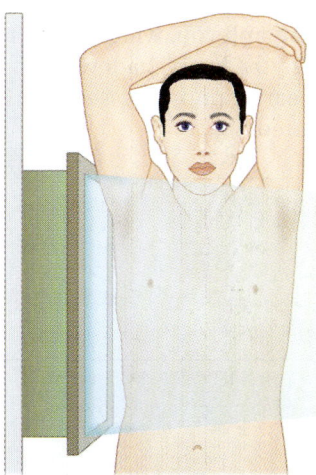

Fig. 12.3: Lateral view.

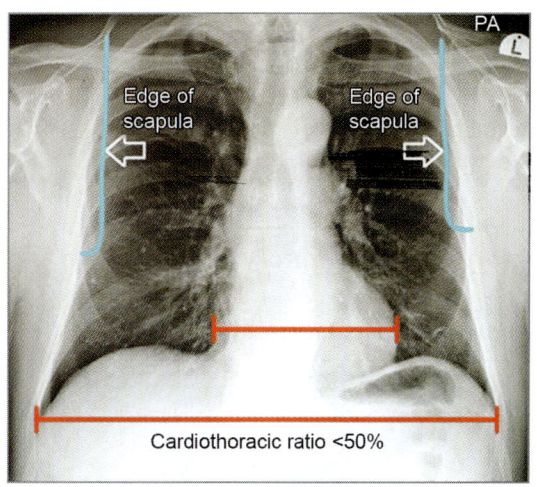

Fig. 12.4: Posteroanterior (PA) view.

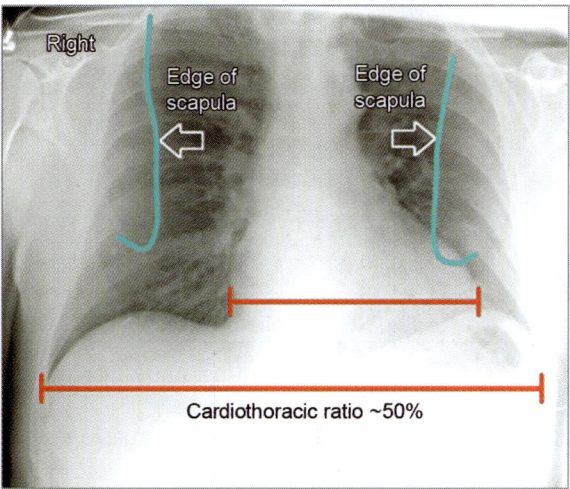

Fig. 12.5: Anteroposterior (AP) view.

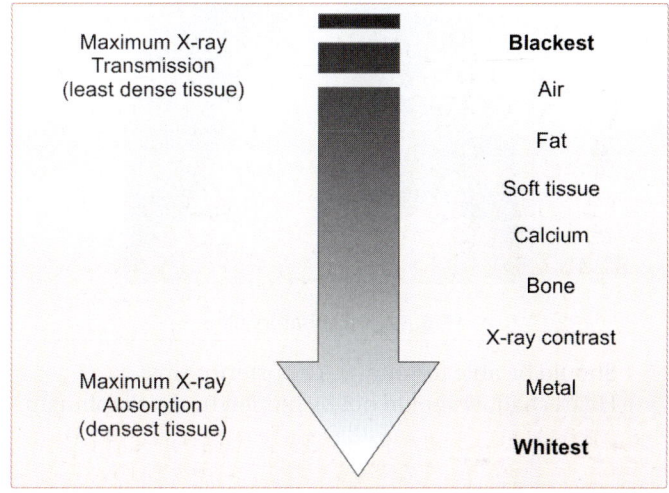

Fig. 12.6: Black and white areas in X-ray.

Exposure/Penetration

Penetration is the degree to which X-ray passes through the body. **Figure 12.6** depicts the grading of shadow in X-ray film.

Criteria of well-penetrated chest X-ray:
- A well-penetrated X-ray is one where the thoracic vertebrae are just visible through the heart shadow, but bony details of spine are not usually seen.

Overpenetrated radiograph (Fig. 12.7)

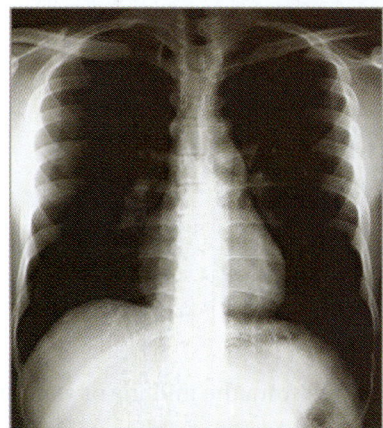

Fig. 12.7: Overpenetrated radiograph.

Underpenetrated radiograph (Fig. 12.8)

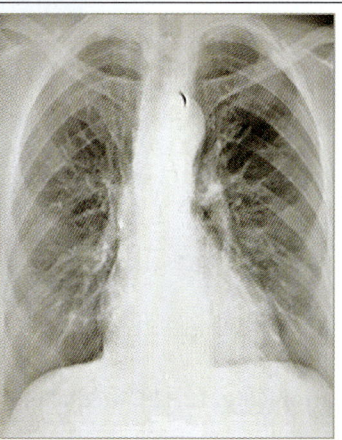

Fig. 12.8: Underpenetrated radiograph.

• In this radiograph, all thoracic vertebrae visible through the heart shadow. • Lung field darker than normal; may obscure subtle pathologies. • Inadequate lung detail.	• In underpenetrated radiograph you, will not able to see thoracic vertebrae through the heart shadow. • Lung tissue behind the heart cannot be assessed. • Hemidiaphragm is obscured.

Inspiratory versus Expiratory Film

Inspiratory film (Fig. 12.9)	Expiratory film (Fig. 12.10)
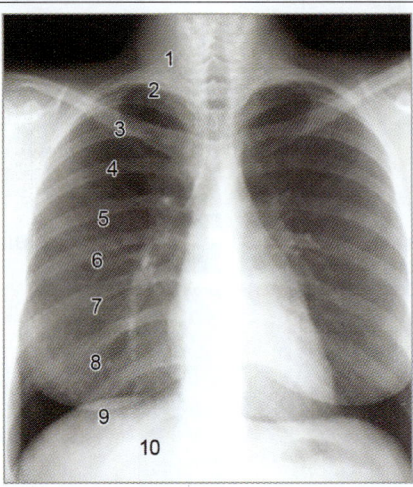 **Fig. 12.9:** Inspiratory film.	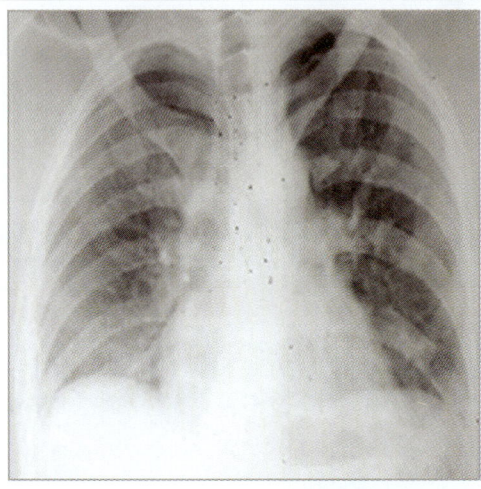 **Fig. 12.10:** Expiratory film.
• Should be able to count 9–10 posterior ribs. • Heart shadow should not be hidden by the diaphragm.	• Poor inspiration can crowd lung markings producing pseudo-airspace disease. • Expiration reduces lung volume, making a small pneumothorax easier to see.

Rotation

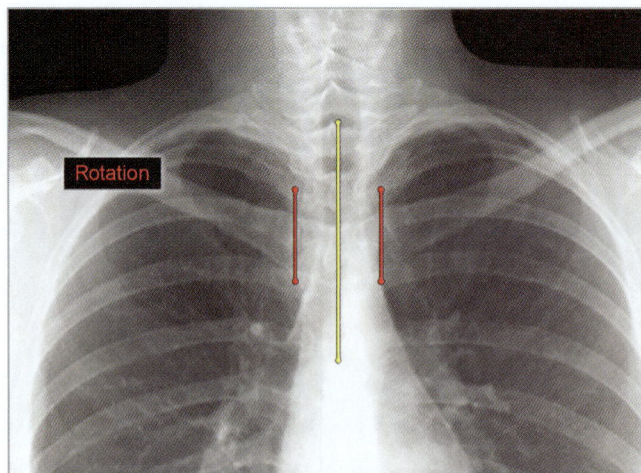

Fig. 12.11: Normal rotation.

- **Normal rotation (Fig. 12.11):** Medial ends of bilateral clavicles are equidistant from the midline or vertebral bodies.

A Systematic Approach to Chest X-rays

Left-rotated film (Fig. 12.12)

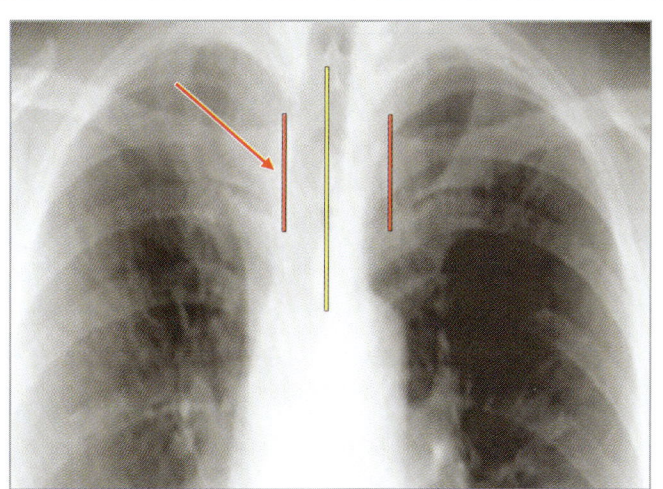

Fig. 12.12: Left-rotated film.

If spinous process appears closer to the right clavicle (red arrow), the patient is rotated toward their own left side.

Right-rotated film (Fig. 12.13)

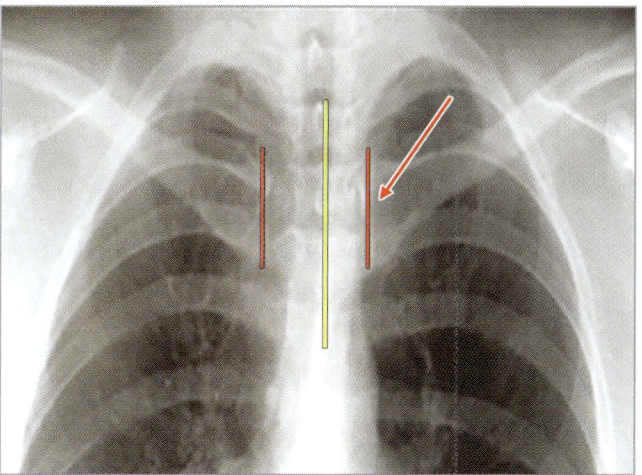

Fig. 12.13: Right-rotated film.

If spinous process appears closer to the left clavicle (red arrow), the patient is rotated toward their own right side.

Angulation

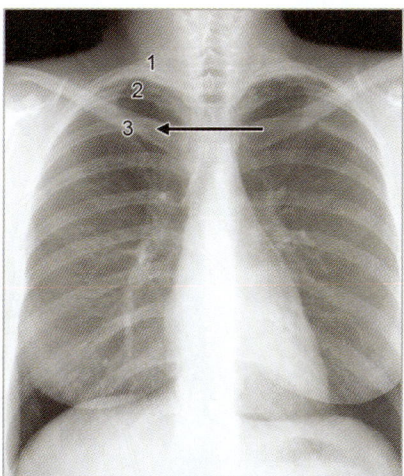

Fig. 12.14: Normal angulation.

Normal angulation (Fig. 12.14): Clavicle should lie over the 3rd rib (posterior end). With proper angulation the apex of lungs are clearly visualized.

Soft Tissues and Bony Structures

Soft Tissues (Fig. 12.15)

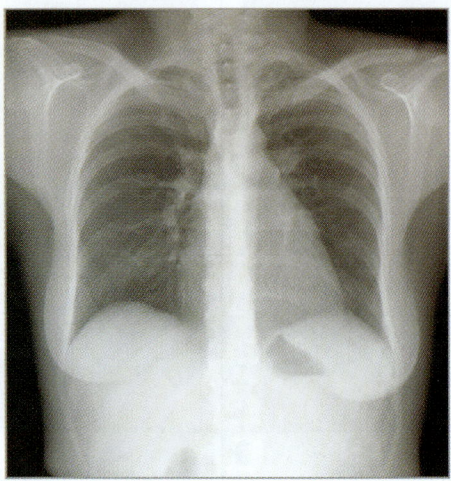

Fig. 12.15: Soft tissues.

Soft Tissues
- Breast shadows
- Supraclavicular areas
- Axillae
- Tissues along the side of breasts

Bony Structures (Fig. 12.16)

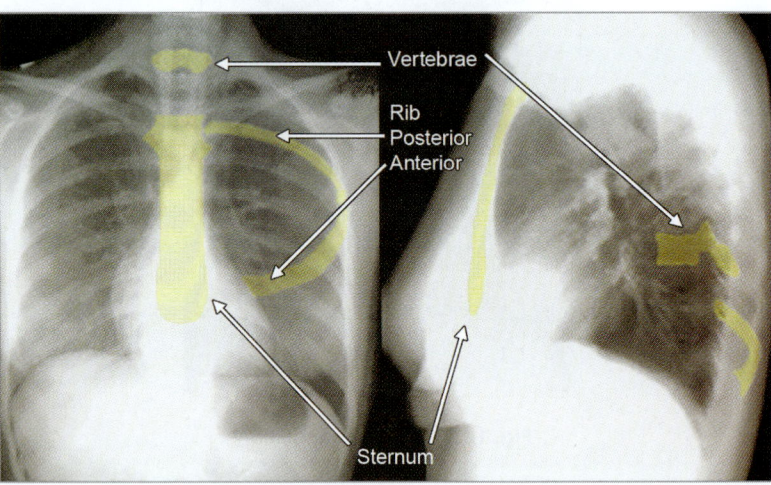

Fig. 12.16: Bony structures.

Bony Structures
- Ribs
- Sternum
- Spine
- Shoulder girdle including the proximal humeri
- Clavicles

Trachea (Figs. 12.17A and B)

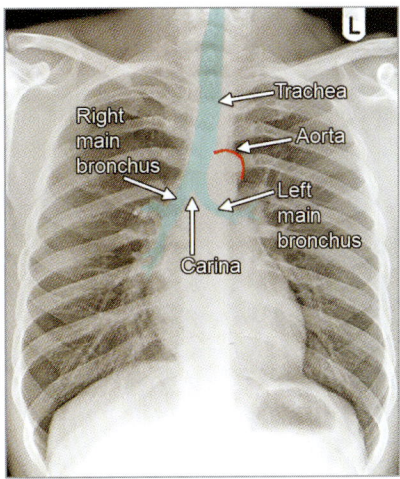

Fig. 12.17A: Trachea (PA view).

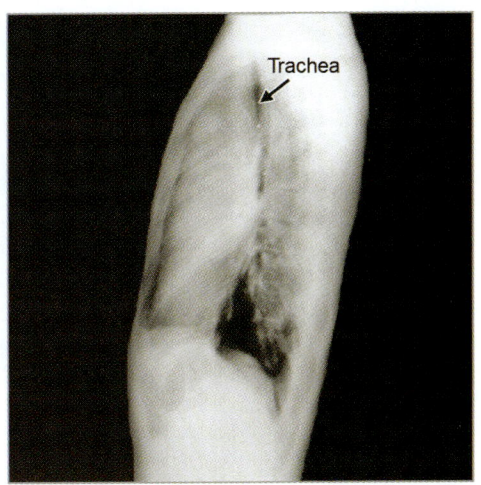

Fig. 12.17B: Trachea (lateral view).

Hilum/Mediastinum (Fig. 12.18)

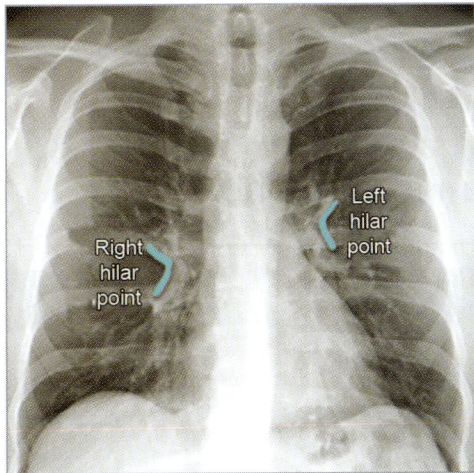

Fig. 12.18: Hilum.

Hilum is the wedge-shaped area on the central portion of each lung where the following structures leave the lung.
- Bronchi
- Pulmonary—arteries, veins and nerves.

Important point:
- Left hilar point is usually higher than right.

Diaphragm (Fig. 12.19)

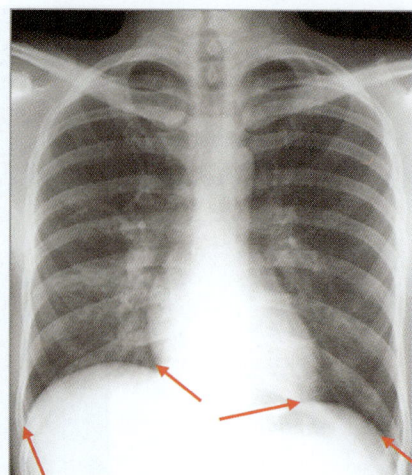

Fig. 12.19: Diaphragm.

Diaphragm
Dome-shaped
- Position:
  - Right hemidiaphragm is located at 9th–10th rib posteriorly or 6th rib anteriorly
  - Right hemidiaphragm is higher than the left by 2 cm because the cardia keeps the left hemidiaphragm down
- Costophrenic angles
- Cardiophrenic angles: Normally the costophrenic and cardiophrenic angles are clear, they are obliterated due to fluid, fat, or fibrosis
- Height—normally 2.5 cm

When do you say diaphragm is flattened (Figs. 12.20A and B)?

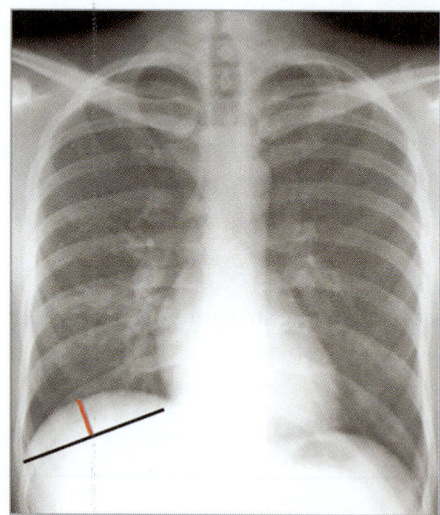

Fig. 12.20A: Normal height of diaphragm.

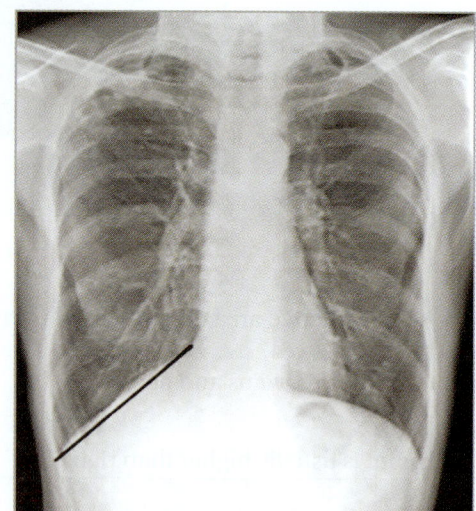

Fig. 12.20B: Flattening of diaphragm.

Draw a line from cardiophrenic angle to costophrenic angle. Now draw a perpendicular onto the line from the highest point of dome of diaphragm. Measure the height of the perpendicular (red line). If the height is <2.5 cm, it suggests flattened diaphragm.

Lung Fields

Lung fields and hilum
- Hilum:
  - Pulmonary arteries
  - Pulmonary veins
- Lungs: Linear and fine nodular shadows of pulmonary vessels
- Blood vessels
- About 40% obscured by other tissue

Segments of the lung	
Right lung	*Left lung*
Superior lobe: Apical, posterior, and anterior **Middle lobe:** Lateral and medial **Inferior lobe:** Superior (apical), medial basal, anterior basal, lateral basal, and posterior basal **Total: 10 segments on right.**	**Superior lobe:** Apicoposterior, anterior, superior lingular, and inferior lingular **Inferior lobe:** Superior (apical), anterior basal, lateral basal, and posterior basal **Total: 8 segments on left side.**

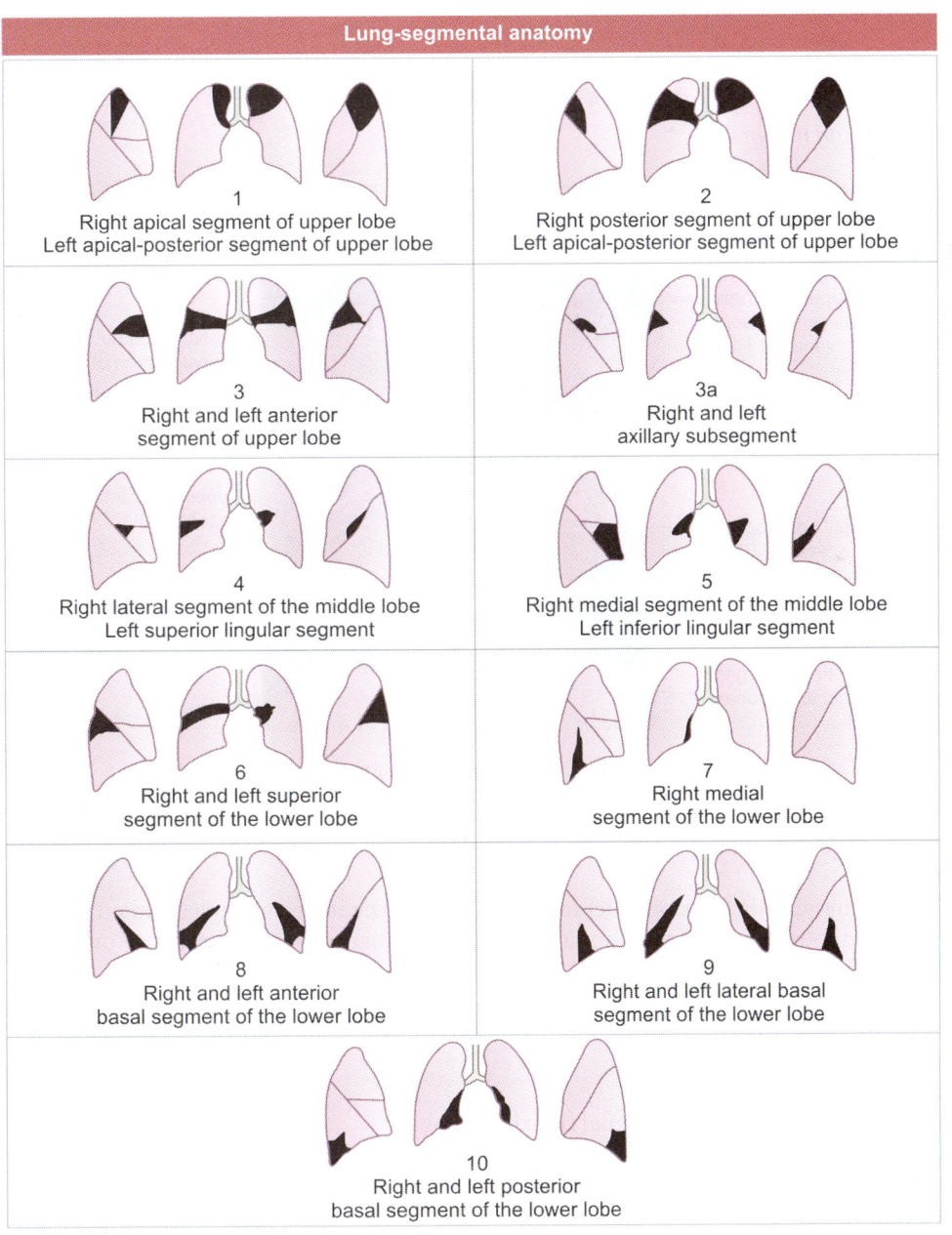

Lung-segmental anatomy

1. Right apical segment of upper lobe / Left apical-posterior segment of upper lobe
2. Right posterior segment of upper lobe / Left apical-posterior segment of upper lobe
3. Right and left anterior segment of upper lobe
3a. Right and left axillary subsegment
4. Right lateral segment of the middle lobe / Left superior lingular segment
5. Right medial segment of the middle lobe / Left inferior lingular segment
6. Right and left superior segment of the lower lobe
7. Right medial segment of the lower lobe
8. Right and left anterior basal segment of the lower lobe
9. Right and left lateral basal segment of the lower lobe
10. Right and left posterior basal segment of the lower lobe

Zones of Lung (Fig. 12.21)

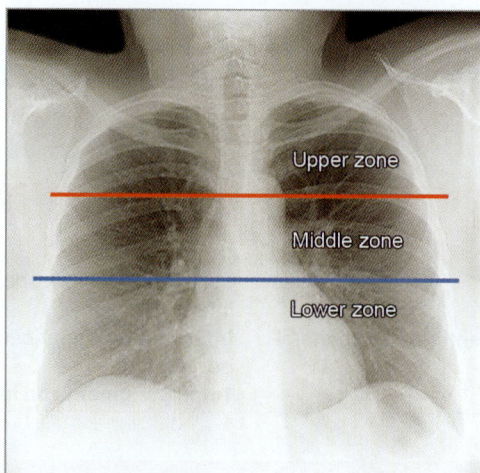

Fig. 12.21: Two lines are drawn one connecting the anteroinferior end of 2nd rib on both sides and 2nd connecting the anteroinferior ends of the 4th rib on both sides.

Note: Zones do not correspond to lobes.

Silhouette Sign (Fig. 12.22)

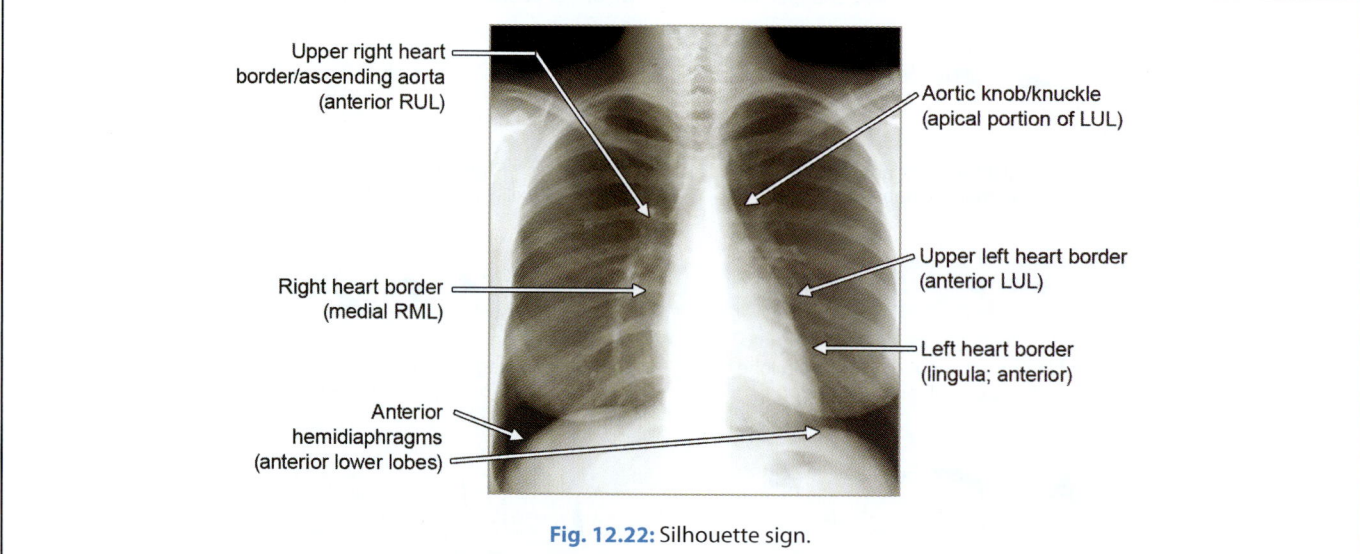

Fig. 12.22: Silhouette sign.

Silhouette sign: It actually denotes the loss of a silhouette; thus, it is sometimes also known as loss of silhouette sign or loss of outline sign.

Felson defined it as "An intrathoracic lesion touching a border of the heart, aorta, or diaphragm will obliterate that border on the roentgenogram. An intrathoracic lesion not anatomically contiguous with a border of one of these structures will not obliterate that border".

Loss of the anatomic border is described as a positive silhouette sign.

Recognition of this sign is useful in localizing areas of consolidation, atelectasis or mass within the lung, with the loss of these normal silhouettes on a PA chest X-ray.
- Right paratracheal stripe: Right upper lobe
- Right heart border: Right middle lobe or medial right lower lobe
- Right hemidiaphragm: Right lower lobe
- Aortic knuckle: Left upper lobe
- Left heart border: Lingular segments of the left upper lobe
- Left hemidiaphragm or descending aorta: Left lower lobe

Cardia (Fig. 12.23)

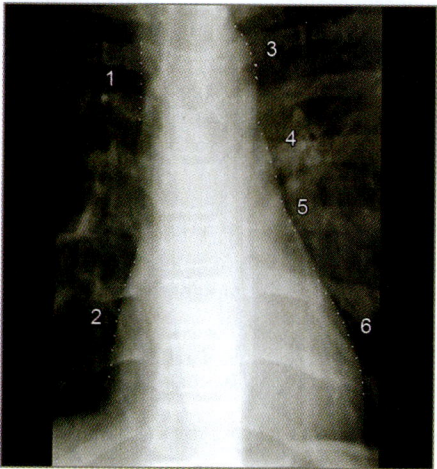

Fig. 12.23: Cardia: (1) Edge of superior vena cava; (2) Right atrium; (3) Aortic arch; (4) Edge of main pulmonary artery; (5) Left atrial appendage; (6) Left ventricle.

Cardiomegaly (Fig. 12.24)

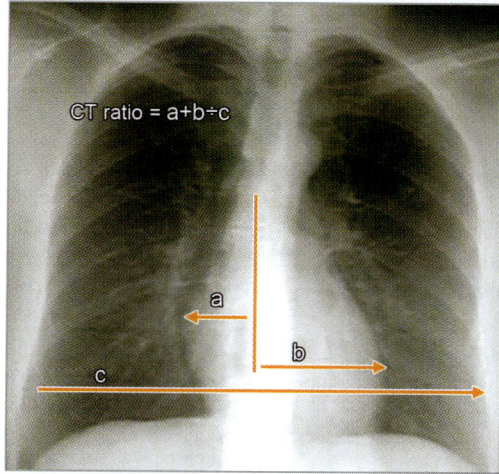

Fig. 12.24: Cardiomegaly.

The cardiothoracic ratio (CTR) is obtained by dividing the transverse cardiac diameter [sum of the horizontal distances from the right and left lateral-most margins of the heart to the midline (spinous processes of the vertebral bodies)] by the maximum internal thoracic diameter.

Cardiomegaly (Fig. 12.24):
- Adults: >0.50
- Neonates and elderly: >0.60

Chicken heart: Cardiothoracic ratio less than 25%. Small sized heart. The causes are:
- Bilateral emphysema
- Anorexia nervosa
- Addison's disease

Approach to Cardiomegaly

Cardiac silhouette		Contour of apex (left cardiophrenic angle)	
Clear	Not clear	Acute (RV contour)	Obtuse (LV contour)
Intrinsic cardiac disease (valvular/muscle)	Extrinsic problem (pericardial effusion)	▪ Mitral stenosis ▪ Atrial septal defect ▪ Chronic obstructive pulmonary disease	▪ Mitral regurgitation ▪ Aortic stenosis ▪ Aortic regurgitation ▪ Hypertension ▪ Cardiomyopathy

Differential diagnosis for gross cardiomegaly (wall-to-wall heart)
1. Pericardial effusion
2. Multivalvular heart disease
3. Severe aortic regurgitation (cor bovinum)
4. Ebstein's anomaly
5. Dilated cardiomyopathy

Chamber/vessel enlargement	Condition seen
Left atrial enlargement	▪ Enlarged left atrial appendage causes filling up of normal concavity between pulmonary artery shadow and the left ventricle. ▪ **Double atrial shadow:** Border of enlarged left atrium together with right atrial border gives an appearance like atrium within an atrium. ▪ **Straightening of left heart border:** Mitralization of heart. ▪ Pushing of left main bronchus upwards causing wide carinal angle (**splaying of carina**). ▪ Pushing esophagus backwards visible in lateral view of chest X-ray. ▪ Left shift of aorta (**Bedford sign**). ▪ **Walking man** sign in lateral X-ray.

Contd...

Pulmonary venous/capillary hypertension	- **Grade 1:** Cephalization (prominence of veins of upper lobe of lung) of pulmonary vasculature (pulmonary venous pressure ≤20 mm Hg) (reverse moustache sign or Stag's antler sign).
	- **Grade 2:** Kerley's lines (A, B, C) (pulmonary venous pressure 20–25 mm Hg), peribronchial, perivascular cuffing.
	  - **Kerley A line:** Linear opacities extending from the periphery to hilum; they are caused by distension of anastomotic channels between periphery and central lymphatics.
	  - **Kerley B line:** Short horizontal lines situated perpendicularly to the pleural surface at the lung base; they represent edema of interlobar septa.
	  - **Kerley C line:** Reticular opacities at lung base, representing Kerley's B line.
	- **Grade 3:** Batwing opacities (pulmonary venous pressure >25 mm Hg).

Pulmonary arterial hypertension	Prominent pulmonary outflow tract: Enlarged pulmonary arteries (diameter of right descending pulmonary artery >14 mm in women and >16 mm in men) + pruning of peripheral pulmonary vessels.
Right ventricle	- Apex forms an acute angle with diaphragm - **Right ventricular hypertrophy:** In presence of cardiomegaly, acute angle is observed between apex of enlarged heart and diaphragm. - **Sternal contact sign:** Earliest and most sensitive sign in the lateral X-ray is obliteration of Holtz neck's space, i.e., retrosternal space.
Right atrial enlargement	- Right border >5.5 cm from midline or 3.5 cm from sternal border. - 2½ intercostal space in its vertical extent. - >50% vertical height compared with mediastinal height.
Left ventricular enlargement	Left ventricular enlargement results in cardiomegaly with obtuse left cardiophrenic angle.

Differential Diagnosis of Consolidation

Based on the chronicity	
Acute	Chronic
- Pneumonia - Aspiration - Edema	- Organizing pneumonia - Malignancy - Alveolar proteinosis - Sarcoidosis - Eosinophilic pneumonia

Based on the content		
Water filled	Pus filled	Blood filled
- Heart failure - ARDS - Renal failure	Pneumonia	- Trauma - Vasculitis (Goodpasture disease, HSP, SLE)

Based on the pattern of involvement	
Diffuse disease	- Pulmonary edema - ARDS - Bronchopneumonia - Diffuse alveolar hemorrhage malignancy - Organizing pneumonia - Hypersensitive pneumonitis
Lobar disease	- Lobar pneumonia - Infarction - Contusion/hemorrhage - Lymphomas
Multiple ill defined	- Bronchopneumonia - Septic emboli - Metastasis - Lymphomas - Wegener's granulomatosis
Bat wing appearance	- Pulmonary edema - *Pneumocystis carinii* pneumonia
Reverse bat wing appearance	- Bronchoalveolar carcinoma - Radiation induced - BOOP - Eosinophilic pneumonia

Differential Diagnosis of Atelectasis

Resorption atelectasis	Relaxation atelectasis
- Mucus plug - Tumor block - Foreign body obstruction	- Pleural effusion - Pneumothorax

Differential Diagnosis of Nodule—Mass

Solitary		Multiple
Nodule <3 cm	Mass >3 cm	
Granulomas	Lung carcinoma	Infections (TB/septic emboli/histoplasmosis)
Lung carcinoma	Metastatic lesions	Metastasis
Metastatic lesions	Hamartomas	Sarcoidosis
Hamartomas		Wegener's granulomatosis
		Rheumatoid nodules

Differential Diagnosis of Interstitial Disease

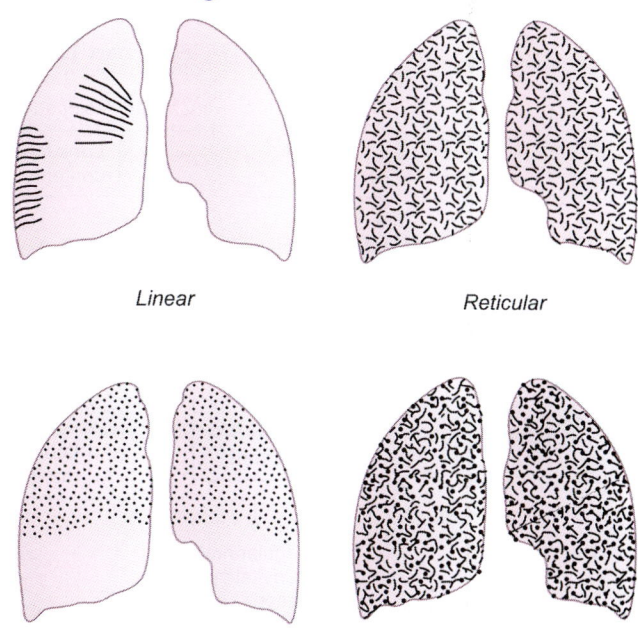

Linear *Reticular*

Nodular *Reticulonodular*

Based on the Pattern

Reticular			Nodular		
Smooth septal	Irregular septal	Honeycombing	Perilymphatic	Centrilobular	Random
- Pulmonary edema - Lymphangitis - Carcinomatosis	- Fibrosis - Lymphangitis - Carcinomatosis	- UIP - Hypersensitive Pneumonitis - Sarcoidosis	- Sarcoidosis - Silicosis - Pneumoconiosis - Lymphangitis Carcinomatosis	- Endobronchial - Infection - Pulmonary edema - Tuberculosis and *Mycobacterium avium* complex (MAC) infections	- Miliary TB - Metastases - Fungal infection

Based on the Attenuation

Low attenuation		High attenuation (ground glass appearance)	
Emphysema	Cystic disease	Acute	Chronic
- Centrilobular - Paraseptal - Panlobular	- Langerhans cell histiocytosis - Pneumatoceles - Lymphangioleiomyomatosis (LAM) - Lymphocytic interstitial pneumonia (LIP)	- Pulmonary edema - Pulmonary hemorrhage - Pneumocystis pneumonia	- Fibrosis - Alveolar proteinosis

Differential Diagnosis of Pleural Opacities

Solitary	Multiple
- Loculated pleural effusion - Loculated empyema - Malignancy	- Pleural plaques (asbestosis) - Loculated pockets of effusions - Sarcoidosis - Silicosis - Metastasis

Differential Diagnosis of Cavitary Lesions (Flowchart 12.1)

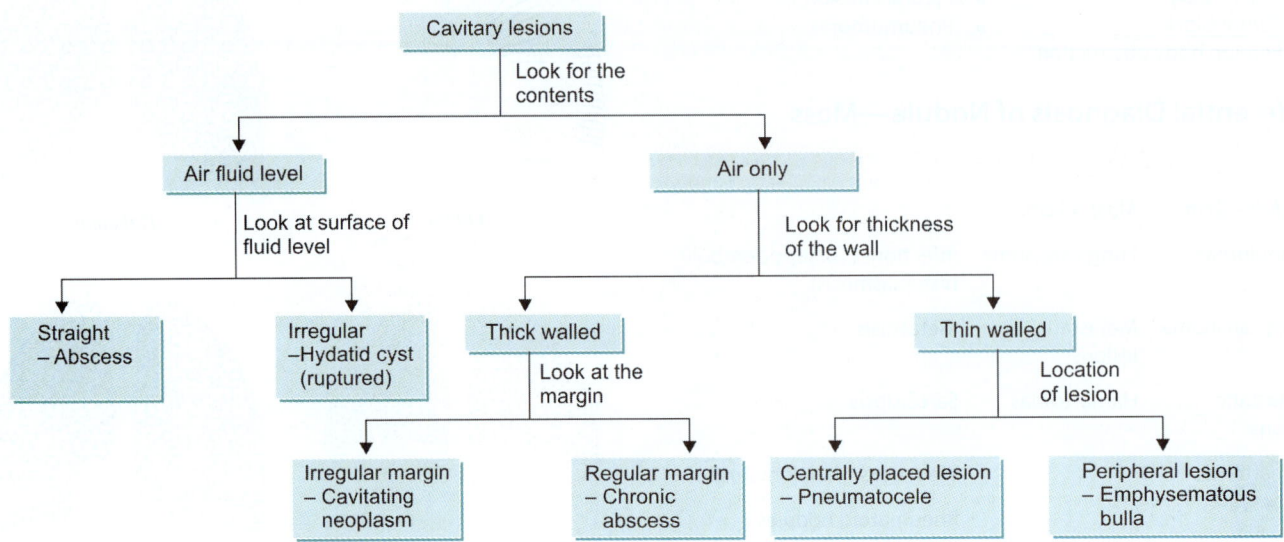

Flowchart 12.1: Diagnosis of cavity lesions.

Differential Diagnosis of Mediastinal Masses (Fig. 12.25)

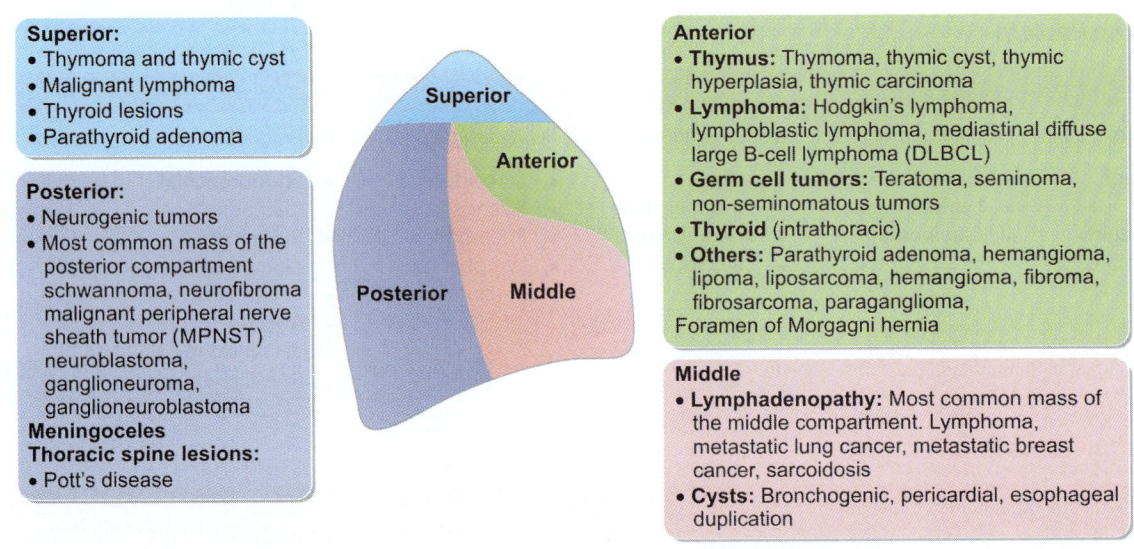

Fig. 12.25: Differential diagnosis of mediastinal masses.

Differential Diagnosis of Hilar Mass

Unilateral	Bilateral
Infections	Sarcoidosis
Tumors	Silicosis
Vascular aneurysm	Lymphomas
	Pulmonary artery hypertension

Hidden Areas of Lung (Fig. 12.26)

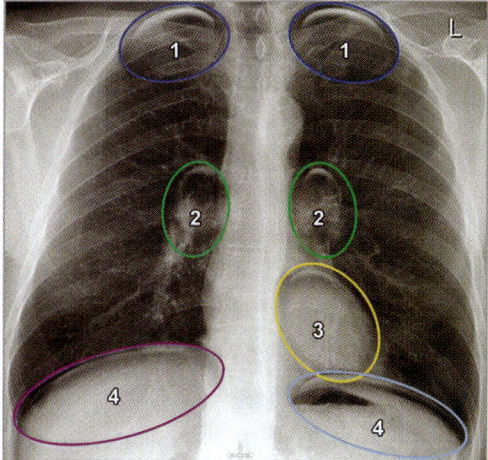

1. Apical zones
2. Hilar zones
3. Retrocardial zone
4. Zone below the dome of diaphragm

Fig. 12.26: Hidden areas of lung.

DISCUSSION ON COMMON X-RAYS (FIGS. 12.27 TO 12.62)

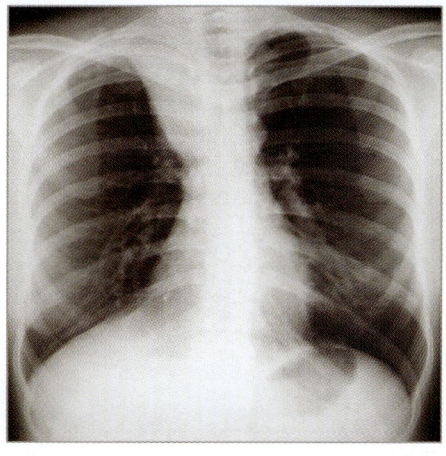

Fig. 12.27: Chest X-ray PA view showing trachea central, cardiophrenic and costophrenic angles are normal, homogeneous opacity in right upper zone with upward shift of horizontal fissure suggestive of **right upper lobe collapse.**

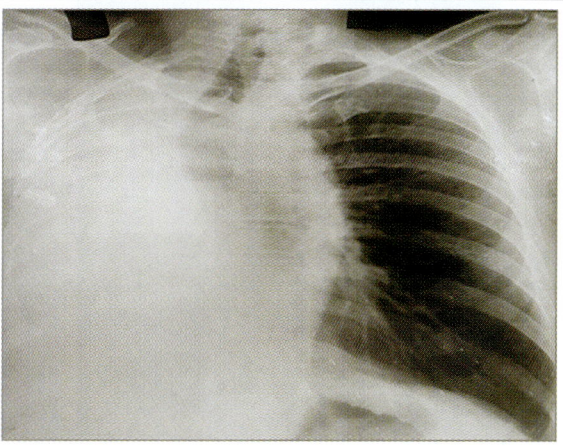

Fig. 12.28: Chest X-ray PA view showing homogeneous opacity on the right hemithorax with trachea shifted to same side suggestive of **right-sided collapse/pneumonectomy**.

Causes of hemithorax white homogeneous opacity/white-out lung:
a. With no mediastinal shift
   1. Consolidation
   2. Mesothelioma
   3. Fibrothorax
b. With mediastinal shift to opposite side
   1. Pleural effusion (moderate to large)
   2. Diaphragmatic hernia
c. With mediastinal shift to same side
   1. Collapse
   2. Postpneumonectomy

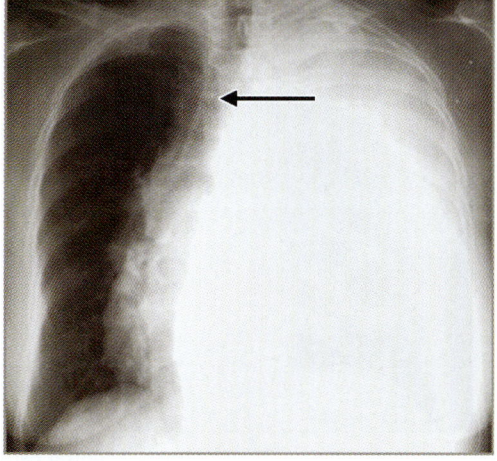

Fig. 12.29: Chest X-ray PA view showing homogeneous opacity on the left hemithorax with trachea shifted to opposite side suggestive of **left-sided massive pleural effusion (arrow)**.

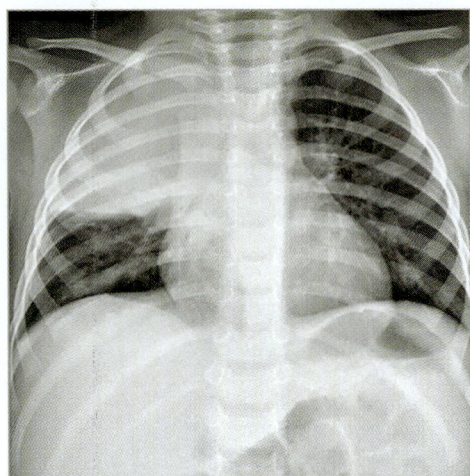

Fig. 12.30: Chest X-ray PA view showing trachea central, cardiophrenic and costophrenic angles are normal, homogeneous opacity in right upper zone with air bronchogram suggestive of **right upper lobe pneumonia**.

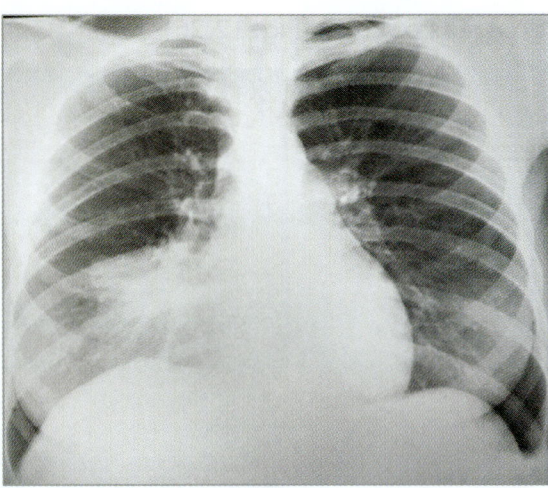

Fig. 12.31: Chest X-ray PA view showing trachea central, cardiophrenic and costophrenic angles are normal, homogeneous opacity in right mid and lower zone with air bronchogram, right heart border is not clear (silhouette sign) suggestive of **right middle lobe pneumonia**.

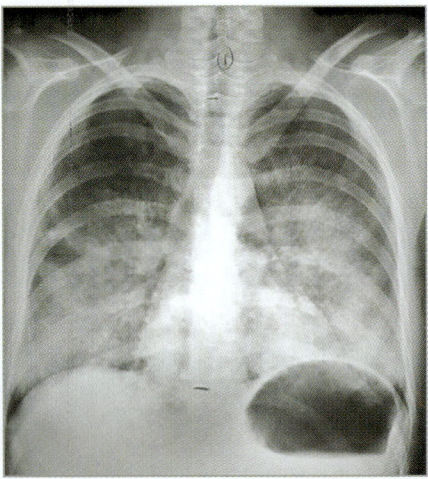

Fig. 12.32: Chest X-ray PA view showing trachea central, cardiophrenic and costophrenic angles are normal, non-homogeneous opacity in bilateral mid and lower zones with air bronchogram suggestive of **bilateral/atypical pneumonia**.

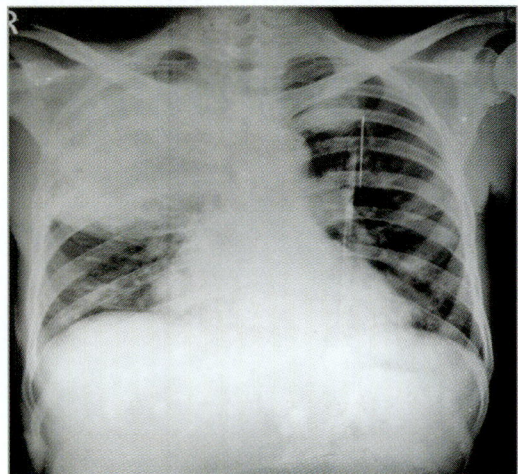

Fig. 12.33: Chest X-ray PA view showing trachea central, cardiophrenic and costophrenic angles are normal, non-homogeneous opacity in right upper zone with air bronchogram and bulging horizontal fissure suggestive of **right upper lobe pneumonia** due to *Klebsiella*.

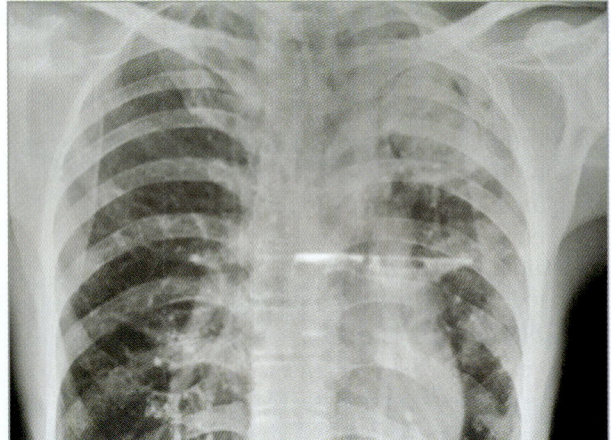

Fig. 12.34: Chest X-ray PA view showing trachea central, cardiophrenic and costophrenic angles are normal, nonhomogeneous opacity in left upper zone with cavity with air crescent sign suggestive of **aspergilloma—crescent sign of Monad**.

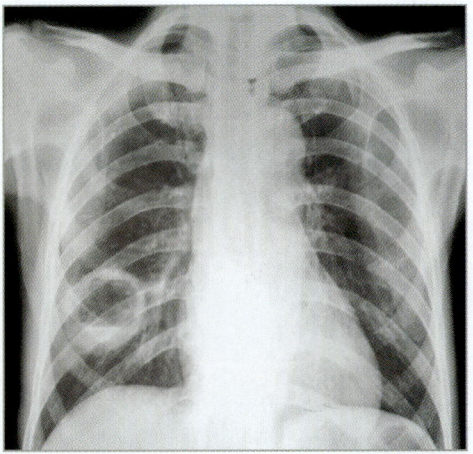

Fig. 12.35: Chest X-ray PA view showing trachea central, cardiophrenic and costophrenic angles are normal, thick-walled cavity with air fluid level in the right lower zone suggestive of **lung abscess**.

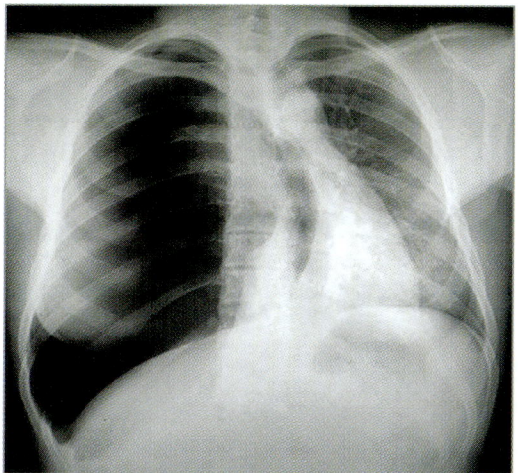

Fig. 12.36: Chest X-ray PA view showing trachea and mediastinum deviated to left, cardiophrenic and costophrenic angles are normal, homogenous hyperlucency in right hemithorax suggestive of **right-sided pneumothorax**.

Causes of unilateral hypertranslucency
- **Technical**
    - Patient rotation
    - Incorrect centering of X-ray beam to grid
- **Chest wall abnormality**
    - Asymmetric soft tissues
    - **Mastectomy**
    - Absent or underdeveloped pectoral muscles (**Poland syndrome**)
- **Skeletal abnormality:** Scoliosis
- **Airway disease**
    - Large pneumothorax
    - Asymmetric emphysema
    - Bronchial obstruction
    - Previous bronchiolitis obliterans (**Swyer–James syndrome = MacLeod's syndrome**)
- **Vascular disease**
    - Pulmonary embolism

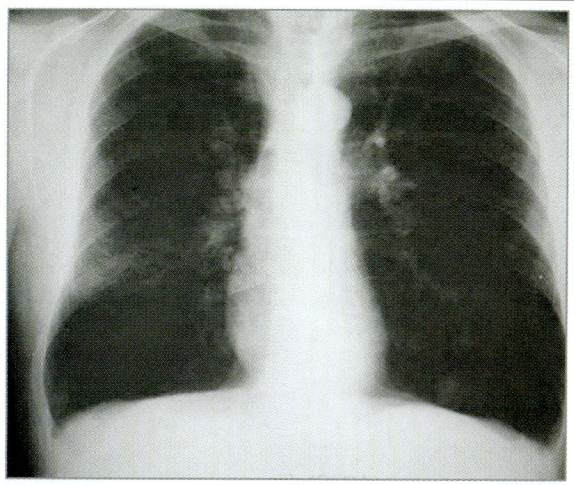

Fig. 12.37: Chest X-ray PA view showing trachea central, cardiophrenic and costophrenic angles are normal, bilateral hyperlucent lung fields with hyperinflation, flattened diaphragm and tubular heart suggestive of **bilateral emphysema**.

Causes of bilateral hyperlucent lung fields
- **Pulmonary emphysema**
- **Pulmonary overinflation**
- **Bilateral pneumothorax**
- Over exposure
- Bilateral congenital lobar emphysema
- Chronic bronchitis
- Cystic fibrosis
- Bronchiectasis
- Asthma

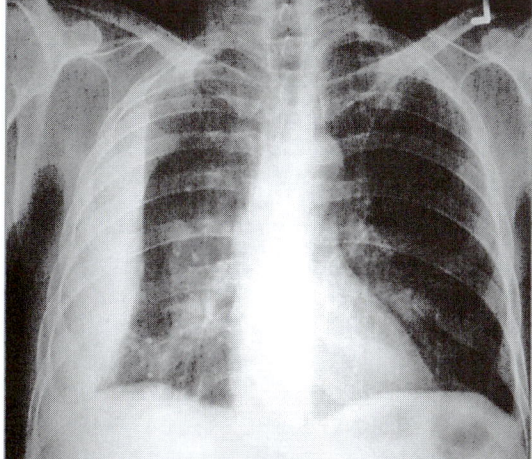

Fig. 12.38: Chest X-ray PA view showing homogeneous opacity in the right hemithorax obliterating the costophrenic angle, pleural based suggestive of **loculated pleural effusion**.

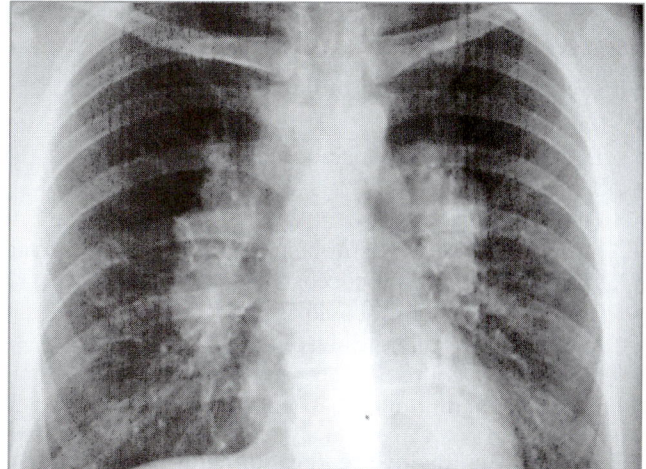

Fig. 12.39: Chest X-ray PA view showing bilateral hilar shadows, lobulated (also subcarinal shadow) suggestive of **lymphadenopathy**. Possible sarcoidosis.

Differential diagnosis—pleural mass/mesothelioma

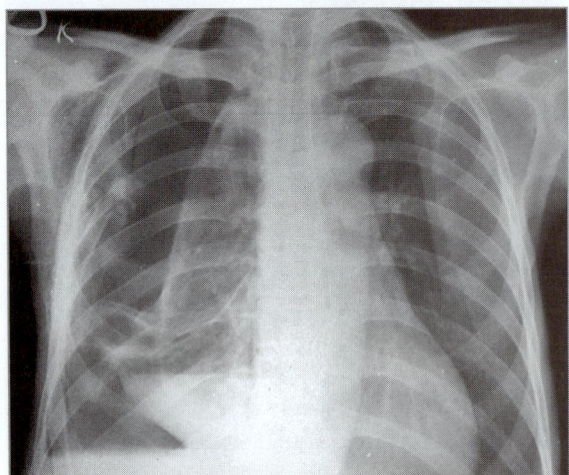

Fig. 12.40: Chest X-ray PA view showing tracheal shift to left, hyperlucency in right hemithorax with collapse lung margin (visceral pleural line) with obliteration of costophrenic angle with multiple air fluid levels suggestive of **hydropneumothorax**.

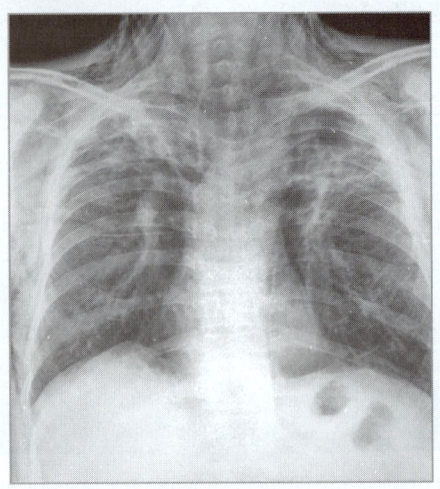

Fig. 12.41: Chest X-ray PA view showing air shadows in the subcutaneous plane in the neck, axilla, anterior chest wall, muscles suggestive of **subcutaneous emphysema**.

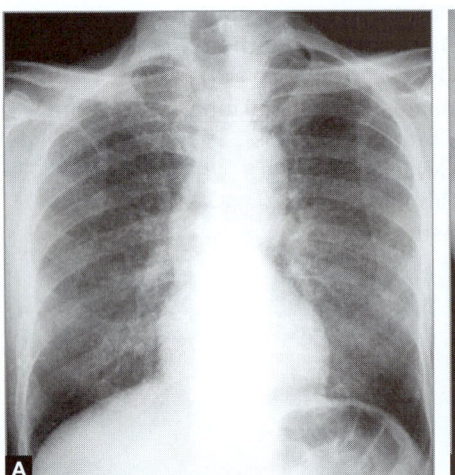
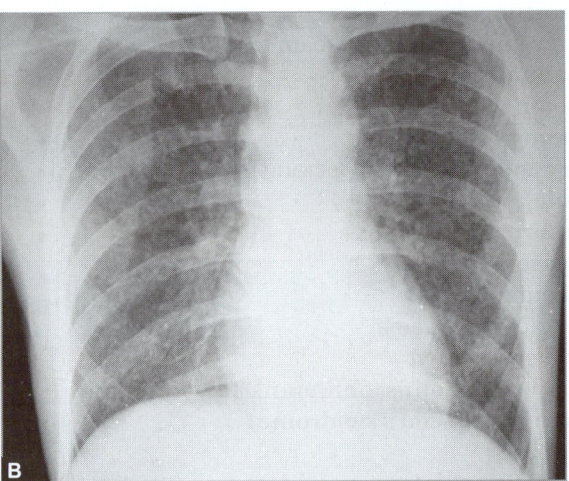

Figs. 12.42A and B: Chest X-ray PA view showing small millet sized (1–3 mm) shadows in bilateral lung fields suggestive of **miliary mottling**.

Differential diagnosis for miliary mottling:
- Miliary tuberculosis
- Tropical pulmonary eosinophilia
- Sarcoidosis
- Pneumocystis
- Fungal diseases: Histoplasmosis, coccidioidomycosis, blastomycosis, cryptococcosis
- Coal miner's pneumoconiosis
- Acute extrinsic allergic alveolitis
- Fibrosing alveolitis
- Varicella pneumonia

Those opacities having greater-than-soft-tissue density:
- Pulmonary hemosiderosis
- Silicosis

Opacities (2–5 mm) tending to remain discrete:
- Miliary/lymphangitis carcinomatosis
- Lymphoma
- Sarcoidosis

Opacities (2–5 mm) tending to coalesce:
- Multifocal pneumonia
- Pulmonary edema
- Extrinsic allergic alveolitis
- Fat emboli

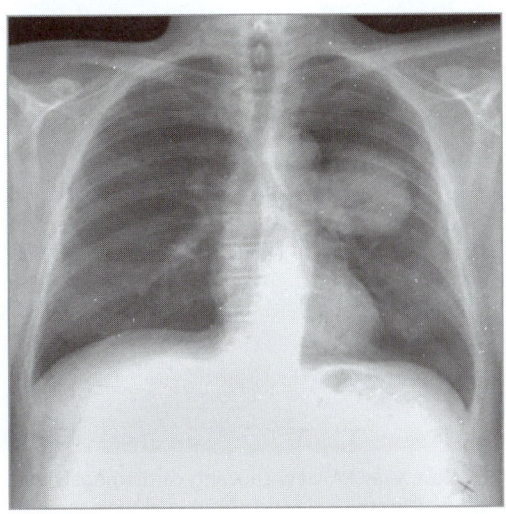

Fig. 12.43: Chest X-ray PA view showing rounded homogeneous lesion in the left mid-zone—**solitary pulmonary nodule.**

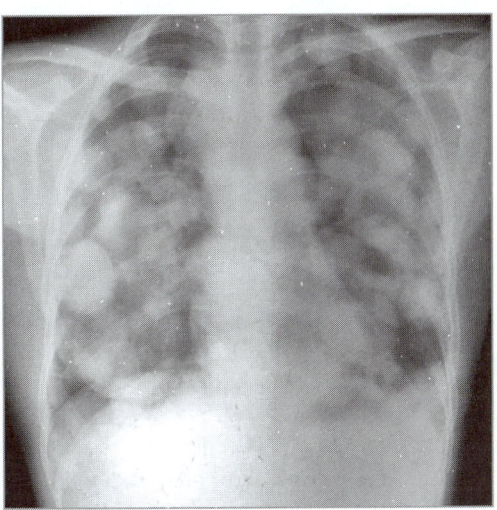

Fig. 12.44: Chest X-ray PA view showing multiple rounded nodular opacities in bilateral lung fields—**cannonball metastasis.**

Possible primary: Breast, thyroid, bowel, testes, renal cell carcinoma (RCC), choriocarcinoma.

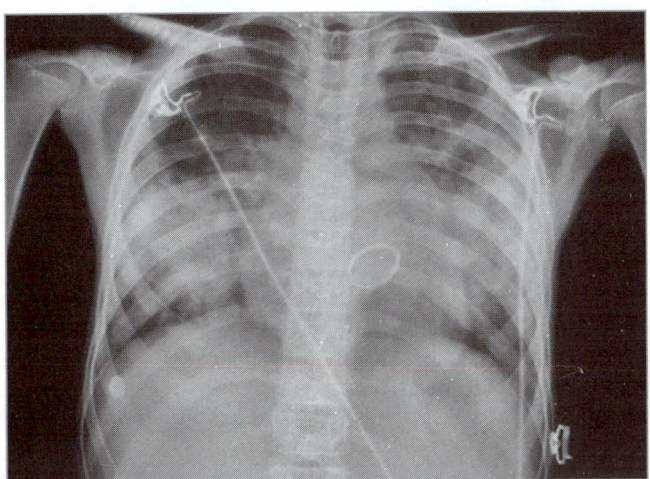

Fig. 12.45: Chest X-ray PA view showing cardiomegaly with bilateral nonhomogeneous opacity in mid and lower zones (bat wing appearance) suggestive of **pulmonary edema.** Also patient has **metallic mitral valve prosthesis.**

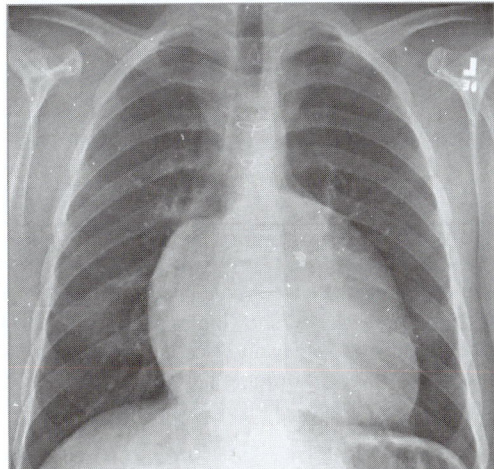

Fig. 12.46: Chest X-ray PA view showing gross cardiomegaly with stenciled heart borders, lungs clear. Suggestive of **pericardial effusion.**

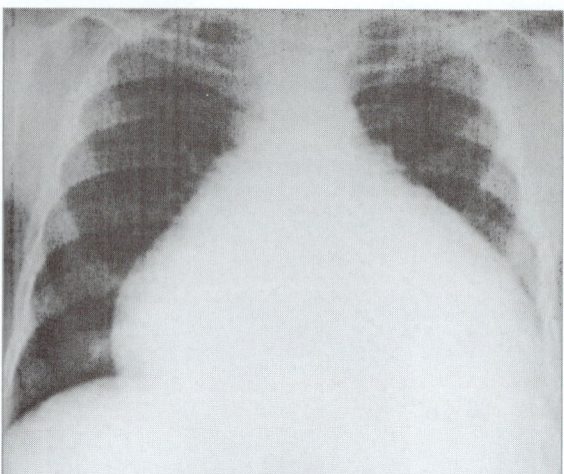

Fig. 12.47: Chest X-ray PA view showing gross cardiomegaly with stenciled heart borders, lungs clear. Suggestive of **pericardial effusion.** Differential diagnosis—Ebstein's anomaly.

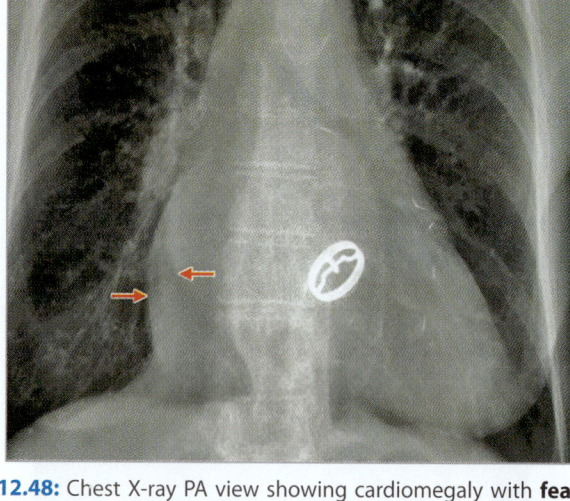

Fig. 12.48: Chest X-ray PA view showing cardiomegaly with **features of mitral valve disease**—splaying of carina, double atrial shadow (red arrows), straightening of left heart border, mitral valve metallic prosthesis.

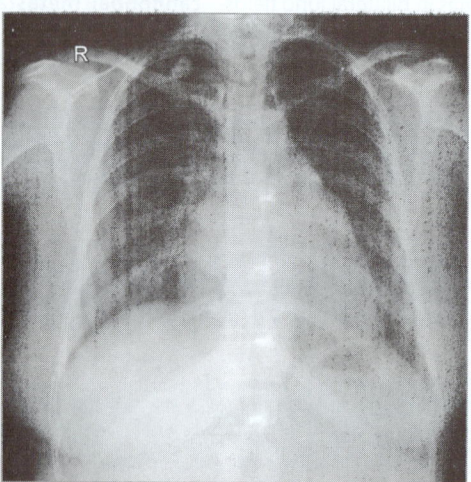

Fig. 12.49: Chest X-ray PA view showing cardiomegaly with **features of mitral valve disease**—splaying of carina, double atrial shadow, straightening of left heart border, enlarged left atrial appendage, prominent pulmonary artery.

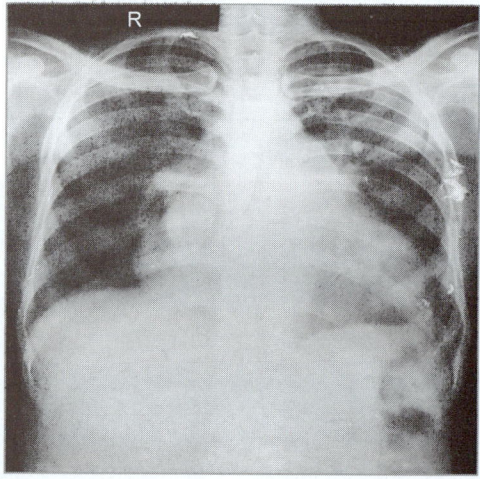

Fig. 12.50: Chest X-ray PA view showing cardiomegaly with **features of mitral valve disease**—splaying of carina, double atrial shadow, straightening of left heart border, mitral valve metallic prosthesis, enlarged left atrial appendage, prominent pulmonary artery, prominent upper lobe veins (stag's antler sign).

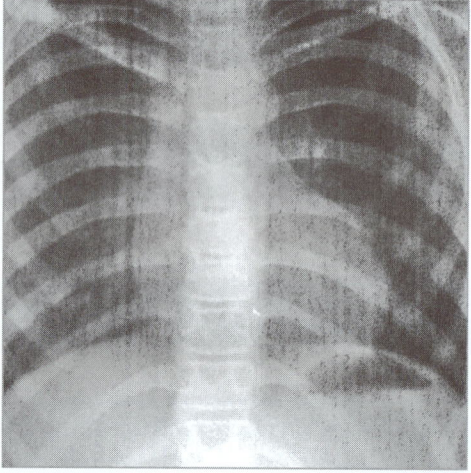

Fig. 12.51: Chest X-ray PA view showing pulmonary oligemia with upturned apex (right ventricle) suggestive of **tetralogy of Fallot (coeur-en-sabot).**

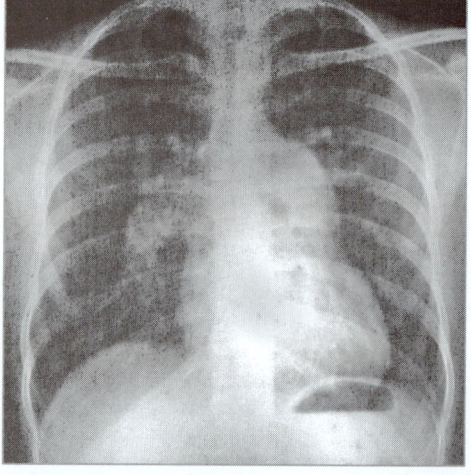

Fig. 12.52: Chest X-ray PA view showing mild cardiomegaly, prominent pulmonary artery, pulmonary plethora, prominent right atrium. Suggestive of **atrial septal defect—jug handle appearance.**

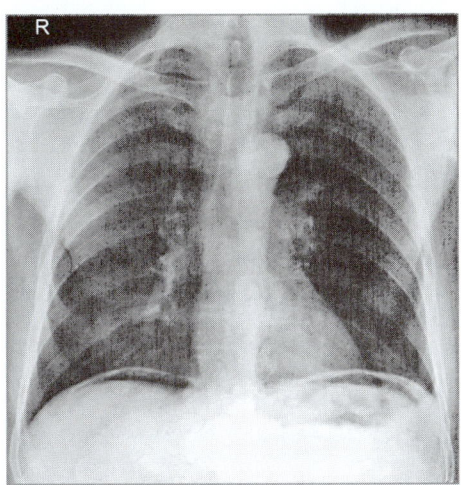

Fig. 12.53: Chest X-ray PA view showing free air under bilateral hemidiaphragm—**pneumoperitoneum**.

Causes:
- Hollow viscus perforation
- Post-laparotomy/laparoscopy
- Subphrenic abscess
- Tubal insufflation (Rubin's test)

Minimum amount of air needed to produce this is 1 cc.

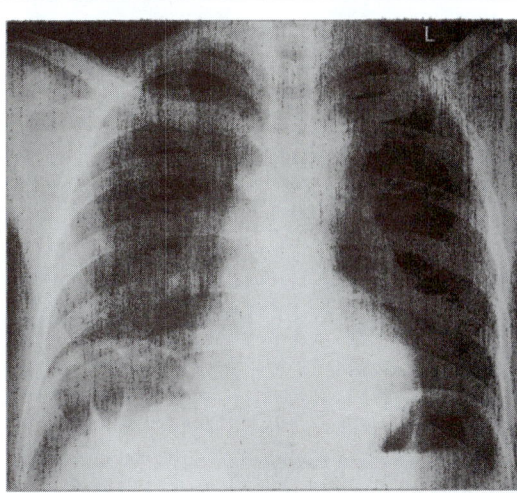

Fig. 12.54: Chest X-ray PA view showing interposition of transverse colon between liver and right hemidiaphragm—**Chilaiditi syndrome**.

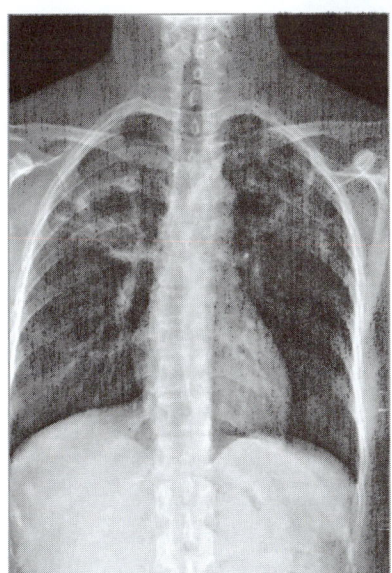

Fig. 12.55: Chest X-ray PA view showing trachea central, cardiophrenic and costophrenic angles are normal, nonhomogeneous opacity in bilateral upper zone with multiple cavities suggestive of **bilateral upper lobe active tuberculosis.**

X-ray signs of active tuberculosis—thin-walled cavities, pleural effusion, interstitial fluffy shadows.

X-ray signs of healed tuberculosis—thick-walled cavities, fibrosis, calcification, pleural thickening.

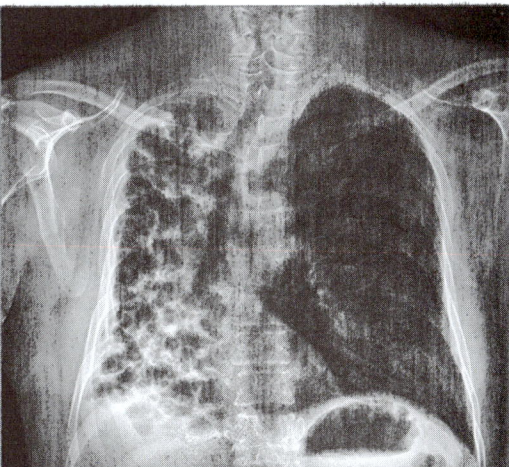

Fig. 12.56: Chest X-ray PA view showing trachea deviated to right, mediastinum pulled to right, decreased size of right hemithorax with rib crowding. Nonhomogeneous opacity in right hemithorax with multiple cystic shadows suggestive of **right-sided fibrosis with cystic bronchiectasis** possibly sequelae of tuberculosis.

A Systematic Approach to Chest X-rays

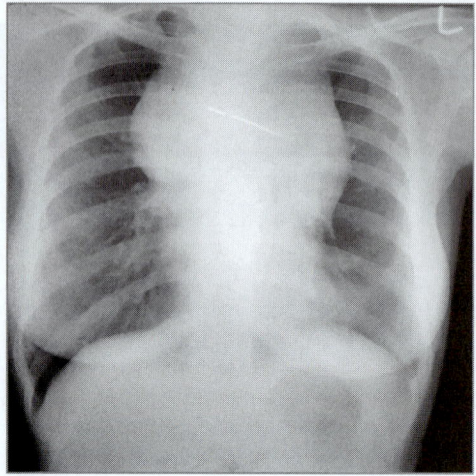

Fig. 12.57: Chest X-ray PA view showing trachea central, cardiophrenic and costophrenic angles are normal, mediastinal widening suggestive of **superior mediastinal mass**.

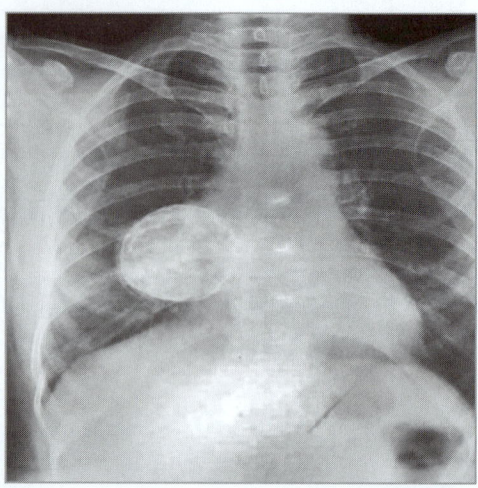

Fig. 12.58: Chest X-ray PA view showing trachea central, cardiophrenic and costophrenic angles are normal, rounded opacity arising from the anterior mediastinum which is **calcified—mediastinal cyst**.

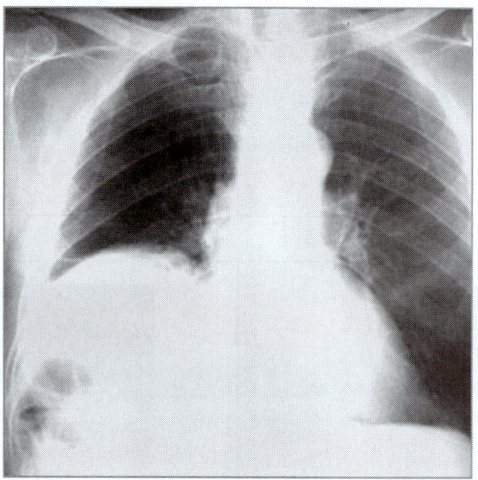

Fig. 12.59: Chest X-ray PA view showing elevated right hemidiaphragm.

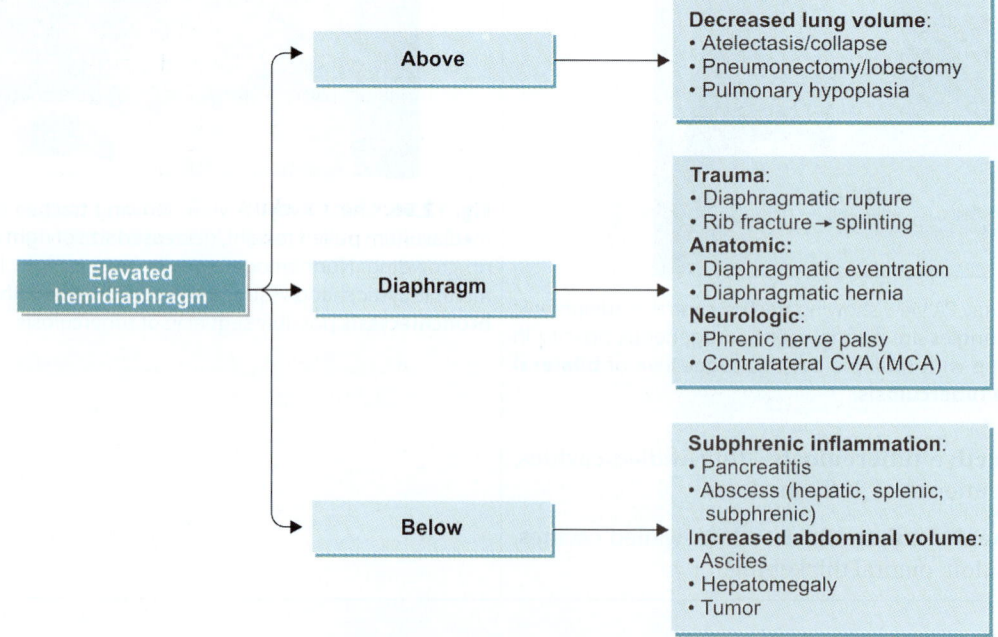

A Systematic Approach to Chest X-rays

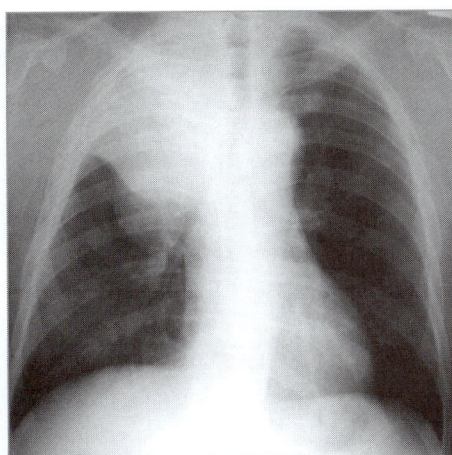

Fig. 12.60: Chest X-ray demonstrates increased density in the right upper hemithorax with loss of volume, and shift of the trachea to the right. A mass is present at the right hilum. Right hilar mass obstructing the right upper lobe bronchus results in collapse of the right upper. This results in a reverse S shape to the pleural edge. It is the typical appearances of a **reverse S sign of Golden**.

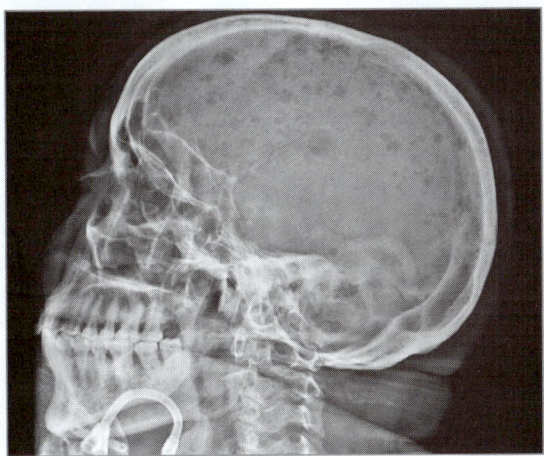

Fig. 12.61: Lateral X-ray of skull showing **multiple punched out lesions**.

Differential diagnosis: Myeloma, metastasis, rarely Langerhans cell histiocytosis.

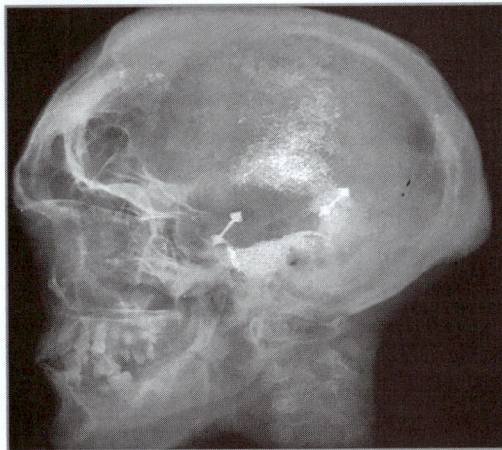

Fig. 12.62: Lateral skull X-ray showing prognathism, thickened skull vault, prominent air sinuses, enlarged sella turcica—**suggestive of acromegaly**.

Chest X-ray Interpretation Template

X-ray Assessment

1. **Type of view: (PA/AP/lateral)**
2. **Orientation**
   - Correct orientation (left and right markers): Yes/No
3. **Inspiratory/expiratory**
4. **Rotation**
   - Clavicles equidistant from spinous processes: Yes/No
5. **Penetration**
   - Spine visible through the heart shadow: Yes/No

Systematic Review

Bony cage and soft tissues

- **Bones**:
  - Ribs: Normal/fractures/lytic lesions/deformities
  - Clavicles: Normal/abnormalities
  - Vertebrae: Normal/abnormalities
- **Soft tissues**:
  - Subcutaneous emphysema: Yes/No
  - Abnormal soft tissue shadows: Yes/No

Trachea

- Midline/deviated
- **Carina and bronchi:** Clear/obstructed
- **Masses or foreign bodies:** Yes/No (describe if present)

Diaphragm

- **Hemidiaphragms:** Normal/elevated/flattened/abnormal contour
- **Costophrenic angles:** Sharp/blunted (indicates effusions)
- **Air under diaphragm:** Yes/No (indicates pneumoperitoneum)

Hilum

- Pulmonary vasculature
- Pulmonary artery: Size—normal/enlarged (>16 mm = pulmonary artery hypertension)
- Pulmonary vein congestion: Present/absent
- Lymph nodes: Present/absent
- Mass or abnormal opacities: Present/absent

Lung zones

- **Lung fields:** Symmetrical/asymmetrical
- **Vascular markings:** Normal/increased/decreased
- **Infiltrates:** Present/absent (describe any opacities, e.g., consolidation, interstitial patterns)
- **Masses:** Present/absent (describe any nodules or masses)
- **Pleura:** Normal/pneumothorax/pleural effusion/pleural thickening

Cardiac and mediastinum

- **Heart size:** Normal/cardiomegaly (cardiothoracic ratio >50% on PA view)
- **Contours:** Normal/abnormal (describe any abnormal contours or masses)
- **Mediastinum:** Normal width/widened/shifted

Additional findings
- **Tubes and lines**: Present/absent (describe position and condition of any medical devices such as endotracheal tube, nasogastric tube, central lines)
- **Foreign bodies**: Present/absent (describe if present)

Clinical correlation
- **Potential diagnoses**

COMPUTED TOMOGRAPHY (FIGS. 12.63 TO 12.67)

Computed Tomography

Types
1. Spiral CT
2. Multislice CT—coronary CT angiography and calcium score

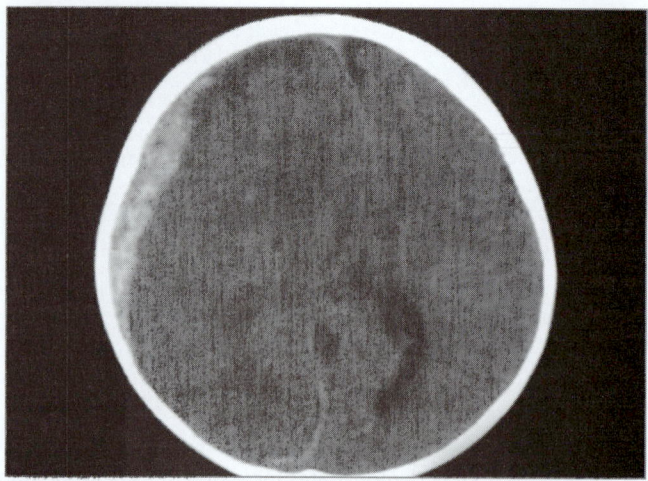

Fig. 12.63: Plain CT head showing hyperdense shadow which is **concavo-convex** in appearance suggestive of **acute right subdural hematoma**.

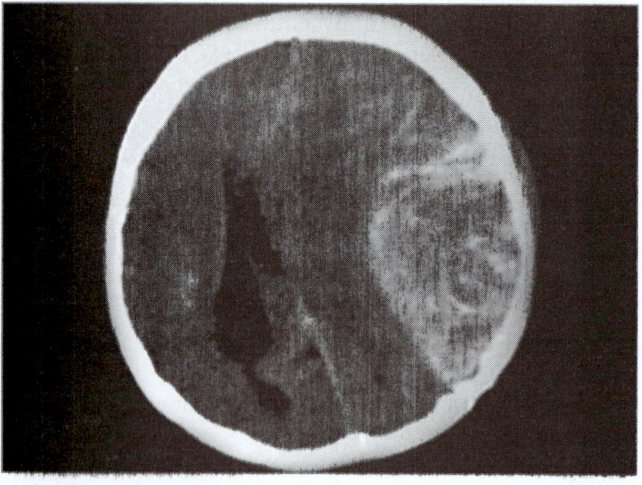

Fig. 12.64: Plain CT head showing hyperdense shadow which **biconvex** in appearance suggestive of **acute left extradural hematoma**.

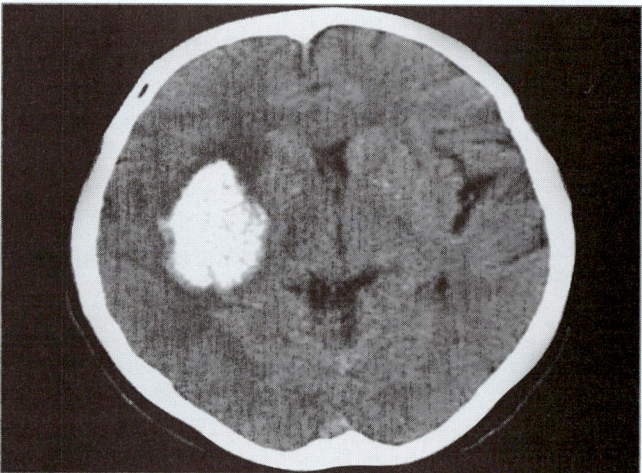

Fig. 12.65: Plain CT head showing hyperdense shadow in the right basal ganglia suggestive of **acute intraparenchymal hemorrhage**.

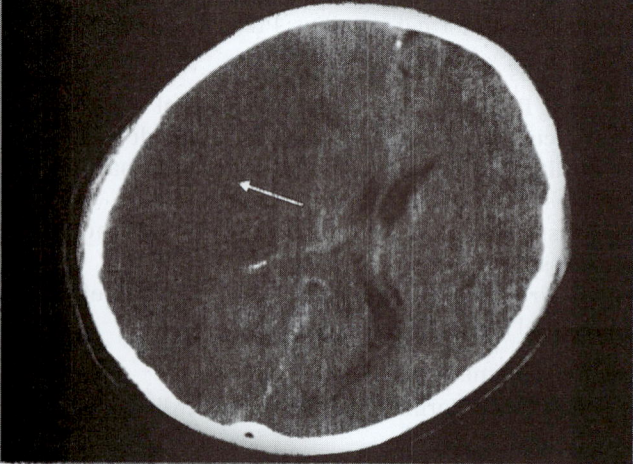

Fig. 12.66: Plain CT head showing hypodense shadow in the right parietotemporal cortex suggestive of **acute infarct** (arrow).

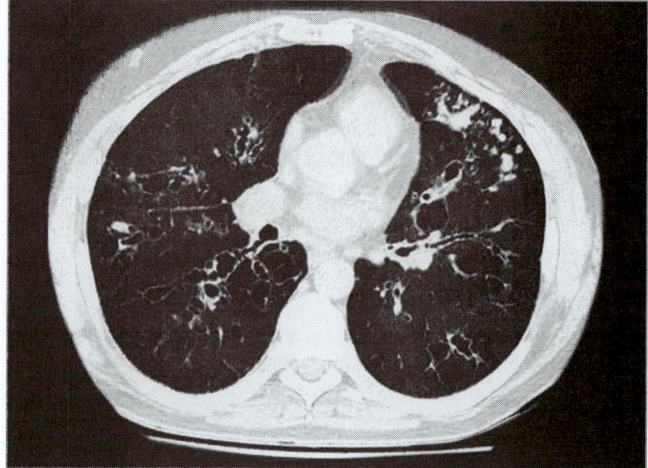

Fig. 12.67: High-resolution computed tomography (HRCT) of chest. Varicose and cystic **bronchiectasis** with mucus plugging in upper lobes.

3. Electron beam CT—faster, used for cardiac application
4. High resolution CT (HRCT)—1–2 mm slices, investigation of choice for ILD and bronchiectasis.

CT density scale—Hounsfield units—range from –1,000 (black) to +1,000 (white).

0—attenuation value of water (considered as reference)

–1,000	Air
–100	Fat
0	Water
+60	Hemorrhage
+1,000	Calcification

MAGNETIC RESONANCE IMAGING (FIGS. 12.68 AND 12.69)

Proton acts as a dipole with magnetic dipole movement and gyromagnetic properties.

Types of MRI Sequences

1. **T1—spin lattice relaxation time**
2. **T2—spin-spin relaxation time**
3. **Fluid-attenuated inversion recovery (FLAIR)**—preferred in CNS demyelinating diseases like multiple sclerosis
4. **Diffusion-weighted images (DWI)**—for detection of early infarcts
5. **Apparent diffusion coefficient (ADC)**

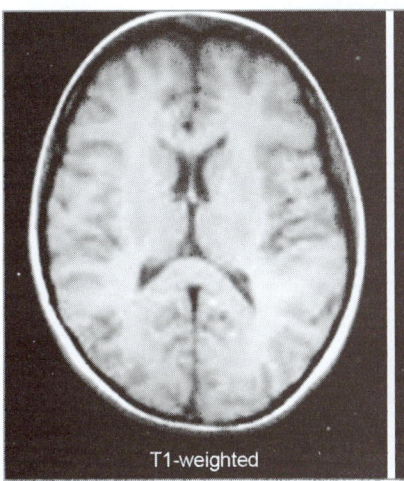 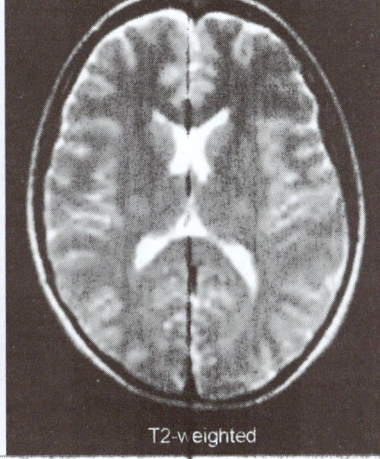 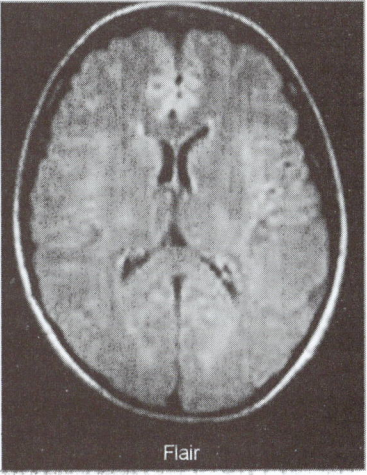

Fig. 12.68: Magnetic resonance imaging.

MR signal characteristics:

	T1	T2
CSF	Hypointense	Hyperintense
Gray matter	Gray	White
White matter	White	Gray
Fat	Hyperintense	Less hyperintense
Tumors (most)	—	Hyperintense
Melanoma	Hyperintense	Hypointense

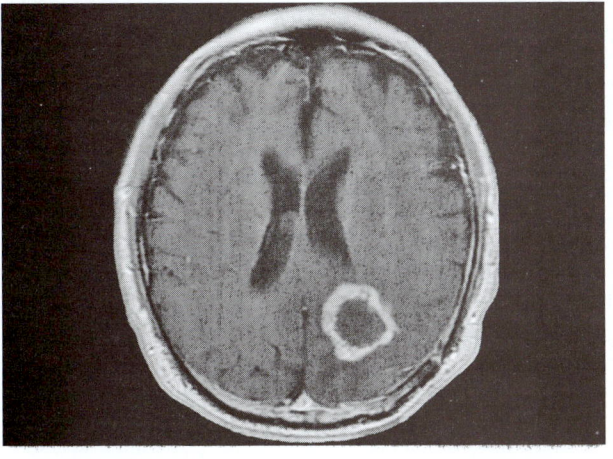

Differential diagnosis:
- Cerebral abscess
- Tuberculoma
- Neurocysticercosis
- Metastasis
- Glioblastoma
- Subacute infarct/hemorrhage
- Demyelination
- Radiation necrosis
- Lymphoma

Fig. 12.69: MRI brain showing ring enhancing lesion.

CONTRAST AGENTS

Contrast for X-ray/CT

Positive contrast agents		Negative contrast agents
Water soluble (Iodine containing agents)	**Water insoluble** (Barium containing agents)	Air water
High osmolar: Urografin, diatrizoate sodium, Conray **Low osmolar:** Optiray, iodixanol		
Note: Low osmolar agents are safer.		

MRI Contrast Agents

Contain paramagnetic metalions, e.g., gadolinium ligated to diethylenetriaminepentaacetic (DTPA).

13 CHAPTER

Basic Instruments and Procedures in Viva

- Student must be able to identify the instrument with its use
- Student must be able to list the indication/s and contraindications for the procedure
- Students must be to briefly describe the procedure and list the complications if any
- Students must be able to interpret the investigation reports

GASTRIC LAVAGE TUBE

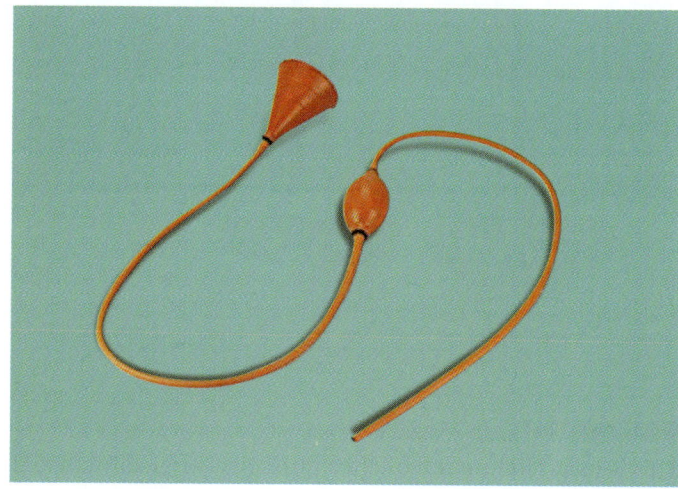

Description

Used for gastric decontamination by removing toxic substances from the stomach by sequential administration and re-aspiration of small volumes of fluid through this tube which can also be sent for analysis.

Helps **clear blood and clots** from the stomach to allow for better visualization during an endoscopy or to monitor ongoing bleeding.

Removes **gas or fluid** in cases like bowel obstruction to reduce pressure.

Other names—Ewald's tube/Boas tube.

Indications

For decontamination after oral consumption of poison.

Contraindications

- Petroleum distillates (e.g., gasoline, furniture polish)
- Corrosives (strong acids, strong bases) (e.g., drain cleaner)
- CNS stimulants, because the act of vomiting may trigger convulsions
- Convulsions
- Cardiac dysrhythmias
- Risk of hemorrhage or GI perforation resulting from pathology or recent surgery
- Others:
  - The poison ingested is not toxic at any dose
  - The poison ingested is adsorbed by charcoal and adsorption is not exceeded by the quantity of ingestion
  - Presented several (46) hours after consumption of the poison
  - A highly efficient antidote, such as N-acetylcysteine (NAC) is available.
  - Unprotected airway where there is decreased level of consciousness.

Technique of Performing Orogastric Lavage (Table 13.1)

TABLE 13.1: The technique of performing orogastric lavage.

Select the correct tube size
Adults and adolescents: 36–40 French
Children: 22–28 French

Procedure

1. If there is a potential airway compromise, endotracheal intubation should precede orogastric lavage
2. The patient should be kept in the left lateral decubitus position. Because the pylorus points upward in this orientation, this positioning theoretically helps prevent the xenobiotic from passing through the pylorus during the procedure
3. Before insertion, the proper length of tubing to be passed should be measured and marked on the tube. The length should allow the most proximal tube opening to be passed beyond the lower esophageal sphincter
4. After the tube is inserted, it is essential to confirm that the distal end of the tube is in the stomach
5. Any material present in the stomach should be withdrawn and immediate instillation of activated charcoal should be considered for large ingestions of xenobiotics that are known to be adsorbed by activated charcoal

Contd...

Contd...

Procedure

6. In adults, 250-mL aliquots of a room temperature saline lavage solution is instilled via a funnel or lavage syringe. In children, aliquots should be 10–15 mL/kg to a maximum of 250 mL.
7. Orogastric lavage should continue for at least several liters in an adult and for at least 0.5–1.0 L in a child or until no particulate matter returns and the effluent lavage solution is clear.
8. After orogastric lavage, the same tube should be used to instill activated charcoal if indicated.

Complications

- Incomplete decontamination leading to severe intoxication despite the procedure
- Pulmonary aspiration of gastric contents (3% of patients)
- Hypoxia
- Laryngospasm
- Mechanical injury to the gastrointestinal tract, esophageal rupture (rare)
- Water intoxication (especially in children)
- Hypothermia
- Bradycardia.

LARYNGOSCOPE

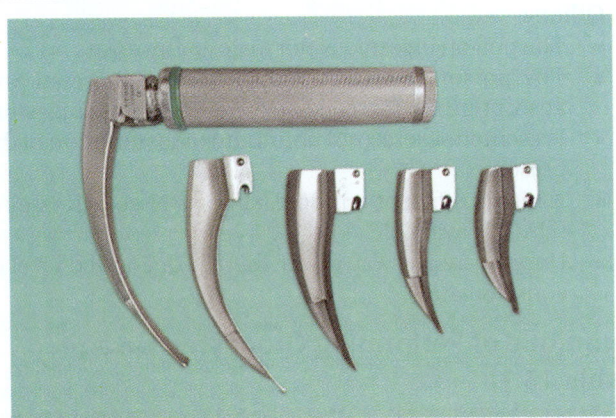

Description

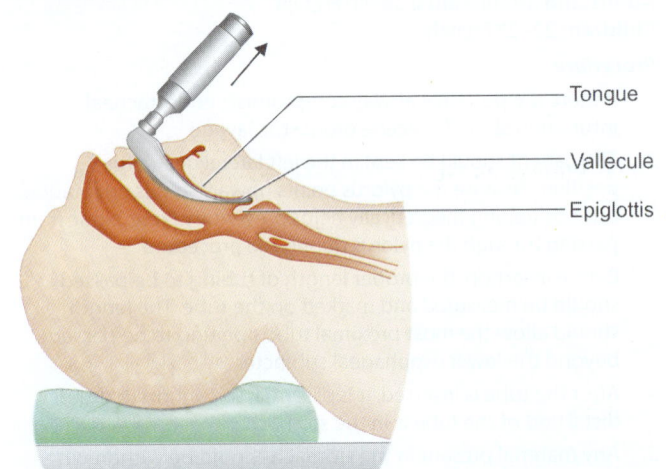

Laryngoscopes are usually left-handed tools designed to facilitate visualization of the larynx. A laryngoscope consists of a handle, a blade, and a light source. The most commonly used blades include the curved Macintosh and the straight Miller blades. Modern advancements have introduced **video laryngoscopes**, which integrate a camera and light source at the blade's tip, projecting real-time images onto a screen.

Indications

- Patients requiring emergent intubation in conditions like acute respiratory failure with inadequate oxygenation and ventilation.
- In patients with altered sensorium for airway protection.
- Nonemergent intubation occurs in the perioperative setting as patients may require general anesthesia.

Contraindications

- Suspected cervical spine injuries
- Patients who have supraglottic or glottic pathology.
- A relative contraindication to laryngoscopy includes patients with anatomy that does not allow successful laryngoscopy use, injuries to the area, or physiologic status that is not conducive to the procedure.

METAL TRACHEOSTOMY TUBE

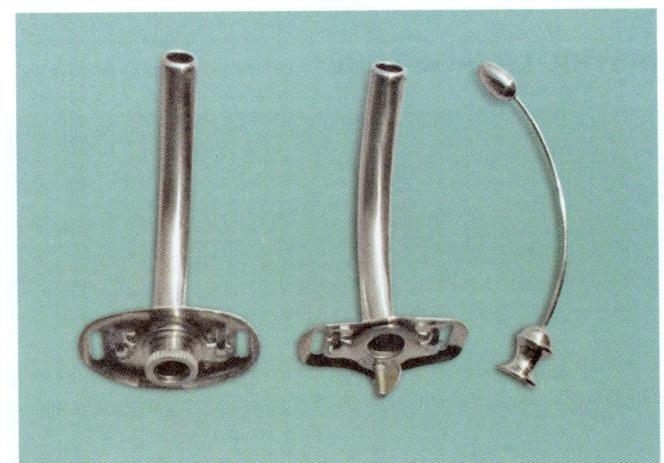

Description

This is inserted into the trachea through a surgically created opening (tracheostomy) in the neck, allowing air to pass directly into the lungs. It consists of three parts:

1. Outer cannula: The main tube that maintains the tracheal opening.
2. Inner cannula: A removable tube within the outer cannula that can be cleaned or replaced without disturbing the outer tube.
3. Obturator: A guide used during insertion to prevent trauma and ensure smooth placement.

Indications

- Upper airway obstruction (e.g., stridor)
- Non-flexible—hence ideal for long-term tracheostomy care.
- Facilitation of ventilation support
- For management of pulmonary secretions.

ENDOTRACHEAL TUBE

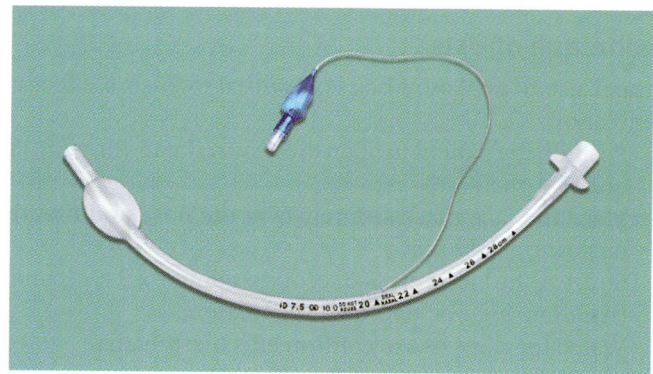

Description

It is a tube constructed of polyvinylchloride (PVC) that is placed between the vocal cords into the trachea to provide oxygen and inhaled gases to the lungs. It also serves to protect the lungs from contamination, such as gastric contents and blood parts of endotracheal (ET) tube.

The Tube

The endotracheal tube (ETT) has a length and diameter. The endotracheal tubes size refers to its internal diameter in millimeters (mm). Generally 7.0–7.5 ETT is appropriate for an average woman and 7.5–8.5 ETT for an average man. PVC is not radio-opaque, and thus a radio-opaque linear material is included throughout the length of the tube to make it easier to visualize the placement on X-ray. Ideally, the distal tip of the ETT is 4 cm (+/−2 cm) above the carina on chest X-ray in adults.

The Cuff

A cuff is an inflatable balloon at the distal end of the ETT. The inflated cuff produces a seal against the tracheal wall; this prevents gastric contents from entering the trachea and facilitates the execution of positive pressure ventilation. The cuff inflates with air by attaching an appropriate size syringe and (10–20 mL for adult ETT) to the pilot balloon.

The Bevel

To facilitate placement through the vocal cords and to provide improved visualization ahead of the tip, the ETT has an angle or slant known as a bevel.

The Murphy's Eye

Endotracheal tubes have a built in safety mechanism at the distal tip known as Murphy's eye, which is another opening in the tube positioned in the distal lateral wall. It provides an alternate gas passage way in case the bevelled tip gets occluded.

The Connector

Endotracheal tube connectors attach the ETT to the mechanical ventilator tubing or an Ambu bag.

Pilot Balloon: Indicates cuff inflation status.

Indications

- Acute respiratory failure, inadequate oxygenation, or ventilation.
- Airway protection in a patient with depressed mental status.
- In the perioperative setting, endotracheal tubes may be placed in many clinical circumstances including patients receiving general anesthesia, surgery involving head and neck where mask ventilation is not possible.
- Prior to urgent aggressive sedation for instance status epilepticus, sustained contractions in tetanus.
- To facilitate thoracic and intra-abdominal interventions that require respiratory control and muscle relaxation.
- Less frequently to manage increased intracranial pressure or to manage copious secretions or bleeding from the airway.

Contraindications

- Severe airway trauma or obstruction that does not allow safe placement of the tube
- Severe cervical spine injury which requires complete immobilization
- Those patients with Mallampati III/IV classification suggesting potentially difficult airway management.

OROPHARYNGEAL AIRWAY

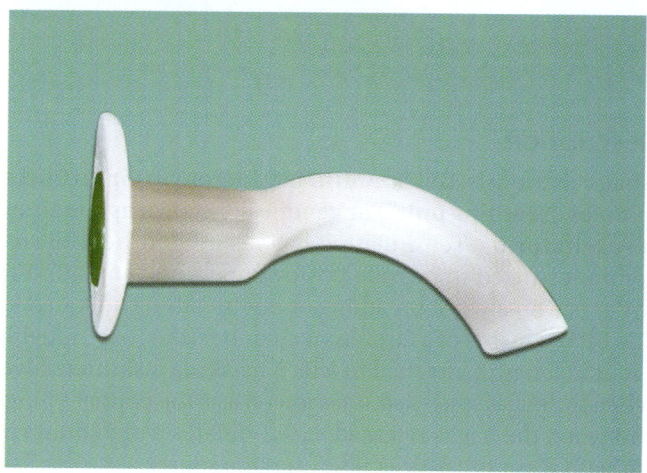

Description

It is also known as Guedel pattern airway and helps to maintain or open a patient's airway by preventing the tongue from falling back against the epiglottis.

It consists of:
1. **Bite block:** A flat, rigid portion at the end that rests on the lips or teeth to prevent biting and occlusion of the airway.
2. **Curved body:** Follows the natural curvature of the tongue and pharynx.
3. **Flange:** A flat portion at the mouth opening that prevents the device from slipping too far into the airway.

The size of the airway can be chosen by measuring the distance between the incisors and the angle of the mouth. The airway is inserted into the mouth of the patient, upside down and once contact is made with the back of the throat, it is rotated 180 degrees. This allows for easy placement and ensures that the tongue is secured.

Indications

Used primarily in **unconscious patients** who are at risk of airway obstruction due to tongue displacement such as cardiopulmonary resuscitation (CPR), general anesthesia, overdose or trauma-related unconsciousness, during bag-valve-mask ventilation

Importantly, it should only be used in patients **without a gag reflex**, as stimulation of the pharynx in a conscious or semiconscious patient can cause vomiting and aspiration.

AMBU BAG

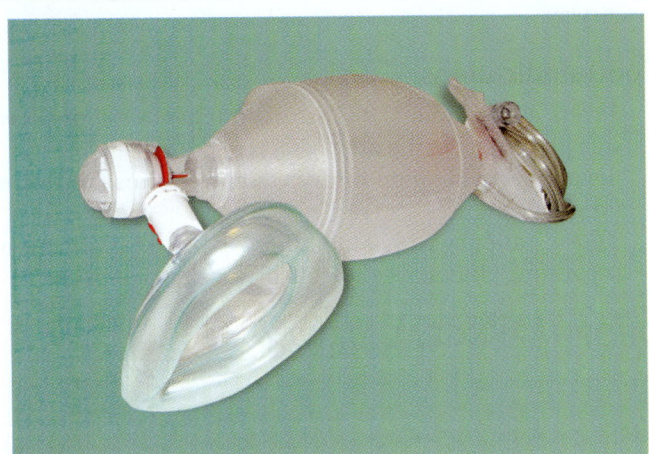

Description

A **bag valve mask (BVM)**, **AMBU bag (acronym for "artificial manual breathing unit")** or generically known as a **manual resuscitator** or "self-inflating bag", is a hand held device commonly used to provide positive pressure ventilation to patients who are not breathing or not breathing adequately. The BVM consists of a flexible air chamber (the "bag", roughly a foot in length), attached to a face mask via a shutter valve. When the bag is squeezed, air is forced into the patient's lungs and when the bag is released, it self-inflates which draws in ambient air or the oxygen flow from the source.

A standard Ambu bag consists of three main parts:
1. **Self-inflating bag:** The squeezable reservoir that delivers air or oxygen to the patient.
2. **One-way valve system:** Ensures that air flows in only one direction—from the bag to the mask or endotracheal tube—and prevents exhaled air from re-entering the bag.
3. **Face mask or airway connector:** Forms a seal over the patient's nose and mouth or connects to an endotracheal tube or tracheostomy.
4. **Oxygen inlet:** Allows connection to an oxygen source for delivering enriched oxygen.

Uses

1. Cardiac or respiratory arrest
2. Respiratory failure
3. Anesthesia induction
4. Transport ventilation

Technique of Use

Proper use of an Ambu bag is essential to ensure effective ventilation:
1. Position the patient to open the airway (head-tilt, chin-lift or jaw-thrust).
2. Place the face mask securely over the nose and mouth, ensuring a tight seal.
3. Squeeze the bag every 5–6 seconds (adults) or 3–5 seconds (children/infants) to provide ventilation.
4. Watch for chest rise to confirm effective breaths.

Complications

- Air inflating the stomach leading to vomiting and possible aspiration of gastric contents.
- Lung injury from overstretching (called volutrauma); and/or
- Lung injury from overpressurization (called barotrauma).

RYLES TUBE—NASOGASTRIC TUBE

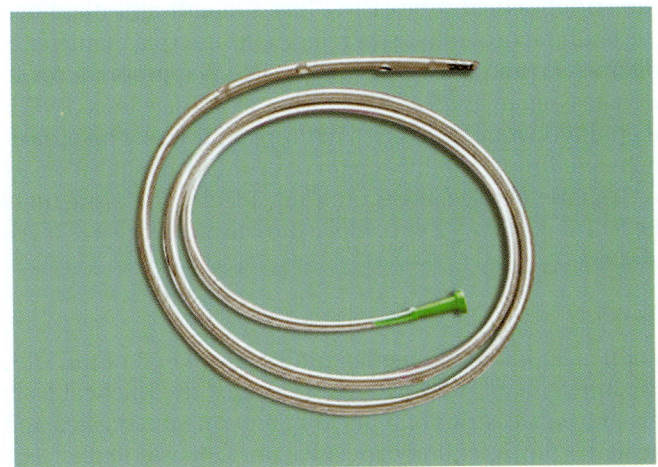

Description

It is a flexible tube made of rubber or nontoxic, medical grade PVC compound, and it has bidirectional potential. It can be used either to feed or remove the contents of the stomach including air, to decompress the stomach or to remove small solid objects and fluid, such as poison from the stomach.

Indications

Diagnostic indications for nasogastric tube (NG) intubation include the following:
- Evaluation of upper gastrointestinal (GI) bleeding (i.e., presence and volume)
- Aspiration of gastric fluid content, e.g., AFB sampling especially patients in whom sputum samples cannot be obtained such as children.
- Identification of the esophagus and stomach on a chest radiograph
- Administration of radiographic contrast to the GI tract.

Therapeutic indications for NG intubation include the following:
- Gastric decompression including maintenance of a decompressed state after endotracheal intubation, often via the oropharynx
- Relief of symptoms and bowel rest in the setting of small bowel obstruction
- Aspiration of gastric content from recent ingestion of toxic material
- Administration of medications in comatose patients
- Feeding when patient is unconscious or when the patient is conscious but unable to swallow voluntarily
- Bowel irrigation.

Contraindications

Absolute contraindications for NG intubation include the following:
- Severe midface trauma
- Recent nasal surgery.

Relative contraindications for NG intubation include the following:
- Coagulation abnormality
- Esophageal varices
- Recent banding of esophageal varices
- Alkaline ingestion (the tube may be kept if the injury is not severe).

Complications
- Nose bleeds, sinusitis, sore throat
- Erosion of the nose
- Esophageal perforation
- Pulmonary aspiration

Verification of Position of Ryles Tube
- Verify proper placement of the NG tube by auscultating a rush of air over the stomach using the 60 mL Toomey syringe or by aspirating gastric content
- Obtaining a chest radiograph
- Colorimetric capnography is another valid method for verifying NG tube positioning in mechanically ventilated patients.

SUCTION CATHETER

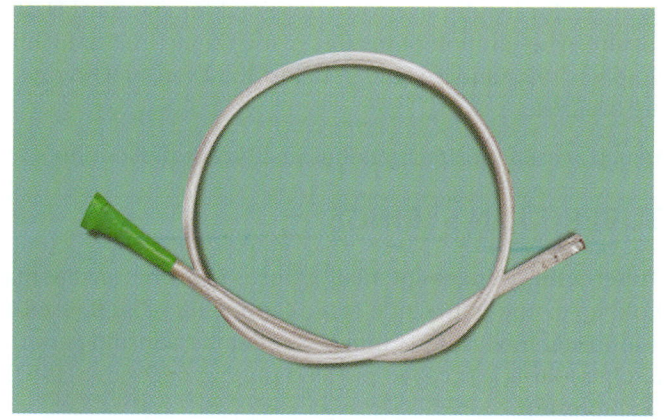

A **suction catheter** is a medical device used to extract bodily secretions, such as mucus or saliva from the upper airway. A suction catheter connects to a **suction machine** or **collection canister**.

Indications
- Prevent aspiration especially if patient is in altered consciousness
- Maintain a patent airway during surgeries, procedures
- Management of chronic respiratory conditions where patients are unable to clear secretions on their own
- Management of airway trauma

FOLEYS CATHETER

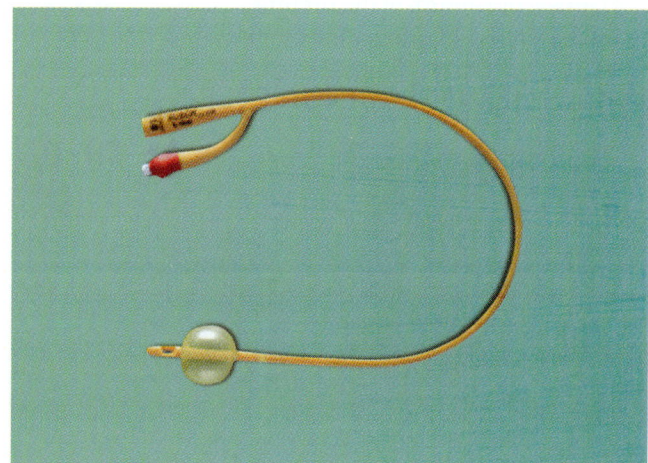

Description

Foley catheter (named for Frederic Foley, who produced the original design in 1929), is made of latex, silicone, or other biocompatible materials and has the following parts:
- **Catheter tube:** A long, flexible shaft that enters the bladder.
- **Drainage lumen:** Allows urine to pass from the bladder to the collection bag.
- **Inflation lumen:** A separate channel used to inflate a small balloon near the tip to keep the catheter in place.
- **Balloon:** Typically holds 5–30 mL of sterile water to prevent the catheter from slipping out.
- **Connector end:** Attaches to a drainage bag to collect urine.

Saline should not be used to inflate the bulb, as it can crystallize within. Air must not be used to inflate as it will float over the urine. Coatings include polytetrafluoroethylene, hydrogel, or a silicon elastomer—the different properties of these surface coatings determine whether the catheter is suitable for 28 days or 3 months indwelling duration. Triluminal Foley catheter is used for bladder irrigation after prostrate surgeries.

Indications
- Acute retention of urine
- Chronic retention of urine with overflow
- In cases of neurogenic bladder

- In surgery involving bladder and prostrate
- In all perineal operations
- Intravesical chemotherapy
- To carry out urethrography
- To monitor urine output
- During induction of labor for extra-amniotic saline infusion

Contraindication

Urethral trauma is the only absolute contraindication to placement of a urinary catheter.

Complications

- Bleeding
- Damage or rupture of the urethra
- Increased risk of urinary infections

SAHLI'S HEMOGLOBINOMETER

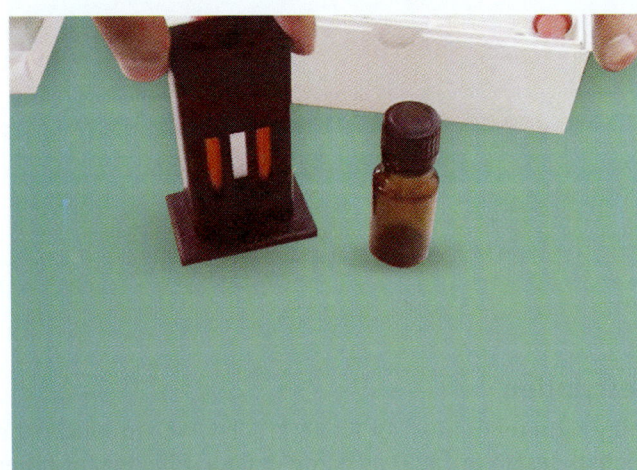

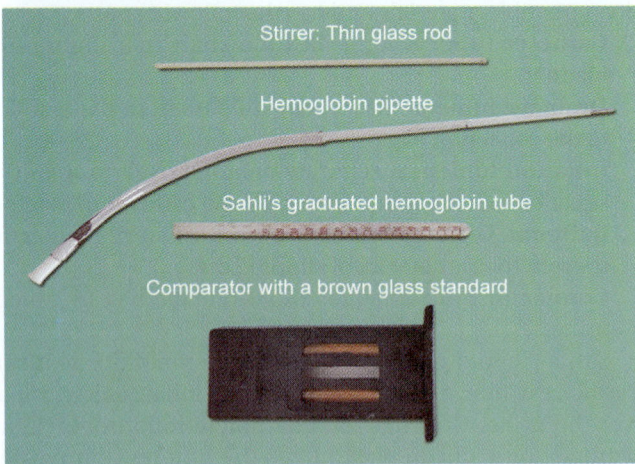

Description

Used to estimate hemoglobin: Method used is acid hematin method. Hydrochloric acid is used to convert hemoglobin to acid hematin which is then diluted until its color matches that of the comparator block. The hemoglobin concentration can then be read from the calibration tube. Although this is a simple and inexpensive technique for hemoglobin estimation, due to interobserver variability, it is often imprecise.

NEUBAUER CHAMBER/HEMOCYTOMETER

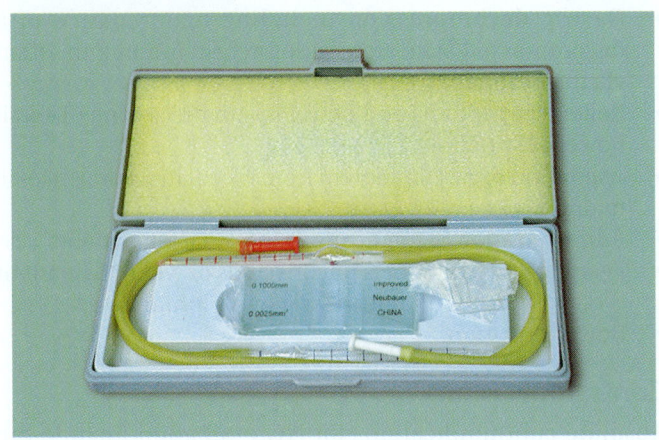

Description

The Neubauer chamber is a thick crystal slide with the size of a glass slide (30 × 70 mm and 4 mm thickness). In a simple counting chamber, the central area is where the cell counts are performed.

Use: Used to count red blood cell/white blood cell (RBC/WBC).

INSULIN SYRINGE

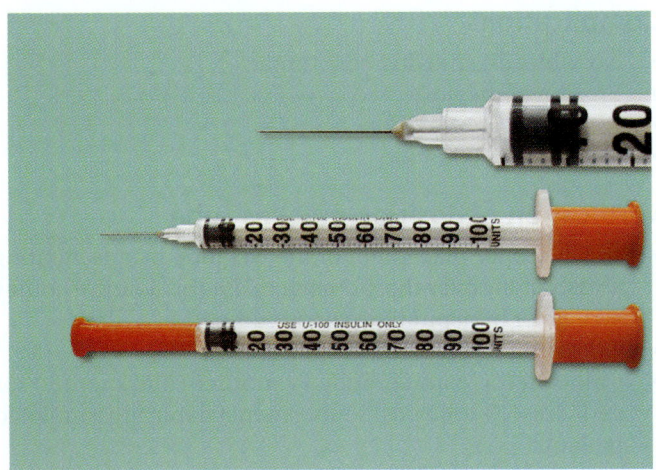

Description

Syringes for insulin users are designed for standard U-100 insulin. The dilution of insulin is such that 1 mL of insulin fluid has 100 standard "units" of insulin. Even 40 IU syringes are available.

Use: It is used for subcutaneous insulin administration.

TUBERCULIN SYRINGE

Tuberculin syringes are small syringes with fine needles that hold up to one-half to one cubic centimeter of fluid, used to administer medication (antigen) under the skin and perform a tuberculosis test called purified protein derivative (PPD)/Mantoux test.

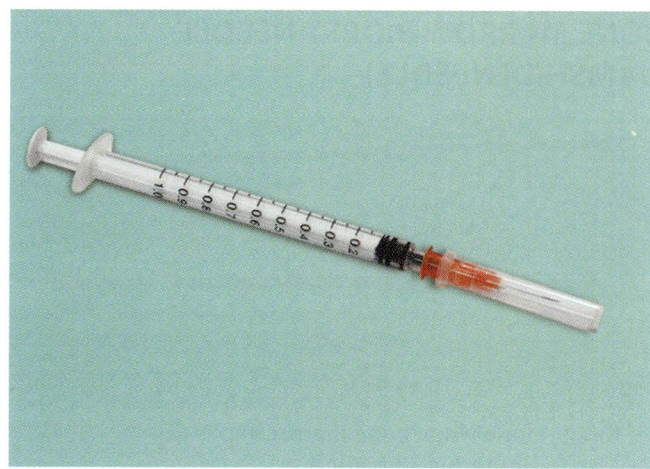

Insulin 40 versus Insulin 100 versus Tuberculin Syringe

U-40 insulin syringes markings on the barrel are up to 40 units, while in U-100 markings are up to 100 units. While in case of 1 mL tuberculin syringes the markings are at zero (0) and each 0.05 mL, e.g., 0.05, 0.1, 0.15, 0.2, 0.25, 0.3, etc.

VIM SILVERMAN LIVER BIOPSY NEEDLE

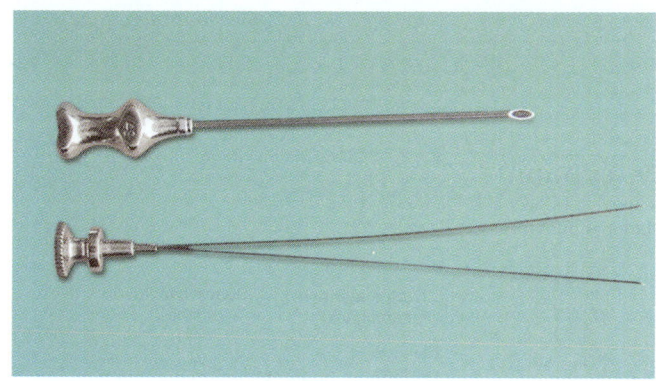

Description

It has **three parts:**
1. Cannula
2. Stylet/trocar
3. Prong/fork/bifid needle—longer than needle and it protrudes out of the needle. It has a very sharp cutting edge and has longitudinal groove. This retains the tissue when the needle and cannula are withdrawn.

Indications for Liver Biopsy

- In evaluation of jaundice
- Liver cirrhosis
- Storage disorders: Glycogen storage disease, hemochromatosis, and Wilson's disease
- Granulomatous lesions like tuberculosis and sarcoidosis
- Infections: Viral [cytomegalovirus (CMV), herpes, and parasitic (amoebic liver abscess where it is both diagnostic and therapeutic)]
- To diagnose benign and malignant neoplasms.
- Evaluation of fever of unknown origin or immunocompromised patients with hepatomegaly or deranged liver enzyme tests.

Contraindications of Liver Biopsy

- Bleeding diathesis
- Hemangiomas
- Hydatid cyst
- Severe ascites.

Complications of Liver Biopsy

- Hemorrhage
- Infection
- Adjacent structures can be injured (gallbladder, colon, and blood vessels)
- Rarely there can be precipitation of hepatic coma.

TRUCUT BIOPSY GUN

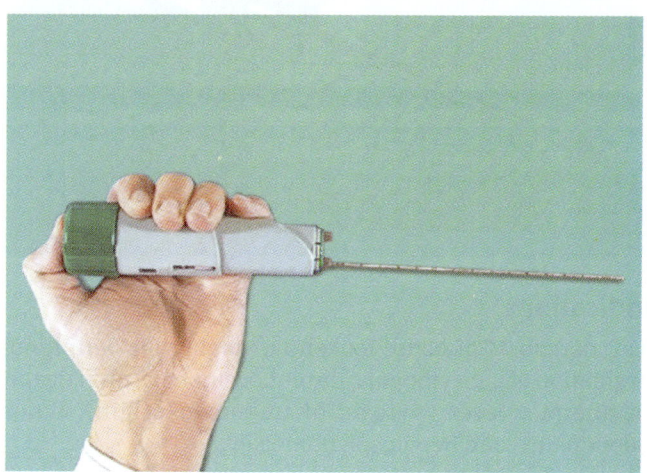

Description

A needle with a gap near its tip is passed into the lesion. A surrounding sheath with a cutting tip is passed down the needle. The sheath cuts a specimen corresponding to the gap in the needle. The needle and sheath with the specimen are then removed from the patient.

It typically consists of the following components:
- **Outer cannula (cutting needle):** A hollow sheath with a sharp edge that cuts the tissue.
- **Inner stylet (sampling needle):** Has a notch at the tip where tissue is collected.
- **Spring-loaded mechanism:** Powers the rapid insertion and cutting action.
- **Trigger or button:** Activates the needle advancement and tissue capture in one or two quick steps.
- **Handle and scale markings:** For grip and depth control during the procedure.

Use: For tissue biopsy—liver/kidney/lymph node/prostate/breast/lung.

BONE MARROW ASPIRATION NEEDLE

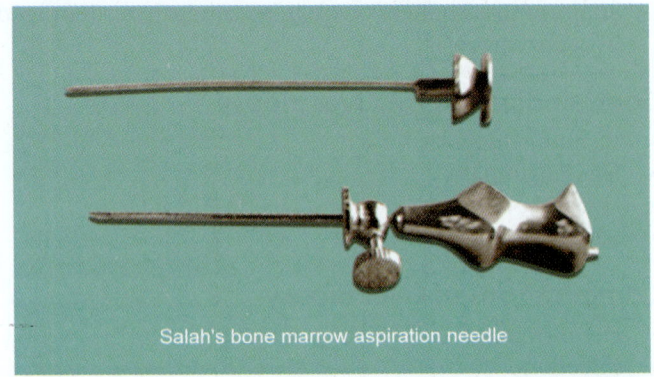
Salah's bone marrow aspiration needle

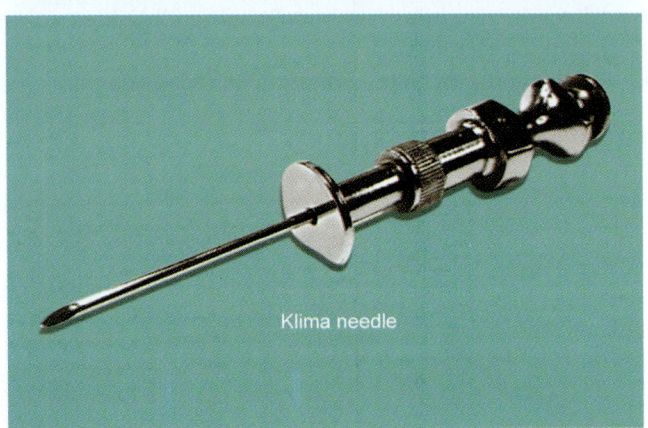
Klima needle

BONE MARROW BIOPSY NEEDLE (JAMSHIDI NEEDLE)

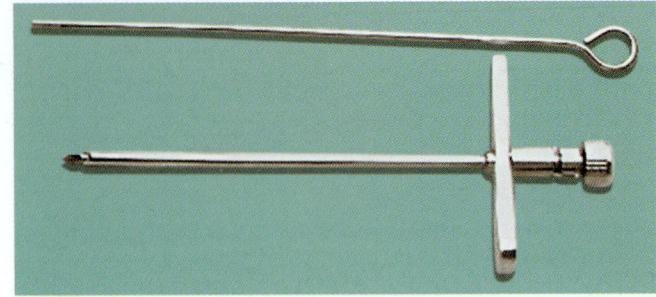

- Biopsy done when bone marrow tap is dry
- Also for infiltrative disorders.

LUMBAR PUNCTURE NEEDLE

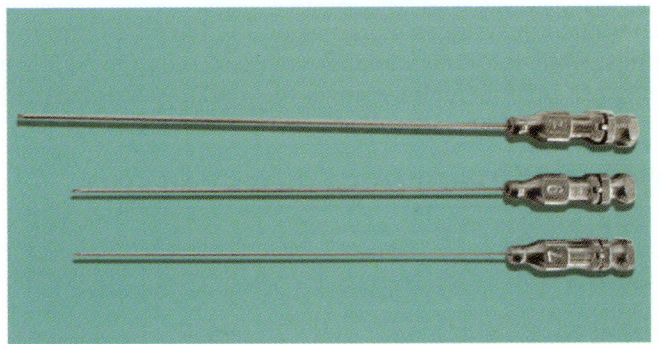

Indications

The diagnosis of acute leukemia, staging for lymphoma, evaluation of pancytopenia, thrombocytopenia, investigation of anemia, fever (pyrexia of unknown origin), lymph adenopathy, and hepatosplenomegaly.

The components of the needle include:
- **Needle shaft (cannula):** A long, hollow tube that is inserted into the bone to collect the marrow sample. It is usually made from stainless steel for strength and durability.
- **Stylet:** A solid rod inside the needle that maintains its shape during insertion and prevents the needle from clogging.
- **Trocar tip:** The pointed end of the needle, which is designed to puncture the bone and create an opening for aspiration.
- **Hub:** The part of the needle that connects to the syringe or aspiration device for collecting the bone marrow sample.
- **Plunger/syringe:** Used to create the suction necessary to extract the marrow.

Contraindications
- Bleeding disorders and coagulopathy
- Local skin infection/osteomyelitis.

Sites
Posterior superior iliac spine, anterior superior iliac spine. sternum, tibial tuberosity.

Description

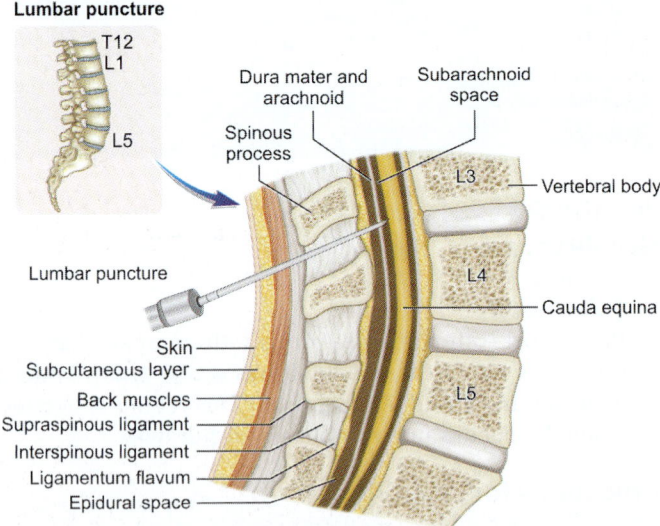

Lumbar puncture is a technique done to obtain cerebrospinal fluid (CSF) sample.

It also provides an indirect measure of intracranial pressure (ICP). It is usually done between L3 and L4 (3rd lumbar space) through the dura and into the spinal canal. The needle pierces in order the following structures; skin, subcutaneous tissue, supraspinous ligament, interspinous ligament, ligamentum flavum, epidural space, dura, arachnoid and finally subarachnoid space.

Indications for Lumbar Puncture

Diagnostic Indications
- Meningitis
- Encephalitis
- Subarachnoid hemorrhage
- Primary or metastatic malignancy (e.g., acute leukemias and lymphoma)
- Demyelinating diseases: Multiple sclerosis
- Subacute sclerosing panencephalitis (SSPE)
- Guillain–Barré syndrome
- Injecting the radioopaque dye for myelography.
- Measuring ICP

Therapeutic Indications
- Spinal anesthesia and epidural analgesia
- Intrathecal injection of chemotherapeutic drugs for CNS prophylaxis/relapse of acute lymphoblastic leukemia (ALL), lymphomas
- Therapeutic CSF drainage in cases of normal pressure hydrocephalus.

Contraindications for Lumbar Puncture
- Raised intracranial pressure, coagulopathy
- Local infective lesion
- Bony deformities at site of puncture.

Complications of Lumbar Puncture
- Post-spinal headache.
- Herniation of cerebellum through the foramen magnum due to raised intracranial pressure.
- Accidental puncture of the aorta or vena cava leading to retroperitoneal hematoma
- Accidental puncture of the spinal cord from being in wrong location
- Infection being introduced into the subarachnoid space
- Pain over the LP site

Xanthochromia is the yellow or pink discoloration of the CSF seen in SAH breakdown of hemoglobin to oxyhemoglobin (pink) and bilirubin (yellow).

Cerebrospinal Fluid Findings in Various Types of Meningitis

	Normal	Bacterial	Viral	Fungal	Tubercular
Opening pressure	6 and 25 cm H_2O	Elevated	Usually normal	Variable	Variable
Appearance	Clear	Cloudy	Clear	Variable	May from coagulum on standing
White blood cell count	<5 cells/µL	≥1,000 per µL	<100 per µL	Variable	Variable
Cell differential	No red cells or neutrophils	Predominance of neutrophils	▪ Several <100/µL mainly mononuclear cells ▪ Predominance of lymphocytes	▪ Occasional mild mononuclear increase ▪ Predominance of lymphocytes	Mixed, mainly mononuclear Predominance of lymphocytes
Protein (g/L)	0.15–0.4	Mild to marked elevation	Normal to elevated	Elevated	Mild to marked elevation
Glucose	50–70% serum	Very low	Usually normal	Low	Low
Other test	Lactate <2.1 mmol/L	Lactate >3.5 mol/L Gram-positive stain	Lactate <2.1 mol/L		Lactate <3.5 mol/L; Ziehl-Neelsen stain acid-fast bacilli

INTRAVENOUS DRIP SET

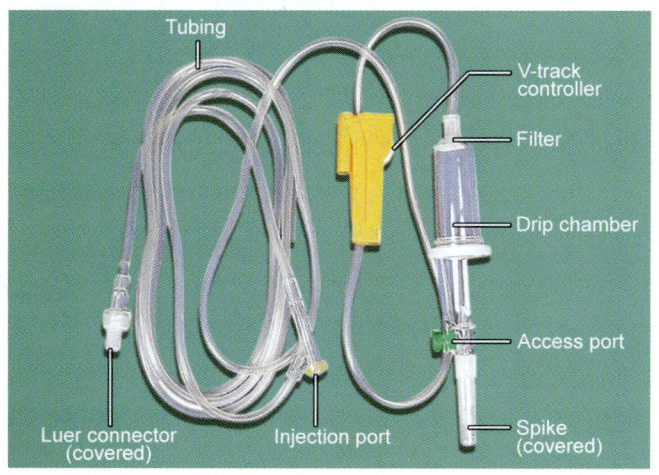

Intravenous Drip Set

Used for administering intravenous fluids, drugs, and blood products.

Intravenous (IV) fluids are administered through thin, flexible plastic tubing called an *infusion set* or **primary infusion tubing/administration set**. The infusion tubing/administration set connects to the bag of IV solution. Primary IV tubing is either a macrodrip solution administration set that delivers 10, 15, or 20 drops/mL, or a microdrip set that delivers 60 drops/mL. Macrodrip sets are used for routine primary infusions. Microdrip IV tubing is used mostly in pediatric or neonatal care, when small amounts of fluids are to be administered over a long period of time (Perry et al., 2014). The drop factor can be located on the packaging of the IV tubing.

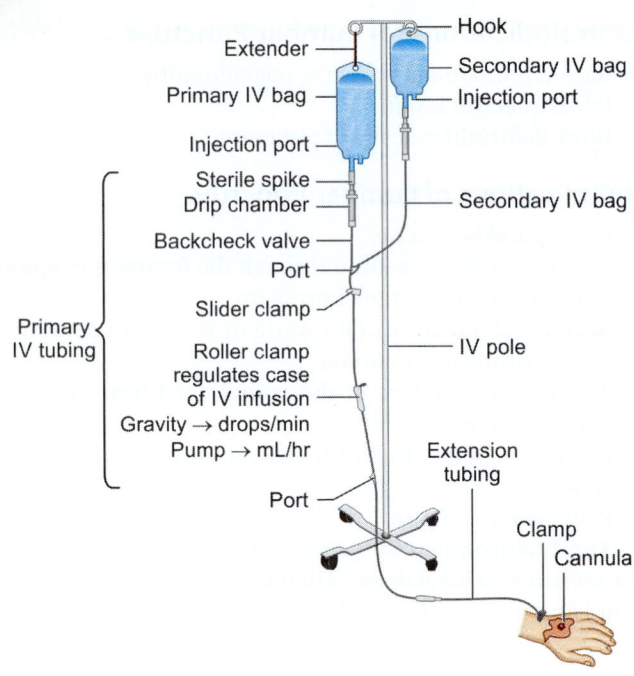

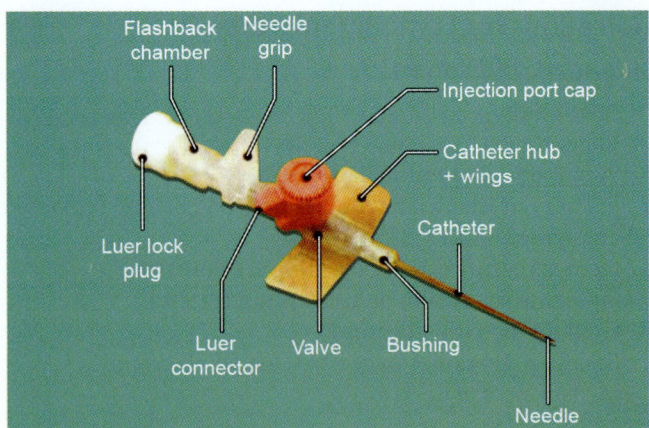

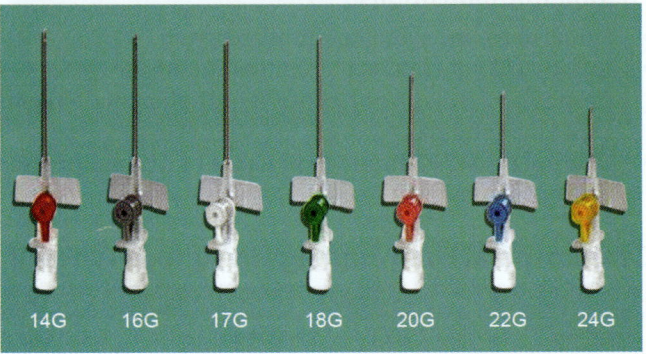

Primary IV tubing is used to infuse continuous or intermittent fluids or medication. It consists of the following parts:
- **Backcheck valve:** Prevents fluid or medication from traveling up the IV.
- **Access ports:** Used to infuse secondary medications and give IV push medications.
- **Roller clamp:** Used to regulate the speed of or to stop and start a gravity infusion.
- **Secondary IV tubing:** Shorter in length than primary tubing with no access ports or backcheck valve; when connected to a primary line via an access port used to infuse intermittent medications or fluids. A **secondary tubing administration set** is used for secondary IV medication.

Flow Rate Calculation

When calculating the flow rate of IV solutions, remember that the number of drops required to deliver 1 mL varies with the type of administration set. Administration sets are of two types:
1. Macrodrip set (delivers 10–20 drops/mL)
2. Microdrip set (60 drops/mL).

Flow rate = Volume of infusion in mL × Drip factor (in drops/mL)/Time of infusion in minutes.

INTRAVENOUS CANNULA

Used for administering intravenous fluids, drugs, and blood products.

Size	Color	Length (mm)	Flow rate (mL/min)	Uses
14G	Orange	45	250–300	▪ Used for adolescent and adult major surgery and trauma ▪ Infusion of large amount of fluids and colloids
16G	Gray	45	150–240	▪ Adolescent and adult major surgery and trauma ▪ Infusion of large amount of fluids or colloids
18G	Green	45	100–120	▪ Adolescent and adult major surgery and trauma ▪ Infusion of large amount of fluids or colloids
20G	Pink	32	55–80	▪ Older children, adolescent, and adult ▪ Ideal for IV Infusion or blood infusion ▪ Medication administration ▪ Emergency management
22G	Blue	25	22–50	▪ Older children, adolescent, and elderly adult ▪ IV Infusion with moderate flow rate ▪ Medication administration

Contd...

Contd...

24G	Yellow	19	23	<ul><li>Infant, toddler, and older children</li><li>Major surgery and trauma among children</li><li>Can administer fluid and medications</li></ul>
26G	Violet	19	10–15	<ul><li>Neonate, infants, and elderly adults</li><li>Suitable for infusion but infusion rate is low</li></ul>

OXYGEN MASK

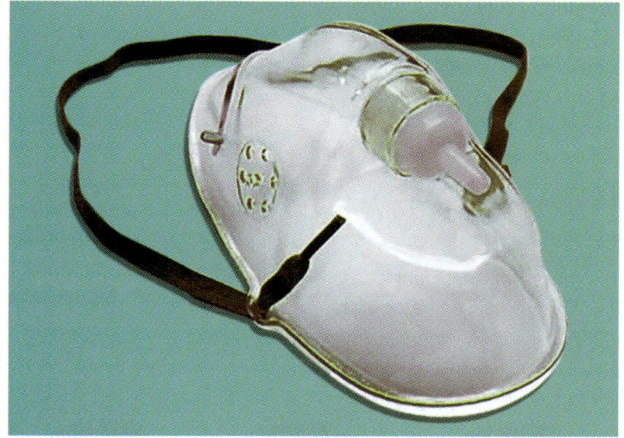

Uses: Used for administering oxygen.

An **oxygen mask** provides a method to transfer breathing oxygen gas from a storage tank to the lungs. Oxygen masks may cover only the nose and mouth (oral nasal mask) or the entire face (fullface mask). They may be made of plastic, silicone, or rubber. The minimum flow rate should be 4 L/min to prevent carbon dioxide accumulation and hence rebreathing. The FiO_2 provided varies between 35% and 60%.

NASAL CANNULA

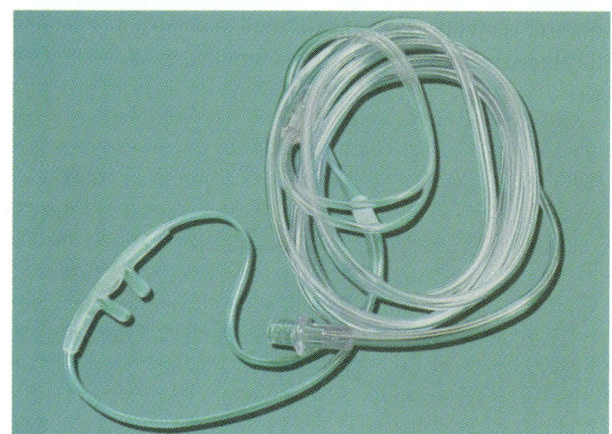

It is an oxygen delivery device. It consists of lightweight tube which on one end splits into two prongs which are placed in the nostrils and delivery a mixture of oxygen and air. The other end of the tube is then connected to an oxygen supply.

It usually provides a low flow rate of oxygen—around 4–6 L/min which equates to an FiO_2 of 37–45%. However, it is easy to use and allows the patient to eat and talk comfortably unlike the other devices.

Higher flow rates can result in drying of the nasal passages making it more uncomfortable and increasing the risk of bleeds from nasal mucosa. The high flow nasal cannula can provide 100% humidified and heated oxygen at flow rates of up to 60 L/min.

VENTURI MASK

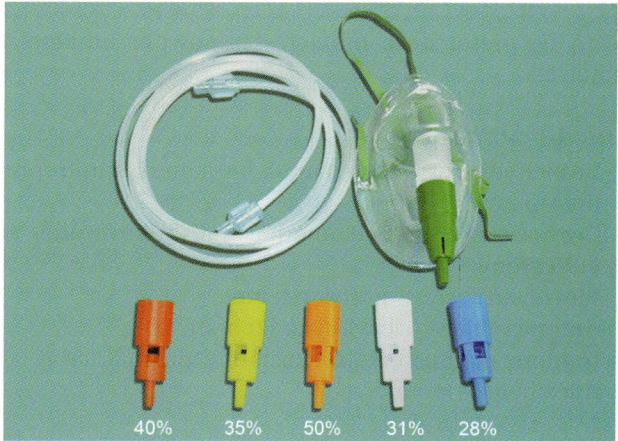

The venturi mask delivers a predetermined and fixed concentration of oxygen to the patient. The different valves have different sixes of constrictions. As air flows through the constriction, negative pressure is created and this causes ambient air to be entrained and mixed with air flow. Hence the smaller the orifice, the more the negative pressure generated and the more ambient air entrained resulting in lower FiO_2. The oxygen concentration can vary between 24% and 60%.

The valves are color coded based on the concentration of oxygen delivered. Due to the high flow rate, the exhaled air is rapidly flushed out of the mask through the holes and hence there is no rebreathing and no increase in dead space.

Venturi masks allow for precise oxygen delivery in patients in whom over ventilation is to be avoided such as COPD patients.

NON-REBREATHER MASK

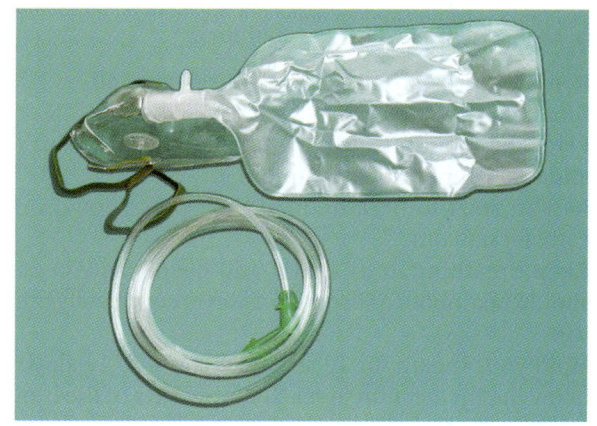

It is also known as Hudsons mask and allows for the delivery of high FiO_2 to a spontaneously breathing patient. Usually delivers FiO_2 between 60% and 90%. It has a reservoir bag that is attached to the fresh gas flow. There is a one-way valve between the reservoir and the patient that prevents exhaled air from entering the reservoir. During expiration the valve also directs the oxygen flow into the reservoir. There should be an adequate air flow rate, usually around 12–15 L/min to ensure the reservoir bag does not collapse during inspiration.

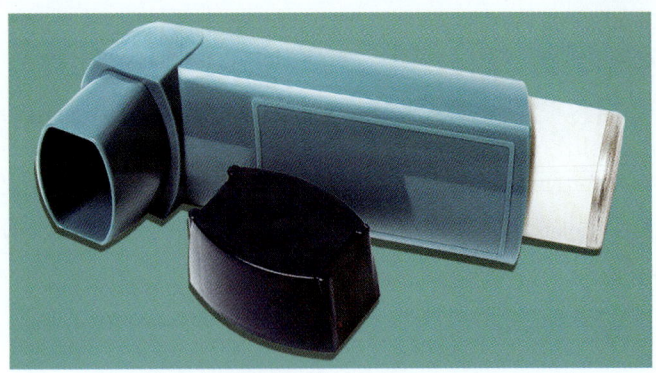

INHALER DEVICES

It can be meter dose inhaler, dry powder inhalers, or nebulizers.

Inhalant Drugs

- Bronchodilators—salbutamol, formeterol, ipratropium, tiotropium
- Corticosteroids—beclomethasone, budesonide, and fluticasone
- Mucolytic agents—acetylcysteine
- Antimicrobials—ribavirin and tobramycin
- Immune modulators—cyclosporine and interferon
- Anesthetics—opioids.

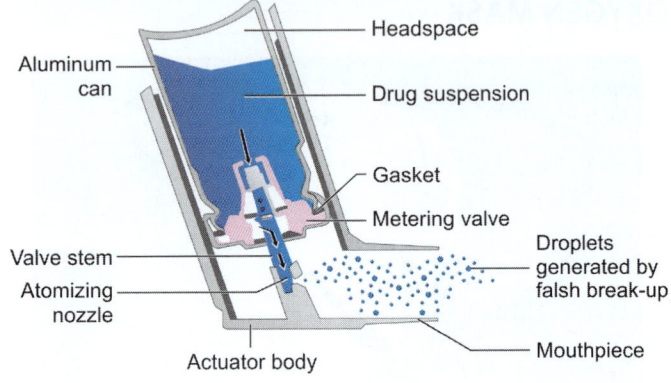

Metered Dose Inhaler

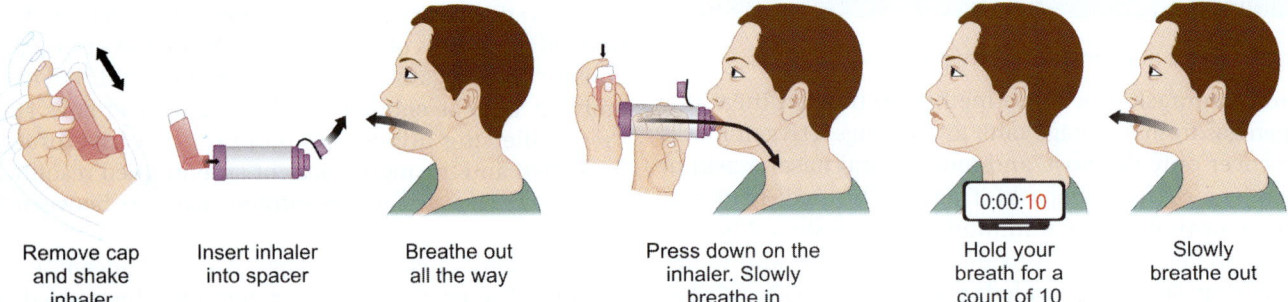

Remove cap and shake inhaler | Insert inhaler into spacer | Breathe out all the way | Press down on the inhaler. Slowly breathe in | Hold your breath for a count of 10 | Slowly breathe out

An metered dose inhaler (MDI) is the most common type of inhaler. It uses a press and breathe method which delivers a specific dose of medication in aerosol form. MDI's use hydrofluoroalkane to propel the medication. Only 20% of the drug will reach the airway if used correctly. The remainder reaches the oropharynx and is then swallowed.

Uses: Using an MDI without a chamber.

- Remove the cap from the MDI and shake well.
- Breathe out all the way.
- Place the mouthpiece of the inhaler between your teeth and seal your lips tightly around it.
- As you start to breathe in slowly, press down on the canister one time.
- Keep breathing in as slowly and deeply as you can (it should take about 5 seconds for you to completely breathe in).
- Hold your breath for 10 seconds (count to 10 slowly) to allow the medication to reach the airways of the lung.
- Repeat the above steps for each puff ordered by your doctor. Wait about 1 minute between puffs.
- Replace the cap on the MDI when finished.

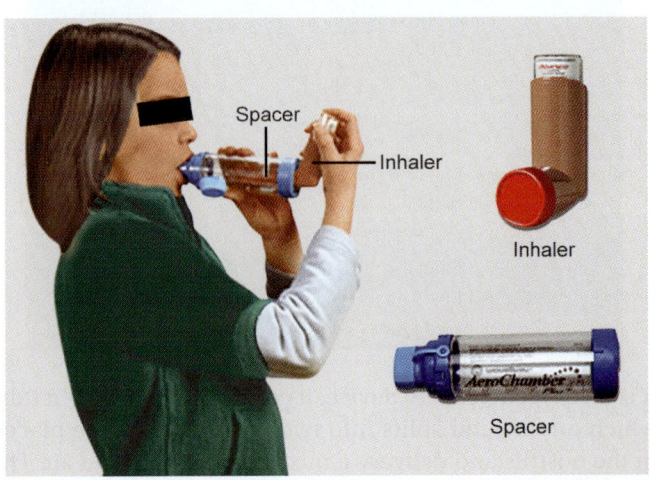

Spacer

A **spacer** is a device used to increase the ease of administering aerosolized medication from a metered dose inhaler (MDI). It adds space in the form of a tube or "chamber" between the mouth and canister of medication. Most spacers have a one way valve that allows the person to inhale the medication while inhaling and exhaling normally; these are often referred to as **valved holding chambers** (VHC).

Metered Dose Inhaler

Advantages	Disadvantages
■ Rapid application ■ Handling ■ Multidose	■ Hand-breath coordination ■ Ineffective use in poor ventilated patients ■ Oropharyngeal deposition and local side effects

Dry Powder Inhalers

Advantages	Disadvantages
■ Less patient coordination required ■ Spacer not necessary ■ Compact, portable ■ No propellant ■ Usually higher lung deposition than a pressurized metered dose inhaler (pMDI)	■ Work poorly if inhalation is not forceful enough ■ Many patients cannot use them correctly ■ Most types are moisture sensitive ■ Need to reload capsule each time

NEBULIZERS

Advantages	Disadvantages
■ Provide therapy for patients who cannot use other inhalation modalities (e.g., MDI and DPI) ■ Allow administration of large doses of medicine ■ Patient coordination not required ■ Effective with tidal breathing ■ Dose modification possible ■ Can be used with ■ Supplemental oxygen	■ Decreased portability ■ Longer set-up ■ Administration time ■ Higher cost ■ Electrical power source required ■ Contamination possible

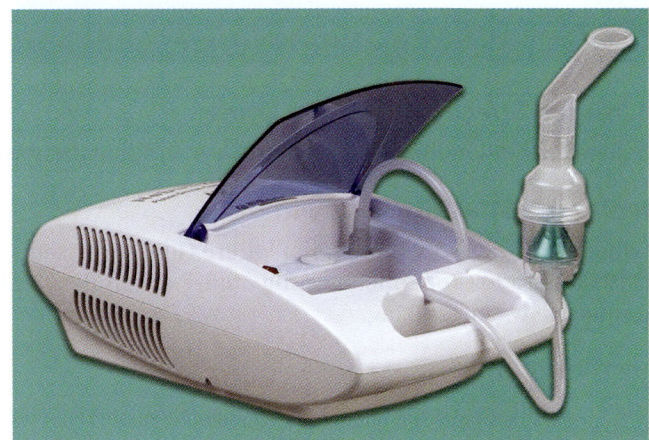

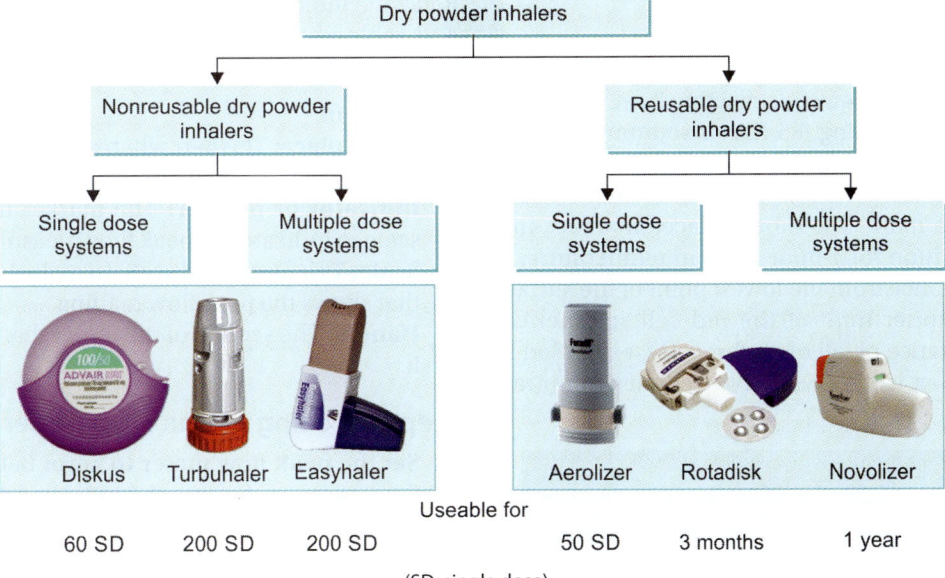

URINOMETER

Urinometer is an instrument used to measure the specific gravity of urine.

There are three parts of urinometer. They are as illustrated in the figure above:
1. **The float:** It is the air containing part
2. **Weight:** The lower end of urinometer
3. **Stem:** It has calibrations with numbers marked to measure the specific gravity.

Normal values of specific gravity are 1.003–1.030. It signifies the relative mass density. Specific gravity of urine is a measure of the concentrating ability of kidneys and is determined to get information about its tubular function.

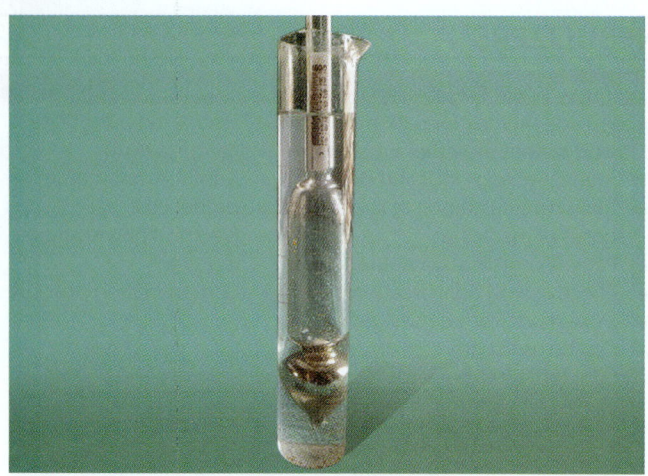

Increased Specific Gravity in Urine
Diabetes mellitus, nephritic syndrome, fever and dehydration.

Decreased Specific Gravity in Urine
Diabetes insipidus, chronic renal failure (low and fixed at 1.010) due to loss of concentrating ability of tubules, and compulsive water drinking.

Isosthenuria
This is condition where there is a fixed specific gravity. The specific gravity of the urine remains at 1.010 regardless of the volume of water consumption by the person. It occurs specifically in chronic renal disease.

WESTERGREN TUBE

The Westergren method requires collecting 2 mL of venous blood into a tube containing 0.5 mL of sodium citrate. It should be stored no longer than 2 hours at room temperature or 6 hours at 4°C. The blood is drawn into a Westergren-Katz tube to the 200 mm mark. The tube is placed in a rack in a strictly vertical position for 1 hour at room temperature, at which time the distance from the lowest point of the surface meniscus to the upper limit of the red cell sediment is measured. The distance of fall of erythrocytes, expressed as millimeters in 1 hour, is the erythrocyte sedimentation rate (ESR).

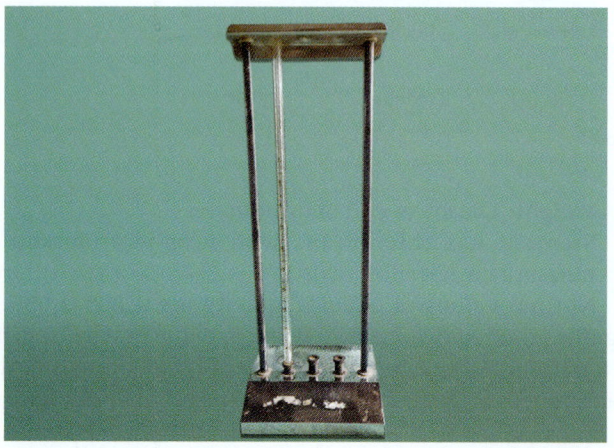

PEAK FLOW METER

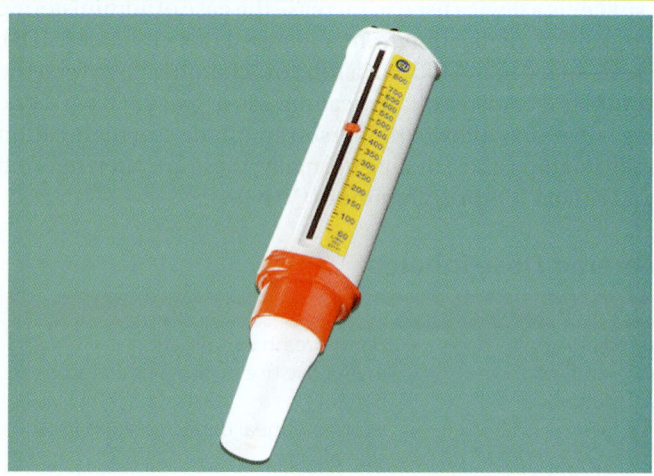

It is a handheld device that shows the amount and rate of air that can be forcefully exhaled out in a single breath. By measuring the air flow through the bronchi, it shows the degree of obstruction. Hence it is useful in asthma patients to assess severity and decide on treatment. The measurements are compared to measurements taken against the general population. The peak expiratory flow rates are classified into three zones of measurement—green, yellow and red. Green indicates normal (80–100% normal or usual flow rate) and good control of asthma symptoms. Yellow is 50–79% of usual or normal flow rates and indicates narrowing of the airways. Red zone indicates less than 50% usual or normal flow rates and requires emergency management of the obstructive disease.

It consists of:
- **Mouthpiece:** The part where the patient places their lips during the measurement.
- **Indicator or pointer:** The marker that moves along a scale to indicate the peak flow measurement.
- **Scale:** The numerical scale (usually in liters per minute) that shows the peak flow reading.
- **Handle:** The section of the meter that is held while using it.

Steps for Using a Peak Flow Meter
1. **Set the peak flow meter to zero:** Before using the peak flow meter, make sure the indicator or pointer is at zero or the baseline reading. If the pointer is not at zero, gently tap or reset it to ensure accurate measurements.
2. **Stand up straight:** For the most accurate results, it is important to stand up straight or sit upright. This ensures that your lungs are fully expanded and you can exhale air efficiently.
3. **Take a deep breath:** Take a **deep breath** in, filling your lungs as much as possible. It is important not to inhale too forcefully, as this may affect the results. Just take a normal, deep breath.
4. **Place the mouthpiece in your mouth:** Place the mouthpiece of the peak flow meter into your mouth.

Be sure to **seal your lips tightly** around the mouthpiece to avoid any air leaks, which could give inaccurate results.

5. **Exhale as hard and fast as you can:** Once the mouthpiece is in place, exhale **as hard and fast as possible** into the meter. You should aim to make a **forceful and quick exhalation** (like blowing out candles on a cake). This action will move the pointer along the scale and give you the peak flow reading.

6. **Record the measurement:** Once you have exhaled completely, record the **peak flow value** shown by the pointer on the scale. This value is usually in liters per minute (L/min).

7. **Repeat the measurement:** It is recommended to perform **three measurements**, waiting about 30 seconds to 1 minute between each one. This helps ensure consistency and accuracy. Record the highest of the three readings, as it is the most reliable indication of your peak flow.

14 CHAPTER

Spotters

In the practical exams 2–3 spotters are kept, where in the student has to observe the patients (inspection) and come to a diagnosis/justify the diagnosis. A few questions regarding the condition will be asked.

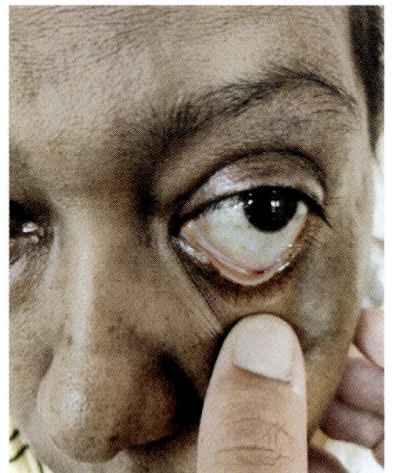

Fig. 14.1: Pallor.

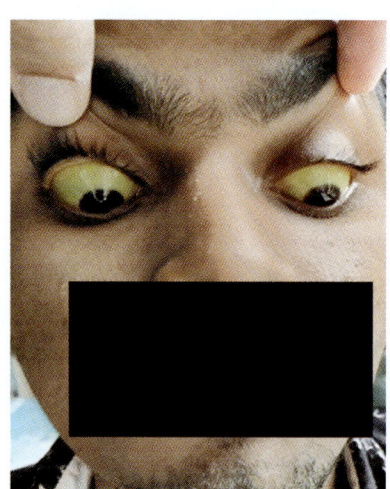

Fig. 14.2: Icterus.

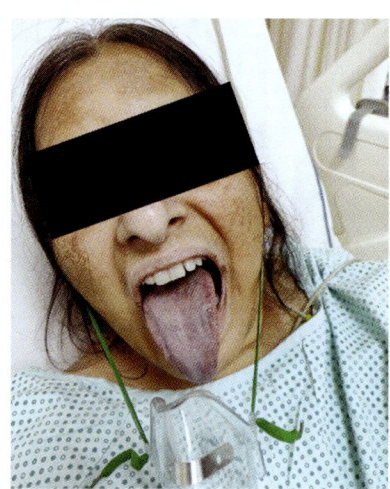

Fig. 14.3: Cyanosis.

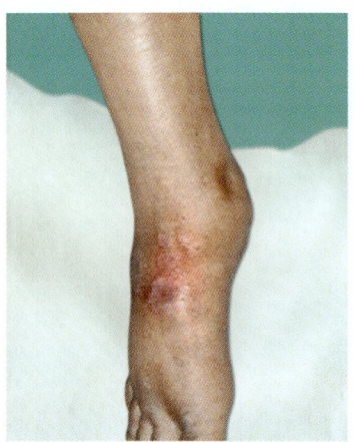

Fig. 14.4: Pitting edema.

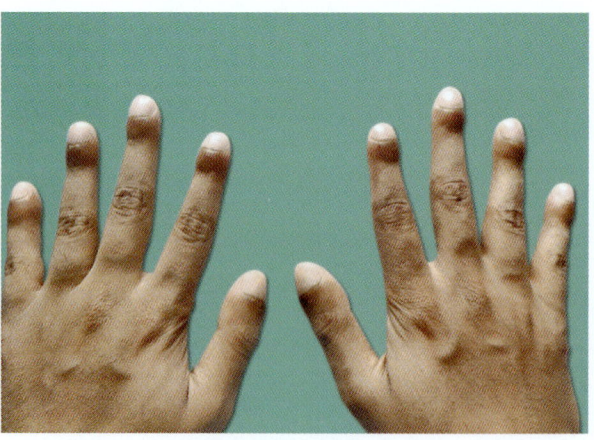

Fig. 14.5: Clubbing.

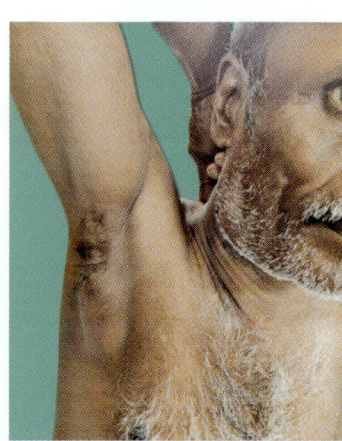

Fig. 14.6: Axillary lymphadenopathy.

Spotters

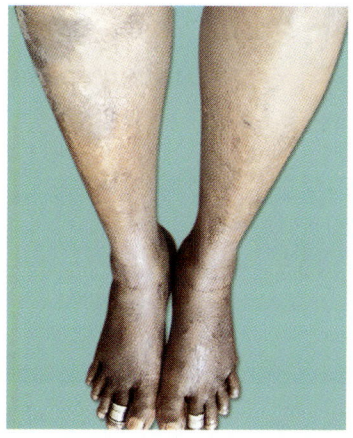

Fig. 14.7: Nonpitting type of pedal edema.

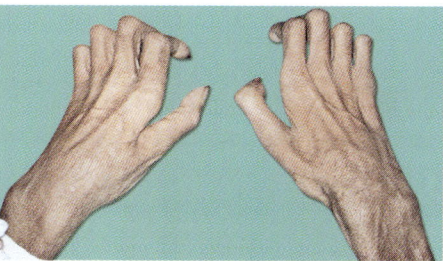

Fig. 14.8: Claw hand.

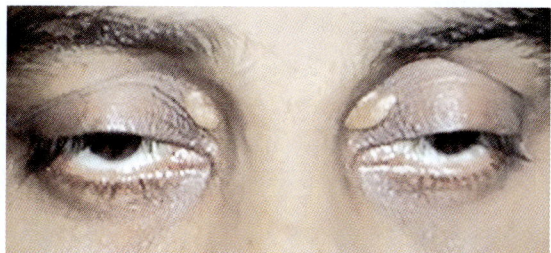

Fig. 14.9: Xanthelasma.

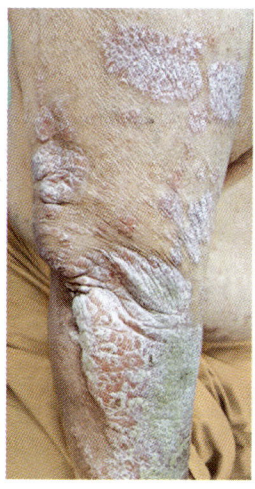

Fig. 14.10: Psoriasis.

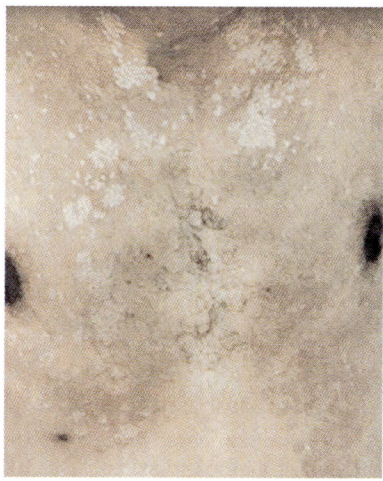

Fig. 14.11: Pityriasis versicolor (tinea versicolor).

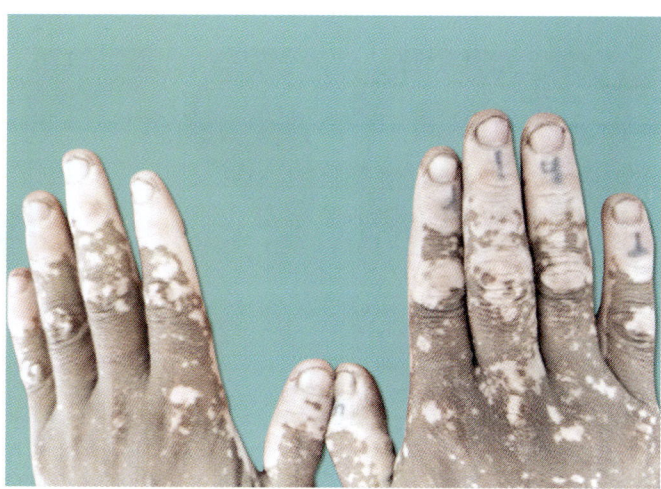

Fig. 14.12: Vitiligo.

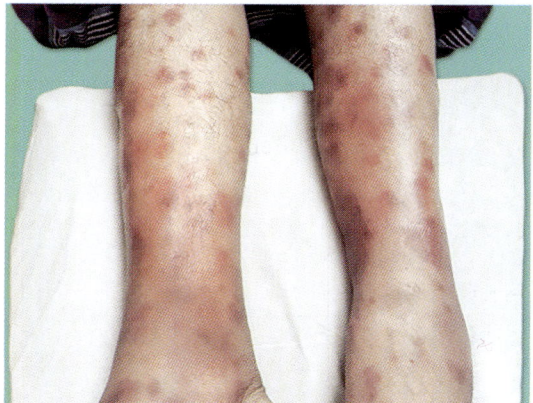

Fig. 14.13: Erythema nodosum.

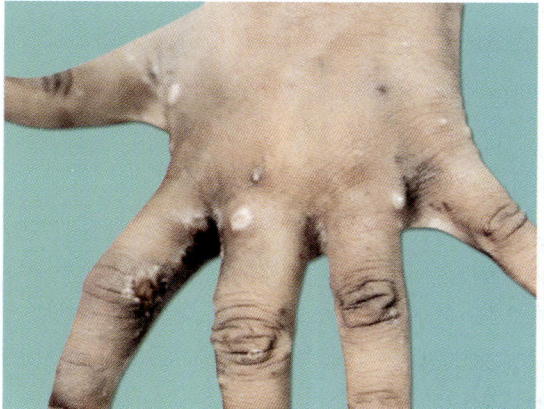

Fig. 14.14: Scabies.

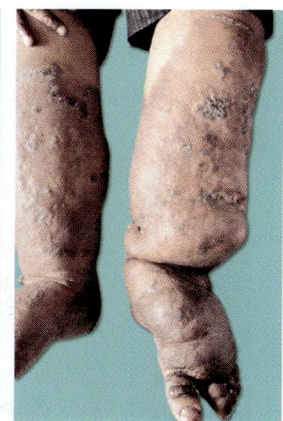

Fig. 14.15: Filariasis.

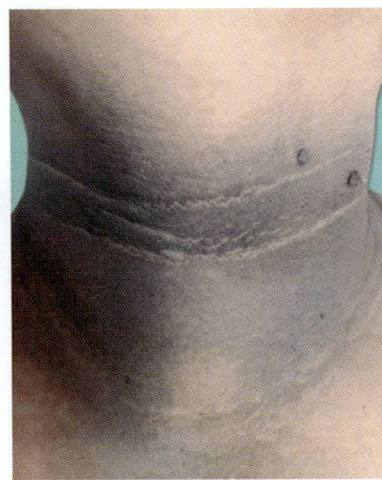

Fig. 14.16: Acanthosis nigricans and skin tags.

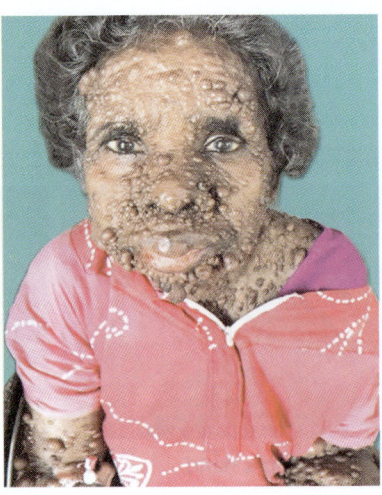

Fig. 14.17: Neurofibromatosis.

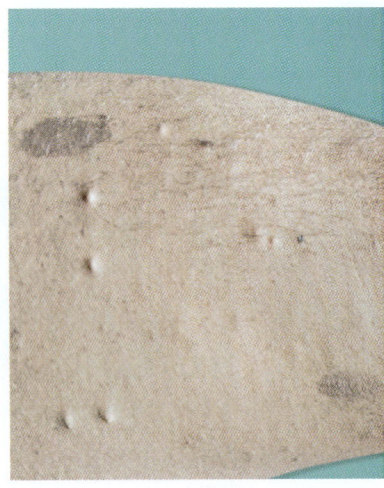

Fig. 14.18: Café-au-lait macules (CALM).

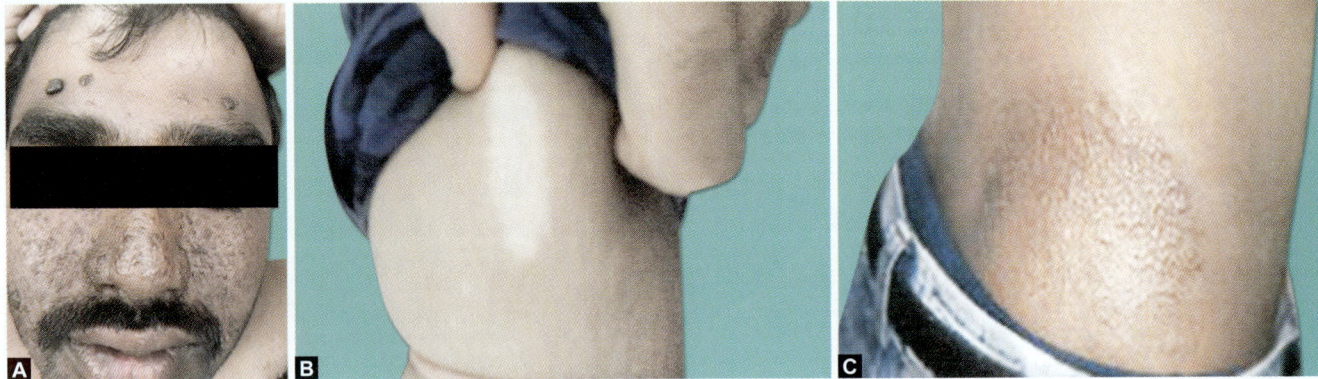

Figs. 14.19A to C: (A) Adenoma sebaceum; (B) Ash leaf-shaped macule is a hypopigmented macule—oval at one end and pointed at the opposite end; (C) Shagreen patches—tuberous sclerosis.

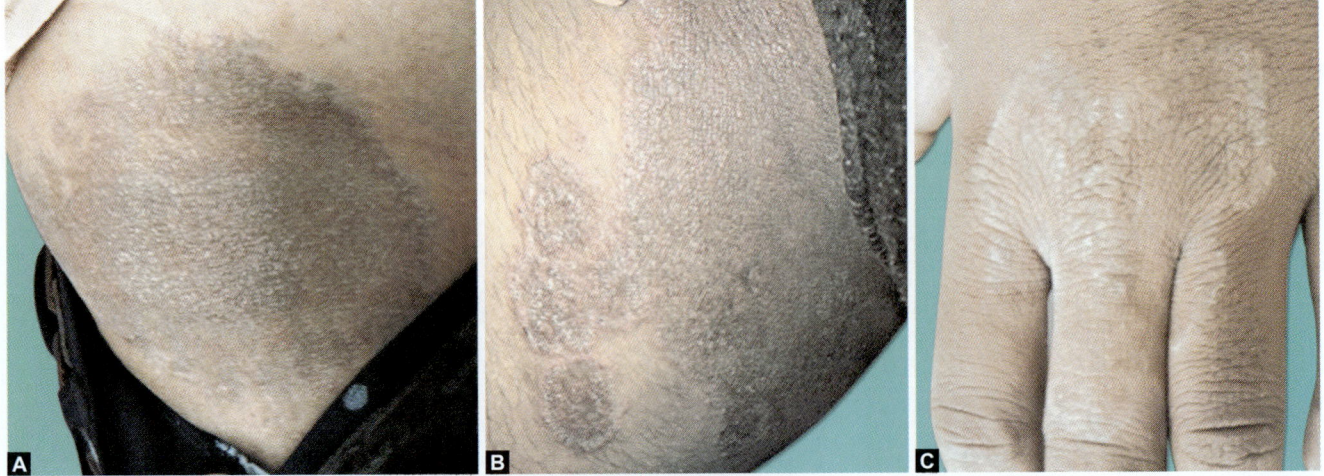

Figs. 14.20A to C: (A) Tinea corporis; (B) Tinea cruris; (C) Tinea manuum.

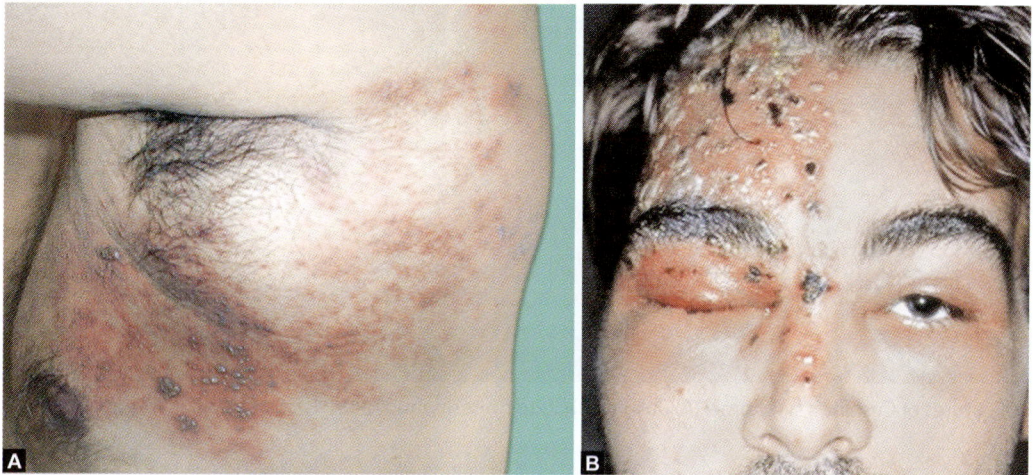

Figs. 14.21A and B: (A) Herpes zoster—dermatomal involvement; (B) Herpes zoster ophthalmicus.

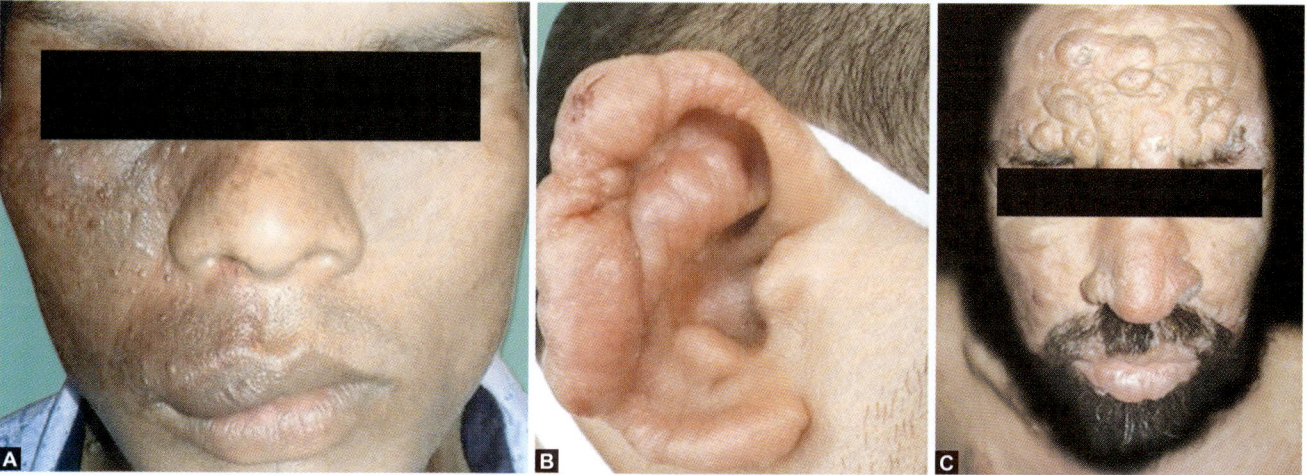

Figs. 14.22A to C: Lesions of lepromatous leprosy. (A) Facial involvement; (B) Nodular lesions on ear; (C) Leonine facies.

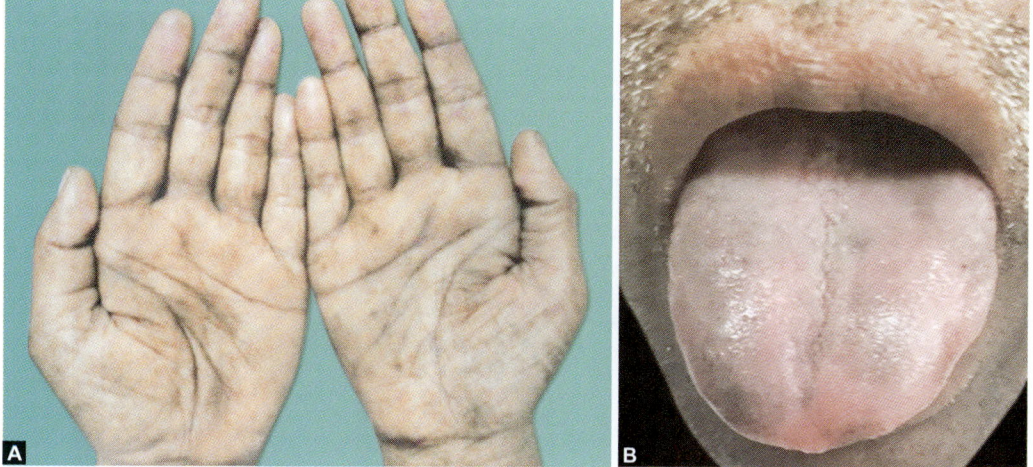

Figs. 14.23A and B: (A) Pigmentation of palms; (B) Oral pigmentation in Addison's disease.

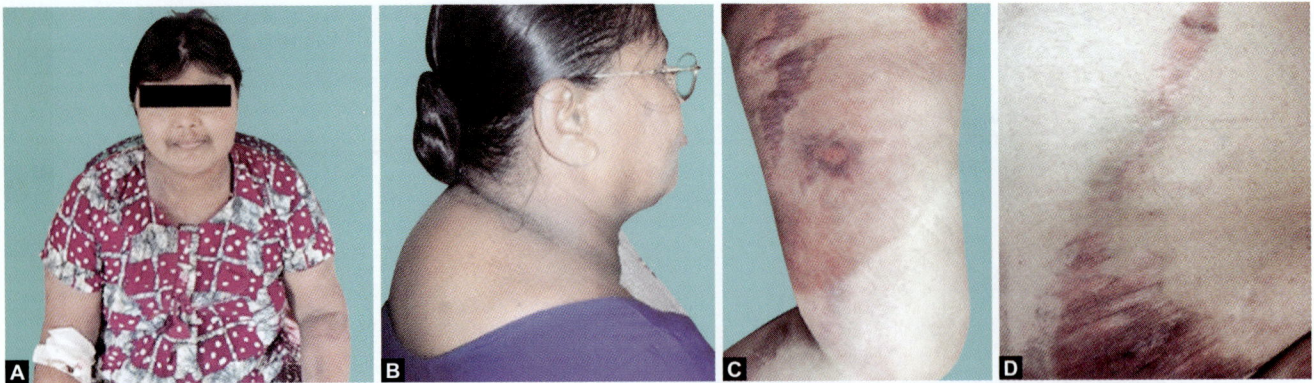

Figs. 14.24A to D: Features of Cushing's syndrome. (A) Cushing's habitus, obesity, and moon facies; (B) Buffalo hump; (C and D) Pigmented striae.

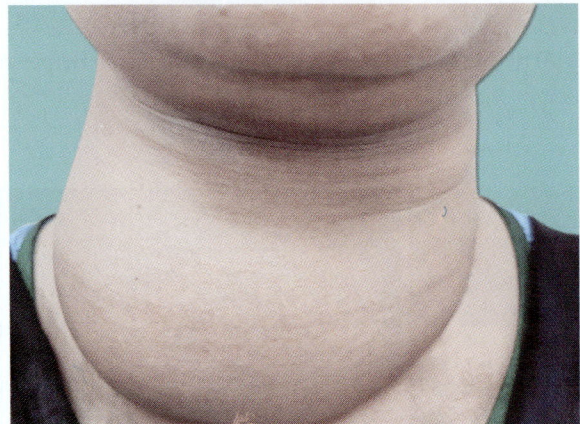

Fig. 14.25: Thyromegaly.

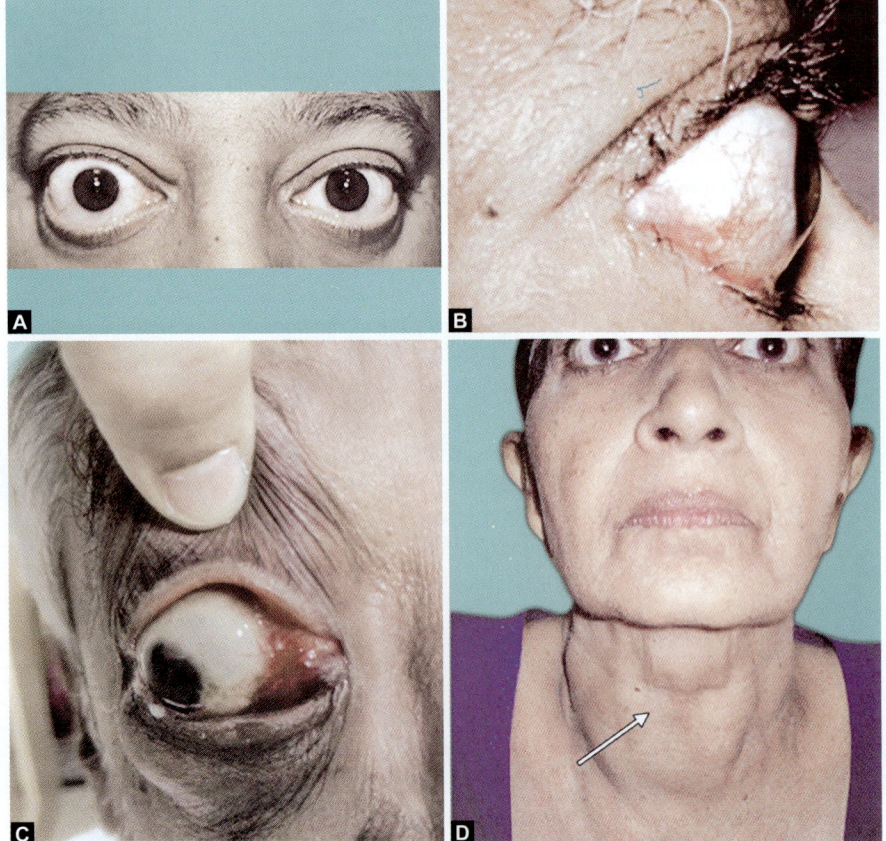

Figs. 14.26A to D: (A and B) Exophthalmos (front and side view); (C) Infiltration of extraocular muscles in hyperthyroidism; (D) Eye signs and enlarged nodular goiter (arrow).

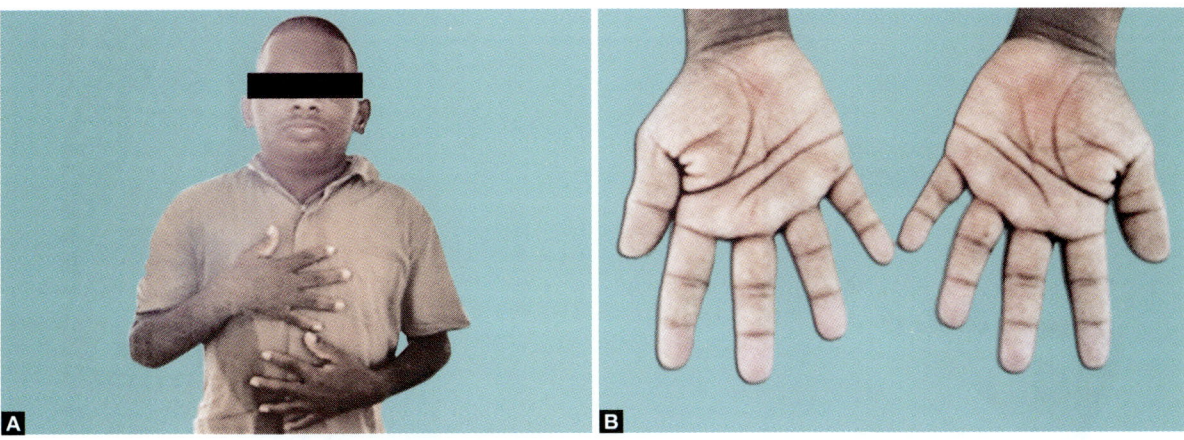

Figs. 14.27A and B: (A) Acromegalic facies; (B) Thick and spade-shaped hands.

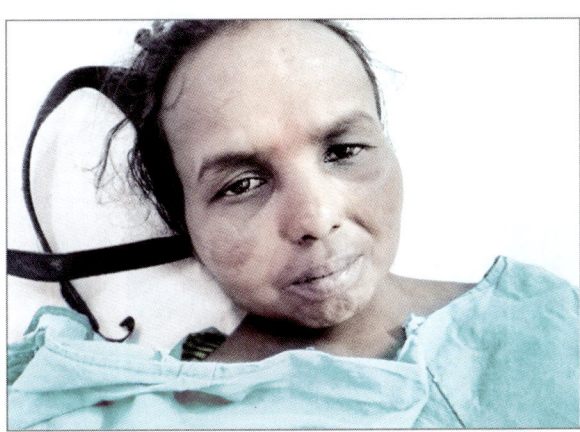

Fig. 14.28: Systemic lupus erythematosus—malar rash, alopecia.

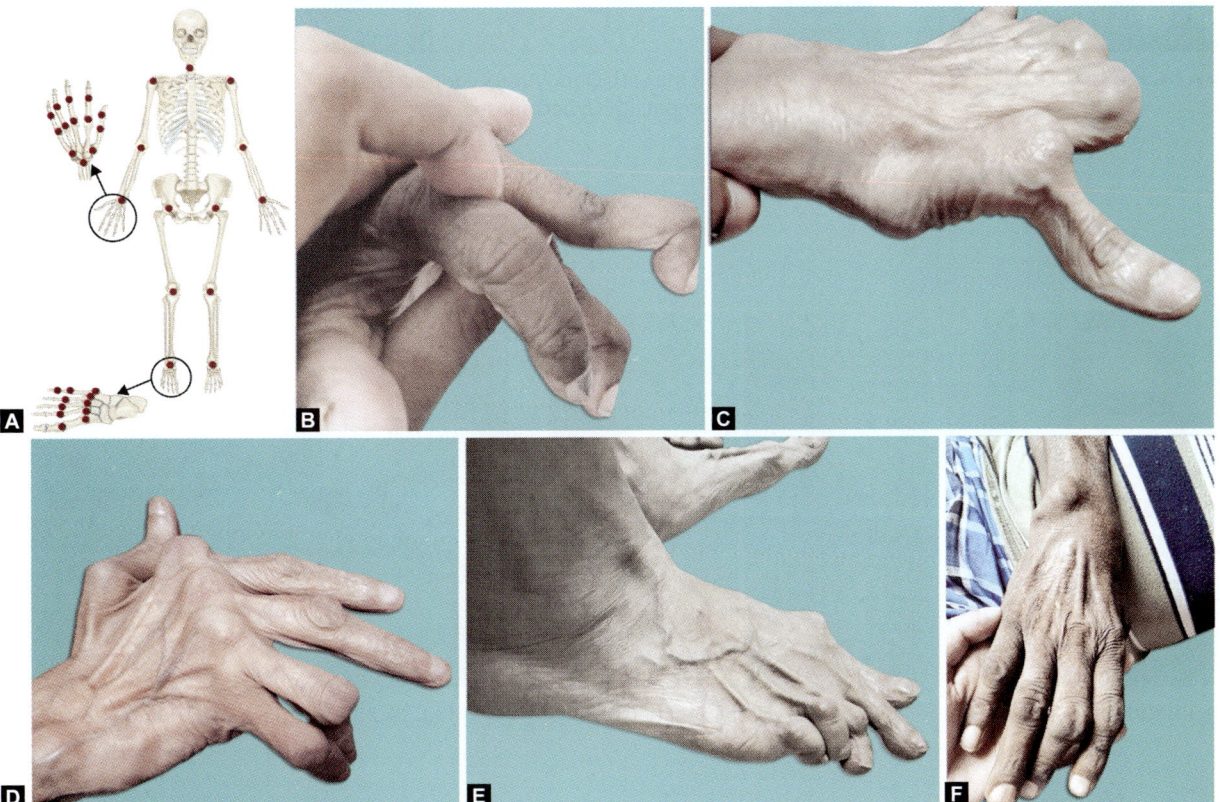

Figs. 14.29A to F: Rheumatoid arthritis. (A) Pattern of joint involvement; (B) Swan neck deformity; (C) Boutonniere deformity; (D) Z deformity and ulnar deviation; (E) Hammer toes and hallux valgus; (F) Bowstring sign.

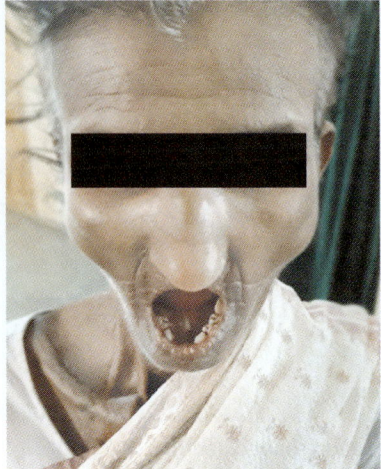

Fig. 14.30: Scleroderma facies.

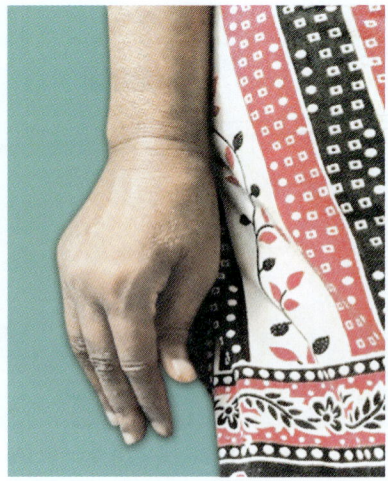

Fig. 14.31: Parkinson's hand tremors.

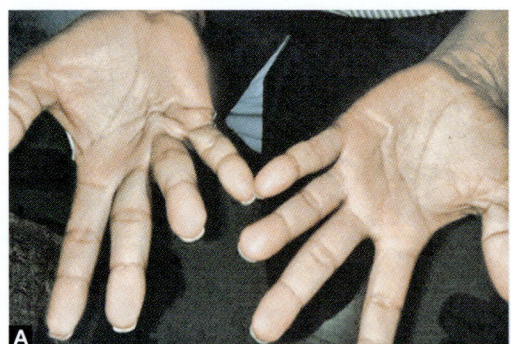
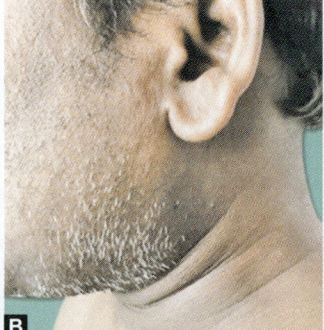
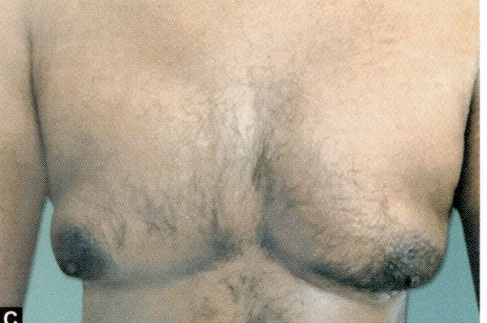

Figs. 14.32A to C: Features of cirrhosis. (A) Palmar erythema with Dupuytren's contracture; (B) Diminished facial hair with parotid enlargement; (C) Gynecomastia.

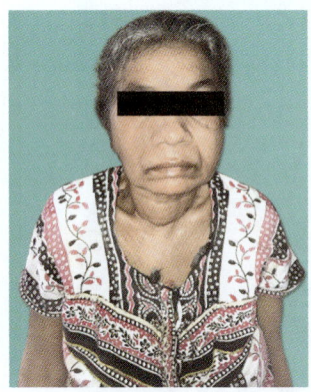

Fig. 14.33: Parkinson's facies.

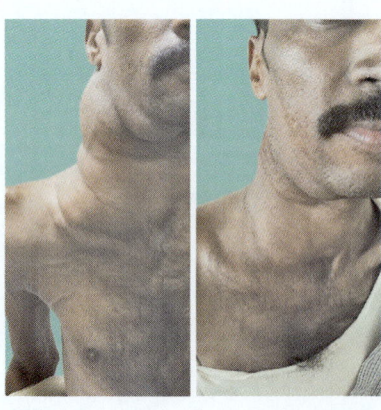

Fig. 14.34: Cervical lymphadenopathy.

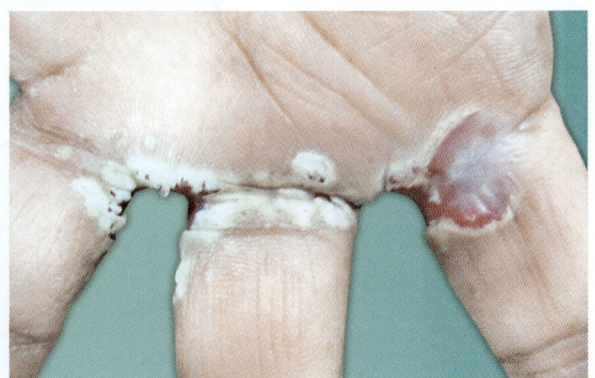

Fig. 14.35: Intertrigo (intertriginous dermatitis).

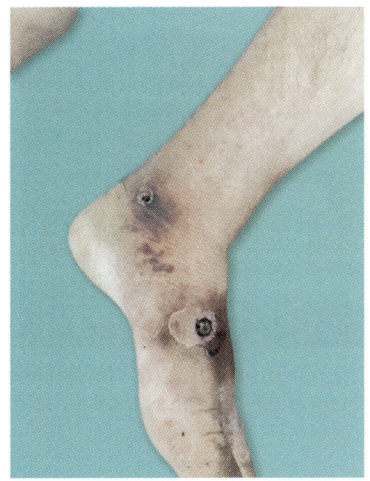

Fig. 14.36: Typhus—eschar with rash.

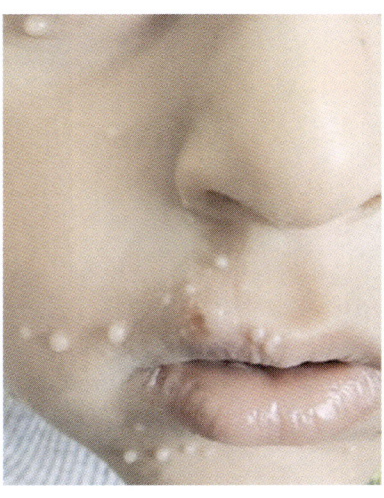

Fig. 14.37: Molluscum contagiosum.

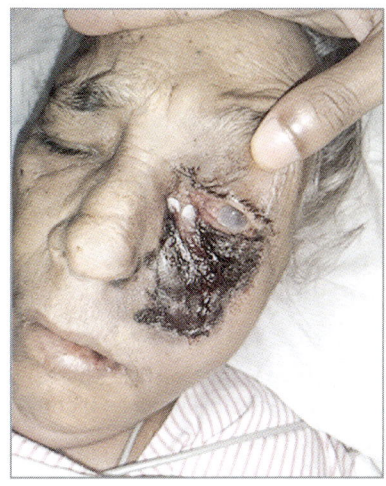

Fig. 14.38: Rhinocerebral mucormycosis.

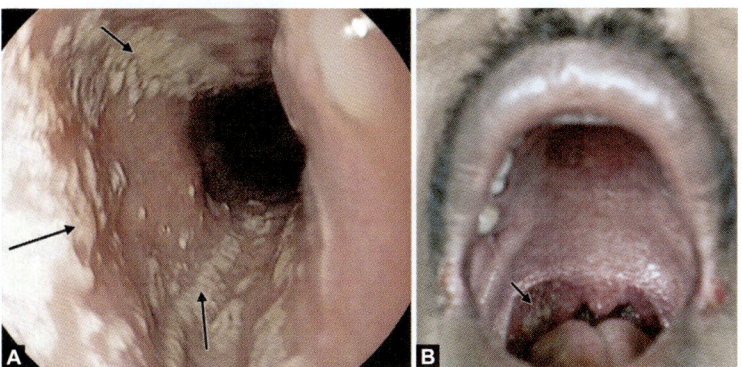

Figs. 14.39A and B: (A) Esophageal candidiasis; (B) Oral candidiasis.

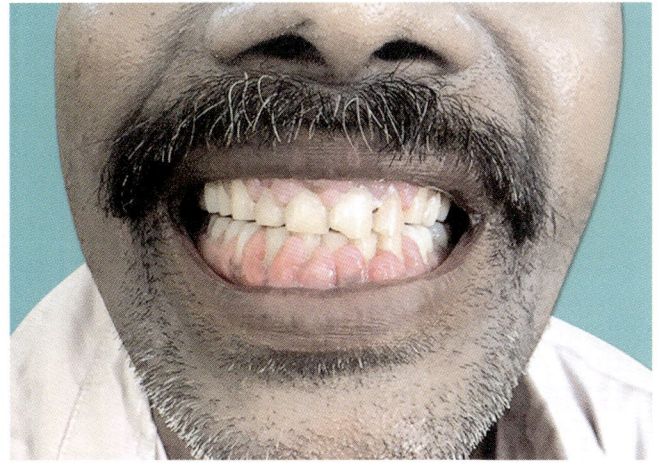

Fig. 14.40: Gingival hyperplasia.

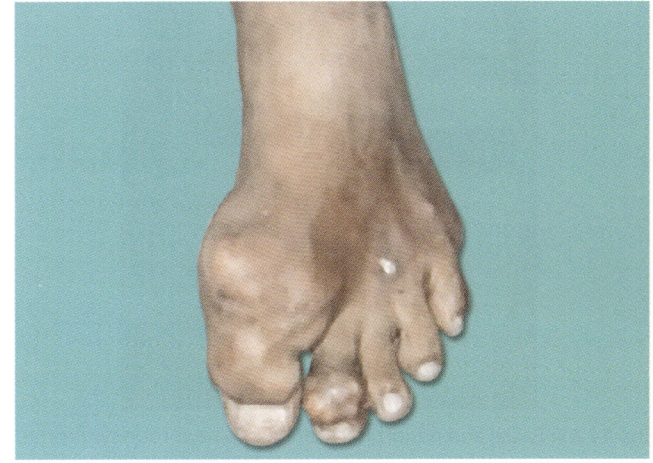

Fig. 14.41: Acute gouty arthritis involving the first metatarsophalangeal (MTP) joint (termed podagra).

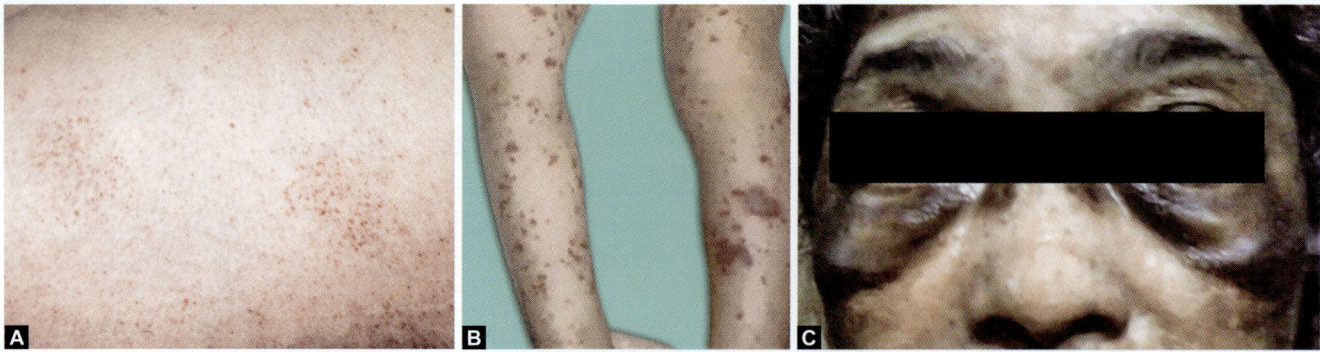

Figs. 14.42A to C: (A) Petechiae which appear as small (1–2 mm in diameter), red to purple hemorrhagic spots in the skin, mucous membranes or serosal surfaces; (B) Purpura—slightly larger (>3 mm) than petechiae; (C) Ecchymoses are larger (>1–2 cm) and result from blood escaping.

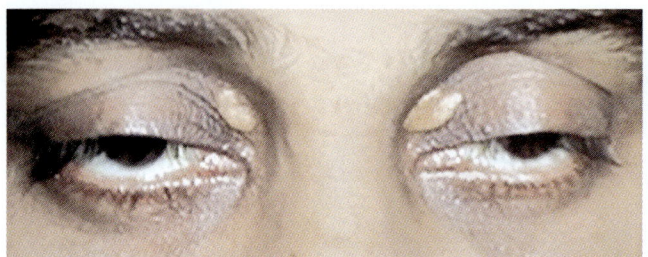

Fig. 14.43: Xanthelasmas around the eyes.

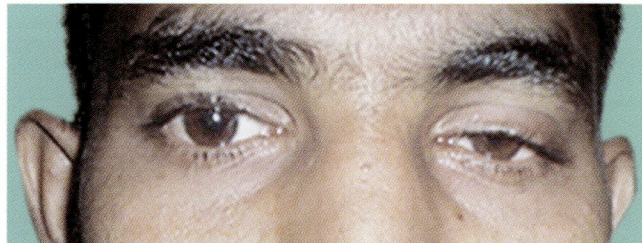

Fig. 14.44: Left Horner's syndrome (ptosis and miosis).

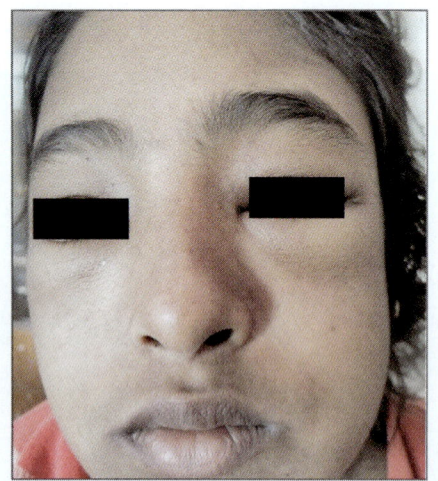

Fig. 14.45: Facial and periorbital puffiness in nephrotic syndrome.

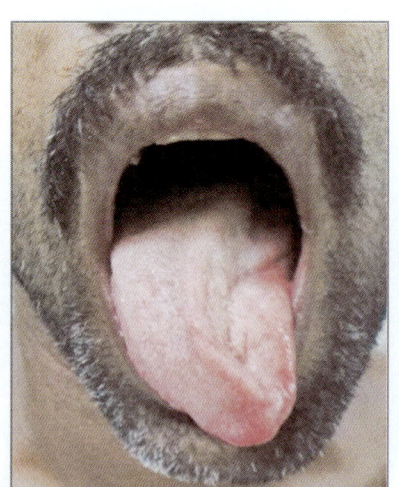

Fig. 14.46: Tongue wasting with deviation.

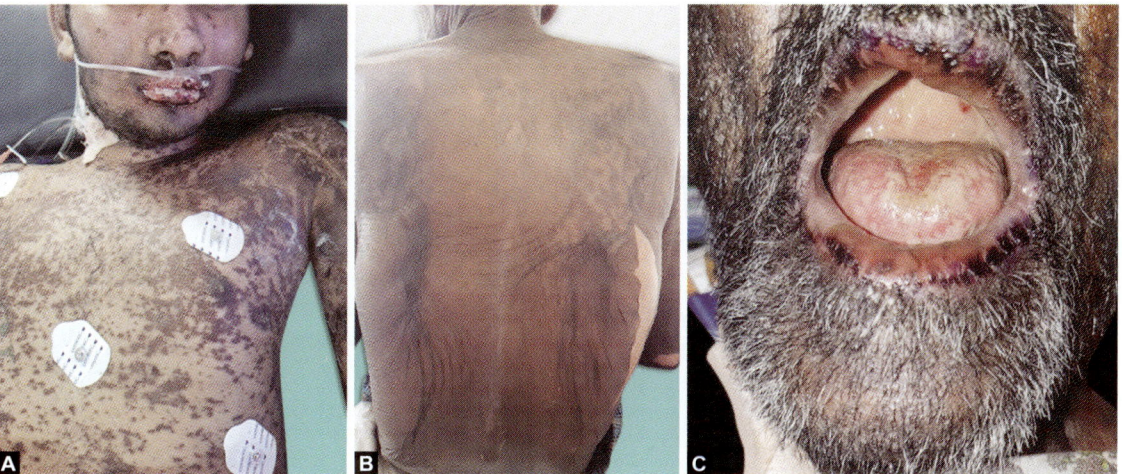

Figs. 14.47A to C: (A) Stevens-Johnson syndrome (SJS)/toxic epidermal necrolysis (TEN); (B) Toxic epidermal necrolysis; (C) Oral lesions in SJS/TEN.

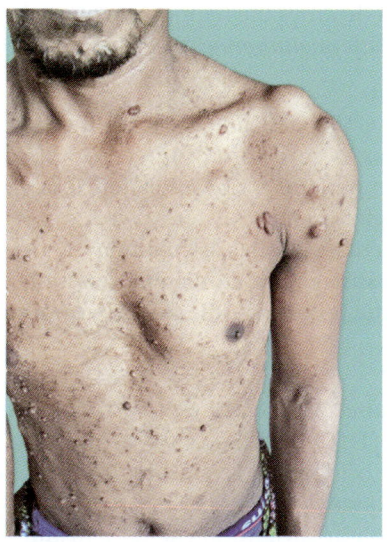

Fig. 14.48: Neurofibromatosis.

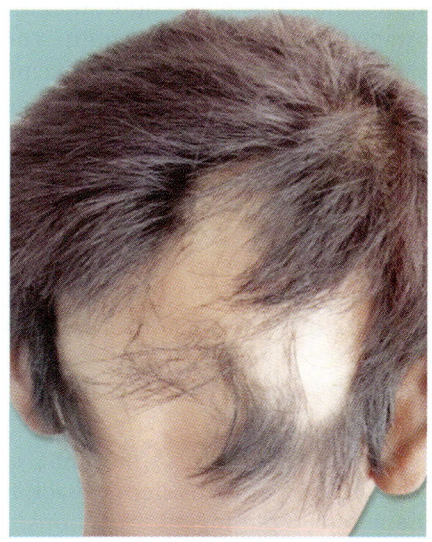

Fig. 14.49: Alopecia areata.

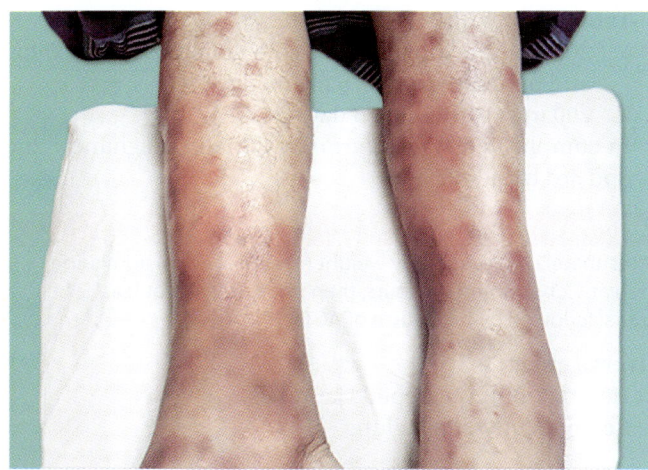

Fig. 14.50: Erythema nodosum on both legs.

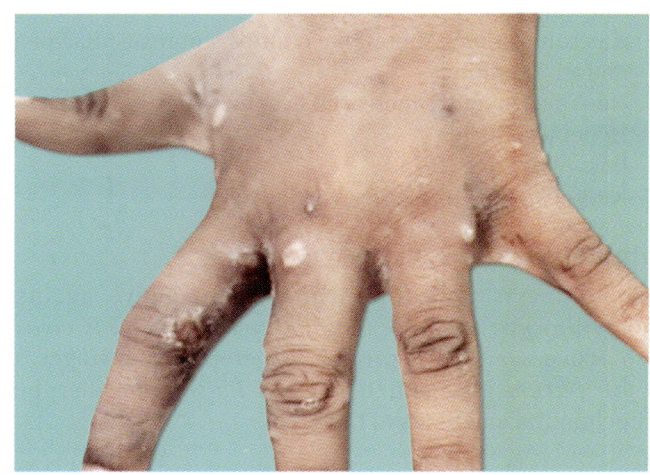

Fig. 14.51: Scabies involving the web spaces of the fingers.

CHAPTER 15: Discussion on Drugs and Medical Emergencies

1. ANTIMALARIALS

Chloroquine

Binds to and inhibits DNA and RNA polymerase; interferes with metabolism and hemoglobin utilization by parasites; inhibits prostaglandin effects; chloroquine concentrates within parasite acid vesicles and raises internal pH resulting in inhibition of parasite growth; may involve aggregates of ferriprotoporphyrin IX acting as chloroquine receptors causing membrane damage; may also interfere with nucleoprotein synthesis.

Indications and dosing:

Type of infection	Suppressive treatment
P. vivax and P. ovale	Chloroquine 25 mg of salt/kg over 36–48 hours
P. malariae and P. knowlesi	Chloroquine 25 mg of salt/kg over 36–48 hours

Chloroquine is also used for treatment of hepatic amebiasis, rheumatoid arthritis, lepra reaction, discoid lupus erythematosus, photogenic reactions, infectious mononucleosis.

Adverse effect:
- Cardiovascular: Atrioventricular block, bundle branch block, cardiac arrhythmia
- Alopecia, bulls eye maculopathy
- Gastrointestinal: Abdominal cramps, anorexia, diarrhea, nausea, vomiting
- Hepatic: Hepatitis, increased liver enzymes
- Hypersensitivity
- Loss of hearing
- Nervous system: Seizures, CNS toxicity

Primaquine

Primaquine is an antiprotozoal agent active against exoerythrocytic stages of *Plasmodium ovale* and *P. vivax*, also active against the primary exoerythrocytic stages of *P. falciparum* and gametocytes of *Plasmodia*; disrupts mitochondria and binds to DNA.

Indications and dosing:
- *P. falciparum:* Primaquine 0.75 mg/kg in single dose as gametocytocidal
  - **Radical cure of malaria due to *P. vivax* and *P. ovale*.**
  - Primaquine is given at a dose of 15 mg daily for 14 days. It destroys the hypnozoite phase in the liver.
- *Pneumocystis pneumoniae* (PCP) in HIV-infected patients

Adverse effect:
- Screen for G6PD deficiency prior to therapy initiation
- Hematologic and oncologic: Anemia, hemolytic anemia (in patients with G6PD deficiency), leukopenia, methemoglobinemia
- Cardiovascular: Cardiac arrhythmia
- Gastrointestinal: Pain, stomach discomfort
- **Primaquine is contraindicated in pregnancy**

Artesunate

Rapidly metabolized to the active metabolite, dihydroartemisinin (DHA). Artesunate and DHA contain an endoperoxide bridge that is activated by heme iron binding, resulting in oxidative stress, inhibition of protein and nucleic acid synthesis, ultrastructural changes, resulting in cell lysis and a decrease in parasite growth and survival.

Indications and dosing: *P. falciparum*
- The ACT used in the national program in India is artesunate + sulfadoxine + pyrimethamine. It is given in **Table 15.1**:
  - 200 mg artesunate along with sulfadoxine 1,500 mg and pyrimethamine 75 mg on day 1.
  - 200 mg artesunate on days 2 and 3.
- In complicated *P. falciparum* malaria in pregnancy: 2nd and 3rd trimester

Table 15.1: Treatment of severe malaria.

Artesunate 2.4 mg/kg body weight (BW) IV or IM on admission; then at 12 hours and 24 hours, then once a day for at least 24 hours, followed by full course of ACT

Adverse effect:
- Hemoglobinuria, hepatic jaundice
- Renal: Acute renal failure

2. ANTITUBERCULAR (TABLE 15.2)

Table 15.2: Tuberculous foci and the drugs acting on them.

Tuberculous foci	Drugs acting on them
Extracellular, in alkaline medium	Streptomycin
Rapidly metabolizing mycobacteria (in a cavity)	Rifampicin
Less actively multiplying bacilli in acidic and closed lesions	Isoniazid
Dormant bacilli (that cause a relapse)	Pyrazinamide

Isoniazid

Isoniazid (INH): It is primarily tuberculocidal drug.

Mechanism of action: Inhibition of mycolic acid cell wall synthesis via O_2-dependent pathways (e.g., catalase-peroxidase reaction). Two gene products labelled InhA and KasA are the targets. Bactericidal against rapidly multiplying and bacteriostatic against resting bacilli. **Active against both extracellular and intracellular organisms.** Resistance occurs spontaneously in 1 in 10^5 bacilli.

Drug (daily dosages)	Adverse reactions	
	Major	Less common (rare)
Isoniazid (H) (5–10 mg/kg)	• Hepatitis • Peripheral neuropathy (preventable and treatable with pyridoxine) • Cutaneous hypersensitivity	Giddiness, seizures, optic neuritis, mental symptoms, hemolytic anemia, aplastic anemia, agranulocytosis, lupoid reactions, arthralgia, and gynecomastia

Tuberculosis Chemoprophylaxis—Isoniazid Preventive Therapy

- **Purpose:** To prevent progression of latent tuberculous infection to active disease.
- **Types:**
  - **Primary or infection prophylaxis:** Drug is given to individuals who have not been infected in order to prevent development of disease (e.g., breastfed infants of sputum-positive mother).
  - **Secondary or disease prophylaxis:** Drug is given to prevent development of disease in individuals already infected.
- **Drugs used: Isoniazid** (H) at the dose of 5 mg/kg/day (not exceeding 300 mg/day) for 6–12 months is used for chemoprophylaxis.

Rifampicin

Mechanism of action: Interrupts RNA synthesis by binding to mycobacterial DNA-dependent RNA polymerase. **Bactericidal against both extracellular and intercellular organisms.**

Drug dosage	Adverse reactions	
	Major	Less common (rare)
Rifampicin (R) (10 mg/kg)	Febrile reactions ("flu" syndrome; more common with intermittent therapy), hepatitis, cutaneous reactions, and gastrointestinal disturbances	Shortness of breath, shock, hemolytic anemia, interstitial nephritis, and thrombocytopenia

Other indications of rifampicin: Anaplasmosis, symptomatic; *Bartonella* spp. infections; brucellosis; cholestatic pruritus; endocarditis, treatment; hidradenitis suppurativa; leprosy; meningococcal disease; mycobacterial (nontuberculous) infection; *Staphylococcus* spp. infections,

Pyrazinamide

Mechanism of action: Inhibition of mycolic acid cell wall synthesis and resembles INH. Bactericidal to slowly metabolizing bacilli in phagosome/granuloma. Most effective in acidic pH

Drug (daily dosages)	Adverse reactions	
	Major	Less common
Pyrazinamide (Z) (20 mg/kg)	Anorexia, nausea, flushing, hepatitis, gastrointestinal disturbance, and hyperuricemia, gout	Vomiting, arthralgia, cutaneous hypersensitivity, loss of diabetes control

Ethambutol

Mechanism of action (MOA): It inhibits arabinose (arabinosyl transferase) involved in arabinogalactan synthesis and is bacteriostatic.

Drug (daily dosages)	Adverse reactions	
	Major	Less common
Ethambutol (E) (15 mg/kg)	Retrobulbar neuritis (dose related) and arthralgia	Peripheral neuropathy and rash

Streptomycin

It is an aminoglycoside, bactericidal antibiotic.

Drug (daily dosages)	Adverse reactions	
	Major	Less common
Streptomycin (S) and other aminoglycosides (15–20 mg/kg)	8th nerve damage, cutaneous hypersensitivity, giddiness, numbness, and tinnitus	Vertigo, ataxia, deafness, hypokalemia, renal damage, aplastic anemia, and agranulocytosis

Second Line Agents

Ethionamide: It is structurally related to INH and acts by inhibiting mycolic acid synthesis. It is effective against bacilli, resistant to other drugs, and is effective in infections due to atypical mycobacteria. It is effective against both intracellular and extracellular organisms.

Cycloserine: It is mainly bacteriostatic and acts by inhibiting the synthesis of the bacterial cell wall. It is effective against bacilli resistant to INH or streptomycin and against atypical mycobacteria. Antitubercular activity is less than that of these two drugs.

Fluoroquinolones: Ciprofloxacin, ofloxacin, levofloxacin, moxifloxacin, and gatifloxacin are active against *M. tuberculosis,* even in cases resistant to other drugs. Given orally or IV. It is useful in treating infections resistant to standard drugs and in relapse cases.

Capreomycin: It is bactericidal and its mechanism of action, pharmacokinetics, and adverse reactions are similar to those of streptomycin. Administer with caution in presence of renal impairment.

Kanamycin and amikacin: Both are bactericidal and are active against bacilli resistant to streptomycin, INH, and cycloserine.

Macrolides: Newer macrolides, azithromycin and clarithromycin, also have action against tubercular bacilli. They are used to treat typical mycobacterial infection as well as in relapse cases.

Newer antitubercular drugs:
- Rifapentin/Rifabutin
- Bedaquiline
- Delaminid
- Sutezolid
- Pretomanid

Drugs	Common adverse effects	Rare adverse effects
Ethionamide (Etm) (10–20 mg/kg)	Anorexia and vomiting	Serious neurologic reactions and hepatitis
Cycloserine (Cys) (10–20 mg/kg)	Headache and somnolence	Psychosis, seizures, and peripheral neuropathy
Quinolones (7.5–15 mg/kg)	GI intolerance and skin rashes	Phototoxicity (with sparfloxacin), dizziness, headache, and insomnia
Thiacetazone (Tzn) (2.5 mg/kg)	Gastrointestinal reactions, cutaneous hypersensitivity, vertigo, and conjunctivitis	Hepatitis, erythema multiforme, exfoliative dermatitis, hemolytic anemia
Para-aminosalicylic acid (PAS) (8–12 g/day)	Gastrointestinal reactions, hepatitis, cutaneous hypersensitivity, and hypokalemia	Acute renal failure, hemolytic anemia, thrombocytopenia, and hypothyroidism

3. ANTIEPILEPTICS (TABLE 15.3)

Table 15.3: Antiepileptic drugs and their mechanism of action, adverse reactions, and uses.

Drug and mechanism of action	Adverse reactions	Uses
Phenytoin: Oldest Nonsedative antiepileptic drug. It alters Na^+, Ca^{2+}, and K^+ conduction	Ataxia and nystagmus, cognitive impairment, hirsutism, gingival hyperplasia, coarsening of facial features, dose-dependent zero order kinetics, exacerbates absence seizures, "Fetal hydantoin syndrome"	Partial seizure, generalized (including tonic-clonic) seizures. Contraindicated in absence seizures. Nonseizure indications include trigeminal neuralgia, manic-depressive disorders
Carbamazepine: Tricyclic, antidepressant (bipolar). Mechanism of action, similar to phenytoin. Inhibits high-frequency repetitive firing (Na^{++})	Autoinduction of metabolism, nausea and visual disturbances, granulocyte suppression, aplastic anemia, exacerbates absence seizures	Partial seizure (including tonic-clonic) seizures. Contraindicated in absence seizures. Nonseizure indications include trigeminal neuralgia, manic-depressive disorders
Oxcarbazepine: Related to carbamazepine. With improved toxicity profile. Less potent than carbamazepine. Active metabolite	Hyponatremia, less hypersensitivity and induction of hepatic enzymes than with carbamazepine	
Phenobarbital: It is the oldest antiepileptic drug. Although considered one of the safest drugs, it has sedative effects. Prolongs opening of Cl^- channels. Blocks excitatory GLU (AMPA) responses. Blocks Ca^{2+} currents (L, N)	Sedation, cognitive impairment, behavioral changes, induction of liver enzymes, may worsen absence and atonic seizures	Useful for partial, generalized tonic-clonic seizures, and febrile seizures
Valproate: Mechanism of action, similar to phenytoin. Increases levels of GABA in brain. May facilitate glutamic acid decarboxylase (GAD). Inhibits GAT-1	Elevated liver enzymes, nausea and vomiting, abdominal pain, heartburn, tremor, hair loss, hepatotoxicity, pancreatitis, teratogen (spina bifida)	A broad-spectrum antiseizure drug effective for partial and generalized seizures, including myoclonic and absence seizures. Non seizure indications include migraine (prophylaxis), bipolar disorder
Gabapentin: Analog of GABA that does not act on GABA receptors. Low potency	Somnolence, dizziness, ataxia, headache, tremor	Used as an adjunct in partial and generalized tonic-clonic seizures, neuropathy
Levetiracetam	Somnolence, incoordination, irritability, mood swings, psychosis	Effective for GTCS, JME. Preferred in elderly

4. ANTIHISTAMINICS

Chlorpheniramine

Competes with histamine for H_1-receptor sites on effector cells in the gastrointestinal tract, blood vessels, and respiratory tract.

Indications:
- Allergic symptoms, allergic rhinitis, urticaria, pruritus: Perennial and seasonal allergic rhinitis and other allergic symptoms including urticaria, pruritus
- Motion sickness

Dose:
- Immediate release: 4 mg every 4 to 6 hours; do not exceed 24 mg/24 h
- Extended release: 12 mg every 12 hours; do not exceed 24 mg/24 h

Adverse effect:
- Central nervous system: Drowsiness (slight to moderate)
- Respiratory: Thickening of bronchial secretions

Contraindication: Narrow-angle glaucoma; bladder neck obstruction; symptomatic prostate hypertrophy; stenosing peptic ulcer; pyloroduodenal obstruction.

Cetrizine

Dose: IV, oral: 10 mg as a single dose

Indications (oral):
- **Allergic rhinitis:** Relief of symptoms associated with allergic rhinitis.
- **Urticaria, chronic spontaneous:** Treatment of uncomplicated skin manifestations of chronic spontaneous urticaria.
- **Atopic dermatitis**
- **Injection:** Urticaria, anaphylaxis

Adverse effect: Cetirizine may cause CNS depression, including sedated state, drowsiness.

Some adverse effects of antihistamines and decongestants:

Antihistamines
Anticholinergic effects
▪ Dry mouth and eyes
▪ Impotence
▪ Urinary hesitancy
▪ Glaucoma
▪ Alteration of bowel habits
Central nervous system effects
▪ Sedation
▪ Rarely stimulation (usually children)
▪ Confusion (older patients)
▪ Cognitive impairment
Miscellaneous effects
▪ Weight gain
▪ Hypersensitivity
▪ Prolonged QT interval

5. ANTIARRHYTHMICS (TABLE 15.4)

Digoxin

Digoxin is a purified glycoside derived from *Digitalis lanata* having cardiac inotropic property.

Pharmacological actions:
- Force of myocardial contraction is increased by a direct action of digitalis.
- **Heart rate:** Decreased and bradycardia is more marked in CHF.
- **Electrophysiological properties:**
  - Prolongs the refractory period of AV node → slows the ventricular rate.
  - Reflex vasodilation in CHF.

Indications:
- **Cardiac arrhythmias:** Supraventricular tachycardia, tachyarrhythmias and atrial fibrillation with a fast ventricular rate.
- Heart failure with reduced ejection fraction (HFrEF)
- Heart failure accompanied by atrial fibrillation or flutter with a rapid ventricular rate.

Dosage and route of administration:
The dosage and route are determined based on the desired action.
- **Rapid digitalizing (loading dose) regimen**
  - **Intravenously:** Initial loading dose of 0.25–0.5 mg followed by 0.25 mg every 6 hour. Careful monitoring of clinical response and toxicity should be performed before each dose.
  - **Orally:** Initial loading dose is 0.5–1 mg followed by 0.25 mg 6 hourly. Careful monitoring of clinical response and toxicity before each dose.
- **Slow digitalization:** Maintenance dose (0.125–0.25 mg/day) given from the beginning. Dose may be increased every 2 weeks depending on clinical response, serum levels of the drug, and toxicity.
- As per ACCF/AHA guidelines, a loading dose to initiate digoxin therapy in patients with heart failure is not required.

Adverse effect:
- **Gastrointestinal (60–80%):** Nausea/vomiting, anorexia, abdominal pain, diarrhea Malaise (30–40%), lethargy, fatigue
- **Neurological (20–30%):** Dizziness, confusion, headache, visual changes (flashing lights, halos, color disturbances in green-yellow spectrum, blurred vision)
- **Cardiac:** Almost any permutations and combinations of heart block (partial to complete), brady and tachydysrhythmias can be produced.
- **Classical:** Paroxysmal atrial tachycardia, ventricular bigeminy, bidirectional ventricular tachycardia, nodal and ventricular extrasystoles.

TABLE 15.4: Vaughan Williams classification of antiarrhythmic drugs.

Class	Mechanism of action	Examples
I. Na⁺ channel blocker	Change the slope of phase 0	Ia: Quinidine, disopyramide, procainamide, and moricizine
		Ib: Lidocaine, phenytoin, and mexiletine
		Ic: Flecainide and propafenone
II. β-blocker	Increased heart rate and conduction velocity	Propranolol, metoprolol, esmolol, and acebutolol

Contd...

Contd...

III.	K+ channel blocker	Action potential duration (APD) or effective refractory period (ERP)	Amiodarone, sotalol, bretylium, dronedarone, Dofetilide, Ibutilide
		Delay repolarization	Vernakalant, azimilide, and tedisamil
IV.	Ca++ channel blocker	Slowing the rate of rise in phase 4 of SA node	Verapamil and diltiazem
	Others		Adenosine, magnesium, digitalis, Isoprenaline, Digoxin, Atropine

Amiodarone

Class III antiarrhythmic agent which inhibits adrenergic stimulation (alpha- and beta-blocking properties), affects sodium, potassium, and calcium channels, prolongs the action potential and refractory period in myocardial tissue; decreases AV conduction and sinus node function.

Indications: Useful in wide range of ventricular and supraventricular arrhythmias.
- Resistant ventricular tachycardia/pulseless VT/Atrial fibrillation/ WPW tachyarrhythmia
- Recurrent ventricular fibrillation
- To maintain sinus rhythm in atrial flutter when other drugs have failed. For patients with heart failure or left ventricular hypertrophy, only amiodarone is recommended.

Duration of action: Long. Hence suitable for long-term prophylactic therapy.

Adverse reactions: These are dose-related and increase with duration of therapy. These reactions include fall in blood pressure, bradycardia, and myocardial depression on IV injection and after drug cumulation. Nausea, gastrointestinal upset with oral medication, photosensitization, and bluish skin discoloration pigmentation may develop in about 10% of patients. Pulmonary alveolitis and fibrosis are serious adverse reactions. Cirrhosis occurs uncommonly. Peripheral neuropathy, and hyperthyroidism (1–2%) or hypothyroidism (2–4%) can be seen.

Dose:
- Oral 400–600 mg/day for few weeks, followed by 100–200 mg for maintenance therapy
- Slow IV injection of 100–300 mg (5 mg/kg) over 30–60 minutes

Adenosine

Antiarrhythmic actions: Slows conduction time through the AV node, interrupting the re-entry pathways through the AV node, restoring normal sinus rhythm.

Dose: Initial—6 mg; if not effective within 1 to 2 minutes, 12 mg may be given; may repeat 12 mg bolus if needed (maximum single dose—12 mg). Follow each dose with 20 mL normal saline flush.

Indications:
Paroxysmal supraventricular tachycardia, Monomorphic wide-complex tachycardia; Narrow-complex regular tachycardia

Adverse effect:
- Cardiovascular: Cardiac arrhythmia (transient and new arrhythmia after cardioversion, e.g., atrial premature contractions, atrial fibrillation, premature ventricular contractions), chest discomfort.
- Central nervous system: Headache, dizziness
- Dermatologic: Facial flushing

6. ANTIANGINAL AND ANTIPLATELETS (TABLE 15.5)

TABLE 15.5: Indications and contraindications of various antianginal drugs.

Drug	Indication	Contraindication
β-blockers	<ul><li>Postmyocardial infarction</li><li>CHF (compensated)</li><li>Ventricular tachycardia</li><li>Supraventricular tachycardia (SVT)</li><li>Systemic hypertension</li><li>Hyperthyroidism</li></ul>	<ul><li>Decompensated HF</li><li>Severe bradycardia or AV block</li><li>Severe depression</li><li>Symptomatic PAD</li><li>Raynaud's phenomenon</li><li>Severe COPD</li></ul>
DHP-CCB	<ul><li>Systemic hypertension</li><li>Raynaud's phenomenon or Prinzmetal's angina</li><li>Severe bradycardia or AV block</li></ul>	Hypotension
Non-DHP-CCB	<ul><li>SVT</li><li>Systemic hypertension</li></ul>	<ul><li>Severe bradycardia</li><li>Significant AV block</li><li>LV dysfunction or HF</li></ul>
Nitrates	LV dysfunction or HF	<ul><li>Severe aortic stenosis</li><li>PDE-5 inhibitor use</li></ul>
Ivabradine	Chronic stable angina with sinus rhythm Inappropriate sinus tachycardia	<ul><li>Bradycardia</li><li>2° AV block</li></ul>
Ranolazine	<ul><li>Bradycardia or AV block</li><li>Low blood pressure</li><li>LV dysfunction</li><li>Possible diabetes</li></ul>	<ul><li>Treatment with QT prolonging agents</li><li>Moderate or severe hepatic dysfunction</li><li>CYP3A4 inhibitors</li></ul>
Nicorandil	Refractory angina	<ul><li>Severe aortic stenosis</li><li>PDE-5 inhibitor use</li></ul>

Nitrates

Short-acting (glyceryl trinitrate (GTN), nitroglycerine) or long-acting (isosorbide dinitrate, isosorbide mononitrate)

Mechanism of action: Nitrates directly act on smooth muscle in the walls of blood vessels and produce dilatation of arteries and veins. This lowers blood pressure, reduces venous return to heart, and produces dilatation of coronary blood vessels. Nitrates cause reduction in myocardial oxygen demand (lower preload and afterload) as well as an increase in myocardial oxygen supply (coronary vasodilatation) predominantly by perfusing the subendocardial region.

Glyceryl trinitrate (GTN):
- **Preparations:** (1) metered-dose aerosol (400 μg per spray) or (2) as a tablet (300 or 500 μg).
- **Action:** Sublingual GTN has a short duration of action and will relieve an attack of angina in 2–3 minutes.

Isosorbide dinitrate (10–20 mg 2 to 3 times daily) has prolonged action and is given by mouth. Headache is a common side effect but tends to diminish if the patient perseveres with the treatment. Tolerance can develop with continuous nitrate therapy which can be avoided by a 6–8-hour nitrate-free period. Hence, doses are given in the morning and afternoon.

Isosorbide mononitrate (20–60 mg once or twice daily) can also be given by mouth.

β-blockers Mechanism (Table 15.6)

These drugs lower oxygen demand of myocardium by reducing heart rate, blood pressure, and myocardial contractility. They inhibit apoptosis by inhibiting beta adrenoceptors, and have antioxidant and antiproliferative properties. They also counteract the direct adverse effects of catecholamines and have antiarrhythmic action. They are useful to control tachycardia, hypertension, and continued angina.

Contraindication: Bronchial asthma, severe bradycardia, second or third degree heart block

Cardioselective β-blockers: These include slow-release **metoprolol** 50–200 mg daily, **bisoprolol** 5–15 mg daily, and **atenolol** (50–200 mg/day). They have fewer peripheral side effects.

Nonselective β-blockers: Propranolol

TABLE 15.6: Uses and contraindications for β-blockers.

Uses of β-blockers	
▪ Angina pectoris	▪ Hypertension
▪ Cardiac arrhythmias	▪ Thyrotoxicosis
▪ Acute myocardial infarction and post myocardial infarction period (to prevent reinfarction)	▪ Pheochromocytoma
	▪ Anxiety with somatic symptoms
▪ Dissecting aortic aneurysm	▪ Chronic open-angle glaucoma
▪ Hypertrophic cardiomyopathy	
▪ Fallot's tetralogy (cyanotic spells)	▪ Portal hypertension
	▪ Migraine prophylaxis
	▪ Essential tremor

Contraindications of β-blockers	
▪ Chronic obstructive pulmonary disease and asthma	▪ Peripheral vascular disease
▪ Cardiac failure	▪ Diabetes mellitus (masks sympathetic signs of hypoglycemia)
▪ Heart block	

Calcium Channel Antagonists (Calcium Channel Blockers)

- **Dihydropyridine calcium antagonists** (e.g., nifedipine, amlodipine, felodipine, nitrendipine, nimodipine, and nicardipine). They produce coronary and peripheral arterial dilatation, and negative inotropy. They often cause a reflex tachycardia.
    - **Nifedipine:** It is a powerful coronary and systemic arteriolar dilator. This can cause marked reflex tachycardia. Short-acting nifedipine are not used because it can increase mortality due to myocardial infarction. Long-acting preparations are given usually along with a β-blocker. Dose is 5–20 mg 3 times daily.
    - **Amlodipine:** Dose is 2.5–10 mg daily. Side effects are ankle edema and reflex tachycardia.
- **Nondihydropyridine calcium antagonists,** e.g., verapamil (phenylalkylamines) and diltiazem (benzothiazepines). They produce coronary and peripheral arterial dilatation and negative inotropy, and also reduce conductivity. Because of its negative inotropic effect, they should be avoided in patients with impaired ventricular function (uncompensated heart failure).
    - **Verapamil:** Dose is 40–80 mg thrice daily. Useful antiarrhythmic properties. Common adverse effect is constipation.
    - **Diltiazem:** 60–120 mg 3 times daily. Similar antiarrhythmic properties to verapamil.

Ivabradine

If channel antagonist: Ivabradine selectively inhibits inward sodium-potassium current [important pacemaking current in the cells sinus (SA) node]. This slows the rate of diastolic depolarization and induces bradycardia ("bradycardic" drug). In contrast to β-blockers and rate-limiting calcium antagonists, it does not have other cardiovascular effects. Thus, it does not affect contractility, AV nodal conduction or hemodynamics.

Aspirin (Box 15.1)

> **Box 15.1: Indications for low-dose aspirin.**
> - Secondary prevention of cardiovascular disease: CAD (coronary artery disease), stroke, post-CABG (coronary artery bypass grafting)
> - Primary prevention of ischemic heart disease
> - Transient ischemic attacks (TIA)
> - Antiphospholipid antibody (APLA) syndrome
> - Pre-eclampsia
> - Essential thrombocytosis, polycythemia vera
> - Venous thromboembolism—prophylaxis

Cyclooxygenase inhibitors:
- Aspirin is cheap, effective and most widely used antiplatelet agent.
- **Mechanism of action:** Aspirin inhibits platelet enzyme cyclooxygenase (COX-1 and COX-2) and prevents the synthesis of thromboxane A_2. This results in impairment of platelet secretion and aggregation.
- **Duration of action:** Effects of aspirin on platelet function develop within an hour and lasts for the whole life span of platelets (~7 days).
- **Indications:** Arthritis, secondary prevention of cardiovascular events (acute coronary syndromes, stable

angina) in patients with coronary artery, cerebrovascular (transient ischemic attack), or peripheral vascular disease (intermittent claudication).
- **Dose:** Usual dose is 75–325 mg once daily.
- **Side effects:** Dyspepsia to erosive gastritis or peptic ulcers with bleeding and perforation.

Other Antiplatelets

Adenosine Diphosphate (ADP) Receptor Antagonists on Platelets

- Thienopyridines are drugs that selectively inhibit ADP-induced platelet aggregation by irreversibly blocking P2Y12.
- Thienopyridines include ticlopidine, **clopidogrel, and** prasugrel.
- Nonthienopyridines include Ticagrelor and Cangrelor
- **Indications:** Reduces the risk of cardiovascular death, MI, and stroke in patients with atherosclerotic disease.
- **Dose:**
  - Ticlopidine: 250 mg twice daily
  - Clopidogrel: 75 mg once daily. Loading dose of 300 mg of clopidogrel is given when rapid ADP receptor blockade is needed such as patients undergoing coronary stenting.
  - Prasugrel: A loading dose of 60 mg, prasugrel produces much more rapid, potent, and consistent inhibition of platelet function than clopidogrel loading dose. It is followed by a maintenance dose of 10 mg once daily.
  - Ticagrelor: A loading dose of 180 mg followed by maintenance dose 90 mg twice daily
- **Side effects:**
  - Ticlopidine: Gastrointestinal and hematologic (neutropenia, thrombocytopenia, and thrombotic thrombocytopenic purpura). These side effects usually occur within the first few months of starting treatment.
  - Clopidogrel and prasugrel: Gastrointestinal and hematologic side effects are rare.
  - Ticagrelor: Hemorrhage, Bradyarrhythmias and respiratory effects like dyspnea, sleep apnea including Cheyne-stokes respiration

Adenosine Reuptake Inhibitors

- **Dipyridamole** is a relatively weak antiplatelet agent.
- **Mechanism of action:** Inhibits phosphodiesterase and blocks the breakdown of cyclic AMP.
- **Dose:** 25–75 mg three to four times a day. Dipyridamole is more commonly used along with aspirin.
- **Indications:** Coronary artery disease, ischemic stroke or transient ischemic attack. Rarely used at present because of dose inconvenience and side effects.
- **Side effects:**
  - Due to **vasodilatory effect**, it can lower the blood pressure and must be used with caution in patients with coronary artery disease.
  - **Others:** Gastrointestinal complaints, headache, dizziness and hypotension.

Glycoprotein IIb/IIIa Receptor Antagonists (Inhibitors)

- **It includes three agents:** Abciximab, eptifibatide, and tirofiban.
- **Uses:** Parenteral GPIIb/IIIa receptor antagonists are used in acute coronary syndromes, unstable angina and non-ST-elevation MI percutaneous coronary interventions.
- **Side effects:** Bleeding tendencies and thrombocytopenia. Eptifibatide may produce hypotension.

7. ANTIPARKINSON

Anticholinergic Drugs

- Nonselective muscarinic antagonists are helpful, especially in **relieving tremor**, e.g., **trihexyphenidyl, benztropine, and orphenadrine.**
- Treatment is started with small dose (2 mg), which is gradually built up until benefit occurs or side effects limit further increments.
- **Adverse effects:** Urinary retention, dry mouth, blurred vision, worsening of glaucoma, constipation, confusion and hallucinosis in elderly. Hence, rarely used as first-line drugs unless patient has severe tremors. They should be avoided in patient above 65 years of age.

Levodopa

- Levodopa, the metabolic precursor of dopamine. It is the single most effective drug available for the treatment. It provides symptomatic benefit in most patients with parkinsonism and is often particularly helpful in relieving bradykinesia. Resolve hypokinesia and rigidity first and tremor later. Levodopa is metabolized by MAO (monoamine oxidase) and COMT (catechol-O-methyl-transferase). Its plasma half-life is around 2 hours. Early use lowers mortality rate. Combined with a dopa decarboxylase inhibitor—benserazide (co-beneldopa) or carbidopa (co-careldopa) to reduce the adverse effects (e.g., nausea and hypotension).
- **Adverse drug reactions:**
  - Postural hypotension, fluctuations in response.
  - Mydriasis, brownish discoloration of the urine, abnormal smell, transient elevations of transaminases and BUN.
  - GIT effects: Nausea and vomiting.
  - Cardiovascular: Tachycardia, ventricular extrasystoles, atrial fibrillation.
  - Dyskinesias, behavioral disturbances.
- **"On-off" effect:** Important late complications of levodopa therapy. It is like a light switch; without warning, all of a sudden, person goes from full control to complete reversion back to bradykinesia, tremor, etc. It lasts from 30 minutes to several hours and then get control again. The on-off phenomenon can be controlled in part by reducing dosing, intervals, administering levodopa 1 hour before meals and restricting dietary protein intake or treatment with dopamine agonists.

MAO-B Inhibitors

- Monoamine oxidase type B **facilitates breakdown of excess dopamine** in the synapse. They produce **asymptomatic motor benefit** when used as a monotherapy and **enhance the efficacy of carbidopa levodopa formulations** when used as adjuncts. e.g., selegiline, rasagiline.
- The addition of selegiline, a monoamine oxidase B inhibitor, reduces the metabolic breakdown of dopamine and may slow down the degeneration in the substantia nigra.

Dopamine Receptor Agonists

- Dopamine receptor agonists are classified as ergot derived (bromocriptine, pergolide and cabergoline) or non ergot-derived (pramipexole, ropinirole, rotigotine and apomorphine).
- **Side effects:** Produce impulse control disorders (e.g., pathological gambling, binge eating and hypersexuality) and daytime somnolence. Dopamine agonists are contraindicated in patients with psychotic disorders and are best avoided in those with recent myocardial infarction, severe peripheral vascular disease, or active peptic ulceration.
- Ergot-derived agonists are no longer recommended because of rare but serious fibrotic side effects including cardiac valvular fibrosis.

COMT Inhibitors

Catechol-O-methyl-transferase produces peripheral breakdown of levodopa (e.g., entacapone and tolcapone). Entacapone prolongs the duration of levodopa by decreasing its peripheral metabolism. The more potent tolcapone is less preferred because of rare but serious hepatotoxicity.

Dopamine Facilitator

- **Amantadine:** It is an antiviral agent that potentiates dopaminergic function by influencing the synthesis, release, reuptake of dopamine. It has a mild antiparkinsonian effect and short-lived effect on bradykinesia. Hence, it is rarely used and are reserved for patients who are unable to tolerate other drugs. Amantadine-either alone or combined with an anticholinergic agent, helpful for mild parkinsonism. It acts by potentiating the release of endogenous dopamine.
- **Adverse effects:** Livedo reticularis, peripheral edema, confusion and other anticholinergic effects.

Peripheral Dopamine Decarboxylase Inhibitors (PDI)

It does not penetrate the blood brain barrier (BBB), reduce the peripheral metabolism of levodopa. Increase plasma levels of levodopa, prolongs the plasma half-life of levodopa, increase available amounts of dopa for entry into the brain and reduce the daily requirement of levodopa by 75%, e.g., **carbidopa, benserazide.**

8. ANTIPSYCHOTICS AND ANTIDEPRESSANTS (TABLE 15.7)

TABLE 15.7: Various types of antidepressants and their side effects.

Group and drug	Side effects
Monoamine oxidase (MAO) inhibitors - *Irreversible inhibitors of MAO-A and B:* Isocarboxazid, phenelzine, tranylcypromine - *Reversible inhibitor of MAO-A (RIMA)s:* Moclobemide and clorgyline	- ↑ appetite (phenelzine) - ↓ appetite (tranylcypromine) - Hepatotoxicity, SLE, drug, and food interactions (cheese reaction)
Tricyclic antidepressants (TCAs) - *NA + 5 HT reuptake inhibitor:* Amitriptyline, imipramine, trimipramine, clomipramine, doxepin, dothiepin, and dosulepin	- Anticholinergic: Dry mouth, bad taste, constipation, epigastric fullness, urinary retention (more common in elderly male), blurred vision, and palpitation - Sedation, mental confusion, and weakness
- *Predominantly NA reuptake inhibitor:* Desipramine, nortriptyline, amoxapine, reboxetine	- Increased appetite and weight, sweating, fine tremors, precipitation of seizures, postural hypotension, cardiac arrhythmias, rashes, and jaundice
Selective serotonin reuptake inhibitors (SSRIs) - Fluoxetine, fluvoxamine, paroxetine, sertraline, citalopram, and escitalopram	- Gastric upset, nausea, interfere with ejaculation, nervousness, restlessness, insomnia, anorexia, headache, diarrhea, epistaxis, ecchymosis, and serotonin syndrome
Selective norepinephrine reuptake inhibitors (SNRIs): Duloxetine, venlafaxine	- Hypertension
Atypical antidepressants - Trazodone, mianserine, mirtazapine, tianeptine, amineptine, and bupropion	- Priapism (trazodone), bone marrow suppression, hepatotoxicity
NMDA (glutamate) antagonists: Ketamine	- Psychosis

Classification of Antipsychotics Drugs

Typical antipsychotics/first generation:
- Phenothiazines (chlorpromazine, perphenazine, fluphenazine, and thioridazine)
- Thioxanthenes (flupenthixol and zuclopenthixol)
- Butyrophenones (haloperidol and droperidol)

Atypical antipsychotics/second generation:
- Aripiprazole, asenapine, brexpiprazole, cariprazine, clozapine, iloperidone, lurasidone, olanzapine, paliperidone, pimavanserin, quetiapine, risperidone, and ziprasidone

Mechanism of action of most first and second-generation antipsychotics: It appears to be postsynaptic blockade of brain dopamine D2 receptors.

Exceptions:
- Aripiprazole and brexpiprazole are D2 receptor partial agonists
- Cariprazine is a D3-preferring D3/D2 receptor partial agonist
- Pimavanserin is a serotonin 5HT2A inverse agonist and antagonist with no dopamine D2 affinity

Antipsychotic Drugs and their Action (Fig. 15.1)
Indications
- Psychomotor agitation: High-potency APMs (haloperidol) parenteral.
- Schizophrenia: Treatment of choice for acute psychotic episodes and for prophylaxis
- Other psychotic disorders: Treatment of psychotic disorders due to general medical conditions and substances, delusional disorder, brief psychotic disorder, schizophreniform disorder, and other rarer psychotic disorders.
- Mood disorders: Treatment of agitation and psychosis during mood episodes.
- Sedation: Useful when benzodiazepines are contraindicated (especially in older patients) or as an adjunct during anesthesia.
- Movement disorders: Treatment of choice for Huntington disease and Tourette disorder.

General Adverse Effects
- **Sedation:** Due to the antihistaminic activity.
- **Hypotension:** Effect is due to alpha-adrenergic blockade and is most common with low potency antipsychotic medications.
- **Anticholinergic symptoms:** Dry mouth, blurred vision, urinary hesitancy, constipation, bradycardia, confusion, and delirium.
- **Endocrine effects:** Gynecomastia, galactorrhea, and amenorrhea (secondary to hyperprolactinemia).
- **Dermal and ocular syndromes:** Photosensitivity, abnormal pigmentation, and cataracts. Thioridazine can cause retinitis pigmentosa.
- **Cardiac conduction abnormalities:** Ziprasidone prolongs QT interval.
- **Agranulocytosis:** Clozapine
- **Movement syndromes:** Tardive dyskinesia (TD)
- **Extrapyramidal syndromes (EPS):** Newer APMs cause minimal or no EPS. Low-potency APMs (e.g., chlorpromazine, thioridazine) cause less EPS than higher potency APMs, but has more sedative effects.
- **Metabolic syndrome:** Weight gain, diabetes, and dyslipidemia
- **Cholestatic jaundice**
- Neuroleptic malignant syndrome

9. ANALGESICS
Nonsteroidal Anti-inflammatory Drugs
Mechanism of NSAID action: Arachidonic acid (AA) is derived from membrane phospholipid and its **metabolism occurs along two major enzymatic pathways namely; cyclooxygenase pathway (**produces prostaglandins by the cyclooxygenase enzyme) (COX) **and lipoxygenase pathway** (produces leukotrienes by 5-lipoxygenase enzyme).

Traditional NSAIDs versus COX-2 Inhibitors
- **Traditional NSAIDs** (e.g., Ibuprofen, diclofenac, and naproxen) exert their anti-inflammatory effect by inhibiting synthesis of prostaglandin from arachidonic acid by blocking both COX enzymes. They do not have a disease-modifying effect in either osteoarthritis or inflammatory rheumatic diseases. Inhibition of COX-1 is required for anti-inflammatory and analgesic effects, but can damage the mucosa of stomach and duodenum and is associated with an increased risk of upper gastrointestinal ulceration, bleeding and perforation. Simultaneous administration of omeprazole (20 mg daily) or misoprostol (200 pg twice or 3 times daily) reduces the risk of NSAID-induced ulceration and bleeding. Other side-effects include fluid retention, renal impairment due to inhibition of renal prostaglandin production, and rashes.
- **COX-2 (cyclooxygenase-2) selective NSAIDs** (e.g., celecoxib, etoricoxib, etodolac, rofecoxib and valdecoxib) selectively inhibit COX-2. They have analgesic and

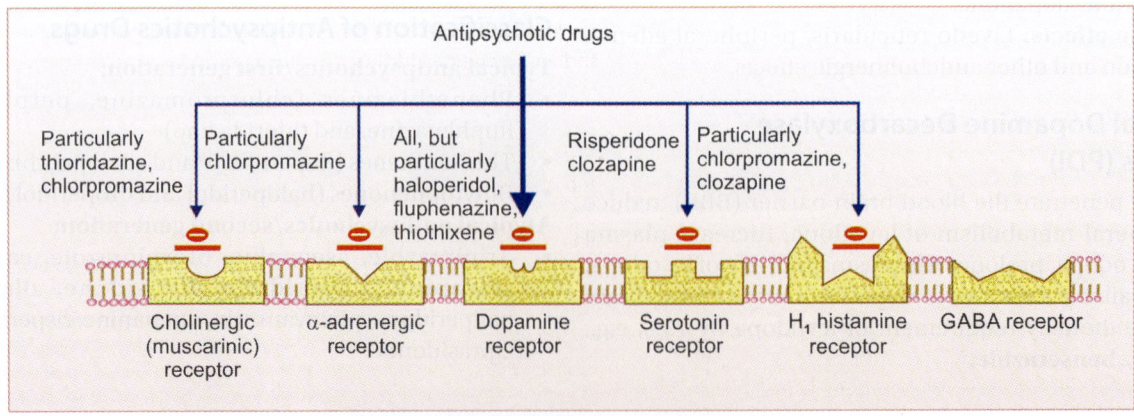

Fig. 15.1: Antipsychotic drugs and their action.

anti-inflammatory properties similar to traditional NSAIDs. However, they are much less likely to cause gastrointestinal toxicity and have minimal antiplatelet effects. Similar to traditional NSAIDs, they can produce significant changes in renal function, and hence, should be cautiously used in patients with diabetes, dehydration and congestive heart failure. They play an important role in the management of inflammation and pain caused by arthritis. It has been observed that there is a higher risk of myocardial infarction and stroke (thromboembolic complications) in patients using COX-2 inhibitors compared to traditional NSAIDs. Hence, two COX-2 inhibitors namely rofecoxib and valdecoxib have been withdrawn. NSAIDs like diclofenac, nabumetone, meloxicam, and etodolac, are also relatively selective for COX-2 at lower doses.

10. DIURETICS (TABLE 15.8)

TABLE 15.8: Summary of diuretics.

Subclass, drug	Site of action	Mechanism of action	Clinical uses	Toxicities	Comments
Loop diuretics					
Furosemide, bumetanide, torsemide (sulfonamide loop diuretics) Ethacrynic acid: Not a sulfonamide but has typical loop activity and some uricosuric action	Ascending limb of Henle's loop	Inhibition of the $Na^+/K^+/2Cl^-$ channel, leading to marked increase in NaCl excretion, K^+ wasting, metabolic alkalosis, increased urine Ca^{2+} and Mg^{2+}	Pulmonary edema, peripheral edema, heart failure, hypertension, acute hypercalcemia, type IV RTA	Ototoxicity, hypovolemia, K wasting, hyperuricemia, hypomagnesemia	Potent diuretics used in diseases associated with significant edema
Thiazides					
Hydrochlorothiazide, metolazone Chlorothiazide: *Only parenteral thiazide available (IV)* Chlorthalidone	Distal convoluted tubule (DCT)	Inhibition of Na/Cl transporter in the distal convoluted tubule leads to increase in NaCl excretion, some K wasting, metabolic alkalosis, decreased urine Ca^{2+}	Hypertension, mild heart failure, nephrolithiasis, nephrogenic diabetes insipidus, osteoporosis	Hyponatremia, hypokalemia, metabolic alkalosis, hyperuricemia, hyperglycemia	Widely used in the treatment of hypertension and less severe edema. Metolazone is commonly used along with loop diuretic for "sequential blockade"
Potassium-sparing diuretics					
Spironolactone Eplerenone	Collecting tubules	Aldosterone antagonists: Reduce Na retention and K wasting in kidney	Cirrhosis of liver (up to 400 mg/day of spironolactone), heart failure with reduced ejection fraction (25–50 mg/day of spironolactone), hypertension associated	Hyperkalemia, gynecomastia (spironolactone, not eplerenone)	Weak diuretics Interaction with other K-retaining drugs such as ACE-I, ARBs, beta-blockers and NSAIDs
Amiloride Triamterene	Collecting tubules	Blocks epithelial sodium channels (ENaC): Reduces Na retention and K wasting	Along with other diuretics to prevent hypokalemia from other diuretics. Prevention of amphotericin-induced hypokalemia and hypomagnesemia Reduces lithium-induced polyuria Liddle's syndrome	Hyperkalemia, metabolic acidosis	
Osmotic diuretics					
Mannitol	Multiple segments	Freely filtered at the glomerulus but not reabsorbed by any part of the tubular system. Retains fluid osmotically within the tubular lumen and limit the extent of sodium reabsorption in multiple segments.	Renal failure due to increased solute load (rhabdomyolysis, chemotherapy), raised intracranial pressure, raised intraocular pressure	Nausea, vomiting, headache	Not used for generalized edema

Contd...

Contd...

		Marked increase in urine flow, reduced brain volume, decreased intraocular pressure, initial hyponatremia, then hypernatremia			
Carbonic anhydrase inhibitors					
Acetazolamide	Proximal convoluted tubule (PCT)	Indirectly inhibits Na$^+$-H$^+$ exchange by reducing the elimination of secreted H$^+$ in the PCT	Glaucoma, mountain sickness, edema with alkalosis	Hyperchloremic metabolic acidosis, hypokalemia, renal stones, may worsen hepatic encephalopathy in cirrhotics	Weak diuretic

11. DRUGS FOR ASTHMA

Bronchodilators

β2-adrenoreceptor Agonists

- **β-adrenoreceptor:** There are two types of β-adrenoreceptor namely, β1 and β2-adrenoreceptors. β1-adrenoreceptors are expressed in the heart and β2-adrenoreceptors are widely expressed in the airways (in bronchial smooth muscles).
- **β2-adrenoreceptors agonists** (β2-agonists) can be divided into **short-acting β2-agonists** (SABAs) (e.g., salbutamol, levosalbutamol, and terbutaline) and **long-acting β2-agonists** (LABAs) (e.g., bambuterol, salmeterol, and formoterol).
    - **Catecholamines:** Catecholamines used are adrenaline, isoprenaline, and isoetharine.
    - **Adrenaline:** Most commonly used agent in this group. However, it is not a β2-selective and produces significant undesirable cardiovascular side effects. The usual dose is 0.3–0.5 mL of a 1:1000 solution administered subcutaneously. It may be repeated thrice at an interval of 20 minutes. They are useful in children.
    - **Salbutamol,** levosalbutamol, **terbutaline, and fenoterol:** These drugs are highly selective for β2-adrenoreceptors and act predominantly on the respiratory tract.
        - Powerful and rapidly but short-acting bronchodilators that relax bronchial smooth muscles.
        - **Routes of administration:** They are active by inhalation, oral, intravenous, subcutaneous route of administration, but the preferred route is inhalation. Inhalation is extremely effective, since, it rapidly decreases airflow obstruction. Intravenous administration has no advantages over inhalation. Other routes of administration are preferably avoided and reserved for selected indications.
        - **Dose:**
            - *Salbutamol:* 2–4 mg thrice a day orally or two puffs of 100 pg each as required.
            - *Terbutaline:* 2.5–5 mg thrice a day or two puffs of 100 μg each as required.
            - *Levosalbutamol:* Two puffs of 50 μg each as required.
        - **Side effects:** Main untoward effects are tremor and palpitation. Prolonged use of β2-adrenoreceptor agonists are preferably avoided because they worsen bronchial hyper-responsiveness. Tachycardia, which is less with levosalbutamol compared to salbutamol.
    - **Bambuterol:** It is a long-acting b2-adrenoreceptor agonist, which is converted into terbutaline in the body.
        - **Dose:** 10–20 mg once a day, orally
        - **Side effects:** More than with inhaled β-agonists and includes tachycardia, palpitations, and tremors
    - **Salmeterol and formoterol:** They are highly selective, potent, and long-acting β2-adrenoreceptor agonist. They are given once or twice a day by inhalation (either as aerosol or dry powder).
        - *Uses:* Routinely used in place of short-acting β2-stimulants when the patient requires regular β2-stimulant therapy. Not to be used as monotherapy but to be used as add-on therapy along with ICS (inhaled corticosteroids) when the response to ICs is suboptimal.
        - Salmeterol has a slow onset of action whereas formoterol has a rapid action. Hence, formoterol is suitable for immediate control of symptoms as well.
        - **Dose:**
            - *Salmeterol:* Two puffs of 25 pg each two to three times a day.
            - *Formoterol:* Two puffs of 6 pg each one to three times a day.

Methylxanthines

They are of little value as monotherapy but they are beneficial as add-on therapy in patients not controlled with inhaled corticosteroids (ICS). Methylxanthines as an add-on therapy are less effective than long-acting inhaled b2-agonists.

Theophylline

- Theophylline is a medium-potency bronchodilator.
- **Actions:** (i) It improves the movement of airway mucus, (ii) improves diaphragm contractility, and (iii) reduces the release of mediators.

- **Route of administration:** Intravenous, oral, or as suppository. Therapeutic plasma concentrations of theophylline range from 10 to 20 pg/mL. However, the dose required to achieve this concentration varies from patient to patient.
- **Type of preparation:**
  - Acute attacks are treated with short-acting theophylline preparations.
  - For maintenance therapy, long-acting theophylline preparations are used. They are given once or twice a day. Single daily dose in the evening controls nocturnal asthma.
- **Dose:** Usual dose is 100–200 mg (of plain preparation) three times/day, and 300 mg twice/day or 450–600 mg once/day for sustained-release preparation.
- **Side effects:** Nervousness, nausea, vomiting, anorexia, and headache. When plasma levels exceed 30 pg/mL, seizures and cardiac arrhythmias can occur.

Aminophylline

- Aminophylline is a bronchodilator that is effective when given orally, intravenously, and as a suppository. The preferred route of administration is intravenous and may have some role in the management of status asthmaticus (severe acute asthma).
- **Mechanism of action:** Bronchodilator effect is by inhibition of phosphodiesterases in airway smooth-muscle cells, which increase cyclic AMP.
- **Dose:** Loading dose of 5 mg/kg is given slowly intravenously over 20 minutes. This is followed by a maintenance dose of 0.5 mg/kg/h delivered as a continuous intravenous infusion. Patients are already on theophylline; loading dose is preferably withheld or in extreme cases, it is given in a reduced amount at 0.5 mg/kg.
- Rapid infusion of the bolus can lead to sudden death due to cardiac arrhythmias.

Inhaled Corticosteroids (ICS)

- Inhaled corticosteroids are the most effective controllers for asthma.
- **Mechanism of action:** Corticosteroids are not bronchodilators, but they are the most effective anti- inflammatory agents used in asthma, which reduce number of inflammatory cells as well as their activation in the airways. They decrease bronchial hyper- responsiveness and relieve or prevent airflow obstruction.
  They also reverse β2-receptor downregulation produced by long-term use of β2-agonists.
- **Uses:** These are beneficial in treating asthma of any severity and age. They are now given as first line of therapy for persistent asthma.
- **Dose:** These are usually given twice daily. Higher doses may be necessary in severe cases.
  - Beclomethasone dipropionate (200 pg), budesonide (200 pg), or fluticasone (125 pg) is given twice daily as aerosols or dry powder form.
  - Ciclesonide is given in a dose of 80–160 pg once a day. Others include flunisolide and mometasone.
- **Advantages:**
  - **Rapid improvement of the symptoms and lung function** (within several days).
    - They are effective in preventing asthma symptoms, exercise-induced asthma (EIA), and nocturnal exacerbations and they also prevent severe exacerbations.
    - Early treatment with ICS can prevent irreversible changes in airway function that develops in chronic asthma.
  - **Reduces airway responsiveness (AHR)**
  - Reduces the number of courses of oral corticosteroid therapy (OCS)
- **Side effects:**
  - **Local:** Hoarseness (dysphonia/husky voice) and oropharyngeal candidiasis. These side effects can be minimized by the use of a spacing device along with the metered-dose inhaler and gargling with water after use.
  - **Systemic:** Relatively free from systemic side effects at conventional doses. Long-term use may result in osteoporosis, skin thinning, and adrenal suppression.

Systemic Corticosteroids

a. **Oral corticosteroids and steroid-sparing agents:**
   - **Oral corticosteroids (OCS):** Oral corticosteroids are necessary in patients controlled by inhaled corticosteroids (ICS).
   - **Dose:** It should be kept as low as possible to minimize side effects. Prednisolone is started as a single morning dose of 40–60 mg orally/day. Thereafter, the dose is reduced by half every 6 hours. Methylprednisolone is given in a dose of 40–125 mg every 6 hours.
   - **Steroid-sparing agents:** Some patients may require continuing treatment with oral corticosteroids. Various immunomodulatory treatments can be used in these patients with severe asthma who have serious side effects with this therapy. Treatment of these patients with low doses of methotrexate (15 mg weekly) can reduce the dose of oral steroids needed to control the disease. Ciclosporin also improves lung function in few steroid-dependent asthmatics.
b. **Parenteral corticosteroids:**
   - Corticosteroids are used intravenously (hydrocortisone or methylprednisolone) for the treatment of acute severe asthma.
   - **Dose:**
     - Hydrocortisone: Loading dose of 4 mg/kg intravenously followed by 2–3 mg/kg every 6 hours
     - Methylprednisolone: 40–125 mg every 6 hours.
     - Indications for corticosteroids in bronchial asthma
   - Acute asthma which does not respond to or even worsen despite bronchodilator therapy
   - Severe acute asthma (status asthmaticus).

Anticholinergics

- Anticholinergics such as atropine sulfate and atropine methyl nitrate were previously used, but they are presently not used because of their systemic side effects.

- Currently used anticholinergics are **ipratropium bromide and tiotropium.** These are nonabsorbable quaternary ammonium compounds with minimal side effects. These are administered as aerosol or in dry powder form. Ipratropium is also given as nebulization solution.
- **Uses:** They are useful in two situations:
  1. Patients with coexisting heart disease, in whom methylxanthines and b2-adrenoreceptor agonists cause significant tachycardia.
  2. In refractory cases, bronchodilator action of b2-adrenoreceptor agonists is enhanced by the addition of ipratropium bromide or tiotropium.
- **Dose:**
  - *Ipratropium:* Two puffs of 20 µg each, four times/day
  - *Tiotropium:* Two puffs of 9 µg each, once a day
  - *Ipratropium:* 250–500 µg nebulization; may be repeated, if necessary
- **Side effects:** Dryness of mouth and bitter taste

Leukotriene modifiers:
- These include leukotriene receptor antagonists—LTRAs (montelukast, zafirlukast, and pranlukast) and 5-lipoxygenase inhibitors (Zileuton).
- **Uses:** Used as add-on therapy.
  - In patients who do not respond to the conventional agents
  - In patients who require high doses of inhaled steroids (ICS). They can be used as a second choice to inhaled corticosteroids in mild persistent asthma.
- **Dose:**
  - *Zafirlukast:* 20 mg BID
  - *Montelukast:* 10 mg once a day in the evening
- **Side effects:** Uncommon and include headache, abdominal pain, skin rashes, angioedema, pulmonary eosinophilia, and arthralgia. Zileuton may cause liver damage.

12. ANTIHYPERTENSIVES (TABLE 15.9)

TABLE 15.9: Various antihypertensive drugs (dose).

Drugs by class	Properties	Initial dose	Dosage range (mg)
β-adrenergic antagonists			
Atenolol	Selective	50 mg PO daily	25–100
Betaxolol	Selective	10 mg PO daily	5–40
Bisoprolol	Selective	5 mg PO daily	2.5–20
Metoprolol	Selective	50 mg PO bid	50–450
Metoprolol XL	Selective	50–100 mg PO daily	50–400
Nebivolol	Selective with vasodilatory properties	5 mg PO daily	5–40
Nadolol	Nonselective	40 mg PO daily	20–240
Propranolol	Nonselective	40 mg PO bid	40–240
Propranolol LA	Nonselective	80 mg PO daily	60–240
Timolol	Nonselective	10 mg PO bid	20–40
Pindolol	ISA	5 mg PO daily	10–60
Labetalol	α- and β antagonist properties	100 mg PO bid	200–1.200
Carvedilol	α- and β antagonist properties	6.25 mg PO bid	12.5–50
Carvedilol CR	α- and β antagonist properties	10 mg PO daily	10–80
Acebutolol	ISA, selective	200 mg PO bid 400 mg PO daily	200–1.200
Calcium channel antagonists			
Amlodipine	DHP	5 mg PO daily	2.5–10
Diltiazem		30 mg PO qid	90–360
Diltiazem LA		180 mg PO daily	120–540
Diltiazem CD		180 mg PO daily	120–480
Diltiazem XR		180 mg PO daily	120–540
Diltiazem XT		180 mg PO daily	120–480
Isradipine	DHP	2.5 mg PO bid	2.5–10
Nicardipine	DHP	20 mg PO tid	60–120
Nifedipine	DHP	10 mg PO tid	30–120
Nifedipine XL (or CC)	DHP	30 mg PO daily	30–90
Nisoldipine	DHP	20 mg PO daily	20–40
Verapamil		80 mg PO tid	80–480
Verapamil SR		120 mg PO daily	120–480
Angiotensin-converting enzyme inhibitors			
Benazepril		10 mg PO bid	10–40
Captopril		25 mg PO bid-tid	50–450
Enalapril		5 mg PO daily	2.5–40
Fosinopril		10 mg PO daily	10–40
Lisinopril		10 mg PO daily	5–40
Moexipril		7.5 mg PO daily	7.5–30
Quinapril		10 mg PO daily	5–80
Ramipril		2.5 mg PO daily	1.25–20
Trandolapril		1–2 mg PO daily	1–4
Perindopril		4 mg PO daily	2–16
Angiotensin II receptor blockers			
Azilsartan		40 mg PO daily	40–80
Candesartan		8 mg PO daily	8–32
Eprosartan		600 mg PO daily	600–800
Irbesartan		150 mg PO daily	150–300
Olmesartan		20 mg PO daily	20–40
Losartan		50 mg PO daily	25–100
Telmisartan		40 mg PO daily	20–80
Valsartan		80 mg PO daily	80–320
Direct renin inhibitor			
Aliskiren		150 mg PO daily	150–300
Diuretics			
Chlorthalidone	Thiazide diuretic	25 mg PO daily	12.5–50
Hydrochlorothiazide	Thiazide diuretic	12.5 mg PO daily	12.5–50
Hydroflumethiazide	Thiazide diuretic	50 mg PO daily	50–100

Contd...

Contd...

Indapamide	Thiazide diuretic	1.25 mg PO daily	2.5–5
Methyclothia-zide	Thiazide diuretic	2.5 mg PO daily	2.5–5
Metolazone	Thiazide diuretic	2.5 mg PO daily	1.25–5
Bumetanide	Loop diuretic	0.5 mg PO daily (or IV)	0.5–5
Ethacrynic acid	Loop diuretic	50 mg PO daily (or IV)	25–100
Furosemide	Loop diuretic	20 mg PO daily (or IV)	20–320
Torsemide	Loop diuretic	5 mg PO daily (or IV)	5–10
Amiloride	Potassium-sparing diuretic	5 mg PO daily	5–10
Triamterene	Potassium-sparing diuretic	50 mg PO bid	50–200
Eplerenone	Aldosterone antagonist	25 mg PO daily	25–100
Spironolactone	Aldosterone antagonist	25 mg PO daily	25–100
α-adrenergic antagonists			
Doxazosin		1 mg PO daily	1–16
Prazosin		1 mg PO bid-tid	1–20
Terazosin		1 mg PO at bedtime	1–20
Centrally acting adrenergic agents			
Clonidine		0.1 mg PO bid	0.1–1.2
Clonidine patch		TTS 1/week (equivalent to 0.1 mg/day release)	0.1–0.3
Guanfacine		1 mg PO daily	1–3
Guanabenz		4 mg PO bid	4–64
Methyldopa		250 mg PO bid-tid	250–2,000
Direct-acting vasodilators			
Hydralazine		10 mg PO qid	50–300
Minoxidil		5 mg PO daily	2.5–100
Miscellaneous			
Reserpine		0.5 mg PO daily	0.01–0.25

- **Angiotensin-converting enzyme inhibitors (ACEI) therapy:**
  - **Mechanism of action:** They prevent the conversion of angiotensin I to angiotensin II. This in turn prevents peripheral vasoconstriction, activation of the sympathetic nervous system, and salt and water retention due to aldosterone release. Thus, they interrupt the vicious circle of neurohumoral activation that is characteristic of moderate and severe heart failure. They also prevent the undesirable activation of the renin-angiotensin system caused by diuretic therapy.
  - **Uses:** ACEIs improve survival in patients in all functional classes (NYHA I—IV) and are given to all patients at risk of developing heart failure. They improve effort tolerance and mortality. They can also improve outcome, prevent the onset of overt heart failure in patients with asymptomatic heart failure following myocardial infarction.
  - **Initiation:** Start low dose; if tolerated then gradual increase in few days to weeks to target dose or maximum tolerable dose with regular blood pressure monitoring. Serum creatinine should be measured concomitantly and potassium-sparing diuretics should be discontinued.
  - **Drugs and dosage:** Captopril (6.25 mg thrice till 50 mg thrice a day), enalapril (2.5 mg twice to 10–20 mg twice a day), lisinopril (2.5–5 mg once to 20–40 mg once a day), and ramipril (1.25–2.5 mg once till 10 mg once a day).
- **Angiotensin II receptor antagonists (ARA)/blockers therapy:**
  - **Indications:** ARAs are indicated as second-line therapy in patients intolerant of ACEI or alternative to ACEI.
  - **Drugs and dosage:** Losartan (25–50 mg once till 50–150 mg once a day), valsartan, and telmisartan. Olmesartan (20–40 mg twice till 160 mg twice).
    - Same initiation and monitoring as ACEI and titration by doubling the dose.
- **Vasodilators and nitrates (hydralazine nitrate combination):**
  - The combination of hydralazine and nitrates reduces afterload and preload. Their use is limited by pharmacological tolerance and hypotension.
  - **Indication:** African-American origin, NYHA III- IV, low EF on ACEI and BB, patients intolerant or contra-indication of ACEI or ARA (e.g., in severe renal failure)
  - **Dose:** 37.5 mg hydralazine and 20 mg and isosorbide dinitrate start one tab TID to increase till two tabs TID.

Centrally Acting Drugs

Reserpine

It is a mild antihypertensive with central and peripheral action.

It is given in the dose of 0.1–0.5 mg daily. Its side effects include nasal congestion, depression, and parkinsonism.
α-methyldopa: It is a precursor of dopamine and noradrenaline.

- **Mechanism of action:** Converted to α-methyl noradrenaline which acts on alpha-2 receptors in brain and causes inhibition of adrenergic discharge in adrenal medulla fall in peripheral vascular resistance and fall in blood pressure.
- **Side effects:** Cognitive impairment, postural hypotension, positive Coombs test, etc. Not used therapeutically now except in hypertension during pregnancy.
- **Dose:** 250–500 mg twice or thrice daily.

Clonidine

Not frequently used because of tolerance and withdrawal hypertension. Side effect is dryness of mouth, rebound hypertension.

Dose: 0.1–1.0 mg daily.

Individualizing Antihypertensive Therapy

Compelling indications (major improvement in outcome independent of blood pressure)	
Diabetes mellitus	ACE inhibitor or ARB
Heart failure with reduced ejection fraction	ACE inhibitor or ARB, beta blocker, diuretic, and aldosterone antagonist
Postmyocardial infarction	ACE inhibitor or ARB, beta blocker, aldosterone antagonist
Proteinuric chronic kidney disease (nondiabetic)	ACE inhibitor or ARB
Angina pectoris	Beta blocker and calcium channel blocker
Atrial fibrillation/flutter rate control	Beta blocker, nondihydropyridine calcium channel blocker
Previous CVA/TIA	ACE inhibitor ± diuretic
Antihypertensive agents with a favorable effect on symptoms in comorbid conditions	
Benign prostatic hyperplasia	Alpha blocker
Essential tremor	Beta blocker (noncardioselective)
Hyperthyroidism	Beta blocker
Migraine	Beta blocker, calcium channel blocker
Osteoporosis	Thiazide diuretic
Raynaud phenomenon	Dihydropyridine calcium channel blocker
Contraindications	
Angioedema	Do not use an ACE inhibitor
Peripheral vascular disease	Avoid beta blocker
Bronchospasm	Do not use a nonselective beta blocker
Liver disease	Do not use methyldopa
Pregnancy	Do not use an ACE inhibitor, ARB, or renin inhibitor
Second or third degree heart block	Do not use a beta blocker, nondihydropyridine calcium channel blocker unless a functioning ventricular pacemaker
Bilateral renal artery stenosis	Avoid ACE inhibitors/ARB/renin inhibitor
Drug classes that may have adverse effects on comorbid conditions	
Depression	Avoid beta blocker, central alpha-2 agonist
Gout	Avoid loop or thiazide diuretic
Hyperkalemia	Avoid aldosterone antagonist, ACE inhibitor, ARB, and renin inhibitor
Hyponatremia	Avoid thiazide diuretic
Renovascular disease	Avoid ACE inhibitor, ARB, or renin inhibitor

Hypertensive Emergencies (Table 15.10)

TABLE 15.10: Drugs used in hypertensive emergencies.

Drug	Administration	Onset	Duration of action	Dosage	Adverse effects and comments
Fenoldopam	IV infusion	<5 min	30 min	0.1–0 µg/kg/min	Tachycardia, nausea, and vomiting
Sodium nitroprusside	IV infusion	Immediate	2–3 min	0.5–10 µg/kg/min (initial dose, 0.25 µg/kg/min for eclampsia and renal insufficiency)	Hypotension, nausea, vomiting, apprehension; risk of thiocyanate and cyanide toxicity is increased in renal and hepatic insufficiency, respectively; levels should be monitored; must shield from light
Diazoxide	IV bolus	15 min	6–12 h	50–100 mg q 5–10 min, up to 600 mg	Hypotension, tachycardia, nausea, vomiting, fluid retention, hyperglycemia; may exacerbate myocardial ischemia, heart failure, or aortic dissection
Labetalol	IV bolus	5–10 min	3–6 h	20–80 mg q 5–10 min, up to 300 mg	Hypotension, heart block, heart failure, bronchospasm, nausea, vomiting, scalp tingling, paradoxical pressor response; may not be effective in patients receiving α or β antagonists
	IV infusion			0.5–2 mg/min	
Nitroglycerin	IV infusion	1–2 min	3–5 min	5–250 mg/min	Headache, nausea, and vomiting. Tolerance may develop with prolonged use
Esmolol	IV bolus IV infusion	1–5 min	10 min	500 µg/kg/min for first 1 min 50–300 µg/kg/min	Hypotension, heart block, heart failure, bronchospasm
Phentolamine	IV bolus	1–2 min	3–10 min	5–10 mg q 5–15 min	Hypotension, tachycardia, headache, angina, and paradoxical pressor response

Contd...

Contd...

Hydralazine (for treatment of eclampsia)	IV bolus	10–20 min	3–6 h	10–20 mg q 20 min (if no effect after 20 mg, try another agent)	Hypotension, fetal distress, tachycardia, headache, nausea, vomiting, and local thrombophlebitis. Infusion site should be changed after 12 h
Methyldopa (for treatment of eclampsia)	IV bolus	30–60 min	10–16 h	250–500 mg	Hypotension
Nicardipine	IV infusion	1–5 min	3–6 h	5 mg/h, increased by 1.0–23 mg/h q 15 min, up to 15 mg/h	Hypotension, headache, tachycardia, nausea, and vomiting
Clevidipine	IV infusion	2–4 min	5–15 min	1–2 mg/h, double dose every 90 seconds up to 16 mg/h	Hypotension, reflex tachycardia
Enalaprilat	IV bolus	5–15 min	1–6 h	0.6255 mg q6h	Hypotension

13. DRUGS ACTING ON AUTONOMIC SYSTEM (TABLE 15.11)

TABLE 15.11: Common sympathomimetic amines used in shock.

Sympathomimetic amine (receptor activated) and dose	Actions
Dopamine: (Dopaminergic+ α + β1) ■ 0.2–1 mg/minute	Vasodilation of renal, mesenteric, cerebral and coronary vessels Increase myocardial contraction, heart rate and cardiac output. Rise in systolic blood pressure
Dobutamine: (β_1) ■ 2–8 µg/kg/minute	Marked increase in myocardial contraction, minimal increase in heart rate and minimal peripheral vessels vasodilatation
Noradrenaline: (α + β_1) ■ 2–8 µg/minute	Increased myocardial contraction, heart rate, cardiac output, and rise in blood pressure vasoconstriction in skin, muscle and splanchnic beds. Coronary vasodilation
Adrenaline: (α + β1+ β_2) ■ 1–8 µg/kg/minute	Increased myocardial contraction, heart rate and cardiac output. Rise in mean blood pressure vasoconstriction in most except skeletal muscles and coronary arteries. Vasodilatation in skeletal muscles and coronary arteries
Isoproterenol: (β1+ β2) ■ 5–10 µg/minute	Increased myocardial contraction, heart rate, cardiac output and rise in systolic blood pressure. Vasodilatation mainly in skeletal muscles
Phenylephrine: (α_1) ■ 30–60 µg/minute	Vasoconstriction

Adrenaline: Indications and Dose

a. **Cardiopulmonary resuscitation (CPR)**
 Adrenaline: Given as a **vasopressor** α-1 effect (not as an inotrope). Dose is 1 mg (0.01 mg/kg) IV every 4 minutes (alternating cycles) while continuing CPR.
 - **Given:** (1) Immediately in nonshockable rhythm (non-VT/VF), (2) In VF or VT given after the 3rd shock.
 - **Repeated** in alternate cycles (every 4 minutes).
b. **Anaphylactic shock**
 Administer adrenaline (epinephrine) intramuscularly into the thigh and is the most critical drug to administer. Earlier administration during the course of an anaphylactic event is better.
 - Adult: 0.3–0.5 mg (0.3–0.5 mL of a 1:1,000 solution) IM in the lateral thigh, repeated at 10- to 15-minute intervals if necessary.

Atropine

Mechanism of action: Blocks the action of acetylcholine at parasympathetic sites in smooth muscle, secretory glands, and the CNS; increases cardiac output, dries secretions. Atropine reverses the muscarinic effects of cholinergic poisoning due to agents with acetylcholinesterase inhibitor activity by acting as a competitive antagonist of acetylcholine at muscarinic receptors. The primary goal in cholinergic poisonings is reversal of bronchorrhea and bronchoconstriction. Atropine has no effect on the nicotinic receptors responsible for muscle weakness, fasciculations, and paralysis.

Indications and dose:
OP Poisoning
- Early use of sufficient doses of atropine is **lifesaving in patients with severe toxicity.** It reverses acetylcholine induced bronchospasm, bronchorrhea, bradycardia, and hypotension.
- **When the diagnosis is uncertain:**
- **Atropine challenge test:** To be performed, if not sure that the patient has consumed OP.
 - **Inject 0.6–1 mg IV atropine:** If pulse rate goes up by 25/minute or skin flushing develops, patient has mild or no toxicity or OP poisoning is unlikely.

Dose and mode of administration of atropine
- **Bolus**
 - Inject 1.8–3 mg (3–5 mL) of atropine bolus.
 - *Check three things after 5 minutes:* Pulse, blood pressure, and chest crepitations.
 - Aim for heart rate >80 beats/minute, SBP >80 mm Hg, and a clear chest.

- If the above-mentioned objectives are not achieved, double the atropine dose every 5 minutes.
- Review patient every 5 minutes. Once these parameters start improving, repeat last same or smaller dose of atropine. If there is persistent and satisfactory improvement in these parameters after 5 minutes, atropine infusion can be planned.
- **Atropine infusion**
  - Calculate total dose of atropine required for rapid atropinization.
  - Start hourly atropine infusion at 10–20% of total dose of atropine required for atropinization
  - Most patients do not need >3–5 mg/h of atropine infusion.
  - Use three-point checklist (**secretions, heart rate, pupils**) to reduce infusion rate by 20% every 4 hourly once the patient is stable.
  - Bronchorrhea is the most important sign for titrating dose of atropine once patient is stable.

Symptomatic AV block
- **Atropine:** Its routine use in **pulseless electrical activity** (PEA) and asystole is not useful. **Indicated** in sinus bradycardia or AV block causing hemodynamic instability. **Dose is 0.5 mg IV.** Repeated up to a maximum of 3 mg (full atropinization).
- **Muscarine-containing mushroom poisoning (IV):** 1 to 2 mg; titrate and repeat as needed to reverse symptoms (i.e., titrate to achieve decreased bronchial secretions)
- **Stress echocardiography (adjunct chronotropic agent)—IV:** 0.25 to 0.5 mg up to a total dose of 1–2 mg until 85% of target heart rate is achieved

Adverse effect:
- Cardiovascular: Atrial arrhythmia
- Gastrointestinal: Bladder distension, abdominal pain, constipation, delayed gastric emptying
- Hypersensitivity reaction
- Confusion, decreased deep tendon reflex, delirium, drowsiness

14. ENDOCRINE

Thyroxine

Treatment of hypothyroidism:
- Hypothyroidism is treated with T4.
- Replacement therapy with **levothyroxine sodium** is given for life as a once daily dosage **(1.6 µg/kg/day).**
- **Initial dose:** It depends upon the severity of the deficiency as well as on the age and fitness of the patient.
  - **For young healthy patients**—1.6 µg/kg/day.
  - **For older patients or those with coronary heart disease**—25–50 µg/day
- **Timing:** Should be taken on an empty stomach with water, ideally an hour before breakfast.
- The patient with symptomatic improvement should be re-evaluated with serum TSH measured in 4–6 weeks. If the TSH remains above the reference range, the dose of T4 can be **increased by 12–25 µg/day in older patients** and in younger patients, it can be increased by a higher dose. The patient will require a repeat TSH measurement in 6 weeks.
- **For patients with heart disease:** 12.5–25 µg/day and increase by 12.5–25 µg/day, if needed, at 6–8 weeks intervals. Few patients with ischemic heart disease may develop angina or worsen with therapy. They require β-blockers, vasodilators or coronary artery bypass graft (CABG) or angioplasty.
- **Dosage adjustments**
  - **Age:** In elderly start with half dose.
  - **Severity and duration of hypothyroidism:** Increase the dose in severe cases
  - **Weight:** 0.5 µg/kg/day increase up to 3.0 µg/kg/day
  - **Malabsorption:** Requires increased dose
  - **Concomitant drug therapy:** Thyroxine only to be taken on empty stomach
  - **Pregnancy:** 25–50% increase in dose, safe in lactating mother
  - **Presence of cardiac disease:** Start low dose or alternate day treatment.
- **Monitoring**
  - **Goal:** It is to **normalize TSH** level regardless of cause of hypothyroidism and to **restore T4 within the normal range.**
  - **Adequacy of replacement: Assessed clinically** and by **thyroid function tests after 6 weeks on a steady dose.**
  - Complete suppression of TSH should be avoided because it may cause atrial fibrillation and osteoporosis.
  - Lifelong therapy is needed.

Antithyroid Drugs

- **Antithyroid drugs (ATD)** may be used initially to control hyperthyroidism (in addition to beta-blockers) prior to definitive therapy with radioiodine or surgery; they may be prescribed for 1–2 years to attain a remission, or may be used long-term.
  - **Indications:** Primary therapy in **pregnancy**, in **children** and **adolescents** and **severe Graves' disease with eye changes**.
  - The drugs include: **Thionamides—methimazole, propylthiouracil, and carbimazole**
  - **Mechanism of action:** Inhibit the function of thyroid peroxidase (TPO) enzyme and prevent binding of iodine to tyrosine (prevents iodination and organification).
    - **Methimazole:** Primary drug to treat.
    Dose:
      - Free T4 1–1.5 times upper limit of normal: begin treatment with 5–10 mg once daily.
      - Free T4 1.5–2 times upper limit of normal: begin treatment with 10–20 mg once daily.
      - Free T4 2–3 times upper limit of normal: begin treatment on 20–40 mg daily in divided doses.
      - The dose is tapered to maintenance levels (5–10 mg/day) as the patient improves.

- **Propylthiouracil:** Preferred during the first trimester of pregnancy.
  Dose: 300 mg daily in 3 equally divided doses; 400 mg daily in patients with severe hyperthyroidism and/or very large goiters; usual maintenance: 100–150 mg daily in 3 divided doses.
- **Carbimazole:** It has additional immuno-suppressive action.
  - **Dose:** Initially 20–60 mg daily given in 2–3 divided doses and maintenance 5–15 mg daily or alternatively 20–60 mg daily. Total duration of treatment: 18–24 months.
  - **Adverse effects:** Rashes, urticaria, fever, arthralgia, blood dyscrasias (agranulocytosis), hepatotoxicity, aplasia cutis in neonates.

Glucocorticoids

Equivalent doses of glucocorticoids (Table 15.12)
- Compared to hydrocortisone, prednisolone has only 25% of mineralocorticoid activity **(Table 15.13).**
- Both dexamethasone and betamethasone have negligible mineralocorticoid activity.
- Adverse effects are given in **Table 15.14**.

TABLE 15.12: Equivalent doses of glucocorticoids (anti-inflammatory potency).

Hydrocortisone (cortisol)	20 mg	Methylprednisolone	4 mg
Cortisone acetate	25 mg	Betamethasone	0.75 mg
Prednisolone	5 mg	Dexamethasone	0.75 mg

TABLE 15.13: Common indications and contraindications of steroids.

Common indications of steroids	
▪ Bronchial asthma ▪ Raised intracranial tension ▪ Cerebral edema ▪ Connective tissue diseases—rheumatoid arthritis and systemic lupus erythematosus ▪ Nephrotic syndrome ▪ Adrenal insufficiency ▪ Shock and septicemia ▪ Transplant rejection and graft versus host disease ▪ Active tuberculosis ▪ Peptic ulcer ▪ Bleeding tendencies	▪ Leukemia, lymphoma ▪ As an adjunct in chemotherapy ▪ Carditis ▪ Demyelinating diseases ▪ Tuberculosis of pericardium and tuberculous meningitis ▪ Bone marrow transplantation ▪ Psoriasis and inflammatory bowel disease ▪ Eye conditions: Scleritis and chorioretinitis ▪ Uncontrolled hypertension

TABLE 15.14: Adverse effects of glucocorticoids.

Immune system	Bones
▪ Increased susceptibility to infections, reactivation of latent tuberculosis ▪ Lymphopenia ▪ Suppression of inflammation impaired wound healing ▪ Suppression of delayed hypersensitivity reaction	▪ Osteoporosis ▪ Avascular necrosis ▪ Bone pains ▪ Fracture

Contd...

Contd...

Gastrointestinal tract	Endocrine
▪ Gastric erosions ▪ Peptic ulceration ▪ Masked perforation ▪ Hemorrhage from stomach and duodenum ▪ Pancreatitis	▪ Growth retardation ▪ Menstrual irregularities ▪ Hypothalamic- pituitary-adrenal axis suppression ▪ Impotence ▪ Acute adrenal insufficiency, Cushingoid features
Skin	Metabolic
▪ Acne rubeosis steriodica ▪ Hirsutism ▪ Striae ▪ Ecchymoses ▪ Thin and fragile skin ▪ Panniculitis (on withdrawal)	▪ Glucose intolerance or frank diabetes mellitus ▪ Weight gain ▪ Hyperlipidemia ▪ Hypokalemia ▪ Alkalosis ▪ Fluid and salt retention ▪ Negative nitrogen balance- muscle wasting
Psychiatric	Cardiovascular
▪ Depression ▪ Insomnia ▪ Euphoria ▪ Steroid psychosis	▪ Hypertension ▪ Fluid retention ▪ Accelerated atherosclerosis ▪ Ischemic heart disease (IHD)
Muscles / Eye	Neurological
▪ Myopathy / ▪ Cataract ▪ Glaucoma	▪ Pseudotumor cerebri

Methylprednisolone: Hematologic (e.g., immune thrombocytopenia, warm autoimmune hemolytic anemia), allergic [e.g., asthma, atopic dermatitis, contact dermatitis, drug hypersensitivity, perennial or seasonal allergic rhinitis (oral only)], serum sickness, transfusion reactions), GI (e.g., Crohn disease, ulcerative colitis), inflammatory, neoplastic, neurologic (e.g., multiple sclerosis), rheumatic [e.g., antineutrophil cytoplasmic antibody-associated vasculitis, dermatomyositis/polymyositis, giant cell arteritis, gout (acute flare), giant cell arteritis, mixed cryoglobulinemia syndrome, polyarteritis nodosa, rheumatoid arthritis, systemic lupus erythematosus]

Dexamethasone: Cerebral edema, COVID-19

Hydrocortisone: Adrenal insufficiency, adrenal crisis, treatment and prevention
- Adrenal insufficiency, chronic
- Asthma, acute exacerbation
- COVID-19, hospitalized patients
- Septic shock
- Thyroid storm

Antidiabetic Drugs (Fig. 15.2)

Insulin (Tables 15.15 and 15.16)

Classes	Types
Rapid acting	Insulin analogs: Lispro, aspart, and glulisine
Short acting	▪ Regular (crystalline, soluble, and plain) ▪ Semilente
Intermediate acting	▪ Isophane insulin (NPH) ▪ Lente (excess zinc ions)
Long acting	▪ Protamine zinc insulin (PZI) ▪ Ultralente ▪ Insulin analogs: Glargine and detemir

Complications:
- **Hypoglycemia during insulin treatment:** It is the most common complication of insulin therapy and causes anxiety for both patients and relatives. It occurs due to imbalance between injected insulin and a patient's normal diet, activity, and basal insulin requirement. The risk of hypoglycemia is more before meals, during the night, and during exercise. Irregular eating habits, unusual exertion, and alcohol excess may precipitate hypoglycemic episodes.
- **At the injection site:**
  - A **shallow injection** causes intradermal (rather than subcutaneous) delivery of insulin resulting in **painful, red lesions** or even scarring. Abscess at injection site is extremely rare.
  - **Local allergic reactions: It may occur at the injection site early in therapy. These include local itching, erythematous and indurated lesions, and discrete subcutaneous nodules. They usually resolve spontaneously.**
  - **Fatty lumps, called as lipohypertrophy, may develop due to overuse of a single injection site due to lipogenic effects of the injected insulin. It may occur with any type of insulin.**
  - **Insulin resistance and anti-insulin antibodies:** Most common cause of mild insulin resistance is obesity.

Insulin resistance may be associated with antibodies directed against the insulin receptor.
- **Weight gain:** Many patients may gain weight on insulin treatment, especially if the insulin dose is increased inappropriately.

TABLE 15.15: Insulin analogs.

Short acting	Long acting
Lispro	Glargine
Aspart	Detemir
Glulisine	Degludec

TABLE 15.16: Indications for insulin therapy.

	Diabetes under following conditions:
- Type 1 DM - Diabetic keto-acidosis (DKA) - Hyperosmolar hyper-glycemic state	- Pregnancy (preferably prior to pregnancy) - Acute severe illness needing hospitalization - Perioperative/intensive care unit setting - Patients with acute coronary syndrome [myocardial infarction (MI)] - Patients on high-dose corticosteroids - Inability to tolerate or contraindication to oral anti glycemic agents - Newly diagnosed type 2 diabetes with significantly elevated blood glucose levels (patients with severe symptoms or DKA) - Patient no longer achieving therapeutic goals on combination of anti glycemic therapy

Profiles of antidiabetic medications

	MET	GLP-1RA	SGLT2I	DPP-4i	AGI	TZD (moderate dose)	SU / GLN	COLSVL	BCR-QR	Insulin	PRAML
Hypo	Neutral	Neutral	Neutral	Neutral	Neutral	Neutral	Moderate/severe / Mild	Neutral	Neutral	Moderate-to-severe	Neutral
Weight	Slight loss	Loss	Loss	Neutral	Neutral	Gain	Gain	Neutral	Neutral	Gain	Loss
Renal/GU	Contraindicated if eGFR <30 mL/min/1.73 m²	Exenatide not indicated CrCl <30 / Possible benefit of liraglutide	Not indicated for eGFR <45 mL/min/1.73 m² / Genital myocotic infections / Possible CKD benefit	Dose adjustment necessary (except linagliptin) / Effective in reducing albuminuria	Neutral	Neutral	More hypo risk	Neutral	Neutral	More hypo risk	Neutral
GI Sx	Moderate	Moderate	Neutral	Neutral	Moderate	Neutral	Neutral	Mild	Moderate	Neutral	Moderate
Cardiac — CHF	Neutral	See #1	See #2	See #3	Neutral	Moderate	Neutral	Neutral	Neutral	CHF risk	Neutral
Cardiac — ASCVD						May reduce stroke risk	Possible ASCVD risk	Benefit	Safe	Neutral	
Bone	Neutral	Neutral	Neutral	Neutral	Neutral	Moderate fracture risk	Neutral	Neutral	Neutral	Neutral	Neutral
Ketoacidosis	Neutral	Neutral	DKA can occur in various stress settings	Neutral	Neutral	Neutral	Neutral	Neutral	Neutral	Neutral	Neutral

- Few adverse events or possible benefits
- Use with caution
- Likelihood of adverse effect

1. Liraglutide—FDA approved for prevention of MACE events.
2. Empagliflozin—FDA approved to reduce CV mortality. Canagliflozin—FDA approved to reduce MACE events
3. Possible increased hospitalizations for heart failure with alogliptin and sexagliptin

Fig. 15.2: Profile of antidiabetic agents.

Oral Hypoglycemic Agents (Table 15.17)

TABLE 15.17: Oral hypoglycemic agents.

	Mechanism of action	Examples	HbA1c reduction (%)	Specific advantages	Specific disadvantages
Oral					
Biguanides	Hepatic glucose production	Metformin	1–2	Weight neutral/ mild weight loss do not cause hypoglycemia, inexpensive	Diarrhea, nausea, lactic acidosis, and vitamin B12 deficiency (0.5%) **(Box 15.2)**
Insulin secretagogues: Sulfonylureas	Insulin secretion	Glibenclamide (glyburide), glipizide, gliclazide, and glimepiride	1–2	Inexpensive	Hypoglycemia, weight gain, and sulfonamide allergies
Insulin secretagogues: Nonsulfonylureas	Insulin secretion	Repaglinide, nateglinide, and mitiglinide	1–2	Short onset of action, lower postprandial glucose	Hypoglycemia
Insulin secretagogues: Dipeptidyl peptidase-4 inhibitors	Prolong endogenous GLP-1 action	Saxagliptin, sitagliptin, vildagliptin, linagliptin, teneligliptin, and evogliptin	0.5–0.8	Do not cause hypoglycemia	Nasopharyngitis, meniscus lesions, headache, contact dermatitis, osteoarthritis, and tremor
α-glucosidase inhibitors	Decreased GI glucose absorption	Acarbose, miglitol, and voglibose	0.5–0.8	Reduce postprandial glycemia	GI flatulence, liver function abnormalities, and contraindicated in kidney disease, inflammatory bowel disease
Thiazolidinediones *Contraindication: CHF and liver disease*	Decreased insulin resistance and Increased glucose utilization	Rosiglitazone and pioglitazone	0.5–1.4	Lower insulin requirements	Peripheral edema, CHF, weight gain, fractures, macular edema; rosiglitazone may increase cardiovascular risk
Sodium-glucose cotransporter 2 (SGLT2) inhibitors	Help eliminate glucose in the urine	Canagliflozin, dapagliflozin, empagliflozin, and remogliflozin	0.4–1.1	No hypoglycemia and weight loss	Genital and urinary infections
Bile acid sequestrants					
Bile acid sequestrants *Contraindications: Elevated plasma triglycerides*	Bind bile acids, mechanism of glucose lowering is not known	Colesevelam	0.5		Constipation, dyspepsia, abdominal pain, nausea, triglycerides interfere with absorption of other drugs, and intestinal obstruction

Box 15.2: Contraindications for metformin.
- Malabsorption or GI disturbances/GI intolerance
- Low BMI <21 kg/m², marked weight loss
- Organ failure: Creatinine: >1.4 mg/dL, eGFR <30 mL/min/1.73 m²
  - Liver failure: Acute/chronic
  - Cardiac failure, hypotension/sepsis
- Active vitamin B_{12} deficiency
- Metabolic acidosis

Parenteral Hypoglycemic Agents (Table 15.18)

TABLE 15.18: Parenteral hypoglycemic agents.

Parenteral					
Insulin	↑Glucose utilization, ↓hepatic glucose production, and other anabolic actions	Refer earlier	Not limited	Known safety profile	Injection, weight gain, and hypoglycemia

Contd...

Contd...

GLP-1 receptor agonists Contraindications: Renal disease, agents that also slow GI motility	↑Insulin, ↓glucagon, slow gastric emptying, and satiety	Exenatide and liraglutide	0.5–10	Weight loss, do not cause hypoglycemia	Injection, nausea, risk of hypoglycemia with insulin secretagogues, pancreatitis, and renal failure
Amylin agonists Contraindication: Agents that also slow GI motility	Slow gastric emptying, ↑glucagon	Pramlintide	0.25–0.5	Reduce postprandial glycemia and weight loss	Injection, nausea, and risk of hypoglycemia with insulin

Statins (Box 15.3)

Competitive inhibitors of hydroxymethylglutaryl (HMG) CoA reductase, the rate-limiting step in cholesterol biosynthesis. They occupy a portion of the binding site of HMG CoA, blocking access of this substrate to the active site on the enzyme.

Examples: Atorvastatin, Rosuvastatin, Simvastatin, Pravastatin, Fluvastatin, Lovastatin, Pitavastatin

Indications:

Familial hypercholesterolemia:
- ACS, acute ischemic stroke
- Primary prevention of CVD
- Secondary prevention in patients with established atherosclerotic cardiovascular disease [e.g., coronary heart disease, cerebrovascular disease (ischemic stroke or transient ischemic attack), peripheral arterial disease]

> **Box 15.3: Major side effects and drug interaction potentials.**
> Muscle-related (e.g., myalgia, myopathy, myositis, rhabdomyolysis); headache; gastrointestinal (e.g., nausea, constipation, dyspepsia, diarrhea); sleep disturbance; elevations in hepatocellular enzymes and alkaline phosphatase.
> Statins are dependent on CYP metabolism and/or transmembrane transporters (e.g., OATP, BCRP) for clearance, subjecting them to a significant number of clinically relevant drug interactions. Coadministration of drugs that alter CYP metabolism or drug transporters often requires dose limitations

Erythropoietin

Mode of action:
- EPO stimulates erythropoiesis by acting on the marrow erythroid progenitors to enhance their survival, proliferation and differentiation.
- EPO may also protect neuronal cells from noxious stimuli.

Recombinant Human Erythropoietin (rHuEPO)

- It has same biological effects of endogenous erythropoietin and is available as erythropoietin-α and erythropoietin-β.
- **Indications:** In the treatment of:
  - Anemia associated with chronic renal failure.
  - Anemia of chronic inflammation.
  - Anemia (hemoglobin <10 g/dL) in cancer patients given chemotherapy.
  - Zidovudine-induced anemia in HIV patients.
  - Anemic patients undergoing nonvascular surgery to reduce the need for allogeneic blood transfusions.
- **Side effects:** Hypertension, bleeding, headache, arthralgia, nausea, edema, diarrhea, increased risk of thrombosis, pure red cell aplasia, and progression of cancers.

Vitamin D

Mechanism of action: Cholecalciferol (vitamin D_3) is a provitamin. The active metabolite, 1,25-dihydroxyvitamin D (calcitriol), stimulates calcium and phosphate absorption from the small intestine, promotes secretion of calcium from bone to blood; promotes renal tubule phosphate resorption.

Indications:
- Hypoparathyroidism
- Hyperparathyroidism

Vitamin D deficiency (oral): 50,000 units (1,250 mg) once weekly (or equivalent dose administered once daily) for 6 to 12 weeks.

15. ANTIBIOTICS

Beta Lactam (Box 15.4, Fig. 15.3 and Table 15.19)

- β-lactam antibiotics have a β-lactam ring structure. They exert a bactericidal action by inhibiting enzymes involved in cell wall synthesis [penicillin binding proteins (PBP)].
- β-lactamases are bacterial enzymes produced by many gram-positive and gram-negative bacteria. Theses enzymes can inactivate β-lactam antibacterials by hydrolysis of β-lactam ring structure and results in infective compounds.
  Production of β-lactamases by these bacteria is the most important factor that contributes to β-lactam antibiotic resistance.

> **Box 15.4: Adverse effects of beta-lactam antibiotics.**
> - Generalized allergy to penicillin
> - Gastrointestinal upset and diarrhea
> - Mild reversible hepatitis
> - Leukopenia, thrombocytopenia and coagulation deficiencies, and interstitial nephritis and potentiation of aminoglycoside-mediated renal damage
> - Thrombophlebitis with parenteral β-lactams

- Many serine-active β-lactamases inhibitors (e.g., clavulanic acid, sulbactam, and tazobactam) in combination with β-lactam antibiotics are used to reduce drug resistance by bacteria containing β-lactamases.

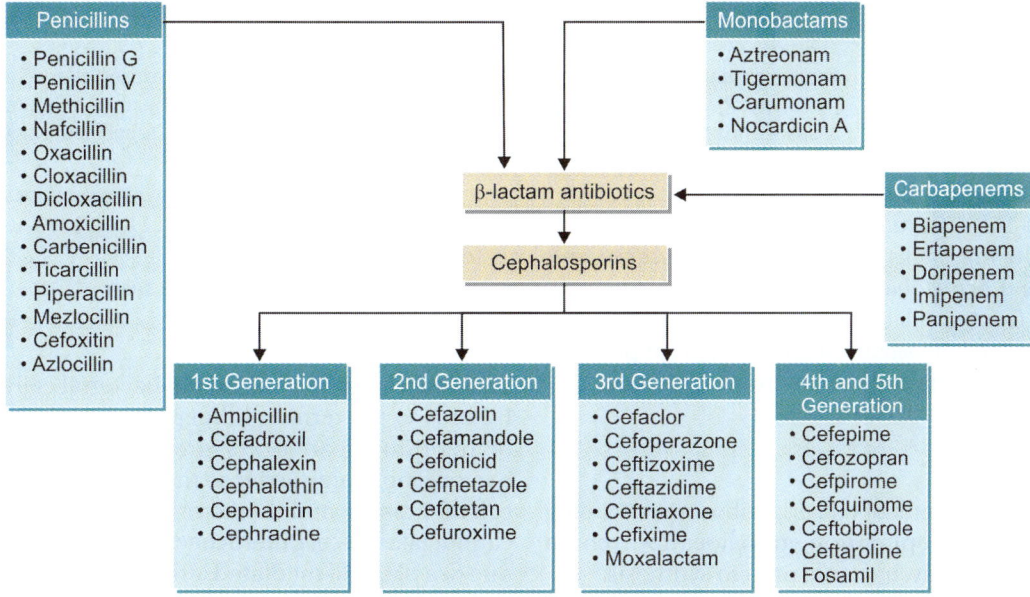

Fig. 15.3: Classification of beta-lactam antibiotics.

TABLE 15.19: Beta lactam antibiotics.				
Subclass, drug	Mechanism of action	Effects	Clinical applications	Pharmacokinetics, toxicities, interactions
Penicillins				
■ Penicillin G	Prevents bacterial cell wall synthesis by binding to and inhibiting cell wall transpeptidases	Rapid bactericidal activity against susceptible bacteria	Streptococcal infections, meningococcal infections, neurosyphilis	IV administration ■ Rapid renal clearance (half-life 30 min, so requires dosing every 4 h) ■ *Toxicity.* Immediate hypersensitivity, rash, seizures
■ Penicillin V: Oral, low systemic levels limit widespread use ■ Benzathine penicillin, procaine penicillin: Intramuscular, long-acting formulations ■ Nafcillin, oxacillin: Intravenous, added stability to staphylococcal β-lactamase, biliary clearance ■ Ampicillin, amoxicillin, piperacillin: Greater activity versus gram-negative bacteria; addition or β-lactamase inhibitor restores activity against many β-lactamase-producing bacteria				
Cephalosporins				
■ Cefazolin	Prevents bacterial cell wall synthesis by binding to and inhibiting cell wall transpeptidases	Rapid bactericidal activity against susceptible bacteria	Skin and soft tissue infections, urinary tract infections, surgical prophylaxis	IV administration ■ Renal clearance (half-life 1.5 h) ■ Given every 8 h ■ Poor penetration into the central nervous system (CNS) ■ *Toxicity.* Rash, drug fever

- **Cephalexin:** Oral, first-generation drug used for treating skin and soft tissue infections and urinary tract infections
- **Cefuroxime:** Oral and intravenous, second-generation drug, improved activity versus *Pneumococcus/ Haemophilus influenzae*
- **Cefotetan, cefoxitin:** Intravenous, second-generation drugs, activity versus *Bacteroides fragilis* allows for use in abdominal/pelvic infections
- **Ceftriaxone:** Intravenous, third-generation drug, mixed clearance with long half-life (6 hours), good CNS penetration, many uses including pneumonia, meningitis, pyelonephritis, and gonorrhea
- **Cefotaxime:** Intravenous, third-generation, similar to ceftriaxone; however, clearance is renal and half-life is 1 hour
- **Ceftazidime:** Intravenous, third-generation drug, poor gram-positive activity, good activity versus *Pseudomonas aeruginosa*
- **Cefepime:** Intravenous, fourth-generation drug, broad activity with improved stability to chromosomal β-lactamases
- **Ceftaroline:** Intravenous, active against methicillin-resistant staphylococci, broad gram-negative activity not including *Pseudomonas aeruginosa*
- **Ceftazidime-avibactam, ceftolozane-tazobactam:** Intravenous, cephalosporin-β-lactamase inhibitor combination drugs, broad activity with improved stability to chromosomal β-lactamase and some extended-spectrum β-lactamases
- **Meropenem, doripenem:** Intravenous, similar activity to imipenem; stable to renal dehydropeptidase, lower incidence of seizures

TABLE 15.20: Carbapenems.

Imipenem-cilastatin	Prevents bacterial cell wall synthesis by binding to and inhibiting cell wall transpeptidases	Rapid bactericidal activity against susceptible bacteria	Serious infections such as pneumonia and sepsis	IV administration - Renal clearance (half-life 1 h), dosed every 6–8 h, cilastatin added to prevent hydrolysis by renal dehydropeptidase - *Toxicity.* Seizures especially in renal failure or with high doses (>2 g/d)

- **Ertapenem:** Intravenous, longer half-life allows for once-daily dosing, lacks activity versus *Pseudomonas aeruginosa* and *Acinetobacter*
- **Faropenem:** Orally available beta lactam antibiotic. Broad spectrum with activity against anaerobes, gram positive, gram negative bacteria and the Enterobacteriaceae.
- **Carbepenems—Table 15.20**

Macrolide

They bind to the 50S subunit of bacterial ribosomes, leading to inhibition of transpeptidation, translocation, chain elongation, and, ultimately, bacterial protein synthesis.

Spectrum

Azithromycin and clarithromycin have a broader spectrum of activity than erythromycin, that includes many gram-negative, atypical, and mycobacterial organisms as well as gram-positive organisms. These agents are therefore used in a variety of infections including infections of the respiratory tract, mycobacterial infections, and sexually transmitted diseases.

Azithromycin is also active against several atypical organisms including *Mycoplasma pneumoniae, Legionella pneumophila, Chlamydophila pneumoniae, Babesia microti*, and *Ureaplasma* spp.

Adverse effect:
- Abnormal liver function tests, hepatitis, cholestatic jaundice, hepatic necrosis, and hepatic failure
- QT interval prolongation and cardiovascular events
- Gastrointestinal toxicity

Linezolid

Inhibits bacterial protein synthesis by binding to bacterial 23S ribosomal RNA of the 50S subunit. This prevents the formation of a functional 70S initiation complex that is essential for the bacterial translation process:

Dose and indications:
- Oral, IV: 600 mg every 12 hours
- Enterococcal infections
- Treatment of pneumonia caused by *Streptococcus pneumoniae*, or *Staphylococcus aureus*

Skin and skin structure infections, anthrax, intracranial abscess (brain abscess, intracranial epidural abscess) and spinal epidural abscess; meningitis, bacterial; osteomyelitis and/or discitis; prosthetic joint infection; septic arthritis; toxic shock syndrome; tuberculosis, drug resistant infections.

Adverse effect:
- Gastrointestinal: Diarrhea
- Hematologic and oncologic: Decreased white blood cell count
- Dermatologic: Pruritus, skin rash

Vancomycin

Vancomycin acts by inhibiting bacterial cell wall synthesis. It hinds to the terminal dipeptide "D-ala-D-ala" sequence of peptidoglycan units prevents its release from the bactoprenol lipid carrier so that assembly of the units at the cell membrane and then cross linking to form the cell wall cannot take place. Enterococcal resistance to vancomycin is due to a plasmid mediated alteration of the dipeptide target site, reducing its affinity for vancomycin.

Systemic use (500 mg 6 hourly or 1 g 12 hourly infused IV over 1 hour) is restricted to serious MRSA infections for which it is the most effective drug, and as a penicillin substitute (in allergic patients) for enterococcal endocarditis along with gentamicin. It is an alternative drug for serious skin, soft tissue and skeletal infections in which gram-positive bacteria are mostly causative. For empirical therapy of bacterial meningitis, IV vancomycin is usually combined with IV ceftriaxone cefotaxime. It is also used in dialysis patients and those undergoing cancer chemotherapy. Penicillin resistant pneumococcal infections and infection caused by diphtheroids respond very well to vancomycin.

Vancomycin is the preferred surgical prophylactic in MRSA prevalent areas and in penicillin allergic patients.

Toxicity: Systemic toxicity of vancomycin is high. It can cause plasma concentration dependent nerve deafness which may be permanent. Kidney damage is also dose related. Other ototoxic and nephrotoxic drugs, such as aminoglycosides, must be very carefully administered when vancomycin is being used. Skin allergy and fall in BP during IV injection can occur. Vancomycin has the potential to release histamine by direct action on mast cells. Rapid IV injection has caused chills, fever, urticaria and intense flushing—called "Red man syndrome".

Nitrofurantoin

Nitrofurantoin is reduced by bacterial flavoproteins to reactive intermediates that inactivate or alter bacterial ribosomal proteins leading to inhibition of protein synthesis, aerobic energy metabolism, DNA, RNA, and cell wall synthesis. Nitrofurantoin is bactericidal in urine at therapeutic doses.

Adverse effects:
- Commonest is gastrointestinal intolerance—nausea, epigastric pain, and diarrhea.
- An acute reaction with chills, fever and leucopenia occurs occasionally.

- Peripheral neuritis and other neurological effects are reported with long term use. Hemolytic anemia is rare, except in G-6-PD deficiency. Liver damage and a pulmonary reaction with fibrosis on chronic use are infrequent events.
- Urine of patients taking nitrofurantoin turns dark brown on exposure to air.

Use: The only indication for nitrofurantoin is uncomplicated lower urinary tract infection not associated with prostatitis, but it is infrequently used now. Acute infections due to *E. coli* can be treated with 50–100 mg TDS (5–7 mg/kg/day) given for 5–10 days. These doses should not be used for 2 weeks at a time. Suppressive long-term treatment has been successful with 50 mg BD or 100 mg at bed time. This dose can also be employed for prophylaxis of urinary tract infection following catheterization or instrumentation of the lower urinary tract and in women with recurrent cystitis.

Aminoglycoside (Box 15.5)

Systemic aminoglycosides	
▪ Streptomycin	▪ Amikacin
▪ Gentamicin	▪ Sisomicin
▪ Kanamycin	▪ Netilmicin
▪ Tobramycin	▪ Paromomycin
Topical aminoglycosides	
Neomycin	Framycetin

Box 15.5: Common properties of aminoglycoside antibiotics.
- All are used as sulfate salts, which are highly water soluble—solutions are stable for months.
- They ionize in solution are not absorbed orally—distribute only extracellularly; do not penetrate brain or CSF.
- All are excreted unchanged in urine by glomerular filtration.
- All are bactericidal and more active at alkaline pH.
- They act by interfering with bacterial protein synthesis.
- All are active primarily against aerobic gram-negative bacilli and do not inhibit anaerobes.
- There is only partial cross resistance among them.
- They have relatively narrow margin of safety.
- All exhibit ototoxicity and nephrotoxicity.

Toxicity
- Nephrotoxicity
- Ototoxicity
- Neuromuscular blockade

Mechanism of action:
The aminoglycosides are bactericidal antibiotics, all having the same general pattern of action which may be described in two main steps:
1. Transport of the aminoglycoside through the bacterial cell wall and cytoplasmic membrane.
2. Binding to ribosomes resulting in inhibition of protein synthesis.

Indications:
- Tularemia
- Plague
- Urinary tract infections due to multidrug resistant (MDR) gram negative organisms
- *Neisseria gonorrhoeae*
- The most frequent clinical use of aminoglycosides (most commonly in combination with other antibacterial agents) is empiric therapy of serious infections, such as septicemia, nosocomial respiratory tract infections, complicated urinary tract infections, complicated intra-abdominal infections, and osteomyelitis.
- Treatment of drug resistant tuberculosis

Tetracycline
Inhibits protein synthesis by binding with the 30S and possibly the 50S ribosomal subunit(s) of susceptible bacteria; may also cause alterations in the cytoplasmic membrane.

Doxycycline

Dose: Oral or IV—100 mg every 12 hours.

Indication:
Doxycycline is a tetracycline antibiotic. It is indicated for many different bacterial infections, such as acne, urinary tract infections, intestinal infections, eye infections, gonorrhea, chlamydia, etc.

Drug	Side effects
Tetracycline	▪ *Dose related:* Epigastric pain, nausea, vomiting, diarrhea, fatty liver, renal damage, phototoxicity, brown discoloration of teeth, antianabolic effect, increased intracranial pressure, and vestibular toxicity ▪ Hypersensitivity ▪ Superinfection

Quinolones

Mechanism of action: Fluoroquinolones are bactericidal antibiotics that directly inhibit bacterial DNA synthesis. All fluoroquinolones bind to complexes of DNA with each of two enzymes that are essential for DNA replication, DNA gyrase and DNA topoisomerase IV, and this binding generates DNA cleavage.

Spectrum:
Fluoroquinolones are broad-spectrum antibiotics with potent activity against aerobic, enteric gram-negative bacilli and many common respiratory pathogens. In addition, some fluoroquinolones are active against *Pseudomonas* species, selected gram-positive organisms, anaerobes, and mycobacteria.

Side effects:

Quinolones/ fluoroquinolones	▪ *GIT:* Nausea, anorexia, vomiting, and bad taste ▪ *CNS:* Dizziness, headache, restlessness, anxiety, insomnia, and tremor ▪ *Skin:* Hypersensitivity, rash, and pruritus ▪ Tendonitis and tendon rupture

16. ANTIVIRAL OSELTAMIVIR

Indications and dose:
- Influenza, seasonal, treatment: Oral: 75 mg twice daily.
- Influenza A, avian (H7N9 or H5N1), prophylaxis; influenza A, avian (H7N9 or H5N1), treatment

Neuraminidase Inhibitors

They **inhibit neuraminidase** which is a glycoprotein on the surface of influenza virus that destroys an infected cell's receptor for viral hemagglutinin. By inhibiting viral **neuraminidase, neuraminidase inhibitor agents decrease the release of viruses** from **infected cells** and, thus, **decrease the spread of virus.** Drugs include **oseltamivir** and zanamivir. Both are effective against both influenza A or B.

Oseltamivir (Tamiflu)

- Must be administered within 48 hours of symptom onset to provide optimal treatment.
- **Adult dose**
  - **Treatment for acute illness:** 75 mg PO BID for 5 days
  - **Prophylaxis:** 75 mg PO OD

Mechanism of action: Oseltamivir, a prodrug, is hydrolyzed to the active form, oseltamivir carboxylate (OC). OC inhibits influenza virus neuraminidase, an enzyme known to cleave the budding viral progeny from its cellular envelope attachment point (neuraminic acid) just prior to release.

Adverse effect: Gastrointestinal—vomiting, nervous system—headache, arrhythmia.

17. ANTIRETROVIRAL (FIG. 15.4 AND TABLE 15.21)

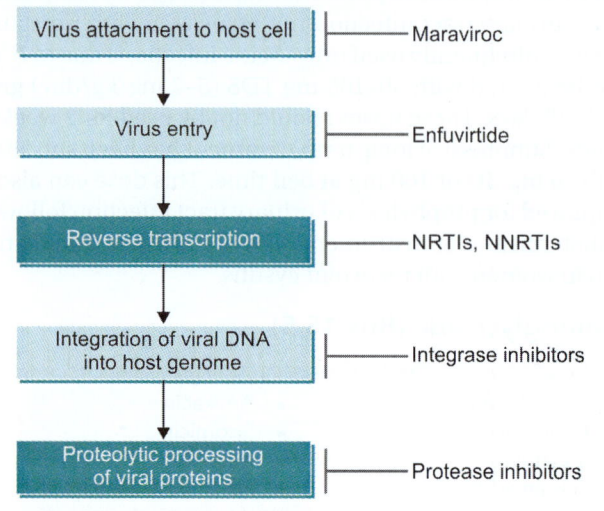

Fig. 15.4: Site of action of antiretroviral therapy (ART).

TABLE 15.21: Antiretroviral therapy.		
Medication and adult dose (normal renal function)	Common side effects	Comments
Nucleoside reverse transcriptase inhibitors (NRTIs): Mechanism: Competitive inhibition of HIV-1 reverse transcriptase. Need to be phosphorylated intracellularly for activity to occur		
Abacavir 300 mg PO BID	Fever and rash	<ul><li>HLA B*5701 testing prior to initiation</li><li>May be used in pregnancy</li><li>Avoid alcohol</li><li>Avoid abacavir in patients with/at risk for cardiovascular disease</li></ul>
Lamivudine 150 mg PO BID or 300 mg PO OD	Rash and peripheral neuropathy. Flare of hepatitis in HBV-coinfected patients who discontinue drug	Do not administer with emtricitabine or zalcitabine
Stavudine 40 mg PO BID	Peripheral neuropathy, pancreatitis, hepatitis, lipoatrophy, rapidly progressive ascending neuromuscular weakness (rare)	<ul><li>Monthly neurologic questionnaire for neuropathy, amylase should be done</li><li>Avoid zidovudine, didanosine, zalcitabine, and isoniazid</li></ul>
Zidovudine (AZT) 300 mg PO BID	Anemia, neutropenia, nausea, headache, lactic acidosis, hepatic steatosis, myopathy (red ragged fibers), nail pigmentation, lipoatrophy, and hyperglycemia	<ul><li>CBC should be done 4–8 weeks after starting AZT</li><li>Monitor RBS and LFTs</li></ul>
Tenofovir disoproxil fumarate (TDF) 300 mg PO OD	<ul><li>Renal dysfunction, proteinuria, glycosuria (Fanconi syndrome), hypophosphatemia, and bone resorption</li><li>Flare of hepatitis in HBV-coinfected patients who discontinue drug</li></ul>	Monitor: <ul><li>Creatinine at baseline, at 2–8 weeks, every 3–6 months; urinalysis and urine glucose and protein at baseline and repeated as clinically indicated; consider bone densitometry</li><li>Avoid atazanavir, didanosine, and probenecid</li></ul>
Nonnucleoside reverse transcriptase inhibitors (NNRTIs): Mechanism: Noncompetitive inhibitors of reverse transcriptase		
Efavirenz 600 mg OD at night	<ul><li>Rash</li><li>Deranged LFTs and lipid profile</li><li>Drowsiness</li><li>Psychiatric manifestations: Abnormal dreams, depression, and dysphoria</li></ul>	Avoid elvitegravir/cobicistat, etravirine, and indinavir

Contd...

Contd...

| Nevirapine 200 mg PO OD × 2 weeks, then 200 mg PO BID | Rash Hepatotoxicity | - Contraindicated with moderate or severe hepatic impairment
- Avoid atazanavir, dolutegravir, and elvitegravir/cobicistat |

Protease inhibitors (PIs): Mechanism: Bind to HIV proteases. This blocks the proteolytic activities of the enzyme, resulting in the inability to form mature, and infectious virions

Atazanavir 400 mg PO OD	- PR prolongation - Transaminase elevations - Nausea and vomiting - Hyperglycemia - Renal stones	- Atazanavir/ritonavir: Atazanavir 300 mg with ritonavir 100 mg OD (given with efavirenz) - Atazanavir/cobicistat: Atazanavir 300 mg with cobicistat 150 mg PO OD - Avoid in severe hepatic insufficiency

Darunavir	- Diarrhea
	- Headache
	- Skin rash
	- Hepatotoxicity
	- Hyperlipidemia
	- Hyperglycemia
		- Avoid in patients with sulfa allergy
		- Darunavir/cobicistat: Darunavir 800 mg and cobicistat 150 mg PO OD
		- Darunavir/ritonavir:
		  • For PI-naïve patients: Darunavir 800 mg and ritonavir 100 mg PO OD
		  • PI-experienced patients: Darunavir 600 mg and ritonavir 100 mg PO BID

Indinavir 800 mg PO TID	- Abdominal pain - Nausea - Hyperbilirubinemia - Fan shaped/Star-burst renal calculi	Avoid efavirenz and etravirine
Lopinavir/ritonavir 400 mg/100 mg PO BD	- Skin rash - Dyslipidemia - Hyperglycemia - Elevated transaminases - Diarrhea - Fatigue	- Separate dosing from didanosine by 1 hour - Avoid darunavir and elvitegravir/cobicistat - Avoid disulfiram and metronidazole with oral solution

INSTI—integrase strand transfer inhibitor (integrase inhibitors):
Mechanism: Blocks the integrase enzyme and prevents the incorporation of viral DNA into the host chromosome

Bictegravir 50 mg orally daily	Diarrhea, nausea, and headache	Used in antiretroviral combination with tenofovir alafenamide 25 mg and emtricitabine 200 mg OD
Dolutegravir Treatment-naive or integrase-naïve patients: 50 mg PO OD	Hypersensitivity, insomnia, fatigue, and headache	- When administered with efavirenz, fosamprenavir/ritonavir, tipranavir/ritonavir, or rifampicin: 50 mg PO BD When administered to integrase-experienced patients with suspected integrase resistance: 50 mg PO BD - Avoid carbamazepine, dofetilide, nevirapine, phenobarbital, and phenytoin

Entry inhibitors (fusion inhibitors):
Mechanism: Binds to gp41 and prevents the conformational changes necessary for the fusion of the viral and cellular membrane

Enfuvirtide 90 mg subcutaneously q12h	- Injection site pain and allergic reaction - Increased rate of bacterial pneumonia	- Indication: ART-experienced patients with HIV replication despite ongoing antiretroviral therapy - It does not inhibit HIV-2

Entry inhibitors (CCR5 inhibitors):
- Mechanism: Selectively binds to the human CCR5 receptor on the cell membrane, and blocks the interaction of the HIV gp120 and the CCR5 receptor for CCR5-tropic HIV
- However, it does not block the viral entry of CXCR4-tropic HIV or HIV that uses both CCR5 and CXCR4 for cell entry

Maraviroc 150 mg PO BD or 300 mg PO BD	- Cough, fever, and rash - Hepatotoxicity - Musculoskeletal symptoms	- Do not administer in patients with severe renal dysfunction - Viral tropism testing should be done before initiation of maraviroc - Cannot be used for CXCR4-tropic HIV or HIV that uses both CCR5 and CXCR4 for cell entry

Entry inhibitors (postattachment inhibitors)

Ibalizumab Single loading dose of 2,000 mg followed by a maintenance dose of 800 mg every 2 weeks IV	Rash, diarrhea, and nausea	- Humanized monoclonal antibody - In combination with other antiretroviral agents in patients with multidrug-resistant HIV-1

18. ANTICOAGULATION (TABLES 15.22 AND 15.23)

TABLE 15.22: Classification of anticoagulants.

Parenteral (rapidly acting)	Clinical situations
- Heparin (unfractionated and low-molecular weight heparins) - Hirudins - Heparinoids - Indirect factor Xa inhibitors (fondaparinux and idraparinux)	- Coumarin derivatives: Warfarin sodium, dicoumarol. These are most commonly used. Bishydroxycoumarin dicoumoral, acenocoumarol (nicoumalone), ethyl biscoumacetate - Indandione derivatives: Phenindione, diphenindione (not used clinically) - Direct thrombin inhibitors: Ximelagatran

TABLE 15.23: Indications for anticoagulant therapy.

Purpose	Clinical situations
Urgent and for long-term anticoagulation: It is initiated with heparin and taken over by oral anticoagulants	Thrombosis and thromboembolism: - Atrial fibrillation and cardiac disorders with thromboembolism - Deep venous thrombosis - Stroke in evolution and resistant transient ischemic attacks - Pulmonary thromboembolism Others: - Unstable angina and non-ST-elevation myocardial infarction - Prosthetic valves - Peripheral vascular disease
Anticoagulants for brief periods: Heparin alone is used	Cardiac bypass surgery: - Hemodialysis - Disseminated intravascular coagulation (DIC)

Contraindications for anticoagulants are given in **Box 15.6**.

Box 15.6: Contraindications for anticoagulant therapy.
- Bleeding disorders, heparin-induced thrombocytopenia
- Severe hypertension, threatened abortion, hemorrhoids, peptic ulcers
- Subacute bacterial endocarditis, tuberculosis
- Ocular and neurosurgery, lumbar puncture
- Chronic alcoholics, cirrhosis, renal failure

Unfractionated Heparin

Mechanism of action: Heparin acts as anticoagulant by activating antithrombin (previously known as antithrombin III) thereby potentiating its action. The activated antithrombin inhibits clotting enzymes, particularly thrombin and factor Xa.
- **Mode of administration:** Heparin is given parenterally. It is usually administered SC or by continuous IV infusion.
- **Dose:** Initial loading dose of 5,000–10,000 units intravenously, followed by maintenance by any one of the following:
  - Continuous intravenous
  - Intermittent intravenous/subcutaneous
- **Methods of anticoagulation:**
  - Total anticoagulation: Continuous intravenous maintenance using an infusion pump at a rate of 1,000 units/hour.
  - Low-dose heparinization (e.g., prophylaxis of DVT): 5,000 units 12 hourly or 8 hourly subcutaneously.
  - For prophylaxis: Fixed doses of 5,000 units SC two or three times daily.
- **Duration of therapy:** Variable, but usually ranges from 7 to 10 days.
- **Monitoring:** Heparin therapy is monitored using activated partial thromboplastin time (aPTT), which is maintained at 1.5 to 2 times the control value.
- **Antidote of heparin:** Protamine sulfate
- **Complications of heparin therapy:** Includes bleeding, heparin-induced thrombocytopenia (HIT), osteoporosis, and osteomalacia (in long-standing therapy). HIT is of two types—type 1 (nonimmune) and type 2 (immune mediated).

Low-molecular Weight Heparins (LMWH)
- LMWH are biologically active forms of conventional heparin. The molecular weights ranging from 3,000 to 8,000 Daltons.
- **Mode of action:** They act as anticoagulant primarily by inhibiting activated factor X (Xa) rather than activated factor II (IIa).
- **Advantages:**
  - Can be administered subcutaneously once or twice/day.
  - Pharmacokinetics is predictable and aPTT monitoring is not needed.
  - Less immunogenic and less likely to produce thrombocytopenia.
  - Many patients with DVT (deep vein thrombosis) can be treated on an outpatient basis.
- **Disadvantage:** Higher cost.
- **Commonly available** LMWH: Enoxaparin, dalteparin and tinzaparin.

Warfarin
- Water-soluble vitamin K antagonist.
- **Mode of action:** Vitamin K is necessary for the synthesis of coagulation factors such as prothrombin (factor II) and

factors VII, IX and X and also protein C and protein S. Warfarin type anticoagulants prevents the conversion of vitamin K to its active hydroquinone form and interferes with the synthesis of the above vitamin K-dependent coagulation factors.
- **Monitoring:** Warfarin therapy is monitored using the **PT.**
- **Dose:**
    - Starting dose: Warfarin is started at a dose of 5 mg oral on the first day. Subsequent daily doses are adjusted according to PT (INR) which is maintained at 1.5–3 times the control value.
    - Maintenance dose: Varies from 2.5 to 7.5 mg/day.
- **Duration of therapy:** Variable and may range from 3 months to lifelong.
- **Side effects:** These include bleeding and rarely skin necrosis.
- **Antidotes of warfarin:** Injections of vitamin K_1, 5 mg intravenously or fresh frozen plasma or prothrombin complex concentrate.
- **Contraindications:**
    - Severe uncontrolled hypertension
    - Severe renal or liver failure
    - Pre-existing hemostatic disorders
    - Pregnancy: It crosses the placenta and can cause fetal abnormalities. Therefore, should not be used during pregnancy.

Novel Oral Anticoagulants (NOACs)

Dabigatran being used for prophylaxis after hip and knee replacement. The major side effect of dabigatran is hemorrhage.

Idarucizumab: *Humanized monoclonal antibody fragment (Fab) indicated in patients treated with dabigatran when reversal of the anticoagulant effects is needed for emergency surgery or urgent procedures, or in the event of life-threatening or uncontrolled bleeding.*

Rivaroxaban and **apixaban** are orally administered drug, factor Xa inhibitor available orally administered direct factor Xa inhibitor that produces its anticoagulant effect through reversible binding with the factor Xa molecule. Rivaroxaban can inhibit both free and thrombus associated factor Xa (Table 15.24).

TABLE 15.24: Potential advantages and disadvantages of NOACs.	
Potential advantages	Potential disadvantages
■ Lower rates of intracranial bleed and hemorrhagic strokes than warfarin ■ No need for routine laboratory monitoring ■ Fewer drug or food interactions than warfarin	■ Higher drug cost; may require prior insurance approval ■ Lack of availability of a reversal agent ■ Increased risk of gastrointestinal bleeding ■ Higher rebound rate of VTE events in patients with poor adherence

19. FIBRINOLYTIC

- **Goal of therapy:** To produce rapid dissolution of thrombus and restore the blood flow.
- Most fibrinolytic or thrombolytic agents are recombinant forms having plasminogen activator activity.
- **Mechanism of action:** They convert the proenzyme, plasminogen to active enzyme plasmin. Plasmin then degrades the fibrin of thrombi and produces soluble fibrin degradation products.
- Currently approved fibrinolytic agents are:
    - Streptokinase (STK):
        - Source: It is obtained from β-hemolytic streptococci. It is not an enzyme and does not directly convert plasminogen to plasmin. Instead it forms a complex with plasminogen, it converts other/additional molecules of plasminogen into plasmin. Since it is obtained from bacteria, it can produce allergic reactions in about 5% of patients.
        - Uses: In acute ST-elevation myocardial infarction and pulmonary embolism.
    - Urokinase (UK): It is used in patients who received STK in the past 6 months and require a thrombolytic agent for MI or pulmonary embolism. It does not produce allergic reaction.
    - Anisoylated plasminogen streptokinase activator complex (APSAC)(anistreplase).
    - Recombinant tissue-type plasminogen activator (rtPA): Also known as alteplase or activase is useful in acute thrombotic strokes (within 3 hours of onset) besides acute MI and pulmonary embolism.
    - Prourokinase (pro-UK) like rtPA.
    - Others: Tenecteplase, desmoteplase and reteplase.
- Indications for use of fibrinolytic agents are listed in **Box 15.7**.

Box 15.7: Indication for use of fibrinolytic or thrombolytic agents.
♦ Acute myocardial infarction ♦ Massive pulmonary embolism with hypotension ♦ Acute ischemic stroke (thrombotic or embolic) ♦ Acute peripheral artery occlusion

20. DISEASE-MODIFYING ANTIRHEUMATIC DRUGS

Conventional Disease-modifying antirheumatic drugs (DMARDs) used in RA (Box 15.8)

Box 15.8: Conventional DMARDs used in RA.
♦ Methotrexate (MTX) ♦ Hydroxychloroquine ♦ Sulfasalazine ♦ Leflunomide ♦ Azathioprine ♦ Gold (auranofin) ♦ Minocycline ♦ D-penicillamine

- Conventional DMARDs exhibit a delayed onset of action and take 2–6 months to exert their full effect.
- Start DMARD therapy early in the disease process. Early in the course of disease, most patients should be started on a combination of DMARDs and analgesics. Before

using DMARDs, complete blood count, serum creatinine, aminotransferases, and screening for hepatitis C, hepatitis B, and latent tuberculosis infection. A chest radiograph should be obtained prior to initiating treatment with MTX.

Methotrexate: Currently, methotrexate is the DMARD of choice (considered as "gold standard" drug) for RA and is the anchor drug for most combination therapies.

- **Mechanism of action** in RA: At the dosages used for RA, methotrexate stimulates extracellular release of adenosine from cells, which has anti-inflammatory and immunomodulatory properties. Enzymes inhibited by methotrexate in RA include **thymidylate synthetase (TS) and 5-aminoimidazole-4-carboxamide ribonucleotide (AICAR) transformylase.** It should not be prescribed in pregnancy.
- **Dose:** Usually given orally in the starting dose of 2.5–7.5 mg/**week** as a single dose. **If there is no positive response** within 4–8 weeks, and there is no toxicity, the dose should be **increased by 2.5–5 mg/week** each month to 15–25 mg/week before considering, the treatment a failure. Oral absorption of methotrexate is variable. If oral treatment is not effective, it is given by subcutaneous injections. It should be monitored with full blood counts and liver biochemistry.
- **Folic acid,** 1 to 4 mg/day (or 5 mg once a week, on the day following methotrexate dose), reduces most methotrexate associated toxicities (e.g., gastrointestinal intolerance, stomatitis, hepatotoxicity, hyperhomocysteinemia, alopecia) without apparent loss of efficacy.

If methotrexate alone does not sufficiently control RA, it is combined with other DMARDs.

- **Antidote** for severe low dose methotrexate toxicity: **Leucovorin (folinic acid)**
- **Glucarpidase** is a bacterial enzyme used in reversing high dose methotrexate toxicity.

Other DMARDs

- **Hydroxychloroquine** is used usually in combination with other DMARDs, particularly methotrexate. It is given orally at a dose of 200–400 mg daily. It is the least toxic DMARD but also the least effective as monotherapy. Regular monitoring (every 6 months to a year) by ophthalmoscopy to detect any signs of retinopathy, bull's eye maculopathy should be done.
- **Sulfasalazine:** It is effective when given in doses of 1–3 g daily. Monitoring of blood cell counts is recommended, particularly WBC counts, in the first 6 months. Combination of sulfasalazine + hydroxychloroquine + methotrexate is referred to as triple therapy.
- **Leflunomide** is a pyrimidine antagonist, also inhibits enzyme **dihydroorotate dehydrogenase,** interfering with cell signal transduction. It has a very long half-life and is given daily in a dose of 10–20 mg. The most common toxicity is diarrhea, which may respond to dose reduction. Leflunomide is teratogenic and hepatotoxic. It is used as monotherapy or in combination with methotrexate and other DMARDs.

21. FOR INFLAMMATORY BOWEL DISEASE

Mesalamine (5-aminosalicylic acid) is the active component of sulfasalazine; the specific mechanism of action is unknown; however, it is thought that mesalamine modulates local chemical mediators of the inflammatory response, especially leukotrienes, and is also postulated to be a free radical scavenger or an inhibitor of tumor necrosis factor (TNF); action appears topical rather than systemic.

- **5-Aminosalicylate (5-ASA) agents (Table 15.25):**
  - Available as oral tablets or topical (enema/suppository) preparation (for rectal and sigmoid disease).
  - These agents include 5-aminosalicylic acid (5-ASA) or mesalazine alone, or combination of 5-ASA with a carrier which releases 5-ASA after splitting by bacteria in colon (sulfasalazine, olsalazine, and balsalazide).

TABLE 15.25: Various oral 5-ASA (5-aminosalicylate agents) preparations used in ulcerative colitis.

Preparation	Dosage
Azo-bond	
Sulfasalazine	3–6 g (acute)
	2–4 g (maintenance)
Olsalazine	1–3 g
Balsalazide	6.75–9 g
Delayed-release	
Mesalamine	2.4–4.8 g (acute)
	1.6–4.8 g (maintenance)
Controlled-release	
Mesalamine	2–4 g (acute)
	1.5–4 g (maintenance)
Delayed and extended-release	
Mesalamine	1.5 g (maintenance)

- Topical mesalamine is the initial preferred agent in mild-to-moderate ulcerative proctitis/proctosigmoiditis, for induction as well as maintenance of remission. It acts as a topical anti-inflammatory within the lumen of the intestine, controls acute exacerbation, maintains remission, and prevents relapses. Maintenance therapy may decrease the risk of colorectal cancer.
- Patients who are unwilling or unable to tolerate topical mesalazine can be started an oral 5-ASA medication. Oral 5-ASA should also be added in those patients who do not show remission after 4 weeks of topical therapy.
- For patients with left-sided or extensive mildly-to-moderately active UC a combination of an oral 5-ASA agent plus rectal mesalazine is used. **Sulfasalazine** and high dose **mesalazine** are the most frequently used oral agents. Sulfasalazine is the combination of a sulfapyridine (acting as a "carrier" that allows 5-ASA to be delivered into the colon) with 5-ASA (active agent). Side effects include: Nausea, dyspepsia, hair loss, headache, worsening diarrhea, and hypersensitivity reactions.
- Sulfa-free aminosalicylate preparations (e.g., olsalazine and balsalazide): They deliver higher amounts of the active ingredient of sulfasalazine

(5-ASA, mesalamine) to the site of active disease in the bowel and have limited systemic toxicity.
- **Azathioprine and 6-mercaptopurine (6-MP):**
  - *Usefulness are as follows:*
    - Patients who require two or more corticosteroid courses within a year.
    - Relapse of disease as the dose of prednisolone is reduced below 15 mg.
    - Relapse within 6 weeks of stopping corticosteroid.
  - *Dosage:* Azathioprine 2–3 mg/kg/day and 6-mercaptopurine 1.5 mg/kg/day.
  - *Disadvantage:* Slow clinical response and may not be evident for as long as 12 weeks.
  - *Side effects:* These include allergic reactions, pancreatitis, myelosuppression, infections, hepatotoxicity, and malignancy (lymphoma).

22. ANTIENCEPHALOPATHY

- **Lactulose therapy:** To reduce plasma ammonia level
  - Actions: Lactulose (beta-galactoside fructose) is a nonabsorbable disaccharide, which acts as an osmotic purgative. In the colon, lactulose and lactitol are catabolized by the bacterial flora to lactic acid and acetic acid. It lowers the colonic pH and favors the formation of the nonabsorbable NH^+ from NH, trapping NH^+ in the colon and thus reducing plasma ammonia concentrations. Other mechanisms of action include: (1) increased incorporation of ammonia by bacteria for synthesis of nitrogenous compounds, (2) modification of colonic flora, resulting in displacement of urease-producing bacteria with non urease-producing bacteria and cathartic effects that improves GI transit, allowing less time for ammonia absorption, (3) increased fecal nitrogen excretion due to the increase in stool volume, and (4) reduced formation of toxic short-chain fatty acids (e.g., propionate, butyrate, valerate).
  - Dose: 15–30 mL three times orally per day. Dose is increased gradually till there are two to three loose stools per day.
- **Rifaximin** semisynthetic, gut-selective, and non-absorbable oral antibiotic, derived from rifamycin and a structural analog of rifampin in the dose of 550 mg twice daily or 400 mg thrice daily is very effective and without any side effects of neomycin or metronidazole. It has only 0.4% systemic absorption.

Probiotics

Definition: Probiotics are defined as live microorganisms which are beneficial to its host. Throughout their journey in the digestive tract, they need to be intact, so they can reach the intestines where they act to give their beneficial effects to the body.

Nature:
- Bacteria: Probiotics are usually bacterial components of the normal intestinal flora of human beings (e.g., *lactobacilli* and *Bifidobacterium infantis*). They produce lactate and short-chain fatty acids (e.g., acetate and butyrate) as end products of metabolism.
- Yeast: *Saccharomyces boulardii* is yeast.

Uses:
- **Malnutrition:** Helps in normalizing the nutritional status of malnourished children. WHO suggested the use of yogurt in nutritional recovery.
- **Lactose intolerance:** Yogurt is preferred.
- **Prevention and treatment of antibiotic-associated diarrhea:** Probiotics containing *Saccharomyces boulardii yeast* may be useful to some extent.
- Irritable bowel syndrome (IBS) and colitis
- Improve immune function/immunity
- Necrotizing enterocolitis in neonates
- Speed treatment of certain intestinal infections
- Prevent and treat eczema in children
- Prevent or reduce the severity of colds and flu
- Prevent and treat vaginal yeast infections and urinary tract infections
- *Reduce bladder cancer recurrence:* Probably reduces the development of carcinoma of colon.

23. COVID-19 DRUGS

Remdesivir

In the SOLIDARITY trial, among hospitalized with COVID-19, there was no difference in overall 28-day mortality between remdesivir group compared to the standard care.

However, in the ACTT-1 trial, among patients who were on oxygen supplementation (but did not require high-flow oxygen or ventilatory support), there was a statistically significant mortality benefit with remdesivir. The study also found a nonstatistically significant trend towards higher mortality among patients who did not require oxygen or ventilatory support.

Hence remdesivir is recommended for those requiring low- flow supplemental oxygen. Dose recommended is 200 mg intravenously on day 1, followed by 100 mg daily for 5 days (with extension to 10 days if there is no clinical improvement and in patients on mechanical ventilation or ECMO).

Remdesivir is not recommended in patients with an estimated glomerular filtration rate (eGFR) <30 mL/min per 1.73 m^2 unless the benefit outweighs the risk.

It is recommended to monitor LFT while on remdesivir. It should be discontinued if alanine aminotransferase (ALT) elevation is >10 times the upper limit of normal.

Baricitinib

An oral Janus kinase inhibitor, baricitinib, which was used for treatment of rheumatoid arthritis, is thought to interfere with the SARS-CoV-2 viral entry. The US-FDA has issued emergency use authorization (EUA) for baricitinib 4 mg orally once daily for up to 14 days to be given in combination with remdesivir, in patients with COVID-19 who require oxygen or ventilatory support.

Adverse effect:
- Hepatic: Increased serum alanine aminotransferase (≥3 × ULN), increased serum aspartate aminotransferase (≥3 × ULN)
- Cardiovascular: Deep vein thrombosis, pulmonary embolism, venous thrombosis

Other Drugs
- **Dexamethasone:** For severely ill patients with COVID-19 who are on supplemental oxygen or ventilatory support (as per RECOVERY trial).
- **Tofacitinib:** Janus kinase inhibitor
- **Tocilizumab:** IL-6 pathway inhibitor is an option for individuals requiring high flow oxygen or more intensive respiratory support.

24. ANTIFUNGAL

Fluconazole

Mechanism of action: Interferes with fungal cytochrome P450 activity (lanosterol 14-α-demethylase), decreasing ergosterol synthesis (principal sterol in fungal cell membrane) and inhibiting cell membrane formation.

Indications: Treatment of candidiasis (esophageal, oropharyngeal, peritoneal, urinary tract, vaginal); systemic candida infections (e.g., candidemia, disseminated candidiasis, pneumonia); and cryptococcal meningitis; and antifungal prophylaxis in allogeneic hematopoietic cell transplant recipients, blastomycosis; candida intertrigo; candidiasis, coccidioidomycosis; tinea.

A single 150 mg oral dose can cure vaginal candidiasis with few relapses.

Oral fluconazole (100 mg/day for 2 weeks) is highly effective in oropharyngeal candidiasis, but is reserved for cases not responding to topical antifungals. Fluconazole (100 mg/day) for 2–3 weeks is the first line treatment for candida esophagitis.

Most tinea infections and cutaneous candidiasis can be treated with 150 mg weekly fluconazole for 4 weeks.

For disseminated candidiasis, cryptococcal/coccidioidal meningitis and other systemic fungal infections the dose is 200–400 mg/day for 4–12 weeks or longer. It is the preferred drug for fungal meningitis, because of good CSF penetration. Long-term oral fluconazole maintenance therapy after initial treatment with IV fluconazole AMB is used in AIDS patients with fungal meningitis.

An eye drop is useful in fungal keratitis.

Fluconazole is ineffective in aspergillosis and mucormycosis, and inferior to itraconazole for histoplasmosis, blastomycosis and sporotrichosis, as well as in tinea unguium.

Posaconazole

Mechanism of action: Interferes with fungal cytochrome P450 (lanosterol-14α-demethylase) activity, decreasing ergosterol synthesis (principal sterol in fungal cell membrane) and inhibiting fungal cell membrane formation.

Aspergillosis
- IV: 300 mg twice daily for 2 doses, then 300 mg once daily
- Delayed-release tablet: 300 mg twice daily for 2 doses, then 300 mg once daily
- IR suspension (off-label use): 200 mg 3 times daily

Amphotericin B

Mechanism of action: Binds to ergosterol altering cell membrane permeability in susceptible fungi and causing leakage of cell components with subsequent cell death. Proposed mechanism suggests that amphotericin causes an oxidation-dependent stimulation of macrophages.

Dose and indications
Intravenous: Adults— 0.3–1.5 mg/kg/day; 1–1.5 mg/kg over 4 to 6 hours every other day may be given once therapy is established; aspergillosis, rhinocerebral mucormycosis, often require 1–1.5 mg/kg/day; do not exceed 1.5 mg/kg/day.

Life-threatening fungal infections: Treatment of patients with progressive, potentially life-threatening fungal infections: Aspergillosis, cryptococcosis (torulosis), blastomycosis, systemic candidiasis, coccidioidomycosis, histoplasmosis, zygomycosis including mucormycosis, candidiasis, endophthalmitis (intravitreal); candidiasis, esophageal, refractory disease, mucocutaneous leishmaniasis.

Adverse effect
- Cardiovascular: Hypotension
- Central nervous system: Chills, headache, malaise, pain
- Endocrine and metabolic: Hypokalemia, hypomagnesemia
- Gastrointestinal: Anorexia, diarrhea, epigastric pain

Anemia
BUN and serum creatinine levels should be determined every other day when therapy is increased and at least weekly thereafter. Renal function (monitor frequently during therapy), electrolytes (especially potassium and magnesium), liver function tests, temperature, PT/PTT, CBC; monitor input and output; monitor for signs of hypokalemia.

25. FOR *H. PYLORI* (TABLES 15.26 AND 15.27)

- **Histamine H2-receptor antagonists:**
  - **Drugs:** These include four agents namely Cimetidine (400 mg BD or 800 mg at night), ranitidine (150 mg BD or 300 mg at night), famotidine (20 mg BD or 40 mg at night), and nizatidine (150 mg BD or 300 mg at night). All are equally effective.
  - **Mechanism of action:** Inhibit acid and pepsin secretion by blocking H_2-receptors.
- **Duration of treatment:**
  - **Duodenal ulcer:** Usually for 4 weeks. Smokers and patients with recent major complications (e.g., hematemesis, perforation), treatment is prolonged to 6–8 weeks.
  - **Gastric ulcer:** For 6 weeks, followed by endoscopy and further treatment if necessary.

TABLE 15.26: First-line treatment of *Helicobacter pylori* infection.

Treatment regimen	Duration
PPI (omeprazole/lansoprazole/pantoprazole/rabeprazole/esomeprazole), clarithromycin 500 mg, amoxicillin 1,000 mg (each twice daily)	10–14 days
PPI, clarithromycin 500 mg, metronidazole 500 mg (each twice daily)	10–14 days
Sequential therapy PPI, amoxicillin 1000 mg (each twice daily) for 5 days **followed by** PPI, clarithromycin 500 mg, tinidazole 500 mg (each twice daily) for next 5 days	10 days
Bismuth subsalicylate 525 mg, metronidazole 500 mg, tetracycline 500 mg (each four times daily) plus PPI or H_2RA (ranitidine twice daily)	10–14 days

TABLE 15.27: Rescue treatment for persistent *Helicobacter pylori* infection.

	Duration
Quadruple therapy: Bismuth subsalicylate 525 mg, metronidazole 500 mg, tetracycline 500 mg (each four times daily) **plus** PPI or H_2RA (twice daily)	14 days

- **Proton pump (H^+, K^+-ATPase) Inhibitors (PPIs)**
    - These agents are substituted benzimidazole derivatives that covalently bind and irreversibly inhibit H^+, K^+-ATPase.
    - They include omeprazole (20 mg/d), esomeprazole (20–40 mg/d), lansoprazole (15–30 mg/d), rabeprazole (20 mg/d), and pantoprazole (40 mg/d). All have similar efficacy in the treatment of various acid-peptic disorders.
    - **Mechanism of action**
        - Proton-pump inhibitors are lipophilic compounds that cross the parietal cell membrane and enter the acidic parietal cell canaliculus.
        - Upon entering the acidic parietal cell, the PPIs are protonated, and trapped within the acid environment of the tubulovesicular and canalicular system. They become activated and bind covalently with the H^+/K^+ ATPase enzyme and potently inhibit all phases of gastric acid secretion by the proton pump.
    - **Side effects:** Headache, diarrhea, abdominal pain, and nausea. The use of PPI may predispose to an increased risk of *Clostridium difficile* infection, community acquired pneumonia, hip fracture, and vitamin B_{12} deficiency.
    - **Advantages:** Superior healing rates, shorter healing time, and faster relief of symptom compared to H_2-blockers.
    - **Indications (Box 15.9)**

Box 15.9: Indications for proton pump inhibitors (PPIs).
- GERD and reflux esophagitis
- Peptic ulcer not responding to other medical measures.
- As an adjunct to anti-*H. pylori* treatment.
- Zollinger-Ellison syndrome

- **Cytoprotective agents**
    - **Sucralfate:** It is a complex sucrose salt insoluble in water and becomes a viscous paste within the stomach and duodenum. It binds to sites of active ulceration. Sucralfate acts as a protective barrier, over the ulcer and increases the mucosal defense and repair. Standard dose 1 g qid.

26. FOR DIARRHEA

Antisecretory Agents: Racecadotril
- Reduces the hypersecretion of water and electrolytes into the intestinal lumen
- Inhibits enkephalinase (an enzyme that degrades enkephalins)
- **Dose:** 100 mg thrice daily. To be given to patients with acute, watery diarrhea only
- **Contraindication:** Renal insufficiency, pregnancy, and breastfeeding

Loperamide
Mechanism of action: Acts directly on circular and longitudinal intestinal muscles, through the opioid receptor, to inhibit peristalsis and prolong transit time; reduces fecal volume, increases viscosity, and diminishes fluid and electrolyte loss; demonstrates antisecretory activity. Loperamide increases tone on the anal sphincter
- **Indication:** Diarrhea, cancer treatment-induced; enterocutaneous fistula, high-output
- **Oral:** Initial—4 mg, followed by 2 mg after each loose stool; maximum: 16 mg/day
- **Adverse effect:** Central nervous system: Dizziness, abdominal cramps

27. TOXICOLOGY (TABLE 15.28)

TABLE 15.28: Toxin-specific antidotes.

Toxin/poison	Specific antidote	Toxin/poison	Specific antidote
Acetaminophen	N-acetylcysteine	Methanol	Ethanol, fomepizole
Anticholinergics	Physostigmine	Methemoglobinemia	Methylene blue
Benzodiazepines	Flumazenil	Glycol	Ethanol, fomepizole
Beta-blockers	Glucagon	Opioid	Naloxone
	Calcium	Oral hypoglycemics	Glucose
	Insulin + dextrose/lipid emulsion therapy	Organophosphate	Atropine/2-PAM (pralidoxime)

Contd...

Contd...

Calcium channel blockers	Glucagon		
	Insulin + dextrose *(hyperinsulinemia euglycemia therapy)*	Snakebites	Snake antivenom
	Calciumm/lipid emulsion therapy	Sulfonylurea	Octreotide + dextrose
Carbamate	Atropine	Tricyclic antidepressants	Sodium bicarbonate
Carbone monoxide	Hyperbaric oxygen	Warfarin	Vitamin K
		Dabigatran	Idarucizumab
		Copper	Penicillamine, dimercaprol, Ca-EDTA
Cyanide	Amyl nitrite pearls	Iron	Desferrioxamine
	Sodium nitrite (3% solution)	Lead	Ca-EDTA, dimercaprol, British anti-Lewisite (BAL)
	Sodium thiosulfate (25%)	Mercury	DMPS (2,3-dimercapto-1-propanesulfonic acid), DMSA (meso-2,3-dimercaptosuccinic acid), BAL
Digoxin	Digoxin antibodies	Arsenic	BAL and derivatives
Heparin	Protamine sulfate	Antimony	BAL and derivatives
Isoniazid	Pyridoxine	Botulism	Botulinum antitoxin
Datura	Physostigmine	Methemoglobinemia-causing agents (copper nitrates dapsone)	Methylene blue

28. INTRAVENOUS FLUIDS

Crystalloids: Solutions that contain small molecular weight solutes (e.g., minerals, dextrose)

Colloids: Solutions that contain larger molecular weight solutes (e.g., albumin and starch)

Balanced IV fluid solutions: Crystalloids or colloids that do not significantly alter the homeostasis of the extracellular compartment.

Crystalloids (Table 15.29)

TABLE 15.29: Common crystalloids used.

Type	Description	Osmolality	Use	Miscellaneous
Saline (NS)	0.9% NaCl in water crystalloid solution	Isotonic (308 mOsm)	Increases circulating plasma volume when red cells are adequate	Replaces losses without altering fluids concentrations Helpful for Na$^+$ replacement
½ Normal saline (½ NS)	0.45% NaCl in water crystalloid solution	Hypotonic (154 mOsm)	Raises total fluid volume	Useful for daily maintenance of body fluid, but is of less value for replacement of NaCl deficit Helpful for establishing renal function Fluid replacement for clients who do not need extra glucose (diabetics)
Lactated Ringer's (LR)	Normal saline with electrolytes and buffer	Isotonic (275 mOsm)	Replaces fluid buffers pH	Normal saline with K$^+$, Ca^{++}, and lactate (buffer) Often seen with surgery
D$_5$W	Dextrose 5% in water crystalloid solution	Isotonic (in the bag) *Physiologically hypotonic (260 mOsm)	Raises total fluid volume. Helpful in rehydrating and excretory purposes	Provides 170–200 calories/1,000 cc for energy Physiologically hypotonic—the dextrose is metabolized quickly so that only water remains—a hypotonic fluid
D$_5$NS	Dextrose 5% in 0.9% saline	Hypertonic (560 mOsm)	Replaces fluid sodium, chloride, and calories	Watch for fluid volume overload
D$_5$ ½ NS	Dextrose 5% in 0.45% saline	Hypertonic (406 mOsm)	Useful for daily maintenance of body fluids and nutrition, and for rehydration	Most common postoperative fluid
D$_5$LR	Dextrose 5% in lactated Ringer's	Hypertonic (575 mOsm)	Same as LR plus provides about 180 calories per 1,000 cc's	Watch for fluid volume overload
Normosol-R	Normosol	Isotonic (295 mOsm)	Replaces fluid and buffers pH	pH 7.4 Contains sodium, chloride, calcium, potassium and magnesium Common fluid for OR and PACU

Colloidal Solutions

- High molecular weight substances that mostly remain confined to the intravascular compartment and thus generate oncotic pressure
- Natural colloids: Albumin, fresh frozen plasma (FFP)
- Artificial colloids: Gelatins, dextrans, hydroxyethyl starch (HES)

COMMON DRUGS USED IN EMERGENCIES (TABLE 15.30)

TAB 15.30: Common drugs used in emergencies.

Drug (concentration) and indication	Dose
Adenosine (3 mg/mL) Acute treatment of supraventricular tachycardia	6 mg IV RAPID push, may give 12 mg IV q 2 minutes if no effect × 2
Atropine (0.1 mg/mL) Organophosphate/carbamate toxicity, bradycardia	<ul><li>Organophosphate/carbamate toxicity: 1–6 mg IV q 3–5 minutes PRN, until dry secretions (can double dose each time until adequate response achieved)</li><li>Pediatric bradycardia: 0.02 mg/kg IV × 1; 0.5 mg maximum single dose; 1 mg maximum cumulative dose</li><li>Adult bradycardia: 0.5 mg IV, 3 mg maximum cumulative dose</li></ul>
Calcium gluconate (100 mg/mL) = 9.4 mg elemental calcium/mL Hyperkalemia, hypocalcemia with dysrhythmia	10% IV solution (gluconate or chloride) contains 1 gram per 10 mL
Dextrose 10% (0.1 g/mL)<ul><li>Hypoglycemia</li><li>Hyperkalemia in combination with insulin</li></ul>	<ul><li>0.2 g/kg/dose IV as D10 W then continuous infusion of D10 W at a rate of 4–8 mg/kg/min. Titrate to attain normoglycemia</li><li>2 mL/kg of dextrose 10% hyperkalemia: Continuous infusion of 0.5 g/kg/h dextrose and 0.1–0.2 units/kg/h regular insulin</li></ul>
Dopamine<ul><li>To give 10 µg/kg/min. @ 1 mL/h: weight × 30 = mg of dopamine (in kg) in 50 mL D_5W/NS</li><li>Hypotension</li></ul>	<ul><li>Begin at 5 µg/kg/min</li><li>May increase in increments of 2.5–5 µg/kg/min, as needed up to 20 µg/kg/min</li></ul>
Epinephrine 1:10,000 (0.1 mg/mL)<ul><li>Resuscitation</li><li>Severe bradycardia</li><li>Short-term use for systemic hypotension</li><li>Anaphylaxis</li></ul>	<ul><li>ACLS: 1 mg 1:10,000 IV</li><li>PALS: 0.01 mg/kg 1:10,000 IV</li><li>Anaphylaxis: 0.1–0.5 mg 1:1,000 IM/SQ (IM preferred)</li><li>Pediatric anaphylaxis/asthma: 0.01 mg/kg 1:1,000 IM/SQ (maximum single dose 0.3 mg)</li><li>Hypotension refractory to IVF: 1–10 µg/min IV</li></ul>
Fentanyl (50 µg/mL)<ul><li>Analgesia</li><li>Sedation</li><li>Anesthesia</li></ul>	25–100 µg IV q 1–2 hours; recommended dose 1 µg/kg
Hydralazine (20 mg/mL) Hypertension by vasodilation	0.1–0.5 mg/kg
Lorazepam (2 mg/mL) Delirium tremens, status epilepticus, serotonin syndrome, agitation	<ul><li>Usual bolus dose: 1–2 mg IV</li><li>Usual continuous infusion: 1–10 mg/h</li></ul>
Morphine (1 mg/mL)<ul><li>Pain</li><li>Sedation</li></ul>	2–10 mg IV q 2–6 hours PRN; recommended dose 0.1 mg/kg IV
Phenobarbital (65 mg/mL) Anticonvulsant	<ul><li>15–20 mg/kg</li><li>For refractory seizures: Additional 5 mg/kg doses, up to a total of 40 mg/kg can be given</li></ul>
Sodium bicarbonate 4.2% (0.5 mEq/mL) Hyperkalemia, TCA toxicity, salicylate toxicity, metabolic acidosis	<ul><li>Hyperkalemia or metabolic acidosis: 50 mEq IV × 1 (1 amp = 50 mEq)</li><li>TCA toxicity: 1–2 mEq/kg IV bolus to achieve a serum pH of 7.45–7.55</li><li>QRS narrowing: Effective serum alkalinization unlikely with continuous infusion</li><li>Salicylate toxicity: 3 amps (150 mEq) in 1 liter D_5W given as 10–20 mL/kg bolus, then 2–3 mL/kg/h; goal urine pH 7.5–8.0</li></ul>
Vecuronium (1 mg/mL) Paralysis Rapid sequence intubation*	0.1 mg/kg

Contd...

Contd...

Volume expanders Red blood concentrate, normal saline - Hypotension - Hypovolemia with evidence of acute blood loss or a decrease in effective volume	- RBCs: 15 mL/kg IV - NS: 10 mL/kg IV
Frusemide Acute pulmonary edema	20–80 mg IV
Naloxone Opioid-induced respiratory depression	- Titrated IV bolus (preferred): 0.1 mg at 1–2 minute intervals - IM (if no IV access): 0.4 mg, repeat every 3 minutes as required (to a maximum of 10 mg)
Glucagon Hypoglycemia	- IV, IM, or SC—adult (and children over 8 years of age) dosage: 1 mg - Children 8 years or under dosage: 0.5 mg
Haloperidol Acute psychosis, mania, severe agitation, severe anxiety or panic attack, delirium	2.5–5.0 mg IM or IV
Amiodarone Pulseless VF/VT, wide complex tachydysrhythmias	- Pulseless VF/VT: 300 mg IV rapid push followed by 150 mg IV rapid push if necessary at next pulse check - Stable wide complex tachycardias: 150 mg IV over 10 minutes, followed by infusion of 1 mg/min × 6 hours, then 0.5 mg/min thereafter
Diltiazem Stable atrial fibrillation with RVR, stable SVT	0.25 mg/kg IV × 1; may give 0.35 mg/kg IV × 1 after 15 minutes; continuous infusion 5–15 mg/h
Enoxaparin PE, NSTEMI, unstable angina	1 mg/kg SQ q 12 hours or 1.5 mg/kg SQ q 24 hours
Esomeprazole Upper GI bleed (nonvariceal)	80 mg IV bolus followed by 8 mg/h
Fosphenytoin Status epilepticus	15–20 mg/kg IV loading dose administered at 150 mg/min
Heparin Thromboembolism; ACS	- Venous thromboembolism: 80 units/kg IV × 1, then 18 units/kg/h - ACS or atrial fibrillation: 60 units/kg IV × 1, then 12 units/kg/h
Hydrocortisone Acute adrenal insufficiency, status asthmaticus, vasopressor refractory septic shock	- Adrenal insufficiency: 100 mg IV bolus, then 50 mg IV q 6 hours × 24 hours followed by a taper - Septic shock: 50 mg IV q 6 hours - Status asthmaticus: 1–2 mg/kg IV q 6 hours × 24 hours followed by a maintenance regimen
Insulin Regular Hyperkalemia, DKA/HHS, CCB overdose	- Hyperkalemia: 5–10 units IV × 1 - CCB overdose: 1 unit/kg bolus given with 25 grams of dextrose if initial BG <250 mg/dL; then initiate insulin drip at 0.1–1 unit/kg/h titrated to SBP along with 0.5 g/kg/h of dextrose titrated to maintain BG 100–200 mg/dL - DKA/HHS: 0.1 unit/kg bolus followed by continuous infusion 0.1 unit/kg/h
Nitroglycerin CHF, angina	5–200 µg/min, increase 10 µg q 3–5 min until desired effect
Nitroprusside Hypertensive emergency	Initiate at 0.3 µg/kg/min IV and titrate to effect; maximum dose 10 µg/kg/min
Octreotide Bleeding esophageal varices, sulfonylurea overdose	- Bleeding esophageal varices: 50 µg IV bolus, then 50 µg/h IV - Sulfonylurea toxicity: 50 µg SQ q 6 hours PRN

CHAPTER 16

Annexures

A. MISCELLANEOUS TOPICS

PEDIGREE ANALYSIS (TABLES 16A.1 AND 16A.2, AND FIGS. 16A.1 TO 16A.4)

A pedigree chart displays a family tree, and shows the members of the family who are affected by a genetic trait.
- Circles represent females and squares represent males.
- Each individual is represented by: A Roman Numeral, which stands for the generation in the family and a Digit, which stands for the individual within the generation.
- A darkened circle or square represents an individual affected by the trait.
- A male and female directly connected by a horizontal line have mated and have children.
- Vertical lines connect parents to their children.
- The "founding family" consists of the two founding parents and their children.

TABLE 16A.1: Examples of autosomal dominant and autosomal recessive disorders.

System	Autosomal dominant disorder	Autosomal recessive disorder
Nervous	Huntington disease Neurofibromatosis Tuberous sclerosis	• Neurogenic muscular atrophies • Friedreich's ataxia • Spinal muscular atrophy
Skeletal	Marfan syndrome Achondroplasia Noonan syndrome	• Alkaptonuria • Ehlers-Danlos syndrome
Metabolic	Familial hypercholesterolemia Intermittent porphyria	Cystic fibrosis, phenylketonuria, lysosomal storage diseases, galactosemia, hemochromatosis, glycogen storage diseases
Hematopoietic	• Hereditary spherocytosis • von Willebrand disease	Sickle cell anemia, thalassemia
Renal	Polycystic kidney disease	Congenital adrenal hyperplasia
Gastrointestinal	Familial polyposis coli	Wilson's disease

TABLE 16A.2: Examples of X-linked recessive disorders.

System	Related X-linked recessive disease
Musculoskeletal	Duchenne muscular dystrophy
Blood	Hemophilia A and B
	Glucose-6-phosphate dehydrogenase deficiency
Immune	Agammaglobulinemia
Metabolic	Diabetes insipidus
Nervous	Fragile-X syndrome

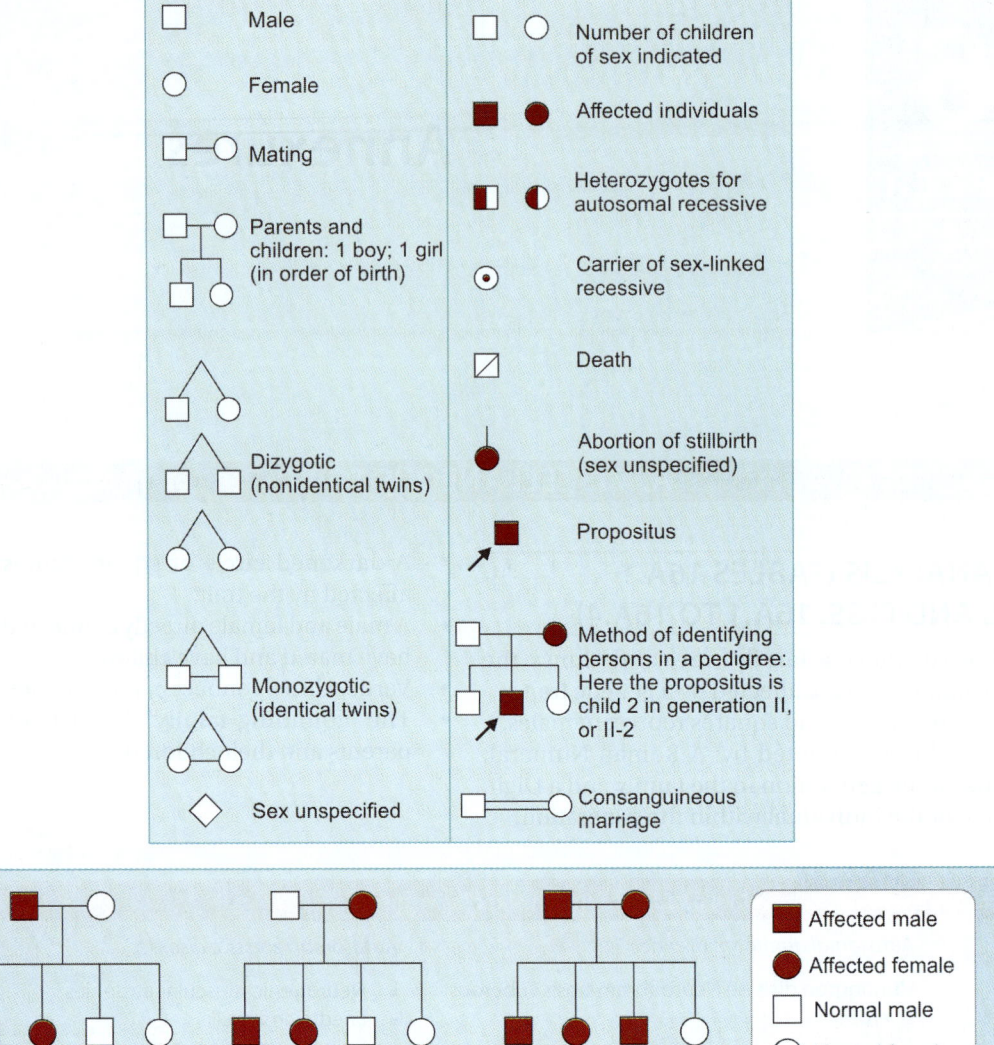

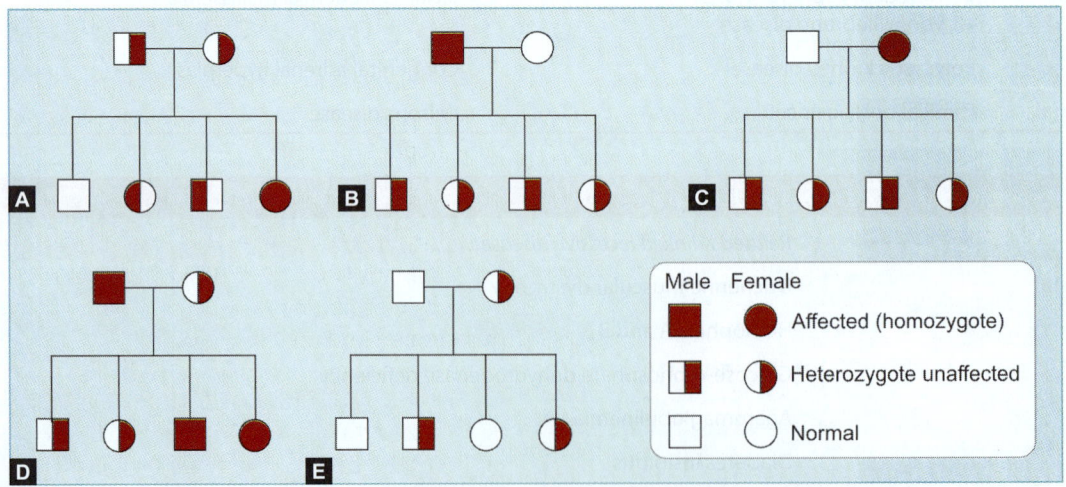

Figs. 16A.1A to C: Pedigree illustrating **autosomal dominant transmission**. (A and B) One parent is affected; (C) Both parents are affected. Note that both males and females are affected equally.

Figs. 16A.2A to E: Pedigree illustrating mechanism of **autosomal recessive transmission**. (A) Both parents are unaffected heterozygotes; (B and C) One parent is sufferer (homozygous) and other is normal; (D) One parent is sufferer and other is unaffected heterozygote; (E) One parent is normal and other is an unaffected heterozygote.

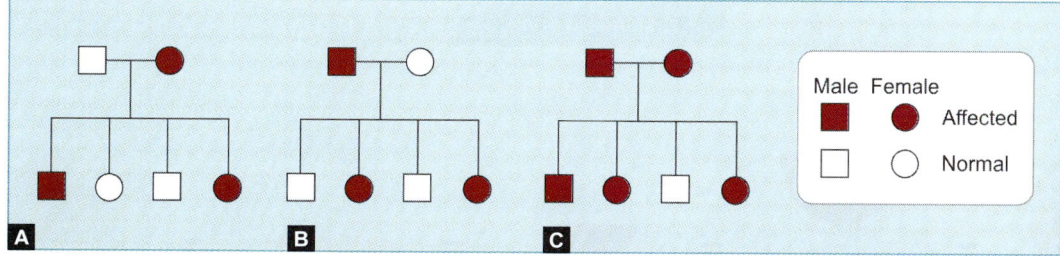

Figs. 16A.3A to C: X-linked dominant transmission. Only females are affected. Usually males who inherit the mutant allele die in utero. (A) Normal male and affected female (sufferer); (B) Affected male and female; (C) Both male and female are affected.

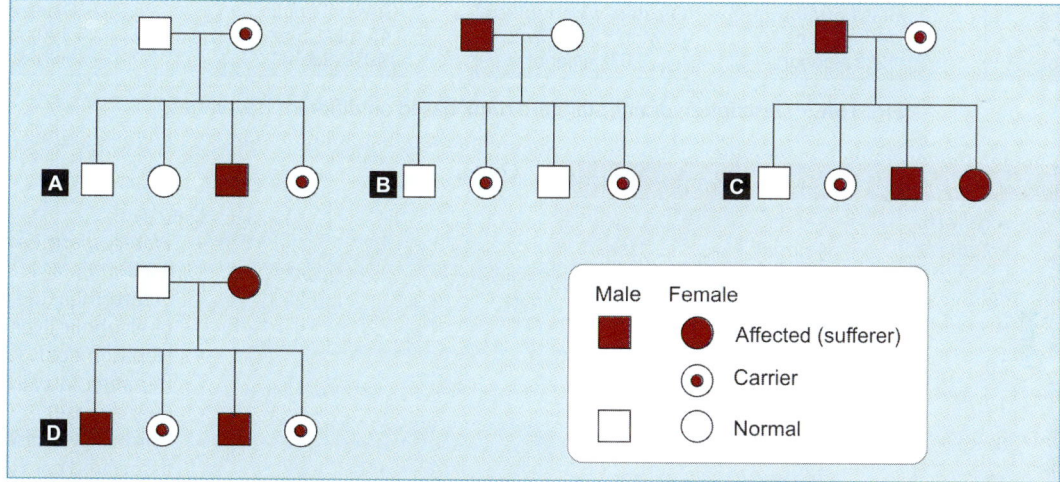

Figs. 16A.4A to D: Mode of **X-linked recessive transmission**. Note the absence of male-to-male transmission. (A) Male is normal and female is a carrier; (B) Male is sufferer and female is normal; (C) Male is a sufferer and female is a carrier; (D) Male is normal and female is sufferer.

ALCOHOL USE (FIG. 16A.5 AND TABLE 16A.3)

One unit of alcohol contains 8 g of ethanol.

A conservative threshold of 14 units/week for both men and women is considered safe.

The risk threshold for developing ALD is variable but begins at 30 g/day of ethanol.

The average alcohol consumption of a man with cirrhosis is 160 g/day for over 8 years.

Some of the risk factors for ALD are:
- **Drinking pattern:** Liver damage is more likely to occur in continuous rather than intermittent or "binge" drinkers, as this pattern gives the liver a chance to recover. It is therefore recommended that people should have at least two alcohol-free days each week.
- **Gender:** The incidence of ALD is increasing in women, who have higher blood ethanol levels than men after consuming the same amount of alcohol. This may be related to the reduced volume of distribution of alcohol.
- **Genetics:** Alcoholism is more concordant in monozygotic than dizygotic twins. The patatin-like *phospholipase domain-containing protein 3 (PNPLA3)* gene, also known as adiponutrin, has been implicated in the pathogenesis of both ALD and NAFLD.
- **Nutrition:** Obesity increases the incidence of liver-related mortality by over five-fold in heavy drinkers. Ethanol itself produces 7 kcal/g (29.3 kJ/g) and many alcoholic drinks also contain sugar, which further increases the calorific value and may contribute to weight gain.

Units of alcohol explained:
A UK unit is 10 milliliters (8 g) of pure alcohol.

For example, most whisky has an ABV (alcohol by volume) of 40%.

One liter (1,000 mL) bottle of this whisky therefore contains 400 mL of pure alcohol. This is 40 units (as 10 mL of pure alcohol = 1 unit).

So, in 100 mL of the whisky, there would be 4 units.

And hence, a 25 mL single measure of whisky would contain 1 unit.

The math is straightforward. To calculate units, take the quantity in milliliters, multiply it by the ABV (expressed as a percentage) and divide by 1,000.

In the example of a glass of whisky (*see* **Fig. 16A.5**), the calculation would be: **25 mL × 40% divided by 1,000 = 1 unit** or for a 250 mL glass of wine with ABV 12%, the number of units is: **250 mL × 12% divided by 1,000 = 3 units**. A 330 mL bottle of lager (ABV 5%) contains: **330 mL × 5% divided by 1,000 = 1.65 units**.

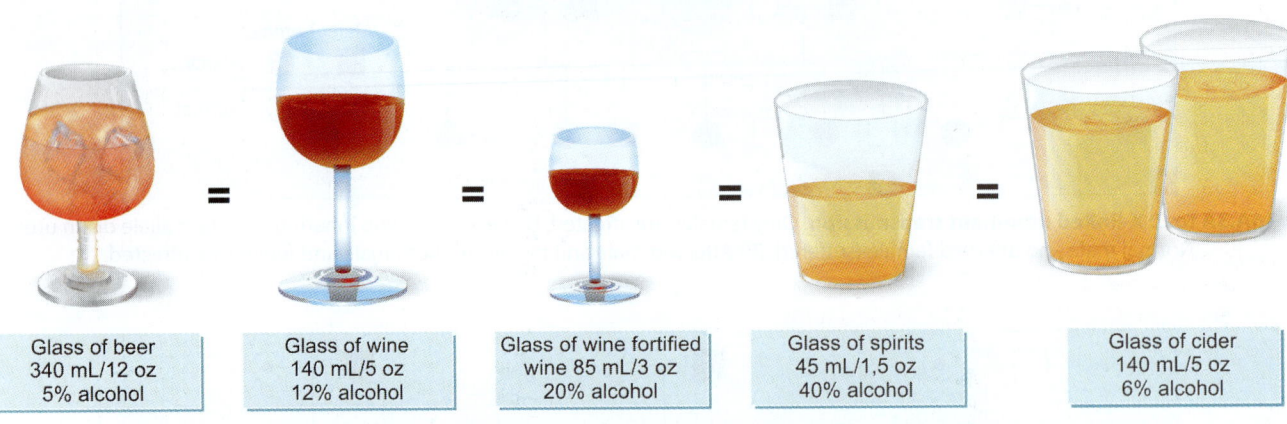

Fig. 16A.5: Description of one standard drink based on different beverages.

TABLE 16A.3: Amount of alcohol in an average drink.			
Alcohol type	Alcohol by volume (%)	Amount	Units*
Beer	3.5	568 mL (1 pint)	2
	9	568 mL (1 pint)	4
Wine	10	125 mL	1
	12	750 mL	9
'Alcopops'	6	330 mL	2
Sherry	17.5	750 mL	13
Vodka/rum/gin	37.5	25 mL	1
Whisky/brandy	40	700 mL	28

*1 unit = 8 g

Complications of Alcohol

Neurologic
- Blackouts
- Withdrawal syndromes (e.g., tremors, hallucinations, rum fits, and delirium tremens)
- Cerebellar degeneration
- Alcoholic dementia
- Alcoholic myopathy
- Autonomic neuropathy
- Peripheral neuropathy
- Marchiafava–Bignami disease (demyelination of corpus callosum)
- Central pontine myelinolysis
- Traumatic brain injury
- Hepatic encephalopathy
- Hemorrhagic stroke
- Seizures

Cardiovascular
- Cardiomyopathy
- Cardiac arrhythmias (holiday heart syndrome), and atrial fibrillation
- Hypertension

Gastrointestinal
- Acute gastric erosions
- GI bleeding—Mallory–Weiss tears, gastric erosions, esophageal varices, and peptic ulcers
- Pancreatitis (acute, recurrent or chronic)

Contd...

Contd...

- Diarrhea
  - Watery diarrhea due to alcohol itself
  - Steatorrhea due to pancreatitis or alcoholic liver disease
  - Hepatomegaly (alcoholic hepatitis, fatty liver, and chronic liver disease)
  - Chronic liver disease and associated complications

Respiratory
Increased susceptibility to pneumonia and tuberculosis

Musculoskeletal
- Increased risk of fractures and osteonecrosis of femoral head
- Increased risk of fall
- Myopathy
- Osteoporosis

Cancers
- Oral cavity
- Oropharynx
- Esophageal
- Colorectal
- Breast
- Hepatocellular carcinoma
- Pancreatic

Metabolic
- Hyponatremia
- Hypoglycemia
- Hypokalemia
- Hypomagnesemia
- Hypocalcemia
- Hypophosphatemia
- Gout
- Hypercholesterolemia
- Ketoacidosis

Psychiatric
- Unipolar depressive disorders
- Anxiety
- Chronic suicidality
- Amnestic disorder
- Psychosis
- Cognitive impairment
- Impulsivity

Behavioral and psychosocial
- Injuries
- Violence
- Crime
- Partner or child abuse
- Tobacco and other drug abuse
- Unemployment
- Legal problems
- Poor hygiene

Hematologic
- Anemia
  - Iron deficiency from blood loss
  - Dietary folate deficiency

Nutritional
- Thiamine deficiency—Wernicke's encephalopathy, Korsakoff psychosis, and peripheral neuropathy
- Niacin deficiency—pellagra
- Folate deficiency

Contd...

Contd...

- B$_{12}$ deficiency with pancreatitis
- Direct toxic suppression of bone marrow
- Sideroblastic anemia
- Zieve's syndrome (hemolytic anemia)
- Thrombocytopenia due to bone marrow suppression or hypersplenism
- Leukopenia

- B$_{12}$ deficiency
- Vitamin D deficiency
- Zinc deficiency

Endocrine
- Diabetes mellitus
- Gynecomastia
- Testicular atrophy
- Amenorrhea
- Infertility

Miscellaneous
- Erectile dysfunction
- Fetal alcohol syndrome
- Spontaneous abortions
- Increased susceptibility to infections like HIV

SMOKING

- Cigarette smoking is the leading preventable cause of mortality, responsible for nearly 6 million deaths worldwide.
- The three major causes of smoking-related mortality are atherosclerotic cardiovascular disease, lung cancer, and chronic obstructive pulmonary disease (COPD).

Pack Years

Pack years = number of packs of cigarettes smoked per day × number of years the patient has smoked

More pack years correlates with higher lung disease risk including lung cancer.

Patients should be considered for screening with low-dose CT if they are ≥55 years with ≥30 pack years history.

Pack years = No. of packs of cigarettes/day × No. of years smoked (each packet = 20 cigarettes)

Smoking Index

Smoking index is defined as the product of average number of cigarettes smoked per day and the total duration of smoking in years.

Example: If a patient is smoking 1 cigarette per day for 10 years the smoking index will be 10.

Smoking index (Si) = No. of cigarettes/day × No. of years smoked
SI <100 = Mild smoker
SI <101–300 = Moderate smoker
SI <300 = Heavy smoker

Lung cancer is common if smoking index more than 300.

Complications of Tobacco Use

Cardiovascular disease
- Premature coronary artery disease
- Peripheral vascular disease and erectile dysfunction
- Cerebrovascular disease
- Aortic aneurysm

Respiratory disease
- Chronic obstructive pulmonary disease
- Cancer of lung, bronchus, and trachea
- Increased incidence of postoperative respiratory complications
- Increased incidence of respiratory infections including tuberculosis
- ILD
- Pneumothorax

Gastrointestinal
- GERD
- Peptic ulceration
- Gallstones and cholecystitis in women
- Pancreatitis
- Crohn's disease

Pregnancy
- Spontaneous abortion
- Abruptio placentae
- Premature rupture of membranes
- Fetal death
- Neonatal death
- Sudden infant death syndrome
- Postpartum venous thromboembolism

Renal
- Increased risk of CKD

Endocrine
- Increased risk of diabetes mellitus

Infections—increased risk of several types of infection including tuberculosis, pneumococcal pneumonia, Legionnaires' disease, meningococcal disease, influenza, and the common cold

Osteoporosis and hip fracture—smoking accelerates bone loss and is a risk factor for hip fracture in women

Neurological
- Dementia and cognitive decline
- Increased risk of amyotrophic lateral sclerosis

Ophthalmological
- Age-related macular degeneration
- Increased risk of cataract

Drug interactions
Induces hepatic microsomal enzyme systems, e.g., increased metabolism of propranolol and theophylline

Other cancers
- Larynx
- Oral cavity and lip
- Nasopharynx, oropharynx, and hypopharynx
- Nasal cavity and paranasal sinus
- Esophagus
- Stomach
- Pancreas
- Colorectal
- Kidney
- Bladder
- Uterine
- Cervix
- Acute myeloid leukemia

B. DEFINITIONS

PULSE

Pulse is the pressure distension wave produced by contraction of left ventricle against a partially filled aorta, which is transmitted to peripheries and is felt on a peripheral artery against a bony prominence.

BLOOD PRESSURE

Arterial blood pressure (BP) can be defined as the lateral pressure exerted by the moving column of blood on the walls of the arteries **(Table 16B.1)**.

$$BP = Cardiac\ output \times Peripheral\ resistance$$

Systolic BP (SBP)
- Defined as the maximum BP in the arteries attainable during systole
- Normal 120+/−20 mm Hg

Diastolic BP (DBP)
- Defined as the minimum pressure that is obtained at the end of the ventricular diastole.
- Normal range 60–90 mm Hg

Pulse pressure (PP)
Denotes the difference between systolic and diastolic pressure.
PP = SBP − DBP = 40 mm Hg

Mean arterial pressure (MAP)
DBP + 1/3 pulse pressure
Normal = 95 mm Hg

TABLE 16B.1: Blood pressure measurement and definitions.

BP measurement	Definition
SBP	First Korotkoff sound
DBP	Fifth Korotkoff sound
Pulse pressure	SBP minus DBP
Mean arterial pressure	DBP pulse one-third pulse pressure
Mid-BP	Sum of SBP and DBP, divided by 2

Reference
Williams B, Mancia G, Spiering W, et al. 2018 ESC/ESH Guidelines for the management of arterial hypertension. Eur Heart J. 2018;39(33):3021-104.

HYPERTENSION

"Hypertension" is defined as the level of BP at which the benefits of treatment (either with lifestyle interventions or drugs) unequivocally outweigh the risks of treatment, as documented by clinical trials.

Reference
Williams B, Mancia G, Spiering W, et al. 2018 ESC/ESH Guidelines for the management of arterial hypertension. Eur Heart J. 2018 1;39(33):3021-104

Hypertension is most commonly defined as systolic blood pressure (SBP) ≥140 mm Hg or diastolic blood pressure (DBP) ≥90 mm Hg, but definitions vary by professional organization.
- ACC/AHA: >130/80
- ESC/ESH: >140/90.

SBP (mm Hg)		DBP (mm Hg)	ESH/ESC 2018	AHA/ACC 2017	Poosition of the DHL, 2017	NICE 2016
<120	and	<80	Optimal	Normal	Optimal	Normal
120–129	and	<80	Normal	Elevated	Normal	Normal
130–139	or	80–89	Upper range of normal	Grade I hypertension	Upper range of normal	Upper range of normal
140–159	or	90–99	Grade I hypertension	Grade II hypertension	Grade I hypertension	Grade I hypertension (≥135/85 mm Hg)
160–179	or	100–109	Grade II hypertension	Grade II hypertension	Grade II hypertension	Grade II hypertension (≥150/95 mm Hg)
≥180	or	≥110	Grade III hypertension	Grade II hypertension	Grade III hypertension	Severe hypertension

RESISTANT HYPERTENSION

Elevated blood pressure despite concurrent use of three antihypertensive drugs of different classes including a diuretic.

Reference
Williams B, Mancia G, Spiering W, et al. 2018 ESC/ESH Guidelines for the management of arterial hypertension. Eur Heart J. 2018;39(33):3021-104.

REFRACTORY HYPERTENSION

A subgroup of patients with resistant hypertension that remains uncontrolled despite maximal medical therapy, often with four or more antihypertensive drugs.

Reference
Rimoldi SF, Scherrer U, Messerli FH. Secondary arterial hypertension: when, who, and how to screen? Eur Heart J. 2014;35(19):1245-54.

PSEUDORESISTANT HYPERTENSION

- Elevated blood pressure measurements due to inaccurate blood pressure measurement techniques such as:
  - Failure to have patient sit quietly for ≥5 minutes before measurement
  - Too small cuff size.
- Poor adherence to medical therapy
- White coat hypertension
- Marked brachial artery calcification
- Clinician inertia.

References
- *Rimoldi SF, Scherrer U, Messerli FH. Secondary arterial hypertension: when, who, and how to screen? Eur Heart J. 2014;35(19):1245-54.*
- *Williams B, Mancia G, Spiering W, et al. 2018 ESC/ESH Guidelines for the management of arterial hypertension. Eur Heart J. 2018;39(33): 3021-104.*

PSEUDOHYPERTENSION

- Defined as cuff diastolic blood pressure ≥15 mm Hg higher than simultaneously measured intra-arterial blood pressure.
- Elevated blood pressure due to arterial stiffening in elderly patients.

Reference
Rimoldi SF, Scherrer U, Messerli FH. Secondary arterial hypertension: when, who, and how to screen? Eur Heart J. 2014;35(19):1245-54.

SECONDARY HYPERTENSION

Hypertension due to an identifiable and potentially curable cause.

MASKED HYPERTENSION

Elevated blood pressure at home or on ambulatory blood pressure monitoring but normal office blood pressure.

WHITE COAT HYPERTENSION

Normal blood pressure at home or on ambulatory blood pressure monitoring but elevated office blood pressure.

HYPERTENSIVE CRISIS

Severe elevations in blood pressure (systolic blood pressure ≥180 mm Hg or diastolic blood pressure ≥120 mm Hg) with impending complications including target end-organ dysfunction.

HYPERTENSIVE EMERGENCY

Severe elevation in blood pressure which is accompanied by end-organ damage.

MALIGNANT HYPERTENSION

Malignant hypertension is term used for patients with severely elevated blood pressure and ischemic end-organ damage usually involving the retina, but may also include the kidneys, heart, arteries, and/or brain.

HYPERTENSIVE URGENCY

Severe elevation in blood pressure which occurs without end-organ damage.

Reference
Whelton PK, Carey RM, Aronow WS, et al. 2017 ACC/AHA/AAPA/ABC/ACPM/AGS/APhA/ASH/ASPC/NMA/PCNA Guideline for the Prevention, Detection, Evaluation, and Management of High Blood Pressure in Adults: A Report of the American College of Cardiology/American Heart Association Task Force on Clinical Practice Guidelines. Hypertension. 2018;71(6):e13-115.

JUGULAR VENOUS PRESSURE

Defined as undulating top of oscillating column of blood in right internal jugular vein that faithfully represents the pressure and volumetric changes in the right side of heart which changes with various stages of cardiac cycle and respiration.

ANEMIA

Anemia is a condition in which the number of red blood cells or their oxygen-carrying capacity is insufficient to meet physiologic needs, which vary by age, sex, altitude, smoking, and pregnancy status.

World Health Organization (WHO) definition of anemia at sea level **(Table 16B.2)**:
- Hemoglobin <13 g/dL (130 g/L) in men ≥15 years old
- Hemoglobin <12 g/dL (120 g/L) in nonpregnant women ≥15 years old or adolescents aged 12–14 years
- Hemoglobin <11.5 g/dL (115 g/L) in children aged 5–11 years
- Hemoglobin <11 g/dL (110 g/L) in pregnant women, or children aged 6–59 months.

ERYTHROCYTOSIS AND POLYCYTHEMIA

Erythrocytosis is an increase in the number of red blood cells (relative to the plasma volume), manifested by a persistent increase in the venous hematocrit, and associated with increased blood viscosity and risk of thrombosis.

TABLE 16B.2: Hemoglobin levels to diagnose anemia at sea level (g/L)±.

Population	Non-anemia*	Anemia* Mild[a]	Moderate	Severe
Children 6–59 months of age	110 or higher	100–109	70–99	Lower than 70
Children 5–11 years of age	115 or higher	110–114	80–109	Lower than 80
Children 12–14 years of age	120 or higher	110–119	80–109	Lower than 80
Nonpregnant women (15 years of age and above)	120 or higher	110–119	80–109	Lower than 80
Pregnant women	110 or higher	100–109	70–99	Lower than 70
Men (15 years of age and above)	130 or higher	110–129	80–109	Lower than 80

±Adapted from references 5 and 6
*Hemoglobin in grams per liter
[a]"Mild" is a misnomer: iron deficiency is already advanced by the time anemia is detected. The deficiency has consequences even when no anemia is clinically apparent.
Reference: WHO.

Erythrocytosis and polycythemia are often used interchangeably; however, erythrocytosis refers exclusively to an increase in erythrocytes, whereas polycythemia more accurately refers to pan-myeloproliferation (as seen in some patients with polycythemia vera).

References
- Lee G, Arcasoy MO. The clinical and laboratory evaluation of the patient with erythrocytosis. Eur J Intern Med. 2015;26(5):297-302.
- McMullin MF, Bareford D, Campbell P, et al. Guidelines for the diagnosis, investigation and management of polycythaemia/erythrocytosis. Br J Haematol. 2005;130(2):174-95.

JAUNDICE

Jaundice (also termed icterus) is a condition of yellow discoloration of the skin, conjunctivae, and mucous membranes, resulting from widespread tissue deposition of the pigmented metabolite bilirubin.

Reference
Feldman M, Friedman L, Brandt L. Sleisenger and Fordtran's Gastrointestinal and Liver Disease. Philadelphia: Saunders; 2015.

CYANOSIS

Cyanosis refers to a bluish discoloration of the skin that is caused by increased amounts of reduced hemoglobin in the subpapillary venous plexus.

Reference
Fishman's Pulmonary Diseases and Disorders.

CLUBBING

Clubbing of the fingers designates the selective bulbous enlargement of the distal segments of the digits due to an increase in soft tissue.

Reference
Fishman's Pulmonary Diseases and Disorders.

FEVER

Fever is "a state of elevated core temperature, which is often, but not necessarily, part of the defensive responses of multicellular organisms (host) to the invasion of live (microorganisms) or inanimate matter recognized as pathogenic or alien by the host."

Reference
Commission for Thermal Physiology of the International Union of Physiological Sciences (IUPS Thermal Commission): Glossary of terms for thermal physiology, 3rd ed. Jpn J Physiol. 2001;51:245-80.

FEVER OF UNKNOWN ORIGIN

Petersdorf and Beeson—"fever higher than 38.3°C (100.9°F) on several occasions, persisting without diagnosis for at least 3 weeks in spite of at least 1 week's investigation in hospital".

REVISED DEFINITION OF FEVER OF UNKNOWN ORIGIN

- Requires fever >38.3°C (101°F)
- Subcategorized by patient immune status and clinical setting:
    - Classic fever of unknown origin (FUO):
        - Fever duration >3 weeks
        - No diagnosis after ≥3 visits or 3 days of hospitalization.
    - Nosocomial (healthcare-associated) FUO:
        - Fever duration >3 days
        - Fever acquired after ≥24 hours in hospital (not present or incubating on admission)
        - No diagnosis after 3 days of appropriate in-hospital investigation.
    - Neutropenic (or immunodeficient) FUO:
        - Fever duration >3 days
        - Neutrophil count ≤500 cells/mm3 with negative cultures after 48 hours
        - No diagnosis after 3 days of appropriate in-hospital investigation.
    - HIV-associated FUO:
        - Confirmed HIV infection
        - Fever duration >3 weeks for outpatients and >3 days for inpatients.

Reference
Wright WF, Mackowiak PA. Fever of unknown origin. In: Mandell GL, Bennett JE, Dolin R, editors. Mandell, Douglas, and Bennett's Principles and Practice of Infectious Diseases, 8th ed. New York, NY: Saunders; 2014:721-31.

HYPERPYREXIA

A fever of >41.5°C is called hyperpyrexia.

Reference
Harrison's Principles of Internal Medicine.

HYPERTHERMIA

An uncontrolled increase in body temperature that exceeds the body's ability to lose heat without a change in the hypothalamic set point. Hyperthermia does not involve pyrogenic molecules.

Reference
- Harrison's Principles of Internal Medicine.

HEATSTROKE

Core body temperature ≥104°F (40°C) with central nervous system dysfunction; can progress to multiple system organ failure.

Reference
Atha WF. Heat-related illness. Emerg Med Clin North Am. 2013;31(4):1097-108.

DYSPNEA

A subjective experience of breathing discomfort that consists of qualitatively distinct sensations that vary in intensity.

Reference
Parshall MB, Schwartzstein RM, Adams L, et al. An official American Thoracic Society statement: update on the mechanisms, assessment, and management of dyspnea. Am J Respir Crit Care Med. 2012;185(4): 435-52.

ORTHOPNEA

Orthopnea signifies dyspnea in the recumbent, but not in the upright or semi-upright position.

Reference
Fishman's Pulmonary Diseases and Disorders.

PAROXYSMAL NOCTURNAL DYSPNEA

Acute episodes of severe shortness of breath and coughing that generally occur at night and awaken the patient from sleep, usually 1–3 hours after the patient retires.

Reference
Harrison's Principles of Internal Medicine.

PLATYPNEA

Platypnea signifies dyspnea induced by assuming the upright position and relieved by recumbency.

Reference
Fishman's Pulmonary Diseases and Disorders.

ORTHODEOXIA

Desaturation of arterial blood when the patient is upright.

Reference
Fishman's Pulmonary Diseases and Disorders.

TREPOPNEA

Dyspnea when the affected side of the chest is in the dependent position, thereby promoting ventilation–perfusion mismatch and resultant hypoxemia.

Reference
Fishman's Pulmonary Diseases and Disorders.

BENDOPNEA

Shortness of breath may be particularly noticeable when bending forward, termed bendopnea.

Reference
Braunwald's Heart Disease: A Textbook of Cardiovascular Medicine.

PALPITATIONS

Palpitations are the awareness of the heartbeat that may be caused by a rapid heart rate, irregularities in heart rhythm, or an increase in the force of cardiac contraction, as occurs with a postextrasystolic beat; however, this perception can also exist in the setting of a completely normal cardiac rhythm.

Reference
Braunwald's Heart Disease: A Textbook of Cardiovascular Medicine.

TACHYCARDIA

An abnormally rapid heartbeat, usually applied to a heart rate above 100 per minute.

Reference ICD-10.

BRADYCARDIA

The National Institutes of Health defines bradycardia as a heart rate <60 bpm in adults other than well trained athletes.

Reference
National Institutes of Health. Pulse. [online] Available from https://medlineplus. gov/ency/article/003399.htm [Last accessed November, 2019].

APEX BEAT

The apex beat or apical impulse is the palpable cardiac impulse farthest away from the sternum and farthest down on the chest wall, usually caused by the LV and located near the midclavicular line (MCL) in the fifth intercostal space.

Reference
McGee S. Palpation of the Heart. Evidence-Based Physical Diagnosis. Netherlands: Elsevier; 2018. pp. 317-26.

ACUTE CORONARY SYNDROME

Definition of Acute Coronary Syndrome(s)

- Acute coronary syndrome includes spectrum of ST-elevation myocardial infarction (STEMI), non-STEMI (NSTEMI), and unstable angina (UA).
- UA/NSTEMI are defined in an appropriate clinical setting (chest discomfort or anginal equivalent), often accompanied by:
  - Electrocardiographic (ECG), ST-segment depression or prominent T-wave inversion and/or
  - Positive biomarkers of necrosis (for example, troponin) in the absence of ST-segment elevation.
- NSTEMI is differentiated from UA by the presence of myocardial necrosis.
- STEMI is diagnosed by ECG in the absence of left ventricular hypertrophy or left bundle branch block

(LBBB) in the presence of new ST elevation (at J point) and either of:
- ≥2 mm [0.2 millivolts (mV)] in men or ≥1.5 mm (0.15 mV) in women in leads V2–V3
- ≥1 mm (0.1 mV) in 2 other contiguous chest leads or limb leads.
- Criteria for acute myocardial infarction:
  - Evidence of acute myocardial injury in clinical setting consistent with acute myocardial ischemia, as evidenced by detection of rise and/or fall of cardiac troponin (cTn) values with ≥1 value >99th percentile of upper reference limit PLUS at least 1 of the following:
    - Symptoms of ischemia
    - New ischemic ECG changes
    - Development of pathological q waves on electrocardiogram (ECG)
    - Imaging evidence of new loss of viable myocardium or new regional wall motion abnormality.
- Cardiac death with symptoms suggestive of myocardial ischemia and presumed new ischemic ECG changes, but death occurring before blood samples obtained or before increases in cardiac biomarkers in blood can be identified.

Reference
European Society of Cardiology, American College of Cardiology, American Heart Association, and World Heart Federation (ESC/ACC/AHA/WHF) 2018 universal definition of myocardial infarction.

PULMONARY HYPERTENSION

Pulmonary hypertension refers to a group of conditions with increased mean pulmonary arterial pressure (mPAP) >20 mm Hg with a PVR ≥3 Wood units (isolated postcapillary PH may have PVR <3 Wood units) as measured by right heart catheterization in supine position at rest.

Reference
Simonneau G, Montani D, Celermajer DS, et al. Haemodynamic definitions and updated clinical classification of pulmonary hypertension. Eur Respir J. 2019;53(1):1801913.

HEART FAILURE

Heart failure is a complex clinical syndrome caused by structural or functional impairment of ventricular filling or ejection of blood, resulting in insufficient perfusion to meet metabolic demands.

Reference
Yancy CW, Jessup M, Bozkurt B, et al. 2013 ACCF/AHA Guideline for the Management of Heart Failure: A Report of the American College of Cardiology Foundation/American Heart Association Task Force on Practice Guidelines. Circulation. 2013;128(16):e240-319.

DILATED CARDIOMYOPATHY

Dilated cardiomyopathy (DCM) refers to a large group of heterogeneous myocardial disorders that are characterized by ventricular dilation and depressed myocardial contractility in the absence of abnormal loading conditions such as hypertension or valvular disease.

Reference
Yancy CW, Jessup M, Bozkurt B, et al. 2013 ACCF/AHA Guideline for the Management of Heart Failure: A Report of the American College of Cardiology Foundation/American Heart Association Task Force on Practice Guidelines. Circulation. 2013;128(16):e240-319.

COUGH

A cough is an explosive expiration that protects the lungs against aspiration and promotes the movement of secretions and other airway constituents upward toward the mouth.

Reference
Fishman's Pulmonary Diseases and Disorders.

MASSIVE HEMOPTYSIS

No clear consensus for definition of massive hemoptysis and criteria have ranged from 100 mL to 1,000 mL of expectorated blood within 24 hours.

Blood loss of 400 mL in 24 hours or 100–150 mL expectorated at one time are considered massive hemoptysis.

Reference
Larici AR, Franchi P, Occhipinti M, et al. Diagnosis and management of hemoptysis. Diagn Interv Radiol. 2014;20(4):299-309.

LUNG SOUNDS (TABLE 16B.3)

TABLE 16B.3: Classification of common lung sounds.

Acoustic characteristics	American Thoracic Society nomenclature	Common synonyms
Discontinuous, interrupted explosive sounds; loud, low in pitch	**Coarse crackle**	Coarse rale
Discontinuous, interrupted explosive sounds; less loud than above and of shorter duration; higher in pitch than coarse crackles or rales	**Fine crackle**	Fine rale, crepitation
Continuous sounds longer than 250 ms, high-pitched; dominant frequency of 400 Hz or more, hissing sound	**Wheeze**	Sibilant rhonchus
Continuous sounds longer than 250 ms, low-pitched; dominant frequency about 200 Hz or less, snoring sound	**Rhonchus**	Sonorous rhonchus

Source: Adapted with permission from Loudon R, Murphy RLH. Lung sounds. Am Rev Respir Dis. 1984;130(4):663-73.

CHRONIC OBSTRUCTIVE PULMONARY DISEASE

Chronic obstructive pulmonary disease (COPD) is a common, preventable, and treatable disease that is characterized by persistent respiratory symptoms and airflow limitation that is due to airway and/or alveolar abnormalities usually caused by significant exposure to noxious particles or gases.

Reference
GOLD, 2018.

CHRONIC BRONCHITIS

Cough and excess sputum production for ≥3 months per year in each of 2 consecutive years.

Reference
GOLD, 2018.

EMPHYSEMA

Pathological term describing destruction of gas exchanging surfaces of lung (alveoli).

Reference
GOLD, 2018.

CHRONIC COR PULMONALE

Right ventricular hypertrophy, dilatation or both as a result of pulmonary hypertension [defined as pulmonary artery mean pressure (PAP) >20 mm Hg] resulting from pulmonary disorders involving lung parenchyma, impaired bellows function or altered ventilatory drive.

Reference
Budev MM, Arroliga AC, Wiedemann HP, et al. Cor pulmonale: an overview. Semin Respir Crit Care Med. 2003;24(3):233-44.

ASTHMA

Asthma is a heterogeneous disease, usually characterized by chronic airway inflammation. It is defined by the history of respiratory symptoms such as wheeze, shortness of breath, chest tightness, and cough that vary over time and in intensity, together with variable airflow limitation.

Reference
GINA 2019.

BRONCHIECTASIS

Persistent or progressive suppurative lung disease characterized by irreversibly dilated bronchi and chronic or recurrent bronchial inflammation and infection.

Reference
Pasteur MC, Bilton D, Hill AT. British Thoracic Society guideline for non-CF bronchiectasis. 2010;65(Suppl 1):i1-58.

UNINTENTIONAL WEIGHT LOSS

Clinical entity whereby the patient does not purposefully set out to lose weight for any reason and when weight loss as a consequence of advanced chronic diseases or their treatments (e.g., diuretics for heart failure) is excluded.

Definition criteria were numerical verification of >5% reduction in usual body weight over the preceding 6–12 months, or, for subjects without numerical documentation, at least two of the following: evidence of change in clothing size, corroboration of the reported weight loss by a relative or friend, and ability to give a numerical estimate of the amount of weight loss.

Reference
Bosch X, Monclús E, Escoda O, et al. Unintentional weight loss: Clinical characteristics and outcomes in a prospective cohort of 2677 patients. PLoS One. 2017;12(4):e0175125.

DYSPHAGIA

Dysphagia is sensation of impaired passage of food from the mouth to stomach.

Reference
Lind CD. Dysphagia: evaluation and treatment. Gastroenterol Clin North Am. 2003;32(2):553-75.

DYSPEPSIA

Dyspepsia is often broadly defined as pain or discomfort centered in the upper abdomen but may include varying symptoms like epigastric pain, postprandial fullness, early satiation, anorexia, belching, nausea and vomiting, upper abdominal bloating, and even heartburn and regurgitation.

Reference
Feldman M, Friedman L, Brandt L. Sleisenger and Fordtran's Gastrointestinal and Liver Disease. Philadelphia: Saunders; 2015.

NAUSEA

Nausea is an unpleasant subjective sensation, most people have experienced at some point in their lives and usually recognize as a feeling of impending vomiting in the epigastrium or throat.

Reference
Feldman M, Friedman L, Brandt L. Sleisenger and Fordtran's Gastrointestinal and Liver Disease. Philadelphia: Saunders; 2015.

RETCHING

Retching consists of spasmodic and abortive respiratory movements with the glottis closed. When part of the emetic sequence, retching is associated with intense nausea and usually, but not invariably, culminates in the act of vomiting.

Reference
Feldman M, Friedman L, Brandt L. Sleisenger and Fordtran's Gastrointestinal and Liver Disease. Philadelphia: Saunders; 2015.

VOMITING

Vomiting is a partially voluntary act of forcefully expelling gastric or intestinal content through the mouth.

Reference
Feldman M, Friedman L, Brandt L. Sleisenger and Fordtran's Gastrointestinal and Liver Disease. Philadelphia: Saunders; 2015.

REGURGITATION

An effortless reflux of gastric contents into the esophagus that sometimes reaches the mouth but is not usually associated with the forceful ejection typical of vomiting.

Reference
Feldman M, Friedman L, Brandt L. Sleisenger and Fordtran's Gastrointestinal and Liver Disease. Philadelphia: Saunders; 2015.

DIARRHEA

Change in normal bowel movement characterized by passage of unusually soft or liquid stools ≥3 times in 24 hours (or >250 g unformed stool/day)

- Acute diarrhea—duration <14 days
- Persistent diarrhea—duration 14-29 days
- Chronic diarrhea—duration ≥30 days.

Reference
DuPont HL. Acute infectious diarrhea in immunocompetent adults. N Engl J Med. 2014;370(16):1532-40.

CONSTIPATION

Constipation defined as unsatisfactory defecation characterized by infrequent stools (fewer than 3 in a week), hard stools, excessive straining or a sense of incomplete evacuation.

Functional Constipation—Rome III Criteria

- ≥2 of the following:
  - Straining during ≥25% of defecations
  - Lumpy or hard stools during ≥25% of defecations
  - Feeling of incomplete evacuation during ≥25% of defecations
  - Feeling of anorectal obstruction or blockage during ≥25% of defecations
  - Manually facilitating defecation during ≥25% of defecations
  - <3 unassisted bowel movements/week.
- Loose stools rarely present without laxatives
- Criteria for irritable bowel syndrome not sufficiently met (although abdominal pain and/or bloating may be present, they are not predominant symptoms)
- Symptoms present for past 3 months with symptom onset ≥6 months before diagnosis.

Reference
Feldman M, Friedman L, Brandt L. Sleisenger and Fordtran's Gastrointestinal and Liver Disease. Philadelphia: Saunders; 2015.

FECAL INCONTINENCE

Fecal incontinence is defined as involuntary passage of fecal matter through the anus or inability to control the discharge of bowel contents.

Reference
Feldman M, Friedman L, Brandt L. Sleisenger and Fordtran's Gastrointestinal and Liver Disease. Philadelphia: Saunders; 2015.

HEMATEMESIS

Hematemesis is defined as vomiting of blood, which is indicative of bleeding from the esophagus, stomach, or duodenum.

Hematemesis includes vomiting of bright red blood, which suggests recent or ongoing bleeding, and dark material (coffee-ground emesis) which suggests bleeding that stopped some time ago.

Reference
Feldman M, Friedman L, Brandt L. Sleisenger and Fordtran's Gastrointestinal and Liver Disease. Philadelphia: Saunders; 2015.

MALENA

Melena is defined as black tarry stool and results from degradation of blood to hematin or other hemochromes by intestinal bacteria. Melena can signify bleeding that originates from a UGI, small bowel, or proximal colonic source and generally occurs when 50-100 mL or more of blood is delivered into the GI tract (usually the upper tract), with passage of characteristic stool occurring several hours after the bleeding event.

Reference
Feldman M, Friedman L, Brandt L. Sleisenger and Fordtran's Gastrointestinal and Liver Disease. Philadelphia: Saunders; 2015.

HEMATOCHEZIA

Hematochezia refers to bright red blood per rectum and suggests active UGI or small bowel bleeding or distal colonic or anorectal bleeding.

Reference
Feldman M, Friedman L, Brandt L. Sleisenger and Fordtran's Gastrointestinal and Liver Disease. Philadelphia: Saunders; 2015.

SEVERE GASTROINTESTINAL BLEEDING

Severe GI bleeding is defined as documented GI bleeding (hematemesis, melena, hematochezia, or positive nasogastric lavage) accompanied by shock or orthostatic hypotension, a decrease in the hematocrit value by at least 6% (or a decrease in the hemoglobin level of at least 2 g/dL), or transfusion of at least 2 units of packed red blood cells.

Reference
Feldman M, Friedman L, Brandt L. Sleisenger and Fordtran's Gastrointestinal and Liver Disease. Philadelphia: Saunders; 2015.

OCCULT GASTROINTESTINAL BLEEDING

Occult GI bleeding refers to subacute bleeding that is not clinically visible.

Reference
Feldman M, Friedman L, Brandt L. Sleisenger and Fordtran's Gastrointestinal and Liver Disease. Philadelphia: Saunders; 2015.

OBSCURE GASTROINTESTINAL BLEEDING

Obscure GI bleeding is bleeding from a site that is not apparent after routine endoscopic evaluation with esophagogastroduodenoscopy (upper endoscopy) and colonoscopy, and possibly small bowel radiography.

Reference
Feldman M, Friedman L, Brandt L. Sleisenger and Fordtran's Gastrointestinal and Liver Disease. Philadelphia: Saunders; 2015.

ACUTE LIVER FAILURE

Acute liver failure is the clinical syndrome of liver dysfunction, coagulopathy and encephalopathy developing within 26 weeks of onset of symptoms in patients without pre-existing liver failure.

Reference
Sherlock's diseases of the liver and biliary system.
Note: One categorization based on clinical patterns and outcome described three groups based on the time interval between the onset of jaundice and encephalopathy:
- Hyperacute liver failure (7 days or less)
- Acute liver failure (ALF) (8–28 days), and
- Subacute liver failure (4–24 weeks).

Reference
Feldman M, Friedman L, Brandt L. Sleisenger and Fordtran's Gastrointestinal and Liver Disease. Philadelphia: Saunders; 2015.

CIRRHOSIS OF LIVER

Cirrhosis is defined as a diffuse disruption of the normal architecture of the liver with fibrosis and nodule formation.

Reference
Sherlock's diseases of the liver and biliary system.

PORTAL HYPERTENSION

Syndrome of increased pressure (>5 mm Hg) in portal venous system due to increased vascular resistance plus increased blood flow.

Reference
Bloom S, Kemp W, Lubel J. Portal Hypertension—Pathophysiology, Diagnosis and Management. Intern Med J. 2015;45(1):16-26.

HEPATIC ENCEPHALOPATHY

Hepatic encephalopathy is a potentially reversible neuro-psychiatric complication of liver failure with a wide variety of clinical manifestations from minimal changes in cognitive function to severe complications of stupor and coma.

Reference
Vilstrup H, Amodio P, Bajaj J, et al. Hepatic encephalopathy in chronic liver disease: 2014 Practice Guideline by the American Association for the Study of Liver Diseases and the European Association for the Study of the Liver. Hepatology. 2014;60(2):715-35.

POLYURIA

The conventional definition of polyuria is a urine volume that is more than 2.5 L/day or

Polyuria is present if the urine flow rate is higher than what is expected in a specific setting.

Reference
Brenner and Rector's The Kidney.

NOCTURIA

The International Continence Society defines nocturia as a urinary storage symptom with the complaint that the individual has to wake one or more times at night to void, with each void being preceded and followed by sleep.

OLIGURIA

- Decreased urine output <300 cc/m^2/24 hours
- <0.5 cc/kg/hour in children
- <1 cc/kg/hour in infants
- Usually <500 cc/day in adults.

Reference
CDC.

ANURIA

- No or minimal urine output
- Usually <100 mL/day

Reference
CDC.

HEMATURIA

Hematuria is defined as three or more erythrocytes per high-power field.

Reference
Brenner and Rector's The Kidney.

MODERATELY INCREASED ALBUMINURIA

Urine albumin levels between 30 mg/day and 300 mg/day. This was previously referred to as microalbuminuria.

Reference
National Kidney Foundation Primer on Kidney Diseases.

SEVERELY INCREASED ALBUMINURIA

Urine albumin levels greater than 300 mg/day. This was previously referred to as macroalbuminuria.

Reference
National Kidney Foundation Primer on Kidney Diseases.

ACUTE KIDNEY INJURY

Acute kidney injury (AKI) is defined as any of the following:
- Increase in SCr by >0.3 mg/dL (>26.5 µmol/L) within 48 hours; or
- Increase in SCr to 1.5 times baseline, which is known or presumed to have occurred within the prior 7 days; or
- Urine volume <0.5 mL/kg/h for 6 hours.

Reference
KDIGO 2012 Guidelines on CKD.

CHRONIC KIDNEY DISEASE

Chronic kidney disease (CKD) is defined as abnormalities of kidney structure or function, present for >3 months with implications for health.

Criteria for CKD (either of the following present for >3 months)	
Markers of kidney damage (one or more)	• Albuminuria (AER >/= 30 mg/24 hours; ACR >/= 30 mg/g • Urine sediment abnormalities • Electrolyte and other abnormalities due to tubular disorders • Abnormalities detected by histology • Structural abnormalities detected by imaging history of kidney transplantation
Decreased GFR	GFR <60 mL/min/1.73 m2 (GFR categories G3a–G5)

Reference
KDIGO 2012 Guidelines on CKD.

NEPHROTIC SYNDROME

Nephrotic syndrome is a clinical syndrome characterized by:
- Proteinuria—adult >3.5 g/day, child >40 mg/h per m^2
- Hypoalbuminemia— <3.5 g/dL
- Edema
- Hypercholesterolemia
- Lipiduria.

Reference

Comprehensive clinical nephrology, John Feehally.

UNCOMPLICATED UTI AND COMPLICATED UTI

Uncomplicated UTI

Uncomplicated urinary tract infection (UTI) refers to acute cystitis or pyelonephritis in nonpregnant outpatient women without anatomic abnormalities or instrumentation of the urinary tract.

Complicated UTI

The term complicated UTI encompasses all other types of UTI.

Reference

Jameson JL, Fauci AS, Kasper DL, et al. Harrison's Principles of Internal Medicine, 20th ed. United States of America: McGraw-Hill Education; 2018.

ASYMPTOMATIC BACTERIURIA

Asymptomatic bacteriuria is defined as the presence of two separate consecutive clean-voided urine specimens, both with 105 or more colony-forming units per milliliter (cfu/mL) of the same uropathogen in the absence of symptoms referable to the urinary tract.

Reference

Johnson RJ, Feehally J. Comprehensive clinical nephrology. US: Mosby; 2000.

NEUTROPENIA AND AGRANULOCYTOSIS

Neutropenia is defined as absolute neutrophil count (ANC) ≤1.5 × 109/L

Agranulocytosis defined as ANC ≤0.2 × 109/L which carries a risk of severe infections with susceptibility to opportunistic organisms.

Reference

Newburger PE, Dale DC. Evaluation and management of patients with isolated neutropenia. Semin Hematol. 2013;50(3):198-206.

FEBRILE NEUTROPENIA

Febrile neutropenia is defined as a single fever [101°F (38.3°C)] or sustained elevated temperature [100.4°F (38°C)] in a patient with a current or anticipated absolute neutrophil count (ANC) <500 cells/mm.

Reference

Freifeld AG, Bow EJ, Sepkowitz KA, et al. Clinical practice guideline for the use of antimicrobial agents in neutropenic patients with cancer: 2010 update by the Infectious Diseases Society of America. Clin Infect Dis. 2011;52(4):e56-93.

LYMPHADENOPATHY

Lymphadenopathy is defined as lymph nodes of:
- Abnormal size, generally >1 cm, although definition of normal size range varies by lymph node regions and age of patient:
  - Jugulodigastric lymph nodes (often the largest of cervical lymph nodes) >1.5 cm are considered abnormal
  - Epitrochlear lymph nodes >5 mm are considered abnormal
  - Any palpable supraclavicular, popliteal, or iliac lymph nodes are considered abnormal
  - Abdominal lymph nodes vary from 6–10 mm; retrocrural lymph nodes >6 mm, retroperitoneal lymph nodes >10 mm, and pelvic lymph nodes >8–10 mm are considered abnormal
  - Inguinal lymph nodes >1.5 cm in diameter are considered abnormal.
- Abnormal dimensions, consistency or mobility.

Reference

Gaddey HL, Riegel AM. Unexplained Lymphadenopathy: Evaluation and Differential Diagnosis. Am Fam Physician. 2016;94(11):896-903.

GENERALIZED LYMPHADENOPATHY

Generalized lymphadenopathy is defined as involvement of ≥2 noncontiguous lymph node groups and is typically indicative of systemic disease.

Reference

Gaddey HL, Riegel AM. Unexplained Lymphadenopathy: Evaluation and Differential Diagnosis. Am Fam Physician. 2016;94(11):896-903.

MASSIVE SPLENOMEGALY

Spleen is massively enlarged when it is palpable >8 cm below the left costal margin or its drained weight is ≥1,000 g.

Reference

Harrison's Principles of internal medicine.

HYPERSPLENISM

Hypersplenism defined as a syndrome comprised of:
- Splenomegaly
- Anemia, leukopenia, and/or thrombocytopenia
- Compensatory bone marrow hyperplasia
- Improvement after splenectomy (if performed).

Reference

Pozo AL, Godfrey EM, Bowles KM. Splenomegaly: investigation, diagnosis and management. Blood rev. 2009;23(3):105-11.

STUPOR

Stupor is a state of baseline unresponsiveness that requires repeated application of vigorous stimuli to achieve arousal.

Reference

Bradley's Neurology in Clinical Practice, 5, 34-50.e1

COMA

Coma is a state of complete unresponsiveness to arousal, in which the patient lies with the eyes closed.

Reference
Bradley's Neurology in Clinical Practice, 5, 34-50.e1

CONFUSION

Confusion is a general term denoting the patient's incapacity to think with customary speed, clarity, and coherence.

Reference
Ropper AH, Samuels MA, Klein JP, et al. Adams and Victor's Principles of Neurology, 11th ed. United States of America: McGraw-Hill Education; 2019.

DEMENTIA

Dementia denotes a deterioration of all intellectual or cognitive functions with little or no disturbance of consciousness or perception.

Reference
Ropper AH, Samuels MA, Klein JP, et al. Adams and Victor's Principles of Neurology, 11th ed. United States of America: McGraw-Hill Education; 2019.

DELIRIUM

The American Psychiatric Association's Diagnostic and Statistical Manual, 5th edition (DSM-5) defines delirium as:
- Disturbance of consciousness with reduced ability to focus, sustain, or shift attention.
- The disturbance develops over a short period of time (usually hours to days) and tends to fluctuate during the course of a day.
- An additional disturbance in cognition (e.g., memory deficit, disorganization, language, visuospatial ability, or perception).
- A change in cognition or development of a perceptual disturbance that is not better accounted for by a pre-existing, established, or evolving dementia.
- There is evidence from history, physical examination, or laboratory findings that the disturbance is caused by medical condition, substance intoxication or withdrawal, (i.e., due to a drug of abuse or to a medication), or exposure to a toxin, or is due to multiple etiologies.

AKINETIC MUTISM

Akinetic mutism refers to a state in which the patient, although seemingly awake remains silent and motionless.

Reference
Brazis P, Masdeu JC, Biller J. Localization in clinical neurology. Philadelphia: Wolters Kluwer Health; 2016.

LOCKED IN SYNDROME

The locked in syndrome refers to a condition in which the patient is mute and motionless but remains awake, alert, aware of self and capable of perceiving sensory stimuli.

Reference
Brazis P, Masdeu JC, Biller J. Localization in clinical neurology. Philadelphia: Wolters Kluwer Health; 2016.

ABULIA

Abulia refers to difficulty in initiating and sustaining spontaneous movements and reduction in emotional responsiveness, spontaneous speech and social interactions.

Reference
Campbell WW. De Jong's The Neurological Examination. Philadelphia: Lippincott Williams & Wilkins; 2012.

ATTENTION AND CONCENTRATION

Attention is the ability to focus on a particular sensory stimulus to the exclusion of others.
Concentration is sustained attention.

Reference
Neurologic history & examination. In: Simon RP, Aminoff MJ, Greenberg DA, editors. Clinical Neurology, 10th ed. New York, NY: McGraw-Hill; 2017.

MEMORY

Memory is the ability to register, store, and retrieve information.

Reference
Neurologic history & examination. In: Simon RP, Aminoff MJ, Greenberg DA, editors. Clinical Neurology, 10th ed. New York, NY: McGraw-Hill; 2017.

AMNESIA

The amnesic state, defined by Ribot possesses two salient features that may vary in severity but are always conjoined:
1. An impaired ability to recall events and other information that has been firmly established before the onset of illness (retrograde amnesia).
2. An inability to acquire new information, learn or form new memories (anterograde amnesia).

Reference
Ropper AH, Samuels MA, Klein JP, et al. Adams and Victor's Principles of Neurology, 11th ed. United States of America: McGraw-Hill Education; 2019.

AGNOSIA

A conceptual inability to recognize objects, persons or sensory stimuli in the absence of a primary deficit in the sensory modality.

Reference
Ropper AH, Samuels MA, Klein JP, et al. Adams and Victor's Principles of Neurology, 11th ed. United States of America: McGraw-Hill Education; 2019.

INSOMNIA

A chronic inability to sleep despite adequate opportunity to do so. It indicates any impairment in the duration, depth or restorative properties of sleep.

Reference
Ropper AH, Samuels MA, Klein JP, et al. Adams and Victor's Principles of Neurology, 11th ed. United States of America: McGraw-Hill Education; 2019.

APHASIA

Loss of the production or comprehension of spoken or written language because of an acquired lesion in the brain.

Reference
Ropper AH, Samuels MA, Klein JP, et al. Adams and Victor's Principles of Neurology, 11th ed. United States of America: McGraw-Hill Education; 2019.

DYSARTHRIA

A defect in articulation of speech with intact mental functions, and comprehension of spoken and written language and normal syntax (grammatical construction of sentences).

Reference
Ropper AH, Samuels MA, Klein JP, et al. Adams and Victor's Principles of Neurology, 11th ed. United States of America: McGraw-Hill Education; 2019.

APHONIA AND DYSPHONIA

A loss (aphonia) or alteration (dysphonia) of voice due to a disorder of the larynx or its innervation.

Reference
Ropper AH, Samuels MA, Klein JP, et al. Adams and Victor's Principles of Neurology, 11th ed. United States of America: McGraw-Hill Education; 2019.

AGRAPHIA/DYSGRAPHIA

Loss of the ability to write, not due to weakness, incoordination, or other neurologic dysfunction of the arm or hand, is called agraphia.

Milder involvement may be referred to as dysgraphia.

Reference
Campbell WW. De Jong's The Neurological Examination. Philadelphia: Lippincott Williams & Wilkins; 2012.

ALEXIA

Loss of the ability to read in the absence of actual loss of vision is alexia.

Reference
Campbell WW. De Jong's The Neurological Examination. Philadelphia: Lippincott Williams & Wilkins; 2012.

ECHOLALIA

Echolalia is the meaningless repetition of heard words.

Reference
Campbell WW. De Jong's The Neurological Examination. Philadelphia: Lippincott Williams & Wilkins; 2012.

PALILALIA

Palilalia is the repetition of one's own speech.

Reference
Campbell WW. De Jong's The Neurological Examination. Philadelphia: Lippincott Williams & Wilkins; 2012.

PERSEVERATION

Perseveration is the persistence of one reply or one idea in response to various questions.

Reference
Campbell WW. De Jong's The Neurological Examination. Philadelphia: Lippincott Williams & Wilkins; 2012.

NEOLOGISMS

Neologisms are new words, usually meaningless, coined by the patient and usually heard in psychotic states or in aphasic patients.

Reference
Campbell WW. De Jong's The Neurological Examination. Philadelphia: Lippincott Williams & Wilkins; 2012.

IDIOGLOSSIA

Idioglossia is the imperfect articulation with utterance of meaningless sounds; the individual may speak with a vocabulary all his own.

Reference
Campbell WW. De Jong's The Neurological Examination. Philadelphia: Lippincott Williams & Wilkins; 2012.

DYSLOGIA

Dyslogia refers to abnormal speech due to mental disease, and it is most often used to refer to abnormal speech in dementia.

Reference
Campbell WW. De Jong's The Neurological Examination. Philadelphia: Lippincott Williams & Wilkins; 2012.

CONFABULATION

The creative falsification of memory in an alert, responsive individual.

Reference
Ropper AH, Samuels MA, Klein JP, et al. Adams and Victor's Principles of Neurology, 11th ed. United States of America: McGraw-Hill Education; 2019.

TONE

Tone is resistance of a muscle to passive movement at a joint.

Reference
Neurologic History & Examination. In: Simon RP, Aminoff MJ, Greenberg DA, editors. Clinical Neurology, 10th ed. New York, NY: McGraw-Hill; 2017.

RIGIDITY

Rigidity is characterized by a plastic resistance to passive movements that affects both agonist and antagonist muscles to a similar extent and that is constant throughout the entire range of movement.

COGWHEEL RIGIDITY

Cogwheel rigidity is characterized by periodic modifications of muscle tone due to the superimposed tremor that can be seen and felt when passively moving the extremity.

Reference
Brazis P, Masdeu JC, Biller J. Localization in clinical neurology. Philadelphia: Wolters Kluwer Health; 2016.

AKATHISIA

Akathisia refers to a feeling of inner restlessness that is often relieved by movement.

Reference
Brazis P, Masdeu JC, Biller J. Localization in clinical neurology. Philadelphia: Wolters Kluwer Health; 2016.

ASTERIXIS

Sudden loss of muscle tone during sustained contraction of an outstretched limb.

Reference
Talley and O'Connor's Clinical examination.

ATHETOSIS

Athetosis is characterized by slow, uncoordinated, twisting, writhing, and involuntary movements of wide amplitude. These predominantly involve the distal appendicular musculature, especially the upper extremities, although face and axial muscles may also be involved.

Reference
Brazis P, Masdeu JC, Biller J. Localization in clinical neurology. Philadelphia: Wolters Kluwer Health; 2016.

CHOREA

Chorea is characterized by sudden, brief, spontaneous, involuntary, purposeless, continuous, irregular, and unpredictable jerks that randomly involve the appendicular, facial, or truncal musculature.

Reference
Brazis P, Masdeu JC, Biller J. Localization in clinical neurology. Philadelphia: Wolters Kluwer Health; 2016.

DYSTONIA

Dystonia is characterized by slow, long sustained, contorting, involuntary movements, and postures involving proximal appendicular and axial muscles.

Reference
Brazis P, Masdeu JC, Biller J. Localization in clinical neurology. Philadelphia: Wolters Kluwer Health; 2016.

HEMIBALLISMUS

Hemiballismus is characterized by occurrence of sudden, paroxysmal, large amplitude, flinging, throwing movements of the arm, and leg contralateral to a lesion in or near the subthalamic nucleus.

Reference
Brazis P, Masdeu JC, Biller J. Localization in clinical neurology. Philadelphia: Wolters Kluwer Health; 2016.

MYOCLONUS

Myoclonus is a movement disorder characterized by unexpected, brief, brisk, shock-like, involuntary, repetitive, synchronous, or asynchronous contractions of a muscle or group of axial or appendicular muscles.

Reference
Brazis P, Masdeu JC, Biller J. Localization in clinical neurology. Philadelphia: Wolters Kluwer Health; 2016.

MYOKYMIA

A repeated contraction of a small muscle group; often involves the orbicularis oculi muscle.

Reference
Talley and O'Connor's Clinical examination.

RESTLESS LEG SYNDROME

Restless leg syndrome refers to a condition in which the patient notes unpleasant crawling sensations of the legs, particularly when sitting and relaxing in the evening which disappear on walking.
Criteria for diagnosis include:
- An intense irresistible urge to move the legs, usually associated with sensory complaints including paresthesia and dysesthesias.
- Motor restlessness.
- Worsening of the symptoms with rest and relief with motor activity.
- Increased severity of symptoms in the evening or at night.

Reference
Brazis P, Masdeu JC, Biller J. Localization in clinical neurology. Philadelphia: Wolters Kluwer Health; 2016.

TICS

Tics are sudden, rapid, usually stereotyped, and predominantly colonic hyperkinesias which may be willfully suppressed for short periods of time and disappear during sleep.

Reference
Brazis P, Masdeu JC, Biller J. Localization in clinical neurology. Philadelphia: Wolters Kluwer Health; 2016.

TREMOR

Involuntary, rhythmic, and oscillatory movements about a fixed point resulting from either alternating or synchronous contractions of reciprocally innervated antagonist muscles.

Reference
Brazis P, Masdeu JC, Biller J. Localization in clinical neurology. Philadelphia: Wolters Kluwer Health; 2016.

AGRAPHESTHESIA

Agraphesthesia is the inability to identify by touch a number written on the hand.

Reference
Neurologic History & Examination. In: Simon RP, Aminoff MJ, Greenberg DA, editors. Clinical Neurology, 10th ed. New York, NY: McGraw-Hill; 2017.

ALLODYNIA

Increase in sensibility to pain; pain in response to a stimulus not normally painful.

Reference
Campbell WW. De Jong's The Neurological Examination. Philadelphia: Lippincott Williams & Wilkins; 2012.

ALLOESTHESIA

Perception of a sensory stimulus at a site other than where it was delivered; tactile allesthesia is feeling something other than at the site of the stimulus.

Visual allesthesia is seeing something other than where it actually is.

Reference
Campbell WW. De Jong's The Neurological Examination. Philadelphia: Lippincott Williams & Wilkins; 2012.

ANALGESIA

Absence of sensibility to pain.

Reference
Campbell WW. De Jong's The Neurological Examination. Philadelphia: Lippincott Williams & Wilkins; 2012.

ASTEROGNOSIS

Absence of spatial tactile sensibility; inability to identify objects by feel.

Reference
Campbell WW. De Jong's The Neurological Examination. Philadelphia: Lippincott Williams & Wilkins; 2012.

ANESTHESIA

Absence of all sensations.

Reference
Campbell WW. De Jong's The Neurological Examination. Philadelphia: Lippincott Williams & Wilkins; 2012.

DYSESTHESIAS

Unpleasant or painful abnormal perverted sensations, either spontaneous or after a normally nonpainful stimulus (e.g., burning in response to touch); often accompanies paresthesias.

Reference
Campbell WW. De Jong's The Neurological Examination. Philadelphia: Lippincott Williams & Wilkins; 2012.

EXTINCTION

Extinction is the failure to perceive a visual or tactile stimulus when it is applied bilaterally, even though it can be perceived when applied unilaterally.

Reference
Neurologic History & Examination. In: Simon RP, Aminoff MJ, Greenberg DA, editors. Clinical Neurology, 10th ed. New York, NY: McGraw-Hill; 2017.

HYPALGESIA

Decrease in sensibility to pain.

Reference
Campbell WW. De Jong's The Neurological Examination. Philadelphia: Lippincott Williams & Wilkins; 2012.

HYPERALGESIA

Increase in sensibility to pain; pain in response to a stimulus not normally painful.

Reference
Campbell WW. De Jong's The Neurological Examination. Philadelphia: Lippincott Williams & Wilkins; 2012.

HYPERPATHIA

Increase in sensibility to pain; pain in response to a stimulus not normally painful.

Reference
Campbell WW. De Jong's The Neurological Examination. Philadelphia: Lippincott Williams & Wilkins; 2012.

KINESTHESIA

The sense of movement.

Reference
Campbell WW. De Jong's The Neurological Examination. Philadelphia: Lippincott Williams & Wilkins; 2012.

PALLESTHESIA

Vibratory sensation.
Hypopallesthesia = decreased vibratory sensation
Apallesthesia = absent vibratory sensation

Reference
Campbell WW. De Jong's The Neurological Examination. Philadelphia: Lippincott Williams & Wilkins; 2012.

PARESTHESIAS

Abnormal spontaneous sensations experienced in the absence of specific stimulation (feelings of cold, warmth numbness, tingling, burning, prickling, crawling, heaviness, compression or itching).

Reference
Campbell WW. De Jong's The Neurological Examination. Philadelphia: Lippincott Williams & Wilkins; 2012.

NEGLECT

Neglect is failure to attend to space or use the limbs on one side of the body.

Reference

Neurologic History & Examination. In: Simon RP, Aminoff MJ, Greenberg DA, editors. Clinical Neurology, 10th ed. New York, NY: McGraw-Hill; 2017.

ANOSOGNOSIA

Anosognosia is unawareness of a neurologic deficit.

Reference

Neurologic History & Examination. In: Simon RP, Aminoff MJ, Greenberg DA, editors. Clinical Neurology, 10th ed. New York, NY: McGraw-Hill; 2017.

CONSTRUCTIONAL APRAXIA

Constructional apraxia is the inability to draw accurate representations of external space, such as filling in the numbers on a clock face or copying geometric figures.

Reference

Neurologic History & Examination. In: Simon RP, Aminoff MJ, Greenberg DA, editors. Clinical Neurology, 10th ed. New York, NY: McGraw-Hill; 2017.

ATAXIA

Ataxia refers to a disturbance in the smooth performance of voluntary motor acts causing muscular incoordination or impaired balance.

Reference

Brazis P, Masdeu JC, Biller J. Localization in clinical neurology. Philadelphia: Wolters Kluwer Health; 2016.

PARALYSIS AND PARESIS

Paralysis means loss of voluntary movement as a result of interruption of one of the motor pathways at any point from the cerebrum to the muscle fiber. A lesser degree of weakness is spoken of as paresis.

Monoplegia refers to weakness or paralysis of all the muscles of one leg or arm.

Hemiplegia refers to weakness or paralysis involving the arm, the leg, and sometimes the face on one side of the body. Paraplegia indicates weakness or paralysis of both legs.

Quadriplegia (tetraplegia) denotes weakness or paralysis of all four extremities.

Reference

Ropper AH, Samuels MA, Klein JP, et al. Adams and Victor's Principles of Neurology, 11th ed. United States of America: McGraw-Hill Education; 2019.

APRAXIA

The term apraxia denotes a disorder in which an attentive patient loses the ability to execute previously learned activities in the absence of weakness, ataxia, sensory loss, or extrapyramidal derangement that would be adequate to explain the deficit.

Reference

Ropper AH, Samuels MA, Klein JP, et al. Adams and Victor's Principles of Neurology, 11th ed. United States of America: McGraw-Hill Education; 2019.

STROKE

Rapidly developing clinical signs of focal (or global) disturbance of cerebral function, lasting more than 24 hours or leading to death, with no apparent cause other than that of vascular origin.

Reference WHO

TRANSIENT ISCHEMIC ATTACK

Transient ischemic attack (TIA) is a transient episode of neurologic dysfunction caused by focal ischemia of the brain, spinal cord, or retina, and without detection of acute infarction on neuroimaging.

Reference

American Heart Association/American Stroke Association 2009 tissue-based definition of TIA.

LACUNAR STROKE

Lacunar stroke (or lacunar infarct) is defined as stroke caused by occlusion of small vessels in the brain.
- Infarcts are generally rounded, ovoid, or tubular in shape, and <20 mm in axial diameter.
- Infarcts result in a small cavity, or lacune, which typically ranges from >3 mm to <15 mm.

Reference

Pantoni L. Cerebral small vessel disease: from pathogenesis and clinical characteristics to therapeutic challenges. Lancet Neurol. 2010;9(7):689-701.

EPILEPTIC SEIZURE

Epileptic seizure—transient occurrence of signs and/or symptoms due to abnormal excessive or synchronous neuronal activity in the brain.

Reference

Berg AT, Berkovic SF, Brodie MJ, et al. Revised terminology and concepts for organization of seizures and epilepsies: report of the ILAE Commission on Classification and Terminology, 2005-2009. Epilepsia. 2010;51(4):676-85.

EPILEPSY

International League Against Epilepsy defines epilepsy as disease of brain defined by any of the following:
- Two or more unprovoked or reflex seizures occurring >24 hours apart.
- Single unprovoked (or reflex) seizure and high risk of recurrence over the next 10 years [similar high risk (≥60%) that occurs after 2 unprovoked seizures].
- Diagnosis of an epilepsy syndrome.

Reference

Berg AT, Berkovic SF, Brodie MJ, et al. Revised terminology and concepts for organization of seizures and epilepsies: report of the ILAE Commission on Classification and Terminology, 2005-2009. Epilepsia. 2010;51(4):676-85.

SYNCOPE

Syndrome of transient loss of consciousness secondary to cerebral hypoperfusion characterized by rapid onset, short duration, and complete spontaneous recovery.

Reference
Brignole M, Moya A, de Lange FJ, et al. 2018 ESC Guidelines for the diagnosis and management of syncope. Eur Heart J. 2018;39(21):1883-948.

METABOLIC SYNDROME

Metabolic syndrome is a cluster of commonly co-occurring metabolic risk factors associated with cardiovascular disease and type 2 diabetes mellitus, including elevated blood pressure, atherogenic dyslipidemia, insulin resistance, and central obesity.

Reference
Alberti KG, Eckel RH, Grundy SM, et al. Harmonizing the metabolic syndrome: a joint interim statement of the International Diabetes Federation Task Force on Epidemiology and Prevention; National Heart, Lung, and Blood Institute; American Heart Association; World Heart Federation; International Atherosclerosis Society; and International Association for the Study of Obesity. Circulation. 2009;120(16):1640-5.

SEPSIS

The Third International Consensus Definitions for Sepsis and Septic Shock (Sepsis-3)
- Sepsis—life-threatening organ dysfunction caused by dysregulated host response to infection.
- Organ dysfunction—acute change in total sequential organ failure assessment (SOFA) score ≥2 points consequent to infection:
  - Assume baseline SOFA score of 0 in patients without known preexisting organ dysfunction
  - SOFA score ≥2 points associated with overall mortality risk of about 10% in general hospital population with suspected infection.
- Septic shock:
  - Sepsis with underlying circulatory and cellular/metabolic abnormalities severe enough to substantially increase mortality
  - Clinically defined as persistent hypotension requiring vasopressors to maintain mean arterial pressure (MAP) ≥65 mm Hg and serum lactate level ≥2 mmol/L (18 mg/dL) despite adequate volume resuscitation

SYSTEMIC INFLAMMATORY RESPONSE SYNDROME

Systemic inflammatory response syndrome (SIRS):
- ≥2 of:
  - Temperature >38.3°C (100.9°F) or <36°C (96.8°F)
  - Heart rate >90 beats/minute
  - Respiratory rate >20 breaths/minute or arterial partial pressure of carbon dioxide ($PaCO_2$) <32 mm Hg
  - White blood cell count (WBC) >12,000/mm² or WBC <4,000/mm³ or >10% immature neutrophils (bands).
- Above abnormalities should represent change from baseline without other known cause (such as leukopenia due to chemotherapy).

Reference
Levy MM, Fink MP, Marshall JC, et al. Society of Critical Care Medicine (SCCM), European Society of Intensive Care Medicine (ESICM), American College of Chest Physicians (ACCP), American Thoracic Society (ATS), and Surgical Infection Society (SIS) 2001. International Sepsis Definitions Conference. Intensive Care Med. 2003;29(4):530-38.

ACUTE RESPIRATORY DISTRESS SYNDROME

Berlin definition of acute respiratory distress syndrome (ARDS):
- Onset within 1 week of known clinical insult or new or worsening respiratory symptoms.
- Bilateral opacities not fully explained by effusions, lobar/lung collapse, or nodules on chest X-ray or computed tomography.
- Respiratory failure not fully explained by cardiac failure or fluid overload (in the absence of risk factors for ARDS, an objective assessment such as echocardiography is required to exclude these causes of hydrostatic edema)
- Oxygenation status:
  - Mild ARDS defined as partial pressure of oxygen in arterial blood (PaO_2) to fraction of inspired oxygen (FiO_2) >200 mm Hg but ≤300 mm Hg with positive end-expiratory pressure (PEEP) or continuous positive airway pressure (CPAP) ≥5 cm H_2O
  - Moderate ARDS defined as PaO_2/FiO_2 >100 mm Hg but ≤200 mm Hg with PEEP ≥5 cm H_2O
  - Severe ARDS defined as PaO_2/FiO_2 ≤100 mm Hg with PEEP ≥5 cm H_2O
  - If altitude >1,000 meters, correction factor is PaO_2/FiO_2 × (barometric pressure/760).

MACULE

A flat, colored lesion, <2 cm in diameter, not raised above the surface of the surrounding skin. A "freckle," or ephelid, is a prototypical pigmented macule.

Reference
Harrison's Principles of Internal Medicine.

PATCH

A large (>2 cm) flat lesion with a color different from the surrounding skin. This differs from a macule only in size.

Reference
Harrison's Principles of Internal Medicine.

PAPULE

A small, solid lesion, <0.5 cm in diameter, raised above the surface of the surrounding skin and thus palpable (e.g., a closed comedone, or whitehead, in acne).

Reference
Harrison's Principles of Internal Medicine.

NODULE

A larger (0.5–5.0 cm), firm lesion raised above the surface of the surrounding skin. This differs from a papule only in size (e.g., a large dermal nevomelanocytic nevus).

Reference
Harrison's Principles of Internal Medicine.

TUMOR

A solid, raised growth >5 cm in diameter.

Reference
Harrison's Principles of Internal Medicine.

PLAQUE

A large (>1 cm), flat-topped, and raised lesion; edges may either be distinct (e.g., in psoriasis) or gradually blend with surrounding skin (e.g., in eczematous dermatitis).

Reference
Harrison's Principles of Internal Medicine.

VESICLE

A small, fluid-filled lesion, <0.5 cm in diameter, raised above the plane of surrounding skin. Fluid is often visible, and the lesions are translucent [e.g., vesicles in allergic contact dermatitis caused by *Toxicodendron* (poison ivy)].

Reference
Harrison's Principles of Internal Medicine.

PUSTULE

A vesicle filled with leukocytes. Note: The presence of pustules does not necessarily signify the existence of an infection.

Reference
Harrison's Principles of Internal Medicine.

BULLA

A fluid-filled, raised, often translucent lesion >0.5 cm in diameter.

Reference
Harrison's Principles of Internal Medicine.

WHEAL

A raised, erythematous, edematous papule or plaque, usually representing short-lived vasodilation and vasopermeability.

Reference
Harrison's Principles of Internal Medicine.

TELANGIECTASIA

A dilated, superficial blood vessel.

Reference
Harrison's Principles of Internal Medicine.

LICHENIFICATION

A distinctive thickening of the skin that is characterized by accentuated skin-fold markings.

Reference
Harrison's Principles of Internal Medicine.

SCALE

Excessive accumulation of stratum corneum.

Reference
Harrison's Principles of Internal Medicine.

CRUST

Dried exudate of body fluids that may be either yellow (i.e., serous crust) or red (i.e., hemorrhagic crust).

Reference
Harrison's Principles of Internal Medicine.

EROSION

Loss of epidermis without an associated loss of dermis.

Reference
Harrison's Principles of Internal Medicine.

ULCER

Loss of epidermis and at least a portion of the underlying dermis.

Reference
Harrison's Principles of Internal Medicine.

EXCORIATION

Linear, angular erosions that may be covered by crust and are caused by scratching.

Reference
Harrison's Principles of Internal Medicine.

ATROPHY

An acquired loss of substance. In the skin, this may appear as a depression with intact epidermis (i.e., loss of dermal or subcutaneous tissue) or as sites of shiny, delicate, and wrinkled lesions (i.e., epidermal atrophy).

Reference
Harrison's Principles of Internal Medicine.

SCAR

A change in the skin secondary to trauma or inflammation. Sites may be erythematous, hypopigmented, or hyperpigmented depending on their age or character. Sites on hair-bearing areas may be characterized by destruction of hair follicles.

Reference
Harrison's Principles of Internal Medicine.

PURPURIC LESIONS

Small, nonblanching, red, or purple areas on skin caused by extravasation of blood from vasculature into skin or mucous membranes.

- Petechiae—spots usually <2 mm in diameter
- Purpura—larger areas of extravasated blood usually 2 mm to 1 cm in diameter
- Ecchymoses—purpuric lesions >1 cm in diameter.

Reference
Leung AK, Chan KW. Evaluating the child with purpura. Am Fam Physician. 2001;64(3):419-28.

GYNECOMASTIA

Gynecomastia refers to enlargement of the male breast.

True gynecomastia is associated with glandular breast tissue that is >4 cm in diameter and often tender.

Reference
Harrison's Principles of Internal Medicine.

C. GRADING SYSTEMS

1952 MRC BREATHLESSNESS SCALE

Grade	Description
Grade 1	Is the patient's breath as good as that of other men of his age and build at work, on walking, and on climbing hills or stairs?
Grade 2	Is the patient able to walk with normal men of own age and build on the level but unable to keep up on hills or stairs?
Grade 3	Is the patient unable to keep up with normal men on the level, but able to walk about a mile or more at his own speed?
Grade 4	Is the patient unable to walk more than about 100 yards on the level without a rest?
Grade 5	Is the patient breathless on talking or undressing, or unable to leave his house because of breathlessness?

Note: "Used with the permission of the Medical Research Council"

MODIFIED MRC DYSPNEA SCALE

Grade	Description
Grade 0	I only get breathless with strenuous exercise
Grade 1	I get short of breath when hurrying on the level or walking up a slight hill
Grade 2	I walk slower than people of the same age on the level because of breathlessness, or I have to stop for breath when walking at my own pace on the level
Grade 3	I stop for breath after walking about 100 meters or after a few minutes on the level
Grade 4	I am too breathless to leave the house or I am breathless when dressing or undressing

Reference: GOLD, 2019.

MRC MUSCLE SCALE

Grade	Description
Grade 0	No contraction
Grade 1	Flicker or trace of contraction
Grade 2	Active movement with gravity eliminated
Grade 3	Active movement against gravity
Grade 4	Active movement against gravity and resistance
Grade 5	Normal power

Grades 4-, 4, and 4+ may be used to indicate movement against slight, moderate, and strong resistance, respectively.

Note: "Used with the permission of the Medical Research Council"

NYHA BREATHLESSNESS

For symptoms or signs in patients with defined or presumed cardiac disease.

Grade	Description
Class I	Without limitations of physical activity. Ordinary physical activity does not cause undue fatigue, palpitations, or dyspnea
Class II	Slight limitation of physical activity. The patient is comfortable at rest. Ordinary physical activity results in fatigue, palpitations, or dyspnea
Class III	Marked limitation of physical activity. The patient is comfortable at rest. Less than ordinary activity causes fatigue, palpitations, or dyspnea
Class IV	Inability to carry on any physical activity without discomfort. Heart failure symptoms are present even at rest or with minimal exertion

Reference: Criteria Committee of the New York Heart Association (NYHA). Nomenclature and Criteria for Diagnosis of Diseases of the Heart and Great Vessels. Boston: Little, Brown & Co; 1994. NYHA classification can be used to grade dyspnea, angina, palpitations, fatigue and syncope.

CANADIAN CARDIOVASCULAR SOCIETY—GRADING OF ANGINA PECTORIS

Grade	Description
Grade 0	Ordinary physical activity does not cause angina, such as walking and climbing stairs. Angina with strenuous or rapid or prolonged exertion at work or recreation
Grade 1	Slight limitation of ordinary activity. Walking or climbing stairs rapidly, walking uphill, walking or stair climbing after meals, or in cold, or in wind, or under emotional stress, or only during the few hours after awakening. Walking more than two blocks on the level and climbing more than one flight of ordinary stairs at a normal pace and in normal conditions
Grade 2	I walk slower than people of the same age on the level because of breathlessness, or I have to stop for breath when walking on my own pace on the level
Grade 3	Marked limitation of ordinary physical activity. Walking one or two blocks on the level and climbing one flight of stairs in normal conditions and at normal pace
Grade 4	Inability to carry on any physical activity without discomfort, anginal syndrome may be present at rest

NINDS MYOTACTIC REFLEX SCALE

Reflex	Description
0	Reflex absent
1	Reflex small, less than normal; includes a trace response or a response brought out only with reinforcement
2	Reflex in lower half or normal range
3	Reflex in upper half of normal range
4	Reflex enhanced, more than normal; includes clonus if present, which optionally can be noted in an added verbal description of the reflex

Reference: Hallett M. National Institute of Neurological Disorders and Stroke (NINDS) myotatic reflex scale. Neurology. 1993;43(12):2723.

FREEMAN AND LEVINE GRADING OF SYSTOLIC MURMUR

Systolic Murmurs

Levine and Freeman grading of systolic murmurs:

Grade	Description	Thrill
Grade 1	Murmur so faint that it can be heard only with special effort. Heard only after a few seconds have elapsed	Absent
Grade 2	Murmur is faint, but is immediately audible	
Grade 3	Murmur that is moderately loud	
Grade 4	Murmur that is very loud	Present
Grade 5	A murmur is extremely loud and is audible with one edge of the stethoscope touching the chest wall	
Grade 6	A murmur is so loud that it is audible with the stethoscope just removed from contact with the chest wall	

Reference: Levine SA. The systolic murmur: its clinical significance. JAMA. 1933;101(6):436-8.

Diastolic Murmurs (by AIMS)

Grade	Description	Thrill
Grade 1	Very soft	Absent
Grade 2	Soft	
Grade 3	Loud	
Grade 4	Very loud	Present

Grading of Pulse

Grade	Description
0	Pulse not palpable
1+	Faint
2+	Slightly diminished pulse than normal
3+	Normal pulse
4+	Bounding pulse

ABCD AND ABCD2 SCORES (TABLE 16C.1)

TABLE 16C.1: ABCD and ABCD2 scores.

	Value	Score
ABCD risk factor		
Age	≥60 years	1
Blood pressure	Systolic blood pressure >140 mm Hg or diastolic blood pressure >90 mm Hg	1
Clinical symptoms	Unilateral weakness	2
	Speech disturbance without weakness	1
Duration of symptoms	>60 minutes	2
	10–59 minutes	1
ABCD2 additional factor		
Diabetes	Oral medication or insulin	1

It is reasonable to hospitalize patients with transient ischemic attack who present within 72 hours of symptoms with:
- ABCD2 score of 3 points or higher
- ABCD2 score of 0–2 points with evidence of focal ischemia
- ABCD2 score of 0–2 points if uncertain that patient can obtain outpatient work-up within 2 days.

Reference: Easton JD, Saver JL, Albers GW, et al. Definition and evaluation of transient ischemic attack: a scientific statement for healthcare professionals from the American Heart Association/American Stroke Association Stroke Council; Council on Cardiovascular Surgery and Anesthesia; Council on Cardiovascular Radiology and Intervention; Council on Cardiovascular Nursing; and the Interdisciplinary Council on Peripheral Vascular Disease. The American Academy of Neurology affirms the value of this statement as an educational tool for neurologists. Stroke. 2009;40(6):2276-93.

BODE INDEX (TABLE 16C.2)

TABLE 16C.2: Variables and point values used for the computation of the body mass index, degree of airflow obstruction and dyspnea, and exercise capacity (BODE) index.*

Variable	Points on BODE index			
	0	1	2	3
FEV_1 (% of predicted)[†]	≥65	50–64	36–49	≤35
Distance walked in 6 minutes (m)	≥350	250–349	150–249	≤149
MMRC dyspnea scale[‡]	0–1	2	3	4
Body mass index[§]	>21	≤21		

* The cutoff values for the assignment of points are shown for each variable. The total possible values range from 0 to 10. FEV_1 denotes forced expiratory volume in 1 second.

† The FEV_1 categories are based on stages identified by the American Thoracic Society.

‡ Scores on the modified Medical Research Council (MMRC) dyspnea scale can range from 0 to 4, with a score of 4 indicating that the patient is too breathless to leave the house or becomes breathless when dressing or undressing.

§ The values for body mass index were 0 to 1 because of the infection point in the inverse relation between survival and body mass index at a value of 21.

- Body mass index
- Obstruction = FEV1 (% of predicted)
- Dyspnea = MMRC dyspnea scale
- Exercise = Distance walked in 6 minutes

Reference: Celli BR, Cote CG, Marin JM, et al. The body-mass index, airflow obstruction, dyspnea, and exercise capacity index in chronic obstructive pulmonary disease. N Engl J Med. 2004;350(10):1005-12.

COPD ASSESSMENT TEST

Example: I am very happy 0 ✗ 2 3 4 5 I am very sad

Statement (low)	Scale	Statement (high)
I never cough	0 1 2 3 4 5	I cough all the time
I have no phlegm (mucus) on my chest at all	0 1 2 3 4 5	My chest is full of phlegm (mucus)
My chest does not feel tight at all	0 1 2 3 4 5	My chest feels very tight
When I walk up a hill or a flight of stairs I am not out of breath	0 1 2 3 4 5	When I walk up a hill or a flight of stairs I am completely out of breath
I am not limited to doing any activities at home	0 1 2 3 4 5	I am completely limited to doing all activities at home
I am confident leaving my home despite my lung condition	0 1 2 3 4 5	I am not confident leaving my home at all because of my lung condition
I sleep soundly	0 1 2 3 4 5	I do not sleep soundly because of my lung condition
I have lots of energy	0 1 2 3 4 5	I have no energy at all

Make sure you print your CAT before visiting your healthcare professional. **Total score**

A COPD assessment test was developed by an interdisciplinary group of international COPD experts with support from GSK. GSK's activities in connection with the COPD assessment test are monitored by a supervisory council that includes external, independent experts, one of which is chair of the council.

CHADS2

Risk factor	Score
Congestive heart failure	1
Hypertension	1
Age ≥75 years	1
Diabetes mellitus	1
Stroke/TIA/TE	2
Maximum score	6

The CHADS2 score for stroke risk in AF.

CHADS-VASC

CHADS-VASc clinical characteristic.

Risk factor	Score
Congestive heart failure	1
Hypertension	1
Age ≥75	2
Age 65–74	1
Diabetes mellitus	1
Stroke/TIA/thromboembolism	2
Vascular disease	1
Sex: Female	1

Reference: https://www.chadsvasc.org/.

HAS-BLED

HAS-BLED clinical characteristic.

Clinical characteristic	Points awarded
Hypertension	1
Abnormal liver function	1
Abnormal renal function	1
Stroke	1
Bleeding	1
Labile INRs	1
Elderly (age >65)	1
Drugs	1
Alcohol	1
Your score	0

Reference: https://www.chadsvasc.org/.

EHRA SCORE

Classification of AF-related symptoms (EHRA score).

EHRA I	No symptoms
EHRA II	Mild symptoms; normal daily activity not affected
EHRA III	Severe symptoms; normal daily activity affected
EHRA IV	Disabling symptoms; normal daily activity discontinued

Reference: https://www.chadsvasc.org/.

CHILD-TURCOTTE-PUGH SCORE

Child-Turcotte-Pugh scoring system and Child-Pugh classification.

Parameter	Numerical score		
	1	*2*	*3*
Ascites	None	Slight	Moderate/severe
Encephalopathy	None	Slight	Moderate/severe
Bilirubin (mg/dL)	<2	2–3	>3
Albumin (g/dL)	>3	2.8–3.5	<2.8
Prothrombin time (seconds increased)	1–3	4–6	>6
Total numerical score	***Child-Pugh class***		
5–6	A		
7–9	B		
10–15	C		

FRAMINGHAM HEART FAILURE CRITERIA

Diagnosis of CHF requires the simultaneous presence of at least 2 major criteria or 1 major criterion in conjunction with 2 minor criteria.

Major Criteria

- Paroxysmal nocturnal dyspnea
- Neck vein distention
- Rales
- Cardiomegaly
- Acute pulmonary edema
- S3 gallop
- Increased central venous pressure (>16 cm H_2O)
- Sustained hepatojugular reflux
- Circulation time ≥25 seconds.

Minor Criteria

- Ankle edema
- Nocturnal cough
- Dyspnea on ordinary exertion
- Hepatomegaly
- Pleural effusion
- Decrease in vital capacity by one-third from maximum recorded
- Tachycardia (heart rate >120 beats/min).
- Major or minor criterion: Weight loss ≥4.5 kg in 5 days in response to treatment.

Minor criteria are acceptable only if they cannot be attributed to another medical condition (such as pulmonary hypertension, chronic lung disease, cirrhosis, ascites, or the nephrotic syndrome).

GCS

Glasgow Coma Scale (GCS)					
Eye opening		*Best verbal response*		*Best motor response*	
				Obeys commands	6
		Oriented and converses	5	Localizes pain	5
Open spontaneously	4	Converses, but disoriented, confused	4	Exhibits flexion withdrawal	4
Open only to verbal stimuli	3	Uses inappropriate words	3	Decorticate rigidity	3
Open only to pain	2	Makes incomprehensible sounds	2	Decerebrate rigidity	2
Never open	1	No verbal response	1	No motor response	1

Maximum score = **15**
Minimum score = **3**
Coma is equal to GCS of less than **8 or less.**

***Mnemonic (GCS → EVM = 4, 5, and 6)**
*In intubated patients, verbal response is denoted as VT.

WEST HAVEN GRADING OF HEPATIC ENCEPHALOPATHY (TABLE 16C.3)

TABLE 16C.3: Clinical stages of hepatic encephalopathy (HE): The West Haven criteria and the proposed classification of the spectrum of neurocognitive impairment in cirrhosis (SONIC).

	West Haven criteria		Sonic			
Grade	Intellectual function	Neuromuscular function	Classification	Mental status	Special tests	Asterixis
0	Normal	Normal	Unimpaired	Not impaired	Normal	Absent
Minimal	Normal examination findings; suitable changes in work or driving	Minor abnormalities of visual perception or on psychometric or number tests	Covert HE	Not impaired	Abnormal	Absent
1	Personality changes, attention deficits, irritability, depressed state	Tremor and incoordination				
2	Changes in sleep-wake cycle, lethargy, mood and behavioral changes, cognitive dysfunction	Asterixis, ataxic gait, speech abnormalities (slow and slurred)	Overt HE	Impaired	Abnormal	Present (absent in coma)
3	Altered level of consciousness (somnolence), confusion, disorientation, and amnesia	Muscular rigidity, nystagmus, clonus, Babinski sign, hyporeflexia				
4	Stupor and coma	Oculocephalic reflex, unresponsiveness to noxious stimuli				

References:
- Ferenci P, Lockwood A, Mullen K, et al. Hepatic encephalopathy—definition, nomenclature, diagnosis, and quantification: final report of the working party at the 11th World Congress of Gastroenterology, Vienna, 1998. Hepatology. 2002;35(3):716-21.
- Bajaj JS, Cordoba J, Mullen KD, et al. Review article: the design of clinical trials in hepatic encephalopathy—an International Society for Hepatic Encephalopathy and Nitrogen Metabolism (ISHEN) consensus statement. Aliment Pharmacol Ther. 2011;33(7):739-47.

CKD STAGES

				Albuminuria categories		
				A1	A2	A3
				Normal to mildly increased	Moderately increased	Severely increased
				<30 mg/g <3 mg/mmoL	30–299 mg/g 3–29 mg/mmoL	≥300 mg/g ≥30 mg/mmoL
GFR stages	G1	Normal or high	≥90	Green	Yellow	Orange
	G2	Mildly decreased	60–90	Green	Yellow	Orange
	G3a	Mildly to moderately decreased	45–59	Yellow	Orange	Red
	G3b	Moderately to severely decreased	30–44	Orange	Red	Red
	G4	Severely decreased	15–29	Red	Red	Deep red
	G5	Kidney failure	<15	Red	Deep red	Deep red

Key to figure:
Colors: Represents the risk for progression, morbidity and mortality by color from best to worst.
Green: Low risk (if no other markers of kidney disease, no CKD)
Yellow: Moderately increased risk
Orange: High-risk
Red: Very high-risk
Deep red: Highest risk

Reference: KDIGO.

2015 REVISED JONES CRITERIA

2015 AHA-Revised Jones criteria for diagnosis of rheumatic fever*	
Major criteria	
Low-risk populations	*Moderate-and high-risk populations*
Carditis (clinical or subclinical†)	Carditis (clinical or subclinical)
Arthritis (polyarthritis only)	Arthritis (including polyarthritis, monoarthritis or polyarthalgia‡)
Chorea	Chorea
Erythema marginatum	Erythema marginatum
Subcutaneous nodules	Subcutaneous nodules
Minor criteria	
Low-risk populations	*Moderate-and High-risk populations*
Polyarthralgia	Monoarthralgia
Fever (>38.5°C)	Fever (>38°C)
ESR >60 mm in the first hour and/or CRP >3.0 mg/dL	ESR >30 mm in the first hour and/or CRP >3.0 mg/dL§
Prolonged PR interval, after for age variability (unless carditis is a major criterion)	Prolonged PR interval, after accounting for age variability (unless carditis is a major criterion)

Joint manifestations are only considered in either the major or the minor category, but not in both categories in the same patient.

* Annual acute rheumatic fever (ARF) incidence of <2 per 1,00,000 school-aged children or all-age rheumatic heart disease (RHD) prevalence of <1 per 1,000 people per year.
† Defined as echocardiographic valvulitis, **Table 16C.4**.
‡ Polyarthralgia should only be considered as a major manifestation in moderate and high-risk populations after exclusion of other causes.
§ C-reactive protein (CRP) value must be greater than the normal laboratory upper limit. In addition, because the erythrocyte sedimentation rate (ESR) might evolve during the course of ARF, peak ESR values should be used.

TABLE 16C.4: The World Heart Federation minimum echocardiographic criteria for diagnosis of pathologic valvular regurgitation caused by rheumatic carditis.	
Pathologic mitral regurgitation*	*Pathologic aortic regurgitation**
<ul><li>Seen in at least two views</li><li>In at least one view, jet length is >2 cm†</li><li>Peak velocity >3 meter/second</li><li>Pansystolic jet in at least one envelope</li></ul>	<ul><li>Seen in at least two views</li><li>In at least one view, jet length is >1 cm†</li><li>Peak velocity >3 meters/ second</li><li>Pandiastolic jet in at least one envelope</li></ul>

* All four Doppler criteria must be met
† A regurgitant jet length should be measured from the vena contracta to the last pixel of regurgitant color (blue or red) on nonmagnified (nonzoomed) images.

Reference: Reményi B, Wilson N, Steer A, et al. World Heart Federation criteria for echocardiographic diagnosis of rheumatic heart disease—an evidence-based guideline. Nat Rev Cardiol. 2012;9(5):297-309.

MODIFIED DUKE'S CRITERIA (TABLE 16C.5)

TABLE 16C.5: Definition of infective endocarditis (IE): Modified Duke's criteria.

Definite infective endocarditis

Pathologic criteria
- Microorganisms demonstrated by results of cultures or histologic examination of vegetation that has embolized, or an intracardiac abscess specimen; or
- Pathologic lesions; vegetation, or intracardiac abscess confirmed by results of histologic examination showing active endocarditis

Clinical criteria
- 2 major criteria, or
- 1 major criterion and 3 minor criteria, or
- 5 minor criteria

Possible infective endocarditis
- 1 major criterion and 1 minor criterion, or
- 3 minor criteria

Contd...

Contd...

Rejected diagnosis of infective endocarditis

Firm alternate diagnosis explaining evidence of suspected IE, or
Resolution of IE syndrome with antibiotic therapy for <4 days, or
No evidence of IE at surgery of autopsy, on antibiotic therapy for <4 days, or
Does not meet criteria for possible IE

Definition of terms used in the modified Duke's criteria for diagnosis of infective endocarditis

Major criteria

Blood culture findings positive for IE

Typical microorganisms consistent with IE from two separate blood cultures:
- Viridans streptococci, *Streptococcus gallolyticus* (formerly known as *S. bovis*), Staphylococcus aureus, HACEK group, or
- Community-acquired enterococci, in the absence of a primary focus, or

Microorganisms consistent with IE from persistently positive blood culture findings, defined as:
- >2 positive culture findings of blood samples drawn >12 hours apart, or
- 3 or more of >4 separate culture findings of blood (with first and last sample drawn >1 hour apart)
- Single positive blood culture for *Coxiella burnetii* or anti-phase I IgG liter >1:800

Evidence of endocardial involvement

Echocardiographic findings positive for IE [TEE recommended in patients with prosthetic valves, rated at least possible IE by clinical criteria or complicated IE (paravalvular) abscess TTE as first test in other patients] defined as follow:
- Oscillating intracardiac mass on valve or supporting structures, in the path of regurgitant jets, or on implanted material in the absence of an alternative anatomic explanation, or
- Abscess, or
- New partial dehiscence of prosthetic valve
- New valvular regurgitation; worsening or changing of pre-existing murmur not sufficient

Minor criteria

- Predisposition, predisposing heart condition, or intravenous drug use
- Fever—temperature >38°C
- Vascular phenomena, major arterial emboli, septic pulmonary infarcts, mycotic aneurysm, intracranial hemorrhage, conjunctival hemorrhages, and Janeway lesions
- Immunologic phenomena: Glomerulonephritis, Osler nodes, Roth spots, and rheumatoid factor
- Microbiologic evidence: Positive blood culture findings but does not meet a major criterion as noted above (excludes single positive culture findings for coagulase-negative staphylococci and organisms that do not cause endocarditis) or serologic evidence of active infection with organism consistent with IE

(TEE: transesophageal echocardiography; TTE: transthoracic echocardiography)
Reference: Li JS, Sexton DJ, Mick N, et al. Proposed modifications to the Duke criteria for the diagnosis of infective endocarditis. Clin Infect Dis. 2000;30(4):633-38.

CAGE QUESTIONNAIRE

- Have you ever felt you should **cut down** on your drinking?
- Have people **annoyed** you by criticizing your drinking?
- Have you ever felt bad or **guilty** about your drinking?
- Have you ever had a drink first thing in the morning to steady your nerves or to get rid of a hangover **(eye opener)**?
- Scoring: Item responses on the CAGE are scored 0 or 1, with a higher score an indication of alcohol problems.
- A total score of two or greater is considered clinically significant.

Reference: Steinweg DL, Worth H. Alcoholism: the keys to the CAGE. Am J Med. 1993;94(5):520-3.

LIGHT'S CRITERIA

These criteria classify an effusion as exudate if one or more of the following are present:

1. The ratio of pleural fluid protein to serum protein is greater than 0.5
2. The ratio of pleural fluid lactate dehydrogenase (LDH) to serum LDH is greater than 0.6
3. The pleural fluid LDH level is greater than two-third of the upper limit of normal for serum LDH.

Reference: Light RW. Clinical practice. Pleural effusion. N Engl J Med. 2002;346(25):1971-7.

qSOFA

A patient is said to have high-risk for developing adverse outcomes if two out of:
- Altered mental status (GCS <15)
- Hypotension (systolic BP ≤100 mm Hg), and
- Tachypnea (respiratory rate ≥22 breaths/min) are present.

SOFA

System	0	1	2	3	4
Respiration PaO_2/FiO_2 mm Hg (kPa)	≥400 (53.3)	<400 (53.3)	<300 (40)	<200 (26.7) with respiratory support	<100 (13.3) with respiratory support
Coagulation platelets (×10³/μL)	≥150	<150	<100	<50	<20
Liver bilirubin μmol/L (mg/dL)	<20 (1.2)	20–32 (1.2–1.9)	33–101 (2.0–5.9)	102–204 (6.0–11.9)	>204 (12.0)
Cardiovascular (catecholamine doses in μg/kg/min for at least 1 hour)	MAP ≥70 mm Hg	MAP <70 mm Hg	Dopamine <5 or dobutamine (any dose)	Dopamine 5.1–15 or adrenaline ≤0.1 or noradrenaline ≤0.1	Dopamine >15 or adrenaline >0.1 or noradrenaline >0.1
Central nervous system Glasgow coma scale score	15	13–14	10–12	6–9	<6
Renal creatinine μmol/L (mg/dL)	<110 (1.2)	110–170 (1.2–1.9)	171–299 (2.0–3.4)	300–440 (3.5–4.9)	>440 (5.0)
Urine output (mL/day)				<500	<200

CURB 65

Confusion of new onset (defined as an AMTS of 8 or less)	1 point
Blood **U**rea nitrogen greater than 7 mmol/L (19 mg/dL)	1 point
Respiratory rate of 30 breaths/min or greater	1 point
Blood pressure less than 90 mm Hg systolic or diastolic blood pressure 60 mm Hg or less	1 point
Age **65** years or older	1 point

The risk of death at 30 days increases as the score increases:
- 0—0.6%
- 1—2.7%
- 2—6.8%
- 3—14.0%
- 4—27.8%
- 5—27.8%

Reference: Lim WS, van der Eerden MM, Laing R, et al. Defining community acquired pneumonia severity on presentation to hospital: an international derivation and validation study. Thorax. 2003;58(5):377-82.

FORREST GRADING OF GASTROINTESTINAL ULCERS

Acute hemorrhage:
- Forrest I a (spurting hemorrhage)
- Forrest I b (oozing hemorrhage)

Signs of recent hemorrhage:
- Forrest II a (pigmented protuberance or nonbleeding visible vessel)
- Forrest II b (adherent clot)
- Forrest II c (flat pigmented spot)

Lesions without active bleeding:
- Forrest III (clean-based ulcer)

Reference: Forrest JA, Finlayson ND, Shearman DJ. Endoscopy in gastrointestinal bleeding. Lancet. 1974;2(7877):394-97.

SEVERITY INDEX FOR ULCERATIVE COLITIS (TABLE 16C.6)

TABLE 16C.6: Truelove and Witts' severity index for ulcerative colitis.

Features	Mild	Moderate	Severe
Bowel movements (number per day)	Fewer than 4	4–6	6 or more plus at least one of the features of systemic upset (marked with below)
Blood in stools	No more than small amounts of blood	Between mild and severe	Visible blood
Pyrexia (temperature greater than 37.8°C)	No	No	Yes
Pulse rate greater than 90 bpm	No	No	Yes
Anemia	No	No	Yes
Erythrocyte sedimentation rate (mm/hour)	30 or below	30 or below	Above 30

D. LABORATORY VALUES OF CLINICAL IMPORTANCE

HEMATOLOGY AND COAGULATION (TABLE 16D.1)

TABLE 16D.1: Hematology and coagulation.

Component (specimen)	Reference value	
	Conventional	SI units
RBCs and hemoglobin		
RBC count		
▪ Males	$4.5–5.5 \times 10^{12}/L$ (mean $5.0 \times 10^{12}/L$)	
▪ Females	$3.8–4.8 \times 10^{12}/L$ (mean $4.3 \times 10^{12}/L$)	
RBC diameter	6.7–7.7 μm (mean 7.2 μm)	
RBC indices (absolute values)		
▪ Mean corpuscular volume (MCV)	82–100 fL	
▪ Mean corpuscular hemoglobin (MCH)	27–32 pg	
▪ Mean corpuscular hemoglobin concentration (MCHC)	31–35 g/dL	
▪ Red cell distribution width (RDW)	11.5–14.0%	
RBC lifespan	120 days	
Erythrocyte sedimentation rate (ESR) (whole blood)		
▪ Westergren, 1st hour		
• Males	0–15 mm 1st hour	
• Females	0–20 mm 1st hour	
• Children	0–10 mm 1st hour	
Wintrobe, 1st hour		
▪ Males	0–9 mm 1st hour	
▪ Females	0–20 mm 1st hour	
Ferritin (serum)		
▪ Males	20–300 ng/mL	20–300 μg/L
▪ Females	15–200 ng/mL	15–200 μg/L
Folate (serum)	3–20 μg/L	3–20 ng/mL
Hematocrit (PCV)		
▪ Males	38–47%	
▪ Females	36–46%	
▪ Infants (cord blood)	45–70%	
Haptoglobin (serum)	40–240 mg/dL	0.4–2.4 g/L
Hemoglobin (Hb)		
▪ Adult hemoglobin (HbA)	95–98%	
▪ Males	13.0–17.0 g/dL	
▪ Females	12.0–15.0 g/dL	
▪ Hemoglobin A_2 (HbA_2)	1.5–3.5%	
▪ Hemoglobin, fetal (HbF) in adults	<0–2%	
▪ HbF, children under 6 months	<5%	
Iron, total (serum)	50–150 μg/dL	7–25 μmol/L
▪ Total iron binding capacity (TIBC)	310–340 μg/dL	45–73 μmol/L
▪ Iron saturation	20–45%	0.20–0.45

Contd...

Contd...

Osmotic fragility		
▪ Slight hemolysis	At 0.45–0.39 g/dL NaCl	
▪ Complete hemolysis	At 0.33–0.36 g/dL NaCl	
▪ Mean corpuscular fragility	0.4–0.45 g/dL NaCl	
Reticulocytes		
▪ Adults	0.5–2.5%	
▪ Infants	2–6%	
▪ Newborn (cord blood)	1–7%	
Transferrin saturation		
▪ Male	25–56%	
▪ Female	14–51%	
Vitamin B_{12} (serum)		
▪ Body stores	10–12 mg	
▪ Daily requirement	2–3 µg	
▪ Serum level	280–1000 pg/mL	
Autohemolysis test (whole blood)	0.4–4.50%	0.004–0.045
Autohemolysis test with glucose (whole blood)	0.3–0.7%	0.003–0.007
Leukocytes		
Differential leukocyte count (DLC)		
▪ P (polymorphs or neutrophils)	40–70% (2,000–7,500/µL)	
▪ L (lymphocytes)	20–40% (1,500–4,000/µL)	
▪ M (monocytes)	2–10% (200–800/µL)	
▪ E (eosinophils)	1–6% (40–450/µL)	
▪ B (basophils)	<1% (10–100/µL)	
Total leukocyte count (TLC)		
▪ Adults	4,000–11,000/µL	
▪ Infants (full term, at birth)	10,000–25,000/µL	
▪ Infants (1 year)	6,000–16,000/µL	
Platelets and coagulation		
Bleeding time (BT)		
▪ Ivy's method	2–7 minutes	
▪ Template method	2–9 minutes	
Clot retraction time (clotted blood)		
▪ Qualitative	Visible in 60 minutes (complete in <24 hours) 48–64%	
▪ Quantitative	(55%)	
Clotting time (CT) Lee and White method	4–11 minutes	
D-dimer (plasma)	220–740 ng/mL	
Fibrinogen (plasma)	200–400 mg/dL	
Fibrin split (or degradation) products (FSP or FDP)	<10 µg/mL	<10 mg/L
Partial thromboplastin time with kaolin (PTTK) or activated partial thromboplastin time (APTT/aAPTT)	30–40 seconds	
Platelet count	150,000–450,000/µL	
Prothrombin time (PT) (Quick's one stage method)	11–16 sec	
Thrombin time (TT)	15–19 sec (control ± 2 sec)	

Clinical Chemistry of Blood (Table 16D.2)

TABLE 16D.2: Clinical chemistry of blood.

Component	Specimen	Reference value	
		Conventional	SI units
Alpha fetoprotein (AFP), adults	Serum	0–8.5 ng/mL	0–8.5 µg/L
Aminotransferases (transaminases) ▪ Aspartate (AST, SGOT) ▪ Alanine (ALT, SGPT)	 Serum Serum	 12–38 U/L 7–41 U/L	 0.20–0.65 µkat/L 0.12–0.70 µkat/L
Amylase	Serum	20–96 U/L	0.34–1.6 µkat/L
Bilirubin ▪ Total ▪ Direct (conjugated) ▪ Indirect (unconjugated)	Serum	 0.3–1.3 mg/dL 0.1–0.4 mg/dL 0.2–0.9 mg/dL	 5.1–22 µmol/L 1.7–6.8 µmol/L 3.4–15.2 µmol/L
CA-125	Serum	0–35 U/mL	0–35 Ku/L
Calcium—ionized	Whole blood	4.5–5.3 mg/dL	1.12–1.32 mmol/L
Calcium—total	Serum	8.7–10.2 mg/dL	2.2–2.6 mmol/L
Chloride	Serum	102–109 mEq/L	102–109 mmol/L
C-reactive proteins	Serum	0.2–3.0 mg/L	0.2–3.0 mg/L
Creatine kinase (CK), total ▪ Males ▪ Females	Serum	 51–294 U/L 39–238 IU/L	 0.87–5.0 µkat/L 0.66–4.0 µkat/L
Creatine kinase MB (CKMB)	Serum	0–5.5 ng/mL	0–5.5 µg/L
Gamma glutamyl transpeptidase (transferase) (γ-GT)	Serum	9–58 IU/L	0.15–1.00 µmol/L
Glucose (fasting) ▪ Normal ▪ Impaired fasting glucose (IFG) ▪ Diabetes mellitus	Plasma	 70–100 mg/dL 101–125 mg/dL >126 mg/dL	 <5.6 mmol/L 5.6–6.9 mmol/L >7.0 mmol/L
Glucose (2-hour postprandial) ♦ Normal ♦ Impaired glucose tolerance (IGT) ♦ Diabetes mellitus	Plasma	 <140 mg/dL 140–200 mg/dL >200 mg/dL	 <7.8 mmol/L 7.8–11.1 mmol/L >11.1 mmol/L
Glycated hemoglobin (HbA$_{1C}$)	Whole blood	4.0–6.0%	20–42 mmol/mol Hb
Lactate dehydrogenase (LDH)	Serum	115–221 U/L	2.0–3.8 µkat/L
Muramidase	Serum	5–20 µg/mL	
5-nucleotidase	Serum	0–11 U/L	0.02–0.19 µkat/L
Phosphatases ▪ Acid phosphatase ▪ Alkaline phosphatase	Serum	 0–5.5 U/L 33–96 U/L	 0.90 µkat/L 0.56–1.63 µkat/L
Prostate-specific antigen (PSA)	Serum	0–4.0 ng/mL	0–4.0 µg/L
Proteins—total ▪ Albumin ▪ Globulins ▪ Albumin/globulin ratio	Serum	6.7–8.6 g/dL 3.5–5.5 g/dL 2.0–3.5 g/dL 1.5–3:1	67–86 g/L 35–55 g/L 20–35 g/L
Rheumatoid factor	Serum	<15 IU/mL	<15 kIU/L
Troponins, cardiac (cTn) ▪ Troponin I (cTnI) ▪ Troponin T (cTnT)	 Serum Serum	 0–0.08 ng/mL 0–0.01 ng/mL	 0–0.8 µg/L 0–0.1 µg/L
Urea nitrogen (BUN)	Blood	7–20 mg/dL	2.5–7.1 mmol/L
Uric acid ▪ Males ▪ Females	Serum	 3.1–7.0 mg/dL 2.5–5.6 mg/dL	 0.18–0.41 µmol/L 0.15–0.33 µmol/L

Lipid Profile (Table 16D.3)

TABLE 16D.3: Lipid profile.

Component	Reference value	
	Conventional	SI units
Total serum cholesterol		
▪ Desirable for adults	<200 mg/dL	<5.17 mmol/L
▪ Borderline high	200–239 mg/dL	5.17–6.18 mmol/L
▪ High undesirable	>240 mg/dL	>6.21 mmol/L
LDL cholesterol		
▪ Desirable range	100–130 mg/dL	<3.34 mmol/L
▪ Borderline high	130–159 mg/dL	3.36–4.11 mmol/L
▪ High	160–189 mg/dL	4.11–4.20 mmol/L
▪ Very high	>190 mg/dL	>4.21 mmol/L
HDL cholesterol		
▪ Low	<40 mg/dL	<1.03 mmol/L
▪ High, protective range	>60 mg/dL	>1.55 mmol/L
Triglycerides	<160 mg/dL	<2.26 mmol/L

Urea and Electrolytes (Table 16D.4)

TABLE 16D.4: Urea and electrolytes.

Analyte	Reference value	
	Conventional	SI units
Sodium	136–146 mEq/L	136–146 mmol/L
Potassium	3.5–5.0 mEq/L	3.5–5.0 mmol/L
Chloride	95–107 mEq/L	95–107 mmol/L
Urea	20–40 mg/dL	3.3–6.6 mmol/L
Creatinine	0.6–1.2 mg/dL	53–106 µmol/L

Thyroid Function Tests (Table 16D.5)

TABLE 16D.5: Thyroid function tests.

Thyroid function tests	Specimen	Reference value	
		Conventional	SI units
Radioactive iodine uptake (RAIU) 24 hours		5–30%	
Thyroxine (T4) total	Serum	5.4–11.7 µg/dL	70–151 nmol/L
Triiodothyronine (T3) total	Serum	77–135 ng/dL	1.2–2.1 nmol/L
Thyroid stimulating hormone (TSH)	Serum	0.4–4.25 µU/mL	0.4–4.25 mU/L

Urine (Table 16D.6)

TABLE 16D.6: Normal urine values.

Component	Reference value
Volume—24 hours	600–1800 mL (variable)
pH	5.0–9.0
Specific gravity, quantitative (random)	1.002–1.028 (average 1.018)
Protein—24 hours urine	<150 mg/day
Protein, qualitative (random)	Negative
Glucose, quantitative—24 hours urine	50–300 mg/day
Glucose, qualitative (random)	Negative
Urobilinogen—24 hours urine	1.0–3.5 mg/day
Microalbuminuria (24 hours)	0–30 mg/24 hours (0–0.03 g/day) (0–30 µg/mg creatinine) (0–0.03 g/g creatinine)

Cerebrospinal Fluid (Table 16D.7)

TABLE 16D.7: Normal values of cerebrospinal fluid.

Component	Reference value	
	Conventional	SI units
CSF volume	120–150 mL	
Appearance	Clear and colorless	
CSF pressure	60–150 mm water	
pH	7.31–7.34	
Total proteins	20–40 mg/dL	0.14–0.45 g/L
Glucose	40–80 mg/dL	2.3–4.5 mmol/L
Chlorides	720–750 mg/dL	
Cells **Polymorphs** **Lymphocytes**	Usually absent 0–5/µL	

E. SHORT LIST OF ROUTINELY USED FORMULAS IN MEDICINE (TABLE 16E.1)

TABLE 16E.1: Short list of routinely used formulas in medicine.

Electrolyte disorders	
Plasma osmolality	2 Na$^+$ (mEq/L) + Serum glucose (mg/dL)/18 + BUN (mg/dL)/2.8
Corrected sodium	Increase Na$^+$ by 1.6 mEq/L for each 100 mg% (when serum glucose >100 mg%)
Total body sodium deficit	(Desired sodium − measured sodium) × Body weight × [0.6 (men) or 0.5 (women)]
Potassium deficit	1 mmol/L decrease → approximately 200–400 mmol loss of total body K$^+$
Urine-plasma electrolyte ratio (in chronic hyponatremia)	Urinary (sodium + potassium)/plasma sodium - >1 (fluid restriction up to less than 500 mL/day) - =1 (500–700 mL/day) - <1 (fluid restriction up to 1 L)
Water deficit (in hypernatremia)	Water deficit = (plasma sodium − 140) × TBW/140
Transtubular potassium gradient (TTKG) in hypokalemia	Urinary potassium × plasma osmolality/serum potassium × urinary osmolality >4 indicates renal loss of potassium
Corrected calcium	0.8 × (4 − serum albumin) + serum calcium
Acid-base disorders	
Anion gap (serum)	(Sodium + potassium) − (bicarbonate + chloride) - 8–16 mEq/L (old methods) - 5–11 mEq/L (new techniques)
Urine anion gap	Urine sodium + potassium − chloride - −25 to −50 (normal range)
Delta ratio	(Serum anion gap − 12)/(24 − serum bicarbonate) - <0.4 hyperchloremic normal anion gap acidosis - <1 high AG and normal AG acidosis - >2 high AG acidosis and a concurrent metabolic alkalosis
Respiratory acidosis	Acute: 10 increase in pCO$_2$ → 1 increase in bicarbonate Chronic: 10 increase in pCO$_2$ → 4 increase in bicarbonate
Respiratory alkalosis	Acute: 10 decrease in pCO$_2$ → 2 decrease in bicarbonate Chronic: 10 decrease in pCO$_2$ → 5 decrease in bicarbonate
Metabolic acidosis	pCO$_2$ = 1.5 (bicarbonate) + 8 ± 2
Metabolic alkalosis	10 increase in bicarbonate → pCO$_2$ increases by 6
Nephrology	
Renal failure index	Urine Na/(Urine Cr/PCr)
Cockcroft-Gault GFR	(140 − Age) × (Body weight in kg) × (0.85 if female)/(72 × Cr)
Fractional excretion of sodium (FENa)	(Serum Cr × Urine Na)/(Serum Na × Urine Cr)%
Hematology	
Corrected reticulocyte count	Reticulocyte % × (Hb/15)
Reticulocyte production index	= Corrected reticulocyte count/maturation time - At a hemoglobin of 15, the maturation time = 1 day - At a hemoglobin of 12, the maturation time = 1.5 days - At a hemoglobin of 8, the maturation time = 2 days - At a hemoglobin of 5, the maturation time = 2.5 days
Mentzer index	(MCV, in fL) divided by (RBC, in millions per μL) - Less than 13, thalassemia is said to be more likely
Parenteral iron in iron deficiency anemia	[2.3 × body weight (kg) × Hb deficit (g/dL)] + 1,000 mg (to replenish stores)
Respiratory system	
A-a gradient	PAO$_2$ − PaO$_2$ (PAO$_2$ = (FiO$_2$ × 713) − PaCO$_2$/0.8; PaO$_2$ is obtained from the ABG)
Cardiology	
Corrected QT	QT/√RR (Bazzett's formula)
MAP	Systolic BP + (2 × diastolic BP)/3
Miscellaneous	
BMI	W/H^2 (W = weight in kg and H = Height in meters)

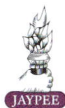
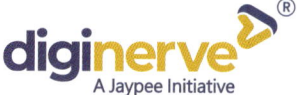

DigiNEET

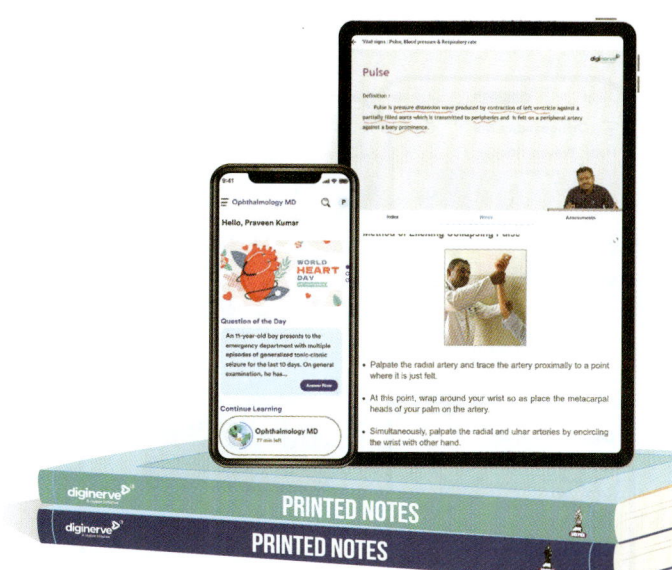

Simplify your undergraduate studies and NEET PG preparation with this comprehensive program covering all 19 subjects. Crafted by India's top faculty, it includes video lectures, printed notes, OSCEs, a QBank, test series, and the innovative Dr. Wise AI Chatbot.

Course Features

1400+ hrs Video Lectures

1500+ Topics in Notes

15000+ Questions in QBank

1800+ GEMS

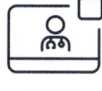
450+ OSCEs

Test Series

Dr. Wise AI Chatbot

Drug Chart

Regular Webinars by Esteemed Faculty

Access Anytime, Anywhere

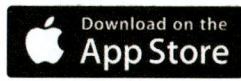
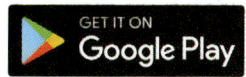

📞 +91-8800-418-418   ✉ marketing@diginerve.com

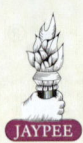 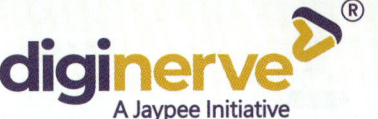

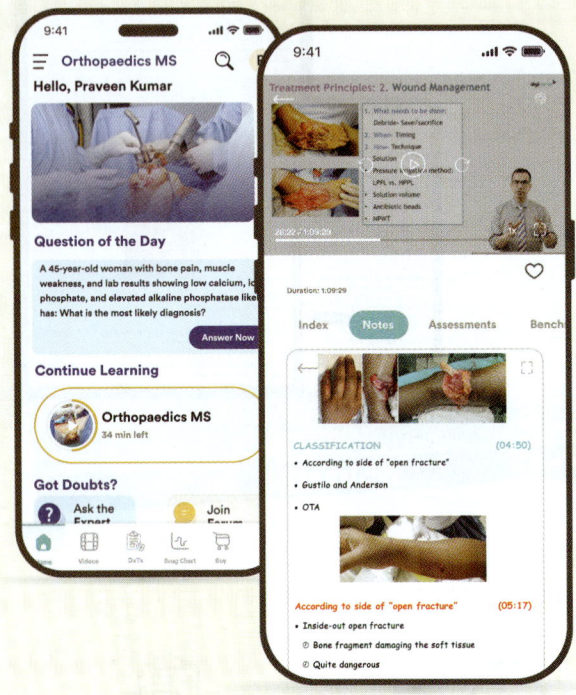

Premium Medical Content, Anytime, Anywhere

Trusted by 150K+ Users

20+ Courses | **3600+** Hrs of Video Content | **790+** Mentors

Available on

A host of features for **UnderGrads, PostGrads** and **Professionals**

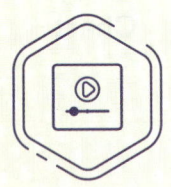 Video Lectures

 Notes

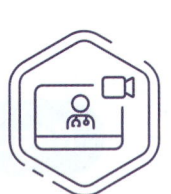 OSCEs

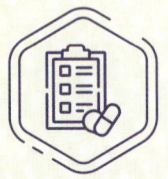 Drug Chart

 Question Bank

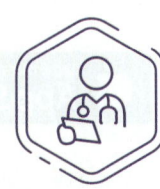 Dr. Wise AI Chatbot

+91-8800-418-418   marketing@diginerve.com

Index

Page numbers followed by *b* refer to box, *f* refer to figure, *fc* refer to flowchart, and *t* refer to table.

A

A wave 23
Abacavir 488
Abdomen
    areas of 159*f*
    four quadrants of 158*f*
    free fluid in 170
    lower 148
    pain in 146
    percussion of 161
    quadrants of 158
    shape of 157*f*
Abdominal angina 104
Abdominal aorta 160, 160*f*
    palpation of 15
Abdominal distension 137
Abdominal irradiation 143
Abdominal movement 17
Abdominal muscles 255, 261*f*
Abdominal obesity 52
Abdominal pain 137
    causes of 148, 149
Abdominal reflex, demonstration of 272*f*
Abdominal swelling 142
Abdominojugular reflux 25, 25*f*, 94
Abducens nerve 184, 184
    palsy 227
Abductor digiti minimi muscle 261*f*
Abductor lurch 296
Abductor pollicis
    brevis 251, 255, 259*f*
    longus 255
Abductor sign 277
Absent pulsus paradoxus 11
Abulia 513
Acanthosis nigricans 456*f*
Acebutolol 476
Acetaminophen 495
Achilles tendon 186
    for swelling, examination of 324
Acid-base disorders 535
Acoustic characteristics 508
Acquired heart disease 97
Acromegalic facies 361*f*, 459*f*
Acromegaly, clinical features of 361*f*
Actinomycosis 163
Acute coronary syndrome 103, 507
Acute kidney injury 178, 511
Acute liver failure 510
Acute respiratory distress syndrome 518
Acyanotic heart disease, congenital 97
Addison's disease 6, 20, 457*f*
Adductor femoris 261*f*
Adductor pollicis 255
Adenine 47
    nucleotides 36

Adenoma sebaceum 197*f*, 456*f*
Adenosine 468, 497
    diphosphate receptor antagonists 470
    reuptake inhibitors 470
Adie's tonic pupil 223
Adjunct chronotropic agent 480
Adrenal insufficiency 149
Adrenaline 474, 479
Adrenergic agents, centrally acting 477
Adrenoreceptor agonists 474
Adult onset Still's disease 40, 332
Advanced diabetic eye disease 214
Aegophony 89
Afferent limb 231
Afferent pupillary defect 223
Ageusia 235
Agitation 354
Agnosia 206, 513
    types of 206
Agranulocytosis 512
Agraphesthesia 516
Agraphia 203, 514
Air
    minimum amount of 433
    sinuses, prominent 435*f*
    under diaphragm 435
Airflow obstruction 64
Airway
    disease 429
    obstruction 18
    partial obstruction of 68
    responsiveness, reduces 475
Akathisia 302, 515
Akinetic mutism 513
Alar chest 74
Albumin gradient, high 171
Albuminuria
    moderately increased 511
    severely increased 511
Alcohol 502
    abuse screening tool 353
    amount of 502*t*
    complications of 502
    type 502
    units of 501
    use 501
        disorder 353
    withdrawal, symptoms of 353
Alcoholic hepatitis 152
Alcoholic liver disease 151
    stigmata of 346
Alcoholism, sign of 154, 156
Alderman's gait 298
Alexia 203, 514
    with agraphia 205
    without agraphia 205
Aliskiren 476

Alkaline phosphatase 34
Allergens 182
Allodynia 283, 516
Alloesthesia 516
Allopurinol 40
Alopecia 315*f*, 459*f*
    areata 463*f*
Alpha fetoprotein 532
Alpha motor neuron 265
Alveolocapillary junction 64
Alzheimer's disease 299, 340
Ambu bag 442
Amikacin 487
Amiloride 477
Aminoacidopathy 294
Aminoglycoside antibiotics 487, 487*b*
Aminophylline 475
Aminosalicylate agents 492
Aminotransferases 432
Amiodarone 34, 468, 498
Amlodipine 476
Amnesia 202, 513
    retrograde 202
Amnestic disorder 352
Amoss's sign 305, 305*f*
Amoxicillin 485
Amphetamine 20
Amphotericin B 494
Ampicillin 485
Amyloidosis 20, 40
Amyotrophic lateral sclerosis 251, 303
Anal reflex 186, 272
Anal sphincter tone 192
Analgesia 283, 516
Analgesics 472
Anasarca 355
Anemia 6, 32, 154, 355, 505, 506
    etiology of 32
Anesthesia 283, 516
Angina 103
    decubitus 103
    functional classification of 104
    pectoris, grading of 522
    sine dolore 104
    types of 103
Angiotensin receptor
    antagonists 477
    blockers 476
Angiotensin-converting enzyme 62, 476, 477
Angulation 417
Anisosphygmia 9
Ankle 186, 267
    brachial index 14, 21, 21*f*, 22*f*
    clonus 271
    joint, examination of 324, 324*f*
    reflex, demonstration of 269*f*, 270*f*
Ankylosing spondylitis 6, 331

Anomia 203
Anorexia 341
Anosmia 209
Anosognosia 206, 208, 517
Antalgic gait 298
Anterograde amnesia 202
Anthropometry 49
Antibiotics 484
Anticitrullinated protein antibodies 328
Anticoagulant therapy 490b, 490t
    classification of 490t
Anticoagulation 490
Anticonvulsants 155
Anticyclic citrullinated peptide antibodies 330
Antidepressants 471
    types of 471t
Antidiabetic agents, profile of 482f
Antidote, specific 495
Antiencephalopathy 493
Antihistamines 467
Antihypertensive agents 478
Antihypertensive therapy, individualizing 478
Anti-inflammatory potency 481t
Anti-insulin antibodies 482
Antinuclear antibodies 329, 330
Antiparkinson 470
Antiplatelets 468, 470
Antipsychotic drugs
    classification of 471
    side effects of 353
Antiretroviral therapy 488, 488f, 488t
    site of action of 488f
Antirheumatic drugs, disease-modifying 330, 491
Antisecretory agents 495
Antitrypsin deficiency, alpha-1 155
Antiviral oseltamivir 488
Anuria 511
Anxiety 20, 105, 354
    disorder, generalized 352
Anxiety-predominant neurotic disorders, types of 352
Aorta 101
    coarctation of 6
Aortic area 95, 115, 116, 118
    auscultation of 130, 130f
Aortic causes 115
Aortic dissection 103
Aortic pulsations 115
Aortic regurgitation 6, 113, 115, 116, 119-122, 126-128, 132, 136
    murmur of 128
    severe 14f, 423
Aortic root dilatation 53f
Aortic stenosis 6, 9, 110, 113, 115, 116, 119, 121, 122, 126-128, 136
Aortic valve closure 124
Apallesthesia 283
Apex
    abnormalities of 113
    beat 507
    contour of 423
    pulse deficit 9, 9f
    systolic retraction of 122
Aphasia 202-204, 204f, 205fc, 514
Aphemia 203
Aphonia 203, 514
Aphthous ulcer 156

Apical area, percussion of 85f
Apical impulse 75, 112
    causing 114
    double 113
    shift, implication of 78
Apical nodes 43
Apixaban 491
Aplastic anemia 32
Apparent cardiomegaly 414
Apparent enophthalmos 225
Appendicitis 148
Appetite 183
Apprehension test, demonstration of 319f
Apraxia 206, 517
    constructional 206, 517
    dressing 206
    gait 206, 293, 296
    gaze 206
    ideational 206
    ideomotor 206
    types of 206
Arcuate fasciculus 204
Argyll Robertson pupil 222, 223, 223f
Arm
    span 50
    swing 298
Arnold's nerve 62
Arrhythmias with regular rhythm 8
Arterial blood pressure 133f, 307
Arterial pulse
    assessment of 8
    graphic recordings of 10
    normal 9
    tracing 10f
Arterial spiders 152
Arteriovenous fistula 113, 126, 358f
Artesunate 464
Arthranesthesia 283
Arthritis 313
    causes of 314
Articulated labials 205
Artificial sweetener 144
Ascites 6, 151, 152f, 170
    assessment for 174
    congestive hepatomegaly with 122
    etiology of 171
    grading systems of 171
    increasing 175f
    praecox 171
    signs of 175f
    without shifting dullness, causes of 174
    without significant edema, causes of 171
Ascorbic acid 47
Aseptic fever 28
Aspartate aminotransferase 34
Aspergilloma 428
Aspergillosis 494
Aspirin 469
    indications for low-dose 469b
Astasia-abasia 298
Asterixis 155, 177, 178, 515, 526
    bilateral 155
    causes of 155
    in hands 155, 155f
    unilateral 155
Asterognosis 516
Asthma 183, 509
    drugs for 474

Asynergia 287
Ataxia 6, 188, 287, 293, 294, 517
    telangiectasia 197
    treatable causes of 294
    types of 293
Ataxic gait 296, 296f
Ataxic speech 205
Atazanavir 489
Atelectasis, differential diagnosis of 425
Atenolol 476
Athetosis 301, 515
Atorvastatin 484
Atrial depolarization 364
Atrial fibrillation 9, 365
Atrial flutter 366
Atrial premature beat 367
Atrial repolarization 364
Atrial septal defect 6, 25, 97, 110, 112, 115, 116, 120, 122, 136, 368, 432f
Atrial shadow, double 423
Atrial tachycardia, multifocal 366
Atrophy 519
Atropine 479, 480, 497
    infusion 480
Auditory agnosia 206
Auditory canal, external 233
Auditory disturbances 354
Auscultatory percussion 83, 174
    Guarino's method of 84, 84f
Ausculto-percussion method 164, 164f
Autoimmune 156
Autonomic dysfunction 192, 308, 308t
Autonomic failure
    preganglionic 308
    primary 20
Autonomic nervous system 187, 306
Autonomic system, drugs acting on 479
Autonomous bladder 192
Autosomal dominant recessive disorders 499, 499t
Autotopagnosia 206
Avibactam 485
Axilla 83, 119
Axillary 57
    area, percussion of 83f
    examination 73
    lymphadenopathy 454f
    temperature 26
Azathioprine 491, 493
Azilsartan 476
Azithromycin 486

B

Babinski
    neurological reflex hammer 266
    reflex 238
    sign 272
Backache 193
Bacterial endocarditis, subacute 6
Bacterial infection 144
Bacteriuria, asymptomatic 512
Balaclava helmet 232f
Balance test 341
Balanoposthitis 356f
Bald tongue 32f
Balint syndrome 293
Ballotability 170

Ballotable 169
Bambuterol 474
Baricitinib 493
Barognosis 283
Baroreflex failure 20
Barré's sign 277
Basal ganglia, right 436f
Bat wing appearance 424
Bazett's formula 371
B-complex 46
Beaus' lines 38
Becker's muscular dystrophy 250
Becks depression inventory 353
Becks hopelessness scale 353
Bedford sign 423
Bedside tests 299
Behavior 201
Bell's phenomenon 235, 236, 238, 238f
Bell's tympany 84
Benazepril 476
Bendopnea 66, 507
Benzathine penicillin 485
Benzodiazepines 354, 495
Bergara-Wartenberg sign 236
Bernheim effect 24
Berry's node 43
Best motor response 201, 525
Best verbal response 201, 525
Beta-blockers 40, 469, 495
    contraindications of 469, 469t
Beta-lactam 484
    antibiotics 485t
        adverse effects of 484b
        classification of 485f
Betaxolol 476
Biceps 254, 267
    examining tone of 252f
    reflex 267f, 268f
        inversion of 277
        supine position 267f
Bifidobacterium infantis 493
Biguanides 483
Bile
    acid sequestrant 483
    duct, common 34
Biliary cirrhosis, primary 155
Bilirubin, unconjugated 34
Bimanual palpation 132, 139, 170
Binet-Kamat test 353
Bing's sign 274f
Binocular diplopia 218
Binocular movements 184
Binswanger's disease 293
Biopsy proven lupus nephritis 330
Biot breathing 17
Biotin 47
Bird index 53
Birmingham paradox 12
Bisoprolol 476
Bite block 441
Bizarre behavior 350
Bladder
    control, loss of awareness of 182
    dysfunction 182, 192
    habits 183
    sensation 192
    size of 192
Blastomycosis 494

Bleeding disorders 6
Blepharospasm 302
Blood 328
    clinical chemistry of 532, 532t
    culture 528
    filled 424
    investigations 343
Blood pressure 18, 70, 94, 138, 151, 183, 195, 310, 336, 504
    category 18
    cuff, placement of 19f
    diastolic 18
    examination 18
    measurement 19, 19f, 504t
    systolic 18, 19
Blood-tinged foamy sputum 63
Body hair, diminished 153
Body mass index 7, 52, 56, 94, 138, 183, 310, 336, 523t
Body myositis, inclusion 299
Body temperature 26, 27
    disorders of increased 29
Bone 481
    infections of 192
    marrow
        aspiration needle 446
        biopsy needle 446
Bony cage 435
Bony structures 418, 418f
Bouchard's nodes 322f
Boutonniere deformity 322f, 459f
Bow legs 325f
Bowel habit 183
    altered 137
Bowel obstruction 149
Bowel sounds 160
    auscultation of 160f
Bowlus-Currier test 286
Bowstring sign 459f
Brachial plexus 251
Brachial pulse, palpation of 14, 15f
Brachioradialis 254, 267
Bradycardia 8, 34, 364, 507
    fever of 27
Bradykinin 36
Brain
    areas in 201
    lesions, bilateral structural 155
    stimulation, direct 354
Brainstem 227, 242
    disorders 17
    nuclei 144
Branham sign 14
Brawny edema 39
Breath sound 57, 90
    bronchovesicular 87
    diminished intensity of 88
    intensity, grading of 87
    tracheal 87
    vesicular 87
Breathing
    abnormal patterns of 17
    advice 87
    increased work of 64
    patterns, type of 18f
    rapid deep 17
    types of normal 87

Breathlessness 67
    acute severe 66b
    classification of 67t
    grading of 66t, 67t
Broadbent's sign 122
Broca's area 204
Broken neck sign 246
Bronchial asthma 6, 65, 355
Bronchial breathing 87
Bronchial carcinoma 6
Bronchial disease 63
Bronchiectasis 6, 509
Bronchitis, chronic 6, 509
Bronchophony 58, 89
Bronchorrhea 63
Brudzinski's leg sign 304, 305f
Brudzinski's neck sign 304, 305f
Bruits 160
Brun's ataxia 206, 293
Buccal mucosa 156
Buccinator, examination of 234f
Buck neurological reflex hammer 266
Bucket handle movement 79f
Budd-Chiari syndrome 156, 163
Bulbar palsy 247
Bulbocavernosus reflex 272, 272f
Bulge sign 323, 324f
Bulging flanks 171
Bulging intercostal spaces 90
Bulla 519
Bumetanide 477
Bundle branch blocks 372
Bursae 311

C

Cachexia 53
Café-au-lait macules 196, 196f, 456f
Calcium
    channel antagonists 469, 476
    channel blockers 469, 496
    gluconate 497
Calf muscle, pseudohypertrophy of 251f
Calorie test 239, 240f
Campbell sign 78
Cancer 335, 503
Candesartan 476
Cannonball metastasis 431f
Capillary hypertension 424
Captopril 40, 476
Carbamate 496
Carbamazepine 40
Carbapenems 486, 486t
Carbimazole 481
Carbone monoxide 496
Carbonic anhydrase inhibitors 474
Cardiac apex, types of 113f
Cardiac arrhythmias 104, 105
Cardiac axis 367
Cardiac causes 9, 23, 37, 104, 105, 115
Cardiac cirrhosis 155
Cardiac condition, associated 124, 131
Cardiac cycle 98, 100, 119, 119f
    duration 119
    pressure changes during 101t
Cardiac defects 110
Cardiac disease 67, 116f, 480
Cardiac dysrhythmias 439

Index

Cardiac failure, congestive 6, 9, 39f
Cardiac impulse, location of 113f
Cardiac silhouette 423
Cardiac syndrome X 103
Cardiac tamponade 25, 103
Cardinal symptoms 61, 102, 142, 189
Cardiomegaly 423
Cardiomyopathy, dilated 6, 423, 508
Cardiopulmonary disease 105, 143
Cardiopulmonary resuscitation 479
Cardiopulmonary symptoms 147
Cardiovascular causes 112, 113
Cardiovascular disease 63, 135, 503
Cardiovascular system 3, 6, 11, 58, 67, 93, 187, 327, 346
    palpation of 111
Carina, splaying of 423, 432f
Carotid artery 119
Carotid pulse 23
    palpation of 14, 15f
Carotid sinus syndrome 20
Carvedilol 476
Castell's method 166
Castell's sign 168f
Castleman's disease 40
Cat scratch disease 46
Catacrotic pulse 10
Catatonia 349
Catecholamines 474
Catechol-O-methyl-transferase inhibitors 471
Catheter 27
    tube 443
Caudal vermis syndrome 294
Caudate lobe 164, 164f
Causalgia 283
Caustic ingestion 146
Cavernous sinus 227
    syndrome 233
    thrombosis 248
Cavitary lesions, differential diagnosis of 426
Cavity 91
    lesions, diagnosis of 426fc
Cefazolin 485
Cefepime 485
Cefotaxime 485
Cefotetan 485
Ceftaroline 485
Ceftazidime 485
Ceftolozane 485
Ceftriaxone 485
Cefuroxime 485
Celiac disease 149, 293
Central facial nerve palsy 238
Central nervous system 3, 189, 228, 346
Central nodes 43
Central nonpleuritic chest pain 66
Central nystagmus 228
Cephalexin 485
Cephalosporins 485
Cerebellar ataxia 293, 294, 296
    causes of 293
Cerebellar disease 253
Cerebellar disorders, signs of 287
Cerebellar dysarthria 288
Cerebellar examination 191
Cerebellar gait 296f
Cerebellar history 182
Cerebellar lesions, localization of 294

Cerebellar signs 6, 186, 294
Cerebellar syndromes 294
Cerebellar system 96
Cerebellopontine angle 236
Cerebellum 287, 294f
    lesions of 296
Cerebral artery, middle 188
Cerebral causes 190
Cerebral disease, evidence of 353
Cerebral dysfunction, evidence of 353
Cerebral hemispheres 207t
    lobes of 207f
Cerebrospinal fluid 447, 534, 534t
Cerebrovascular accident 188
Cerebrovascular disease 6
Cervical
    lymph nodes 40, 41
    lymphadenopathy 460f
    pleura 70
    spine 311
    venous hum 31, 31f
Cetrizine 467
Chaddock's method 273
Chaddock's sign 274f
CHARGE syndrome 110
Cheek sign 304
Cheese reaction 20
Chemoreceptors 64
Chest
    anterior 83
    barrel-shaped 74, 74f
    circumference 57
    deformities of 74, 112
    diameters, measurements of 80
    examination of 73
    expansion 57, 90
        examination of 81f
    flat 74
    flip-flopping in 105
    lower
        anterior 79
        posterior 79
    movements, causes of decreased 80
    pain 55, 68, 93, 102
        causes of 102, 102f, 103, 103t
        differential diagnosis of 102, 102t
    percussion of anterior 83f
    posterior of 83
    radiograph, reading into 414
    rapid fluttering in 105
    respiratory movements 79f, 80f
    upper
        anterior 78
        posterior 79
    wall abnormality 429
    wall with breast 44
    X-ray 62b, 414
Chilaiditi syndrome 433f
Childhood autism rating scale 353
Child-Turcotte-Pugh score 525
Chipmunk facies 33f
Chloroquine 34, 211, 464
Chlorpheniramine 466
Chlorpromazine 34
Chlorthalidone 476
Cholecalciferol 46
Chorea 253, 277, 301, 515
Choreiform gait 298

Chromium 47
Chronic inflammatory demyelinating
    polyneuropathy 6
    polyradiculoneuropathy 293
Chronic kidney disease 6, 355, 357, 357f, 511
Chronic liver disease, peripheral signs of 151
Chronic obstructive
    airway disease 94, 137, 183
    pulmonary disease 62, 65, 113, 355, 368, 508, 524
Chylous 171
Cingulotomy 354
Circumduction gait 295f
Cirrhosis 460f
    cause of 152f
    complications of 177, 177t
    etiology of 155
    of liver 141, 152f, 511
        signs of 151
    portosystemic anastomosis in 179f
    signs pointing etiology of 155
Cisplatin 293
Clarithromycin 486
Clasp knife phenomenon 253
Classical vasovagal syncope 105
Clavicles 414
Claw hand 6, 455f
Clear blood and clots 439
Clevidipine 479
Clinical disease activity index 333f
Clock drawing test 340
Clonidine 477
    patch 477
    withdrawal 20
Clonus 271
Clostridium difficile 4
Coanda effect 9, 135
Coarse leathery crepitations 89
Coat hanger headache 306
Cocaine 20
    bugs 348
Coccidioidomycosis 494
Cochlear component 239, 242
    testing 240
Cognition assessment tool 202
Cognitive behavior therapy 354
Cognitive functions 348
Cogwheel
    examining for 253f
    rigidity 253, 515
Coin test 90, 90f
Collagen vascular diseases 28
Collapsing pulse 13f
    causes of 13,
Collapsing weakness 277
Collet-Sicard syndrome 248
Colloidal solutions 497
Colloids 496
Colonic bleeding 143
Color vision 211
    Ishihara chart for 212f
    method of examining 212f
Colorectal cancer 149
Columbia suicide severity scale 353
Coma 347, 513
    pupillary abnormalities in 224f
Common autonomic symptoms 306
Complex motor activities 206

Comprehensive geriatric assessment 6, 335, 337, 338, 338f
Compulsive disorder 352
Concomitant drug therapy 480
Conjugated bilirubin 34
Conjunctival reflex 231, 232f
Conjunctival rim pallor 31, 31f
Connective tissue
   disease 308
   disorders 156
Consciousness 200
   abnormalities of 347
   altered state of 181, 189
   level of 346
Consensual reflex 231, 232
Constipation 145, 149, 510
   etiology of 145
Constrictive pericarditis 9, 11, 25, 25f, 26, 122
Convergence retraction nystagmus 228
Copper 47
   wiring 215f
Cor bovinum 423
Cor pulmonale 71, 509
Cord compression 6
Core body temperature 26
Corneal anesthesia, bilateral 233
Corneal reflex 231, 232f, 235, 238
Cornelia de Lange's syndrome 110
Cornell response 273
Coronary artery
   affected 374
   disease 116, 122
Coronary insufficiency 20
Corrigan's pulse 13
Cortical sensation 186, 278, 281
Corticosteroids, inhaled 475
Costophrenic angles 435
Costovertebral angle 170f
   tenderness 170
Cotrimoxazole 40
Cotton
   wisp of 278
   wool spots 215f
Cough 55, 61, 62, 66, 182, 508
   acute 62
   barking 62
   based on duration of 62
   bovine 62
   chronic 62, 62b
   classification of 62t
   dry 62
   gander 62
   hacking 62
   otogenic 62
   paroxysmal 62
   production, mechanism of 61
   productive 62
   reflex 61fc
   spluttering 62
   subacute 62
   types of 62t
Courvoisier's law 169
Cover-uncover test 221
COVID-19 drugs 493
Coxalgic gait 298, 298f
Cracked pot resonance 84
Cranial nerve 96, 184, 209, 210, 215, 228, 239, 243-246, 248
   disorders of 244

   dysfunction 181, 189
   examination of 6
   palsy 222f
      multiple 248
   X, disorders of 244
C-reactive protein 328, 532
Crescent sign of Monad 428, 428f
Creutzfeldt-Jakob disease 340
Crohn's disease 145, 503
Cross fluctuation sign 323, 324f
Cruveilhier-Baumgarten venous hum 129
Cryptococcosis 494
Crystalloids 496, 496t
Cuff 441
Currant-Jelly and Sticky sputum 63
Cushing's habitus 360f
Cushing's syndrome 6, 49, 359, 360f, 458f
Cyanide 496
Cyanosis 34, 70, 94, 151, 454f, 506
   admixture 35
   atypical presentation of 35
   cardiac 35
   central 34, 35, 35f, 154
   cyclical 35
   distributive 35
   hypoxic 35
   intermittent 35
   iron
      deplete 35
      replete 35
   mixed 34
   peripheral 34, 35
   pigment 34
   pulmonary 35
   replacement 34, 35
   reverse differential 35
   tardive 34, 35
   theories of 35
   true 34
Cystic disease 425
Cystic fibrosis 72
Cystitis 148
Cytoprotective agents 495

D

D'espine sign 46
Dahl's sign 76
Daily living, activities of 339
Damoiseau's curve 86
Dangling jaw 230
Darunavir 489
Deep flipped T waves 412
Deep tendon reflex 186, 266, 272
   reinforcement maneuvers for 266
Delirium 200, 347, 352, 513
   confusion assessment method for 353
Delphian node 43
Delta wave 369
Delusion 206, 347, 350
   types of 206, 347
Delusional disorder 351
Dementia 335, 339, 340, 352, 353, 513
   causes of 340, 340b
Deoxyribonucleic acid, double-stranded 330
Depression 335, 353
Dermatological disorders 156
Detemir 482

Detrusor
   areflexia 192
   hyperreflexia 192
   sphincteric dyssynergia 192
Dexamethasone 481, 494
Dextrose 497
Diabetes mellitus 6, 183, 355
Diabetic maculopathy 214
Diabetic neuropathies 278
Diabetic papillopathy 214
Diabetic retinopathy
   nonproliferative 214, 356f
   stages of 214
Diaphragm 127, 420, 420f, 435
   flattening of 420f
   normal height of 420f
Diaphragmatic movements 80, 80f
Diarrhea 144, 145, 495, 509
   causes of 67t, 144t, 145t
   chronic 144
   fatty 145
   large-volume 144
   overflow 145
   treatment of 493
   types of 144
Diazoxide 478
Diffuse disease 424
Digeorge syndrome 110
Digestive disorder 144
Digital index 38
Digitalis 211
Digoxin 467, 496
Dihydroorotate dehydrogenase 492
Diltiazem 476, 498
Dipeptidyl peptidase-4 inhibitors 483
Diplegia 189
Diplopia 218, 220, 221
   assessment of 218
   constant 219
   examination of 220
Direct-acting vasodilators 477
Disease, nature of 188
Dissociated rhythm, nystagmus of 228
Distal wasting 251
Distractibility 351
Diuretics 473, 473t, 476
Diverticulitis 148
Diverticulosis 149
Dobutamine 479
Doll's eye oculocephalic reflex 242
Dome pulse 10
Dopamine 479, 497
   decarboxylase inhibitors, peripheral 471
   facilitator 471
   receptor agonists 471
Dorello's canal 227
Doripenem 485
Dorsalis pedis artery 15
   palpation of 15, 16f
Double quotidian fever 27
Double simultaneous stimulation 282
Down beat nystagmus 228
Down syndrome 110, 111, 111f, 253
Downstroke 87
Doxazosin 477
Doxycycline 487
D-penicillamine 491
Drainage lumen 443

Drooping of shoulder, examination of 75
Dropped head syndrome 246
Drowsy 347
Drug
    and medical emergencies 464
    antianginal 468*t*
    antiarrhythmic 467, 467*t*
    anticholinergic 470, 475, 495
    antidiabetic 481
    antiepileptic 466, 466*t*
    antihypertensive 476*t*
    antipsychotic 471, 472, 472*f*
    antithyroid 480
    centrally acting 477
    fever 28
    inhalant 450
    interaction potentials 484*b*
    malignancy 156
Dry powder inhalers 451
Duchene's muscular dystrophy 250
Duke's criteria, modified 527, 527*t*, 528
Dullness, paravertebral triangle of 86
Duodenal causes 142
Duodenal ulcer 494
Dupuytren's contracture 154, 154*f*, 460*f*
    causes of 154
Dysarthria 203, 205, 287, 294, 514
    types of 205
Dysdiadochokinesia 287, 288, 291, 291*f*
Dyselectrolytemia 155
Dysesthesias 516
Dysgraphia 514
Dyslogia 514
Dysmetria 287, 288
Dyspepsia 145, 509
    causes of 145*t*
Dysphagia 146, 509
Dysphonia 514
Dyspnea 6, 55, 64, 66, 67, 67*t*, 105, 507, 523*t*
Dystonia 302, 515

E

Ear, nodular lesions on 457*f*
Eating, disorders of 350
Ebstein's anomaly 423, 432*f*
Echolalia 202, 514
Ectopic atrial tachycardia 366
Edema 6, 38, 39, 70
    drug-induced 39
    examination of 38
    variability of 106
Efferent limb 231
Effusion, moderate 90
Egophony 58, 90
Ehlers Danlos syndrome 110
Ehra score 525
Eisenmenger's syndrome 6
Ekbom's syndrome 302
Elbow 186
    examination of 319
    flex-ex sign 277
    palpation of 319*f*
Electrocardiogram 373, 376
    12-lead 378, 379, 380, 381, 382, 383, 384, 385, 386, 387, 388, 389, 390, 391, 392, 393, 394, 395, 396, 397, 398, 399, 400, 401, 402, 403, 404, 405, 406, 407, 408, 409, 410, 411

    basic interpretation of 412
    grid 363*f*
    leads 363
    waveforms 100, 362
Electrolyte 376, 533, 533*t*
    disorders 535
    disturbances 277
Elemental calcium 497
Elicitation 272, 273, 275
Eliciting collapsing pulse, method of 13
Eliciting pedal edema, method of 38*f*
Eliciting pulsus
    bisferiens, method of 13
    paradoxus, method of 11
Ellis-Van Creveld syndrome 49
Ellsberg phenomenon 181, 190
Emergencies, common drugs used in 497*t*
Emotional facial paresis 238
Emotional fibers checking 185
Emotional function, testing for 235
Emphysema 6, 91, 425, 429*f*, 509
Empyema 6
Enalapril 476
Enalaprilat 479
Encephalopathy 525
Endocardial cushion defect 110
Endocarditis
    definite infective 527
    signs of infective 97, 109, 109*f*
Endocrine 6, 49, 480, 481
    changes 153
Endocrinology 328
Endotracheal tube 441
Engorged neck veins 23*f*
Enophthalmos 184, 216
Enoxaparin 498
Enteric infections 143
Enterogenous 34
Eosinophilic granulomatosis with polyangiitis 72
Epigastric pulsations 115, 115*f*
    causes of 115
Epigastrium 119, 161*f*
Epilepsy 517
Epileptic seizure 517
Epinephrine 497
Episodic angina 103
Episodic memory 202
Epistaxis 72
Epitrochlear lymph nodes, palpation of 46*f*
Epitrochlear lymphadenopathy, systemic causes of 46
Eplerenone 477
Eprosartan 476
Epsilon wave 369
Equinus gait 298
Erb's
    maneuver 119, 130*f*
    neoaortic area 95, 119
    palsy 250
Erosion 519
Erotomanic delusions 206
Ertapenem 486
Erythema nodosum 316*f*, 455*f*, 463*f*
Erythrocyte sedimentation rate 328
Erythrocytosis 505
Erythropoietin 484
Esmolol 478

Esomeprazole 498
Esophageal cancer 142, 146
Esophageal candidiasis 461*f*
Esophageal causes 142
Esophageal dysphagia, causes of 146*t*
Esophageal ulcers 142
Esophageal varices 142
Ethacrynic acid 477
Ethambutol 211, 465
Europids 52
Excoriation 519
Exercise 250
    effect of 9
Exophthalmos 184, 216, 458*f*
Expiratory crepitations 89
Explicit memory 201, 349
Extensor carpi
    radialis longus 254, 257*f*
    ulnaris 254, 258*f*
Extensor digitorum 254, 258*f*
    brevis 263*f*
    longus 263*f*
Extensor hallucis longus 263*f*
Extensor pollicis brevis 255
Exteroceptive system, examination of 278
Extradural hematoma, acute left 436*f*
Extrahepatic portal hypertension 171
Extraocular movements 184, 217*f*
Extraocular muscles 216
Extrapyramidal disorders 244
Extrasystolic palpitations 105
Eye 481
    changes 316
    closed 288
    dryness of 316
    open 201, 288, 525
    signs 458*f*
    stimulus 231
    to eye contact 347
Eyeball
    at rest, position of 216
    non-nystagmus oscillations of 228
Eyelids 184, 215

F

Facial canal 236
Facial edema 39
Facial expressions 347
Facial hair, diminished 155*f*
Facial motor function 238
Facial muscles 238
Facial nerve 184, 233
    innervation by 237*f*
    lesion 232
    palsy 6, 236, 239
    pathway 236*f*
Facial numbness 232
Facial palsy 205
    peripheral 236
    syndromes 239
Facial weakness 238
Facilitatory paratonia 253
Facioscapulohumeral dystrophy 251*f*
Familial hypercholesterolemia 484
Familial mediterranean fever 40
Family, type of 345

Far vision 210
    Snellen's chart for 210f
Fascicular lesion 235
Fasciculations 246, 303
Fasciculus, medial longitudinal 227
Fat 142
Fatal growth 142
Fatigability 94, 191
Fatty
    lumps 482
    stools 144
Febrile neutropenia 512
Fecal incontinence 145, 510
Feces 142
Feet drop 6, 295
Feet pat test 292
Feet
    position of 288
    small muscles of 186
    tapping 292f
        test 264, 292
    touching 292
Femoral artery, palpation of common 15
Femoral pulse, site of examination of 15f
Fenoldopam 478
Fenoterol 474
Fentanyl 497
Ferritin 36
Festinant gait 297
Fetor hepaticus 155
Fetus 142
Fever 27, 55, 151, 195, 355, 506
    based on duration, types of 27
    clinical pattern of 28f
    continuous 27
    defervescence, nature of 28
    grading of 27
    named 29
    of unknown origin 27, 506
    patterns of 27
    relapsing 27
    remittent 27
    tertian 27
    type of 27
Fibrinolytic agents, use of 491b
Fibromyalgia 331, 331f
Fibrosis 91
Fibrothorax 6
Figure-of-4 test 326
Filariasis 40f, 455f
Finger
    flexion reflex, demonstration of 270f
    flexion test 267
    nose test, demonstration of 290f
    web spaces of 463f
Fingertip
    light touch of 278
    localizing apex with 112f
Finger-to-nose test 288, 290
Fissure 73f
Fitz-Hugh-Curtis syndrome 161
Flaccid 205
Flail chest 74
Flange 441
Flapping tremor 155
Flesche test 325, 325f
Flexor carpi
    radialis 254, 258f
    ulnaris 255, 258f
Flexor digiti minimi 255
Flexor digitorum
    longus 263f
    profundus 255, 260f
    sublimis 255, 260f
Flexor pollicis longus 252, 255
Floating nail sign 37
Floppy head syndrome 246
Fluconazole 494
Fluid
    amount of 174
    in lung, presence of 85
    thrill, demonstration of 174f
Fluid-attenuated inversion recovery 437
Fluvastatin 484
Focal brain lesions 155
Focal neurological deficit 350
Foleys catheter 443
Folic acid 47
Folinic acid 492
Foodborne illness 149
Forearm rolling test 264, 264f
Foreign bodies 435, 436
Formoterol 474
Fosinopril 476
Fosphenytoin 498
Foster-Kennedy syndrome 210
Fothergill's disease 232
Foul smelling sputum 63
Frailty syndrome 339
Framingham heart failure criteria 525
Framycetin 487
Frey syndrome 233
Friction fremitus 82
Friedreich's sign 25, 86
Frontal lobe ataxia 293
Frontalis 185
Frusemide 498
Full bladder 142
Fundic gas shadow 414
Fundus examination 212
Furosemide 477
Fusion inhibitors 489

G

Gaenslen maneuver 326
Gaenslen test, demonstration of 326f
Gaertner's method 25
Gag reflex 243, 247
    components of 243
    examination of 243f
    testing of 243
Gait 187, 288, 295
    abnormalities 182, 191, 295, 298
    ataxia 294
    cycle, normal 295, 295f
    initiation 298
    painful 298
    speed 299
    type of 296
Gallbladder 139
    examination of 169
Gallivardian phenomenon 130
Gamma glutamyl transpeptidase 532
Gamma motor neuron 265
Ganglionic disorders 308
Garland's triangle 86
Gastric causes 142
Gastric lavage tube 439
Gastric ulcer 494
Gastroenterology 151
Gastroesophageal reflux disease 62, 148
Gastrointestinal bleeding 142, 510
Gastrointestinal causes 37
Gastrointestinal disease 156
Gastrointestinal symptoms 94
Gastrointestinal system 3, 6, 58, 96, 137, 187, 327, 346
Gastrointestinal tract 132, 481
    perforation of 149
Gastrointestinal ulcers, Forrest grading of 529
Gaze palsies 226, 227
Gaze-evoked nystagmus 294
Geniculate ganglion 236
Geniculocalcarine tract 211
Genitourinary 306
    symptoms 147
    system 328
Gentamicin 487
Genu valgus 325f
Genu varus 325f
Gerhardt's sign 86
Geriatric giants 339
Geriatric problems 341
Ghent criteria, modified 54
Gibson's area 119
Gilles de la Tourette syndrome 302
Gingival hyperplasia 461f
Give-way weakness 277
Glabellar tap 275, 276f
Glargine 482
Glasgow coma scale 201, 525
Glomerulonephritis 6
Glossopharyngeal nerve 185, 243
Glucagon 498
Glucarpidase 492
Glucocorticoids 481
    doses of 481, 481t
Glulisine 482
Glutamic acid decarboxylase 293
Gluteus maximus 262f
Gluteus medius gait 296
Glycoprotein 470
Gordon's sign 273
Gordon's technique 274f
Gouty arthritis, acute 325f, 461f
Gradenigo's syndrome 233
Graduated Rydel-Seiffer tuning fork 280
Grandiose delusions 206
Granulomas 425
Graphesthesia 282, 282f
Grasp reflex 276, 277f
Graves' disease 6, 39
Gray matter 437
Great arteries, transposition of 121
Great toe, vibration over proximal 280f
Greater auricular nerve 198f
Grocco's triangle 86
Ground glass appearance 425
Guanfacine 477
Guillain-Barré syndrome 6, 182, 246, 308
Gum 156
Gum hypertrophy 156
Gunn phenomenon, reversed 233
Gustatory hallucination 348

Gynecomastia 153, 153f, 460f, 520
    causes of 153
    male 112
    palpation breast bud in 153f

H

Hackett's grading system 165, 165f
Hair, loss of 153
Halitosis 137
Hallucination 206, 207, 348, 350
Hallux valgus 459f
    deformity 325f
Hallux varus deformity 325f
Haloperidol 498
Hamartomas 425
Hamilton anxiety rating scale 353
Hamilton depression rating scale 353
Hamman's mediastinal crunch 90
Hammer toes 459f
Hamstrings 262f
Hand
    deformities of 321
    grip 9, 186
    hygiene 4
    muscle wasting, causes of 251
    push patella 324f
    small muscle wasting of 251f
    squeeze test of 320f
    ulnar deviation of 322f
Handedness 200, 346
Harvey's sign 175f
Head to toe signs 138
Headache 182, 354
Head-up tilt-table testing 307
Hear distorted labials 205
Hearing 336
    loss, conductive 240
Heart
    base of 115
    block 370
    border 57
        determination of 117
        percussion of 118f
    conduction system of 362, 362f
    palpation of 111
    topographical areas of 112, 119
Heart disease 335, 480
    congenital 97, 110, 112
    cyanotic 34
        congenital 13
    multivalvular 6, 423
    structural 104
Heart failure 6, 508
    congestive 65, 66
    severe 26
    symptoms of 107
Heart rate 133, 133f, 412
    calculation of 364f
    determining 364
Heart sound 114f, 119, 120, 120f, 121f, 122, 124, 136
    auscultation of 124
    frequency 119
    palpable 115
Heat stroke 29, 507
Heberden's nodes 322f
Heel knee test 288, 289f
Heel-to-shin test 288, 293
Helicobacter pylori 494, 495t
    infection, treatment of 495t
Hematemesis 64, 64t, 142, 510
Hematochezia 142, 510
Hematological disorders 63
Hematology 6, 530, 530t, 535
Hematuria 511
Hemiballismus 301, 515
Hemidiaphragm 434t, 435
Hemiplegia 238, 250
    causes of 190
Hemisensory loss 191
Hemispheric syndrome 294
Hemithorax 81
    circumference 81f
    movement, decreased 81
    right 57, 427f
    white homogeneous opacity, causes of 427
Hemochromatosis 155
Hemoglobin 35, 444
    levels 506t
Hemolytic anemia 32
Hemoptysis 63, 64, 64t, 93
    causes of 63t
    clinical clues of 63t
Henoch-Schönlein purpura 315f
Heparin 496, 498
    antidote of 490
    therapy, complications of 490
    unfractionated 490
Hepatic bruit 160, 160f
Hepatic causes 115
Hepatic encephalopathy 177, 511
    clinical stages of 526t
    types of 177, 178f
Hepatic friction rub 161
Hepatobiliary system 151
Hepatojugular reflux 25
Hepatomegaly 6, 151
    causes of 164, 164f
    painless 163
Hepatopulmonary syndrome 152
Hepatorenal syndrome 178
Hepatosplenomegaly 6
    causes of 168, 168f
Herpes zoster 457f
Hiccoughs 68
Hiccups 137
Hilar mass, differential diagnosis of 426
Hilum 419, 419f, 421, 435
Hip 186
    circumference 52
    fracture 503
    joint
        deformities 325f
        examination 323
Hippocrates fingers 35
Hippocrates succussion 90
Hippus 224
Hirschfelder wave 99
Histamine H2-receptor antagonists 494
Histoplasmosis 494
Hitchhiker's thumb 322f
Hoffman's reflex 275, 275f
Holistic care 1
Holmes-Adie syndrome 277
Holt-Oram syndrome 110
Homocystinuria 50
Homogeneous opacity 427f
Honeycombing 425
Hooking maneuver 166
Hooking method, demonstration of 166f
Hoover's sign 277
Horn cell disease, anterior 251
Horner's syndrome 225, 225f, 226f, 462f
Horseshoe dullness 171, 171f
House-Brackmann grading system 237
Human immunodeficiency virus 46, 308, 340
Hungup knee jerk 277
Huntington's chorea 226
Huntington's disease 340
Hurler's syndrome 49
Hutchinson's index 74
Hutchinson's pupil 224
Hydralazine 40, 477, 479, 497
    nitrate combination 477
Hydrochlorothiazide 476
Hydrocortisone 481, 498
Hydroflumethiazide 476
Hydropneumothorax 6, 86f, 91, 430f
Hydroxychloroquine 491, 492
Hydroxymethylglutaryl, competitive inhibitors of 484
Hypalgesia 516
Hyperalgesia 283, 516
Hypercalcemia 376
Hyperesthesia 283
Hyperestrogenism, causes of 153
Hyperglycemia 153
Hyperkalemia 376
Hyperkinetic dysarthria 205
Hyperkinetic gait 298
Hyperkinetic states 13
Hyperlucent lung fields, causes of bilateral 429
Hypermagnesemia 253, 376
Hyperoxia test 35
Hyperpathia 283, 516
Hyperpyrexia 28, 29, 506
Hypersomnia 351
Hypersplenism 512
Hypertension 6, 115, 183, 335, 355, 356, 504
    diagnosis, thresholds for 21
    factitious 20
    malignant 505
    masked 20, 505
    nocturnal 20
    renovascular 20
    secondary 505
Hypertensive crisis 505
Hypertensive emergencies 478, 478t, 505
Hypertensive retinopathy 214, 357f
Hypertensive urgency 505
Hyperthermia 29, 506
Hyperthyroidism 20, 303
Hypertonia 253
    causes of 253
Hypertrophic cardiomyopathy 6, 116, 122
Hypertrophic obstructive cardiomyopathy 110, 113, 122, 125, 128
Hypertrophy 250, 372
Hyperventilation 64
Hypnagogic hallucinations 207
Hypnopompic hallucinations 207
Hypoalbuminemia 171

Index

Hypoalgesia 283
Hypocalcemia 376
Hypochondrial pain, right 94
Hypoesthesia 283
Hypogeusia 235
Hypoglossal muscle, left 247f
Hypoglossal nerve 185, 246
    location of 247f
Hypoglycemia 20, 482
Hypogonadism 50
Hypokalemia 376
Hypomagnesemia 376
Hypomastia, female 112
Hypopituitarism 6, 20
Hypotension 20
Hypothermia 29
Hypothyroid myopathy 246
Hypothyroidism 6, 250, 253, 294
    severity and duration of 480
    treatment of 480
Hypotonia 253, 287
Hypovolemia 9
Hysterical weakness, signs to identify 277

I

Ibalizumab 489
Ice pack test 216, 217f
Icterus 32, 33f, 70, 151, 195, 454f
    dark yellow 34f
Idarucizumab 491
Idioglossia 514
Idiopathic edema 39, 106
Iliac bruit 160, 161f
Iliopsoas 261f
Illusions 207, 348
Immune system 481
Impingement test, demonstration of 319f
Incontinence, type of 192
Indapamide 477
Indinavir 489
Infection 40, 503
    acute 168
    chronic 168
    type of 464
Infectious colitis 148
Infectious esophagitis 146
Infective endocarditis 94, 527, 527t
    diagnosis of 528
Inflammatory bowel disease 145, 147, 492
Inflammatory diarrhea 144, 145
Inflammatory disease 143, 313
Inflammatory myopathy 246
Inflation lumen 443
Infranuclear lesions 246
Infranuclear ophthalmoplegia 226, 228
Infranuclear palsy, etiology of 227
Infranuclear processes 244
Infusion tubing, primary 447
Inguinal lymph nodes 46
Inhaler devices 450
Inhibitors, post-attachment 489
Inhibitory neuron 265
Initiation of emesis, mechanism of 144
Inositol 47
Insinuate middle finger 78f
Insomnia 336, 351, 513
Inspiration, normal 80
Inspiratory crepitations 89
Inspiratory dyspnea, causes of 67
Inspiratory film 416f
Insulin 445, 481, 483
    analogs 482t
    regular 498
    resistance 482
    secretagogues 483
    syringe 444
    therapy, indications for 482t
    treatment 482
Intellectual ability 349
Intellectual disability 353
    stigmata of 346
Intellectual function 526
Intelligence assessment 353
Intensity 87, 131
Intention tremor 288
Intercostal muscles 64
Intercostal retraction 77, 77f
Intercostal space 113, 115, 116, 119
Intercostal widening 82, 83
Interlobar fissure, right minor 73f
Interlocking flexed fingers 266
Intermittent fever 27
Inter-morbid personality 346
Internal auditory meatus 236
Internal jugular vein, right 22f
International personality disorder examination 353
Internuclear ophthalmoplegia 226, 227, 227f
Interphalangeal joint 38f, 321, 328, 328f
    examination of 321f
Interstitial disease, differential diagnosis of 425
Interstitial lung disease 6, 37, 62
Intertriginous dermatitis 460f
Intertrigo 356f, 460f
Intracerebral disorders 143
Intracranial pressure, raised 182
Intracranial tension, raised 144
Intrahepatic portal hypertension 171
Intraparenchymal hemorrhage, acute 436f
Intravenous cannula 448
Intravenous drip set 447
Intravenous fluids 496
Inverse jaw winking 233
Inverted brachioradialis reflex 277
Involuntary movements 6, 182, 191
Iodine 47
Ipratropium bromide 476
Irbesartan 476
Iris nodules 196f
Iron 47
    deficiency anemia 32
Irregular rhythm, causes of 8
Irritable bowel syndrome 149
Ischemia 375
Ischemic cardiac pain 102, 102t
Ischemic heart disease 94, 183
Ischemic noncardiac pain 102, 102t
Isolation aphasia 204
Isometric hand grip test 308
Isoniazid 465, 496
    preventive therapy 465
Isoproterenol 479
Isosthenuria 452
Isradipine 476
Ivabradine 469

J

J wave 369
Jacobson's neuralgia 244
Jacod syndrome 248
Jamshidi needle 446
Janus kinase inhibitor 494
Jaundice 33, 34, 137, 142, 151, 506
    type of 33
Jaw deviation 184
Jaw jerk 184, 186, 231, 248
    examination of 231f
Jaw winking phenomenon 233
Jendrassik maneuver 266, 266f
Jerk nystagmus 228
Joint 328
    examination of 310, 327
    motion 279
    movement of 318f
    pain 309
    position 191
    sense, examination of 279f
Jones criteria, revised 527
Jug handle appearance 432f
Jugular foramen, lesions of 244
Jugular vein, internal 22
Jugular venous
    pressure 23, 26, 70, 94, 99f, 109, 138, 184, 310, 195, 505
        causes of raised 23
        examination of 23, 23f
        method of measuring 23f
        waveforms of 23, 25f, 99
    pulse 22, 23, 24f, 138, 184, 310
        waveform 94
    system 22
Jugulodigastric lymph nodes 42f
Jugulo-omohyoid lymph nodes 42f
Juvenile rheumatoid arthritis 40

K

Kallmann syndrome 210
Kanamycin 487
Katz-Wachtel phenomenon 373
Kawasaki disease 40
Keith-Wagener-Barker classification 214
Keratitis 317f
Kerley line 424
Kernig's sign 304, 304f
Ketoacidosis 149
Kidney 139, 170
    enlargement 169
    examination of 169
    palpation of right 169, 169f
Kikuchi-Fujimoto disease 40
Kimura disease 40
Kinesia paradoxa 12
Kinesthesia 279, 516
Kirby's method examination 349
Klebsiella 428f
Klinefelter's syndrome 50
Klumpke's paralysis 251
Knee 186, 267
    jerk 269f
    joint
        deformities 325f

examination of 323
 palpation of 323f
 reflex, inversion of 277
Knock knees 325f
Knuckle pigmentation 33f
Kocher-Debré-Semelaigne syndrome 250
Koilonychia 32f
Korotkoff sounds 18
Korsakoff's psychosis 202
Kronig's isthmus 57, 85f
Kugelberg Welander spinal muscular atrophy 250
Kussmaul's sign 26, 122

L

Labetalol 476, 478
Labile hypertension 20
Labiodentals 205
Labyrinthine disease 143
Lacrimal gland enlargement 154
Lacrimation hyperacusis 185
Lactate dehydrogenase 34
Lactobacilli 493
Lactose intolerance 149, 493
Lacunar stroke 517
Lamivudine 488
Langerhans cell histiocytosis 435
Language
 and brain 203f
 domains of 204
Laryngeal fixation 78
Laryngeal nerve, superior 243
Laryngoscope 440
Lateral cavernous sinus syndrome 248
Lateral thoracotomy 116
Latissimus dorsi 254
Leflunomide 491, 492
Left ankle clonus, demonstration of 271f
Left anterior group lymph nodes 45f
Left apical group lymph nodes 45f
Left atrial enlargement 115, 423
Left atrium 101, 115, 126
Left bundle branch block 120, 122, 372
Left carotid pulse, palpation of 15f
Left eye, fundus examination of 213f
Left heart border
 percussion of 118f
 straightening of 423
Left hemithorax 57
Left kidney 170
 examination of 169
 palpation of 169f
Left major interlobar fissure 73f
Left parasternal pulsation 114
Left patellar clonus, demonstration of 271f
Left upper lobe 70
Left vagal nerve stimulation 354
Left ventricle 101
Left ventricular
 apex 114
 enlargement 114, 424
 failure 34, 62, 116
 hypertrophy 110, 113, 372
 types of 373
Left-rotated film 417f
Leg
 flapping tremors in 155f
 ulcers on 315f

Leonine facies 457f
Leopard syndrome 110
Lepromatous leprosy, lesions of 457f
Leprosy, lesions of 278
Lesion 204f, 307
 location 235
 peripheral 246
 site of 191, 192, 204, 211, 212f, 232, 301
Lethargy 200
Leucovorin 492
Leukocytes 531
Leukodystrophy 294
Leukonychia 154f
Leukotriene modifiers 476
Levator anguli oris 234, 234f
Levator palpebrae superioris, paralysis of 215
Levator sign 236
Levine 126
Levodopa 470
Levosalbutamol 474
Levothyroxine sodium 480
Lewy body disease 340
Lichenification 519
Lid retraction 216
Liebermister rule 8
Life-threatening fungal infections 494
Ligaments 311
Light breakfast 5
Light reflex 221
 pathway 222f
Light's criteria 528
Limb
 ataxia 294
 attitude of 250
 stiffness of 182, 191
 weakness 94
Linea nigra 158
Linezolid 486
Linked angina 103
Lipid profile 533, 533t
Lipohypertrophy 482
Lips 156
Lisch nodules 196f
Lisinopril 476
Lispro 482
Litten's sign 76
Livedo reticularis 316f
Liver 170
 abscess 6
 biopsy 445
 cell failure 34, 138
 disease 141, 483
 disorders 152
 dullness 57, 117f
 examination of 161
  hooking method of 162
 palm 152
 palpation 162f
  in ascites, method of 162, 163f
 projecting from right lobe, anomalous lobe of 164f
 span 57, 162, 163, 163f
Lobar disease 424
Lobe 73f, 207
 left side 72
Local allergic reactions 482
Locomotor system examination 310
Loculated pleural effusion 429f

Loop diuretics 473
Loperamide 495
Lorazepam 497
Losartan 476
Lovastatin 484
Low albumin gradient 171
Low back pain, red flags for acute 193
Low cardiac output, symptoms of 107
Low pitch 119
Lower gastrointestinal bleeding 143, 143f
Lower limb 39, 187, 250, 255
 bilateral 250
 distal 191
 examination of 323
 reflexes, reinforcement of 266f
 tactile extinction in 283f
 tone in 252f
Lower motor neuron 238, 253
 facial palsy
  causes of 237
  signs of 236
 palsy, bilateral 238
Lower respiratory tract 56, 72, 77, 83, 86
Low-molecular weight heparins 490
Low-risk populations 527
Ludwig's angina 104
Lumbar puncture 447
 needle 446
Luminal gastrointestinal tract 145
Lung 421
 abscess 6, 428f
 carcinoma 425
 collapse of 6
 disease, unilateral 66
 fields 421, 435
 fissures 73f
  and lobes 72f
 function 475
 hidden areas of 427, 427f
 large airways of 87
 left 421
 lower margin of 73f
 lymphatic drainage of 70
 parenchymal disease of 63
 resonance 84
 right 421
 segments of 421
 sounds 508
  classification of 508t
 topographical percussion of 85
 tumor 66
 vascular diseases of 63
 white-out 427
 zones 435
Lyme's disease 294
Lymph node 40, 41f, 43, 43f, 44, 44f, 45f
 enlargement, causes of posterior triangle 43
 mesenteric 46
 occipital 43f
 postauricular 42f
 preauricular 42f
 right posterior group 44f
 submandibular 42f
 supraclavicular 42f, 43
Lymphadenopathy 6, 40, 70, 151, 195, 429f, 512
Lymphangitis carcinomatosis 430

Lymphatic drainage 71f
Lymphoma 430
Lysergic acid diethylamide 20

M

Macleod's syndrome 429
Macruz index 368
Malabsorption syndromes 145
Malar rash 315f, 459f
Malaria, treatment of severe 464t
Malena 510
Malignancy 37, 40
    external markers of 71
Mallory-Weiss tear 142
Malnutrition 493
Mandibular reflex 231
Marcus-Gunn
    phenomenon 233
    pupil 223, 223f
Marfan's syndrome 50, 53f, 54, 110
Marin-Amat sign 233
Mask 449
Masses 435
Masseter muscle 230f
Massive ascites 170, 174
Massive effusion 90
Massive hemoptysis 64, 508
    causes of 64b
Massive pleural effusion, left-sided 427f
Mastectomy 429
May's sign 25
May-Thurner syndrome 39
Mediastinal cyst 434f
Mediastinal lymph nodes 46
Mediastinal mass 434f
    differential diagnosis of 426, 426f
Mediastinal pleura 70
Mediastinum 419, 435
Medical palsy 218
Medications disorders 143
Megaloblastic anemia 32
Melanoma 437
Melena 142
Memory 201, 335, 349, 513
    classification of 201
    declarative 201, 349
    implicit 201
    recall 336
    systems, concept of 202
    types of 201
Meningeal irritation, signs of 187, 304
Meningeal signs 96, 192, 304
Meningeal stiffness 304
Meningism 305
Meningitis 182
    types of 447
Menstrual cycle 27, 182
Menstrual history 138, 310, 346
Mental function, higher 181, 184, 189, 200
Mental imagery 348
Mental state and cognition 181, 189
Mental status 526
    examination 342, 346
Mercaptopurine 493
Meropenem 485
Mesalazine 492
Mesence-Phalic nuclei 229

Mesenteric ischemia 149
Metabolic disorders 143
Metabolic syndrome 52, 518
Metacarpophalangeal joint 320, 320f, 328, 328f
Metal
    pollutants, heavy 303
    tracheostomy tube 440
Metastatic lesions 425
Metatarsophalangeal joint 324, 324f, 325f, 328, 461f
Metered dose inhaler 450, 451
Metformin, contraindications for 483b
Methimazole 480
Methotrexate 156, 491, 492
Methyclothiazide 477
Methyldopa 477, 479
Methylprednisolone 481
Methylxanthines 474
Metolazone 477
Metoprolol 476
Michigan alcoholism screening test 353
Microaneurysms 214
Microvascular angina 103
Micturition syncope 20
Midaxillary line 73
Midclavicular line 73, 113
Middleton's maneuver 165, 166
    percussion 167f
Migraine headaches 20
Miliary mottling 430, 430f
Miller-Fisher syndrome 293
Mimic meningism 305
Mimic paralysis 238
Minerals 47
Minimal hepatic encephalopathy, diagnosis of 178
Minocycline 34, 491
Minoxidil 477
Miosis 221, 462f
Mirror movements 302
Misnomer 11
Mitochondrial encephalomyopathies 294
Mitral area 119
    auscultation of 130f
Mitral regurgitation 6, 113, 115, 116, 119, 120, 122, 125-128, 136
Mitral stenosis 6, 9, 116, 119, 120, 122, 123, 126-129, 130f, 136
    murmur of 128
Mitral valve
    disease 432f
    metallic prosthesis 432f
    prolapse 128
    prosthesis 431f
Modern geriatric giants 339f
Moexipril 476
Mogigraphia 302
Molluscum contagiosum 461f
Moniz's sign 273, 274f
Monoarthritis 314
Monocular diplopia 218
Monoplegia affecting
    lower limb, causes of 190
    upper limb, causes of 190
Montelukast 476
Montreal cognitive assessment 340

Mood 348
    and affect 348
    disorders 351, 351f
    disturbance 351
    symptoms 350
Morphine 497
Morquio's syndrome 49
Morris index 368
Motility disorders 146
Motivation, stage of 343
Motor atonic bladder 192
Motor behavior, abnormal 347
Motor component 229, 230
Motor disorder 253
Motor dysfunction 181, 189, 232
Motor function, examination of 233
Motor neuron disease 6, 251, 303
Motor nuclei 229
Motor power 254
Motor system 96, 185
    examination 6, 250
Motor tics 302
Mouth, deviation of angle of 237f
Movement disorders 300, 300fc, 303
Movement fluidity 299
Mucosal ulcers 315f
Müller's maneuver 133
Multiple lentigines syndrome 49
Multiple punched out lesions 435f
Multiple sclerosis 6
Multiple system atrophy 293
Murmur 116, 124-126, 127f
    Austin Flint 129
    Cabot-Locke 129
    cardiac 99, 99f
    Carey Coombs 129
    changing 130
    Cole-Cecil 129
    continuous 126
    Cruveilhier-Baumgarten 160, 161f
    diastolic 126, 522
    docks 129
    early diastolic 126, 128, 136
    ejection-systolic 136
    Gibson's 129
    grading of 126
    Graham-Steel 129
    heart 131
    innocent 128, 129
    Key-Hodgkin 129
    maximum intensity of 128
    mid-diastolic 119, 126, 127, 130f, 136
    mid-systolic 125
    mill wheel 129
    palpable 115
    pansystolic 119, 125, 136
    pontains 129
    presystolic 126
    radiation of 127f
    right-sided 128
    Roger's 129
    Rytand's 129
    stills 129
    systolic 125, 126, 522
    systolic-diastolic 126
    timing of 125f
Murphy's eye 441
Murphy's kidney punch 170

Murphy's sign 169
Muscarine-containing mushroom poisoning 480
Muscle 185, 221, 481
   accessory 17
   bilateral weakness of 230
   bulk 250
      loss of 182, 191
   disease 251
   fiber and pathways 265f
   function, impaired 64
   hypertrophy, causes for 250
   spindles 64
   swelling, localized 250
   tested 233
   tone 252
   wasting, causes of 251
Musculoskeletal complaint 314
Musculoskeletal system, examination of 310, 317
Mutism 203
Myasthenia gravis 6, 246
Myasthenic dysarthria 205
Mydriasis 221
Myeloma 435
Myerson's sign 275
Myocardial infarction 148, 374
Myocardial ischemia 376
Myoclonus 302, 515
Myoedema 254
Myokymia 302, 515
Myopathic gait 296
Myopathy 6
Myotonia 253
   congenita 250
   demonstration of 254f
Myotonic dystrophy 251
Myxedema 39, 39f, 358f

N

Nadolol 476
Nafcillin 485
Nail
   black 38
   blue 38
   changes 38, 48, 48f, 154, 316
   Muehrcke's 154
   plummer 38
   psoriatic 322f
   red 38
   white 38, 154f
Naloxone 498
Nasal cannula 449
Nasal discharge 72
Nasal mucosa, color of 72
Nasal reflex 231
Nasogastric tube 442
Nausea 137, 143, 509
   causes of 143t
Near vision 210
   Jaeger's chart for 210f
Nebivolol 476
Nebulizers 451
Neck 185
   circumference 52
   extensor of 254, 256f
   flexion of 254, 255f
   height ratio 53
   muscle of 182, 191, 254
   pain 192
   pounding in 105
   stiffness, examination of 304f
Negro's sign 236
Neologism 202, 514
Neomycin 487
Neoplasm 142
Nephrolithiasis 148
Nephrology 535
Nephrotic syndrome 6, 462f, 512
Nerve 197
   dysfunction, causes of 242
   lesion, peripheral 236
   palsies, etiology of 218
   root 251
   thickening 197
      causes of 198
   trunk 242
Nervous system 6, 58, 96, 132, 181, 188, 195, 327
   examination 184, 200
Netilmicin 487
Neubauer chamber 444
Neuraminidase inhibitors 488
Neuritis, peripheral 487
Neurocardiogenic syncope 105
Neurocutaneous syndromes 195
Neurodevelopmental disorders 350
Neurofibromas 195f
Neurofibromatosis 195, 196, 456f, 463f
Neurogenic bladder, causes of 192t
Neurogenic edema 39
Neurogenic ptosis 216f
Neuroleptic malignant syndrome 29
Neurological causes 37
Neurological diseases, pathology of 189
Neurological disorder 345
Neurological examination 336
Neurological history 189
Neurological symptoms, common 182
Neuromuscular causes 76, 146
Neuromuscular disorders 146
Neuromuscular function 526
Neuronopathy 308
Neuropathy 6, 188, 308
Neurosis 350
Neurotic disorders 350, 352
Neurovascular syncope 105
Neutropenia 512
Nevirapine 489
Nevus Araneus 152
Niacin 47
Nicardipine 476, 479
Nicoladoni-Israel-Branham sign 14
Niemann-Pick disease 40, 226
Nifedipine 476
Night sweats, fever of 27
Nihilistic delusions 206
Nisoldipine 476
Nitrates 468, 477
Nitrofurantoin 486
Nitroglycerin 478, 498
Nitroprusside 498
Nixon's method 167f, 168, 168f
Nocturia 511
Nocturnal angina 103
Nocturnal blood pressure dipping patterns 21f
Nodular goiter, enlarged 458f
Nodule, differential diagnosis of 425
Noisy breathing 68
Noisy restrictive dyspnea, causes of 67
Nonaffective psychosis 350
Noncardiac causes 23, 67, 105, 113
Noncardiac pain 102
Noncardiovascular causes 112
Nondiscriminative touch 284
Nonejection clicks 123
Non-Hodgkin's lymphoma 46
Nonhomogeneous opacity 433f
Noninflammatory disease 313
Nonlife-threatening causes, common 102
Nonnucleoside reverse transcriptase inhibitors 488
Nonpulsatile neck vein 23
Nonrespiratory causes 62, 67
Nonspinal infection 193
Non-ST-elevation myocardial infarction 376
Nonsteroidal anti-inflammatory drugs 62, 472
Nonsulfonylureas 483
Noonan's syndrome 49, 110
Noradrenaline 479
Normal apical impulse, mechanism of 113
Nose 72
Nose-finger-nose test 290, 290f
Novel oral anticoagulants 491, 491t
Nuchal rigidity 304
Nuclear lesions 244
Nuclear ophthalmoplegia 226, 228
Nuclear processes 244
Nucleoside reverse transcriptase inhibitors 488
Nucleus 215, 229
   tractus solitarius 61
Numb cheek syndrome 233
Numb chin syndrome 233
Nutrition 250, 501
Nutritional assessment 46
Nutritional deficiencies 46
   signs of 195
Nystagmus 184, 228, 287
   pendular 228
   physiological 228
   testing for 239
   types of 228

O

Obesity 6, 355
   hypoventilation syndrome 70
Obsession, themes of 348
Obstetric history 138, 310
Obstructing disorders 143
Occipital pole 211
Occipitofrontalis, frontal belly of 234f
Occult gastrointestinal bleeding 510
Octreotide 498
Ocular bobbing 228
Ocular dipping 228
Ocular flutter 228
Ocular movement 217
   testing 218, 218f
Oculomotor dysfunction 288
Oculomotor nerve 184, 218f
   palsy 227
Oculosympathetic palsy 225

Odor 63
Odynophagia 146
    causes of 146t
Olfaction, disturbances in 209
Olfactory nerve 209, 209f
Olfactory pathway 209
Oligoarthritis 314
Oliguria 511
Oliver's sign 78, 78f, 117, 117f
Olivopontocerebellar ataxia 226
Olmesartan 476
Openheim's and plantar strike 275f
Openheim's technique 274f
Ophthalmoplegia 226, 219f
    painful 228
Oppenheim method 273
Opponens pollicis 255
Opsoclonus 228
Optic ataxia 293
Optic atrophy, causes of 214
Optic nerve 210
Optic tract 211
Optokinetic nystagmus 228
Oral candidiasis 461f
Oral cavity examination 70, 156
Oral corticosteroids 475
Oral hypoglycemic agents 483, 483t
Oral lesions 463f
Oral mucosa
    bluish discoloration of 35f
    pigmentation of 156
Oral ulcers, causes of 156
Orbicularis oculi 185
    examination of 234f
    reflex 235
    weakness of 237f
Orbicularis oris 185
    reflex 235
Orbital apex syndrome 248
Organic mental disorders 350
    types of 352
Organic psychosis 350
Organophosphorus poisoning 303
Orogastric lavage, technique of
        performing 439, 439t
Oromandibular dystonia 302
Oropharyngeal airway 441
Oropharyngeal dysphagia, causes of 146t
Oropharynx 72
Orthocyanosis 35
Orthodeoxia 507
Orthopnea 65, 65t, 507
    pathophysiology of 65
Orthostatic hypotension 20, 105
Osborn wave 369
Oseltamivir 488
Osler's nodes 109f
Osmotic diarrhea 144
Osmotic diuretics 473
Osteoarthritis 313, 330, 330f
Osteogenesis imperfecta 49
Osteoporosis 503
Oxacillin 485

P

P wave 368, 412
Pacemaker, artificial 367

Pachydermoperiostosis 37
Pain 29, 106, 191, 278, 284
    acute 146
    assessment
        model 30f
        scales 30
    chronic 146
    description of 146
    disorders of 283
    referred 149f
    site of 148
    spontaneous 182
    types of 30
Palatal myoclonus 244
Palatal paralysis 205
Palatal tremor 294
Palate 156
Palilalia 514
Pallanesthesia 283
Pallesthesia 280, 516
Palliation 147
Pallor 31, 31f, 34, 70, 151, 195, 454f
    grading of 31
    over conjunctiva, demonstration of 31f
Palm
    flat on chest, palpating apex with 112f
    hyperpigmentation of 33f
    pigmentation of 457f
Palmar erythema 152, 460f
Palmar interossei, card test for 260f
Palmomental reflex 235, 275, 276f
Palpable gallbladder 34
Palpable nerves 197t, 198f
Palpable splenomegaly 165
Palpation 57, 77, 91, 95, 138, 161
Palpebral oculogyric reflex 235
Palpitations 104, 507
    causes of 104, 104t
    frequency of 105
    types of 105
Palsy
    response in 233
    surgical 218
Pancerebellar syndrome 294
Pancoast tumor 251
Pancreaticobiliary disorders 146
Pancreatitis 148
Pandysautonomia, acute 308
Panic disorder 20, 352
Panretinal photocoagulation 214f
Pantothenic acid 47
Papilledema 213, 213f
    causes of 214
Papule 518
Para-aortic lymphadenopathy 46
Paradoxical hypertension 20
Paradoxical respiration 12, 76
Parageusia 235
Paralysis 517
Paramedian pontine reticular formation 227, 228
Paraneoplastic disorders 293
Paraphasia 202
Paraplegia 250
    causes of 190
Parasitic infection 144
Parasitic infestations 168
Parasternal area, palpable sounds in 116

Parasternal heave 114f
Paratonia 253
Parenchymal lung disease, diffuse 6
Parenteral corticosteroids 475
Parenteral hypoglycemic agents 483, 483t
Paresis 517
Paresthesia 182, 283, 516
Parietal drift 187
Parietal pleura 44, 70
Parietotemporal cortex, right 436f
Parkinson's disease 188, 226, 299, 340
Parkinson's facies 460f
Parkinson's gait, stages of 297f
Parkinson's hand tremors 460f
Parkinsonism 6
Paromomycin 487
Parotid gland enlargement 154
Paroxysmal hypertension 20
Paroxysmal nocturnal dyspnea 65, 65t, 507
Paroxysmal positional vertigo, benign 239
Passive leg raising 128
Patellar clonus 271
Patellar tap test 323
Patent ductus arteriosus 6, 110, 113, 115, 116, 118, 119, 125, 126, 136
Pathologic aortic regurgitation 527
Pathologic mitral regurgitation 527
Pathologic valvular regurgitation,
        diagnosis of 527t
Patient-doctor privilege 4
Patrick's test 326, 326f
Pectoral reflex 270f
Pectoralis major 254
Pectus
    carinatum 74, 75f, 112
    excavatum 74, 75f, 112
Pedal edema 93, 106, 107fc, 137, 151, 195, 355, 358f
    type of 39f
        nonpitting 40f, 455f
        pitting 39f
Pedigree analysis 499
Pel-Ebstein's fever 27
Pendular movement 269f
Penicillin 485
Pentaplegia 189
Peptic ulcer disease 148
Perceptual abnormalities 348
Percussion
    over posterior chest 83f
    types of 83
Perianal sensation 192
Pericardial effusion 423, 431f
Pericardial knock 122
    early mid-diastolic 124
Pericardial rub 123
Pericarditis 25, 103
Perindopril 476
Peripheral arteries 10
Peristalsis, direction of 159
Peritoneal causes 171
Peritonitis, dialysis-related 149
Permanent junctional reciprocating
        tachycardia 366
Peroneal nerve, common 198f
Persecutory delusions 206
Persistent vegetative state 200

Personality 353
    disorders of 350
        classification of 353
    factor test 353
Pes cavus, diagnose 299
Pes planus, diagnose 299
Petroleum distillates 439
Petrous apex 227
PHACE syndrome 197
Phakomatoses 195
Phalangeal depth ratio 38
Phantom limb pain 283
Pharmacokinetics 485
Pharynx 87, 156
Phenobarbitone 293
Phentolamine 478
Phenylephrine 479
Phenytoin 40, 293
Pheochromocytoma 20
Phobic anxiety disorder 352
Phonation 202
Phonic tics 302
Phthinoid chest 74
Phylloquinone 46
Pick's disease 340
Pickwickian syndrome 70
Pill-induced injury 146
Pin prick sensation, examination of 278*f*
Pindolol 476
Piperacillin 485
Pitavastatin 484
Pitting edema 454*f*
    grading of 38, 39*f*
Pituitary giants 50
Pityriasis versicolor 455*f*
Placing ulnar border 114*f*
Plantar reflex 272, 273*f*
Plantar response, variants of 273
Plaque 519
Platelets 531
Platypnea 66, 507
Platysma 185, 234, 234*f*
    sign of Babinski 236
Pleura 435
    diaphragmatic 70
    lymphatic drainage of 70
    parts of 71*f*
Pleural effusion 6, 66, 90, 91
Pleural opacities, differential diagnosis of 425
Pleural rub 89
Pleuritic chest pain 66, 68
Pneumoconiosis 37
Pneumonectomy 427*f*
Pneumonia 428*f*
Pneumoperitoneum 433*f*
Pneumothorax 6, 91, 103
    bilateral 429
    right-sided 429, 429*f*
Poison 495
    oral consumption of 439
Poland syndrome 429
Polyarthritis 314
Polycystic kidney disease 6
Polycythemia 70, 505
Polymyositis 246
Polypharmacy 336
Polysynaptic reflexes 272
Polyuria 511

Pons 235
Popliteal artery, palpation of 15, 16*f*
Popliteal lymphadenopathy 46
Portal hypertension 511
    classification of 179, 179*f*
Portosystemic anastomosis, sites of 179
Posaconazole 494
Positive contrast agents 438
Positive pronator drift 264
Posterior column sensations, disorders of 283
Postganglionic disorders 308
Postherpetic neuralgia 232
Postprandial hypotension 20
Post-tussive crepitations 89
Postural hypotension 20
Posture 347
    induced crackles 89
Potassium 376*f*
    sparing diuretics 473
Potentially life-threatening causes 102
Pott's spine 49
Pout reflex 276, 276*f*
Prader's orchidometer 154*f*
Pravastatin 484
Prayer sign, demonstration of 320*f*
Prazosin 477
Precipitating incidents 345
Precordial bulge 112
Precordial R wave progression 369
Premature ventricular
    complexes 367
    contraction 122, 128
Premorbid personality 342, 346
Present illness, history of 3, 55, 181, 309, 342, 345
Pressor functional tests 308
Presyncope 105
Primaquine 464
Primidone 40
Primitive reflexes 186, 275
Principle sensory nucleus 229
Probiotics 493
Procaine penicillin 485
Procedural memory 349
Profile sign, demonstration of 36*f*
Progressive supranuclear palsy 226*f*
Projectile vomiting 144
Proliferative diabetic retinopathy 214, 214*f*, 356*f*
Pronation sign 277
Pronator drift 187
Propranolol 476
Proprioceptive system, examination of 279
Propylthiouracil 481
Prosody 208
Prosopagnosia 206
Prostaglandins 36
Protease inhibitors 489
Protein deficiency 47
Proton pump inhibitors, indications for 495*b*
Proximal wasting 251
Pseudo-athetosis 281*f*
Pseudo-bulbar palsy 247
Pseudo-cyanosis 34
Pseudo-diarrhea 145
Pseudo-Foster-Kennedy syndrome 210
Pseudo-gynecomastia 153
Pseudo-hallucination 206, 348

Pseudo-hemoptysis 64
Pseudo-hypertension 20, 505
Pseudo-hypertrophy 250
Pseudo-papilledema 214
Pseudo-polymelia 206
Pseudo-ptosis 216
Pseudo-resistant hypertension 505
Pseudo-syncope, causes of 106, 106*b*
Pseudo-tumor cerebri 214
Psoriasis 455*f*
    nail changes in 316*f*
Psoriatic arthritis 322*f*, 331
    classification of 331
Psychiatric disorder 345, 350
    diagnosis of 350
    management of 354
Psychiatric illness 143, 342, 350*f*
Psychiatric management 354
Psychiatry
    assessment tools used in 353
    diagnosis of 350
Psychological management 354
Psychomotor
    activity 347
    agitation 351
    disturbances 352
    retardation 351
Psychosis 350
    types of 350, 351
Psychosomatic disorders 104
Psychotic disorders 349, 350
Psychotic symptoms 353
Pterygoid muscle 230*f*
Ptosis 184, 215, 216, 217*f*, 462*f*
    partial 225
Puddle sign 174
Pulled trachea syndrome 86
Pulmonary area 95, 115, 118, 119
Pulmonary artery 101, 110, 118
    hypertension 97, 118, 424
    prominent 432*f*
    temperature-sensing 27
Pulmonary capillaries 101
Pulmonary communication, systemic to 126
Pulmonary compliance, decreased 64
Pulmonary congestion during recumbency 65
Pulmonary edema 431*f*
Pulmonary embolism 67, 103
Pulmonary emphysema 429
Pulmonary hemosiderosis 430
Pulmonary hypertension 115, 121, 122, 508
    symptoms of 107
Pulmonary infarction 67
Pulmonary oligemia 432*f*
Pulmonary overinflation 429
Pulmonary pulsations 115
Pulmonary stenosis 110, 115, 116, 121, 128, 136
Pulmonary vasculature 435
Pulmonary venous 424
Pulsatile liver 132, 132*f*
Pulsatile neck vein 23
Pulsatility 164
Pulsations 115
Pulse 8, 94, 138, 151, 183, 195, 310, 336, 504
    character of 9, 10
    collapsing 11
    deficit 9

grading of 9, 523
normal contour of 9
oximetry saturation 94
palpation of 111f
peripheral 14, 14f
pressure 9, 18
rate 8
wave 10, 10f
waveform 9, 10f
Pulseless electrical activity 480
Pulsus
    alternans 11, 12, 12f
    anacroticus 10
    bigeminus 11
    bisferiens 11, 14f
    celer 11
    dicroticus 11
    magnus 9
    paradoxus 11, 12
    parvus et tardus 10
Pump handle movement 79f
Pupil 184, 221
    large 216, 221
    reactivity score 201
    unreactive to light 201
Pupillary abnormalities 222, 224f, 225f
Purpuric lesions 519
Pursed lip breathing 17, 76, 77f
Pursuits 217
Pus filled 424
Pustule 519
Pyelonephritis 148
Pyramidal gait 295
Pyrazinamide 465
Pyrexia of unknown origin 6
Pyridoxine 47

Q

Q waves 369
QRS
    axis 412
    complex 363, 369, 412
qSOFA 528
QT interval 363, 371, 412
Quadriceps femoris 262f
Quadriceps weakness gait 298
Quadriplegia, causes of 190, 190t
Quadruple therapy 495
Quantitative sudomotor axon reflex test 307
Quartan fever 27
Queen square neurological reflex hammer 266
Quinapril 476
Quinidine 146
Quinolones 487
Quotidian fever 27

R

Racecadotril 495
Rachitic chest 74
Racing thoughts 351
Radial artery, method of palpation of 8, 8f
Radiation 103, 127, 131
    sickness 28
Radio-femoral delay 16, 16f
Radio-radial delay 16
Raeder's paratrigeminal syndrome 233

Ramipril 476
Ramus internus 245
Rapid finger tapping test 264
Recombinant human erythropoietin 484
Rectal temperature 26
Recti, divarication of 159, 159f
Recurrent laryngeal nerve 243
    palsy 245
Reflex 96, 184, 186, 217, 231, 235, 265, 267,
    275, 277, 304, 305f, 522
    causes of altered 277
    direct 231, 232
    generation, mechanism of 265
    grading of 265
    pathway, accommodation of 223f
    perverted 277
    superficial 186, 272
    types of 265
Reflux esophagitis, severe 146
Refractory angina 103
Refractory hypertension 505
Regurgitation 509
Rehabilitation 354
Reinke's dysphonia 68
Reitan's number connection test 178, 178f
Relaxation atelectasis 425
Remdesivir 493
Renal angle 170, 170f
Renal artery bruit 160, 160f
Renal failure, chronic 28
Renal function, normal 488
Renin inhibitor, direct 476
Reserpine 477
Residual urine 192
Resistant hypertension 505
Resorption atelectasis 425
Respiration 16, 310
    movement with 159, 170
    muscles of 17
    type of 17, 17f
    variation with 128
Respiratory causes 37, 62, 68
Respiratory disease 78, 503
    common 91
    with emaciation 70
Respiratory failure 60, 71
Respiratory movements, examination of 78
Respiratory muscle function, impaired 64
Respiratory rate 16, 70, 94, 138, 183
    method of calculating 17f
Respiratory system 3, 6, 11, 67, 91, 132, 187,
    327, 335, 346
    abnormal signs in 76
    examination 55, 72
Restless leg syndrome 302, 515
Restricted chest expansion 64
Retching 509
Retinol 46
Rheumatic carditis 527t
Rheumatic fever 6
    diagnosis of 527
    signs of 109
Rheumatoid arthritis 6, 251, 313, 328, 328f,
    329f, 330, 459f
    classification for 328
Rheumatoid factor 328
Rheumatoid nodules 425
Rheumatological diseases 328

Rheumatological disorders 327
Rheumatology 6, 309
    skin changes in 314
Rhinocerebral mucormycosis 461f
Rhomboids 254
Rhonchi 88
Rhythm 8, 412
Rib 414
    crowding 82, 82f, 83
Riboflavin 47
Rickets 49
Riedel's lobe 164
Rifampicin 465
Rifaximin 493
Right ankle clonus 271f
Right atrial enlargement 424
Right atrium 101
    connection 126
Right axillary lymph nodes, examination of 44
Right bundle branch block 120, 122, 372
Right eye, fundus examination of 213f
Right heart
    border 117, 117f
    connection, systemic to 126
Right middle lobe pneumonia 428, 428f
Right patellar clonus 271f
Right ventricle 101, 424
Right ventricular
    apex 114
    dilatation 71
    enlargement 114
    failure 71
        severe 25
    hypertrophy 115, 372, 424
    infarction 26
Right-rotated film 417f
Ring enhancing lesion 437f
Rinne's and Weber's test 240
Rinne's test 185, 240, 241f, 242f
Rivaroxaban 491
Rivero-Carvallo sign 128
Roger's area 119
Roger's sign 233
Romberg's sign 281, 281f
Romhilt-Estes score 373
Rooting reflex 276, 276f
Rorschach inkblot technique 353
Rosai-Dorfman syndrome 40
Rostral vermis syndrome 294
Rosuvastatin 484
Rotational test 239
Roth spots 109f
Rubella syndrome 110
Rust-colored purulent sputum 63
Ryles tube 442, 443

S

Saccades 217
Saccadic dysmetria 294
Saccharomyces boulardii yeast 493
Sacroiliac joint 311
Sahli's hemoglobinometer 444
Salbutamol 474
Salmeterol 474
Samter's triad 72
Sarcoidosis 28, 37, 40, 429f, 430
Sarcopenia 341

Index

Scabies 455f, 463f
Scalene lymph nodes 43, 43f
Scanning speech 205, 287
Scapula 414
Scar 116, 519
    surgical 116f
Schaeffer's sign 273
Schaeffer's technique 274f
Schamroth's sign 36f, 37f
Schizoid 353
Schizophrenia 351
    types of 350
Schizophreniform disorder 351
Schober's test 326, 326f
    modified 326, 326f
Scissoring gait 297, 297f
Sclera
    blue 32f
    unexposed 33
Scleroderma facies 460f
Scoliosis, causes of 76
Scorbutic rosary 74
Scratch sign 90
Scrivener's palsy 302
Scrotum 177
Secretory diarrhea 144
Secretory function 235
Seesaw nystagmus 228
Seizure 183
    disorder 20
Selenium 47
Sella turcica, enlarged 435f
Semantic memory 202
Semilong cases 355
Semmes-Weinstein monofilament 278
Sensation 186, 284
Sense 191
    position 280
Sensitive sweat test 307
Sensorimotor functions, altered 143
Sensorineural hearing loss 240
Sensorium 71
Sensory 184, 185, 233, 293
    ataxia 293, 297, 298f
    atonic bladder 192
    component 229
    dermatomes 284
    dysfunction 182, 191, 232
        clinical patterns of 286f
    homunculus 283f
    part 229
    pathway 283f
Sensory loss
    ascending 191
    clinical patterns of 283
    descending 191
    dissociative 191
    functional 285
    graded 191
    nonorganic 285
    pattern of 182, 191
Sensory system 96, 186
    examination 6, 234, 278
    Sherrington classification of 278
Sepsis 518
Sequential electrocardiogram changes 375
Sequential inspiratory wheeze 88
Serum
    bilirubin 33, 34
    enzymes 34
    sickness 40
Serum-ascites albumin gradient 171
Severity of disease, scoring systems for 332
Sexual precocity, severity index for 50
Shagreen patch 197f, 456f
Shield-like chest 74
Shifting dullness 57, 85, 86, 171, 173f
Shock 26, 479t
    anaphylactic 479
    septic 481
Short stature 6, 49
    cause of 49
Shoulder 185
    drooping 75f
    examination of 319
    joint 319f
Silastic sweat imprint 307
Sildenafil 211
Silent restrictive expiratory dyspnea, causes of 67
Silhouette sign 422, 422f, 428f
Silicosis 430
Simultanagnosia 206
Simvastatin 484
Singer's nodules 68
Sinoatrial node re-entrant tachycardia 366
Sinus 77
    bradycardia 365
    pause 365
    rhythm 365
    tachycardia 365
Sisomicin 487
Situational syncope 20
Sjogren's syndrome 40, 293, 308, 316
Skeletal abnormality 429
Skin 481
    hands, and eyes, examination of 314
    segment innervation 284f, 285f
    tags 456f
Skinfold
    calipers, types of 51f
    thickness 51
Skull 187, 304
    examination of 306
    radiograph 197
Sleep
    deprivation 182
    disorders of 350
Slit-lamp examination 317f
Slurred speech 94, 203
Small fiber, chronic 308
Small intestinal bleeding 143
Small pupil 216, 221
Smell
    impaired 210
    persistent loss of 209
Smoking 503
    index 503
Smooth septal 425
Sneeze reflex 231
Snoring 68
Snout reflex 235, 276
Social skills 354
Sodium
    bicarbonate 497
    nitroprusside 478
Sodium-glucose cotransporter 2 inhibitors 483
Soft brush 278
    tactile sensation with 279f
Soft neurological signs 187
Soft tissues 418, 418f, 435
Sokolow index 369
Solitary pulmonary nodule 431f
Somatic delusions 206
Sotos syndrome 50
Sound
    adventitious 58, 88, 88fc
    alveolar 205
    articulated 205
    low frequency 116
    nonejection 124
    production 87, 205
Spastic paraplegia 6
    causes of 190t
Spectrum 486
Speech 202, 248, 347
    disorganized 350
    genesis of 203f
Spider angiomas 152
Spider nevi 138, 152, 152f, 153f
Spider telangiectasia 152
Spinal accessory nerve 185, 245
    anatomy of 245f
    testing 245
Spinal causes 190
Spinal cord
    disease 188, 278
    posterior column of 293
    transverse lesion in 190
Spinal joints, arthritis of 192
Spinal muscular atrophy 251
Spinal nucleus 229
Spinal part 245
Spine 177, 187, 304, 414
    deformities 74, 76f, 327, 327f
    examination of 75, 306, 311, 325
    extensors of 261f
    movements of 306f, 311
Spinoacromial distance 57
Spinoacromion distance, examination of 82, 82f
Spinoscapular distance 57
    examination of 81, 82f
Spinothalamic tract 278
Spironolactone 477
Spleen 139, 170
    examination of 165
    palpation 166f
    surface marking of 165f
Splenic enlargement 165
Splenic percussion, Castell's method of 167f
Splenic rub 161
Splenomegaly 6, 34
    causes of 168
    grading of 165f
    severe 165, 168
Split hand plus 252
Split hand sign 251
Spontaneous bacterial peritonitis 149
Spoon test 307
Sporotrichosis 46
Spotters 454
Sputum 62
Square root sign 26

Index

Square wave jerks 294
Squint 221
    types of 221
ST segment
    depression, causes of 374
    elevation, causes of 374
Stable angina 103
Staccato speech 205, 287
Stag's antler sign 432f
Stamping gait 297
Stapedius reflex 235
Statins 484
Status anginosus 103
Steatohepatitis, nonalcoholic 151
Stepping gait, high 296f
Stereognosis 282
    with coin 282f
Sternal contact sign 424
Sternoclavicular joint 115, 327, 327f
Sternoclavicular pulsations 115
Sternocleidomastoid muscle 245f
Sternotomy, median 116
Sternutatory reflex 231
Steroids
    common indications of 481
    contraindications of 481t
    indications of 481t
    sparing agents 475
Stevens-Johnson syndrome 463f
Stiffness 182
Stimulus
    direction of 273f
    real external 348
Stony dullness 84
Strabismus 221
Straight back syndrome 112
Straight leg raising test 326, 326f
Straight line walking 292f
Stransky method 273
Streptomycin 465, 487
Stress 182
    echocardiography 480
    incontinence 340
Stride 293
Stridor 89
Stroke 517
Structural cardiac disease 105
Strümpell's phenomenon 273
Stupor 200, 347, 349, 512
Sturge-Weber
    disease 233
    syndrome 196, 197f
Subarachnoid space 227
Subconjunctival hemorrhage 109f
Subcutaneous emphysema 82, 430f
Subcutaneous nodules, differential diagnosis 316
Subdural hematoma, acute right 436f
Substance
    induced disorder 345
    use disorders 343, 350, 354
Subtle hemiparesis, examination for 263, 263f
Succussion splash 90, 90f, 161
Sucking reflex 235, 276, 276f
Sucralfate 495
Suction catheter 443
Sudomotor 306, 307
    function 307

Suicidal attempt, assessment of lethality of 353
Suicidal ideation, Becks scale for 353
Suicide 353
Sulfasalazine 491, 492
Sulfonylureas 483
Sunset sign 226
Superior orbital fissure 227
    syndrome 233, 248
Superior vena cava, edge of 423f
Supinator 267
    reflex, demonstration of 268f
Supraclavicular fossa 131, 177
Supraclavicular lymphadenopathy, mechanism of left 43
Supranuclear lesion 235, 244
Supranuclear ophthalmoplegia 226, 228
Supraorbital nerve 198f
Suprapatellar pouch 323f
Suprasegmental component 265
Supraspinatus 256f
Suprasternal pulsations 115
Supraventricular tachycardia 366
Sustained handgrip test 307
Suzman's sign 116
Swan-neck deformity 321f, 459f
Swelling over Achilles tendon 324f
Swyer-James syndrome 429
Sympathomimetic amine 479, 479t
Symphyseal sign 304, 305f
Symptomatology 313
Syncope 105, 518
    causes of true 105, 105t
    classification of 106
Syndromic lymphadenopathy 40
Synkinesis 302
Synovium 311
Syphilis, secondary 46
Syringobulbia 232f
Syringomyelia 251
Systemic aminoglycosides 487
Systemic candidiasis 494
Systemic capillaries 101
Systemic corticosteroids 475
Systemic hypertension 115, 121, 122
Systemic illness, history of 106
Systemic inflammatory response syndrome 518
Systemic lupus erythematosus 6, 40, 308, 315, 328, 330, 330f, 459f
Systemic sclerosis 6, 315f
Systolic murmur
    Freeman and Levine grading of 522
    Freeman grading of 126
Systolic pulsation 132

T

T wave 369, 412
    inversions, causes of 369
Tachycardia 364, 507
    atrioventricular re-entrant 366
    relative 8
Tachycardiac palpitations 105
Tachycardic rhythm originating 366
Tachypnea 90
Tactile
    disturbances 354

    extinction 282
    fremitus 82, 90
    hallucination 348
    sensation 278, 279f
Tall stature 50
    causes of 50
Tall T waves 369, 412
Tamiflu 488
Tamponade 25
Tandem walking 292, 292f
Tarsal muscle, paralysis of 215
Taste
    impaired 235
    sensation 235f, 238
Taylor hammer 266
Tazobactam 485
Tectal pupils 225
Teeth 156
    clenching 266, 266f
Telangiectasia 519
Telmisartan 476
Temperature 8
    circadian variation of 27
    disorders of 283
Temporal elements 147
Temporal lobe 242
Temporal temperature 26
Temporomandibular joint 327, 327f
Tender hepatomegaly 163
Tendons 311
Tenesmus 145
Tenofovir disoproxil fumarate 488
Tense ascites 170, 174
Terazosin 477
Terbutaline 474
Test device 191
Testicular atrophy 153
Tetany, trousseau sign of 43
Tetracycline 487
Tetralogy of Fallot 6, 110, 432f
Thalamic hemorrhage 226
Thalamic pain 283
Thematic apperception test 353
Thenar muscles compared, dysfunction of 252
Theophylline 474
Thermanalgesia 283
Thermhyperesthesia 283
Thermhypoesthesia 283
Thermometers 26
Thermoregulatory sweat test 307
Thiamine 46
Thiazides 473
Thiazolidinediones contraindication 483
Thomas test 323, 323f
Thomson's disease 250
Thoracic movement 17
Thoracolumbar spine 311
Thought
    continuity 347
    formation 347
    possession 347
    stream 347
Throat 72
Throckmorton's sign 273
Thrombolytic agents, use of 491b
Thrombotic paradox 12
Thumb
    abduction 259f

extension 259f
flexion 259f
sign 53f
Z-shaped deformity of 322f
Thyroid
   disorders 355
   function tests 533, 533t
   storm 481
Thyromegaly 458f
Thyrotoxicosis 6, 50
Thyroxine 480
Tibial artery, palpation of posterior 15
Tibial pulse, palpation of posterior 16f
Tibialis
   anticus 262f
   posticus 262f
Tic 302, 515
   types 302
Tidal percussion 57, 85, 85f
Tidal wave 9
Timed up-and-go test, principle of 340
Timolol 476
Tinea
   corporis 456f
   cruris 456f
   infections 494
   manuum 456f
   versicolor 455f
Tiotropium 476
To-and-fro murmurs 126, 127f
Tobacco use, complications of 503
Tobramycin 487
Tocilizumab 494
Tocopherol 46
Toe finger test 289, 289f
Toe-walking 298
Tofacitinib 494
Tolosa-Hunt syndrome 248
Tone 185, 514
   abnormalities of 253
   in arms, testing for 252
   in legs, testing for 252
Tongue 156
   bluish discoloration of 35f
   deviation 246
   motor power of 247f
   numbness 233
   palpation of 247f
   paralysis 205
   wasting with deviation 462f
Topical aminoglycosides 487
Topognosis 282
Torsades de pointes 366
Torsemide 477
Total anomalous pulmonary venous connection 126
Total ophthalmoplegia 226
Touch, disorders of 283
Toxic epidermal necrolysis 463f
Toxicity 473, 485-487
Toxicology 495
Toxin 495
   specific antidotes 495t
Trachea 75, 77, 419, 419f, 435
   large airways of 87
Tracheal rales 89
Tracheal tug sign 78, 117
Tracing trachea down with middle finger 78f

Trail sign 75
Trandolapril 476
Transaminases 532
Transcortical aphasia, mixed 204
Transcortical motor 204
Transcortical sensory 204
Transient ischemic attack 517
Transverse myelitis 6
Trapezius muscle 246f
Traube's space 57, 139, 167, 168f
   obliteration of 86, 167
   percussion of 85, 85f, 167, 167f
Trauma 251
Traveler's diarrhea 144
Tremor 287, 301, 354, 515
Trendelenburg
   gait 296, 298f
   sign 323f
   test 323
Trepopnea 66, 507
Triamterene 477
Triceps reflex 268f, 269f, 277
Triceps skinfold 51, 51f
Tricuspid area 95, 119
   auscultation of 129
Tricuspid regurgitation 25, 113, 115, 116, 119, 120, 125-128, 130f, 132, 136
Tricuspid stenosis 25, 115, 116, 119, 120, 127, 128, 132
Trigeminal lesion 231
Trigeminal nerve 184, 228
   causes of 232
   disorders 233
   divisions of 229f
   mandibular division of 230f
   maxillary division of 230f
   motor component of 230f
   sensory component of 229f
Trigeminal neuralgia 232
Triplegia 189
Tripod
   position 76, 77f
   sign 305, 305f
Trisection method 9
Trochlear nerve 184
   palsy 227
Troisier's sign 43
Tromner's neurological reflex hammer 266
Tromner's reflex 275, 275f
Trousseaus syndrome 43
Trucut biopsy gun 445
Trumpet player's neuropathy 233
Trunk 182, 186
   muscles 255
Tuberculin syringe 444, 445
Tuberculosis 37, 60, 94, 183, 433
   chemoprophylaxis 465
   choroid tubercles in 213f
   disseminated 46
   external markers of 70
   sequelae of 433f
Tuberculous foci 465, 465t
Tuberous sclerosis 196, 456f
   complex 196t
Tumor 192, 519
   plops, early mid-diastolic 124
Turner syndrome 49, 111, 111f, 210
Twin beating pulse 11

Tympanic membrane 242f
Tympanic temperature 26
Typhoid fever 29f
Typhus 461f

U

U waves 369
Ulcer 519
Ulcerative colitis 145, 492t, 529, 529t
Ulnar deviation 459f
Ulnar nerve 198f
Ulnar paradox 12
Unidigital clubbing 38
Uninhibited bladder 192
Uniocular movements 184, 217
Unstable angina 103
Up-and-go test, timed 340f
Upper extremity 186
Upper gastrointestinal bleeding, causes of 143f
Upper limb 39, 44, 250, 253f, 254, 281f
   distal 182, 190
   examination of 319
   proximal 182, 190
   reflexes 266f, 275
   tactile extinction in 282f
Upper lobe 436f
   active tuberculosis 433f
   pneumonia, right 428, 428f
Upper motor neuron 190, 190t, 238
   disease 253
   palsy, bilateral 238
Upper respiratory tract 72
   examination 56, 72
Urea 533, 533t
Urge incontinence 182, 340
Urinary incontinence, types of 340
Urinary retention 148, 182
Urinary tract infection 512
Urine 452, 533
   bilirubin 34
   gravity in 452
   urobilinogen 34
   values, normal 533t
Urinometer 451
Urogenital system 3
Uvula, deviation of 243f

V

V wave 24, 99
Vagal ganglia 244
Vagal lesion, unilateral 244
Vagal paralysis, bilateral complete 244
Vagus nerve 244
Valsalva maneuver 132, 133f
   modified 133
   phases of 133, 307
Valsalva ratio 307
Valsartan 476
Valvular disease 122, 128
Valvular heart disease, acquired 97
Vancomycin 486
Variant angina 103
Vascular disease 429
Vascular spiders 152
Vasodepressor syncope 105

Vasovagal syncope 105
Vaughan Williams classification 467t
Vecuronium 497
Velcro crepitations 89
Venous hum 160
Venous paradox 12
Ventricular activation time 369
Ventricular fibrillation 366
Ventricular premature complexes 9
Ventricular septal defect 6, 110, 113, 115, 116, 119, 122, 125, 126, 128, 136, 368
Ventricular tachycardia 366
Verapamil 476
Vernet jugular foramen syndrome 248
Vertebral bruit 183
Vertigo 228
    testing for 239
Vessel wall, condition of 13
Vestibular ataxia 293
Vestibular component 239, 242
Vestibular disease 299
Vestibular ganglia 239
Vestibular nerve 239, 242
Vestibulocochlear nerve 185
Vibration over medial malleolus 280f
Vim Silverman liver biopsy needle 445
Vincent's angina 103
Vineland social maturity scale 353
Viral gastroenteritis 149
Viral infection 144
Virchow's node 43
Visible mass 159
Visible peristalsis 159
Visible pulsation 77, 115
Visible scars 77
Vision 336
    changes before headache 182
Visual acuity 210
Visual agnosia 206
Visual disturbances 354
Visual field
    defect 211, 212f
    testing 210
Vital examination 7, 8, 70, 94
Vital signs 29, 346
Vitamin
    A 46
    B_1 46
    B_{12} deficiency 294
    B_2 47
    B_3 47
    B_4 47
    B_5 47
    B_6 47
    B_7 47
    B_8 47
    B_9 47
    C 46, 47
    D 46, 484
    deficiency 46
    E 46, 294
    fat-soluble 46
    K 46
    water-soluble 46
Vitiligo 455f
Vocal cord polyps 68
Vocal fremitus 82, 82f
Vocal resonance 58, 89
Vocalization 202
Voice, hoarseness of 68
Vomiting 137, 143, 509
    causes of 143t
    type of severe 144
von Grey's hairs 278
von Hippel-Lindau disease 197

W

Waddling gait 296, 296f
Waist circumference 52
Waist-hip ratio 52, 52f
Walking man sign 423
Warfarin 490
    antidotes of 491
Wartenberg's reflex 275
Wartenberg's sign 275f
Water
    attenuation value of 437
    filled 424
    hammer pulse 11
Watery diarrhea 144, 145
Watson's water hammer pulse 13
Watsons pulse 11
Wavy impulse 113
Weakness 190
    distribution of 181, 189
    progression of 181
    qualitative assessment of 254
Weber's test 185, 240, 241f, 242f
Weber-Dimitri disease 233
Wegener's granulomatosis 72, 425
Weight gain 482
Weight loss 53, 137, 509
Wernicke's area 204
Wernicke's encephalopathy 202, 226, 294
Wernicke's hemianopic pupil 223
Weschler's adult intelligence scales 353
Westergren tube 452
Wet test 299
    and appearance 299f
Wheeze 55, 66, 88
    classification of 88
Whispering pectoriloquy 89
White chalky 154
White coat hypertension , 505
White matter 437
Wiggers diagram 100f
William's syndrome 110
William's tracheal resonance 86
Wilson's disease 156, 294
Winterbottom sign 43
Wintrich's sign 86
Woods, node of 43
Wrist 186
    clonus 271
    joint, examination of 319, 320f
    sign 53f
Writer's cramp 302

X

X nerve 243
X wave 23, 25, 99
Xanthelasma 138, 455f
    around eyes 462f
Xanthoma 155
Xiphisternum 139
X-linked recessive
    disease 499
    disorders 499t

Y

Y descent 25
Y wave 25, 99
Yamaguchi's criteria 332
Yeast 493
Yes-no test 286
Young's syndrome 72
Youngs mania rating scale 353

Z

Z deformity 459f
Zafirlukast 476
Zidovudine 146, 488
Zieve's syndrome 154
Zinc 47
Zygomycosis 494